Grossman's Cardiac Catheterization, Angiography, and Intervention

SEVENTH EDITION

Grossman's Cardiac Catheterization, Angiography, and Intervention

SEVENTH EDITION

EDITOR

▬ DONALD S. BAIM, MD

Professor of Medicine, Harvard Medical School
Director, Center for Integration of Medicine and Innovative Technology
Brigham and Women's Hospital
Boston, Massachusetts

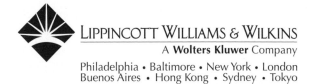

LIPPINCOTT WILLIAMS & WILKINS
A **Wolters Kluwer** Company

Philadelphia • Baltimore • New York • London
Buenos Aires • Hong Kong • Sydney • Tokyo

Acquisitions Editor: Fran DeStefano
Managing Editor: Joanne P. Bersin
Project Manager: David Murphy
Design Manager: Teresa Mallon
Manufacturing Manager: Ben Rivera
Marketing Manager: Kathy Neely
Production Services: TechBooks
Printer: Edwards Brothers

© 2006 by LIPPINCOTT WILLIAMS & WILKINS
530 Walnut Street
Philadelphia, PA 19106 USA
LWW.com

Library of Congress Cataloging-in-Publication Data

Grossman's cardiac catheterization, angiography, and intervention / editor, Donald S. Baim.—7th ed.
   p. ; cm.
Includes bibliographical references and index.
ISBN 0-7817-5567-0
1. Cardiac catheterization 2. Angiography. I. Baim, Donald S. II. Grossman, William, 1940– III. Title: Cardiac catheterization, angiography, and intervention.
   [DNLM: 1. Heart Catheterization. 2. Angiography—methods. 3. Heart Diseases—diagnosis. 4. Heart Diseases—therapy. 5. Heart Function Tests—methods. WG 141.5.C2 G878 2005]
  RC683.5.C25C38 2005
  616.1′207572—dc22   2005018112

Care has been taken to confirm the accuracy of the information presented and to describe generally accepted practices. However, the authors, editors, and publisher are not responsible for errors or omissions or for any consequences from application of the information in this book and make no warranty, expressed or implied, with respect to the currency, completeness, or accuracy of the contents of the publication. Application of this information in a particular situation remains the professional responsibility of the practitioner.

The authors, editors, and publisher have exerted every effort to ensure that drug selection and dosage set forth in this text are in accordance with current recommendations and practice at the time of publication. However, in view of ongoing research, changes in government regulations, and the constant flow of information relating to drug therapy and drug reactions, the reader is urged to check the package insert for each drug for any change in indications and dosage and for added warnings and precautions. This is particularly important when the recommended agent is a new or infrequently employed drug.

Some drugs and medical devices presented in this publication have Food and Drug Administration (FDA) clearance for limited use in restricted research settings. It is the responsibility of the health care provider to ascertain the FDA status of each drug or device planned for use in their clinical practice.

To purchase additional copies of this book, call our customer service department at (800) 638-3030 or fax orders to (301) 824-7390. International customers should call (301)714-2324.

Visit Lippincott Williams & Wilkins on the Internet: at LWW.com. Lippincott Williams & Wilkins customer service representatives are available from 8:30 am to 6 pm, EST.

10 9 8 7 6 5 4 3 2 1

To my friend, mentor, and colleague—Bill Grossman—recognizing his vision and persistence in creating and then sustaining this textbook over the past 25 years.

And to my wife and children, for bearing with me over the many months of night and weekend work that were required to create this seventh edition.

Contents

DVD Table of Contents   ix
Preface to the 7th Edition   xi
Preface to the DVD Companion to Grossman's
   7th Edition   xiii
Contributing Authors   xv

SECTION I: GENERAL PRINCIPLES   1

1.   Cardiac Catheterization
     History and Current Practice Standards   3
     Donald S. Baim

2.   Cineangiographic Imaging, Radiation Safety, and
     Contrast Agents   14
     Stephen Balter and Donald S. Baim

3.   Complications and the Optimal Use of Adjunctive
     Pharmacology   36
     Donald S. Baim and Daniel I. Simon

SECTION II: BASIC TECHNIQUES   77

4.   Percutaneous Approach, Including Trans-septal
     and Apical Puncture   79
     Donald S. Baim and Daniel I. Simon

5.   Brachial Cutdown Approach   107
     Ronald P. Caputo and William Grossman

6.   Diagnostic Catheterization in Childhood and
     Adult Congenital Heart Disease   118
     Michael J. Landzberg and James E. Lock

SECTION III: HEMODYNAMIC PRINCIPLES   131

7.   Pressure Measurement   133
     William Grossman

8.   Blood Flow Measurement: Cardiac Output and
     Vascular Resistance   148
     William Grossman

9.   Shunt Detection and Quantification   163
     William Grossman

10. Calculation of Stenotic Valve Orifice Area   173
     Blase A. Carabello and William Grossman

SECTION IV: ANGIOGRAPHIC TECHNIQUES   185

11. Coronary Angiography   187
     Donald S. Baim

12. Cardiac Ventriculography   222
     Donald S. Baim

13. Pulmonary Angiography   234
     Nils Kucher and Samuel Z. Goldhaber

14. Angiography of the Aorta and
     Peripheral Arteries   254
     *Michael R. Jaff, Briain D. MacNeill,
     and Kenneth Rosenfield*

SECTION V: EVALUATION OF CARDIAC FUNCTION   281

15. Stress Testing During Cardiac Catheterization:
     Exercise and Pacing Tachycardia   283
     William Grossman

16. Measurement of Ventricular Volumes, Ejection
     Fraction, Mass, Wall Stress, and Regional Wall
     Motion   304
     Michael A. Fifer and William Grossman

17. Evaluation of Systolic and Diastolic Function
     of the Ventricles and Myocardium   315
     William Grossman

SECTION VI: SPECIAL CATHETER TECHNIQUES   333

18. Evaluation of Myocardial Blood Flow and
     Metabolism   335
     Morton J. Kern and Michael J. Lim

19   Intravascular Imaging Techniques   371
     Yasuhiro Honda, Peter J. Fitzgerald, and Paul G. Yock

20. Endomyocardial Biopsy   395
     Kenneth L. Baughman and Donald S. Baim

21. Intra-Aortic Balloon Counterpulsation and Other
     Circulatory Assist Devices   412
     Daniel Burkhoff

SECTION VII: INTERVENTIONAL TECHNIQUES 431

22. **Percutaneous Balloon Angioplasty and General Coronary Intervention** 433
    Donald S. Baim

23. **Coronary Atherectomy, Thrombectomy, and Embolic Protection** 467
    Campbell Rogers and Donald S. Baim

24. **Coronary Stenting** 492
    Gregg W. Stone

25. **Percutaneous Therapies for Valvular Heart Disease** 543
    Ted Feldman

26. **Peripheral Intervention** 562
    Briain D. MacNeill and Kenneth Rosenfield

27. **Intervention for Pediatric and Adult Congenital Heart Disease** 604
    Robert J. Sommer

SECTION VIII: PROFILES OF SPECIFIC DISORDERS 635

28. **Profiles in Valvular Heart Disease** 637
    Ted Feldman and William Grossman

29. **Profiles in Coronary Artery Disease** 660
    Jeffrey J. Popma and Judith L. Meadows

30. **Profiles in Pulmonary Embolism and Pulmonary Hypertension** 677
    Samuel Z. Goldhaber, Nils Kucher, and Michael J. Landzberg

31. **Profiles in Cardiomyopathy and Congestive Heart Failure** 694
    James C. Fang and Andrew C. Eisenhauer

32. **Profiles in Pericardial Disease** 725
    John F. Robb and Roger J. Laham

33. **Profiles in Congenital Heart Disease** 744
    Michael J. Landzberg and Robert J. Sommer

34. **Profiles in Aortic and Peripheral Vascular Disease** 759
    Stephen R. Ramee, José A. Silva, and Christopher J. White

DVD Table of Contents

CASE 1–Coronary angio–Simulated angiographic projection viewer

CASE 2–Coronary angio–Posterior LM origin, value of RAO caudal

CASE 3–Coronary angio–Anomoloushigh anterior origin of RCA

CASE 4–Coronary angio–Anomolous Cx from the RCA -1

CASE 5–Coronary angio–Anomalous Cx from RCA- 2

CASE 6–Coronary angio–Superdominant RCA

CASE 7–Coronary angio–Anomalous left coronary from RCA

CASE 8–Coronary angio–Separate ostia of the LAD and Cx

CASE 9–Coronary angio–Coronary fistula

CASE 10–Coronary angio–Vascuar left atrial myxoma

CASE 11–Coronary angio–Coronary ectasia

CASE 12–Coronary angio–Atherosclerotic coronary aneurysm

CASE 13–Coronary angio–Coronary aneurysm–Kawasaki-1

CASE 14–Coronary angio–Coronary aneurysm–Kawasaki-2

CASE 15–Coronary angio–Non-obstructive coronary disease

CASE 16–Coronary angio–Small coronary clot, use of pressure wire for borderline lesion

CASE 17–Coronary angio–Ostial left main and RCA lesions

CASE 18–Coronary angio–Lucent left main due to eccentric lesion

CASE 19–Coronary angio–Borederline left main–IVUS evaluation

CASE 20–Coronary angio–Muscle bridge

CASE 21–Coronary angio–Coronary spasm

CASE 22–Coronary angio–Coronary spasm post stent

CASE 23–Coronary angio–Catheter tip-induced spasm

CASE 24–Coronary angio–Pleating artifact–RCA

CASE 25–Coronary angio–Pleating artifact–LAD

CASE 26–Coronary angio–Spontaneous and catheter-induced dissections

CASE 27–Coronary angio–Left main dissection–stent rescue

CASE 28–Coronary angio–Bridging collaterals

CASE 29–Coronary angio–Kugel collateral

CASE 30–Coronary angio–Vieussens collateral

CASE 31–Coronary angio–LAD collaterals

CASE 32–Aorta and aortic valve–Aortic dissection

CASE 33–Aorta and aortic valve–Aortic dissection-2

CASE 34–Aorta and aortic valve–Traumatic aortic transection

CASE 35–Aorta and aortic valve–Aortic dissection fenestration

CASE 36–Aorta and aortic valve–Right sinus of Valsalva aneurysm

CASE 37–Aorta and aortic valve–Left sinus of Valsalva aneurysm

CASE 38–Aorta and aortic valve–Aortic regurgitation

CASE 39–Aorta and aortic valve–Peri-valve aortic regurgitation

CASE 40–Aorta and aortic valve–Aortic stenosis–crossing issues

CASE 41–Aorta and aortic valve–Aortic valvular and sub-valvular stenosis

CASE 42–Aorta and aortic valve–Balloon aortic valvuloplasty

CASE 43–Aorta and aortic valve–Percutaneous aortic valve replacement–PVI-Edwards

CASE 44–Aorta and aortic valve–Aortic valve replacement–Corevalve

CASE 45–Aorta and aortic valve–Aortic coarctation stent repair

CASE 46–Aorta and aortic valve–Patent Ductus Arteriosis–Amplatz closure

CASE 47–Aorta and aortic valve–Patent Ductus Arteriosis–coil closure

CASE 48–LV angio–Cardiomyopathy

CASE 49–LV angio–Lateral MI with mitral regurgitation

CASE 50–LV angio–LV aneurysm with remodelling

CASE 51–LV angio–True aneurysm

CASE 52–LV Angio–Pseudoaneurysm

CASE 53–LV angio–Post-MI VSD

CASE 54–LV angio–Post-MI VSD–StarFlex closure

CASE 55–LV angio–Tako-tsubo-1

CASE 56–LV angio–Tako-tsubo-2

CASE 57–LV angio–IHSS alcohol septal ablation

CASE 58–LV angio–Mitral prolapse

CASE 59–LV angio–Papillary muscle rupture

CASE 60–Mitral Valve–Transseptal Puncture

CASE 61–Mitral valve–Balloon mitral valvotomy

CASE 62–Mitral Valve–Edge to edge repair–evalve

CASE 63–Mitral valve–Annuloplasty approaches

CASE 64–Pericardial–Heart border in tamponade

CASE 65–Pericardial–Balloon pericardiostomy

CASE 66–Pulmonary–Congenital valvular pulmonic stenosis

CASE 67–Pulmonary–Pulmonary Embolus

CASE 68–Pulmonary–Selective balloon pulmonary angio

CASE 69–Pulmonary–IVC Filters

CASE 70–Congenital–Coil closure of pulmonary AV fistula

CASE 71–Congenital–Patent foramen ovale, and RV biopsy from below

CASE 72–Congenital–Patent Foramen Ovale–CardioSEAL closure

CASE 73–Congenital–VSD- AR, RVH

CASE 74–Congenital–Mustard Baffle Obstruction

CASE 75–Noninvasive angiography–magnetic resonance

CASE 76–Noninvasive angiography–computerized tomography

CASE 77–IVUS–Basics

CASE 78–IVUS–Hematoma

CASE 79–IVUS–Incomplete Stent Apposition

CASE 80–IVUS–Left Main Assessment

CASE 81–IVUS–Plaque Assessment

CASE 82–Stent issues–3-vessel drug-eluting stent

CASE 83–Stent issues–Ostial Cx plaque shift

CASE 84–Stent issues–Origin LAD stent

CASE 85–Stent issues–Cx bifurcation stent crush

CASE 86–Stent issues–Bifurfcation kissing stents

CASE 87–Stent issues–Left Main stent–alternative approaches

CASE 88–Stent issues–Force-focused angioplasty approaches

CASE 89–Stent issues–Cutting balloon and brachytherapy for restenosis

CASE 90–Stent issues–Re-stenting of stent margin restenosis

CASE 91–Stent issues–Restenosis of Kissing left main stent

CASE 92–Stent issues–Failures of crush and T-stent for bifurcations

CASE 93–Post-CABG–Engagement of LIMA and SVG to RCA

CASE 94–Post-CABG–LAD endarterectomy with LIMA touchdown stenosis

CASE 95–Post-CABG–SVG venous valve

CASE 96–Post CABG–Ostial lesion in grafted OM

CASE 97–Post CABG–Complex native intervention for graft failure

CASE 98–Post-CABG–LIMA stent

CASE 99–Post-CABG–Percusurge embolic protection

CASE 100–Post CABG–FilterWire embolic protection

CASE 101–Post-CABG–Proxis embolic protection

CASE 102–Post-CABG–Rapid progression of SVG disease

CASE 103–Post-CABG–Total occlusion of SVG

CASE 104–Post-CABG–Complex SVG lesion

CASE 105–Post-CABG–SVGno reflow

CASE 106–Post-CABG–Native vessel no reflow

CASE 107–Post-CABG–total native LAD instead of SVG

CASE 108–Post-CABG–Fistula from SVG to coronary sinus

CASE 109–Total occlusion–Conventional stiff wires

CASE 110–Total occlusion–ILT SafeCross wire

CASE 111–Total occlusion in stent restenosis–Lumend

CASE 112–Thrombus–SVG AngioJet

CASE 113–Thrombus–Thrombectomy and atherectomy animations

CASE 114–Thrombus–AMI AngioJet for large thrombus

CASE 115–Thrombus–Primary PCI, with in stent restenosis

CASE 116–Atherectomy–DCA and stent

CASE 117–Atherectomy–Calcified LAD, Rotablator, balloon withdrawal issue

CASE 118–Atherectomy–Rotablator of calcified LAD

CASE 119–Atherectomy–Rotablator of calcified RCA

CASE 120–Atherectomy–Calcified ostial LAD Rota

CASE 121–Atherectomy–Excimer laser for failure to cross

CASE 122–Complications–Coronary angio dye stain–VF

CASE 123–Complications–Coronary air embolism

CASE 124–Complications–Massive fatal coronary air embolism

CASE 125–Complications–Guiding catheter dissection into sinus of Valsalva

CASE 126–Complications–Left sinus of Valsalva dissection

CASE 127–Complications–DCA left main dissection–stented

CASE 128–Complications–LAD perforation–covered stent

CASE 129–Complications–Left main perforation

CASE 130–Complications–Subacute stent thrombosis, retroperiotoneal bleed

CASE 131–Complications–Thrombus on the guidewire

CASE 132–Complications–Retrieval of fractured pacemaker lead

CASE 133–Complications–Early post-CABG misadventures

CASE 134–Complications–Cerebral embolus–Neurovascular rescue

CASE 135–Vascular access–General issues

CASE 136–Vascular access–Calcified femoral, occluded iliacs, radial catheterization

CASE 137–Vascular access–Femoral tips and misadventures

CASE 138–Vascular access–High stick–retroperitoneal bleed

CASE 139–Vascular access–Hypogastric artery laceration vs. ureter

CASE 140–Vascular access–Iliac laceration

CASE 141–Vascular access–Femoral arterio-venous fistula

CASE 142–Vascular access–Thrombin injection of femoral pseudoaneurysm

CASE 143–Vascular access–Puncture of an AO-bifemoral graft

CASE 144–Vascular access–Groin Closure Animations

CASE 145–Vascular access–Thrombosis of an AngioSeal site

CASE 146–Peripheral–Renal artery stent–1

CASE 147–Peripheral–Renal artery stent–2

CASE 148–Peripheral–CHF with renal and subclavian stenosis

CASE 149–Peripheral–Renal accessory artery stent

CASE 150–Peripheral–Renal transplant stent

CASE 151–Peripheral–Renal fibromuscular dysplasia

CASE 152–Peripheral–Iliac and Subclavian interventions

CASE 153–Peripheral–Subclavian occlusion with steal

CASE 154–Peripheral–Total occlusion of subclavian–ILT wire

CASE 155–Peripheral–Carotid Case 1

CASE 156–Peripheral–Carotid case 2

CASE 157–Peripheral–Carotid Case 3

CASE 158–Peripheral–SFA Intervention 1

CASE 159–Peripheral–Infra-popliteal atherectomy

Preface to the 7th Edition

This seventh edition of Grossman's *Cardiac Catheterization, Angiography, and Intervention* represents a major milestone in the history of this text: After 30 years of brilliantly shaping this book since the publication of the first edition of *Cardiac Catheterization and Angiography* in 1974, William Grossman has stepped down as its coeditor. His legacy, however, remains clear in the title of the book, in the content of the hemodynamic chapters, and hopefully in a lucid style that always seeks to balance theory and evidence-based medicine with practical technical tips.

The basic structure of recent editions has been retained, with sections devoted to general principles, basic techniques, hemodynamic principles, angiographic techniques, evaluation of cardiac function, special catheter techniques, interventional techniques, and profiles of specific disorders. But in accord with the major and ongoing shifts from the use of the cardiac catheter as a purely diagnostic tool to an important therapeutic tool, the emphasis in this 7th edition of Grossman's has been shifted even further toward interventional techniques.

The returning reader will find many major enhancements throughout this edition. Some examples are the updated treatment of digital x-ray systems and radiation biology, the enhanced treatment of complications and adjunctive pharmacology, the fuller discussion of percutaneous radial artery approach to left heart catheterization, and the strengthened treatment of both pediatric and adult congenital heart disease. Several chapters have been recast, including those relating to pulmonary angiography and pulmonary embolism, endomyocardial biopsy, circulatory assist devices, as well as profile chapters on coronary artery disease, cardiomyopathy and heart failure. In addition, the interventional section has been totally revamped as pertains to atherectomy, thrombectomy, and distal embolic protection devices; bare metal and drug-eluting stents; percutaneous valve therapies (including new approaches to catheter-based reduction of mitral regurgitation and percutaneous valve replacement for aortic stenosis); and the interventional treatment of pediatric and adult congenital heart disease. The coverage of peripheral vascular disease has continued in three chapters devoted to the head-to-foot review of diagnostic methods, interventional techniques, and case examples.

These represent only a few of the most prominent changes introduced in an attempt to capture the major progress made in this field since the publication of the sixth edition in 2000. We have also revised and expanded the companion DVD-ROM compared with that of the previous edition—it now includes more than 50 digital cases that show a full spectrum of normal anatomy, anatomic variations, diagnostic and interventional procedures, and a variety of complications. This companion DVD-ROM also includes more than 20 animations that illustrate the principle of action of various invasive and interventional devices. These materials are an important supplement and significant extension of the printed text, and are intentionally encoded in unprotected standard media formats to enable their extraction for use in teaching materials or presentations.

The growing clinical use and rapid evolution of interventional techniques, and the ongoing introduction of important new methods all underscore the importance of providing a comprehensive, balanced, and up-to-date resource in this field. It is my sincere hope that this text will be one such resource, and prove valuable to both new entrants to invasive and interventional cardiology (Fellows and new catheterization laboratory staff) and to the more than 10,000 practitioners of this specialty worldwide. Because the pace of development in this area is continuing to accelerate, readers are encouraged to monitor new publications and trial results frequently or keep abreast of new developments in this area through such resources as Up-to-date www.uptodate.com/index.asp.

Even while working to provide the latest current information, I have tried not to lose the incremental (layer on layer) historical flavor and theoretical background (including approaches that were tried and abandoned) that have been such an integral part of this textbook. I believe that this context adds significantly to the reader's overall understanding and can be particularly valuable as discarded procedures reenter mainstream practice (e.g., trans-septal puncture)! Most important, I hope that my efforts and those of the contributing authors to describe the scope and depth of invasive and interventional cardiology will translate into the better patient care, as invariably stems from an improved understanding on the part of those who perform and interpret cardiac catheterization procedures.

Beyond the list of contributing authors, I wish to thank my many colleagues across the country and throughout the world whose shared experiences have been woven into much of the material contained in the book, as well as several generations of our Cardiology Fellows for their questions and research efforts that have led to many of the principles and techniques described throughout this book.

Donald S. Baim, M.D.
Boston, Massachusetts

Preface to the DVD Companion to Grossman's 7ᵗʰ Edition

The previous (6ᵗʰ) edition of this text included a companion CD-ROM that contained roughly 40 full-motion cases illustrating various types of coronary anomalies, interventional procedures, and complications. At that time, most cases were captured onto 35 mm cine film and then transferred to electronic media. During the past 5 years, virtually all cardiac catheterization laboratories have converted from 35 mm film to DICOM-standard digital recording (as discussed in Chapter 2), which allows far easier and higher-quality image migration into secondary (i.e., non-DICOM) electronic formats. There has also been progressive penetration of DVD-ROM technology, with its 8-fold greater memory capacity than the traditional CD-ROM.

For the current (7ᵗʰ) edition of *Grossman's*, we have taken advantage of both of those technologic advances, to provide a companion DVD-ROM that contains more than 150 cases covering an even-broader range of classic findings, specific procedures (including percutaneous valve and other new therapies), anomalies, and complications. We have also revised the presentation format to the now prevalent electronic slide show containing imbedded movies. Most cases conclude with a summary of important teaching points, and references to the particular chapters in the printed textbook.

The cases were generally performed by one of us (DSB or JJP) unless otherwise noted.

We cannot predict how you may choose to view these cases—some readers may find it most useful to review the clusters of these cases that pertain to certain chapters of the printed book as they read them, other readers may wish to review specific case examples related to actual procedures that they have just or are about to perform, while some very experienced operators (or those preparing for certifying exams) may choose to use them as a series of "unknowns" to test their ability to recognize various findings. Either way, we can assure you of 2 things: 1) there are procedures, findings, and complications that even the most experienced operators have never encountered, and 2) failure to delve into these case examples will limit the overall educational benefit provided by the 7ᵗʰ edition!

Please feel free to transfer any of the case examples from the DVD to your own computer for use in educational formats such as cath lab teaching conferences or presentations at meetings, as long as you acknowledge their source.

Donald S. Baim
Jeffrey J. Popma
Boston, MA

Contributing Authors

DONALD S. BAIM, MD
Professor of Medicine, Harvard Medical School
Director, Center for Integration of Medicine
and Innovative Technology
Brigham and Women's Hospital
Boston, Massachusetts

STEPHEN BALTER, PhD
Medical Physicist
Columbia University Medical Center
New York, New York

KENNETH L. BAUGHMAN, MD
Professor of Medicine
Harvard Medical School
Director, Advanced Heart Disease Section
Brigham and Women's Hospital
Boston, Massachusetts

DANIEL BURKHOFF, MD
Adjunct Associate Professor of Medicine
Columbia University
Adjunct Associate Attending
New York Presbyterian Hospital
New York, New York

RONALD P. CAPUTO, MD
Assistant Clinical Professor of Medicine
State University of New York Health Science Center, Syracuse
Chief of Cardiology Research
St. Joseph's Hospital Health Care Center
Syracuse, New York

BLASE A. CARABELLO, MD
Professor of Medicine
Baylor College of Medicine
Medical Care Line Executive
Veterans Affairs Medical Center
Houston, Texas

ANDREW C. EISENHAUER, MD
Assistant Professor of Medicine
Harvard Medical School
Director, Interventional Cardiovascular Medicine Service
Associate Director, Cardiac Catheterization Laboratory
Brigham and Women's Hospital
Cardiovascular Division
Boston, Massachusetts

JAMES C. FANG, MD
Associate Professor of Medicine
Harvard Medical School
Medical Director, Heart Transplantation and Circulatory Assist
    Program
Director, Cardiovascular Fellowship Training Program
Brigham and Women's Hospital
Cardiovascular Division
Boston, Massachusetts

TED FELDMAN, MD, FSCAI, FACC
Professor of Medicine
Northwestern University Feinberg Medical School
Director, Cardiac Catheterization Laboratory
Evanston Hospital
Cardiology Division
Evanston, Illinois

MICHAEL A. FIFER, MD
Associate Professor of Medicine
Harvard Medical School
Director, Coronary Care Unit
Massachusetts General Hospital
Boston, Massachusetts

PETER J. FITZGERALD, MD, PhD
Associate Professor of Medicine (Cardiology)
Associate Professor of Engineering
Director, Cardiovascular Core Analysis Laboratory
Codirector, Center for Research in CV Intervention
Stanford University Medical Center
Cardiovascular Intervention
Stanford, California

SAMUEL Z. GOLDHABER, MD
Associate Professor of Medicine
Harvard Medical School
Staff Cardiologist
Director, Venous Thromboembolism Research Group
Director, Anticoagulation Service
Brigham and Women's Hospital
Boston, Massachusetts

WILLIAM GROSSMAN, MD
Meyer Friedman Distinguished Professor of Medicine
University of California, San Francisco, School of Medicine
Chief, Division of Cardiology
UCSF Medical Center
San Francisco, California

YASUHIRO HONDA, MD
Research Associate, Stanford School of Medicine
Codirector, Cardiovascular Core Analysis Laboratory
Stanford University
Stanford, California

MICHAEL R. JAFF, DO
Kirksville College of Osteopathic Medicine
Director, Vascular Medicine
Massachusetts General Hospital
Boston, Massachusetts

MORTON J. KERN, MD
Clinical Professor of Medicine, Cardiology, Keck School of
   Medicine
University of Southern California
Director of Clinical Research
Interventional Cardiologist for Pacific
Cardiovascular Associates
Costa Mesa, CA

NILS KUCHER, MD
Department of Medicine
Cardiovascular Division
University Hospital Zurich
Zurich, Switzerland

ROGER J. LAHAM, MD
Associate Professor of Medicine
Harvard Medical School
Director, Basic Angioplasty Research
Beth Israel Deaconess Medical Center
Boston, Massachusetts

MICHAEL J. LANDZBERG, MD
Assistant Professor of Medicine
Harvard Medical School
Director, Boston Adult Congenital Heart (BACH) and
   Pulmonary Hypertension Group
Brigham and Women's Hospital and Children's Hospital
Boston, Massachusetts

MICHAEL LIM, MD
St. Louis University Hospital
St. Louis, Missouri

JAMES E. LOCK, MD
Alexander S. Nadas Professor of Pediatrics
Harvard Medical School
Physician-in-Chief
Chairman, Department of Cardiology
Children's Hospital Boston
Boston, Massachusetts

BRIAIN D. MacNEILL, MD
Instructor in Medicine
Harvard Medical School
Clinical Associate in Medicine
Massachusetts General Hospital
Knight Catheterization Laboratory
Boston, Massachusetts

JUDITH L. MEADOWS, MD
Clinical Fellow
Harvard Medical School
Brigham and Women's Hospital
Boston, Massachusetts

JEFFREY J. POPMA, MD
Associate Professor of Medicine
Harvard Medical School
Director, Interventional Cardiology
Brigham and Women's Hospital
Boston, Massachusetts

STEPHEN R. RAMEE, MD
Cardiology, Section Head
Department of Cardiology
Ochsner Clinic
Director, Cardiac Catheterization Laboratory
New Orleans, Louisiana

JOHN F. ROBB, MD, FACC, FSCAI
Associate Professor of Medicine
Dartmouth Medical School
Director, Cardiac Catheterization Laboratories
Dartmouth-Hitchcock Medical Center
Lebanon, New Hampshire

CAMPBELL ROGERS, MD, FACC
Associate Professor of Medicine
Harvard Medical School
Director, Cardiac Catheterization Laboratory
Director, Experimental Cardiovascular Interventional
   Laboratory
Brigham and Women's Hospital
Boston, Massachusetts

KENNETH ROSENFIELD, MD
Director of Cardiac & Vascular Invasive Services
Massachusetts General Hospital
Boston, Massachusetts

JOSÉ A. SILVA, MD
Staff, Interventional Cardiologist
Alton Oschsner Medical Foundation
New Orleans, Louisiana

DANIEL I. SIMON, MD
Associate Professor of Medicine
Harvard Medical School
Associate Director, Interventional Cardiology
Brigham and Women's Hospital
Boston, Massachusetts

ROBERT J. SOMMER, MD
Associate Clinical Professor of Medicine/Pediatrics
Columbia University College of Physicians and
   Surgeons
Director, Adult Invasive Congenital Heart Services
Milstein Hospital
New York, New York

GREGG W. STONE, MD
Professor of Medicine
Columbia University School of Medicine
Director of Cardiovascular Research and Education
Center for Interventional Vascular Therapy
New York Presbyterian Hospital
New York, New York

CHRISTOPHER J. WHITE, MD
Chairman, Department of Cardiology
Ochsner Clinic
New Orleans, Louisiana

PAUL G. YOCK, MD
Martha Meier Weiland Professor of Medicine
Stanford University
Director, Center for Research in Cardiovascular Interventions
Stanford University Medical Center
Stanford, California

General Principles

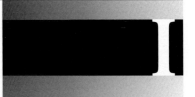

Cardiac Catheterization History and Current Practice Standards

Donald S. Baim[a]

Our concepts of heart disease are based on the enormous reservoir of physiologic and anatomic knowledge derived from the past 70 years' of experience in the cardiac catheterization laboratory. As Andre Cournand remarked in his Nobel lecture of December 11, 1956, "the cardiac catheter was . . . the key in the lock." (1). By turning this key, Cournand and his colleagues led us into a new era in the understanding of normal and disordered cardiac function in humans.

According to Cournand (2), cardiac catheterization was first performed (and so named) by Claude Bernard in 1844. The subject was a horse, and both the right and left ventricles were entered by a retrograde approach from the jugular vein and carotid artery. In an excellent review of the history of cardiac catheterization, angiography, and interventional cardiology, Mueller and Sanborn (3) describe and cite references for experiments by Stephen Hales and others whose work antedates that of Claude Bernard. Although Claude Bernard may not have been the first to perform cardiac catheterization, his careful application of scientific method to the study of cardiac physiology using the cardiac catheter demonstrated the enormous value of this technical innovation. An era of investigation of cardiovascular physiology in animals then followed, resulting in the development of many important techniques and principles (pressure manometry, the Fick cardiac output

method), which awaited direct application to the patient with heart disease.

Werner Forssmann usually is credited with performing the first cardiac catheterization of a living person—himself (4). At age 25, while receiving clinical instruction in surgery in Germany, he passed a catheter 65 cm through one of his left antecubital veins, guiding it by fluoroscopy until it entered his right atrium. He then walked to the radiology department (which was on a different level, requiring that he climb stairs), where the catheter position was documented by a chest roentgenogram (Fig. 1.1). During the next 2 years, Forssmann continued to perform catheterization studies, including six additional attempts to catheterize himself. Bitter criticism, based on an unsubstantiated belief in the danger of his experiments, caused Forssmann to turn his attention to other concerns, and he eventually pursued another catheter-related career as a urologist (5). Nevertheless, for his contribution and foresight he shared the Nobel Prize in Medicine with Andre Cournand and Dickinson Richards in 1956.

Forssmann's primary goal in his catheterization studies was to develop a therapeutic technique for the direct delivery of drugs into the heart. He wrote:

> If cardiac action ceases suddenly, as is seen in acute shock or in heart disease, or during anesthesia or poisoning, one is forced to deliver drugs locally. In such cases the intracardiac injection of drugs may be life saving. However, this may be a dangerous procedure because of many incidents of laceration of coronary arteries and their branches leading to cardiac tamponade, and death. . . . Because of such

---

[a] William Grossman authored this chapter in previous editions and contributed much of the historical information.

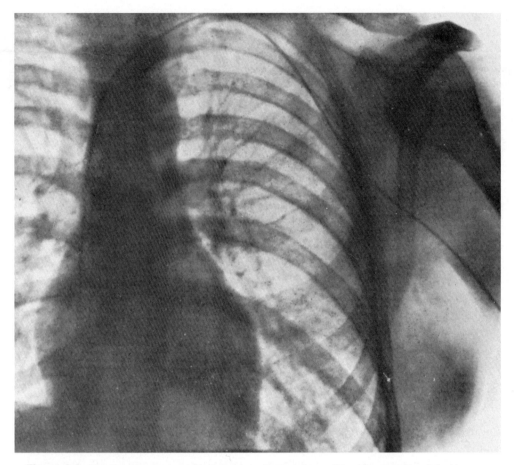

Figure 1.1   The first documented cardiac catheterization. At age 25, while receiving clinical instruction in surgery at Eberswalde, Werner Forssmann passed a catheter 65 cm through one of his left antecubital veins until its tip entered the right atrium. He then walked to the radiology department where this roentgenogram was taken. (*Klin Wochenschr* 1929;8:2085. Springer-Verlag, Berlin, Heidelberg, New York).

incidents, one often waits until the very last moment and valuable time is wasted. Therefore I started to look for a new way to approach the heart, and I catheterized the right side of the heart through the venous system" (4).

Others, however, appreciated the potential of using Forssmann's technique as a diagnostic tool. In 1930, Klein[6] reported 11 right heart catheterizations, including passage to the right ventricle and measurement of cardiac output using Fick's principle. In 1932, Padillo and coworkers reported right heart catheterization and measurement of cardiac output in two subjects (2). Except for these few early studies, application of cardiac catheterization to study the circulation in normal and disease states was fragmentary until the work of Andre Cournand and Dickinson Richards, who separately and in collaboration produced a remarkable series of investigations of right heart physiology in humans (7–9). In 1947, Dexter reported his studies on congenital heart disease and passed the catheter to the distal pulmonary artery, describing "the oxygen saturation and source of pulmonary capillary blood" obtained from the pulmonary artery "wedge" position (10). Subsequent studies

from Dexter's laboratory (11) and by Werko (12) elaborated the use of this pulmonary artery wedge position and reported that the pressure measured at this position was a good estimate of pulmonary venous and left atrial pressure. During this exciting early period, catheterization was used to investigate problems in cardiovascular physiology by McMichael and Sharpey-Shafer in England (13), Lenègre and Maurice in Paris (14), and Warren, Stead, Bing, Dexter, Cournand, and others in the United States (15–23).

Further developments came rapidly in the 1950s and 1960s. Retrograde left heart catheterization was first reported by Zimmerman and others (24) and Limon-Lason and Bouchard (25) in 1950. The percutaneous (rather than cutdown) technique was developed by Seldinger in 1953 and was soon applied to cardiac catheterization of both the left and right heart chambers (26). Trans-septal catheterization was first developed by Ross (27) and Cope (28) in 1959 and quickly became accepted as a standard technique. Selective coronary arteriography was reported by Sones and others in 1959 and was perfected to a remarkable excellence over the ensuing years (29,30). Coronary angiography was modified for a percutaneous approach by Ricketts and Abrams (31) in

1962 and Judkins (32) in 1967. In 1970 Swan and Ganz introduced a practical balloon-tipped, flow-guided catheter technique enabling the application of catheterization outside the laboratory (33). Better radiographic imaging techniques and less toxic radiographic contrast agents have been developed progressively, as the number of diagnostic catheterizations has exceeded 2,000,000 per year.

INTERVENTIONAL CARDIOLOGY

The biggest change in the last 25 years has been the return to the therapeutic potential of the cardiac catheter. In 1977 Grüntzig and others introduced the technique of balloon angioplasty, generally known as percutaneous transluminal coronary angioplasty (PTCA) (34, 35). With rapid evolving technology and expanding indications, PTCA grew to equal stature with coronary artery bypass grafting (CABG) as the number of annual PTCA procedures grew to 300,000 by 1990 (see Chapter 22). Encouraged by the success of PTCA but challenged by its shortcomings, physician and engineer inventors have developed and introduced into clinical practice a panoply of new percutaneous interventional devices over the past decade. This includes various forms of catheter-based atherectomy, bare metallic stents, and drug-eluting stents, which together have largely solved earlier problems relating to elastic recoil, dissection, and restenosis of the treated segment (see Chapters 23 and 24). These newer techniques are usually subsumed (along with conventional balloon angioplasty) under the broader designation of percutaneous coronary intervention (PCI). Similar techniques have also developed in parallel for the treatment of peripheral arterial atherosclerotic disease, which is a common cause of morbidity and even mortality in patients with coexisting coronary disease (see Chapters 14 and 26).

The development of percutaneous coronary intervention has also stimulated the development of other techniques for the treatment of *structural heart disease.* Catheter devices developed to close intracardiac shunts in pediatric patients have now been adapted to close adult congenital and acquired defects (see Chapter 27). Balloon valvuloplasty was developed in the mid-1980s and remains successful for the treatment of rheumatic mitral stenosis, but because of early recurrence is now used as a treatment for aortic stenosis only in patients who are not candidates for aortic valve replacement surgery. Newer technologies for percutaneous aortic valve replacement and percutaneous reduction of mitral regurgitation are now entering clinical testing (see Chapter 25).

In essence, these new procedures have made interventional cardiology a new field in cardiovascular medicine, whose history is well summarized by Spencer King (36), and the interested reader is referred there for further historical details. But it is thus clear in the 21st century that interventional cardiology—by virtue of its new technologies, potent adjunctive drug therapies, expanding indications, and improving results—has blossomed. In many ways, these therapeutic modalities (rather than purely diagnostic techniques) have now become the centerpiece within the broad field of cardiac catheterization. *Although the emphasis thus lies appropriately on this dynamic field of catheter-based intervention, we can ill afford to lose sight of the basic principles of catheter insertion, hemodynamic measurement, high-quality angiography, and integration of catheterization findings with the overall clinical scenario as the foundations on which all current interventional techniques are built and from which future evolution of cardiac catheterization will proceed.*

INDICATIONS FOR CARDIAC CATHETERIZATION

As performed today, cardiac catheterization is a combined hemodynamic and angiographic procedure undertaken for diagnostic and often therapeutic purposes. As with any invasive procedure, the decision to perform cardiac catheterization must be based on a careful balance of the risk of the procedure against the anticipated benefit to the patient. Indications for the use of catheterization and coronary intervention in the management of stable angina, unstable angina, and ST-elevation myocardial infarction (MI) have been developed by the American College of Cardiology and the American Heart Association (37–39), and are available online at <http://www.acc.org/clinical/topic/topic.htm>. As an example, a summary of the indications for cardiac catheterization in patients with stable angina is given in Table 1.1.

The basic principle is that cardiac catheterization is recommended to confirm the presence of a clinically suspected condition, define its anatomic and physiologic severity, and determine the presence or absence of associated conditions when a therapeutic intervention is planned in a symptomatic patient. The most common indication for cardiac catheterization today thus consists of a patient with an acute coronary ischemic syndrome (unstable angina or acute myocardial infarction) in whom an invasive therapeutic intervention is contemplated. The goal of cardiac catheterization in such patients is to identify the culprit lesions and then to restore vessel patency via PCI. In a few such patients, the diagnostic portion of the catheterization procedure may reveal other features (e.g., complex multivessel or left main coronary disease, severe associated valvular disease), which provide critical information for the decision and planning of open heart surgery.

Although few would disagree that consideration of heart surgery is an adequate reason for the performance of catheterization, clinicians differ about whether *all* patients being considered for heart surgery should undergo preoperative cardiac catheterization. Many young patients with echo-proven valvular disease and no symptoms of myocardial ischemia are sometimes operated on using only noninvasive data, but the risks of catheterization in such

---

TABLE 1.1

INDICATIONS FOR CARDIAC CATHETERIZATION IN STABLE ANGINA

Class I
1. Patients with disabling (Canadian Cardiovascular Society [CCS] classes III and IV) chronic stable angina despite medical therapy. (Level of Evidence: B)
2. Patients with high-risk criteria on noninvasive testing [Table 23 in source] regardless of anginal severity. (Level of Evidence: B)
3. Patients with angina who have survived sudden cardiac death or serious ventricular arrhythmia. (Level of Evidence: B)
4. Patients with angina and symptoms and signs of CHF. (Level of Evidence: C)
5. Patients with clinical characteristics that indicate a high likelihood of severe CAD. (Level of Evidence: C)

Class IIa
1. Patients with significant LV dysfunction (ejection fraction less than 45%), CCS class I or II angina, and demonstrable ischemia but less than high-risk criteria on noninvasive testing. (Level of Evidence: C)
2. Patients with inadequate prognostic information after noninvasive testing. (Level of Evidence: C)

Class IIb
1. Patients with CCS class I or II angina, preserved LV function (ejection fraction greater than 45%), and less than high-risk criteria on noninvasive testing. (Level of Evidence: C)
2. Patients with CCS class III or IV angina, which with medical therapy improves to class I or II. (Level of Evidence: C)
3. Patients with CCS class I or II angina but intolerance (unacceptable side effects) to adequate medical therapy. (Level of Evidence: C)

Class III
1. Patients with CCS class I or II angina who respond to medical therapy and who have no evidence of ischemia on noninvasive testing. (Level of Evidence: C)
2. Patients who prefer to avoid revascularization. (Level of Evidence: C)

Class I: Conditions for which there is evidence or general agreement that a given procedure or treatment is useful and effective.
Class II: Conditions for which there is conflicting evidence or a divergence of opinion about the usefulness/efficacy of a procedure or treatment.
Class IIa: Weight of evidence/opinion is in favor of usefulness/efficacy.
Class IIb: Usefulness/efficacy is less well established by evidence/opinion.
Class III: Conditions for which there is evidence and/or general agreement that the procedure/treatment is not useful/effective and in some cases may be harmful.
With permission from Gibbons RJ, Abrams J, Chatterjee K, et al. ACC/AHA 2002 guideline update for the management of patients with chronic stable angina. *J Am Coll Cardiol*. 2003;41:159–68.

---

patients are extremely small, particularly compared to the risk of embarking on cardiac surgery on a patient for whom an incorrect clinical diagnosis or the presence of an unsuspected additional condition greatly prolongs and complicates the planned surgical approach. By providing the surgical team with a precise and complete road map of the course ahead, cardiac catheterization can permit a carefully reasoned and maximally efficient operative procedure. Furthermore, information obtained by cardiac catheterization may be invaluable in the assessment of crucial determinants of prognosis, such as left ventricular function, status of the pulmonary vasculature, and the patency of the coronary arteries. For these reasons, we recommend cardiac catheterization (or at least coronary angiography) in nearly all patients for whom heart surgery is contemplated, even if the severity of valve disease and ventricular function have been determined by preoperative echocardiography.

Catheterization data can also inform other nonsurgical therapeutic considerations. For example, the decision for pharmacologic intervention with heparin and/or a thrombolytic agent in suspected acute pulmonary embolism, the use of high-dose beta-blocker and/or calcium antagonists in suspected hypertrophic subaortic stenosis (versus catheter-based alcohol septal ablation) might well be considered of sufficient magnitude to warrant confirmation of the diagnoses by angiographic and hemodynamic investigation prior to the initiation of therapy. Although a clinical diagnosis of primary pulmonary hypertension can often be made by echocardiography, cardiac catheterization is usually required (a) to confirm the diagnosis and (b) to assess potential responsiveness to pharmacologic agents, such as epoprostenol (40). Catheterization can also be used to optimize pharmacologic therapy for advanced congestive heart failure.

Another broad indication for performing cardiac catheterization is to aid in the diagnosis of obscure or confusing problems, even when a major therapeutic decision is not imminent. A common instance of this indication is presented by the patient with chest pain of uncertain cause, about whom there is confusion regarding the presence of obstructive coronary artery disease. Both management and prognosis of this difficult problem are greatly simplified when it is known, for example, that the coronary arteries are widely patent. Another example within this category is the symptomatic patient with a suspected diagnosis of cardiomyopathy. Although some may feel satisfied with a clinical diagnosis of this condition, the implications of such a diagnosis in terms of prognosis and therapy (such as long-term bed rest or chronic anticoagulant therapy) are so important that we feel it worthwhile to be aggressive in ruling out potentially correctable conditions (e.g., hemochromatosis, pericardial effusive-constrictive disease) with certainty, even though the likelihood of their presence may appear remote on clinical grounds.

Research

On occasion, cardiac catheterization is performed primarily as a research procedure. Although research is conducted to some degree in many of the diagnostic and therapeutic studies performed at major medical centers, it usually relates to the evaluation of new therapeutic devices (e.g., new stent designs) in patients who would be undergoing diagnostic and therapeutic catheterization in any event. All such studies (41) require prior approval of the Food and Drug Administration (FDA) in the form of an Investigational Device Exemption, of the local Committee on Human Research at the institution (Institutional Review Board, or IRB), and attainment of informed consent after the details of the risks and potential benefits of the procedure and its alternatives have been thoroughly explained. Doing such research also requires meticulous attention to protocol details, inclusion/exclusion criteria, data collection, and prompt reporting of any complications.

Even so, this is quite different from a catheterization that is performed solely for the purpose of a research investigation (as a 6-month follow-up angiogram after a new stent might be). Such studies should be carried out only by or under the direct supervision of an experienced investigator who is expert in cardiac catheterization, using a protocol that has been carefully scrutinized and approved by the Institutional Review Board (Human Use Committee) at the investigator's institution.

Contraindications

Although it is important to carefully consider the indications for cardiac catheterization in each patient, it is equally important to discover any contraindications. Over the years, our concepts of contraindications have been modified by the fact that patients with acute myocardial infarction, cardiogenic shock, intractable ventricular tachycardia, and other extreme conditions now tolerate cardiac catheterization and coronary angiography surprisingly well.

At present, the only *absolute* contraindication to cardiac catheterization is the refusal of a mentally competent patient to consent to the procedure. But a long list of relative contraindications must be kept in mind, including all intercurrent conditions that can be corrected and whose correction would improve the safety of the procedure. Table 1.2 lists these relative contraindications. For example, ventricular irritability can increase the risk and difficulty of left heart catheterization and can greatly interfere with interpretation of ventriculography; therefore, it should be suppressed if possible prior to or during catheterization. Hypertension increases predisposition to ischemia and/or pulmonary edema and should be controlled before and during catheterization. Other conditions that should be controlled before elective catheterization include intercurrent febrile illness, decompensated left heart failure, correctable anemia, digitalis toxicity, and hypokalemia. Allergy to radiographic contrast agent is a relative contraindication to cardiac angiography, but proper premedication and use of a newer nonionic low osmolar contrast agent can substantially reduce the risks of a major adverse reaction, as discussed in Chapter 2. Even so, severe allergic reactions or even anaphylaxis can occur, and the operator and catheterization laboratory staff should be well versed in managing the procedure.

Anticoagulant therapy is more controversial as a contraindication. Heparin (unfractionated or low molecular weight), direct thrombin inhibitors (bivalirudin), and antiplatelet agents such as aspirin, clopidogrel, or the platelet glycoprotein IIb/IIIa receptor blockers are widely used in the precatheterization management of acute coronary syndromes and are part and parcel of any coronary intervention. But the use of heparin for simple diagnostic

TABLE 1.2

RELATIVE CONTRAINDICATIONS TO CARDIAC CATHETERIZATION AND ANGIOGRAPHY

1. Uncontrolled ventricular irritability: the risk of ventricular tachycardia/fibrillation during catheterization is increased if ventricular irritability is uncontrolled
2. Uncorrected hypokalemia or digitalis toxicity
3. Uncorrected hypertension: predisposes to myocardial ischemia and/or heart failure during angiography
4. Intercurrent febrile illness
5. Decompensated heart failure: especially acute pulmonary edema, unless catheterization can be done with the patient sitting up
6. Anticoagulated state: prothrombin time >18 seconds
7. Severe allergy to radiographic contrast agent
8. Severe renal insufficiency and/or anuria: unless dialysis is planned to remove fluid and radiographic contrast load

coronary angiography, once felt to lower the incidence of thromboembolic complications during coronary angiography (42), is now uncommon (43). These agents may be continued through and after the catheterization, particularly with the use of groin puncture closure technology, with only a small increase in the risk of local bleeding. If a complication arises, these agents can often be reversed (protamine, platelet transfusion) or allowed to wear off. But the view regarding oral anticoagulants (e.g., warfarin) is that it is best to reverse the prolonged prothrombin time to a prothrombin time of <18 seconds or an international normalized ratio (INR) of <2 before cardiac catheterization represents a more complex problem. This is best done by withholding warfarin for 3 to 5 days before the procedure, potentially switching to subcutaneous low–molecular-weight heparin or intravenous heparin for a strong antico-agulant indication (e.g., a mechanical heart valve). If more rapid reversal of oral anticoagulation is required, we favor administration of fresh-frozen plasma rather than vitamin K, which can occasionally trigger a hypercoagulable state with thrombosis of prosthetic valves or thrombus formation within cardiac chambers, arteries, or veins.

Factors Influencing Choice of Approach

Of the various approaches to cardiac catheterization, certain ones have only historical interest (transbronchial approach, posterior transthoracic left atrial puncture, suprasternal puncture of the left atrium). In this book, we will discuss in detail catheterization by percutaneous approach from various sites (including femoral or radial arteries, femoral internal or jugular veins, trans-septal catheterization of the left heart, and apical puncture of the left ventricular puncture; Chapter 4). Although it has largely been supplanted by the percutaneous approach, we will also discuss catheterization by direct surgical exposure of the brachial artery and vein (the so-called Sones technique, Chapter 5).

The great vessels and all cardiac chambers can be entered in nearly all cases by any of these approaches; thus the choice depends on patient issues (aortic occlusion, morbid obesity), procedural issues (need for use of larger bore catheters), and patient/operator preference. Ideally, the physician performing cardiac catheterization should be well versed in several of these methods (at least one upper extremity approach as well as the femoral approach).

DESIGN OF THE CATHETERIZATION PROTOCOL

Every cardiac catheterization should have a protocol, that is, a carefully reasoned sequential plan designed specifically for the individual patient. This protocol may be so common (e.g., left heart catheterization with coronary angiography, annual transplant evaluation) that the operator and support staff are already in synch with the plan. If

anything beyond this approach is planned, it is helpful to map this out, even preparing and posting a written protocol in the catheterization suite so that all personnel in the laboratory understand exactly what is planned and anticipate the needs of the operator.

Certain general principles should be considered in the design of a protocol if it includes hemodynamic measurements. First, hemodynamic measurements should generally precede angiographic studies, so that crucial pressure and flow measurements may be made as close as possible to the basal state. Second, pressures and selected oxygen saturations should be measured and recorded in each chamber "on the way in," that is immediately after the catheter enters and before it is directed toward the next chamber. If a problem should develop during the later stages of a catheterization procedure (atrial fibrillation or other arrhythmia, pyrogen reaction, hypotension, or reaction to contrast material), it will be beneficial to have the pressures and saturations already measured in advance, rather than waiting until the time of catheter pullback. Third, measurements of pressure and cardiac output (using true Fick, Fick with estimated oxygen consumption, or thermodilution, Chapter 8) should be made as simultaneously as possible.

Beyond these general guidelines, the protocol will reflect differences from patient to patient and factor in changes when unexpected findings are encountered (e.g., finding an unexpected marked elevation of left ventricular end diastolic pressure may cause addition of a right heart catheterization to the protocol). It is important to be selective about the inclusion of angiographic studies beyond the coronaries to limit total contrast volume for the study (the upper limit is 3 mL/kg divided by the serum creatinine). In a patient with an elevated creatinine in whom coronary intervention is anticipated, the left ventricular angiogram should be replaced by a noninvasive evaluation of ventricular function and even the number of baseline coronary injections should be limited. With regard to angiography, it is important to keep Sutton's law in mind (When asked why he robbed banks, Willie Sutton is reported to have replied, "because that's where the money is."), and limit contrast injections to the most important diagnostic considerations in a given patient.

Preparation and Premedication of the Patient

It goes without saying that both the medical and the emotional preparation of the patient for cardiac catheterization are the responsibility of the operator. This includes a full explanation of the proposed procedure in such terms that the patient can give truly informed consent. This should include a candid but general discussion of the potential risks, particularly if the patient's condition or the nature of the procedure increases them above the boilerplate information in the preprinted consent form: "There is a less than 1% risk of serious complications (stroke, heart attack, or death) and a similar risk of other complications including bruising or bleeding at the catheter site, plus less than 1 in 1,000 risk of a complication requiring emergency surgery." Otherwise, it is not necessary to go into intricate detail of each of the component risks unless the patient and family indicate a desire for more information. We try to accurately state the moderate amount of discomfort involved, the duration of the procedure, and the postprocedure recovery—failure to do so risks one's credibility. A study of psychologic preparation for cardiac catheterization (44) found that patients who received careful psychologic preparation had lower levels of autonomic arousal both during and after cardiac catheterization than did control subjects.

It is our practice to have the patient fasting (except for oral medications) after midnight, but some laboratories allow a light tea and toast breakfast without ill effects. Complete vital signs should be recorded before the patient leaves the floor (for inpatients), or shortly after arriving at the Ambulatory Center (for outpatients), so that the procedure may be reconsidered if a change has occurred in the patient's condition since he or she was last seen.

Once the question of indications and contraindications has been dealt with and the patient's consent obtained, attention can be directed toward the matter of premedications. We do not administer antibiotics prophylactically before cardiac catheterization, and we know of no controlled studies to support their use, but we may give a dose of intravenous cephalosporin (plus two follow-up doses 8 and 16 hours later) if there have been any breaks in sterile technique or if a groin closure device is being used (particularly in a patient with diabetes mellitus). Various sedatives have been used for premedication. We no longer routinely order premedication to be given before the patient is sent to the Catheterization Laboratory, but instead assess the patient's state of alertness and need for sedation once he or she is on the catheterization table. Per conscious sedation guidelines, we usually administer small repeated doses of midazolam (Versed) 0.5 to 1 mg intravenously and/or fentanyl 25 to 50 mg intravenously to maintain a comfortable but arousable state. With appropriate prior counseling, good local anesthesia, and a reassuring presence by the operator and team throughout, a cardiac catheterization should be an easily tolerated procedure.

THE CARDIAC CATHETERIZATION FACILITY

A modern cardiac catheterization laboratory requires an area of 500 to 700 ft^2, within which will be housed a conglomeration of highly sophisticated electronic and radiographic equipment. Reports of the Inter-Society Commission for Heart Disease Resources on optimal resources for cardiac catheterization facilities have appeared in 1971, 1976, 1983, and 1991 (45). The American College of Cardiology (ACC) and the Society of Cardiac Angiography and

Interventions published a clinical consensus document of cardiac catheterization laboratory standards in 2001 (43). These reports deal with issues regarding lab construction, staffing, quality assurance, and more controversial topics such as the following:

1. Traditional versus nontraditional settings for a cardiac catheterization laboratory; location within a hospital versus freestanding
2. Ambulatory cardiac catheterization: indications and contraindications
3. Ethical issues related to self-ownership of laboratories, self-referral of patients, and advertising
4. Optimal annual caseload for physicians and for the laboratory
5. Safety issues during conduct of the procedure (sterile technique, heparin)
6. Physical arrangements and space requirement
7. Radiation safety and radiologic techniques

Certain points, however, are worth discussing here.

Location Within a Hospital Versus Freestanding

The issue of whether cardiac catheterization laboratories should be hospital based, freestanding, or mobile has been the subject of much debate (45–47). Performance of catheterization in a freestanding or mobile unit should be limited to diagnostic procedures in low-risk patients. In its 1991 report, the ACC/AHA (American Heart Association) Task Force "generally found that in freestanding catheterization laboratories, access to emergency hospitalization may be delayed, and appropriate oversight may be lacking. Additionally, opportunities for self-referral may be fostered and the perception of commercialism and entrepreneurial excess in practice created" (45). Immediately available cardiac surgical backup is particularly critical for laboratories that perform diagnostic catheterization on unstable or high-risk patients, as well as for those that perform coronary angioplasty, endomyocardial biopsy, or trans-septal catheterization. Some states, however, have recently allowed performance of acute MI and even elective coronary intervention in hospitals without on-site cardiac surgery as long as it is performed by operators active at other sites and with a formal plan (e.g., an ambulance standing by, and an agreement with a nearby surgical facility to provide timely backup if needed).

Outpatient Cardiac Catheterization

Outpatient cardiac catheterization has been demonstrated by a variety of groups to be safe, practical, and highly cost efficient, and is now widely practiced throughout the world. Outpatient catheterization can be accomplished by the radial, brachial, or femoral approaches, which allow the patient to be ambulatory within minutes of the completion of the catheterization study (48–51). For femoral procedures, hemostasis can be obtained by manual compression for 10 minutes over the femoral artery, followed by a pressure dressing and bed rest for 2 to 4 hours, or use of a femoral closure device (see Chapter 5) with 1 to 2 hours of bed rest before discharge.

TRAINING STANDARDS

Training in the performance and interpretation of hemodynamic and angiographic derived from cardiac catheterization is an important part of fellowship training in Cardiovascular Disease. The current Accreditation Council for Graduate Medical Education (ACGME) training guidelines call for a minimum of 4 months of diagnostic catheterization experience (100 cases), with an additional 4 months of catheterization experience (100 additional cases) for individuals wishing to perform *diagnostic catheterization* in practice, within the basic 3-year Cardiovascular Disease fellowship (52). Although many cardiologists in the past were jacks-of-all-trades performing office evaluation, noninvasive imaging, pacemaker implantation, and diagnostic cardiac catheterization, the current trends toward ad hoc coronary intervention as an adjunct to diagnostic catheterization (see Chapter 22) make it less likely that new practitioners will be seeking to establish practices that are limited to diagnostic cardiac catheterization.

As the field continues to evolve, it is thus increasingly likely that an *invasive cardiologist* (one who performs cardiac catheterization) will also be an *interventional cardiologist* (one who performs percutaneous coronary intervention). In the first 20 years of coronary intervention (1977–1997), one's designation as an interventional cardiologist was at first based on an expressed interest in the field and attendance at one or more informal training symposia. Subsequently, most interventional cardiologists completed a 1-year fellowship at a center that performed interventional procedures (53).

In 1999, however, the ACGME established the structural, content, and faculty requirements for creating an accredited fellowship in interventional cardiology, requiring an additional 12 months beyond the 3-year general cardiovascular training period, during which at least 250 interventional procedures should be performed (52,54). As of 2005, there were 116 accredited interventional programs with 231 positions (compared with 169 accredited general cardiovascular disease programs with 2,117 positions).

In parallel, the American Board of Internal Medicine (ABIM) recognized the body of knowledge subsumed by interventional cardiology by offering a voluntary one-day proctored examination to individuals who met certain eligibility requirements—documented prior performance of 500 coronary interventions (the practice pathway, no

---

TABLE 1.3
SAMPLE TOPICS THAT MAY BE INCLUDED IN THE INTERVENTIONAL BOARD EXAM

Case selection and management
    Choice of intervention or surgery in patient with chronic ischemic disease
    Intervention in acute myocardial infarction and acute ischemic syndromes
    Drug and device management of hemodynamic compromise
    Selection of patients for percutaneous versus surgical valve therapy
    Management of adult congenital heart disease
    Diagnosis and selection of therapy for peripheral vascular disease
Procedural techniques
    Planning and execution of an interventional plan and backup plans
    Selection and use of guiding catheters, balloons, stents, etc.
    Knowledge of catheter techniques and risks
    Use of antithrombotic agents in interventional procedures
    Management of procedural complications
Basic Science
    Vascular biology of plaque formation, vascular healing, reperfusion
    Platelet function and the clotting cascade, including drug effects
    Coronary anatomy and physiology (flow dynamics, collaterals, perfusion)
Pharmacology
    Biologic effects and use of drugs (vasoactive, sedatives, antiarrhythmics, etc)
    Biologic effects of contrast agents
Imaging
    Use of angiography and ultrasonography (intravascular and intracardiac)
    Radiation physics and radiation safety
Miscellaneous
    Ethical issues and risks of diagnostic and therapeutic techniques
    Statistics, epidemiology, and economic issues of intervention

TABLE 1.4

ACC/AHA TASK FORCE GUIDELINES FOR CATHETERIZATION LABORATORY AND PHYSICIAN CASELOADS

Category	Cases Per Year
Adult catheterization laboratories	300
Pediatric catheterization laboratories	150
Physician caseload*	
Adult diagnostic catheterizations	≥150 but ≤1,000
Adult PTCA procedures	75
Pediatric catheterizations	50
Electrophysiology procedures	100

* The report indicates that physicians with extensive experience (e.g., more than 1,000 independently performed catheterizations) can perform fewer catheterizations to maintain their skill levels.

  Pepine CJ, Allen HD, Bashore TM, et al. ACC/AHA Guidelines for Cardiac Catheterization and Cardiac Catheterization Laboratories. American College of Cardiology/American Heart Association Ad Hoc Task Force on Cardiac Catheterization. *Circulation.* 1991;84: 2213, 2247, and updated in 2001 (see reference 45).

longer open after 2003), or completion of an ACGME-approved interventional fellowship (the fellowship pathway). Candidates able to pass this examination receive Board Certification via a Certificate of Additional Qualification in Interventional Cardiology. An example of the type of content tested in this exam is given in Table 1.3. At this writing, more than 4,000 interventional cardiologists have received the Certificate of Additional Qualification in interventional cardiology, which may soon include the performance of computer-simulated procedures for both training and certification. On the other hand, several thousand individuals continue to perform interventional procedures without the benefit of such certification.

As the field of interventional cardiology expands, it is increasingly recognized that knowledge and skill in coronary intervention does not necessarily confer the ability to safely perform *peripheral* vascular intervention. Some content relating to peripheral vascular procedures is tested in the interventional exam, but individuals interested in performing complex lower extremity or carotid intervention are increasingly undertaking an additional training period after their interventional fellowship to gain the necessary skills and experience (55,56). This training usually includes some degree of training in vascular medicine and noninvasive testing for peripheral vascular disease. At this time, additional board certification has been discussed but not implemented.

As is evident from the range of topics discussed in the remainder of this text, the knowledge and experience base that is now required to perform invasive and interventional cardiology procedures is quite extensive and changes continuously with the serial introduction of new devices and procedures. Staying current in this field thus requires more than completion of a training program and demonstrating an adequate fund of knowledge at one point in

time, but rather it requires an ongoing involvement with a sufficient number of procedures (see below) and serial exposure to new procedures and didactic content through review of new clinical trial literature, attendance at one or more lecture and live-case demonstration courses each year, and participation in FDA-mandated industry training programs on significantly novel interventional devices. *We hope that this text will also be an important part of the effort to stay current in this clinically important field!*

Physician and Laboratory Caseload

Use levels and optimal physician caseload are important issues in invasive cardiology. Earlier reports have recommended 300 diagnostic catheterization cases per year for the laboratory and 150 cases per year for each operator to maintain cost-effectiveness, skills, and favorable outcome (Table 1.4) (45,53). At the same time, a cardiologist should not have such an excessive caseload that it interferes with proper precatheterization evaluation of the patient and adequate postcatheterization interpretation of the data, report preparation, patient follow-up, and continuing medical education. More recent guidelines, however, have pointed out the exceptionally low incidence of complications from diagnostic catheterization and questioned the need for minimum individual operator volumes as long as outcome data collection and quality assurance programs are in place (see below) (43).

For interventional cardiology, the guidelines call for the laboratory to perform a minimum of 200 procedures (more than 400 being ideal), and each operator to perform a minimum of 75 cases per year, to remain proficient (43,53). In actuality, these numbers are generally not enforced except at the level of hospital privileging (compliance with minimal volumes is required in some states, however), and a segment of the interventional community still performs as few as 25 to 50 interventions per year. Outcomes data suggest that higher-volume operators working in higher-volume interventional centers do have greater procedural success and fewer adverse complications. But contradictory data suggest that lower-volume operators can still practice safely, at least if they work side-by-side with more-experienced operators in high-volume centers and if they limit the complexity of the procedures they attempt. With the current very low rate of major complications associated with interventional procedures and the difficulties in accurately adjusting outcomes for differences in case complexity, it would be very difficult to draw statistically valid conclusions about this issue. But as in other areas of procedural medicine, there is a compelling truth to the adage that "practice makes perfect."

The Catheterization Laboratory Director and Quality Assurance

An important check on the appropriateness of procedural indications, the safety of procedural outcomes, and the quality of cath lab report documentation, is the existence of a qualified director in each functioning catheterization laboratory. There are some published general guidelines (43), but my (DSB) comments below are also drawn from more than 20 years of experience in this role.

The director should have at least 5 years of postfellowship experience in procedural performance and should ideally be board certified in both Cardiology and Interventional Cardiology (i.e., the Certificate of Additional Qualification as described above). Important roles of the director include selection and upkeep scheduling of all equipment, oversight of device ordering systems and procedural policies, training supervision of ancillary personnel (nurses, cardiovascular technicians, and radiographic technicians), and development of an equitable case scheduling methodology. The director usually also has fiduciary responsibilities to the hospital for the safe and efficient use of catheterization lab time, personnel, and supplies, as well as oversight of the hospital billing activity for catheterization procedures. In exchange, the director often receives partial salary support from the hospital to cover time taken away from remunerative clinical practice.

But one of the most important roles of the catheterization laboratory director is the systematic collection of outcomes data (using a home-grown database, or increasingly, one of several commercial software packages) and periodic (at least annual) reporting of laboratory volumes, procedure mix, and major adverse outcomes (43). This usually includes periprocedural death, myocardial infarction (usually using the definition of total creatine kinase [CK] greater than twice the upper limit of normal), emergency cardiac surgery, stroke, local vascular complications, and renal failure (see Chapter 3). These are best presented to the clinical cardiology and cardiac surgery staffs in a joint conference, during which laboratory-wide solutions to certain problems can be introduced and their effectiveness monitored in subsequent conferences (so-called Continuous Quality Improvement methodology). The director should also organize didactic conferences for the fellows and faculty as well as a periodic "cath conference" in which interesting cases, complications, and cases performed with new technologies are presented. In short, the director is responsible for overseeing the safe, effective, and up-to-date operation of the laboratory, with the commitment to provide the best patient care.

PERFORMING THE PROCEDURE

Having carefully considered indications and contraindications, chosen a method of approach, designed the catheterization protocol, and prepared the patient, the next step is to perform the cardiac catheterization itself and thereby gain the anatomic and physiologic information needed in the individual case. Benchmarking from 82,548 procedures across 53 catheterization laboratories

in 1997–1998 (57) showed that the average left heart catheterization took 64 minutes of lab time, including 25 minutes of procedure time. Adding a right heart catheterization increased lab time to 84 minutes and procedure time to 32 minutes. Interventional procedures averaged 117 minutes, with a procedure time of roughly 70 minutes. Of course, the actual procedure time varies with operator experience and patient complexity, but these data serve as useful benchmarks.

In individual cardiac catheterization procedures, the choice of procedure components will draw selectively on the techniques that are described throughout this text. Detailed descriptions of catheter insertion and hemodynamic measurements are contained in Section II (Chapters 4 through 6) and Section III (Chapters 7 through 10), with description of angiographic and interventional techniques in Section IV (Chapters 11 through 14) and Section VII (Chapters 22 through 27). Methods for evaluation of cardiac function and special catheter techniques used only in selected situations are described in Section V (Chapters 15 through 17) and VI (Chapters 18 through 21). Interventional techniques are described in Section VII (Chapters 22 through 27).

Our readers should note that the techniques that are described throughout this text are not proposed as the only correct approaches to cardiac catheterization (many laboratories and operators take different approaches, and still obtain excellent results). Rather, they are the methods that have consistently been found to be safe, successful, and practical. Moreover, their strengths and weaknesses are well characterized, and they therefore constitute an excellent point of reference as one's personal practice continues to evolve based on new clinical trial data and individual preference.

REFERENCES

1. Cournand AF. Nobel lecture, December 11, 1956. In *Nobel lectures, physiology and medicine 1942–1962*. Amsterdam: Elsevier, 1964:529.
2. Cournand A. Cardiac catheterization. Development of the technique, its contributions to experimental medicine, and its initial application in man. *Acta Med Scand Suppl* 1975;579:1–32.
3. Mueller RL, Sanborn TA. The history of interventional cardiology: Cardiac catheterization, angioplasty, and related interventions. *Am Heart J* 1995;129:146.
4. Forssmann W. Die Sondierung des rechten Herzens. *Klin Wochenschr* 1929;8:2085.
5. Forssmann, W. *Experiments on myself; memoirs of a surgeon in Germany*. New York, St. Martin's Press. 1974.
6. Klein O. Zur Bestimmung des zerkulatorischen minutens Volumen nach dem Fickschen Prinzip. *Munch Med Wochenschr* 1930;77:1311.
7. Cournand AF, Ranges HS. Catheterization of the right auricle in man. *Proc Soc Exp Biol Med* 1941;46:462.
8. Richards, DW. Cardiac output by the catheterization technique in various clinical conditions. *Fed Proc* 1945;4:215.
9. Cournand AF, et al. Measurement of cardiac output in man using the technique of catheterization of the right auricle or ventricle. *J Clin Invest* 1945;24:106.
10. Dexter L, et al. Studies of congenital heart disease. II. The pressure and oxygen content of blood in the right auricle, right ventricle, and pulmonary artery in control patients, with observations on the oxygen saturation and source of pulmonary "capillary" blood. *J Clin Invest* 1947;26:554.

11. Hellems HK, Haynes FW, Dexter L. Pulmonary "capillary" pressure in man. *J Appl Physiol* 1949;2:24.

12. Lagerlöf H, Werkö L. Studies on circulation of blood in man. *Scand J Clin Lab Invest* 1949;7:147.

13. McMichael J, Sharpey-Schafer EP. The action of intravenous digoxin in man. *Q J Med* 1944;13:1123.

14. Lenègre J, Maurice P. Premiers recherches sur la pression ventriculaire droits. *Bull Mem Soc Med d'Hôp Paris* 1944;80:239.

15. Stead EA Jr, Warren JV. Cardiac output in man: Analysis of mechanisms varying cardiac output based on recent clinical studies. *Arch Intern Med* 1947;80:237.

16. Stead EA Jr, Warren JV, Brannon ES. Cardiac output in congestive heart failure: Analysis of reasons for lack of close correlation between symptoms of heart failure and resting cardiac output. *Am Heart J* 1948;35:529.

17. Bing RJ, et al. Catheterization of coronary sinus and middle cardiac vein in man. *Proc Soc Exp Biol Med* 1947;66:239.

18. Bing RJ, et al. Measurement of coronary blood flow, oxygen consumption, and efficiency of the left ventricle in man. *Am Heart J* 1949;38:1.

19. Bing RJ, Vandam LD, Gray FD Jr. Physiological studies in congenital heart disease. I. Procedures. *Bull Johns Hopkins Hosp* 1947;80:107.

20. Burchell HB. Cardiac catheterization in diagnosis of various cardiac malformations and diseases. *Proc Mayo Clin* 1948;23:481.

21. Wood EH, et al. General and special techniques in cardiac catheterization. *Proc Mayo Clin* 1948;23:494.

22. Burwell CS, Dexter L. Beri-beri heart disease. *Trans Assoc Am Physicians* 1947;60:59.

23. Harvey RM, et al. Some effects of digoxin upon heart and circulation in man: digoxin in left ventricular failure. *Am J Med* 1949;7:439.

24. Zimmerman HA, Scott RW, Becker ND. Catheterization of the left side of the heart in man. *Circulation* 1950;1:357.

25. Limon-Lason R, Bouchard A. El Cateterismo Intracardico; Cateterizacion de las Cavidades Izquierdas en el Hombre. Registro Simultaneo de presion y Electrocardiograma Intracavetarios. *Arch Inst Cardiol Mexico* 1950;21:271.

26. Seldinger SI. Catheter replacement of the needle in percutaneous arteriography: A new technique. *Acta Radiol* 1953;39:368.

27. Ross J Jr. Transseptal left heart catheterization: A new method of left atrial puncture. *Ann Surg* 1959;149:395.

28. Cope C. Technique for transseptal catheterization of the left atrium: Preliminary report. *J Thorac Surg* 1959;37:482.

29. Sones FM Jr, Shirey EK, Prondfit WL, Westcott RN. Cinecoronary arteriography. *Circulation* 1959;20:773 (abstract).

30. Ryan TJ. The coronary angiogram and its seminal contribution to cardiovascular medicine. Circulation 2002; 106:752–756.

31. Ricketts JH, Abrams HL. Percutaneous selective coronary cine arteriography. *JAMA* 1962;181:620.

32. Judkins MP. Selective coronary arteriography: A percutaneous transfemoral technique. *Radiology* 1967;89:815.

33. Swan HJC, et al. Catheterization of the heart in man with use of a flow directed balloon-tipped catheter. *N Engl J Med* 1970;283:447.

34. Grüntzig A, et al. Coronary transluminal angioplasty. *Circulation* 1977;56(II):319 (abstract).

35. Grüntzig A, Senning A, Siegenthaler WE. Nonoperative dilatation of coronary artery stenoses. Percutaneous transluminal coronary angioplasty. *N Engl J Med* 1979;301:61.

36. King SB III. The development of interventional cardiology. *J Am Coll Cardiol* 1998;31:64B.

37. Gibbons RJ, Abrams J, Chatterjee K, et al. ACC/HA 2002 guideline update for the management of patients with chronic stable angina.

38. Braunwald E, Antman EM, Beasley JW, et al. ACC/AHA 2002 guideline update for the management of patients with unstable angina and non-ST segment elevation myocardial infarction. A report of the American College of Cardiology/American Heart Association Task Force on Practice Guidelines (Committee on the Management of the Patients with Unstable Angina). 2002. American College of Cardiology Web site. Available at: *http://www.acc.org/clinical/guidelines/unstable/incorporated/index.htm*. Accessed October 17, 2002.

39. Antman EM, Anbe DT, Armstron PW, et al. ACC/AHA guidelines for the management of patients with ST-elevation myocardial infarction. *J Am Coll Cardiol* 2004;44:671–719.

40. Shapiro SM; Oudiz RJ; Cao T, et al. Primary pulmonary hypertension: improved long-term effects and survival with continuous intravenous epoprostenol infusion. *J Am Coll Cardiol* 1997;30: 343–9.

41. Kaplan AV, Baim DS, Smith JJ. Medical device development: from prototype to regulatory approval. *Circulation* 2004;109:3068–3072.

42. Green GS, McKinnon CM, Rosch J, Judkins MP. Complications of selective percutaneous transfemoral coronary arteriography and their prevention. *Circulation* 1972;45:552.

43. Bashore TM, Bates ER, Berger, et al. American College of Cardiology/Society of Cardiac Angiography and Interventions clinical expert consensus document of cardiac catheterization laboratory standards. *J Am Coll Cardiol* 2001;37:2170–214.

44. Anderson KO, Masur FT. Psychological preparation for cardiac catheterization. *Heart Lung* 1989;18:154–163.

45. Pepine CJ, et al. ACC/AHA Guidelines for Cardiac Catheterization and Cardiac Catheterization Laboratories. American College of Cardiology/American Heart Association Ad Hoc Task Force on Cardiac Catheterization. *Circulation* 1991;84:2213.

46. Conti CR. Presidents' page: cardiac catheterization laboratories: Hospital-based, free-standing or mobile? *J Am Coll Cardiol* 1990; 15:748.

47. Elliott CM, Bersin RM, Elliott AV, et al. Mobile Cardiac Catheterization Laboratory. *Cathet Cardiovasc Diagn* 1994;31:8–15.

48. Fierens E. Outpatient coronary arteriography. A report on 12,719 studies. *Cathet Cardiovasc Diagn* 1984;10:27.

49. Block PC, Ockene I, Goldberg RJ, et al. A prospective randomized trial of outpatient versus inpatient cardiac catheterization. *N Engl J Med* 1988;319:1251.

50. Kern MJ, Cohn M, Talley JD, et al. Early ambulation after 5 French diagnostic cardiac catheterization: Results of a multi-center trial. *J Am Coll Cardiol* 1990;15:1475.

51. Pink S, Fiutowski L, Gianelly RE. Outpatient cardiac catheterizations: analysis of patients requiring admission. *Clin Cardiol* 1989;12:375–378.

52. Beller GA, Bonow RO, Fuster V. ACC revised recommendations for training in adult cardiovascular medicine core cardiology training II (COCATS 2). *J Am Coll Cardiol* 2002;39:1242–1246.

53. Hirshfeld JW, Ellis SG, Faxon DP, et al. Recommendations for the assessment and maintenance of proficiency in interventional procedures. *J Am Coll Cardiol* 1998;31:722–743.

54. Hirshfeld JW, Banas JS, Cowley et al. American College of Cardiology training statement on recommendations for the structure of an optimal adult interventional cardiology training program. *J Am Coll Cardiol* 1999;34:2141–2147.

55. Creager MA, Goldstone J, Hirshfeld JW Jr, et al. ACC/ACP/SCAI/SVMB/SVS clinical competence statement on vascular medicine and catheter-based peripheral vascular intervention. *J Am Coll Cardiol* 2004;44:941–957.

56. Rosenfield K, Babb JD, Cates CU, et al. Clinical competence statement on carotid stenting: training and credentialing for carotid stenting—multidisciplinary consensus recommendation. *J Am Coll Cardiol* 2005:165–174.

57. Becker ER, Cohen D, Culler SD, et al. Benchmarking cardiac catheterization laboratories—the impact of patient age, gender and risk factors on variable costs, total time and procedural time. *J Invasive Cardiol* 1999;11:533–542.

Cineangiographic Imaging, Radiation Safety, and Contrast Agents

2

Stephen Balter   *Donald S. Baim*

In addition to mastering clinical, pharmacologic, and technical knowledge (see Chapter 1), an interventional cardiologist must also have a good working knowledge of the physical, engineering, and radiobiologic principles underlying fluoroscopic-cineangiographic equipment and radiation safety. This applies to both selection and quality maintenance of complex imaging equipment, as well as to its correct operation to provide optimal images while protecting both patients and staff from unnecessary radiation. Safety is more than a theoretical concern, because severe radiation injuries have occured as a result of prolonged interventional procedures with fluoroscopy times >30 minutes (1–3). The introduction of beta- and gamma-brachytherapy into the catheterization laboratory (see Chapter 22) has further broadened the operator knowledge requirements about radiation biology and radiation safety, and formal documentation of radiation competency is now expected of interventional cardiologists. The qualifying examination for the Certificate of Additional Qualification in Interventional Cardiology thus assigns 15% of the examination to imaging and radiation safety (4). A current intersociety clinical competency statement outlines the necessary body of knowledge (5), with similar guidance available in Europe (6).

This chapter consists of major sections devoted to basic x-ray physics, fluoroscopic imaging technology, radiopathology, patient radiation management, staff radiation safety, and iodinated contrast agents. It is current at the time of its writing, but those seeking more detailed technical information are referred to standard textbooks in the field (7–9).

BASIC X-RAY PHYSICS

X-rays are a form of electromagnetic radiation, like their longer wavelength cousins, radio waves and visible light. Like light, the x-ray beam can also be viewed as a stream of particles (photons, i.e., discrete packets of electromagnetic radiation that each contain a defined amount of energy. By virtue of its very short wavelength and related very high frequency, each x-ray photon contains thousands of times the energy of a photon of visible light. This explains why x-ray photons can pass through solid matter and why different and more potent biologic effects occur when an x-ray photon is absorbed or scattered from living tissue.

X-Ray Dose and Its Measurement

There are many ways to measure radiation units, and a full explanation of all of the current dose definitions, and those of related older units, is available in the literature. This chapter focuses on those dosimetric units that are of importance in the interventional laboratory (Table 2.1).

Exposure is the radiation level at a point in space, commonly measured with an ionization chamber in units of air kerma (*k*inetic *e*nergy *r*eleased in *ma*terial; dose delivered to air). The older unit was the roentgen, R, defined as 2.58×10^{-4} coulombs per kilogram of air. By itself, exposure gives no direct information regarding how much radiation energy is delivered to a person or the biologic effects that irradiation might have.

TABLE 2.1
CLINICALLY IMPORTANT DOSIMETRIC DEFINITIONS

Dose (to a defined substance) Unit is the gray.	The concentration of radiation energy locally absorbed by the defined substance. Under almost all circumstances, the dose delivered by an x-ray beam varies from point to point in the patient. 1 Gy (specific substance) = 1 joule (absorbed)/kg (specific substance)
Air kerma (exposure) Unit is the gray.	The dose delivered to air at a point in space. Fluoroscopic output is usually stated in terms of air dose at a reference point. This value can then be used to calculate patient-related dosimetric quantities. 1 Gy (air) = 1 joule (absorbed)/kg (air)
Effective dose Unit is the sievert.	A calculated quantity based on the physical dose delivered to each of the patient's tissues and modified by the sensitivity of that tissue to cancer induction. It is therefore a measure of the risk of cancer induction caused by that irradiation. Radiation protection guidelines are often expressed in terms of effective dose. ED (Sv) = Σ [Dose to a volume of tissue (Gy)] $\times$ Radiosensitivity of that tissue
Skin dose Unit is the gray.	The dose delivered to a portion of the patient's skin during a procedure. It is the sum of the dose delivered by the imaging beam and the dose delivered by x-ray photons backscattered from the patient toward the entrance surface. Backscatter adds approximately 30% to the entrance dose delivered by the fluoroscope in typical invasive cardiology settings.
Peak skin dose Unit is the gray.	The maximum dose delivered to any portion of a patient's skin during a fluoroscopic procedure. Deterministic radiation injuries, such as skin burns, are produced if the peak skin dose exceeds a threshold value.
Dose–area product (DAP) Unit is the gray cm^2.	The product of the air dose at a certain distance from the x-ray tube and the cross sectional area of the x-ray beam at the same distance. DAP is actually independent of distance; as distance increases, air dose decreases and beam size increases in an exactly offsetting manner. Because most of the x-ray beam is absorbed by the patient, DAP is a conveniently measurable surrogate for effective dose. Most currently used interventional fluoroscopes include a DAP meter.
Cumulative dose Unit is the gray (air kerma).	The air dose delivered to the interventional reference point during an entire procedure. It includes both fluoroscopic and cinefluorographic contributions to the total. It represents the skin dose from that procedure only if the beam does not move during the procedure.
Dose at the interventional reference point (DIRP) Unit is the gray (air kerma).	The air dose delivered to a defined reference point. This point is selected to be representative of the entrance skin surface of an average sized patient's skin for a fixed x-ray beam. Under these circumstances, DIRP provides a reasonable estimate of peak skin dose.

Dose refers to the local concentration of energy absorbed by tissue from the x-ray beam when the exposure interacts with the individual atoms in the tissue. Specifically, dose is the amount of energy absorbed from the radiation field by a small volume of tissue, divided by the mass of the tissue. This is currently measured in gray (Gy, or 1 joule per kilogram), which corresponds to a very large radiation dose. Accordingly, dose is more often expressed as centigray (cGy, 1/100 Gy), equal to the older unit of dose known as the *rad* or radiation absorbed dose or milligray (mGy, 1/1000 Gy). Because the dose delivered by an x-ray beam is almost always nonuniform (owing to absorption of incoming photons by the more superficial tissues with fewer photons available to deliver dose to deeper tissues), the highest dose is generally delivered to the skin where the beam enters the patient (entry dose). There are also tissue-to-tissue differences in absorbed dose for the same exposure (the principle on which x-ray imaging is based), with water absorbing 0.9 rad (9 mGy) per 1 R of exposure, compared with bone absorbing 4 rad (40 mGy) per 1 R of exposure.

Different types of radiation produce different degrees of damage (i.e., alpha particles versus x-rays), which is taken into account by an absorbed *equivalent* dose expressed in units of sievert (in older units, the unit was rem [radiation equivalent in man] with 10 mSv equal to 1 rem). Although this distinction is important for certain types of radiation, the distinction between Gy and Sv (or between rad and rem) is largely semantic, because they (Gy and Sv) are essentially equivalent for diagnostic x-rays. In 1987, the National Council on Radiation Protection (NCRP) introduced a new term, the effective dose equivalent (EDE, also measured in Sv or rem), which is a weighted average that takes into account the physical distribution of radiation and the relative radiosensitivity of different organs.

Clinical Measurement of Radiation

Two important locations at which to measure dose are the patient's entrance skin and the entrance to image receptor (Fig. 2.1). Measurements at the patient's entrance surface provide information needed to calculate the radiogenic risk to the patient, whereas measurements at the image receptor entrance define the number of photons available for image formation and determine image noise. Direct

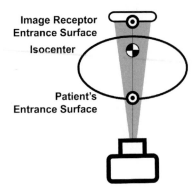

Image Receptor
Entrance Surface

Isocenter

Patient's
Entrance Surface

Figure 2.1 Patient and image receptor dose measuring points. Dose measurements referenced to the point at which the x-ray beam enters the patient are useful for estimating patient radiation risks. Measurements referenced to the image receptor entrance can be used to manage image quality.

measurements of patient entrance dose during a procedure are not compatible with clinical routine, so fluoroscopic systems provide a variety of indirect measurements that can be used to estimate actual skin dose. The most basic of these is fluoroscopic time, the time (in minutes) when the x-ray beam is "on" during a procedure. This was a useful tool for the manually controlled fluoroscopes available in the 1950s, but it is of limited value now because it neither keeps track of cine usage nor reflects the effect on patient entrance dose owing to tissue thickness. Most modern cardiovascular fluoroscopes thus incorporate software to estimate the *dose–area product (DAP)*. DAP includes both fluoro and cine exposure and reflects the influence of tissue thickness on skin dose. But because the same DAP can be delivered as either a high dose to a small field size or as a low dose to a large field size, it cannot be used directly to predict the possibility of a skin injury (which would be significantly higher in the former case). Rules of thumb, however, do allow DAP meters to be used to manage skin risk with reasonable accuracy, as discussed below.

Interventional systems compliant with the International Electrotechnical Commission's (IEC) standard on Interventional Fluoroscopic Safety (10) also provide a measurement of estimated dose at the entrance surface of a normal-sized patient under typical angiographic conditions. This may overestimate or underestimate skin dose for a real patient and assumes that the beam entry point is constant during a procedure. It thus overestimates actual skin dose when there is considerable beam movement during a procedure, as in performing angiography from different angles.

X-Ray Production

X-rays are produced when high-energy electrons are decelerated by interacting with a metallic target (in our case, tungsten). For that reason, the principal method of x-ray production is usually called *bremsstrahlung* (breaking radiation). The resulting x-ray photons have a spectrum of photon energies, from approximately 20 KeV up to the maximum voltage applied to the x-ray tube (usually 70 to 120 KeV). Some additional x-ray production occurs when the incoming electrons interact with the orbital electrons of the target's atoms. Because the emerging x-ray photons produced by this means carry a particular energy characteristic reflecting the energy levels of the target's atomic orbits, these are called characteristic x-rays.

X-Ray Image Formation

An x-ray beam traveling through a uniform material would carry little information. When the beam travels through tissues with different x-ray absorbance, different fractions of the incident radiation are absorbed (Fig. 2.2); thus the beam leaving the patient is modulated by the pattern of differential absorbance. The modulated beam exits from the patient and is detected by an image receptor. An object can be delineated in the image only if its x-ray absorbance is sufficiently different from that of its surrounding structures to produce sufficiently different exit beam intensity in that location, as a function of the atomic number of the attenuating material, x-ray photon energy, physical density (gm/cc) of the object, and the thickness of the object.

Natural differences in absorbance between tissues can be enhanced by using a contrast agent—a material of markedly different absorbance than the tissue—which can be delivered or concentrated in an anatomic structure of interest. In the catheterization laboratory, the intravascular contrast agents described later in this chapter are based on iodine, whose high atomic number and x-ray spectrum (it absorbs intensely at 40 to 75 KeV) allow visualization of even small (submillimeter) vessels on the x-ray image when the iodine-containing contrast agent displaces lower-density water (blood) during angiography.

Unfortunately, when higher energy x-ray spectra (>100 KeV) are used to image the heart through long tissue paths, the difference between iodine or steel (i.e., a stent or guidewire) and the water density of surrounding tissue is reduced substantially. This is one of the reasons why stents and contrast media vary in visibility from view to view and from patient to patient.

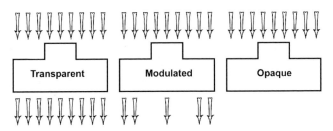

Figure 2.2 Beam modulation. Total transmission of the x-ray beam produces a uniform signal. Total attenuation produces a silhouette. Image formation requires attenuation of a portion of the x-ray beam. Thus patient dose is unavoidable (see reference 5).

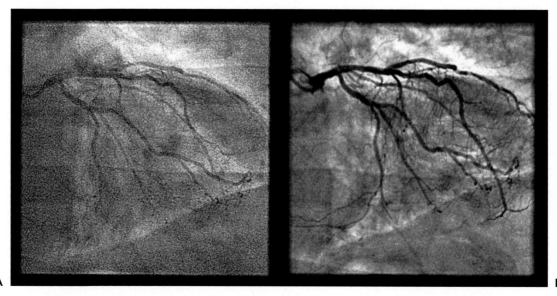

A   B

Figure 2.3 Image receptor dose, system settings, and image quality. The image on the left is a fluoroscopic last image hold (LIH). The image on the right is a cine frame. The increased noise in the LIH results from less dose used in its production. The increase contrast in the cine results from system programming to a lower kVp.

Image Noise

A radiographic image of even a uniformly dense object will have random point-to-point variations in brightness over time. These random fluctuations are called *image noise* (commonly referred to as *quantum mottle*). As the x-ray dose striking the image receptor decreases (Fig. 2.3), the amount of image noise increases (fewer imaging photons equals a noisier image). Noise reduces the ability to detect low-contrast structures, but this can be overcome by increasing the dose, thereby suppressing noise and increasing our ability to resolve such structures. On the other hand, the desire for a low-noise image always must be balanced against the fact that increasing dose also increases patient x-ray exposure.

Scattered Radiation

Scattered radiation is produced when the x-ray beam interacts with the patient and is redirected rather than absorbed completely. If scattered radiation reaches the image receptor, it contributes to noise and reduces the image contrast created as the primary x-ray beam interacts with the anatomic structures. Scattered radiation is also the principal source of exposure for the patient's body parts that lie outside the field of the primary x-ray beam and also for the laboratory staff. The amount of scatter increases with increases in the intensity of the x-ray beam and the size of the x-ray field.

Optimizing the Exposure Parameters and Image Quality

From the discussion above, it is clear that the goal of producing a usable x-ray image requires a number of trade-offs.

Ideal x-ray imaging parameters must appropriately balance the requirements for contrast (needed to detect the object), sharpness (needed to characterize it, including image noise), and patient dose. The dose must be chosen at the minimum level that will generate an image with an acceptable degree of noise, to minimize patient exposure. Increasing *kVp* (using more energetic photons) can penetrate a large patient more easily and thus reduce patient exposure, but it decreases image contrast significantly. Decreasing the *image receptor input dose* reduces patient exposure, but increases image noise. Thus, for a given patient size, there is an optimal balance that provides acceptable image contrast at an acceptable image noise level while minimizing patient dose. In most modern cinefluorographic units, programs installed at system setup are designed to give a clinically useful balance between these parameters automatically, although some configurable settings can be programmed by the user if flexibility is desired.

THE OPERATION OF A CINEFLUOROGRAPHIC SYSTEM

The main functions of an x-ray cinefluorographic system are to produce a collimated x-ray beam of appropriate intensity and quality, to project that beam through the patient at a desired angle, to detect the modulated x-ray beam after it passes through the patient, and to transduce the modulated x-ray beam into a usable visible light image. These components are schematically illustrated in Fig. 2.4.

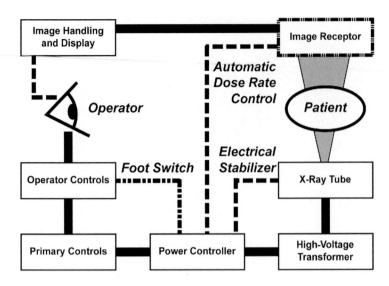

Figure 2.4 Generator and feedback schematic. Modern generators rely on a large number of feedback loops to manage radiation dose and stabilize image quality. The operator provides the final control loop by managing system resources.

Radiation Production and Control

Generators

The cinefluorographic x-ray generator controls and delivers electrical power to the x-ray tube. It heats the x-ray tube's filament to produce a beam of electrons at a current between 1 and 1,000 milliamperes (mA). These electrons are accelerated toward the target anode by high voltage between 40 and 125 DC kilovolts (kVp), applied by the generator. The flow of high-energy electrons toward the anode is not continuous, but is separated into pulses whose duration ranges from 1 to 10 milliseconds (mS) and whose repetition rate ranges from 15 to 60 pulses per second.

Most new x-ray generators use the incoming electrical power to drive a power oscillator operating in the audio frequency range. Voltage is increased by means of a step-up transformer, and the output is rectified (converted to DC) and smoothed before being applied to the x-ray tube. A second circuit supplies a nominal 10 volts to heat the filament of the x-ray tube. Switching circuits effectively turn the electron flow through the x-ray tube on or off to provide beam pulsing. The operator instructs the generator to initiate beam generation at either fluoroscopic or cinefluorographic levels through a pair of foot pedals.

Although beam pulsing was always part of cineangiography to minimize motion and lack of sharpness, earlier systems used continuous x-ray generation during fluoroscopy. In contrast, current digital systems use *pulsed fluoroscopy*, in which the x-ray beam is briefly turned on (pulsed for 1 to 10 mS) once during the recording of each video frame. The fluoroscope must deliver enough radiation dose during each pulse to ensure appropriate image quality, with the video detector storing that image until it is read out and displayed. Digital systems provide gap-filling images to

eliminate visual flicker that would otherwise result from frame rates of 15 images per second. Although higher rates may be needed when tachycardia is present, they clearly increase patient dose.

Juggling and optimizing these various x-ray parameters is necessary as angles change and as the beam is moved (panned) across the heart. This is well beyond the manual capabilities of a technologist and therefore requires circuitry in the generator that continuously measures the actual voltage across the x-ray tube, the current flowing through it, the pulse width, and the amount of light generated at the image receptor. These data are used to adjust the input parameters—voltage (kVp), current (mA), and pulse width (mS)—for proper operation.

X-Ray Tubes

The x-ray tube is a device that converts a portion of the electrical energy delivered by the generator into x-rays. The x-ray tube consists of an evacuated glass or metal housing that contains a tungsten filament (housed in a focusing cup), and an anode disc (tungsten alloy, 100 to 200 mm in diameter), which rotates at more than 10,000 rpm (Fig. 2.5). Electrons are emitted from the filament by thermionic emission. The number of emitted electrons, and thereby the tube current (mA), is controlled by adjusting the filament temperature. These electrons accelerate toward the anode under the influence of the electric field (~100 kV) supplied by the generator. The sudden deceleration caused by interactions with the tungsten atoms in the anode produces x-ray photons by the bremsstrahlung (braking) process, as described above. For sharpest imaging, the point of impact of the electron beam on the target should be as small as possible, so that x-ray emission appears to come from a single "point" focal spot.

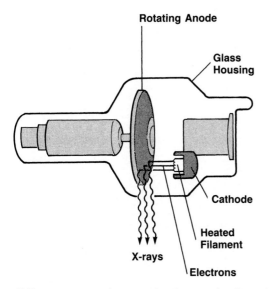

Figure 2.5 Rotating anode x-ray tube. See text for discussion.

The actual size of the focal spot represents a balance between the requirements for sharp and fast imaging and the need to avoid melting the target. X-ray tubes have two filaments and hence two focal spots. The smaller (typically 0.3 to 0.5 mm) is used for fluoroscopy. A larger focal spot (typically 0.8 to 1.0 mm) is used to accommodate the higher power requirements of adult cine. In addition, the anodes rotate at high speed to spread the heating over a long focal track instead of concentrating it on a small point.

X-ray generation is extremely inefficient from the standpoint of energy transformation. Less than 1% of the electrical energy applied to the tube is converted to x-rays. The remainder is deposited in the tube as heat. This creates an important heat dissipation challenge for X-ray tube design. Too much heat delivered in too short a time will melt the anode. Present tube designs are capable of dissipating several times as much heat as those of the early 1990s. Thus, these tubes can deliver significantly more radiation to patients without overload than was possible a decade or so ago. A tube heat warning occurring during a procedure is a clinical indicator that substantial amounts of radiation may have been delivered to the patient.

X-Ray Beam Filtration and Shaping

Although the maximum x-ray photon energy is set by the acceleration voltage supplied by the generator (kVp), the beam contains a spectrum of lower energies as well. These low-energy x-ray photons are easily absorbed by the patient's superficial tissues and thus do not contribute to image formation. To avoid nonproductive entry site exposure, it is good practice to remove (filter) these low-energy photons from the beam before they enter the patient. An aluminum plate placed in the x-ray tube's beam port preferentially absorbs the low-energy photons and increases

the effective penetrating power of the resulting beam (beam hardening). Many modern interventional fluoroscopes offer a copper filter as well as the required aluminum filter, because the higher atomic number of copper relative to aluminum produces even more beam hardening than does aluminum. High-power x-ray tubes, copper filters, and appropriate fluoroscopic system programming can be combined to produce an x-ray spectrum that has a large fraction of its photons just beyond the K-absorption edge of iodine (~40 KeV), to provide significant skin dose reduction without adversely affecting iodine visibility (11).

But too much beam filtration can be a liability by discarding too much of the generated x-ray beam. The x-ray tube and generator have clear limits on input power delivery that make it impossible to overcome excessive filtering by increased beam generation. Copper filters of any appreciable thickness are thus too attenuating for adult cine and are automatically removed when the cine pedal is selected. In some systems, the automatic dose rate control system may automatically add and remove filters during fluoroscopy, depending on beam angulation and the patient size. Small changes in path length can thus result in large changes in skin dose rate if one is working near such a transition point. Operators should be aware of the filter operating strategy for the systems and clinical modes in which they work.

The x-ray beam is spatially limited so that only the field of view (FOV) seen by the operator on the monitor is irradiated. Absolute beam limitation requirements are specified in national regulations and international standards. The primary beam port is equipped with lead shutters, which are adjusted automatically as the system tracks the active FOV and distance between the focal spot and the image receptor, to adjust these shutters to appropriately limit the irradiated area. The functionality of this device needs to be checked periodically. The lead shutters can also be manually closed to less than the full FOV. Such collimating of the beam has a beneficial effect on image quality (reducing scatter) while simultaneously reducing both patient and staff irradiation.

Many systems also have movable semitransparent copper shutters (also called *wedges*) that can be positioned over the lung field up to the heart border in each projection to improve overall image quality by reducing excessive image brightness over the lungs. These shutters also help minimize unnecessary patient and staff irradiation.

Imaging Modes

X-ray cinefluorographic units operate in two modes: fluoroscopy and acquisition (cine or image recording). The purposes and x-ray generator operating parameters of the two modes are different, particularly in terms of the input x-ray dose delivered and in image quality. Figure 2.3 shows single-frame images acquired at fluoroscopic and acquisition doses.

Fluoroscopy

Fluoroscopy provides a real-time x-ray image with adequate quality for guiding manipulations. The physiology of vision effectively integrates several frames; this reduces perceived image noise, so greater image noise can be tolerated allowing fluoroscopic x-ray input dose rates that are significantly lower than those used for acquisition.

Current fluoroscopic systems have two or more operator selectable fluoroscopic dose rates. The higher dose rates provide less image noise at the cost of greater patient and operator exposure. Many systems offer variable fluoroscopic frame rates. Decreasing the frame rate saves dose at the expense of visual smoothness of the transition between frames. Because of persistence of vision effects, lowering frame rates does not linearly lower required dose rates (12) Many operators find 15 frames per second (fps) to be satisfactory for digital cardiac fluoroscopy.

Acquisition (Cine)

The acquisition mode generates images of sufficient quality for single-frame viewing. Higher x-ray input dose rates are needed to reduce image noise and optimize clinical visualization, and most x-ray cinefluorographic units are calibrated such that the per-frame dose for acquisition is approximately 15 times greater than for fluoroscopy. A single frame acquired in acquisition mode thus delivers about the same patient dose as one second of pulsed fluoroscopy at 15 fps.

The optimal acquisition mode input dose per frame is that which achieves the best balance between image noise and image quality. The cine dose rate is also directly proportional to the acquisition frame rate. As with fluoroscopy, digital gap-fill can achieve flicker-free image displays at any frame rate, but the image presentation may become increasingly jerky at frame rates below 15 fps despite such gap-fill. The typical acquisition frame rate for adult studies is 15 fps.

Feedback

The x-ray beam is attenuated as it passes through tissue. The degree of attenuation varies with tissue density and other factors such as the projection angle and the distance between the x-ray tube and the image receptor. Feedback circuits measure the brightness of the image generated by the image receptor. This feedback signal is used to modulate the output of the generator in response to changes in patient density and position. This is accomplished by an automatic dose rate control (ADRC) circuit that is designed to maintain a constant brightness level of the image-intensifier output signal. The normal function of this circuit has a profound influence on patient skin dose. X-ray intensity is increased if the detector measures too dim a signal and decreased if the signal is too bright. This means that the patient entrance port skin dose increases substantially when compound projection angles with cranial or caudal skewing are used (Fig. 2.6).

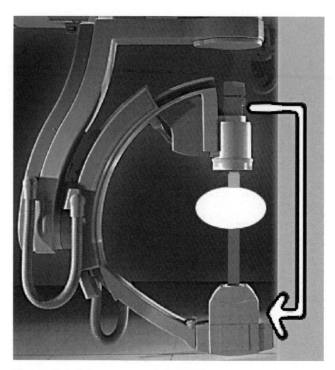

Figure 2.6 Patient size profoundly affects patient dose. Fluoroscopic systems continuously adjust x-ray output to account for differences in patient size and beam angulation. This is accomplished by using feedback circuits that maintain constant image receptor dose by adjusting the x-ray tube's electrical inputs. Skin dose will double for every 4- to 6-cm increase in path length through the patient. (Photo of gantry courtesy of Philips.)

The ADRC can control the tube voltage (kV), tube current (mA), pulse width (expressed in mS), and beam filtration. Different makes and models of fluoroscopes are likely to have different ADRC strategies. Most machines offer different ADRC modes of operation. For example: When the system is set to cine coronary arteries, the ADRC remains functional throughout the entire cine run; when the same system is set to LV lock, however, the ADRC establishes a level early in the run and then maintains that level during the contrast injection phase of the ventriculogram.

X-Ray Detection and Recording

Image Detection

The x-ray image formed by the interaction of the x-ray beam and the patient must be detected and transformed into a visible format. The fluorescent screen was the original x-ray detector used by Roentgen. It was the only fluoroscopic detector available from the discovery of x-rays in 1895 until the development of the x-ray image intensifier in the 1950s. The image intensifier was the enabling technology for coronary angiography (13). At the start of the new millennium, solid-state detectors are now beginning to replace the conventional image intensifier.

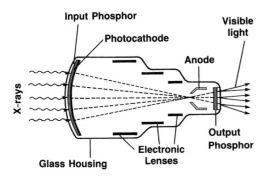

Figure 2.7 X-ray image intensifier. See text for discussion.

Image Intensifier

The structure of a single-mode image intensifier is shown in Fig. 2.7. The modulated x-ray beam emerging from the patient enters the image intensifier and is detected by a cesium iodide (CsI) fluorescent layer. The visible light image emerging from the CsI is converted into an electron image by a photocathode. Focusing electrodes in the tube accelerate and converge the electrons onto a small output window. The electron image is then converted back into a visible light image when these electrons interact with an output screen. The combination of acceleration of the electrons and minifying of the output image relative to the input produces the 100,000-fold brightness gain provided by the image intensifier.

Cardiac image intensifiers offer several magnification modes. These tubes contain a separate set of focusing electrodes for each magnification mode. When a specific magnification is selected, the corresponding set of electrodes is energized. This focuses a larger or smaller portion of the input screen onto the fixed size output screen. The minifying gain of the tube (ratio of active input screen area to the fixed output screen area) decreases as the tube is zoomed; therefore smaller fields of view require higher input dose rates than do larger fields of view.

Cardiac image intensifiers have a typical maximum physical FOV of 23 to 25 cm. For any magnification, the actual FOV can be somewhat smaller if the optics are set up to overframe the image. Smaller FOVs (typically around 17 and 12 cm) provide better spatial resolution at the expense of requiring an increased dose rate. Patient dose can be minimized by working at the largest FOV consistent with appropriately seeing the structures of image. Visibility can sometimes be improved in heavy patients by increasing the FOV and collimating the beam because of the increased minifying gain associated with large FOVs.

Vascular image intensifiers are available with FOVs exceeding 40 cm. When these tubes are operated using a typical 17-cm cardiac FOV, they require a significantly higher dose rate than smaller cardiac image intensifiers. In addition, the larger size of vascular tubes limits beam angulation. Moving the image intensifier farther from the patient to obtain the necessary angles further increases patient dose.

Image intensifiers degrade over time. Service adjustments can compensate for these losses. Eventually the brightness gain deteriorates such that x-ray dose rates must be increased simply to obtain adequate brightness. This will often happen between 3 and 10 years after installation. When the service engineer informs you that the system is at the limits of its adjustment range, it is time to replace the image intensifier.

Cine Camera and Associated Optics

The technology for recording coronary images has almost totally migrated from the cine-film camera to the digital domain. However, film-based technology still merits a brief review both to provide an understanding of older systems and to demonstrate the migration of imaging requirements from film to digital.

Cine cameras are electronically synchronized with the hospital's AC power supply. The usual adult filming speed was 30 fps in the United States and 25 fps in Europe. Most of the cine-film systems built in the late 20th century incorporated pulsed x-ray beams. These systems were programmed to produce x-ray pulse widths in the 2- to 10-mS range. These single-frame exposure times are short enough to freeze cardiac motion.

An optical system coupled the image intensifier to the cameras. Adjustable optical diaphragms were used to balance radiation dose and camera light levels. These diaphragms also allow service compensation for image intensifier degradation over time. The focal length of the optical system determines framing mode—the way in which the round output phosphor is represented on the rectangular cine frame (Fig. 2.8). Most laboratories used some form of overframing, in which the recorded field is less than the full active image intensifier area. In all such systems, it is essential to verify that only the recorded area of the patient is irradiated. In film-based systems, the ultimate quality of the recorded image depends nearly as much on the selection of cine film and its processing parameters as on the elements within the image chain.

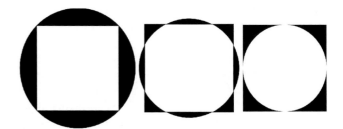

Figure 2.8 Image framing. The focal length of the lens between the image intensifier and the video camera determines the visualized fraction of the output screen. Full overframing is shown on the left, partial in the center, and exact framing on the right. The choice determines the relative use of the image intensifier's physical field of view.

Video

Real-time fluoroscopic visualization is the enabling technology for invasive and interventional procedures. Video cameras and displays are the conduit between the image receptor and the observer's eye. Since the 1960s, this has been accomplished by placing a television camera in a position where it can (along with the 35-mm cine camera) view the output phosphor of the image intensifier. Solid-state charge-coupled device (CCD) television pickups have displaced analog video cameras in the last decade. The outputs of the video camera are converted into a digital television image and processed to enhance image quality before being stored or displayed. When the intent of imaging is simply to position a catheter or to perform a test injection, the cine camera need not operate, and the generator need provide only a low dose rate of radiation that is adequate to create a television image. Fluoroscopy thus involves <10% of the x-ray beam intensity that is used for permanent image recording (cineangiography). However, because fluoroscopic times are much longer than cine times, fluoroscopy typically provides more than half of the patient's total dose.

Older analog systems used the same interlaced scanning and display format as for broadcast television. Newer analog and all CCD systems use a progressive scanning and display format to allow higher video line rates (e.g., 1,024 versus 512 scan lines) and frame refresh rates. Therefore, video clips produced by such systems are not directly compatible with broadcast video components and recorders, although scan converters can be used to translate the video back to broadcast formats and standards.

Flat-Panel X-Ray Detectors

The image intensifier/video camera combination is currently being displaced by integrated digital image receptors (flat-panel detectors). Indirect detectors incorporate a charge-coupled device or photodiode visible light detector array in direct contact with the input phosphor. Direct detectors use a selenium layer to directly convert x-rays into an electron signal. Both designs generate a digital video signal with fewer intervening stages than described above for the phosphor image intensifier/video camera systems. Figure 2.9 schematically illustrates the structure of both flat-panel detectors.

The dose efficiency of a flat-panel detector is grossly similar to that of a modern image intensifier, so patient doses delivered by two fluoroscopes—one a flat-panel and the other an image intensifier—will be similar. However, flat-panel fluoroscopic systems often have a broader dynamic range and better dosimetric performance than older image intensifier–based systems owing to better dose management hardware and software in other parts of the fluoroscope.

The imaging behavior of a flat-panel system differs from an image intensifier/digital video system in one important respect. As shown in Fig. 2.10, when an image intensifier is

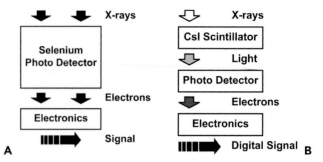

Figure 2.9 Indirect and direct digital (flat-panel) image receptors. The indirect (left) detector uses a CsI scintillator, virtually identical to that in an image intensifier, to convert the x-ray signal into light. A photodetector converts the light into an electron signal. This signal is then digitized. The direct detector (right) uses a selenium layer to directly convert the x-ray signal into an electrical charge distribution. This signal is then digitized.

zoomed, less and less of the patient is imaged by the tube's fixed-size output screen. Therefore each pixel in the zoomed image is smaller (relative to the patient) than for the unzoomed case; i.e., spatial resolution increases with zoom. In the flat-panel case, zooming simply uses fewer of the available pixels, so that the intrinsic spatial resolution does not increase with zoom. However, the digitally magnified image on the monitor may provide better detail coupling to the observer's eye, increasing the clinically effective resolution as a flat-panel system is zoomed.

Image Display and Processing

Digital images are processed before they are displayed (14). Image processing techniques include gray-scale transformations (changes contrast level), edge enhancement (improves the visibility of small high-contrast structures), smoothing (reduces the effect of noise in a single frame at the expense of image sharpness), and temporal averaging. This last function combines several image frames. It reduces noise while maintaining the sharpness of non-moving structures. However, temporal averaging may blur moving objects. The type and extent of applied image processing can be configured by the service engineer and partially controlled by the operator.

Digital video facilitates functions such as fluoroscopic last-image-hold and instant replay of fluoroscopic and cinefluorographic images. Reviewing stored images instead of continuing fluoroscopy is an excellent means of patient and staff dose reduction.

DICOM PACS

Digital cardiac fluoroscopic and cinefluorographic images are typically produced using a nominal 1,024 × 1,024 pixel matrix. The bit depth can range from 8 to 12 bits (256 to 4,098 shades of gray). In the laboratory, these images are usually stored and displayed at full resolution. For archiving images, the 1995 DICOM standard

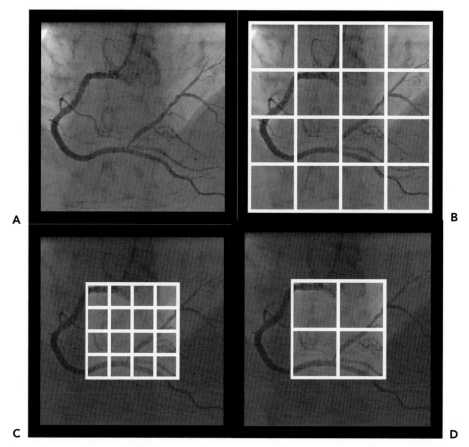

Figure 2.10 Zoom differences between image intensifiers and flat-panel detectors. The image before digitization **(A)**; full-field digitization for both systems—typically a matrix size of 1,024 × 1,024 **(B)**. When the image intensifier is zoomed **(C)**, the same matrix covers a smaller field of view; this reduces the effective pixel size. When a first-generation flat-panel is zoomed **(D)**, the pixel size remains the same; fewer pixels are used. Displays are usually electronically zoomed to fill the monitor. This does not increase physical resolution, but may improve the visibility of detail.

specified a 512 × 512 × 8 bit image format so that most studies would fit onto a single CD-ROM disc. The image standard has proved to be acceptable for most purposes over the decade since its release. Laboratory images are thus usually downscanned from their internal format into 512 × 512 × 8 bit before writing the study to a CD or transmitting it over a network for storage or remote viewing. Thus, image resolution when viewed in the laboratory is somewhat better than when the same cine run is recalled from storage. Higher-resolution images can be transmitted and stored at the expense of increased transmission time and storage space, and a general DICOM cine format maintains the same logical structure while permitting archiving of higher resolution images. Digital storage devices are available with an online capacity of tens of terabytes (TB). A 10-TB archive can store 20,000 to 30,000 cardiac cine studies in the 512 × 512 × 8 DICOM format. The cost of storage continues to decline by 10 to 30% per year, so online storage for all of a laboratory's archives is both technically and economically achievable.

DICOM images can be compressed (reduced in size) to save digital resources. Compression can be either reversible (the original image can be reconstructed exactly) or nonreversible. Reversible compression has been used in cardiology since the early 1990s, and the latest ACC document (15) specifically does not recommend the use of nonreversible compression for clinical decision making. Ongoing increases in device speeds, storage capacity, and network bandwidth have made the need for compression less urgent. It should be noted that common computer and Internet tools (MPEG, AVI) often lose much in compression, and they should be viewed with caution for diagnosis if DICOM images are available.

Image quality can be significantly degraded by poor viewing monitor performance. In DICOM terms, the world is divided into diagnostic workstations and review stations. The expectation is that primary medical decisions are made using images displayed only on diagnostic workstations. Facilities' quality programs are expected to include routine quality assurance of diagnostic workstations. Good practice dictates that a physician should have appropriate confidence in the quality of any image display used for critical clinical decisions. Test procedures and images can be used to validate the performance of any imaging workstation.

THE ANGIOGRAPHIC ROOM

Size, Shape, Layout

The angiographic room must have sufficient space to house the fluoroscope and ancillary equipment as well as patient care, work, and storage areas. The minimum recommended size is 50 m^2 (500 ft^2) with a ceiling height of 3m (10 ft). Where possible, the bulky components that constitute the generator and its associated electronics should be in a well-ventilated but visually and acoustically isolated space. The architectural arrangement must meet cable length limitations and should permit unimpeded access between the procedure room and electronics area for installation and service purposes. Room lighting must be sufficient to facilitate each of the multitudes of tasks associated with an interventional procedure. However, the lighting should not interfere with optimum viewing of the fluoroscopic images (perhaps by switching from high-level to lower-level lighting when the x-ray beam is on).

The angiographic room requires appropriate structural radiation shielding. Specifications are based on the laboratory's anticipated workload, the nature of the occupancy of adjacent areas (including above and below), and local regulatory requirements. Structural shielding includes the doors to the laboratory and the observation window between the control and procedure rooms. Additional portable shielding may be required for gamma-brachytherapy, when performed. For radiation protection purposes, support personnel should work at a distance from the x-ray gantry and be positioned behind x-ray shielding (fixed lead or rolling lead-acrylic partitions) whenever not delivering direct services to the patient. An appropriately sized lead-shielded control room should be provided outside of the procedure room, housing instrumentation for patient monitoring. Design elements should optimize staff access as well as verbal and visual communications between the procedure and control rooms.

Gantry and Table

The centerpiece of the cardiac catheterization laboratory is the floor-mounted or ceiling-suspended gantry that holds the x-ray tube and the image intensifier in correct alignment and provides a full range of two-dimensional rotation (left to right anterior oblique) and skew (cranial to caudal) of the direction with which the x-ray beam passes through the patient. The two axes of rotation meet at a single point (the isocenter of the gantry), so that an object (the patient's heart) placed at that point in space will remain centered on the screen even as the beam direction is changed. The patient is supported in that position on an adjustable-height, flat-top table. The table top can be panned in the left-right or head-foot direction to move the patient relative to the x-ray beam.

A second complete imaging chain is provided in some laboratories to provide simultaneous viewing of cardiac structures from two angles. Biplane imaging is indispensable when indicated for certain patients and procedures, but is not required for most invasive cardiology procedures.

Other Equipment

The other piece of indispensable fixed equipment is the physiologic monitor (including an in-laboratory display). Means for electronically time-stamping and recording all events during the procedure may be included in the physiologic monitor's computer. Online access to old studies (images, reports, physiologic data) is often desirable.

Various additional fixed or mobile equipment is found in the modern laboratory, including defibrillators, ultrasound imaging systems, interventional devices, pulse oximetry and noninvasive blood pressure monitors. All such devices must meet patient electrical safety regulations, with specific rules for line- or battery-operated equipment that might come in contact with the patient (or anything conductive attached to the patient) under normal or emergency circumstances.

Equipment Quality Assurance

The proper functioning of the imaging equipment can be ensured only if it is tested on acceptance for compliance with its published specifications. Testing includes verification of compliance with local regulatory requirements as well as an evaluation of imaging performance and patient dose (16–18). Image performance and patient dose aspects of the protocol need to be rechecked on a periodic basis. The NEMA XR-21 phantom, jointly developed with SCAI (19) can serve as the basis for much of the constancy test protocol.

Images are viewed on any one of a variety of video displays (either CRT or LCD). These range from dedicated in-laboratory displays, through dedicated PACS workstations, to office PCs and laptops. Any display used for clinical decision making should be included in the laboratory's quality assurance protocol (20,21).

BIOLOGIC EFFECTS OF RADIATION (GENERAL)

The average person in the United States is irradiated by a variety of natural and human-made sources (Fig. 2.11), and radiation is arguably the best studied of all environmental

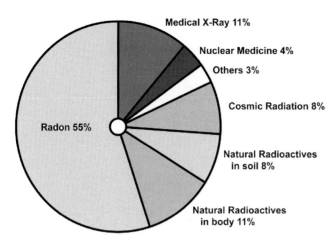

Figure 2.11 Average annual effective dose in the United States. More than 80% of the effective dose is delivered by natural sources. Medical use of radiation supplies most of the remaining amount.

"pollutants" (22–24). A typical annual effective dose equivalent from natural background, including radon, is around 3 mSv (300 mrem) (25,26). The actual amount of natural background varies depending on where individuals live, housing construction, and other factors. The major cause of human-made exposure is medical *imaging* (27). Presuming that radiologic imaging procedures are clinically justified and technically optimized, the expected clinical benefits of using radiation outweigh the radiation risks of the procedures. For the interventional staff, radiation exposure is a byproduct of the procedure, and the occupational dose received during all such procedures should be minimized to the extent possible without compromising appropriate patient care—referred to as ALARA (*as low as reasonably achievable*).

Radiation injuries are induced by one of two mechanisms. The *stochastic* mechanism of action is caused by unrepaired radiation damage to the DNA of even a single viable cell. In contrast, the *deterministic* mechanism is caused by radiation acutely killing off large numbers of cells. Radiation management differs for these two mechanisms.

Stochastic Effects

The word *stochastic* is defined as involving chance or probability. Stochastic effects are presumably induced by a single photon causing unrepaired injury to the DNA of a single viable cell. Depending on their type, damaged cells can proliferate to produce a malignancy in the irradiated individual or a genetic disorder in future generations. The severity of the resultant injury, caused by propagation of a single (unrepaired) damaged cell, is independent of the dose that started the process (22, 24). But the linear nonthreshold (LNT) model often used for radiation protection calculations states that the probability of injury increases linearly with dose. Risk coefficients are small for radiation

injuries, and direct evaluation of that risk at background radiation levels or even at levels corresponding to most imaging procedures is a statistical impossibility. Instead, the coefficients are obtained by looking at available populations exposed to high levels of radiation (i.e., atomic bomb survivors) and extrapolating back to lower doses. Because manifestation of the injury requires cellular propagation, stochastic effects are typically seen years to decades after irradiation. Radiation-induced leukemia thus occurs between 2 and 25 years after irradiation, whereas solid radiogenic cancers have a latent period of 5 to 20 years.

Cancer

For the purposes of this chapter, the risk coefficients for cancer induction in staff and patients are 5 and 10% per Sv of effective dose (28). The difference between the two values is the presence of repair, which reduces the risk of an exposure if it is delivered over a lifetime rather than acutely. The patient coefficient applies to adults and is higher for pediatric patients and perhaps for procedures in which the premenopausal female breast is directly irradiated. The error bars in these estimates are as large as the values. Moreover, 1 Sv is quite a large radiation dose that would correspond to receiving a maximal occupational dose (5,000 mrem equals 50 mSv) each year for 20 years, and it is difficult to detect any increase in cancer rates above the significant cancer risk in the nonradiated population.

Heritable Abnormalities

The risk for radiation-induced heritable effects is also estimated to be less than 10% per sievert of dose delivered to the gonads (22). Interventional cardiac procedures seldom expose the gonads to significant amounts of radiation. Even this small risk is applicable only to patients who become future parents. Thus, the main concerns for radiation-induced genetic damage should be focused on pediatric and young adult patients. Patient risk can be managed by reducing total patient dose while minimizing pelvic irradiation. Staff risk is reduced by most actions taken to reduce staff dose.

Deterministic Effects

Deterministic effects occur when a significant number of existing cells are sufficiently damaged so as to cause observable injury. Immediate injury is either owing to massive cell killing or a prompt biochemical tissue response to radiation. Delayed injuries become manifest when injured cells die without being replaced. The threshold dose for a deterministic effect depends on the fraction of cells that need to be killed before tissue loses viability, whereas the time course is dependent on the nature of the tissue and its

TABLE 2.2		
DETERMINISTIC INJURY THRESHOLDS		
Effect: Single-Dose	**Threshold (Gy)**	**Onset**
Early transient erythema	2	Hours
Main erythema	6	~10 days
Temporary (permanent) epilation	3 (7)	~3 weeks
Dry (moist) desquamation	14 (18)	~4 weeks
Secondary ulceration	24	>6 weeks
Ischemic dermal necrosis	18	>10 weeks
Dermal atrophy (2nd phase)	10	>1 year
Late dermal necrosis	>12?	>1 year
Skin cancer	stochastic	>5 years

Food and Drug Administration. *FDA Public Health Advisory: Avoidance of Serious X-Ray-Induced Skin Injuries to Patients During Fluoroscopically Guided Procedures.* 1994 (see reference 37).

cellular kinetics. Table 2.2 reviews the threshold doses required to induce different effects and the time between irradiation and the emergence of the injury. The threshold doses apply to the entire dose being delivered in 1 day. Tissue can tolerate a greater total dose if the irradiation is divided over several sessions instead of being delivered at once, assuming that they are separated by enough time for repair to occur. The necessary time intervals are not well known and may range from a day to several months. Thus, the radiobiologic effect of skin irradiation cannot be predicted by simply adding the dose (delivered to the same skin area) from multiple procedures.(8)

Following moderate radiation doses, repair processes gradually replace nonviable cells with normal tissue or scar. Repair is seldom complete, and chronic radiation injury reflects incomplete repair. In that setting, the tissue (i.e., the patient's skin) may have a lower threshold than that shown for a single dose.

Patient Radiation Risks

Skin Injuries

Radiation-induced skin injury is the most common deterministic effect that occurs as a consequence of fluoroscopic procedures. Because the doses required to cause these injuries are large (usually >60 minutes of fluoroscopy time and entry doses >2 Gy), they are rare complications of invasive cardiac procedures. The Food and Drug Administration (FDA) has received about 100 reports, mostly as the result of electrophysiology ablations or complex coronary artery interventions. A severe skin injury obtained from the FDA web site is illustrated in Fig. 2.12. Many additional cases are reported in the literature (3,29–37). The skin at the site where the fluoroscopic beam enters the patient receives the largest radiation dose and is the organ at greatest risk.

Radiation-induced skin injury can usually be identified by the temporal pattern of its development in relation to the time of irradiation and by the location of the injury at the beam entrance site. If the beam is positioned over a single skin site for a prolonged time and the collimation is not changed, the lesion will be well demarcated with a square or rectangular shape consistent with that of the collimated beam. The appropriate management of several major injuries was delayed because the prompt erythema was initially attributed to other causes (e.g., allergic reaction to a defibrillator pad). If the patient fails to mention the x-ray exposure when a dermatologist is consulted, a skin biopsy may be performed resulting in a chronic nonhealing of the radiation-damaged tissues. The patient's state of health may modify the normal response of skin to radiation (30,35) with collagen vascular disease, diabetes mellitus, and hyperthyroidism making the patient more susceptible to injury. Various chemical and pharmaceutic agents have also been associated with increased risk for skin injury.

Because of incomplete repair, patients who have previously undergone fluoroscopically guided procedures or radiation therapy may have a lower threshold for radiation injury in subsequent procedures. The literature reports several cases of chronic skin changes associated with multiple procedures irradiating the same portion of skin (3,36). Such factors need to be considered when planning a follow-on intervention.

Induced Neoplasm in Adults

A typical diagnostic coronary angiogram (DAP of 40 Gy/cm^2) will deliver approximately 8 mSv to the patient (38–40). The resultant cancer risk is likely to be less than 0.1%. The cancer risk resulting from a complex intervention in a heavy patient (DAP of 200 Gy/cm^2) is unlikely to be increased by as much as 1%. By way of comparison, a

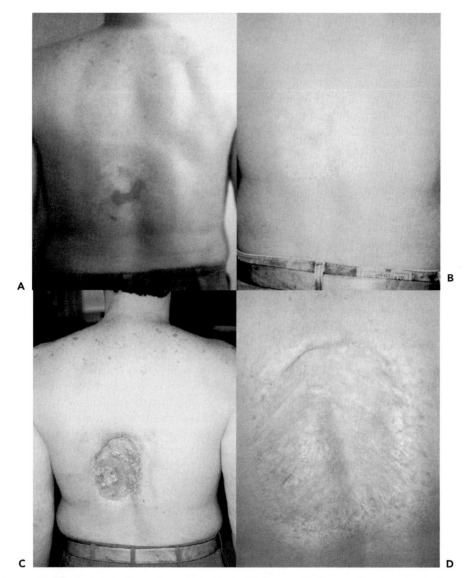

Figure 2.12 Time line of a major radiation injury (Reference 1). Early erythema and blistering at approximately 8 weeks is seen in **(A)**. This has resolved by approximately 20 weeks **(B)**; however the tissue is necrotic. The tissue has broken down by 20 months **(C)**. A skin graft was required **(D)**. A fuller explanation of this sequence is available in a 1995 publication at http://www.fda.gov/cdrh/rsnaii.html (last accessed 17 Mar 05)

60-year-old cancer-free male with no special risk factors has a 16% probability of being diagnosed with cancer in the next 10 years of his life. The stochastic risk of neoplasm from an invasive procedure is thus small in comparison with the natural incidence of cancer.

Risk of Neoplasm in Children

Radiation risk management in children is different than that for adults. Radiogenic neoplasm is importantly related to age at exposure and is gender dependent (22). Females are more susceptible than males because of greater breast and thyroid sensitivity. Additionally, because of a smaller body, a greater portion of a child's radiosensitive tissues are in close proximity to the x-ray beam during cardiologic

procedures. Fortunately, because of the small body, radiation penetrates small children more readily, so dose rates and total doses are relatively low. Caution is indicated when working with almost-adult-size children.

The Pregnant Patient

Radiation risks associated with pregnancy are thoroughly reviewed elsewhere (41). At low fetal doses, the principal risk is radiation-induced cancer. The lifetime risks induced by an in utero exposure are likely to be similar to the newborn risk. Fetal doses >100 mSv place the child at risk for deterministic effects such as central nervous system damage, growth retardation, malformation, or miscarriage. The specific risks are determined by actual fetal dose and gestation age. Fetal doses in this range seldom happen unless the uterus is directly irradiated.

Fluoroscopic procedures on pregnant women may be justifiable in an emergent situation. Procedures that involve structures above the diaphragm are unlikely to induce fetal deterministic effects (malformations), because direct irradiation of the fetus can usually be avoided and the fetus then receives only radiation scattered from the irradiated area. The carcinogenic risk to the child is the principal concern, and this risk must be weighed in relation to the anticipated clinical benefits to the mother. Minimizing the total use of radiation, applying good collimation, and avoiding unnecessary direct irradiation of the uterus during pregnancy contribute to minimizing fetal injury. Protective measures including avoiding extreme cranial angulations and using an arm approach reduce fetal radiation risk. A consultation with a medical physicist regarding fetal dose management prior to the procedure can be helpful.

Patient Radiation Management

Radiation-induced injury must be considered in the overall risk–benefit decision making process. How much radiation can be safely used before stopping? What are the benefits of splitting a procedure? Several factors enter into the decision of stopping or continuing a procedure: These include an adequate knowledge of the pathophysiology of radiation, appropriate patient consent, information on prior radiation usage, and the clinical requirements for continuing the procedure.

The quantity of radiation used in a simple diagnostic study performed on an average-sized patient is well below the threshold of deterministic injury or significant stochastic risk. But radiation dose increases with increasing complexity and patient size and may increase these risks to reach clinical significance. Under these circumstances the operator should proceed with caution, and only if the operator is certain that proceeding is essential to the patient's health and no other practical alternatives exist.

Equipment and Technique Selection for Dose Management

Equipment features and user-selectable operational modes provide fair control over x-ray dose rates. Operators should thus know the location and function of available dose management controls on each piece of equipment that they use and use them as needed to ensure minimal patient and personnel exposure. Common operator-selectable parameters include fluoroscopic pulse and dose rate and acquisition frame rate. Other factors may or may not be under the operator's control, including acquisition dose rate, x-ray beam energy (kVp), and beam filtration.

Images generated at lower dose per frame and at lower frame rates can be of lesser absolute quality, but may still be sufficient for clinical needs (42). However, too low a dose or frame rate may paradoxically increase total dose. This is because increased irradiation time is needed to allow the operator to make clinical decisions. The lowest total-dose operating conditions that meet procedural requirements should be selected.

Different types of imaging equipment are available in most laboratories. The operator should have sufficient knowledge of the equipment's dosimetric characteristics to select the most appropriate room for each patient. For example, a laboratory equipped with a large FOV image intensifier (needed for peripheral procedures) is less dose efficient at cardiac FOVs than a dedicated cardiac laboratory. The operator should consider another available laboratory if the use of substantial amounts of radiation is probable.

Effects of Patient Size on Patient Dose

As patient size increases, the input dose of radiation required for sufficient penetration of the x-ray beam through the patient to the image receptor increases rapidly. In most systems, increased penetration is achieved by using a higher kVp. This results in lower primary image quality because of reduced subject contrast. Large patients also generate more scattered radiation. This degrades image contrast and signal-to-noise ratio. The reduced image quality may increase the procedure's technical difficulty, potentially prolonging it and consequently requiring an even greater total radiation input.

Positioning of the Gantry Relative to the Patient

It is convenient to perform a coronary interventional procedure with the target lesion located at the fluoroscopy unit's isocenter. This minimizes the need to reposition the patient when the x-ray projection angle is changed. However, this strategy often shortens the distance between the x-ray tube and the patient, increasing the patient's entrance port skin dose. On the other hand, positioning the x-ray tube too far from the patient entrance may require an excessive increase in beam kVp, potentially degrading image quality. Where clinically possible, the beam angulations should be changed during a long intervention to minimize the irradiation of any particular portion of the patient's skin.

Beam Collimation

Collimating the x-ray beam to less than the working FOV is an important radiation management technique. Although this maneuver does not reduce skin dose per se, it does decrease the total radiation load on the patient. Less scatter is produced in comparison to an uncollimated beam. This has two beneficial effects: Image quality is improved and less scatter by the patient reduces staff exposure. The semitransparent lung shutter provides similar benefits: Image burnout over the lung is reduced when it is used, and the total radiation flux reaching the patient is reduced, thereby reducing scatter with a consequent reduction in staff exposure.

Clinical Dose Monitoring

Intraprocedural radiation dose monitoring is a responsibility of the operating physician. The operator needs to be aware of beam orientation, x-ray field size, and output dose rates to achieve this goal. By way of analogy, the use of radiation should be monitored and managed as well as the dose of iodinated contrast agents. The goal of intraprocedural dose monitoring is to avoid unintentionally crossing of deterministic dose thresholds for the skin. Ideally, this can be accomplished by displaying a real-time map of the dose distribution on the patient's skin, but no technologies are commercially available to provide an accurate real-time display of peak skin dose (43,44).

Instead, catheterization laboratories have traditionally relied on fluoroscopic time as a primary dose measure. Although this was of marginal value for diagnostic studies, it is a very poor clinical metric in the interventional era, since it does not account for cine usage or the variations in x-ray output attributable to patient size or other variables (45). Most interventional fluoroscopic systems are now equipped with DAP meters, which can be used to estimate skin dose, but DAP readings do not account for the distance between the x-ray tube and the patient's skin nor for beam motion during the procedure. Systems compliant with the IEC interventional fluoroscopy standard are equipped with a cumulative dose monitor. This instrument reports the cumulative dose delivered during a procedure to a reference point defined relative to the x-ray system. It is at its most accurate when the beam does not move and the reference point coincides with the patient's skin. Intraprocedural and patient follow-up trigger levels based on cumulative dose have an improved correlation with peak skin dose. Laboratory policies should use this metric if it is available.

Incorporating dose monitoring results into the laboratory's continuous quality improvement (CQI) program is beneficial, because periodic review of all dose data will yield important information regarding equipment and operator performance. This information can be used to improve both equipment and operator dose efficiency.

Considerations Regarding Multiple Procedures

Dose fractionation reduces the deterministic risk of a given total radiation dose. However, the LNT model states that stochastic radiation risk depends on the total dose accumulated by a patient during his or her lifetime. Thus the cancer risk is presumed to increase with each additional procedure.

Patient Education, Consent, and Follow-up

It is appropriate to include the possibility of radiation injury when obtaining informed consent from a patient who is at increased risk. Such patients include those who are expected to undergo a particularly long complex procedure, a patient who has had multiple recently performed procedures, or a patient who is extremely obese. An appropriate postprocedure discussion and follow-up plan is applicable to all patients where substantial amounts of radiation were used. A combination of patient size and available dose measuring tools can be used to establish a follow-up policy that is likely to detect significant injuries. In high-dose patients; rashes appearing within 30 days or so at the beam entry point should be presumed to be radiogenic, and the interventional cardiologist should take an active role in arranging appropriate follow-up for all such cases.

Staff Radiation Safety

Staff radiation safety has a different benefit–risk analysis than patient radiation safety (46). Acute deterministic effects (cataracts, skin burns) should never happen in an interventional setting, because the operator should never be in the primary beam and should receive scattered radiation exposure only. There are a few reports of chronic deterministic effects (e.g., hair loss on the legs below the lead apron) in individuals who have spent decades in the laboratory, but future occurrences of these effects can be avoided by extending the basic principles of radiation protection discussed in this section.

Cancer induction is a topic of real concern to staff members. But repeated studies of radiation workers of all types, including interventional cardiologists, over the last 30 years have produced only anecdotal reports with no confirmed evidence of increased cancer incidence in these populations (47–49). Nevertheless, interventional staff members are clearly exposed to radiation in the course of their duties, and the LNT model predicts a small increased risk of which workers should be aware.

Stochastic Risk

Staff stochastic risk is a function of the effective dose actually received by a staff member. (This reflects the whole-body dose and not the raw reading from a film badge worn outside the lead apron (50))! The most highly irradiated operators in a properly functioning interventional laboratory probably receive an effective dose of a few mSv/year. Most lab staff receive <1 mSv/year. By way of comparison, the natural background radiation level in Denver exceeds that in New York City by about 1 mSv/year. With a risk of fatal cancer estimated at 4% per sievert of exposure (even without considering the effect of appropriate shielding), the allowable occupational dose of 50 mSv/year would add only a 0.2% per year increment (to the background 20% spontaneous incidence) of developing a fatal neoplasm.

Staff Deterministic Injury

Acute deterministic effects (cataracts, skin burns) should never happen in an interventional setting. Nevertheless, radiation cataracts have been recently reported (51). Routine cinefluorographs documenting the operator's hand are seen with some frequency. Such incidents are almost always owing to poor understanding and technique as well as violations of the basic laws of radiation protection. The lens of the eye has been reported to be relatively insensitive to radiation. In a well-documented study of the effects of low-voltage radiation therapy treatments of the head and neck (52), the cataract threshold was demonstrated to be 2,000 mSv for a single exposure, rising to 4,000 mSv for a 30-day course of therapy. At the present regulatory limit for eye exposure of 150 mSv/year, it would take more than 25 years of dose accumulation at the regulatory limit to exceed the 30-day threshold. However, a very recent preliminary study has shown evidence of lenticular changes at lower levels, and use of eye shielding (lead glasses or a portable lead-acrylic shield) should be considered.

Basic Principles of Reducing Staff Radiation Exposure

Most patients undergo only a few catheterization studies in their lifetime, but staff have daily exposure. The operator can use several methods to reduce his or her exposure to radiation (53–57), the most important of which is to minimize patient dose—the ultimate source of exposure of the operator and staff. One of the most important means of reducing radiation exposure is reducing the amount of fluoroscopy and cine time to the clinically required minimum. It is important to avoid the "lead foot" syndrome; the operator must learn to depress the fluoroscopy pedal briefly when it is necessary to confirm a catheter position and to reflexively take his or her foot off the pedal whenever looking away from the television monitor. Similarly, cineangiographic runs should be selected carefully to show important findings, and each run should be terminated as soon as the necessary information is recorded.

The other cardinal measures used to reduce the operator's x-ray dose are *increasing distance* and the *use of shielding*. The operator should stand as far from the beam as possible to take advantage of the inverse square law—one or two steps farther away from the x-ray tube may cut the dose in half. A wraparound apron should be provided to individuals in the laboratory who have occasion to turn their back toward the patient. A wide variety of designs, materials, and lead thicknesses are available for tailoring radiation garments, but 0.5 mm lead equivalent provides roughly 95% shielding from diagnostic x-ray scatter.

Additional radiation protection can be gained from wearing separate thyroid collars and wraparound leaded eyeglasses. Too much lead is detrimental to the operator's musculoskeletal system, but pull-down and table-side shields serve to protect the staff from radiation without the necessity of wearing heavy lead.

Laboratory staff needs to know when radiation is being produced. Modern digital systems give few clues in this regard. A "beam on" light is often installed in the procedure room. This is helpful if it can be seen. Oftentimes, the nurse is asked to attend to the patient's needs during a procedure. These duties can occur in a potentially high radiation zone, and the operator should refrain from irradiating when staff is close to the patient.

Effect of Beam Orientation

This is particularly important during angulated shots such as the left lateral or left anterior oblique cranial projections, which place the operator in close proximity to the beam entry point (Fig. 2.13).

Staff Radiation Monitoring

There is no substitute for having each operator measure his or her own exposure (58–61), and a radiation monitor should be worn at all times when working in the cardiac catheterization laboratory. A collar badge should be worn on the left shirt collar outside the lead apron. This gives a good measurement of eye exposure. Current recommendations also call for a second waist badge, which is worn on the operator's belt just beneath the lead apron. These two badges should be of different colors (e.g., red for the collar and yellow or green for the waist) to avoid misplacement. Standard formulas allow an estimate of effective dose for the one- and two-badge cases. Each month, badges should be turned in for processing and replaced with fresh units. The resulting reports should be reviewed to confirm that no individual's collar badge dose exceeded 1 mSv/month (100 mrem/month) without further investigation. These dose levels should be observed only on busy operators. Recorded doses need to be studied regularly to ensure that occupational exposures remain below the prescribed limits.

BRACHYTHERAPY ISSUES

In-stent restenosis was a vexing clinical problem prior to the release of drug-eluting stents in 2003 (see Chapter 24). Mechanical retreatment still carried high (>50%) subsequent recurrence rates. It was then shown that intracoronary radiation therapy (also known as *brachytherapy* in reference to the short distance between the source and the target tissue) delivered at the time of mechanical retreatment of the in-stent restenosis markedly reduced (by nearly 70%) the chance of subsequent recurrence (62–64). Both beta and gamma radiation were effective when

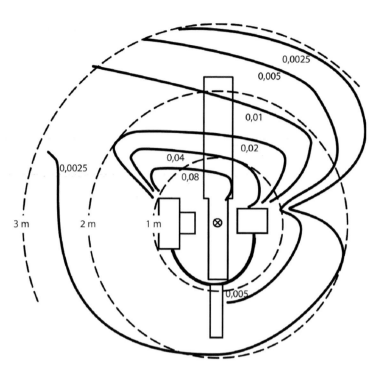

Figure 2.13 Scatter isodose curves around an interventional fluoroscope. This figure illustrates the radiation scatter levels 1 m above the floor from a full lateral beam. The asymmetry is caused by backscatter from the patient coupled with attenuation by the patient and equipment. (Figure courtesy of Philips Medical Systems.)

roughly 2,000 rads (20 Gy) was delivered to the vessel wall from radioactive seeds positioned within a catheter lying inside the treated segment. Several beta isotopic sources were used, including Sr-Y-90 and P-32, and proved to be convenient in terms of the short (3-minute) exposure times required; also, the low penetration of beta radiation made additional shielding unnecessary beyond the precaution of using a remote afterloader delivery system and avoiding operator hand contact with the catheter during source advancement. In contrast, the gamma radiation emitted from the Ir-192 source is very energetic (0.2 to 1.0 MeV, or roughly 10 times the energy of diagnostic x-ray) and would require 3 mm of lead or 2 inches of concrete for even 50% shielding (65,66). Special precautions in terms of thick portable lead shields and removal of staff from the room were required during the roughly 30-minute dwell time of the isotopic seeds in the treated arterial segment. When dealing with high-exposure sources such as these, the collaboration of both a radiation oncologist and a radiation physicist is required by NRC regulations to confirm dosing, to monitor safe handling and confirm retrieval of the source seeds, and to supervise radiation safety.

INTRAVASCULAR CONTRAST AGENTS

Shortly after publication of the classic papers by Roentgen in the 1890s, the search began for effective and nontoxic contrast agents to define vascular anatomy. Although early experimentation involved a number of heavy metals (bismuth, barium, thorium), all modern contrast agents are based exclusively on *iodine*, which by virtue of its high atomic number and chemical versatility has proved to be an excellent agent for intravascular opacification. Inorganic iodine (sodium iodide), however, cause marked toxic reactions. Experiments in 1929 thus explored an organic iodide preparation (Selectan) that contained one iodine atom per benzoic acid ring. In the 1950s, a series of substituted *tri-iodobenzoic acid* derivatives were developed, which contain three iodine atoms per ring. These agents differ from each other in terms of the specific side chains used in positions 1, 3, and 5 (Fig. 2.14), influencing both solubility and toxicity.

Ratio-1.5 ionic compounds are substituted ionic tri-iodobenzoic acid derivatives that contain three atoms of iodine for every two ions (that is, the substituted benzoic acid ring and the accompanying cation). Included in this family of high-osmolar contrast agents are agents such as Renografin (Bracco), Hypaque (Nycomed), and Angiovist (Berlex), which are mixtures of the meglumine and sodium salts of diatrizoic acid. Functionally similar agents are based on iothalamic acid (Conray [Mallinckrodt]) or metrizoic acid (Isopaque). These agents have a sodium concentration roughly equal to blood, pH titrated between 6.0 and 7.0, and a low concentration (0.1 to 0.2 mg/mL) of calcium disodium EDTA. Higher or lower sodium concentrations may contribute to ventricular arrhythmias during coronary injection, and calcium binding by sodium citrate may cause greater myocardial depression (67). To have an iodine concentration of 320 to 370 mg I/mL, as is required for left ventricular and coronary contrast injection, solutions of these agents are markedly hypertonic (with an osmolality >1,500 mOsm/kg, roughly six times that of blood).

Class	Structure	Examples	Iodine	Osm	Viscosity@37°
High-Osmolar Ionic Ratio 1.5 (3:2)	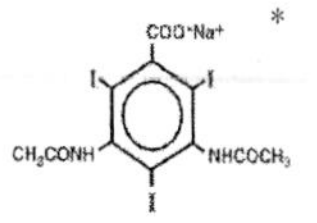	Diatrizoate (Renografin, Hypaque, Angiovist) Iothalmate (Conray) Metrizoate (Isopaque)	370 325 --	2076 1797	8.4 2.8
Low-Osmolar Nonionic Ratio 3 (3:1)		Iopamidol (Isovue) Iohexol (Omnipaque) Ioversol (Optiray) Ioxilan (Oxilan)	370 350 350 350	796 844 792 695	9.4 10.4 9.0 8.1
Low-Osmolar Ionic Dimer Ratio 3 (6:2)	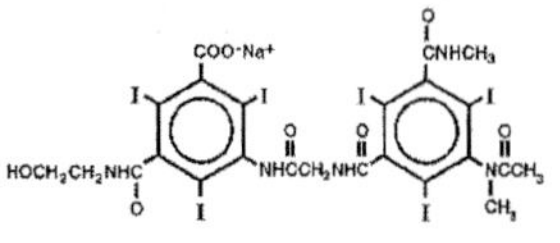	Ioxaglate (Hexabrix)	320	600	7.5
Iso-Osmolar Nonlonic Dimer Ratio 6 (6:1)	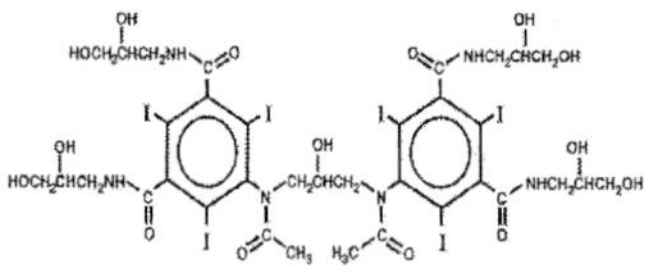	Iodixanol (Visipaque)	320	290	11.8

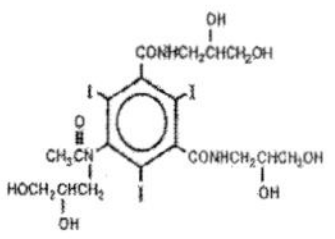

Figure 2.14 Sample structures and properties of current available contrast agents. The traditional high-osmolar ionic contrast media (HOCM or ratio 1.5) are Na+/meglumine salts of substituted tri-iodobenzoic acid, which have three iodine atoms per anion/cation pair, with six times the osmolality of blood. Two types of low-osmolality contrast media (LOCM or ratio 3) are also shown: the true nonionic agents and the Na+/meglumine salt of an ionic dimer, which have three iodine atoms per nonionic molecule or six iodine atoms per anion/cation pair, with an osmolality two to three times that of blood. The newest class of iso-osmolar contrast medium (IOCM or ratio 6) is a nonionic dimer with six iodine atoms per molecule and an osmolarity equal to that of blood. Also included are the iodine contents (in mg I/mL), the osmolarity (Osm, in mOsm/kg-H_2O), and the viscosity at 37°C. *Mixed sodium and meglumine salt; see text for details.

In the mid-1980s, the first *ratio-3* lower-osmolality contrast materials (LOCM) were introduced. Although it is still ionic (as a mixture of meglumine and sodium salts), ioxaglate (Hexabrix [Mallinckrodt]) is a ratio-3 agent by virtue of its unique dimeric structure that includes six molecules of iodine on the dimeric ring (three atoms of iodine for every one ion). To achieve an iodine concentration of 320 mg I/mL, Hexabrix has an osmolality roughly twice that of blood and contributes to a lower incidence of undesirable side effects related to hypertonicity (68).

A more significant modification in the late 1980s, however, was the introduction of true *nonionic ratio-3* contrast agents. These low-osmolality contrast agents are water-soluble in a noncharged form, without an associated cation. Examples include iopamidol (Isovue [Bracco]), iohexol (Omnipaque [Nycomed]), metrizamide (Amipaque, [Winthrop]), ioversol (Optiray [Mallinckrodt]), and ioxilan (Oxilan [Cook]), each of which contains three atoms of iodine for every molecule (69). With calcium disodium EDTA as a stabilizer and tromethamine (1.2 to 3.6 mg/mL) as a buffer, an iodine content of 320 to 370 mg I/mL can be achieved with an osmolality of 600 to 700 mOsm/kg, between two and three times that of blood. Their viscosity

(which influences ease of injection through small-lumen catheters) is roughly 6 to 10 times that of water.

More recently, a *ratio-6* nonionic dimeric compound (iodixanol, Visipaque [Nycomed]) has been released as an *iso-osmolar* contrast agent. This agent requires the addition of sodium and calcium chloride to bring its osmolarity up to that of blood (290 mOsm/kg) (70). Randomized comparisons of iodixanol to the low-osmolar contrast, ioxaglate, show that iodixanol has a significantly lower incidence of allergic reactions ($<$1% versus 3%) and no increase in adverse coronary events (thrombosis, vessel closure, or periprocedural myocardial infarction) (71,72). There are also data suggesting a reduction in nephrotoxicity with this agent, although the magnitude of this benefit is still unresolved (73).

As is clear from the discussion above, the low-osmolar contrast materials are definitely better tolerated by patients undergoing coronary and peripheral angiography. They produce fewer episodes of bradycardia and hypotension, precipitate less angina, and cause less nausea and sensation of heat than traditional high-osmolar contrast agents (74,75). There is also evidence that the nonionic ratio-3 and ratio-6 agents produce fewer allergic side effects (72) and may be less nephrotoxic in human studies (73,76). For all of these reasons, most coronary angiography is now performed with a low-osmolar contrast. Some early studies, however, suggested that the true nonionic agents might predispose patients to thrombotic events (77). We have not seen practical clinical problems related to nonionic contrast use, which is consistent with more recent studies (71,72) that have failed to confirm any increase in deleterious thrombotic complications. The only other issue that limits the universal use of the low-osmolar and iso-osmolar agents is cost (78). These agents were once 10 times more expensive than the high-osmolar agents, and although randomized trials comparing high- and low-osmolar agents in routine angiography have shown a clear reduction in minor side effects, they have failed to show any significant net clinical benefit in terms of serious side effects that would justify across-the-board use of a more expensive agent. Some institutions have thus confined their use to the roughly 25% of patients who have two or more of the following characteristics—age older than 65 years, left ventricular end diastolic pressure >15 mm Hg, New York heart Association functional class IV symptoms, or a history of previous contrast reaction—who would benefit most from the lower side effect profile (78). But with increasing competition among nonionic contrast agents, there has been a marked reduction in price, such that most nonionic low-osmolar agents cost only slightly more than a high-osmolar ionic agent. At such a low incremental cost, the clear reduction in minor side effects compared to the high-osmolar contrast agents may be sufficient to justify more liberal use of low-osmolar nonionic contrast.

It should be emphasized that even the best current radiographic contrast agents still have complications in terms of allergic reactions and kidney injury (radiocontrast nephropathy, or RCN) (79,80) (see also Chapter 3). The volume of contrast that may be used in a given procedure is thus limited, and patients with preprocedure risk factors (especially with abnormal preprocedure renal function or diabetes mellitus) (81) need aggressive preprocedure hydration, a renoprotective drug regimen (82–85), hemofiltration, (86) as well as careful limitation of the total contrast load. In the highest-risk patients, iodinated contrast agents may even be mixed with gadolinium-containing contrast agents designed for magnetic resonance imaging (Magnevist, Berlex), (87,88), or CO_2 angiography may be performed in the peripheral vasculature (89).

REFERENCES

1. Shope TB. Radiation-induced skin injuries from fluoroscopy. *Radiographics* 1996;16:1195–1199.
2. Park TH, Eichling JO, Schechtman KB, Bromberg BI, Smith JM, Lindsay BD. Risk of radiation induced skin injuries from arrhythmia ablation procedures. *Pacing Clin Electrophysiol* 1996;19: 1363–1369.
3. Dehen L, Vilmer C, Humiliere C, et al. Chronic radiodermatitis following cardiac catheterisation: a report of two cases and a brief review of the literature. *Heart* 1999;81(3):308–312.
4. ABIM. Interventional Board Requirements. http://abim.org/resources/eiblue.shtm.
5. Hirshfeld JW, Balter S, Brinker JA, ACCF/AHA/HRS/SCAI clinical competence statement on optimizing patient safety and image quality in fluoroscopically guided invasive cardiovascular procedures. *J Am Coll Cardiol* 2004;44:2259–82.
6. European-Union. *Guidelines for Education and Training in Radiation Protection for Medical Exposures*. Brussels: 2000. http://europa.eu.int/comm/environment/radprot/116/rp-116-en.pdf.
7. Balter S. *Interventional Fluoroscopy, Physics, Technology, Safety*. New York: John Wiley; 2001.
8. Hall EJ. *Radiobiology for the Radiologist*. 4th ed. Philadelphia: JB Lippincott,1994.
9. Bushberg J, Seibert JA, Ledidholdt EM, Boone JM. *The Essential Physics of Medical Imaging*. 2nd ed. Baltimore: Williams & Wilkins; 2002.
10. International Electrotechnical Commission. Medical electrical equipment, pt 2-43: particular requirements for the safety of X-ray equipment for interventional procedures. In: *IEC Report 60601 (2000)*. Geneva: 2000.
11. den Boer A, de Feyter PJ, Hummel WA, Keane D, Roelandt JR. Reduction of radiation exposure while maintaining high-quality fluoroscopic images during interventional cardiology using novel x-ray tube technology with extra beam filtering. *Circulation* 1994;89:2710–2714.
12. Aufrichtig R, Xue P, Thomas CW, Gilmore GC, Wilson DL. Perceptual comparison of pulsed and continuous fluoroscopy. *Med Phys* 1994;21(2): 245–256.
13. Sones FM Jr. Cine-cardio-angiography. *Pediatr Clin North Am* 1958;5:945–979.
14. Balter S. Digital images. *Catheter Cardiovasc Interv* 1999;46:487–496.
15. Bashore TM, Bates ER, Berger PB, et al. American College of Cardiology/Society for Cardiac Angiography and Interventions Clinical Expert Consensus Document on cardiac catheterization laboratory standards. A report of the American College of Cardiology Task Force on Clinical Expert Consensus Documents. *J Am Coll Cardiol* 2001;37:2170–2214.
16. European Union. Health protection of individuals against the danger of ionizing radiation in relation to medical exposure. In: European Directive 97/43/EURATOM (1997).; http://europa.eu.int/comm/energy/nuclear/radioprotection/doc/legislation/9743_en.pdf (last accessed 17 Mar 05).
17. Nickoloff EL, Strauss KJ, Austin BT, et al. *AAPM Report No. 70 Cardiac Catheterization Equipment Performance, Report of Task Group #17 Diagnostic X-ray Imaging Committee, 2001* Madison WI Medical Physics Publishing.
18. Shepard SJ, Lin PP, Boone JM, et al. *AAPM REPORT NO. 74 QUALITY CONTROL IN DIAGNOSTIC RADIOLOGY Report of Task Group #12 Diagnostic X-ray Imaging Committee, 2002*, Madison WI. Medical Physics Publishing.
19. Balter S. A new tool for benchmarking cardiovascular fluoroscopes. *Radiat Prot Dosimetry* 2001;94(1-2):161–166.
20. Samei E, Badano A, Chakraborty D, et al. Assessment of Display Performance for Medical Imaging Systems. Draft Report of the American Association of Physicists in Medicine (AAPM) Task Group 18, Version 10.0, August 2004 http://deckard.mc.duke.edu/~samei/tg18#_DOCUMENT_THE_PUBLIC (last accessed 17 Mar 05).
21. Ly CK. SoftCopy Display Quality Assurance Program at Texas Children's Hospital. *J Digit Imaging* 2002;15(suppl 1):33–40.
22. Committee on the Biological Effects of Ionizing Radiation (BEIR V). *Health Effects of Exposure to Low Levels of Ionizing Radiation*. Washington, DC: National Academy of Science, National Research Council, 1990.
23. United Nations Scientific Committee on the Effects of Atomic Radiation. *UNSCEAR 2000 Report to the General Assembly, with scientific annexes*. Vol I: *SOURCES*. 2000; New York, NY, United Nations.
24. United Nations Scientific Committee on the Effects of Atomic Radiation. *UNSCEAR 2000 Report to the General Assembly, with scientific annexes*. Vol II: *EFFECTS*. 2000; New York, NY, United Nations.
25. National Council on Radiation Protection and Measurements. *Report 94. Exposure of the Population in the United States and Canada from Natural Background Radiation*. Bethesda, MD: National Council on Radiation Protection and Measurements; 1988.
26. National Council on Radiation Protection and Measurements. *Report 93. Ionizing Radiation Exposure of the Population of the United*

States. Bethesda, MD: National Council on Radiation Protection and Measurements; 1987.

27. National Council on Radiation Protection and Measurements. *Report 100. Exposure of the U.S. Population from Diagnostic Medical Radiation.* Bethesda, MD: National Council on Radiation Protection and Measurements; 1989.

28. National Council on Radiation Protection and Measurements. *Report 115. Risk Estimates for Radiation Protection.* Bethesda, MD: National Council on Radiation Protection and Measurements; 1993.

29. Rosenthal LS, Beck TJ, Williams J, et al. Acute radiation dermatitis following radiofrequency catheter ablation of atrioventricular nodal reentrant tachycardia. *Pacing Clin Electrophysiol* 1997;20: 1834–1839.

30. Koenig TR, Wolff D, Mettler FA, Wagner LK. Skin injuries from fluoroscopically guided procedures, pt 1: characteristics of radiation injury. *AJR Am J Roentgenol* 2001;177(1):3–11.

31. Mettler FA Jr, Koenig TR, Wagner LK, Kelsey CA. Radiation injuries after fluoroscopic procedures. *Semin Ultrasound CT MR* 2002; 23(5):428–442.

32. Barnea Y, Amir A, Shafir R, Weiss J, Gur E. Chronic radiodermatitis injury after cardiac catheterization. *Ann Plast Surg* 2002;49: 668–672; discussion 672.

33. Aerts A, Decraene T, van den Oord JJ, et al. Chronic radiodermatitis following percutaneous coronary interventions: a report of two cases. *J Eur Acad Dermatol Venereol* 2003;17(3):340–343.

34. Monaco JL, Bowen K, Tadros PN, Witt PD. Iatrogenic deep musculocutaneous radiation injury following percutaneous coronary intervention. *J Invasive Cardiol* 2003;15(8):451–453.

35. Wagner LK, McNeese MD, Marx MV, Siegel EL. Severe skin reactions from interventional fluoroscopy: case report and review of the literature. *Radiology* 1999;213:773–776.

36. Vano E, Goicolea J, Galvan C, et al. Skin radiation injuries in patients following repeated coronary angioplasty procedures. *Br J Radiol* 2001;74:1023–1031.

37. Food and Drug Administration. *FDA Public Health Advisory: Avoidance of Serious X-Ray-Induced Skin injuries to Patients During Fluoroscopically Guided Procedures.* 1994. http://www.fda.gov/cdrh/fluor.html (last accessed 17 Mar 05).

38. van de Putte S, Verhaegen F, Taeymans Y, Thierens H. Correlation of patient skin doses in cardiac interventional radiology with dose-area product. *Br J Radiol* 2000;73:504–513.

39. Betsou S, Efstathopoulos EP, Katritsis D, Faulkner K, Panayiotakis G. Patient radiation doses during cardiac catheterization procedures. *Br J Radiol* 1998;71:634–639.

40. Bor D, Sancak T, Olgar T, et al. Comparison of effective doses obtained from dose-area product and air kerma measurements in interventional radiology. *Br J Radiol* 2004;77:315–322.

41. International Commission on Radiological Protection. Pregnancy and medical radiation. *Ann ICRP* 2000;30(1):iii–viii, 1–43.

42. Kuon E, Glaser C, Dahm JB. Effective techniques for reduction of radiation dosage to patients undergoing invasive cardiac procedures. *Br J Radiol* 2003;76):406–413.

43. den Boer A, de Feijter PJ, Serruys PW, Roelandt JR. Real-time quantification and display of skin radiation during coronary angiography and intervention. *Circulation* 2001;104:1779–1784.

44. Miller DL, Balter S, Cole PE, et al. Radiation doses in interventional radiology procedures: the RAD-IR study, pt II: skin dose. *J Vasc Interv Radiol* 2003;14:977–990.

45. Miller DL, Balter S, Wagner LK, et al. Quality improvement guidelines for recording patient radiation dose in the medical record. *J Vasc Interv Radiol* 2004;15(5): 423–429.

46. National Council on Radiation Protection and Measurements. *Report 105. Radiation Protection for Medical and Allied Health Personnel.* Bethesda, MD: National Council on Radiation Protection and Measurements; 1989.

47. Berrington A, Darby SC, Weiss HA, Doll R. 100 years of observation on British radiologists: mortality from cancer and other causes 1897–1997. *Br J Radiol* 2001;74:507–519.

48. Mohan AK, Hauptmann M, Linet MS, et al. Breast cancer mortality among female radiologic technologists in the United States. *J Natl Cancer Inst* 2002;94:943–948.

49. Niklason LT, Marx MV, Chan HP. Interventional radiologists: occupational radiation doses and risks. *Radiology* 1993;187: 729–733.

50. National Council on Radiation Protection and Measurements. *Report 122. Use of Personal Monitors to Estimate Effective Dose Equivalent and Effective Dose to Workers for External Exposure to LOW-LET Radiation.* Bethesda, MD: National Council on Radiation Protection and Measurements; 1995.

51. Vano E, Gonzalez L, Beneytez F, Moreno F. Lens injuries induced by occupational exposure in non-optimized interventional radiology laboratories. *Br J Radiol* 1998;71:728–733.

52. Merriam GR Jr, Focht EF. A clinical study of radiation cataracts and the relationship to dose. *Am J Roentgenol Radium Ther Nucl Med* 1957;77:759–785.

53. National Council on Radiation Protection and Measurements. *Report 134. Operational Radiation Safety Training.* Bethesda, MD: National Council on Radiation Protection and Measurements; 2000.

54. National Council on Radiation Protection and Measurements. *Report 127. Operational Radiation Safety Program.* Bethesda, MD: National Council on Radiation Protection and Measurements; 1998.

55. National Council on Radiation Protection and Measurements. *Report 105. Radiation Protection for Medical and Allied Health Personnel.* Bethesda, MD: National Council on Radiation Protection and Measurements; 1989.

56. Balter S. Radiation safety in the cardiac catheterization laboratory: basic principles. *Catheter Cardiovasc Interv* 1999;47(2):229–236.

57. Balter S, Sones FM Jr, Brancato R. Radiation exposure to the operator performing cardiac angiography with U-arm systems. *Circulation* 1978;58:925–932.

58. McKetty MH. Study of radiation doses to personnel in a cardiac catheterization laboratory. *Health Phys* 1996;70:563–567.

59. Renaud L. A 5-y follow-up of the radiation exposure to in-room personnel during cardiac catheterization. *Health Phys* 1992;62(1): 10–15.

60. Bashore T. Fundamentals of X-ray imaging and radiation safety. *Catheter Cardiovasc Interv* 2001;54(1):126–135.

61. Balter S., Guidelines for Personnel Radiation Monitoring in the Cardiac Catheterization Laboratory, Laboratory Performance Standards Committee of the Society for Cardiac Angiography and interventions; *Cath. and Cardiov. Diag.* 1993;30:277–279.

62. Leon MB, Teirstein PS, Moses JW, et al. Localized intracoronary gamma-radiation therapy to inhibit the recurrence of restenosis after stenting (GAMMA I). *N Engl J Med* 2001;344:250–256.

63. Waksman R, Raizner AE, Yeung AC, Lansky AJ, Vandertie L. Use of localized intracoronary beta radiation in treatment of in-stent restenosis: the INHIBIT randomised controlled trial. *Lancet* 2002;359:551–557.

64. Popma JJ, Suntharalingam M, Lansky AJ, et al. Stents And Radiation Therapy (START) Investigators. Randomized trial of 90Sr/90Y beta-radiation versus placebo control for treatment of in-stent restenosis. *Circulation* 2002;106:1090–1096.

65. Jani SK, Steuterman S, Huppe GB, et al. Radiation safety of personnel during catheter-based Ir-192 coronary brachytherapy. *J Invasive Cardiol* 2000;12:286–290.

66. Bass BG. Radiation safety requirements for cardiovascular brachytherapy. *Cardiovasc Radiat Med* 1999;1:297–306.

67. Zuckerman LS, Frichling TD, Wolf NM, et al. Effect of calcium binding additives on ventricular fibrillation and repolarization changes during coronary angiography. *J Am Coll Cardiol* 1987;10:1249.

68. Piao ZE, Murdock DK, Hwang MH, et al. Hemodynamic abnormalities during coronary angiography: comparison of Hypaque-76, Hexabrix, and Omnipaque-350. *Cathet Cardiovasc Diagn* 1989;16:149.

69. Ritchie JL, Nissen SE, Douglas JS Jr, et al. Use of non-ionic or low osmolar contrast agents in cardiovascular procedures (ACC Position Statement). *J Am Coll Cardiol* 1993;21:269.

70. Hill JA, Cohen MB, Kou WH, et al. Iodixanol, a new isosmotic nonionic contrast agent compared with iohexol in cardiac angiography. *Am J Cardiol* 1994;74:57.

71. Sutton AG, Ashton VJ, Campbell PG, et al. A randomized prospective trial of ioxaglate 320 (Hexabrix) vs. iodixanol 320 (Visipaque) in patients undergoing percutaneous coronary intervention. *Catheter Cardiovasc Interv* 2002;57:346–352.

72. Bertrand ME, Esplugas E, Piessens J, et al. Influence of a non-ionic, iso-osmolar contrast medium (iodixanol) versus an ionic,

low-osmolar contrast medium (ioxaglate) on major adverse cardiac events in patients undergoing percutaneous transluminal coronary angioplasty. *Circulation* 2000;101:131–136.

73. Aspelin P, Aubry P, Fransson SG, et al. Nephrotoxic effects in high-risk patients undergoing angiography (iodixinol). *N Engl J Med* 2003;348:491–499.

74. Matthai WH, Kussmaul WG 3rd, Krol J, et al. A comparison of low- with high-osmolality contrast agents in cardiac angiography—identification of criteria for selective use. *Circulation* 1994;89:291.

75. Barrett BJ, Parfrey PS, Vavasour HM, et al. A comparison of nonionic, low-osmolality radiocontrast agents with ionic, high-osmolality agents during cardiac catheterization. *N Engl J Med* 1992;326:431.

76. Schwab SJ, Hlatkey MA, Pieper KS, et al. Contrast nephrotoxicity—a randomized controlled trial of a nonionic and an ionic radiographic contrast agent. *N Engl J Med* 1989;320:149.

77. Piessens JH, Stammen F, Vrolix MC, et al. Effects of an ionic versus a nonionic low osmolar contrast agent on the thrombotic complications of coronary angioplasty. *Cathet Cardiovasc Diagn* 1993;28:99.

78. Steinberg EP, Moore RD, Powe NR, et al. Safety and cost effectiveness of high-osmolality as compared with low-osmolality contrast agents in patients undergoing cardiac angiography. *N Engl J Med* 1992;326:425.

79. Murphy SW, Barrett BJ, Parfrey PS. Contrast nephropathy. *J Am Soc Nephrol* 2000;11:177–182.

80. Gami AS, Garovic VD. Contrast nephropathy after coronary angiography. *Mayo Clin Proc* 2004;79:211–219.

81. Bartholomew BA, Harjai KJ, Dukkipati S, et al. Impact of nephropathy after percutaneous coronary intervention and a method for risk stratification. *Am J Cardiol* 2004;93:1515–1519.

82. Cox CD, Tsikouris JP. Preventing contrast nephropathy: what is the best strategy? A review of the literature. *J Clin Pharmacol* 2004;44:327–337.

83. Faddy SC. Significant statistical heterogeneity in a meta-analysis of the usefulness of acetylcysteine for prevention of contrast nephropathy. *Am J Cardiol* 2004;94:414.

84. Stone GW, McCullough PA, Tumlin JA, et al. Fenoldopam mesylate for the prevention of contrast-induced nephropathy: a randomized controlled trial. *JAMA* 2003;290:2284–2291.

85. Merten GJ, Burgess WP, Gray LV, et al. Prevention of contrast-induced nephropathy with sodium bicarbonate: a randomized controlled trial. *JAMA* 2004;291:2328–2334.

86. Marenzi G, Marana I, Lauri G, et al. The prevention of radiocontrast-agent-induced nephropathy by hemofiltration. *N Engl J Med* 2003;349:1333–1340.

87. Spinosa DJ, Angle JF, Hartwell GD, et al. Gadolinium-based contrast agents in angiography and interventional radiology. *Radiol Clin North Am* 2002;40:693–710.

88. Sarkis A, Badaoui G, Azar R, et al. Gadolinium-enhanced coronary angiography in patients with impaired renal function. *Am J Cardiol* 2003;91:974–975.

89. Huber PR, Leimbach ME, Lewis WL, et al. CO_2 angiography. *Catheter Cardiovasc Interv* 2002;55:398–403.

Complications and the Optimal Use of Adjunctive Pharmacology

Donald S. Baim   *Daniel I. Simon*[a]

Because all cardiac catheterizations involve the insertion of foreign objects (i.e., cardiac catheters) into the circulatory system, it should not be surprising that a variety of adverse events (complications) can ensue. These complications range from minor problems with no long-term sequelae (e.g., transient bradycardia during coronary contrast injection), to major problems (e.g., cardiac perforation, abrupt closure of a coronary artery during percutaneous transluminal coronary angioplasty [PTCA]) that may require immediate interventional or surgical attention, to major and irreversible damage (e.g., stroke, myocardial infarction, renal failure, or death). Fortunately, the risk of producing a major complication during most procedure types is generally well below 1%, a level at which the risk–benefit ratio still favors the performance of cardiac catheterization to investigate or treat cardiac disorders that are themselves life threatening or symptom limiting. Because the many complications are treated pharmacologically, or their incidence is either increased or decreased by drug treatment, we have included a new section on the use of adjunctive pharmacology in this chapter, which emphasizes current anticoagulant and antiplatelet agents but also includes other vasoactive, antiarrhythmic, and sedative agents commonly used in the cardiac catheterization laboratory.

OVERVIEW

The most important determinants of the risk for dying or sustaining a complication on an invasive procedure are clinical rather than procedural. The risk thus varies widely depending on demographics (age, gender), the cardiac anatomy (left main coronary artery disease, severe aortic stenosis, diminished left ventricular function), the clinical situation (unstable angina, acute myocardial infarction, cardiogenic shock). Other variations in risk are based on the type of procedure being performed (diagnostic catheterization, coronary intervention, and so on) and to some extent on the type of lesions being treated via percutaneous intervention (see Chapter 22).

By considering all these factors, the physicians and support staff can arrive at a fairly accurate estimate of the level of risk entailed in any given procedure. Familiarity with those risks can be of immeasurable value in the following: (a) anticipating increased risks of complication, (b) taking extra precautions to avoid them (e.g., placing a prophylactic pacemaker in a patient prior to rotational atherectomy of a right coronary artery lesion), (c) promptly recognizing complications when they occur (e.g., perforation of the right atrium during a trans-septal puncture), and (d) taking corrective and potentially life-saving action (e.g., pericardiocentesis for perforation-induced tamponade).

Before proceeding with any procedure, the details of the planned procedure and its anticipated risks must be discussed

---

[a] Some material was contributed by William Grossman in his role as a coauthor of this chapter in prior editions.

candidly with the patient and family. This discussion should include which specific procedures are planned, what benefits are hoped for, the attendant risks and their probabilities, and how the risks and benefits of the planned procedure compare with those of any possible alternatives (e.g., bypass surgery instead of percutaneous coronary intervention). By covering these cornerstones of informed consent clearly and candidly, the patient and family will be realistically prepared should a complication occur. Such a discussion should be documented in the patient's chart, and that documentation should specify the type of procedure that is planned, the potential major complications, and their estimated risk of occurrence (e.g., "death, MI, or stroke <1%; vascular injury requiring transfusion or surgical repair <2%").

If a significant major complication does occur, the patient and family should be informed of same as soon as the procedure has been completed (or when a delayed complication occurs, as soon as it is recognized). This discussion should describe the nature of the complication (without placing blame on anyone), indicate whether any long-term consequences are expected, and outline what corrective actions have been and will continue to be pursued. The catheterizing physician should also continue daily inpatient follow-up visits to any patient who has sustained a significant complication, because a patient's feeling abandoned by an uncaring physician tends to foster a desire for retribution (i.e., a malpractice suit).

For these reasons, all individuals performing cardiac catheterization should be intimately knowledgeable about the potential complications of the procedures they perform, as detailed in this and other chapters. In addition, the catheterization laboratory director should collect information about the frequency of these complications on at least a yearly basis and should review those data with the physician staff to identify where the laboratory as a whole (or an individual operator) is performing below expected standards. The types of complications that are routinely tracked in this process are shown in Table 3.1. This type of data collection, analysis (including breakdown by procedure type and by individual operator), reporting, and subsequent adjustment in laboratory policy and procedures (1,2) is one of the most important jobs of any catheterization laboratory director and has now become a reporting requirement in several states.

DEATH

Death as a Complication of Diagnostic Catheterization

Death as a complication of diagnostic catheterization has declined progressively over the last 30 years. Whereas a 1% mortality was seen with diagnostic catheterization in the 1960s, (3), the first Society for Cardiac Angiography registry of 53,581 diagnostic catheterizations performed in 1979–1981 showed a 0.14% procedure-related mortality (4). By the second registry of 222,553 patients catheterized in 1984–1987 (5), procedure-related mortality for diagnostic catheterization had fallen further, to 0.1% (i.e., 1 in 1,000). The small size of this reduction in mortality, however, belies the fact that the second registry included many more patients who fell into a high-risk subgroup for the procedure. Based on variables identified from the 218 deaths in the second registry (age older than 60 years, New York Heart Association (NYHA) functional class IV, left ventricular ejection fraction <30%, or left main disease), the mortality for such patients fell by half between the first and second registry (6). A third registry of 58,332 patients studied in 1990 showed an even lower overall mortality of 0.08%, with a 1.5% incidence of any major complication (7). A number of baseline variables (including NYHA class,

---

> **TABLE 3.1**
>
> **MAJOR COMPLICATIONS OF CARDIAC CATHETERIZATION AND INTERVENTION TO BE TRACKED IN EACH CATHETERIZATION LABORATORY**

Death
Myocardial infarction
   Q-wave
   Non-Q-wave with CPK > 2× normal or CK-MB > 5× normal
Stroke
Emergency bypass surgery
Cardiac perforation
Major arrhythmia requiring countershock or pacing
Local vascular injury requiring surgery or transfusion
Contrast-induced renal failure
Allergic reactions (anaphylaxis)

multivessel disease, congestive heart failure, and renal insufficiency) were identified in this registry, whose presence predicted an up to eightfold increase in major complication rates (from 0.3% in patients with none of these factors, to 2.5%) (8). Several of the major factors are discussed below.

Left Main Disease

Although there has been a progressive reduction in the overall mortality of diagnostic cardiac catheterization over the last 25 years, patients with severe left main coronary disease remain at increased risk. Their mortality was 6% in the 1976 report by Bourassa (9), and 2.8% in the study by Hillis and others performed between 1978 and 1992 (compared with a mortality of 0.13% in patients without such disease) (10). Although the mortality of such patients had fallen to 0.86% in the first Society for Cardiac Angiography registry, this was still more than 20 times higher than the 0.03% mortality seen in patients with single-vessel disease (4).

Because roughly 7% of patients undergoing coronary angiography have significant left main disease, the protocol used for coronary angiography (see Chapter 11) should always begin with careful catheter entry into the left coronary ostium to facilitate early recognition of ostial left main disease through catheter pressure damping or performance of a test "puff" immediately after engagement. Even without these early warnings of left main disease, we routinely perform the first left coronary injection in the right anterior oblique (RAO) projection with caudal angulation to screen for mid and distal left main disease and get the maximal anatomic information on the first injection. If ostial left main stenosis is suspected, a straight anterior (AP) injection may be performed. If severe left main disease is present, the only other left coronary injection needed is an RAO projection with cranial angulation (to see the left anterior descending and its diagonal branches). If angiography shows a borderline lesion (30 to 70%), additional diagnostics including intravascular ultrasound (IVUS; Chapter 19) or pressure wire (Chapter 18) can be performed after completing diagnostic coronary angiography to inform the subsequent management decision. But performing a large number of superfluous contrast injections in a patient with a critical left main disease offers little more in the way of important anatomical information and increases the risk of triggering the vicious cycle of ischemia/hypotension/more ischemia that may lead to irreversible collapse.

Careful attention to all other aspects of technique is essential, since even an otherwise minor complication (e.g., a vasovagal reaction or arrhythmia) may have fatal consequences in this situation. If a patient with severe left main disease exhibits any significant instability during the procedure, we usually opt to place an intra-aortic balloon pump (see Chapter 21) and arrange for prompt bypass surgery. When the hemodynamics are markedly compromised and the patient is a poor surgical candidate, emergency coronary stenting should be performed if a trained operator and the necessary equipment are available (see Chapter 22). A similar consideration regarding the use of hemodynamic support applies to any patient with an unstable ischemic syndrome or acute myocardial infarction who behaves in a brittle fashion under the stresses of catheter placement and contrast injection.

Left Ventricular Dysfunction

Patients with cardiogenic shock in the setting of acute myocardial infarction or severe chronic left ventricular dysfunction (ejection fraction <30%) also have a several-fold increased risk of procedural mortality (5), particularly when reduction in ejection fraction is associated with a baseline pulmonary capillary wedge pressure >25 mm Hg and a systolic arterial pressure <100 mm Hg. An effort should generally be made to bring such congestive heart failure under control before cardiac catheterization is attempted.

Although right heart catheterization is no longer routine (see Chapter 4), I believe that it should always be performed before angiography in a patient with poor ejection fraction, because it provides valuable data about baseline hemodynamic status and allows ongoing monitoring of pulmonary artery pressure as an early warning about hemodynamic decompensation before frank pulmonary edema ensues. If the baseline pulmonary capillary wedge pressure is >30 mm Hg, every effort should be made to improve hemodynamic status before angiography is attempted. This may entail administration of a potent intravenous diuretic (furosemide), supplemental oxygen, a vasodilator (intravenous nitroglycerine or sodium nitroprusside) when the mean arterial pressure is >65 mm Hg, or a positive inotrope (dopamine, dobutamine, milrinone) when the mean arterial pressure is <65 mmHg or when severe congestive heart failure hemodynamics persist despite vasodilator treatment (see below). When frank cardiogenic shock is present or develops during a cardiac catheterization, prompt placement of an intra-aortic balloon pump in the contralateral groin may be required to get the patient safely though the procedure. More potent forms of temporary hemodynamic support are now available (see Chapter 21). The availability of low-osmolar contrast agents that produce less myocardial depression than traditional high-osmolar agents, however, has greatly enhanced our ability to perform necessary angiography without precipitating hemodynamic decompensation in such unstable patients (see Chapter 2).

Valvular Heart Disease

Despite the preponderance of coronary artery disease as the indication for diagnostic cardiac catheterization patients with severe valvular heart disease are also at increased risk for dying during cardiac catheterization. The VA Cooperative Study on Valvular Heart Disease (11) thus showed a 0.2% mortality among 1,559 preoperative catheterizations performed in patients with valvular heart disease, with one death in a patient with mitral regurgitation and two deaths in patients with aortic stenosis. With current noninvasive methods for assessing the severity of valvular lesions, there is some debate about whether it is necessary to cross severely stenotic valves in the course of preoperative cardiac catheterization (12).

Prior Bypass

Patients who have previously undergone coronary bypass surgery make up a growing subgroup (up to 20% in our laboratory) of diagnostic and interventional catheterizations. They are typically 5 years older, have more diffuse coronary and generalized atherosclerosis, worse left ventricular function, and require a more lengthy and complex procedure to image both native coronary arteries and all grafts. Despite these adverse risk factors, the Post CABG Trial (13) looked at 2,635 diagnostic angiograms performed in stable patients and found 0% mortality, with major complications in 0.7% (myocardial infarction 0.08%, stroke 0.19%, vascular trauma requiring transfusion or surgery 0.4%).

Pediatric Patients

Pediatric patients may be at higher risk (see Chapter 6). One review of 4,952 patients (median age 2.9 years) studied at the Hospital for Sick Children in Toronto (14) found a mortality of 1.2% confined to patients younger than age 5 years (half in critically ill neonates <30 days of age). Although the risk was lower for diagnostic than electrophysiologic or interventional procedures, there were three deaths (0.1%) among the 3,149 diagnostic procedures.

Death in the Course of an Interventional Procedure

Because they involve the use of more aggressive catheters, superselective cannulation of diseased coronary arteries, and brief interruption of coronary or even systemic flow (see Chapter 25), interventional procedures tend to carry higher mortality than purely diagnostic catheterizations. In the first 1,500-patient coronary angioplasty registry sponsored by the National Heart, Lung, and Blood Institute (NHLBI) from 1979 to 1982, the mortality of elective angioplasty was 1.1% (15). This was relatively unchanged at 1.0% in the second NHLBI registry of 1,802 patients treated at 15 centers between 1984 and 1987, mainly because the second registry included more

patients with adverse features (advanced age, poor ventricular function, multivessel disease, prior bypass surgery, and so on) (16). In fact, the mortality for single-vessel procedures fell from 1.3 to 0.2% between the first and second registry.

With the introduction of newer devices (e.g., stents, atherectomy, laser) to treat high-risk lesions preemptively or reverse abrupt closure following attempted conventional balloon angioplasty, the overall mortality for elective coronary intervention has fallen further (Chapter 22), but the extension of intervention to other high-risk subsets, including patients with acute myocardial infarction undergoing primary angioplasty, has kept overall mortality close to 1% (17)—roughly 10-fold higher than purely diagnostic catheterization (i.e., 1% versus 0.1%). Several multivariable models that predict procedural mortality (range 0 to 35%) have been developed based on age, ejection fraction, treatment for acute myocardial infarction/shock, urgent/emergent priority, and so on (17–20) (Fig. 3.1; see also Chapter 22). There is thus such a wide variation in risk of death in the course of coronary intervention—based on patient comorbidities, clinical indication, and procedure type—that these "average" risks should be quoted only to "average" patients, whereas patients with one or more adverse risk factors should be told candidly during the informed consent process that their expected risks are somewhat higher than these averages.

MYOCARDIAL INFARCTION

Although transient myocardial ischemia is relatively common during diagnostic catheterization and occurs routinely during coronary intervention, myocardial infarction is an uncommon but important complication of diagnostic cardiac catheterization. In the late 1970s, data from the Coronary Artery Surgery Study showed a myocardial infarction rate of 0.25% for coronary angiography (21). In the first, second, and third registries conducted by the Society for Cardiac Angiography (4,5,7), the risk of myocardial infarction fell progressively, from 0.07%, to 0.06%, to 0.05%. However, the risk of precipitating myocardial infarction during diagnostic catheterization is clearly influenced by patient-related factors that include the extent of coronary disease (0.06% for single-vessel disease, 0.08% for triple-vessel disease, and 0.17% for left main disease) (5), the clinical indication (e.g., unstable angina or recent subendocardial infarction), and the presence of insulin-dependent diabetes. The progressive reduction in overall risk of myocardial infarction since the 1970s likely reflects greater attention to catheter flushing, pressure damping—all nuances that are now considered to be integral parts of coronary angiography (see Chapter 11), as well as the potential benefits of interval adoption of systemic heparinization for coronary angiography (22). It should

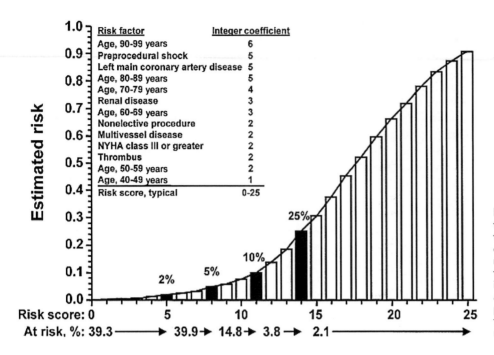

Figure 3.1 Mayo clinic risk score for mortality after coronary intervention assigns integer coefficients for each named clinical variable and reads the estimated mortality risk that corresponds to the total of the integer coefficients from the curve and the valve on the Y-axis. The 2% of patients with a total score over 14 thus have an expected procedural mortality of 25%!

Interventional Procedures

Coronary interventions may produce myocardial infarction by a variety of mechanisms that include dissection, abrupt vessel closure, "snowplow" occlusion of side branches, spasm of the epicardial or arteriolar vessels (no reflow), thrombosis, or distal embolization (see Chapter 22). Q-wave myocardial infarction was reported in 4.8% of patients in the first NHLBI registry and 3.6% in the second NHLBI registry (16). This includes roughly half of the 6% of PTCA patients who were sent for emergency bypass surgery owing to abrupt vessel closure (15). Over the last decade, experience with coronary stenting has led to marked reduction in the need for emergency bypass surgery (to roughly 0.2%; see Chapter 22), and accordingly the incidence of Q-wave infarction has fallen to roughly 1%.

Largely as a spin-off of trials conducted with the platelet glycoprotein IIb/IIIa receptor blockers in the mid 1990s, however, the official definition of periprocedural myocardial infarction has now been broadened to include non–Q-wave infarctions (more properly called non–ST-elevation myocardial infarctions) detected by elevation of the total creatine kinase (CK) to more than

twice normal, or elevation of the CK-MB fraction to more than three times normal—even if the total CK is not elevated (23). Using these more sensitive definitions, roughly 20% of patients experience some increase in CK-MB fraction after an otherwise successful intervention (24). Patients with these low-level enzyme elevations are more likely to have some degree of chest discomfort, but this finding is common also in patients without enzyme elevation, where it presumably represents stimulation of adventitial pain receptors by local stretching at the treatment site (25).

Although elevation of CK-MB above five or eight times normal corresponds to a significant amount of myocardial necrosis and carries the same adverse impact on long-term prognosis as a Q-wave infarction, considerable debate still exists about the meaning of such CK elevations in patients who have had otherwise successful interventional procedures (26) (Fig. 3.2A). Yet long-term follow-up of patients from several multicenter trials (27) has shown that patients with even low-level (one to three times normal) elevation of postprocedural CK after PCI have a greater incidence of late adverse outcomes (Fig. 3.2B). In my mind (DSB), the question is whether any such relationship is cause and effect, or simply an association of both periprocedural CK elevation and late events with a common confounding variable (such as the diffuse underlying atherosclerosis) (28,29). In any event, there does not seem to be an increase in early mortality with low-order CK elevation, so there is no need to prolong hospitalization beyond what is necessary to document that the CK curve has peaked and begun to fall, nor to institute any specific therapy other than the usual postintervention antiplatelet and lipid-lowering therapies.

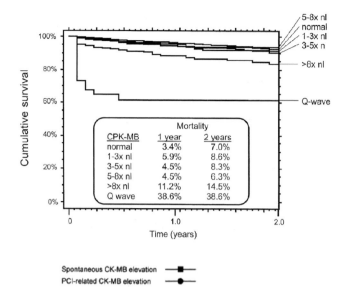

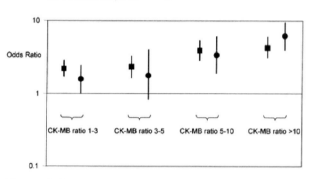

Figure 3.2 Mortality analysis for CK-MB elevation postintervention shows clear effect only for CK-MB greater than five to eight times normal. However, some other analyses suggest that lower-order CK elevations are also associated with increased mortality. (Top, See reference 26. bottom, from Akkerhuis KM, et al. Minor Myocardial Damage and Prognosis: Are Spontaneous and Percutaneous Coronary Intervention—Related Events Different? *Circulation* 2002;105: 554–556).

CEREBROVASCULAR COMPLICATIONS

Cerebrovascular accidents (strokes) are uncommon but potentially devastating complications of diagnostic cardiac catheterization. Early experience showed an incidence as high as 0.23% in the 1973 study of Adams and others (30), compared with the 0.07% incidence for the more recent diagnostic catheterizations included in the Society for Cardiac Angiography registries (4,5). Every invasive cardiologist should be familiar with potential etiologies, preventive strategies, and treatments for catheterization-related stroke, and should develop the routine habit of speaking with the patient directly at the end of the procedure. If the patient is less alert, has slurred speech, and either visual, sensory, or motor symptoms during or after a left heart procedure, there should be a low threshold for performing a screening neurologic exam or obtaining an urgent stroke neurology consultation. For major hemispheric events, an urgent carotid angiogram and neurovas-

cular rescue should be considered (usually with a prior computed tomography [CT] or magnetic resonance [MR] scan to exclude hemorrhage), in the hope that neurovascular rescue will minimize the risk of major long-term neurologic deficit or death (if a qualified neurointerventionalist is available) (31).

The risk of stroke is somewhat higher with coronary intervention, as expected based on the use of guiding catheters, multiple equipment exchanges in the aortic root, aggressive anticoagulation, and longer procedure times. A recent review of 12,407 patients who underwent PCI at the Washington Hospital Center (32), showed a 0.38% risk of per-procedural stroke (roughly half hemorrhagic and half embolic). Risk factors included age older than 80 years, use of an intra-aortic balloon pump, and saphenous vein graft intervention. Patients who sustained a stroke had a 37% in-hospital and 56% 1-year mortality, compared with 1.1% in-hospital and 6.5% 1-year mortality in patients who did not sustain a stroke.

Although cerebral hemorrhage must always be excluded, the main cause of catheterization-related strokes seems to be embolic. There is some evidence that many such emboli are dislodged from unsuspected aortic plaque or diffuse atherosclerosis, given the observation that atherosclerotic debris is liberated from the wall of the aorta in 40 to 60% of cases during advancement of large-lumen guiding catheters over a 0.035-inch guidewire (33). Sensitive measures such as transcranial Doppler monitoring of the middle-cerebral artery shows common high-intensity transients during contrast injections or catheter movements (34), and diffusion-weighted magnetic resonance imaging (MRI) before and after retrograde left heart catheterization shows ≤20% incidence of scan defects (but only a 3% neurologic event rate) when aortic stenotic valves are crossed (35). Most neuro-ophthalmologic complications (i.e., retinal artery embolization) (36), and the syndrome of diffuse cholesterol embolization (37) also appear to be caused by emboli released by disruption of unrecognized plaques on the walls of the aorta, liberating cholesterol crystals, calcified material, or platelet-fibrin thrombus into the aortic root.

So beyond paying careful attention to flushing and injection technique, and minimizing dwell time of guidewires in the aortic root of patients who are not fully anticoagulated, we have begun routinely advancing our end hole (i.e., coronary angiographic or, particularly, guiding) catheters around the arch to the ascending aorta over the guidewire, and before removing the wire, flushing and clearing the catheter with contrast (see Chapter 4). We believe that the benefit of advancement over a guidewire in reducing trauma to arch atheroma offsets the risk of introducing debris, clot, or air into the aortic root by performing the first catheter flush in the ascending rather than in the descending aorta. There can be no excuse, however, for contributory technical malfeasance such as sloppy catheter flushing, introduction of air bubbles during contrast injection, inadvertent placement of wires and catheters into the arch vessels, prolonged (>3 minutes) wire dwell times during attempts to cross a stenotic aortic valve, or failure to carefully wipe and immerse guidewires in heparinized saline before their reintroduction during left-sided heart catheterization.

In addition to aortic root sources, embolic material may also originate in the cardiac chambers, thrombotic coronary arteries, or the surface of cardiac valves. One should thus avoid placing the pigtail catheter fully out to the left ventricular apex in patients with suspected aneurysm or recent myocardial infarction, since either condition may be associated with potentially dislodgeable mural thrombus. A clot contained in an occluded native coronary artery or vein graft can also be inadvertently withdrawn or propelled out of that vessel and into the aortic root during attempted coronary intervention or forceful injection of contrast through a distal superselective catheter. Care must also be taken to avoid trans-septal catheterization or mitral valvuloplasty in patients with left atrial thrombus, which may increase the incidence of clinical stroke. Even avoiding such patients, there is an unexpectedly high incidence of new hyperintense brain lesions by MRI after percutaneous balloon mitral valvuloplasty (38) suggesting that small subclinical emboli may occur more commonly than previously suspected. In patients with right-to-left shunting (including atrial septal defects with Eisenmenger physiology and patients with right ventricular infarction and a patent foramen ovale), paradoxic embolization may also lead to stroke. In such patients, the same level of care regarding flushing catheters and sheaths that is routine during left heart procedures should also be extended to right heart procedures.

The question of embolic risk also invariably comes up when it is necessary to perform catheterization on patients with endocarditis of left-sided (aortic and mitral) heart valves. Although these vegetations look friable and can embolize spontaneously, they have already withstood repeated trauma from opening and closing of the affected valves without dislodgment. In a series of 35 patients with active endocarditis who underwent left-sided cardiac catheterization (5 of whom had prior spontaneous systemic emboli), none had a catheterization-induced embolic event (39). With current noninvasive techniques for assessing the left ventricle and mitral valve, it generally is not necessary to enter the left ventricle in a patient with left-sided endocarditis, however (see Chapter 12).

Beyond cerebrovascular emboli from intracardiac, arterial, or catheter sources, patients receiving aggressive anticoagulation, antiplatelet, or thrombolytic therapy are also prone to spontaneous intracerebral bleeding as a potential cause for postprocedure neurologic complications. If any doubt exists, and particularly if thrombolytic therapy or intensive anticoagulation is being considered as treatment for a presumptive cerebrovascular embolus, neurologic consultation and CT or MRI scanning are advis-

able. The distinction is critical, because there have been reported cases of resolution of embolic strokes that occurred during cardiac catheterization after selective infusion of a thrombolytic into the occluded cerebral vessel (31), as well as successful treatment of patients with posterior fossa bleeds as the result of prompt recognition and neurosurgical evacuation.

LOCAL VASCULAR COMPLICATIONS

Local complications at the catheter introduction site are among the most common problems seen after cardiac catheterization procedures, and probably are the single greatest source of procedure-related morbidity. Specific problems include vessel thrombosis, distal embolization, dissection, or poorly controlled bleeding at the puncture site. Ongoing bleeding may be owing to a poorly placed puncture, vessel laceration, excessive anticoagulation, or poor technique in either suture closure (brachial approach, see Chapter 5), mechanical groin compression, or use of a puncture-sealing device (femoral approach, see Chapter 4).

With the femoral approach, poorly controlled bleeding may present as free hemorrhage, femoral or retroperitoneal hematoma, false aneurysm, or arteriovenous fistula. Although frank hemorrhage and hematoma are generally evident within 12 hours of the procedure, the diagnosis of false aneurysm may not be evident for days or even weeks after the procedure. Given the common and troublesome nature of postprocedure vascular complications, all cardiac catheterization operators must understand vascular access and closure techniques completely to recognize and treat each type of complication. Early experience with the femoral approach by Judkins and others reported a 3.6% local complication rate (40), but the Society for Cardiac Angiography registries reported a 0.5 to 0.6% incidence of vascular complication for diagnostic catheterization, which was similar for the brachial and femoral approaches (7). Brachial complications (see Chapter 5) tend to be thrombotic whereas femoral complications tend to be hemorrhagic, but exceptions to this general rule can and do occur.

Femoral artery thrombosis can occur in patients with a small common femoral artery lumen (peripheral vascular disease, diabetes, female gender), in whom a large-diameter catheter or sheath (e.g., an intra-aortic balloon pump) has been placed, particularly when the catheter dwell time is long or when prolonged postprocedure compression is applied. Such patients have a white painful leg with impaired distal sensory and motor function, as well as absent distal pulses. If this develops during the catheterization procedure and is not corrected promptly by sheath removal, a flow-obstructing dissection or thrombus at the femoral artery puncture site or a distal arterial embolus should be suspected. This requires urgent attention via vascular surgery consultation (for exploration and correction of any local dissection or plaque avulsion and Fogarty embolectomy of the distal vessel as needed to restore distal pulses). Alternatively, operators skilled in peripheral intervention may be able to puncture the contralateral femoral artery, cross over the aortic bifurcation, and address a common femoral occlusion percutaneously (41) (Fig. 3.3). Either way, failure to restore limb flow within 2 to 6 hours may result in extension of thrombosis into smaller distal branches, with muscle necrosis requiring fasciotomy or even amputation.

Femoral venous thrombosis and pulmonary embolism are rare complications of diagnostic femoral catheterization (Fig. 3.4). A small number of clinical cases have been reported, however, particularly in the setting of venous compression by a large arterial hematoma, sustained mechanical compression (see Chapter 4), or prolonged procedures with multiple venous lines (e.g., electrophysiologic studies) (42). The actual incidence of thrombotic and pulmonary embolic complications may, however, be substantially under-reported, since most are not evident clinically. Asymptomatic lung scan abnormalities have thus been described in up to 10% of patients after diagnostic catheterization (43). (See also Chapters 13 and 30.)

Although thrombotic complications do occur, poorly controlled bleeding from the arterial puncture site is a more common problem after cardiac catheterization by the femoral approach (44). Uncontrollable free bleeding around the sheath suggests laceration of the femoral artery. If such free bleeding does not respond to replacement with the next larger diameter sheath, the bleeding should be restricted by manual compression around the sheath until the procedure is completed. Anticoagulation may be reversed, and an attempt made to remove the sheath and control bleeding with prolonged (30- to 60-minute) compression or to place a femoral closure device (see Chapter 4). But blood should be typed and cross-matched for transfusion, and the vascular surgeons should be consulted regarding operative repair should the bleeding continue.

Formation of a hematoma—a collection of blood within the soft tissues of the upper thigh—is more common than free bleeding. It tends to cause a tender mass the size of a baseball or softball. If ongoing bleeding stops with manual compression, the hematoma will usually resolve over 1 to 2 weeks as the blood gradually spreads and is reabsorbed from the soft tissues. Instances of femoral or lateral cutaneous nerve compression from groin hematomas, however, may lead to sensory or motor deficits that may take weeks or even months to resolve (45). Larger hematomas may require transfusion, but surgical repair of a hematoma (as opposed to a false aneurysm, see below) is generally not required. Given the discomfort caused by large hematomas, and the potential of such hematomas to evolve into false aneurysms, accurate puncture and puncture site compression or closure technique to

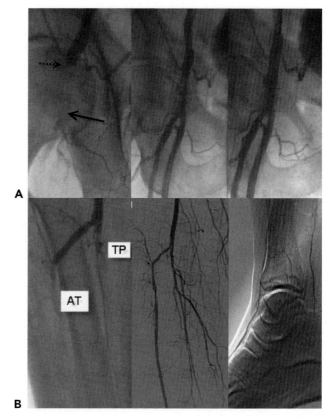

Figure 3.3 Femoral artery thrombosis. The morning after AngioSeal closure of the right femoral artery, this patient experienced sharp pain and swelling at the site, managed by 30 minutes of compression. After that, he reported severe pain and loss of sensation in a white limb. **Upper left.** Crossover from the contralateral side showed occlusion of the common femoral with reconstitution. **Upper center.** After balloon dilation, there was a prominent filling defect consistent with thrombus. **Upper right.** After AngioJet thrombectomy, the filling defect has decreased in size. **Lower left.** Distal injection, however, showed thrombotic occlusion of both the anterior tibial (AT) and the tibioperoneal (TP) trunk. **Lower center.** After catheter suction, patency of these vessels was restored. **Lower right.** Distal angiogram shows filling of both the dorsalis pedis and posterior tibial vessels. (Case courtesy of Dr. Andrew Eisenhauer, Brigham and Women's Hospital.)

minimize hematoma formation are essential parts of good catheterization technique.

Retroperitoneal bleeding may occur if the front or back wall of the femoral artery was punctured above the inguinal ligament, allowing the resulting hematoma to extend into the retroperitoneal space (46,47). Such bleeding is not evident from the surface, but should be considered whenever a patient develops unexplained hypotension (particularly if it responds only briefly to aggressive volume loading), fall in hematocrit, or ipsilateral flank pain following a femoral catheterization procedure. The diagnosis may be confirmed by CT scanning or abdominal ultrasound (Fig. 3.5), but the treatment is usually expectant (transfusion, bed rest) rather than surgical. The best prevention for retroperitoneal bleeding is careful identification of the puncture site to avoid entry of the

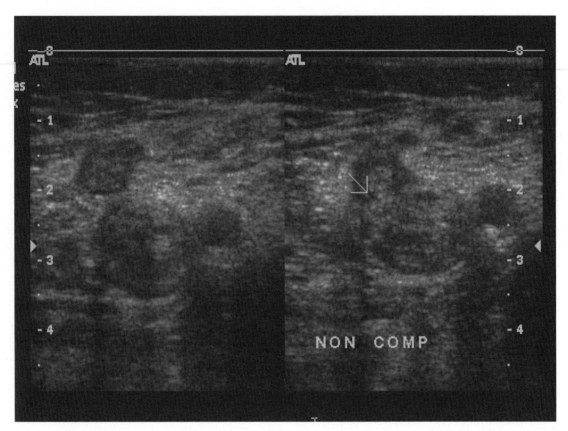

Figure 3.4 Deep venous thrombosis postcatheterization. This 63-year-old man had an 8-F AngioSeal device used to close the arterial puncture site in the right groin. When the patient sat up 18 hours after the procedure, he developed acute pain and swelling in the right groin. Manual pressure was held during 20 minutes for suspected groin hematoma. Ultrasound was performed for the presence of a bruit and showed that the femoral vein was not compressible (**right panel,** *arrow*), indicating femoral thrombosis. In addition to therapy with aspirin and clopidogrel, anticoagulation was initiated with enoxaparin until adequately anticoagulated with oral warfarin. (Case provided courtesy of Dr. Marie Gerhard-Herman, Brigham and Women's Hospital.)

common femoral near or above the inguinal ligament. Effective catheter-based interventions include an ipsilateral (or contralateral if the problem is low in the iliac) approach for localization and tamponade of the retroperitoneal bleeding site, using a peripheral angioplasty balloon followed by placement of a covered stent, as possible alternatives (41,47,47a). This is particularly relevant when the cause is a sheath-induced laceration of a tortuous iliac artery, bleeding from which can be fatal within a matter of minutes without such catheter-based control (Fig. 3.6).

A pseudoaneurysm may develop if a hematoma remains in continuity with the arterial lumen (i.e., following dissolution of the clot plugging the arterial puncture site; Fig. 3.7). Blood flowing in and out of the arterial puncture expands the hematoma cavity during systole and allows it to decompress back into the arterial lumen in diastole. Since the hematoma cavity contains no normal arterial wall structures (i.e., media or adventitia), this condition is referred to as false or pseudoaneurysm. It can often be distinguished from a simple hematoma on physical examination by the presence of pulsation and an audible bruit over

the site, but Duplex ultrasound scanning is confirmatory (48). Since all but the smallest (<2-cm diameter) false aneurysms tend to enlarge and ultimately rupture, we usually have the vascular surgeons repair them (generally under local anesthesia) when they are detected (44). Less invasive alternatives to vascular surgical repair include ultrasound-guided compression of the narrow neck through which blood exits the femoral artery for 30 to 60 minutes, which may permanently close the track and eliminate the need for surgery (49), or injection of the false aneurysm cavity with procoagulant solutions or embolization coils during ultrasound or contralaterally inserted balloon occlusion of the aneurysm neck (50) (Fig. 3.8). False aneurysms smaller than 2 cm in diameter may be followed expectantly, since up to half close before a 2-week follow-up ultrasound (51).

The keys to avoiding pseudoaneurysm formation are accurate puncture of the common femoral artery and effective initial control of bleeding after sheath removal. Punctures of the superficial femoral or profunda artery (i.e., puncture below the bifurcation of the common femoral)

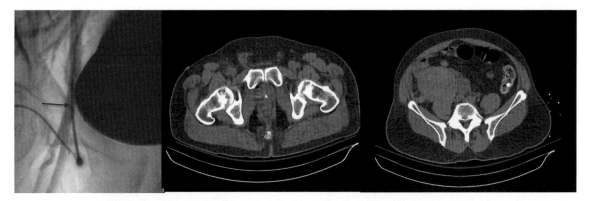

Figure 3.5 Retroperitoneal bleed. A 67-year-old man underwent coronary intervention. **Left.** The sheath injection shows a relatively high puncture entering the common femoral artery at the top (rather than the middle) of the femoral head. The next day after AngioSeal closure, he felt a pop and pain in his groin and became hypotensive, responding only briefly to atropine and fluids, with a fall in hematocrit from 42 to 35%. **Center.** A CT scan at the level of the femoral neck shows the common femoral artery bilaterally. **Right.** A CT scan slice in the lower abdomen shows a large right retroperitoneal bleed obliterating the psoas muscle. With continued fall in his hematocrit, he was taken to the operating room, where active bleeding was found from the anterior wall of the external iliac artery, from which the closure device had dislocated. He was discharged on day 9 after a total of 15 units of packed red cells.

are significantly more likely to lead to false aneurysm formation because of the smaller caliber of the artery and the lack of a bony structure against which to compress after sheath removal (52). Fluoroscopic localization of the skin nick to overlie the inferior border of the femoral head effectively avoids this error (see Chapter 4). Effective initial control is also essential, because allowing a hematoma to form makes effective control more difficult and initiates natural thrombolytic activity in the hematoma that may dissolve the early fibrin plug at the puncture site.

An arteriovenous fistula results from ongoing bleeding from the femoral arterial puncture site that decompresses into an adjacent venous puncture site (Fig. 3.8). This can be recognized by a to-and-fro continuous bruit over the puncture site, and may not be clinically evident until days after a femoral catheterization procedure (53). These fistulae may enlarge with time, but at least one third close spontaneously within 1 year, after which surgical repair should be entertained (54). The most common findings at surgery are a low puncture (i.e., of the superficial femoral

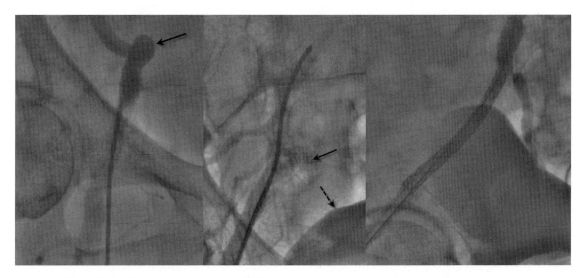

Figure 3.6 Iliac artery laceration. **Left.** Baseline sheath insertion angiogram shows marked tortuosity of the right iliac artery (*arrow*), which led to the placement of a long sheath past the area of tortuosity. **Center.** After the coronary intervention, the patient complained of abdominal pain and became progressively hypotensive, with sheath reinjection showing extravasation of contrast from the iliac and compression of the right dome of the bladder, consistent with free retroperitoneal bleeding. **Right.** Via contralateral crossover access, a covered WALLGRAFT was placed in the external iliac to seal the laceration. (Case provided courtesy of Dr. Paul Teirstein, Scripps Clinic.)

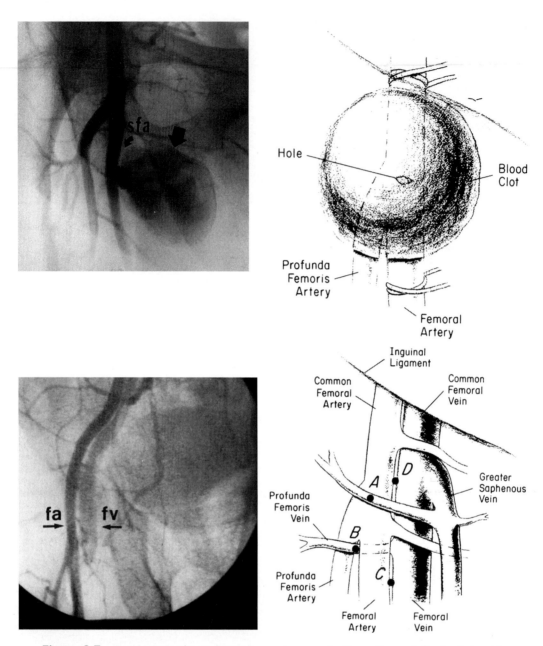

Figure 3.7   Common significant femoral vascular complications. **Upper left.** Angiographic appearance of a false aneurysm of right femoral artery (*arrow*) that developed 4 to 5 days following percutaneous retrograde femoral arterial catheterization complicated by a significant local hematoma after groin compression. Note that the arterial puncture had been made in the superficial (rather than common) femoral artery. **Upper right.** Schematic diagram showing the surgical approach to the false aneurysm cavity and the underlying puncture. **Lower left.** Angiographic appearance of an arteriovenous fistula with simultaneous filling of the femoral artery (left) and vein (right). **Lower right.** Diagram showing the potential anatomic situations (overlying arterial and venous branches) that may underlie fistula formation after femoral puncture (reference 44, with permission).

or profunda, transecting a small venous branch), emphasizing the importance of careful puncture technique in avoiding this femoral vascular complication.

The level of anticoagulation and antiplatelet therapy as well as increased sheath size, female gender, and advanced age all increase the risk of hemorrhagic complications described above (1,53). During the era (1990–1996) when

uninterrupted transition from intravenous heparin to oral warfarin was used for stenting, vascular complications were as high as 10% (see Chapter 24) (55). Even before the switch to less aggressive anticoagulant protocols (aspirin and ticlopidine or clopidogrel), second-generation stents that permit use of smaller 6 F sheaths, and the widespread use of puncture-closure devices, the incidence

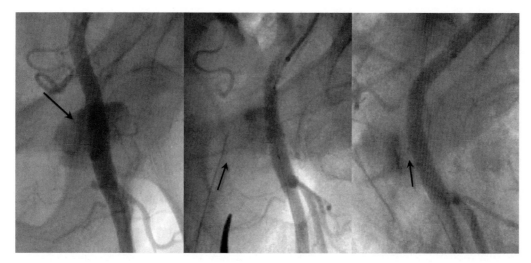

Figure 3.8 Femoral pseudoaneurysm. **Left.** To evaluate a pulsatile mass in the left groin following a catheterization, crossover angiography was performed from the right groin showing a large pseudoaneurysm over the common femoral artery. **Center.** An angioplasty balloon was positioned under the prior puncture site as a needle (*arrow*) was advanced to puncture the pseudoaneurysm cavity confirmed by contrast injection. **Right.** After occlusion of the common femoral by inflation of the angioplasty balloon, thrombin was injected through the needle into the pseudoaneurysm cavity, causing it to clot, as shown by the absence of further contrast flow into it on the postprocedure angiogram (*arrow*). (Case provided courtesy of Dr. Andrew Eisenhauer, Brigham and Women's Hospital.)

of hemorrhagic access site complications after stenting remains at 1 to 2% (see Chapter 4). The tendency of platelet glycoprotein IIb/IIIa blockers to increase local hemorrhagic complications (see below), however, has been tempered by lower levels of heparinization and the growing use of femoral puncture-sealing devices (see Chapter 4). Various approaches for collagen plugging or percutaneous suture-mediated closure of the femoral arterial puncture site have been introduced in the last several years (see Chapter 4). Although these devices avoid the discomfort of prolonged manual or mechanical compression and allow earlier or even immediate ambulation, clinical trials have failed to demonstrate significant reduction of major vascular complications compared with compression (56). Ultimately, however, it is likely that this class of devices will improve sufficiently to make closure of the femoral artery puncture site so reliable as to eliminate the 1 to 2% incidence of complication. Until that time, operators must be prepared to recognize and repair them when they occur or to work from other access sites such as the radial artery (where hemorrhagic complications are unheard of, and thrombosis [with a negative Allen test] is usually inconsequential) (57) (see Chapter 4), in patients at high risk for a femoral complication.

ARRHYTHMIAS OR CONDUCTION DISTURBANCE

Various cardiac arrhythmias (tachycardia or bradycardia) or conduction disturbance may occur during the course of diagnostic or therapeutic cardiac catheterization. Most, like ventricular premature beats (VPBs) during catheter entry into the right or left ventricle, are devoid of clinical consequence. Others, like asystole or ventricular fibrillation, pose immediate risk. Finally, some rhythm disturbances (like atrial fibrillation) are well tolerated in most patients, but may trigger profound hemodynamic decompensation in patients with severe coronary disease, aortic stenosis, or hypertrophic cardiomyopathy by excessively increasing heart rate or eliminating the atrial "kick" needed to maintain diastolic filling of a stiff left ventricle.

An important part of safe cardiac catheterization is thus for the operator and the nurses/technicians to monitor the surface electrocardiogram on the same physiologic monitor used to display the pressure tracings. The monitoring equipment typically also generates an audible beep with each QRS complex to serve as another information modality while the operator is intent on watching the fluoroscopic image. The technicians should be trained to call out any disturbance in rhythm such as VPBs that may otherwise escape the operator's attention. The tools to treat these rhythm disorders—including a defibrillator capable of synchronized or asynchronous countershock, temporary transvenous pacing leads and pacemaker generator, and the full array of antiarrhythmic drugs—must be immediately accessible in any cardiac catheterization laboratory (58) (see below). The ability to promptly recognize and reverse major rhythm disturbances (e.g., by promptly countershocking ventricular fibrillation, sometimes even before the patient fully loses consciousness) can avoid progression to full cardiopulmonary arrest that would require the institution of CPR. Still, all operators and cardiac catheterization support staff should be current in their basic and advanced cardiac life support (ACLS) certification, including the newest guidelines published in 2000 (59) and prepared to institute ventilatory and circulatory support without delay, when necessary. Duplication of those guidelines here would be beyond the scope of this text, but the following comments about arrhythmias during cardiac catheterization are in order.

Ventricular Fibrillation

Ventricular ectopy or even brief (three- to five-beat) runs of ventricular tachycardia are not uncommon during passage of catheters into the right or left ventricle. Even balloon-flotation right heart catheterization may cause such brief runs of ventricular tachycardia in up to 30% of patients, with sustained ventricular tachycardia in 3% and ventricular fibrillation in 0.7% of cases (60). This emphasizes the importance of controlling the catheter position in the right ventricle and smooth passage through the right ventricular outflow tract; similar issues relate to careful positioning of the pigtail catheter free in the midportion of the left ventricle (see Chapter 12). If a sudden increase in ectopic activity is noted, or if a run of ventricular tachycardia is initiated, the offending catheter must be repositioned immediately so that baseline cardiac rhythm is restored. The same holds true for ventricular ectopy precipitated when the tip of a guidewire is placed into a small intramyocardial branch (usually a septal branch of the left anterior descending) during coronary intervention. The guidewire should be withdrawn slightly and repositioned in the main vessel. Other than these mechanical stimuli, ventricular fibrillation can also be induced by catheter transmission of "leakage" electrical currents into the heart. This problem has been effectively eliminated, however, by the adoption of standards for grounding systems in the cardiac catheterization laboratory that ensure a maximum leakage current of 20 μA between any two exposed conductive surfaces (58).

Although ventricular tachycardia and ventricular fibrillation may result from catheter manipulation, the most common is intracoronary injection (particularly using an ionic [high-osmolar] contrast agent) into the right coronary artery. Although this is less common with the current low-osmolar agents (see Chapter 2), it can still occur if the contrast injection is prolonged or performed with a partially damped catheter pressure (see Chapter 11). But changes in injection technique and the formulation of contrast agents used for coronary angiography have progressively reduced the incidence of this complication from 1.28% in the 1973 publication of Adams (30), to 0.77% in the 1970–1974 series from the Montreal Heart Institute (9), to less than 0.4% in the Society for Cardiac Angiography registry (7), and now to 0.1% with the routine use of nonionic low-osmolar agents (see Chapter 2). The incidence of ventricular fibrillation may be somewhat higher, however, in patients with baseline prolongation of the QT interval (61).

Some of the most refractory ventricular ectopy is seen in the setting of profound transmural ischemia or early myocardial infarction. Ventricular fibrillation or unstable ventricular tachycardia should be treated with prompt countershock, whereas lower-grade ventricular ectopy may respond to loading with intravenous lidocaine (1 to 1.5 mg/kg over 1 minute, with a second bolus of 0.75 mg/kg 3 to 5 minutes later), amiodarone (300 mg over 20 minutes, with additional boluses of 150 mg over 10 minutes for breakthrough ectopy, followed by a drip of 1 gm/24 hours), or procainamide (15 mg/kg over 20 minutes, watching for fall in blood pressure or broadening of QT or prolongation of QRS intervals), or (see below). Although amiodarone is very effective for ischemic ventricular ectopy, it is so lipid soluble that it must be combined with a detergent (Tween-80) that may cause arterial hypotension (62). Magnesium sulfate (1 to 2 gm intravenously over 2 minutes) may be given for suspected hypomagnesemia or torsades de pointes). But it is rare for witnessed and promptly treated ventricular fibrillation as occurs in the catheterization laboratory to result in a prolonged arrest. In that case, however, the full ACLS protocol (59) should be initiated. Of course, precordial compression and bag/mask ventilation should be begun as arrangements for endotracheal intubation are made, in the case of ventricular fibrillation that does not respond immediately to countershock.

Atrial Arrhythmias

Atrial extrasystoles are common during catheter advancement from the right atrium to the superior vena cava, or during looping of the catheter in the right atrium to facilitate passage in a patient with enlargement of the right-sided heart chambers. These extrasystoles usually subside once the catheter is repositioned, but they may progress to atrial flutter or fibrillation in sensitive patients. Both rhythms tend to revert spontaneously over a period of minutes to hours, but may require additional therapy if they produce ischemia or hemodynamic instability. Atrial flutter can be treated by a brief (15-second) but rapid (300- to 400-beats per minute) burst of right atrial pacing, following which reversion to sinus rhythm or onset of atrial fibrillation (with a more controlled ventricular response) can be expected (63). Care must be taken, however, to ensure a stable atrial pacing location, since catheter migration into the ventricle during burst pacing may trigger ventricular fibrillation.

Atrial flutter or atrial fibrillation are generally benign during catheterization, but may cause clinical sequelae if the ventricular response is rapid (>100) or if the loss of the atrial kick causes hypotension in a patient with mitral stenosis, hypertrophic cardiomyopathy, or diastolic left ventricular dysfunction. If tolerated poorly in such individuals, atrial fibrillation or flutter may require synchronized DC cardioversion. If no significant hemodynamic dysfunction occurs, intravenous beta-blockers (Inderal [Propranolol] 1 mg, or esmolol (64) [Brevibloc] at a loading dose of 500 mcg/kg per minute for 30 seconds, followed by an infusion of 50 to 250 mcg/kg per minute) or a calcium channel blocker (diltiazem, or verapamil 5 mg) may be given and up-titrated until adequate control of the ventricular response is achieved. Once the ventricular response is controlled, chemical conversion to normal sinus rhythm can usually be accomplished by administration of intravenous procainamide (15 mg/kg over 20 minutes) or ibutilide (1 vial equals 1 mg, given over 10 minutes) (65). Because the latter agent can cause QT prolongation and torsade, it should not be given to patients who are on other QT-prolonging drugs, have reduced potassium or magnesium concentrations, bradycardia, or baseline QTc intervals >440 milliseconds. If there is significant hemodynamic instability from either atrial flutter or atrial fibrillation, however, the most rapid and reliable therapy is synchronized cardioversion (starting at 35 to 50 watt-seconds, after appropriate intravenous sedation).

Other narrow complex tachycardias such as paroxysmal supraventricular tachycardia can be treated with vagal maneuvers (carotid sinus massage), intravenous adenosine, verapamil, or adenosine). Synchronized DC cardioversion should be reserved for prolonged episodes with hemodynamic compromise. In the setting of Wolf-Parkinson-White syndrome, however, these agents should be avoided in preference to amiodarone.

Bradyarrhythmias

Transient slowing of the heart rate occurs commonly during coronary angiography, particularly at the end of a right coronary artery injection performed using a high-osmolar ionic contrast agent. Since forceful coughing helps to clear contrast from the coronaries, support aortic pressure and cerebral perfusion during asystole, and restore normal cardiac rhythm, patients should be warned at the beginning of the procedure that they may be asked to cough forcefully and that they must do so without hesitation when asked. This problem is far less common now with the widespread use of low-osmolar agents (see Chapter 2).

Vasovagal reactions, in which bradycardia is associated with hypotension, nausea, yawning, and sweating, should be suspected when bradycardia is more prolonged. This is one of the more common complications (with a roughly 3% incidence) seen in the cardiac catheterization laboratory (1), triggered by pain and anxiety, particularly in the setting of hypovolemia. Some elderly patients may exhibit the hypotensive findings of a vasovagal reaction without the hallmark finding of bradycardia (66). In the study by

Landau et al. (67), more than 80% of such reactions occurred as vascular access was being obtained, with 16% occurring during sheath removal. This highlights the importance of adequate preprocedure sedation and adequate administration of local anesthetic before catheter insertion is attempted. The treatment for vasovagal reaction consists of the following: (a) cessation of the painful stimulus, (b) rapid volume administration (elevation of the legs on a linen pack and hand pumping of saline through the sidearm of the venous sheath or peripheral intravenous line), and (c) atropine (0.6 to 1 mg intravenously). If hypotension persists, additional pressor support (Levophed or Neo-Synephrine) may be needed. Although the vasovagal episode itself tends to be benign, patients with critical valvular heart disease may undergo severe and even irreversible decompensation if they are allowed to remain hypotensive from an indolently treated vasovagal reaction. When the vasovagal constellation occurs during catheter manipulation (instead of sheath insertion or removal), it should still be treated as outlined above, but the operator should be aware that vagal stimulation is one of the earliest findings in cardiac perforation (see below) as the pericardium is irritated by blood.

Conduction disturbances (bundle branch block or complete AV block) are an uncommon but potentially serious cause of bradycardia during cardiac catheterization (68). They may be precipitated when the catheter impacts the area of the right bundle during right-sided heart catheterization. This may cause a transient change in complex on the monitor electrocardiogram (ECG), but requires no treatment except in the patient with pre-existing left bundle branch block (69). With right bundle branch block superimposed on pre-existing left bundle branch block, asystole and cardiovascular collapse may ensue unless an adequate escape rhythm (i.e., a junctional escape) takes over. The same scenario may be seen when left bundle branch block is produced as the aortic valve is crossed in a patient with pre-existing right bundle.

When complete heart block develops, atropine is rarely helpful in the setting of inadequate junctional escape and hemodynamic deterioration, but should be given anyway, since it has few adverse effects. Coughing may help support the circulation and maintain consciousness as a temporary pacing catheter is inserted. Isuprel can be helpful, but is rarely indicated in the cardiac catheterization laboratory where temporary pacing can be rapidly initiated. At one time, temporary pacing catheters were placed prophylactically in patients with bundle branch block or planned right coronary intervention, but this has been abandoned because frank asystole is rare and there is generally adequate time for insertion of a pacing catheter. The only procedures for which we currently place prophylactic right-sided heart catheters are rotational atherectomy or rheolytic thrombectomy (particularly in the right and circumflex coronary arteries; see Chapter 23).

PERFORATION OF THE HEART OR GREAT VESSELS

Perforation of the cardiac chambers, coronary arteries, or the intrathoracic great vessels is fortunately a rare event in diagnostic catheterization. In the Cooperative study from 1968 (3), 100 patients (0.8%) had perforation during diagnostic catheterization. Most involved the cardiac chambers, particularly the right atrium (33 cases), right ventricle (21 cases), left atrium (10 cases), and the left ventricle (10 cases). Most (30 of 33) right atrial perforations involved trans-septal catheterization. The right ventricle was the most common site for perforation in the remaining (non-trans-septal) diagnostic procedures, related to the use of stiff catheters (woven Dacron right heart catheters [i.e., Cournand], endomyocardial biopsy, or temporary pacing catheters). Elderly women (age older than 65 years) seem particularly susceptible, because the walls of the right-sided heart chambers tend to be thinner.

When cardiac perforation does occur, it is usually heralded by bradycardia and hypotension owing to vagal stimulation (see vasovagal reaction, above) (70,71). As blood accumulates in the pericardium, the cardiac silhouette may enlarge and the normal pulsation of the heart borders on fluoroscopy will become blunted. Hemodynamic findings of tamponade may develop in the form of arterial paradox and elevation of the right atrial pressure with loss of the "y" descent (see Chapter 32). If the patient is hemodynamically stable, a portable transthoracic echocardiogram may help document the presence of blood in the pericardial space, but if hemodynamic compromise is severe or progressive, immediate pericardiocentesis should be performed via the subxiphoid approach. We use a disposable kit containing an 18-gauge needle, a J-tip guidewire, and a tapered catheter with multiple side holes, which is immediately available in the catheterization laboratory. Once pericardiocentesis has stabilized the situation, the operator must decide whether or not emergency surgery will be needed to oversew the site of perforation. Most perforations, in fact, will seal so that surgery is unnecessary, as illustrated in an 18-year review from the Mayo Clinic (71). During this period, 92 patients (0.08% of invasive procedures) developed tamponade, including 1.9% of valvuloplasties, 0.23% of electrophysiology studies, 0.08% of coronary angioplasties, and 0.006% of diagnostic catheterizations. Most (57%) patients were in frank hemodynamic collapse (systolic pressure <60 mm Hg) at the time of pericardiocentesis. Echo-guided pericardiocentesis was successful in 91 cases, as was the only therapy required in 82% of cases (the remaining 18% also required surgical intervention). There were no procedural deaths in this series, but there were three major complications (pneumothorax, intercostal artery injury, and right ventricular laceration), and seven patients (8%) died within 30 days of the procedure.

In the modern interventional laboratory, however, the most common cause of tamponade is perforation or rupture of a coronary artery. This was unheard of in the era of diagnostic catheterization and was a reportable rare complication with conventional balloon coronary angioplasty (72). With the use of or hydrophilic-coated guidewire, platelet IIb/IIIa receptor blockers, and more aggressive atherectomy technologies, the incidence of coronary perforation may be as high as 1% (73–75). Some perforations, particularly those limited to deep injury to the vessel wall with localized perivascular contrast staining, can simply be observed. But such patients are at risk for delayed tamponade during the several hours following the procedure and must be monitored expectantly. In contrast, free perforations may lead to the development of frank tamponade within seconds to minutes (Fig. 3.9), particularly when the patient is well anticoagulated or has received a IIb/IIIa blocker. The first countermeasure is to seal the site of leakage by inflation of a balloon catheter that spans the perforated segment. If available, a perfusion balloon catheter can be used to maintain antegrade flow to the myocardium as the site of perforation is effectively sealed, but speed of sealing is of the essence. Once this is done, anticoagulation

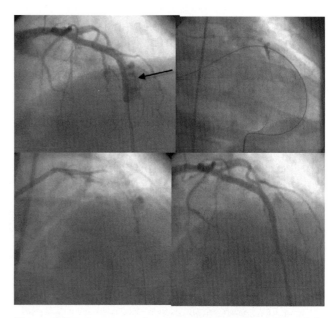

Figure 3.9 Coronary perforation and management. **Upper left.** Immediately after 18 atm postdilation of a mid LAD stent through a 6F catheter, coronary perforation with free extravasation of contrast was noted (*arrow*). **Upper right.** The patient became hypotensive within minutes, and the angioplasty balloon was reinflated within the area of perforation to seal the leak as pericardiocentesis was performed via the subxiphoid route. **Lower left.** Via the contralateral groin, an 8F guiding catheter was engaged in the left coronary ostium, and a wire and Jomed covered stent were advanced to the point of perforation. **Lower right.** After this stent was deployed, there was no further extravasation, and the heparin was not reversed as the platelet glycoprotein IIb/IIIa receptor blocker was continued to protect the patency of the stents that had been placed in the right and proximal left anterior descending coronary arteries.

should generally be reversed (i.e., giving protamine 1 mL equals 1 mg for each 1,000 units of heparin) if possible. Pericardiocentesis may also be necessary if hemodynamic embarrassment is present. Although many localized coronary perforations will seal with just prolonged balloon inflation and reversal of anticoagulation, ongoing bleeding is the rule for free perforations. Nonsurgical options then include coil embolization if the bleeding site is in a small distal branch, or placement of a covered stent (see Chapter 24) to seal the perforation site in a larger proximal vessel. A free perforation with ongoing leakage, however, is a strong indication for emergent surgical repair (73–74).

Perforation of the great vessels (aorta or pulmonary artery) is extremely rare. The aorta is sufficiently elastic to resist perforation, except in the case of weakening by ascending aortic dissection or aneurysm. Aortic puncture may occur, however, during attempted transseptal puncture with too anterior a needle orientation (see Chapter 4). Ascending aortic dissection can also result from vigorous use of a guiding catheter or extension from a proximal coronary dissection (75). If the dissection remains localized angiographically, and is confined to the first few centimeters of the aortic root, it can usually be managed medically and will resolve within weeks (Fig. 3.10).

Rupture of the pulmonary artery is also rare, but care must be taken not to use stiff-tip guidewires in these thinner-walled vessels. Perforation of the branch pulmonary arteries has been reported when balloon flotation catheters are inflated while positioned in a distal branch (rather than in the left or right main pulmonary artery) (76). Patients typically develop massive hemoptysis of bright red

blood and respiratory distress. This requires tamponade of the proximal pulmonary artery, embolization of the bleeding branch, and placement of a double-lumen endotracheal intubation to protect the noninjured lung (or even emergency lobectomy or pneumonectomy). Placement of the patient with the lacerated pulmonary artery down may help maintain aeration of the uninjured lung until the double-lumen tube is placed. To avoid this serious complication, a balloon-tip catheter should never be inflated in a distal position under fluoroscopy or at the bedside without a clear pulmonary artery trace, and then only in a slow gradual fashion just until the waveform changes shape (i.e., from pulmonary artery to pulmonary capillary wedge).

INFECTIONS AND PYROGEN REACTIONS

Because cardiac catheterization is an inherently sterile procedure, infection is extremely unusual. Recommended technique includes shaving and cleaning the catheter introduction site with povidone-iodine (Betadine), use of a nonporous drape, and adequate operator clothing (including a scrub suit, gown, and sterile gloves) (77). Endocarditis prophylaxis is not usually recommended when cardiac catheterization is performed with standard sterile precautions, but bacteremia has been reported after long or complex PCI interventions (78). Administration of a cephalosporin (e.g., Kefzol 1 gm on call and every 8 hours for 24 hours) should thus be considered when a delayed intervention is

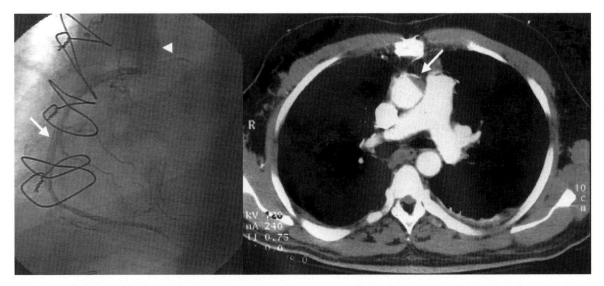

Figure 3.10 Guiding catheter dissection of right coronary artery extending into the aortic root. **Left.** During attempted angioplasty of the right coronary artery, an extensive coronary dissection was produced (*arrow*) with contrast extending into the wall of the aortic root (*arrow head*). **Right.** CT angiogram showed a localized hematoma in the right side of the aorta (*arrow*), which was managed expectantly and resolved on follow-up CT studies. (From Goldstein JA, et al. Aortocoronary dissection complicating a percutaneous coronary intervention. *J Invasive Cardiol* 2003;15:89–92.)

performed by exchanging sheaths placed in an earlier diagnostic procedure, in a patient at high risk (prosthetic valve) undergoing a complex procedure, or when any break in sterile technique is suspected. When performing a repeat procedure within 2 weeks of an initial diagnostic procedure, the contralateral groin should be used since an increased infection rate has been reported with early reuse of the same groin site (79). Special care should also be taken when performing catheterization through a femoral graft since such grafts appear more prone to infection with potentially disastrous consequences (80), and when implanting a foreign body (e.g., a femoral closure device, see Chapter 5).

The AHA/ACC task force does not insist that the operator performs a surgical scrub or wears a surgical cap and mask during femoral procedures (58). These precautions are, however, recommended for catheterization by the brachial approach, where the risk of infection is 10 times higher than for the femoral approach (0.62% versus 0.06%). Full sterile precautions (hand scrub, cap, and mask including a splash shield) are also strongly recommended for the femoral approach when the procedure is prolonged, when the sheath will remain in place for any period, when a stent or permanent pacemaker is being implanted, or when a vascular graft is punctured. Although some operators choose not to wear hats or masks, there have now been isolated reports of life-threatening stent, groin, or disseminated infections (78), which were presumably seeded in the cardiac catheterization laboratory. Although some might accuse us of overkill, we have elected to use these precautions on all catheterization procedures in our laboratory, partially to protect the patient and partially to protect the operator from blood contamination, as recommended under the universal precaution guidelines of the Occupational Safety and Health Administration (OSHA).

Even with these precautions, exposure to blood through splashes, glove punctures, and needle sticks is one of the greatest risks of working in the cardiac catheterization environment. Care should be taken in recapping needles and in segregating all "sharps" on the back table so that they are not found inadvertently by the operator or support staff breaking the table down following a procedure. Vaccination for hepatitis B is encouraged for all laboratory personnel (80a), and anyone who suffers a puncture or laceration should report the event to the laboratory director and employee health where they should be given the option to implement anti-HIV therapy. Therapy with two nucleoside analog reverse transcriptase inhibitors (usually zidovudine and lamivudine) plus a protease inhibitor (either indinavir or nelfinavir) should be initiated within hours of a puncture with a hollow access needle contaminated with blood from an HIV-positive patient and continued for 4 weeks to reduce the risk of subsequent infection (81).

To eliminate the risk of patient-to-patient contamination, we also avoid the multiuse drug vials and clean the room thoroughly between procedures. With the precautions described above, it is relatively unlikely that infection is the cause of a postprocedure fever. Although the patient should undergo the usual fever evaluation (chest radiograph, urine analysis, complete blood count, blood cultures), two other causes should be considered: Phlebitis may develop after brachial catheterization, with low-grade fever and a warm tended cord overlying the affected vein. Pyrogen reactions may present with shaking chills during or within the first hour after a catheterization, with a brief fever spike as high as 102°F. These previously common reactions were caused by the presence of contaminating materials that remained on incompletely cleaned catheter surfaces (82), but have been virtually eliminated by the switch to disposable single-use commercial catheters.

ALLERGIC AND ANAPHYLACTOID REACTIONS

Cardiac catheterization may precipitate allergic or anaphylactoid reactions to three materials: (a) local anesthetic, (b) iodinated contrast agent, or (c) protamine sulfate. True allergies to local anesthetic do occur, but are more common with older ester agents (e.g., procaine) than with newer amide agents (lidocaine, bupivacaine) (83). Some purported allergic reactions to these agents are actually vasovagal episodes or reactions to preservatives. For patients who claim this history, preservative-free anesthetic (bupivacaine or mepivacaine) or the use of other class (amide vs. ester) are practical alternatives to performing the procedure without local anesthetic.

The most common allergic reactions ($\leq 1\%$ of procedures) are triggered by iodinated contrast agents. In contrast to true anaphylactic reactions (which are mediated by IgE), reactions to contrast appear to involve degranulation of circulating basophils and tissue mast cells by direct complement activation (i.e., an anaphylactoid reaction) (84). Release of histamine and other agents causes the clinical manifestations (sneezing, urticaria, angioedema of lips and eyelids, bronchospasm, or in extreme cases, shock with warm extremities owing to profound systemic vasodilation). Risk of such reactions is increased in patients with other atopic disorders, allergy to penicillin, or allergy to seafood (which contains organic iodine) and may be as high as 15 to 35% in patients who have had a prior reaction to contrast. Premedication of patients with a seafood allergy or prior contrast reaction using the combination of prednisone (20 mg three times a day for 24 to 48 hours), an H1 antihistamine (diphenhydramine 25 mg three times a day), and an H2 blocker (cimetidine or ranitidine) can reduce the incidence of a second reaction to 5 to 10% and that of severe reactions (bronchospasm or shock) to <1%. The availability of newer low- and iso-osmolar nonionic contrast agents (see Chapter 2) adds a further margin of safety, since the rate of severe cross-reactions in patients with prior reaction to an ionic contrast agent is also <1% (85,86). For this indication, the true nonionic agents are preferable to an ionic low-osmolar agent such as Hexabrix, to which cross-reactions may still occur. In patients with a severe prior allergic reaction to contrast, use of a nonionic contrast agent can be combined with steroid and antihistamine premedication, although even then breakthrough allergic reactions may occur (87-88). (see Chapter 2).

When a patient with a well-documented prior severe contrast reaction needs to undergo repeat catheterization, aortic pressure should be recorded before the catheter is cleared with contrast, since even this small amount of contrast can cause significant histamine release. The "money shots" of the coronaries should be obtained first, since a severe contrast reaction to the left ventriculogram may preclude further angiography. If a severe reaction occurs, it can be reversed with an intravenous injection of dilute epinephrine (89): 1 mL of 1:10,000 epinephrine (i.e., 0.1 mg of epinephrine per mL) is drawn up from the syringe on the crash cart, diluted further to a total volume of 10 mL (10 mcg/mL), and labeled so that it is not mistaken for flush. The epinephrine is administered into the right-sided heart catheter in boluses of 1 mL (or 10 mcg) every minute, until arterial pressure is restored. It is rare to have to give more than 10 mL (100 mcg) in total, and excessive doses should be avoided, since they may precipitate life-threatening hypertension, tachycardia, or even ventricular fibrillation.

Although reactions to contrast are the most common allergic reaction in the cardiac catheterization laboratory, reactions to protamine sulfate, a biologic product derived from salmon eggs, can also occur. These reactions seem to be more common in insulin-dependent diabetics who have received NPH insulin (that contains protamine) (89). In current practice, with no heparin given for most diagnostic catheterizations and widespread use of puncture-closure devices, it is rare to administer protamine in the catheterization laboratory.

Another allergic reaction that should be considered—even though it is rarely seen in the cardiac catheterization laboratory itself—is heparin-induced thrombocytopenia (HIT) (90,91) (see also below). Up to 10% of patients will have a fall in platelet count to <50,000 after 4 days of heparin exposure owing to a direct nonimmune mechanism (so called HIT-1). But a much smaller number (<1 %) will exhibit a more profound fall in platelets combined with arterial and venous thrombosis owing to an antibody that binds to the complex of heparin with platelet factor 4 and causes platelet activation (HIT-2, or HITT {heparin-induced thrombocytopenia and thrombosis})(91a). This usually does not develop until day 5, unless there has been prior sensitization to heparin, and can be diagnosed by blood testing, which should be done in any postprocedure patient who develops thrombocytopenia. If positive, an alternative nonheparin (i.e., neither unfractionated nor low–molecular-weight heparin) anticoagulant agent should be used (see below). If thrombocytopenia develops after a coronary interventional procedure, the assay for heparin antibodies is particularly important to distinguish it from the thrombocytopenia that develops in 1 to 3% of

patients treated with a IIb/IIIa receptor blocker (see below).

RENAL DYSFUNCTION

Temporary or permanent renal dysfunction is a serious potential complication of cardiac angiography. The potential mechanisms of contrast-induced nephropathy (CIN) include vasomotor instability, increased glomerular permeability to protein, direct tubular injury, or tubular obstruction. At least 5% of patients experience a transient rise in serum creatinine (>0.5 mg/dL or a relative increase of 25%) following cardiac angiography (92), making CIN the third most common cause of hospital-acquired renal failure. It may occur in 15% of the general cath population, or ≤50% of patients who have risk factors including diabetes, preexisting renal dysfunction, multiple myeloma, volume depletion, or other drug therapy (e.g., gentamicin, angiotensin-converting enzyme inhibitors, nonsteroidal anti-inflammatory drugs [NSAIDs]). Most such creatinine elevations are nonoliguric, peak within 1 to 2 days, and then return to baseline by 7 days, but may rarely go on to require chronic dialysis. The occurrence of CIN increases length of hospital stay and is associated with a fivefold increase in in-hospital mortality (93). If dialysis is required, there is a further increase in mortality (from 1.1 to 7.1% with CIN to 35.7% with CIN plus dialysis).

The main defense against contrast-induced nephropathy is limitation of total contrast volume to 3 mL/kg (or 5 mL/kg divided by serum creatinine, in patients with elevated baseline creatinine). In the 1990 Society for Cardiac Angiography and Intervention (SCA&I) registry, the mean volume of contrast administered during diagnostic cardiac catheterization was 130 mL for diagnostic procedures and 191 mL for angioplasty procedures, indicating that staying within 3 mL/kg limit for patients with normal renal function (7) should usually be possible. In patients with reduced renal function and especially with diabetes, extra attention must be paid to limiting unnecessary angiographic views and multiple contrast puffs during interventional wire and device placement, which may drive up the total contrast volume. There is some experience with using gadolinium (Magnevist, Amersham GE) as a substitute or diluent for iodinated contrast (see Chapter 2). Animal data suggest that low-osmolar contrast agents may have lower renal toxicity; prospective trials comparing high- and low-osmolar contrast agents have generally failed to show consistent benefit (94,95). Trials with the iso-osmolar agent iodixanol (Visipaque), however, have tended to show benefit (96).

Adequate prehydration is also critically important in any patient with impaired baseline renal function. In one classic study (97), 26% of patients with a mean baseline serum creatinine of 2.1 mL/dL had a rise in serum creatinine by >0.5 mg/dL. Hydration with 1/2 normal saline for 12 hours before and after the contrast procedure provided the best protection against creatinine rise (which then occurred in

11%), but 26 to 28% of patients who received hydration in combination with either furosemide or mannitol had such a rise. There may be some benefit to the use of sodium bicarbonate (154 mEq/L) rather than saline for prehydration (98). Postprocedure hemofiltration in the intensive care unit has also been reported to reduce the incidence of contrast nephropathy in one study, presumably by direct contrast removal and consequent shortened renal exposure (99).

The free-radical scavenger n-acetyl cysteine (600 mg orally before and twice a day after contrast exposure) has shown some benefit (100), although other trials have failed to show benefit (101). A meta-analysis of seven randomized trials, however, does suggest benefit (102), and the agent is generally quite benign.

There is also some support for afferent arteriolar vasoconstriction as a mechanism for contrast nephropathy, but renal-range dopamine actually worsens contrast nephropathy (103). The selective DA-1 receptor, fenoldopam, provides more potent afferent arteriolar vasodilation and had positive results in a pilot trial (104). But benefit of systemic infusion was evident however, in the 300-patient CONTRAST trial in which 28% of fenoldopam patients and 24% of placebo patients had a 0.5 mL/dL increase in serum creatinine at 96 hours postcatheterization (105). A device that allows selective simultaneous infusion of fenoldopam into both renal arteries (Be*nephit*™ Infusion System, FlowMedica, Fremont CA) allows more profound renal vasodilation with little or no systemic hypotension, is now under investigation for CIN.

Another cause of renal failure following cardiac catheterization is systemic cholesterol embolization (106). This clinical syndrome is seen in 0.15% of catheterizations, but cholesterol emboli can be identified pathologically in many more patients. Patients at greatest risk are those with diffuse atherosclerosis or abdominal aortic aneurysm, in whom insertion of a guiding catheter will frequently produce a shower of glistening particles on the table drape (33). The hallmarks of cholesterol embolization are evidence of peripheral embolization (including livido reticularis, abdominal or foot pain, and purple toes). Episodic hypertension or systemic eosinophilia may be apparent well before the other manifestations develop. Renal failure due to cholesterol embolization tends to develop slowly (over weeks to months, rather than over 1 to 2 days as is seen with contrast nephropathy). Half of the patients with this syndrome progress to frank renal failure. Renal biopsy can confirm the presence of cholesterol clefts, but is seldom necessary for diagnosis. Treatment is purely supportive.

OTHER COMPLICATIONS

Hypotension

Reduction in arterial blood pressure is one of the most common problems seen during catheterization. This reduc-

tion represents the final common manifestation of a variety of conditions including the following: (a) hypovolemia, owing to inadequate prehydration, blood loss, or excessive contrast-induced diuresis; (b) reduction in cardiac output, owing to ischemia, tamponade, arrhythmia, or valvular regurgitation; or (c) inappropriate systemic arteriolar vasodilation, owing to vasovagal, excessive nitrate administration, or a vasodilator response to contrast or mixed inotrope-vasodilator drugs such as dopamine or dobutamine. Few places, however, are as well equipped as the cardiac catheterization laboratory to recognize, diagnose, and treat hypotension. If routine right heart catheterization has not been done, evolving hypotension is certainly an adequate reason to insert such a catheter to differentiate among hypovolemia, high output syndrome (including sepsis), and cardiogenic shock.

Low filling pressures mandate rapid volume administration through the peripheral intravenous line and the side arm of the venous sheath (500 to 1,000 mL of normal saline can be given in 5 minutes by this route) and consideration of potential sites of blood loss (expanding thigh hematoma, retroperitoneal bleeding). If low filling pressures are combined with inappropriate bradycardia, atropine should be given for a potential vasovagal reaction. High filling pressures, however, suggest primary cardiac dysfunction and should prompt consideration of ischemia, tamponade, or sudden onset of valvular regurgitation. Such patients should be supported empirically by inotropic agents (dopamine, dobutamine, milrinone), vasopressors (Levophed or Neo-Synephrine), or circulatory support devices (see Chapter 21), as a more precise cause is uncovered and treated. The operator also must decide whether the precipitating problem will require surgical intervention or whether a corrective intervention should be performed in the cardiac catheterization laboratory. If bradycardia is present and does not respond to atropine, consideration should be given to atrial (or AV) sequential pacing to preserve the atrial kick in such patients.

One of the most common oversights in managing hypotension is the failure to assess the cardiac output through thermodilution or measurement of pulmonary arterial oxygen saturation. On several occasions, high pulmonary arterial saturation in a hypotensive patient has signaled coexistent sepsis, contrast reaction, or an idiosyncratic vasodilator reaction to dopamine infusion. The essential importance of initial empiric and then definitive correction of hypotension and its causes—before hypotension leads to secondary ischemia and an irreversible spiral of left ventricular dysfunction—cannot be overemphasized in salvaging patients who might otherwise go on to have major complications.

Volume Overload

Patients in the cardiac catheterization laboratory are prone to volume overload owing to the administration of hypertonic contrast agents, myocardial depression or ischemia induced by contrast, poor baseline left ventricular function, as well as their supine position and attempts to volume load patients at risk for contrast-induced renal dysfunction. The best treatments are prevention by optimizing volume status before or early during the procedure and by use of low-osmolar contrast agents. The support measures described above (inotropes, diuretics, vasodilators, balloon pumping) should also be applied in a progressive manner before the patient goes into frank pulmonary edema with the resultant agitation and desaturation. Once pulmonary edema develops, even more aggressive treatment is warranted. Allowing the patient to sit up partially while morphine and nitroprusside are administered to bring filling pressures down may be necessary. If respiratory failure seems imminent, anesthesia support should be requested early enough to allow intubation before a full arrest develops.

Anxiety/Pain

Cardiac catheterization procedures should be well tolerated with oral sedative pretreatment (diazepam [Valium] 5 to 10 mg, and diphenhydramine [Benadryl] 25 to 50 mg) and liberal use of local anesthetic at the catheter insertion site. However, the amount of discomfort, level of anxiety, and tolerance for either vary widely from patient to patient. The first effort should be to understand why the patient is having pain (vascular complication, perforation, coronary occlusion, ischemia) and whether anything can be done to reverse the problem. In the meantime, the catecholamine surge associated with pain and anxiety may worsen the condition of a patient who came to the cardiac catheterization laboratory with unstable angina, aortic stenosis, congestive heart failure, or hypertrophic myopathy. It is thus routine practice also to manage such complaints symptomatically by administering small intravenous doses of fentanyl (25 to 50 mg) and midazolam (Versed 0.5 to 1 mg). Care must be taken, however, not to oversedate the patient or to overlook an important and treatable cause for patient complaints. Guidelines for monitoring conscious sedation require monitoring of blood pressure, respiratory rate, and pulse oximetry after such medications are administered. The antagonist drugs—naloxone (Narcan) for opiates and flumazenil (Mazicon) for benzodiazepines—should also be stocked wherever the agonist drugs are used for conscious sedation.

Respiratory Insufficiency

Problems with adequate ventilation or oxygenation are not uncommon in the cardiac catheterization laboratory; they may result from pulmonary edema, baseline lung disease, allergic reaction, obstructive sleep apnea, or oversedation. Patients are monitored throughout the procedure with a finger pulse oximeter to detect progressive desaturation. Data from such monitoring show that low-flow supplemental oxygen (2 L per minute via nasal prongs) helps avoid episodes of desaturation (saturation <90%) that otherwise occur with surprising frequency during cardiac catheterization (34%) or coronary angioplasty (56%) (107). If oxygen consumption is to be measured as part of a calculation of cardiac output by the Fick method, supplemental oxygen administration should not be begun until after that measurement (or should be interrupted for at least 10 minutes before the oxygen consumption is measured). In most labs, however, the oxygen consumption is assumed at 125 mL/m^2 rather than measured, under which circumstance there is absolutely no reason to discontinue supplemental oxygen administration during a Fick measurement of cardiac output.

Retained Equipment

Although diagnostic and therapeutic cardiac catheters have a high degree of reliability, failures can and do occur whereby devices knot (108), become entrapped (109), or leave fragments in the circulation (110–111). Most of these events are precipitated when such devices are stressed beyond their design parameters, e.g., when a coronary angioplasty guidewire is rotated multiple times in a single direction while its tip is entrapped in a total occlusion, or when a bare-mounted coronary stent cannot be advanced across a lesion and strips off the delivery balloon during attempted withdrawal. Operators should thus be familiar with device performance limits and avoid placing devices into situations that promote failure. Operators should also be familiar with the use of vascular snares, bioptomes, baskets, and other devices and techniques that can be used to recover the errant fragments (111) when devices do fail (Fig. 3.11).

ADJUNCTIVE PHARMACOLOGY FOR CARDIAC CATHETERIZATION

It is clear from the above discussion that an important part of interventional catheterization involves mastery of a broad range of drugs. This includes anticoagulant, antiplatelet, vasoactive, sedative, and antiarrhythmic agents. There is little doubt that refinements in antiplatelet adjunctive pharmacology (e.g., glycoprotein IIb/IIIa inhibitors and thienopyridine class of ADP receptor blockers) have contributed significantly to the improvements in PCI success, safety, and durability over the last decade, and this section will focus on evidence-based recommendations for antithrombotic therapy during PCI based on clinical presentation (Table 3.2), highlighting the guidelines from the ACC/AHA (112,113) and 7th ACCP Consensus Conference on Antithrombotic Therapy (114).

Aspirin

Acetylsalicylic acid (ASA) is one the most valuable medications used in cardiovascular medicine today and exerts its

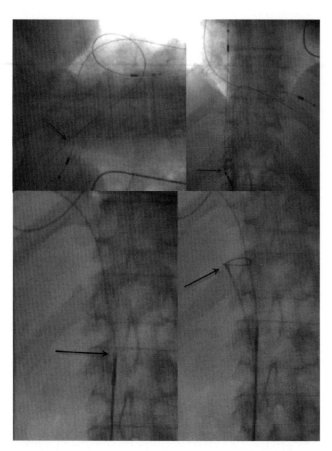

Figure 3.11 Retrieval of fractured pacemaker lead. When this biventricular pacemaker ceased to pace the atrium, the fractured end of the lead was found free in right ventricle **(upper left,** *arrow*), the loop of this lead was grasped with a deflectable mapping catheter **(upper right,** *arrow*), and the free end was pulled down into the inferior vena cava. The free end was grasped with a bioptome **(lower left,** *arrow*), and a goose-neck snare was advanced over the lead to allow it to be removed though a 12 F femoral venous sheath **(lower right).** (Case provided courtesy of Dr. Laurence Epstein, Brigham and Women's Hospital.)

TABLE 3.2
ANTITHROMBOTIC THERAPY DURING PCI

Aspirin, 81–325 mg at least 2 hr prior to PCI
UFH using weight-adjusted dosing:
   50–70 U/kg bolus (+GP IIb/IIIa) with ACT target 200–250 sec
   70–100 U/kg bolus (−GP IIb/IIIa) with ACT target 250–350 sec
Bivalirudin, 0.75 mg/kg bolus followed by 1.75 mg/kg per hour
   infusion during PCI only
LMWH
   0.5–0.75 mg/kg IV (+GP IIb/IIIa)
   1.0 mg/kg IV (−GP IIb/IIIa)
Eptifibatide, 180 mcg/kg bolus,repeated 10 minutes later, and
   followed by 2 mcg/kg per minute infusion for 18 hrs post PCI
Abciximab, 0.25 mg/kg IV bolus followed by 0.125 mcg/kg
   per minute infusion for 12 hrs post PCI
Clopidogrel, 300–600 mg load, 75 mg daily
Ticlopidine, 500 mg load, 250 mg twice daily

The 7th ACCP consensus conference on antithrombotic and thrombolytic therapy. (Modified from Popma, JJ, et al. Antithrombotic therapy during percutaneous coronary intervention. *Chest* 2004;126:576S–599S.)

---

effect primarily by irreversibly inhibiting cyclo-oxygenase to block platelet synthesis of arachidonic acid–derived thromboxane A2—a promoter of platelet aggregation (115). It causes a measurable inhibition of platelet function within 60 minutes (116). Although the optimal dose for PCI has not been firmly established, randomized trials have shown antithrombotic effect between 50 and 100 mg/day. When given in combination with warfarin or thienopyridine class of antiplatelet agents (e.g., clopidogrel), the ASA dose should probably be lowered to 80 to 100 mg based on a post hoc analysis of data from the Clopidogrel in Unstable angina to prevent Recurrent Events (CURE), which showed similar efficacy but less major bleeding with the low dose (<100 mg) of ASA (117).

The benefits of ASA in reducing cardiovascular death, MI, and stroke in patients with coronary artery disease (118) has led to the near universal use of this medication for patients undergoing PCI. The initial studies involving ASA in PCI included combined antiplatelet regimens with dipyri-

damole, which reduced the incidence of periprocedural MI during PCI by 77% compared with patients receiving placebo when administered 24 hours prior to balloon angioplasty and continued for 4 to 7 months (119). Dipyridamole, however, provides no additional benefit beyond ASA (120). ASA has been shown to be effective in patients undergoing intracoronary stent placement, especially in combination with ticlopidine or clopidogrel (121).

Several studies have suggested that 5 to 60% of patients may not respond to ASA (122,123). This concept of ASA nonresponsiveness or resistance is based on variable definitions, including inability to protect against thrombotic complications, failure to cause prolongation of bleeding time, failure to inhibit platelet aggregation, or failure to inhibit platelet TXA2 production. The precise mechanism of ASA resistance is unknown, but it may include cellular, clinical, and genetic factors, as well as concomitant use of nonsteroidal anti-inflammatory drugs (NSAIDs), which may inhibit the clinical benefits of ASA by competing for a common docking site on COX-1 (124).

There is emerging clinical evidence that ASA resistance is associated with an increased risk of major adverse cardiovascular events. Five studies in patients with coronary, peripheral, and/or cerebrovascular disease have reported 1.8- to 10-fold increased risk of thrombotic events (125–129). Using a bedside point-of-care device, Wang et al. (30) reported the incidence of ASA nonresponsiveness in a prospective multicenter registry to be 23% and determined a history of coronary artery disease to be associated with twice the chance of being nonresponder (odds ratio [OR], 2.01, 95% confidence interval [CI] 1.189 to 3.411, $P = .0009$). This point-of-care determination of ASA nonresponsiveness appears to have important clinical implications in the PCI setting, with a significant increased risk of periprocedural myocardial infarction in ASA-nonresponsive patients compared with ASA-sensitive patients (130).

Allergic reactions to ASA include generalized urticaria, maculopapular rash, asthma, angioedema, and anaphylaxis. ASA-allergic patients with coronary disease undergoing PCI may be treated with a thienopyridine (e.g., clopidogrel) alone or in combination with cilostazol. Some interventional cardiologists favor ASA desensitization using escalating doses of oral ASA challenge prior to known coronary interventions. This can be done safely and likely reduces the ischemic complications of PCI without ASA pretreatment (131,132).

Guideline Recommendations for ASA

The ACC/AHA guidelines recommend that ASA should be administered as soon as possible after presentation with acute coronary syndrome and continued indefinitely (Class I, Level of evidence: A) (112). According to ACCP guidelines (114), pretreatment with aspirin, 75 to 325 mg, is recommended for all patients undergoing PCI (Grade 1A). For long-term treatment after PCI, aspirin, 75 to 162 mg/day, is recommended (Grade 1). For long-term treatment after PCI in patients who receive antithrombotic agents such as clopidogrel or warfarin, lower-dose aspirin, 75 to 100 mg/day, is advised (Grade 1C+).

Thienopyridines

The thienopyridine derivatives—ticlopidine and clopidogrel—selectively and irreversibly inhibit the P2Y12 ADP receptor, which plays a critical role in orchestrating platelet activation and aggregation (133), and are synergistic with ASA in providing greater inhibition of platelet aggregation than either agent alone (134). Both agents are inactive in vitro, but are metabolized by hepatic cytochrome P450-3A4 to produce active metabolites (135). Clopidogrel differs structurally from ticlopidine by the addition of a carboxymethyl group, is six times more potent than ticlopidine, and does not share any common metabolites with ticlopidine (38). The inhibition of platelet aggregation by ticlopidine and clopidogrel is present after 2 to 3 days of therapy with ticlopidine 500 mg/day or clopidogrel 75 mg/day, and platelet function recovers in 5 to 7 days after discontinuation owing to the synthesis of new platelets (136).

Pretreatment with clopidogrel prior to PCI improves 30-day outcomes compared with those not pretreated (137–139), reducing death and MI by nearly 39% (Fig. 3.12). To achieve this benefit, patients must be treated between 6 and 12 to 15 hours prior to PCI, although use of a 600-mg clopidogrel load may reduce the required pretreatment period to as short as 2 hours prior to PCI. The thienopyridines and ASA in combination offer fivefold reductions in acute and subacute stent thrombosis compared with either ASA alone, warfarin, heparin, or long-term LMWH (121,140) (Fig. 3.13).

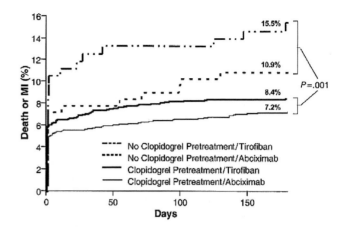

Figure 3.12 Pretreatment with clopidogrel in the TARGET study demonstrated a significant reduction in death or MI regardless of GP IIb/IIIa inhibitor therapy. (From Chan AW, et al. A device that allows selective simultaneous infusion of fenoldopam into both renal arteries (Benephit™ Infusion System, FlowMedica, Fremont CA) allows more profound renal vasodilation with little or no systemic hypotension, is now under investigation for CIN. *J Am Coll Cardiol* 2003;42:1188–1195.)

Longer-term clopidogrel after PCI reduces subsequent adverse events. In the CURE study, 12,562 patients received ASA and clopidogrel 300-mg bolus, followed by 75 mg daily, versus ASA and placebo (47). The clopidogrel group had a significant reduction (9.3% versus 11.4%, relative risk reduction 20%, P < 0.001) in the primary end point (death from cardiovascular cause, nonfatal myocardial infarction, or stroke) in the group receiving clopidogrel. This benefit was noted early (within 24 hours of treatment), was sustained at 1 year, and was observed in all patients with acute coronary syndromes regardless of their level of risk (141). CURE patients who underwent PCI and were randomized to clopidogrel had a 31% relative risk reduction in death and myocardial infarction compared with placebo-treated PCI patients. Furthermore, long-term (9 to 12 months) compared with short-term (4 weeks) clopidogrel therapy

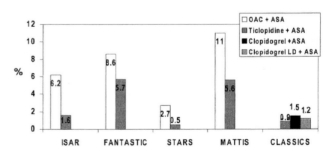

Figure 3.13 Comparison of major adverse clinical events (MACE %) after bare-metal stenting in the ISAR, FANTASTIC, STARS, MATTIS, and CLASSICS trials. These events largely reflect the incidence of subacute stent thrombosis. OAC, oral anticoagulants; ASA, acetylsalicylic acid (aspirin); LD, loading dose. (From Bertrand ME, et al. Double-blind study of the safety of clopidogrel with and without a loading dose in combination with aspirin compared with ticlopidine in combination with aspirin after coronary stenting: the clopidogrel aspirin stent international cooperative study (CLASSICS). *Circulation* 2000;102:628.)

post-PCI was associated with a 31% lower rate of cardiovascular death, MI, or revascularization ($P = .03$).

Similar benefits of clopidogrel were seen in the CREDO trial (138), which studied a more stable population undergoing stenting. Patients were randomly assigned to receive a 300-mg clopidogrel loading dose or placebo 3 to 24 hours before PCI, followed by clopidogrel 75 mg daily for 28 days post PCI. The group loaded with clopidogrel were continued on active drug from day 28 through 12 months while the control group received placebo. There was a significant 27% ($P = .02$) reduction in death, myocardial infarction, or stroke in patients receiving clopidogrel, suggesting that clopidogrel therapy should be continued in addition to ASA for a minimum of 9 months post PCI.

Clopidogrel does cause a significant increase in major bleeding. In CURE, those receiving clopidogrel had bleeding rates of 3.7% versus 2.7% ($P = .001$), most notably in those patients requiring CABG (142). In CREDO, there was only a trend toward more TIMI (Thrombolysis in Myocardial Infarction [study]) major bleeding (8.8 versus 6.7%, $P = .07$) and no excess bleeds among patients undergoing CABG (138). In light of these findings, it is recommended to delay elective CABG for 5 days after stopping clopidogrel, and possibly to avoid preloading of clopidogrel in unstable angina/non–ST elevation myocardial infarction (UA/NSTEMI) patients until after the coronary anatomy is identified and the need for CABG excluded, although this decision needs to take into account the consistent and substantial benefit of clopidogrel pretreatment in reducing the risk of death and myocardial infarction (Fig. 13.12) versus the fact that revascularization by PCI is more likely than CABG. Other noncardiac surgery should also be postponed until adequate passivation of the coronary vessel and stented segment occurs, allowing the clopidogrel to be stopped. In a series of 207 patients who had clopidogrel stopped prior to noncardiac surgery within 6 weeks of stent placement, 4% died, suffered an MI, or developed stent thrombosis (143). In the era of DES, the period of obligatory clopidogrel therapy should be extended to 3 to 6 months depending on the type of stent, with continuation of dual antiplatelet therapy in the preoperative, perioperative, and postoperative setting whenever possible.

Although the original stent thrombosis data were obtained with ticlopidine, its use has been virtually abandoned in the United States owing to its increased risk of neutropenia. Four randomized clinical trials (144–147) have directly compared ticlopidine and clopidogrel in combination with ASA after stenting. A meta-analysis demonstrated that clopidogrel was associated with a significant reduction in the incidence of major adverse cardiac events (OR, 0.50; $P = .001$) and mortality (OR, 0.43; $P = .001$) compared with ticlopidine, and the safety and tolerability of clopidogrel were superior to that of ticlopidine. This includes less rash and fewer gastrointestinal side effects, as well as fewer hematologic complications than seen with ticlopidine (neutropenia with ticlopidine is 1.3 to 2.1% compared with 0.10% with clopidogrel).

The clearance of ticlopidine is reduced by 50% with concomitant cimetidine use, and there is interindividual variability in platelet inhibition by clopidogrel; the occurrence of clopidogrel resistance has been documented in ≤30% of patients by several groups (148). In one study of patients undergoing PCI for ST elevation myocardial infarction (STEMI), clopidogrel resistance was associated with a significant increased risk of atherothrombotic events over the next 6 months (149).

Guidelines for Thienopyridines

For patients who undergo stent placement, the combination of aspirin and a thienopyridine derivative is recommended over systemic anticoagulation therapy (Grade 1A). Clopidogrel is recommended over ticlopidine (Grade 1A), with a loading dose of 300 mg given at least 6 hours prior to planned PCI (Grade 1B). If clopidogrel is started <6 hours prior to PCI, a 600-mg loading dose of clopidogrel is suggested (Grade 2C). After PCI, aspirin and clopidogrel (75 mg/day) is recommended for at least 9 to 12 months (Grade 1). In patients with low atherosclerotic risk, such as those with isolated coronary lesions, clopidogrel is recommended for at least 2 weeks after placement of a bare-metal stent (Grade 1A), for 2 to 3 months after placement of a sirolimus-eluting stent (Grade 1C+), and 6 months after placement of a paclitaxel-eluting stent (Grade 1C).

Unfractionated Heparin

Unfractionated heparin (UFH) is the most commonly used anticoagulant during PCI. Its effect is monitored by the activated clotting time (ACT) because the required level of anticoagulation for PCI is beyond the range that can be measured using the activated partial thromboplastin time (aPTT) (150,151). At least two studies have retrospectively related ACT values to clinical outcomes after PCI (152,153), and a third retrospective analysis suggested that ischemic complications of PCI were 34% lower with an ACT in the range of 350 to 375 seconds than they were with an ACT between 171 and 295 seconds ($P = .001$) (154). However, this was at the cost of progressively increased bleeding from 8.6% at ACTs <350 seconds to 12.4% at ACTs 350 to 375 seconds. When heparin is given in the absence of adjunctive GP IIb/IIIa inhibition, the recommended dose is 70 to 100 IU/kg with a target ACT between 250 and 350 seconds. When heparin is given in conjunction with a GP IIb/IIIa inhibitor, the recommended dose is 40 to 60 IU/kg with a target ACT of 200 to 250 seconds. In either case, removal of the femoral sheath should be delayed until the ACT is between 150 and 180 seconds, unless a puncture-closure device is used (see Chapter 4). Intravenous heparin is no longer routinely used after PCI, because several randomized studies have shown that prolonged heparin infusions do not reduce ischemic complications and are associated with a higher rate of bleeding at the catheter insertion site (155) (see Chapter 22).

Guidelines for UFH

In patients receiving a GP IIb-IIIa inhibitor, a heparin bolus of 50 to 70 IU/kg to achieve a target ACT >200 seconds is recommended (Grade 2C). In patients not receiving a GP IIb-IIIa inhibitor, heparin should be administered in a dose of 60 to 100 IU/kg sufficient to produce an ACT of 250 to 352 seconds (Grade 1C+). In patients after uncomplicated PCI, routine postprocedural infusion of heparin is not recommended (Grade 1A).

Low–Molecular-Weight Heparins

Low–molecular-weight heparins (LMWHs) are fragments of UFH produced by controlled chemical or enzymatic depolymerization processes that yield chains with a mean molecular weight of about 5,000 daltons. Like heparin, they work by binding to antithrombin-3, causing a conformational change that accelerates the interaction of

antithrombin with thrombin and activated factor X (factor Xa) 1,000-fold (156). The LMWHs differ from UFH in that their anti-Xa activity predominates over their anti-IIa activity. The most widely studied LMWHs are enoxaparin (mean molecular weight of 4,200 daltons with anti-Xa:anti-IIa ratio of 3.8) and dalteparin (mean molecular weight of 6,000 daltons and anti-Xa:anti-IIa ratio of 2.7).

The use of the LMWH as an alternative anticoagulant to UFH in the PCI setting has been driven largely by earlier trials showing superiority of enoxaparin compared with UFH in the medical treatment of patients with acute coronary syndromes. As the result of this front-end use of LMWH in unstable patients, many patients now come to the catheterization laboratory on this therapy and present a dilemma in subsequent anticoagulation (Fig. 3.14). Several randomized studies (157–159) have been performed comparing the safety and efficacy of UFH with enoxaparin during PCI. In the Coronary Revascularization Using Integrilin and Single bolus Enoxaparin (CRUISE)

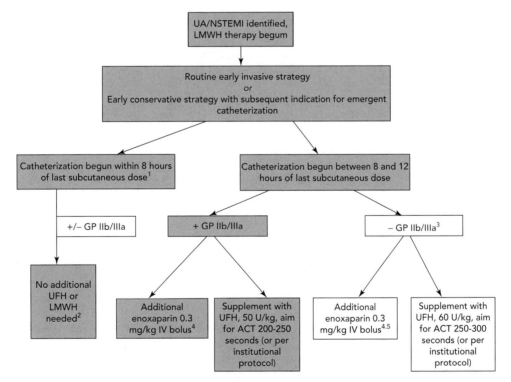

Figure 3.14 Strategies for the transition from medical therapy to procedural anticoagulation in patients receiving low–molecular-weight heparin. UA/NSTEMI, unstable angina/non-ST elevation myocardial infarction; LMWH, low–molecular weight. (From Kereiakes DJ, et al. Low-molecular weight heparin therapy for non-ST-elevation acute coronary syndromes and during percutaneous coronary intervention: an expert consensus. *Am Heart J* 2002;144:621).
Note:
1. For PCI, wait at least 30 to 60 minutes after SC injection, depending on molecular weight of the agent (30 minutes for enoxaparin, 60 minutes for dalteparin).
2. Insufficient data are available to guide heparinization in patients who have received only 1 dose of SC LMWH.
3. Fewer data are available on patients treated with SC enoxaparin and no GP lib/IIia receptors antagonists undergoing PCI.
4. If the patient has been receiving dalteparin, switch to UFH, as there are no available data on transitioning from medical to interventional therapy when the last SC dose of dalteparin was given 8 to 12 hours before PCI.
5. Consideration can be given to enoxaparin 0.5 mg/kg in those patients not receiving concomitant GP IIb/IIIa receptor antagonist therapy.

study, researchers randomized patients undergoing elective or emergent PCI to eptifibatide and enoxaparin or eptifibatide plus UFH (79), and demonstrated comparable safety and efficacy of enoxaparin to UFH during PCI in a randomized controlled study. The Integrilin and Enoxaparin Randomized Assessment of Acute Coronary syndrome Treatment (INTERACT) study randomized 746 patients with high-risk ACS to receive eptifibatide plus either enoxaparin (1 mg/kg twice daily subcutaneously for 48 hours) or weight-adjusted UFH for 48 hours (80). Cardiac catheterization and coronary revascularization were performed at the discretion of the investigator (63% of patients underwent angiography, 28.5% underwent PCI). Compared with UFH, enoxaparin significantly reduced the rate of non-CABG related major bleeding (3.8% versus 1.1% at 48 hours, $P = .014$; and 4.6% versus 1.8% at 96 hours, $P = .03$). The rate of the secondary end point, death or MI, was significantly lower in the enoxaparin group than in the UFH group (5% versus 9%, $P = .03$), and recurrent ischemia determined by continuous electrocardiographic monitoring was significantly lower in the enoxaparin group during the initial 48 hours (14.3% versus 25.4%; $P = .0002$) and from 48 to 96 hours (12.7% versus 25.9%; $P < .0001$).

In Superior Yield of the New strategy of Enoxaparin, Revascularization and Glycoprotein IIb/IIIa inhibitors (SYNERGY) trial, 10,027 high-risk ACS patients were randomized to enoxaparin (1mg/kg twice daily subcutaneously) or UFH (60 U/kg bolus followed by 12 U/kg per hour infusion) with a goal of early invasive therapy (82). The primary composite clinical end point of all-cause death or nonfatal MI during the first 30 days occurred in 14.0% of patients assigned to enoxaparin and 14.5% of patients assigned to unfractionated heparin (OR, 0.96; 95% CI, 0.86 to 1.06). No differences in ischemic events during PCI were observed between enoxaparin and unfractionated heparin groups in terms of abrupt closure, threatened abrupt closure, unsuccessful PCI, or emergency coronary artery bypass graft surgery. More bleeding was observed with enoxaparin using one definition (TIMI major bleeding, 9.1% versus 7.6%, $P = .008$) but not another (GUSTO severe bleeding 2.7% versus 2.2%, $P = .08$, with similar transfusion rates of 17.0% versus 16.0%, $P = .16$). Subgroup analysis suggests that cross-over therapy and protocol violations contributed adversely to bleeding complications.

In summary, enoxaparin appears to be equally effective as UFH during PCI at preventing a major adverse clinical event (MACE) with modest excess of major bleeding. Difficulties associated with monitoring the anticoagulation intensity of enoxaparin during PCI have led to empiric dosing algorithms and consensus statements guiding its use based on pharmacokinetic and registry data (160) (Fig. 3.14.). It is important to note that steady state anticoagulation without intravenous bolus of enoxaparin (0.3 mg/kg) requires three subcutaneous doses. A rapid, point-of-care assay designed for estimating the anticoagulant activity of enoxaparin has been developed (enoxaparin clotting time, ECT) and evalu-

ated in a clinical trial to define optimal range of anticoagulation with respect to efficacy and safety outcomes (161), with a target ECT of 260 to 450 seconds prior to PCI and <180 seconds for sheath removal. But because many interventional cardiologists favor rapid triage to the cardiac catheterization laboratory in STEMI (door-to-balloon less than 90 minutes) and increasingly in UA/NSTEMI as well (door-to-cath lab <6 hours based on the results of ISAR-COOL (162)), intravenous UFH and the direct thrombin inhibitors are likely to remain the anticoagulants of choice for the catheterization laboratory at the present time.

Guidelines for LMWH

In patients who have received LMWH prior to PCI, the administration of additional anticoagulation therapy depends on the timing of the last dose of LMWH (Grade 1C). If the last dose of enoxaparin was administered ≤8 hours prior to PCI, no additional anticoagulant therapy is recommended (Grade 2C). If the last dose of enoxaparin was administered between 8 hours and 12 hours before PCI, a 0.3 mg/kg bolus of intravenous enoxaparin at the time of PCI is suggested (Grade 2C). If the last enoxaparin dose was administered >12 hours before PCI, conventional anticoagulation therapy during PCI is advised (Grade 2C; Table 3.2, Fig. 3.14).

Direct Thrombin Inhibitors

Direct thrombin inhibitors (DTIs) offer a number of theoretical advantages over UFH including: activity against fibrin-bound thrombin, less nonspecific protein binding, direct action without a cofactor, absence of known inhibitors, and less platelet binding. These benefits ultimately result in more effective and reliable thrombin inhibition, less platelet activation, less thrombocytopenia, and a more predictable pharmacokinetic profile obviating the need to measure ACTs. Of the current agents (hirudin, bivalirudin, and argatroban), bivalirudin has been the most extensively studied (163–165). Although the anticoagulant effect of bivalirudin dissipates quickly owing to its short half-life of 25 minutes, there is no rapid reversal agent available in the event of life-threatening bleeding. Furthermore, in patients with severe impairment of renal function, the half-life may be increased significantly. Following PCI with bivalirudin, sheath removal should be delayed for 2 hours for patients with normal renal function and up to 8 hours for patients on dialysis.

The Bivalirudin Angioplasty Trial (BAT) randomized 4,098 high-risk patients with ACS undergoing PCI to high-dose heparin bolus (175 IU/kg bolus followed by a 15 IU/kg per hour infusion for 18 to 24 hours) or bivalirudin (1.0 mg/kg bolus followed by an infusion of 2.5 mg/kg per hour for 4 hours, reduced to 0.2 mg/kg per hour for the next 14 to 20 hours). Bleeding complications were reduced with bivalirudin and ischemic complications were lower in the subset of patients with post infarction angina, with reanalysis using a contemporary combined end point (death, MI, or repeat revascularization) showing a significant reduction with bivalirudin (6.2% versus 7.9%, P = .039) (165).

The Randomized Evaluation in PCI Linking Angiomax to reduced Clinical Events (REPLACE-2) trial assigned 6,010 patients undergoing PCI to intravenous bivalirudin (0.75 mg/kg bolus plus 1.75 mg/kg per hour infusion for the duration of PCI) with provisional GP IIb/IIIa inhibition, or heparin (65 U/kg bolus) plus GP IIb/IIIa inhibition (abciximab or eptifibatide) (164). The primary composite end point (30-day incidence of death, MI, urgent repeat revascularization, or in-hospital major bleeding) occurred among 9.2% of patients in the bivalirudin group and 10.0% of patients in the heparin plus GP IIb/IIIa group (OR, 0.92; 95% CI 0.77 to 1.08; P = .32). The secondary composite end point of death, MI, or urgent revascularization occurred in 7.6% of patients in the bivalirudin group versus 7.1% of patients in the heparin plus GP IIb/IIIa group (OR, 1.09; 95% CI 0.90 to 1.32; P = .40). Bivalirudin with provisional GP IIb/IIIa blockade was thus statistically noninferior to heparin plus planned GP IIb/IIIa blockade and by historical comparisons was statistically superior to heparin alone in suppressing acute ischemic end points with less associated bleeding. Although in-hospital major bleeding rates were significantly reduced by bivalirudin (2.4% versus 4.1%; P <.001), it is important to note that the heparin dosing in this trial resulted in higher ACTs (317 seconds, interquartile range 263 to 373 seconds) than reported in prior GP IIb/IIIa trials, which may have contributed to the excess bleeding complication in patients assigned to treatment with UFH and GP IIb/IIIa inhibitors. But the trial data still favor the use of bivalirudin in patients at increased bleeding risk (e.g., elderly, renal insufficiency, bleeding disorders, and immediate postoperative state). Bivalirudin is likely to become the anticoagulant of choice in patients undergoing PCI with a known prior history of HIT, and clinical trials evaluating the use of bivalirudin in STEMI and UA NSTEMI/ USA are currently underway.

Guidelines for Bivalirudin

For patients undergoing PCI who are not treated with a GP IIb-IIIa antagonist, bivalirudin (0.75 mg/kg bolus followed by an infusion of 1.75 mg/kg per hour for the duration of PCI) is recommended over heparin during PCI (Grade 1A). In PCI patients who are at low risk for complications, bivalirudin is recommended as an alternative to heparin as an adjunct to GP IIb-IIIa antagonists (Grade 1B). In PCI patients who are at high risk for bleeding, bivalirudin is recommended over heparin as an adjunct to GPIIb-IIIa antagonists (Grade 1B).

Intravenous GP IIb/IIIa Inhibitors

Platelet GP IIb/IIIa receptors mediate the final common pathway of platelet aggregation by binding fibrinogen and other adhesive proteins that bridge adjacent platelets, and have thus served as a primary focus of pharmacologic antiplatelet strategies. Three parental agents—abciximab (ReoPro), eptifibatide (Integrilin), and tirofiban (Aggrastat)—are currently approved for clinical use by FDA.

Abciximab is a humanized Fab fragment engineered from murine monoclonal antibody 7E3 directed against GP IIb/IIIa (166). Unlike the small-molecule agents, abciximab interacts with the GP IIb/IIIa receptor at sites distinct from the ligand-binding RGD sequence site and is a noncompetitive inhibitor (167). Most of the drug is cleared from plasma within 26 minutes, but the clearance from the body is much slower, with a functional half-life up to seven days (168). Because of the high affinity of abciximab for GP IIb/IIIa receptors, more abciximab molecules are bound to platelets than are free in the plasma pool of the drug for the duration of treatment—platelet-associated abciximab can be detected for >14 days after the infusion is stopped (169).

The cyclic heptapeptide eptifibatide is based on barbourin, a 73-amino acid peptide isolated from the venom of the Southeastern pygmy rattlesnake *Sistrurus m. barbouri* (170). The recommended bolus (180 mcg/kg followed by a second 180-mcg/kg bolus 10 minutes later) and infusion (2 mcg/kg per minute) regimen, provides peak plasma levels shortly after the bolus dose and slightly lower concentration throughout the infusion. Plasma concentration decreases rapidly after the infusion is discontinued with a predominantly renal elimination half-life of 2.5 hours (171). A lower infusion dose (1 mcg/kg per minute) of eptifibatide is thus recommended in patients with creatinine clearance <50 mL/minute. Substantial recovery of platelet aggregation is apparent within 4 hours of discontinuing the infusion.

Tirofiban, a peptidometic inhibitor, occupies the binding pocket on GP IIb/IIIa and thereby competitively inhibits platelet aggregation mediated by fibrinogen or von Willebrand factor (172). The stoichiometry of both eptifibatide and tirofiban is >100 molecules of drug per GP IIb/IIIa receptor needed to achieve full platelet inhibition (most circulating unbound in the plasma). This compares with a stoichiometry of 1.5 molecules of abciximab for each receptor. Like eptifibatide, substantial recovery of platelet aggregation is apparent within 4 hours of stopping the infusion (171).

Preclinical and clinical pharmacodynamic studies suggest that the target for clinically effective antiplatelet activity should be 80% inhibition of platelet aggregation by light-transmission aggregometry (173). The level of platelet inhibition varies between the three GP IIb/IIIa inhibitors following the recommended bolus and infusions (174). In general, the bolus and infusion regimen of abciximab and the double bolus and infusion regimen of eptifibatide are associated with rapid and profound inhibition of platelet function (174–176), but the FDA-approved bolus and infusion regimen for tirofiban achieves suboptimal levels of platelet inhibition for up to 4 to 6 hours that likely accounted for inferior clinical results in the PCI setting

(176) including in TARGET (Tirofiban And ReoPro Give similar Efficacy Trial) (177). Increasing the tirofiban bolus 2.5-fold (25 mcg/kg) appears to enhance platelet inhibition and improve PCI outcomes compared with the FDA-approved dosing regimen (178).

The landmark trial with balloon angioplasty that demonstrated the efficacy of GP IIb/IIIa inhibition is the Evaluation of IIb/IIIa platelet receptor antagonist 7E3 in Preventing Ischemic Complications (EPIC) trial (179). In this study, high-risk patients undergoing balloon angioplasty were randomized to abciximab bolus and infusion versus abciximab bolus alone versus placebo. The group treated with abciximab bolus and infusion had a 35% lower rate of death, MI, or unplanned urgent revascularization at 30 days compared with the placebo group (8.3% versus 12.8%, $P = .008$). Major bleeding complications occurred in an unacceptably high proportion of patients treated with abciximab compared with placebo (major bleeding 14% versus 7%, transfusion 15% versus 7%, respectively). Procedural modifications, including performing front-wall arterial access only, reducing arterial sheath size from 8F to 6F, reducing heparin dosing to target ACT 200 to 250 seconds rather than >300 seconds, removing sheaths as soon as possible (ACT <180 seconds) rather than overnight pretension, and abandoning the use of routine venous sheaths successfully reduced major bleeding complications to <1 to 1.5% in subsequent trials.

The benefit of GP IIb/IIIa inhibition patients undergoing elective stent placement has been shown in two large, randomized controlled trials (180,181) The Evaluation of Platelet IIb/IIIa Inhibition in Stenting Trial (EPISTENT) trial (180) randomized 2,399 patients to stent plus placebo, stent plus abciximab, or balloon angioplasty plus abciximab. The primary 30-day end point, a combination of death, MI, or urgent revascularization, occurred in 10.8% of patients in the stent plus placebo group, 5.3% of those in the stent plus abciximab group (hazard ratio 0.48; $P < .001$), and 6.9% in the group undergoing balloon angioplasty plus abciximab (hazard ratio 0.63; $P = .007$). These benefits were maintained at 1 year (182), with a reduction in 1-year mortality in patients treated with stent plus abciximab compared with stent without the IIb/IIIa inhibitor (2.4% versus 1.0%, $P = .037$). No significant differences in bleeding complications were noted among the various groups.

The Enhanced Suppression of the Platelet IIb/IIIa Receptor with Integrilin Therapy (ESPRIT) trial randomized 2,064 patients undergoing stenting to eptifibatide (180 mcg/kg bolus followed by a 2.0 mcg/kg per hour infusion, with a second bolus of 180 mcg/kg given 10 minutes after the first bolus) (181,183) or placebo. In this trial, patients were administered a loading dose of clopidogrel or ticlopidine on the day of the procedure. The primary end point—composite of death, MI, urgent revascularization, or thrombotic bailout at 48 hours—was reduced by 37% with eptifibatide (10.5% versus 6.6%, $P = .0017$). Death or MI at 48 hours was significantly reduced with eptifibatide compared with placebo (5.5% versus 9.2%,

RRR = 40%, $P = .0013$), and these benefits were maintained at 6 months (113) and 1 year (184). Major bleeding was rare, but occurred more frequently in patients receiving eptifibatide compared with placebo (1.3% versus 0.4%, respectively; $P = .027$).

In patients with UA/NSTEMI undergoing PCI, three large, randomized clinical trials have evaluated each of the three GP IIb/IIIa inhibitors. In the Chimeric c7E3 Fab Antiplatelet Therapy in Unstable angina Refractory to standard treatment trial (CAPTURE), patients were randomly assigned to receive abciximab 18 to 24 hours prior to PCI and for 1 hour after completion of the procedure or placebo (185). MACE was reduced in the abciximab group compared with placebo (15.9% versus 11.3%, $P = .012$, respectively), although there was a significant increase in major bleeding (1.9% versus 3.8%, $P = .043$) and the need for transfusion (3.4% versus 7.1%, $P = .005$). In the Platelet Receptor Inhibition in ischemic Syndrome Management in Patients Limited by Unstable Sign and symptoms (PRISM-PLUS) trial, patients with UA/NSTEMI were randomized to tirofiban alone, tirofiban plus heparin, or placebo infusion plus heparin (186). The combination of tirofiban and heparin led to a 32% risk reduction in the rate of death, MI, or recurrent refractory ischemia at 7 days compared with heparin alone (12.9% versus 17.9%, respectively, $P = .004$), including the subgroup of patients undergoing PCI (RRR of death or MI at 30 days = 0.44). In the Platelet glycoprotein IIb/IIIa in Unstable angina: Receptor Suppression Using Integrilin Therapy (PURSUIT) trial, patients with UA/NSTEMI were randomized to eptifibatide or placebo. The primary end point of 30-day death or MI was reduced in those patients receiving eptifibatide versus placebo (14.2% versus 15.7%, $P = .042$, respectively) and was most pronounced among patients undergoing PCI within 72 hours of presentation (11.6% versus 16.7%, $P = .01$, respectively). Moderate or severe hemorrhage was more common in the eptifibatide group (12.8% versus 9.9%, $P < .001$, respectively).

In patients undergoing primary PCI for STEMI, several trials support the use of abciximab in reducing MACE at 30 days by 35 to 54%. In the Abciximab before Direct angioplasty and stenting in Myocardial Infarction Regarding Acute and Long-term follow-up (ADMIRAL) trial, 300 patients with STEMI were randomized to abciximab plus stenting or stenting alone prior to angiography (187). At 30 days, the primary end point—composite of death, reinfarction, or urgent revascularization of the target vessel—occurred in 6.0% of the patients in the abciximab group, as compared with 14.6% of those in the placebo group ($P = .01$). This beneficial effect was sustained at 6 months (7.4% versus 15.9%, $P = .02$) in ADMIRAL, but not in two other trials (188,189).

Because there is an inevitable 60- to 90-minute delay in performing primary PCI (see chapter 22), an optimal pharmacologic strategy is needed to bridge this period. Several studies have been performed to assess the safety and efficacy of combination therapy using half-dose thrombolytic therapy and various GP IIb/IIIa inhibitors pre-PCI to improve

TABLE 3.3

OUTCOMES OF PATIENTS RECEIVING GLYCOPROTEIN IIb/IIIa INHIBITORS

Meta-analysis of 20 trials involving 20,137 patients shows >35% reduction in periprocedural MI (using a CK-MB greater than three times normal definition), with a parallel reduction in the composite outcome including death, myocardial infarction (MI), or revascularization (note: MI was the most prevalent component and therefore drove the reduction in the composite end point).

| Outcome | No. of Studies (n) | Total Events/Patients (%) | | RR (95% cl) |
		Active Treatment	Control Arm	
MI (30 days)	20 (20,137)	537/11,676 (4.6)	585/8,461 (6.9)	0.63 (0.56–0.70)
MI (6 months)	13 (15,250)	481/8,485 (5.7)	550/6,765 (8.1)	0.67 (0.60–0.76)
Composite* (30 days)	20 (20,137)	926/11,676 (7.9)	978/8,461 (11.6)	0.65 (0.59–0.72)
Composite* (6 months)	13 (15,250)	1,817/8,485 (21.4)	1,624/6,765 (24.0)	0.85 (0.80–0.90)
Major bleeding	20 (20,137)	531/11,676 (4.6)	273/8,461 (3.2)	1.26 (1.09–1.46)
Hemorrhagic stroke[†]	18 (19,612)	14/11,373 (0.1)	10/8,239 (0.1)	0.89 (0.46–1.72)

*The composite outcome includes death, myocardial infarction (MI), or revasculartization. For the last component, we used any target vessel revascularization, except for studies where this was not a trial outcome, in which case, urgent or all revascularizations were counted.
[†]The ADMIRAL and ERASER trials provided no data on hemorrhagic stroke. There was no statistically significant heterogeneity, and random effects estimates were vary similar (data not shown), except for the composite outcome at 30 days (p=0.04 for heterogeneity, and random effects RR 0.66 [95% Cl 0.57–0.75]) and major bleeding (P=0.08 for heterogeneity, random effects RR 1.19 [95% Cl 0.96–1.48])
Modified from Karvouni E., et al. Intravenous giycoprotein IIb/IIIa receptor antagonists reduce mortality after percutaneous coronary /interventions. *J Am Coll Cardiol* 2003;41:26–32.

baseline angiographic patency of the infarct-related artery. Each of these trials has demonstrated improved early patency of the infarct-related artery compared with full-dose thrombolytic therapy alone, at the expense of increased major bleeding. The Facilitated Intervention with Enhanced Reperfusion Speed to Stop Events (FINESSE) (190) study has been designed to test the hypothesis that facilitated PCI would be more effective than primary PCI and is currently randomizing approximately 3,000 patients with STEMI undergoing primary PCI to receive upstream abciximab, upstream half-dose reteplase plus abciximab, or abciximab at the time of PCI, with a primary end point of 90-day all-cause mortality or complications of MI.

GP IIb/IIIa inhibitors have been shown to reduce major adverse cardiac events (death, MI, and urgent revascularization) by 35 to 50% in patients undergoing PCI (191) Table 3.3). Although no single study demonstrated a significant reduction in mortality alone with GP IIb/IIIa inhibitors, meta-analysis suggests that these agents as a class reduce death by 20 to 30% (Fig. 3.15). The mechanism by which an 18-hour infusion of a GP IIb/IIIa inhibitor might reduce long-term mortality cannot be explained solely by its ability to reduce periprocedural death or myocardial infarction (other than in conventional balloon angioplasty, where this translates directly to morbid events such as emergency surgery), and is thus unclear and speculative at this time (see also Chapter 22).

GP IIb/IIIa and Thrombocytopenia

In a meta-analysis of eight clinical trials, abciximab increased the incidence of mild thrombocytopenia (>50,000, <100,000) compared with the placebo group (4.2% versus 2.0%, $P < .001$; OR, 2.13) (192), whereas eptifibatide or tirofiban did not increase mild thrombocytopenia compared

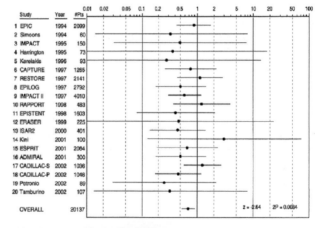

A   Favors Treatment   Favors Control

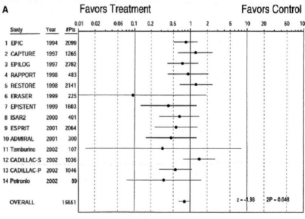

B   Favors Treatment   Favors Control

Figure 3.15 Meta-analysis of GP IIb/IIIa inhibitors and mortality reduction. Mortality at 30-day (**A**) and 6-month (**B**) follow-up. Risk ratios and 95% confidence intervals are shown for each study and for the random effects summary. S, stenting; P, PTCA. (From Karvouni E, et al. Intravenous glycoprotein IIb/IIIa receptor antagonists reduce mortality after percutaneous coronary interventions. *J Amer Coll Cardiol* 2003;41:30.).

64

Section I: General Principles

with placebo (OR, 0.99). The incidence of severe thrombocytopenia (platelet count 20 to 50,000) was doubled by abciximab (1.0% versus 0.4%, *P* = .01; OR, 2.48), but not changed by eptifibatide or tirofiban compared with heparin alone (0.3% versus 0.2%, *P* = .16). Although uncommon, severe and profound (<20,000) thrombocytopenia requires immediate cessation of GP IIb/IIIa therapy. An algorithm for the evaluation and management of these patients has been proposed (Fig. 3.16 A and B) (193). Pseudothrombocytopenia secondary to platelet clumping as well as HIT needs to be ruled out. The platelet count usually returns to normal within 48 to 72 hours. Severe and profound thrombocytopenia from GP IIb/IIIa receptor inhibitors are infrequent, more commonly associated with abciximab use. Regardless of its cause, thrombocytopenia in patients undergoing PCI is associated with more ischemic events, bleeding complications and transfusions (194).

Guidelines for GP IIb/IIIa Inhibitors

American College of Chest Physicians (ACCP) guidelines recommend the use of a GP IIb-IIIa antagonist (abciximab or eptifibatide) for all patients undergoing PCI, particularly those undergoing primary PCI, or those with refractory UA or other high-risk features (Grade 1A). ACC/AHA guidelines recommend that a platelet GP IIb/IIIa antagonist should be administered along with ASA and heparin to patients with UA/NSTEMI in whom catheterization and PCI are planned (Class I, Level of evidence: A) (33). Eptifibatide or tirofiban (but not abciximab) should be administered in addition to ASA and LMWH or UFH to patients with continuing ischemia, an elevated troponin, or with other high-risk features in whom an invasive management strategy is not planned (Class IIa, Level of evidence: A) (33).

In patients with STEMI (Class IIa, Level of evidence: B), it is reasonable to start treatment with abciximab as early as possible before primary PCI (with or without stenting). Treatment with tirofiban or eptifibatide may be considered before primary PCI (Class IIb, Level of evidence: C) (2).

For patients with UA/NSTEMI who are designated as moderate-to-high risk based on TIMI score, the upstream use of a GPIIb-IIIa antagonist (either eptifibatide or tirofiban) is recommended as soon as possible prior to PCI (Grade 1A). In UA/NSTEMI patients who receive upstream treatment with tirofiban, it is recommended that PCI be deferred for at least 4 hours after initiating the tirofiban infusion (Grade 2C). With planned PCI in UA/NSTEMI patients with an elevated troponin level, we recommend that abciximab be started no earlier than 24 hours prior to the intervention (Grade 1A). For patients with UA/NSTEMI who are designated as moderate-to-high risk based on the TIMI risk score, upstream use of a GP IIb/IIIa antagonist (either eptifibatide or tirofiban) should be started as soon as possible prior to PCI (Grade 1A). If upstream treatment with tirofiban is used, PCI should be deferred for at least 4 hours after initiating the infusion.

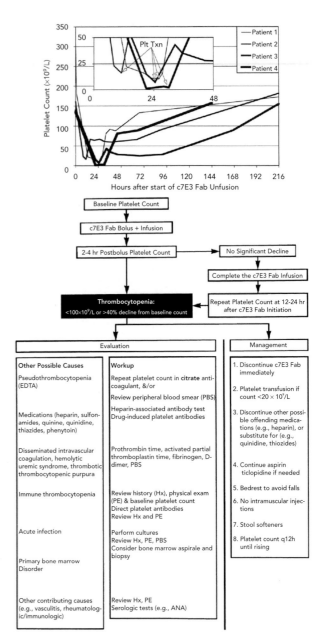

Figure 3.16 Time course and evaluation of thrombocytopenia following administration of abciximab. **Top.** Platelet counts before and during therapy and after recovery in four patients who developed acute profound thrombocytopenia after receiving c7E3 Fab bolus plus infusion. The inset focuses on the platelet counts during the first 48 hours and notes the first platelet transfusion (Plt Txn) given. **Bottom.** Evaluation and management of thrombocytopenia with c7E3 Fab therapy. ANA, antinuclear antibody; EDTA, ethylene diamine tetra-acetic acid. (From Berkowitz SD, et al. Acute profound thrombocytopenia after C7E3 Fab (abciximab) therapy Circulation 1997;95:811.).

Other Pharmacologic Agents

Although a review of vasoactive, sedative, and antiarrhythmic drugs used in the cardiac catheterization laboratory is beyond the scope of this book, the following table of drug doses used at the Brigham and Women's Hospital is provided as a quick reference. There is some variability in drug dosing based on package inserts, published data, guidelines,

TABLE 3.4

COMMONLY USED CATH LAB PHARMACOLOGY AT THE BRIGHAM AND WOMEN'S HOSPITAL

Drug Class	Agent	Dosing and Comments
Anticoagulants	Heparin, unfractionated (UFH)	IV bolus and infusion: • Initial bolus 70–100 IU/kg for PCI without IIb/IIIa, to ACT 250–300 sec • Reduce bolus to 50–60 IU/kg for PCI with IIb/IIIa blocker, to ACT 200–250 sec • If procedure longer than 1 hr, recheck ACT and rebolus (1,500–2,000 units) as needed • May be reversed with protamine sulphate (1 mL = 10 mg, reverses 1000 Units of heparin); maximum dose 50 mg
	Low–molecular-weight heparin (Enoxaparin)	Subcutaneous dose: • 1 mg/kg BID SC for 2 to 8 days, administered with aspirin • Reduce to 0.5 mg/kg BID if renal insufficiency IV dose for PCI • For full anticoagulation without IIb/IIIa blocker: 1.0 mg/kg • With a IIb/IIIa blocker: reduce bolus to 0.5–0.75 mg/kg for full anticoagulation • To supplement SC dose given 8–12 hours previously: 0.3 mg/kg intravenous bolus; also consider 0.3 mg/kg IV bolus if patient not at steady state anticoagulation with SC dosing (i.e., <3 doses) • Does not prolong ACT owing to high Xa/IIa ratio • Partial reversal with protamine: 1 mg protamine/1 mg enoxaparin <8 hours last SC dose; 0.5 mg protamine/1 mg enoxaparin 8–12 hr
	Direct thrombin inhibitor: bivalirudin (Angiomax)	• Loading dose: 0.75 mg/kg IV • Infusion: 1.75 mg/kg per hr for the duration of PCI (note: short half-life 25 min) • Reduce dose to 0.25 mg/kg per hr for dialysis-dependent patients • Estimate CCr (mL/min) as ((140-age) × weight (kg)) / (72 × serum Cr) [times 0.85 for female] and reduce infusion to 1 mg/kg per hour for renal insufficiency • Can monitor ACT, usually >350 sec after dose; no reversal agent, but half life ~25 min
Antiplatelet Agents	Aspirin 160–325-mg tablets	• 160 mg to 325 mg tablet taken as soon as possible (chewing is preferable) • Higher doses (1,000 mg) interfere with prostacyclin production and may limit benefits
Thienopyridines	Clopidogrel 75-mg tablets (Plavix)	• 300 mg loading dose, given 6 hr before a known procedure if possible (600 mg loading dose option) • 75 mg/day maintenance • 2–4 weeks for bare-metal stents; 3–6 months for drug-eluting stents; lifetime for brachytherapy
	Ticlopidine 250-mg tablets (Ticlid)	• 750 mg oral loading dose • 250 mg BID oral maintenance • Duration as for clopidogrel above • Monitor for thrombocytopenia and neutropenia if duration >2 weeks • Plavix is preferred unless there is clear allergy to that agent
IIb/IIIa inhibitors	Abciximab (ReoPro)	PCI or acute coronary syndromes with planned PCI within 24 hr: • 0.25 mg/kg IV bolus (10–60 min before procedure), then 0.125 mcg/kg per min (maximum of 10 mcg/min) IV infusion, × 18–24 hr • Check platelets at 4 hr of infusion to monitor for thrombocytopenia
	Eptifibatide (Integrilin)	For PCI: • 180 mcg/kg IV bolus • Repeat the same dose in 10 min • Infuse 2 mcg/kg per min for 18 hr • Reduce infusion to 1 mcg/kg per min for creatinine clearance <50 mL/min • Maximum dose (reached at patient weight of 121 kg): 22.6 mg IV bolus × 2, then maximum infusion of 242 mcg/min
	Tirofiban (Aggrastat)	Acute coronary syndromes • 0.4 mcg/kg per min IV for 30 min, then 0.1 mcg/kg per min IV infusion • Not recommended for PCI

(continued)

TABLE 3.4
(continued)

Drug Class	Agent	Dosing and Comments
Arrhythmia Bradycardia	Atropine sulfate	For vasovagal or symptomatic sinus bradycardia • 0.5 to 1.0 mg IV every 3–5 min as needed • Do not exceed total dose of 0.04 mg/kg
	Isoproterenol	IV Infusion for bradycardia owing to infranodal block with slow ventricular escape: • Mix 2 mg in 250 mL D5W • Infuse at 2–10 mcg/min, titrated to adequate heart rate • In torsades de pointes, titrate to increase heart rate until VT rhythm is suppressed
Atrial fibrillation or flutter	Dofetilide	IV infusion dose for atrial fibrillation or flutter • Single infusion of 8 mcg/kg over 30 min • Not approved for use in U.S.
	Ibutilide	IV dose for atrial fibrillation or flutter (for adults ≥60 kg) • 1 mg (10 mL) administered IV (diluted or undiluted) over 10 min. A second dose may be administered at the same rate 10 min after completion of first dose • For atrial fibrillation or flutter
Supraventricular tachycardia	Adenosine	IV rapid push to convert SVT (see vasodilator below for use in no-reflow or FFR measurement) • Initial bolus of 6 mg given rapidly over 1–3 sec followed by normal saline bolus of 20 mL; then elevate the extremity • Repeat dosage of 12 mg in 1–2 min if needed • A third dose of 12 mg may be given in 1–2 min if needed
Ventricular	Lidocaine	For stable VT, wide-complex tachycardia or uncertain type, significant ectopy: • 1.0 to 1.5 mg/kg IV push • Repeat 0.5–0.75 mg/kg every 5–10 minutes; maximum total dose: 3 mg/kg • Maintenance infusion 1–4 mg/min (30–50 mcg/kg per min)
	Amiodarone	For VF • IV push 300 mg • Repeat 150 mg over 2–5 minutes, if necessary For VEA or stable VT • Rapid infusion: 150 mg in 50 mL over 10 min, repeat every 10 min as needed • Slow infusion: 360 mg IV over 6 hr (1 mg/min) • Maintenance infusion: 540 mg IV over 18 hr (0.5 mg/min)

	Procainamide	Recurrent VF/VT:
		• 20 mg/min IV infusion (maximum total dose: 17 mg/kg)
		• In urgent situations, up to 50 mg/min may be administered to total dose of 17 mg/kg
		• Suspend loading infusion if one of the following occurs:
		  –Arrhythmia suppression
		  –Hypotension
		  –QRS widens by >50%.
		• Maintenance infusion 1–4 mg/min

	Magnesium sulfate	Cardiac arrest (for hypomagnesemia or torsades de pointes): • 1–2 g (2–4 mL of a 50% solution) diluted in 10 mL of D5W IV push Torsades de pointes (not in cardiac arrest): • Loading dose of 1–2 g mixed in 50–100 mL of D5W over 5–60 min IV • Follow with 0.5 to 1.0 g/h IV (titrate dose to control the torsades) for up to 24 hr
	Sodium bicarbonate	For prolonged cardiac arrest—IV bolus • 1 mEq/kg IV bolus • Repeat half this dose every 10 min thereafter • If rapidly available, use arterial blood gas analysis to guide bicarbonate therapy (calculated base deficits or bicarbonate concentration) • An acute change in $PaCO_2$ of 1mm Hg is associated with an increase or decrease in pH of 0.008 U (relative to normal pH of 7.4)

(continued)

TABLE 3.4
(continued)

Drug Class	Agent	Dosing and Comments
Beta-blockers	Esmolol	• 0.5 mg/kg over 1 min, followed by continuous infusion at 0.05 mg/kg per min (maximum: 0.3 mg/kg) • Titrate to effect—note esmolol has a very short half-life (2–9 min)
	Atenolol	• Initial IV dose: 5 mg slow IV (over 5 min) • Wait 10 min, then give second dose of 5 mg slow IV (over 5 min) • In 10 min, if tolerated well, may start PO; then give 50 mg PO BID
	Metoprolol	• Initial IV dose: 5 mg slow IV, repeat at 5-min intervals to a total of 15 mg • Oral regimen to follow IV dose: 50 mg BID for 24 hr, then increase to 100 mg BID
	Propranolol	• Total dose: 0.1 mg/kg by slow IV push, divided in 3 equal doses at 2–3-minute intervals • Do not exceed 1 mg/min, watching for excessive bradycardia or hypotension • Nonselective beta-1 and beta-2 agent (use with care in asthmatic patients)
	Labetalol	For severe hypertension: • 10 mg labetalol IV push over 1 to 2 min • May repeat or double labetalol every 10 min to a maximum dose of 150 mg, or give initial bolus dose and start labetalol infusion at 2 to 8 mg/min
Calcium channel blockers	Diltiazem	Acute rate control (see vasodilator section for use in no-reflow): • 15 to 20 mg (0.25 mg/kg) IV over 2 min • May repeat in 15 min at 20–25 mg (0.35 mg/kg) over 2 min • Maintenance infusion 5 to 15 mg/h, titrated to heart rate
	Verapamil	Acute rate control (see vasodilator section for use in no-reflow) • 2.5–5.0 mg IV bolus over 2 min • Second dose: 5 mg bolus every 15 min to total dose of 30 mg
Conscious sedation	Fentanyl	• 25–50 mcg intravenously • Repeat as needed every 5 min • Monitor vital signs, oximety, and state of consciousness as per conscious sedation guidelines
	Versed	• 0.5–1 mg IV • Repeat as needed every 5 min • Monitor vital signs, oximetry, and state of consciousness per conscious sedation guidelines
	Morphine sulfate	• 2–4 mg IV (over 1 to 5 min) every 5–30 min • Monitor vital signs, oximetry, and state of consciousness as per conscious sedation guidelines
Reversal agents	Flumazenil (Romazicon, "Re-versed")	For oversedation with benzodiazepines • Dosage: 0.2 to a maximum dose of 1 mg • Administer in 0.2-mg increments over 15 sec; may repeat in 1-min intervals to 1 mg • Maximum dose: 1 mg/dose and 3 mg/hr • Monitor closely for re-sedation for at least 2 hr
	Naloxone hydrochloride (Narcan)	For oversedation with narcotics • Dilute 0.4 mg (1 mL) with 9 mL NS (0.04 mg/mL) • Administer 0.04 mg or 1 mL every 2-3 min PRN to increase respiratory rate and alertness • Onset 1 min, duration 30–40 min • Monitor closely for re-sedation for at least 2 hr

(continued)

TABLE 3.4
(continued)

Drug Class	Agent	Dosing and Comments
"Unconscious" sedation* *Use only with anesthesiologist	Propafol (Diprivan)	Induction of general anesthesia: • Healthy adults <55 years of age: 40 mg every 10 sec until induction onset (2–2.5 mg/kg) • Elderly, debilitated, ASAIII/IV patients: 20 mg every 10 sec until induction onset (1–1.5 mg/kg) Maintenance of general anesthesia: • Healthy adults <55 years of age: 100–200 mcg/kg per min (3–6 mg/kg per hr) • Elderly, debilitated, ASAIII/IV patients: 50–100 mcg/kg per min (3–6 mg/kg per hr)
Neuromuscular blocker* *Use only with anesthesiologist	Cisatracurium besylate (Nimbex)	• Dosage must be individualized • Skeletal muscle relaxation: initial, 0.15–0.20 mg/kg IV bolus as component of a propofol/nitrous oxide/oxygen induction-intubation technique • Skeletal muscle relaxation: maintenance, 0.03 mg/kg IV • Skeletal muscle relaxation: maintenance, initial continuous IV infusion rate of 3 mcg/kg per min may be required to rapidly counteract spontaneous recovery from initial bolus dose; thereafter, 1–2 mcg/kg per min continuous IV infusion; in ICU, infusion range of 0.5–10.2 mcg/kg per min
	Vecuronium bromide (Norcuron)	• Dosage must be individualized • Skeletal muscle relaxation: initial, 0.08–0.1 mg/kg IV bolus • Skeletal muscle relaxation: maintenance, 0.01–0.015 mg/kg IV 25–40 min after initial dose, repeat every 12–15 min as needed • Skeletal muscle relaxation: 1 mcg/kg per min continuous IV infusion 20–40 min after initial intubation dose, after early evidence of spontaneous recovery; then adjust to maintain 90% suppression of twitch response; range 0.8–1.2 mcg/kg per min
Contrast nephropathy	Hydration	For prevention of contrast-induced nephropathy • Normal saline 1 ml/kg per hr for 12 hr pre and 12 hr post contrast exposure • Alternative normal saline 3 ml/kg over 1 hr preprocedure, then 1 ml/kg per hr for 6 hr post-procedure • Alternative sodium bicarbonate (154 mEq/L) in D5W • Limit infusion and monitor closely in CHF patients • Do not add Lasix, mannitol, dopamine, fenoldopam (systemic) • Consider use of iodixanol (Visipaque), iso-osmolar contrast; limit contrast volume
	N-acetylcysteine	• 600 mg orally BID, start 6 hr prior to contrast exposure • Continue for 24 hr post contrast exposure
Contrast allergy or toxicity	Prednisone	• Pretreat 60 mg PO daily for 24–48 hr • May use Solu-Medrol 100 mg IV just before the procedure
	Benadryl	• H1 blocker • 25–50 mg PO before the procedure • May also be given as 25 mg IV for intraprocedural allergic reactions
	H2-blocker Ranitidine (Zantac)	• Needed to prevent histamine-induced vasodilation • 150 mg PO prior to procedure • Alternative, 50 mg IV, given over 5 min
	Epinephrine	For anaphylaxis, bronchospasm, cardiovascular collapse • 0.1 mg (1 mL of 1:10,000) epinephrine given in small divided doses until response • Monitor closely for tachycardia or hypertensive overshoot • May repeat or use IV infusion as noted below
	Ondansetron HCl (Zofran)	For prevention or treatment of periprocedural nausea and vomiting • 2–4 mg undiluted IV over 4 min

(continued)

TABLE 3.4
(continued)

Drug Class	Agent	Dosing and Comments
Diuretic	Furosemide (Lasix)	IV infusion: • 0.5–1.0 mg/kg given over 1 to 2 min • If no response, double dose to 2.0 mg/kg, slowly over 1 to 2 min
	Bumetanide (Bumex)	IV infusion • Bolus 0.5–1 mg is equivalent to 40 mg of furosemide
Inotrope	Dobutamine (Dobutrex)	IV infusion: • Dilute 500 mg (20 mL) in 250 mL D5W • Usual infusion rate is 2–20 mcg/kg per min • Titrate so heart rate does not increase by >10% of baseline
	Dopamine	IV infusion • Mix 400–800 mg in 250 mL normal saline, lactate Ringer solution, or D5W • Continuous infusions (titrate to patient response) • Low dose: 1–5 mcg/kg per min—gamma (dopaminergic) stimulation • Moderate dose: 5–10 mcg/kg per min ("cardiac doses"—beta stimulation) • High dose: 10–15 mcg/kg per min ("vasopressor doses"—alpha stimulation)
	Amrinone (now inamrinone)	IV loading dose and infusion for severe pump failure: • Loading dose 0.75 mg/kg, given over 10 to 15 min • Follow with infusion of 5–15 mcg/kg per min to clinical effect • Optimal use requires hemodynamic monitoring • Note: Amrinone and Milrinone inhibit PDE and do not depend on beta-adrenergic receptors
	Milrinone (Primacor)	IV loading dose and infusion for severe pump failure: • Supplied as 200 mcg/mL • Loading dose 50 mcg/kg over 10 min • Follow with infusion 0.5–0.75 mcg/kg per min • Reduce infusion for renal insufficiency (e.g., 0.33 mcg/kg per min for CCr 30 mL/min)
	Epinephrine	Cardiac arrest: • Note: Available in 1:1,000 (1 mg/mL) and 1:10,000 (0.1 mg/mL) concentrations! • IV dose: 1 mg (10 mL of 1:10,000 solution) every 3–5 min during resuscitation • Higher doses (up to 0.2 mg/kg) may be used if 1-mg dose fails • Continuous infusion: 30 mg epinephrine (30 mL of 1:1,000 solution) to 250 mL normal saline, run at 100 mL/hr and titrate to response Profound bradycardia or hypotension: • 2 mg in 500 mL NS • 2–10 mcg/min infusion (add 1mg of 1:1,000 to 500 mL normal saline; infuse 1–5 mL/min)
	Glucagon	To treat excessive bradycardia from beta-blockers • 1–5 mg over 2–5 min
	Calcium chloride	IV slow push in cardiac arrest: • 100 mg/mL in 10 mL vial (total equals 1g; a 10% solution) • 8–16 mg/kg (usually 5–10 mL) IV for hyperkalemia and calcium channel blocker overdose • May be repeated as needed • 2–4 mg/kg (usually mL) IV for prophylaxis before IV calcium channel blockers
	Digoxin	IV infusion (for rate control in atrial fibrillation/flutter (note beta- or calcium channel blocker preferred): • 0.25 mg/mL or 0.1 mg/mL supplied in 1 or 2 mL ampule (totals equal 0.1–0.5 mg) • Loading doses of 10–15 mcg/kg lean body weight—therapeutic effect with minimum toxicity • Maintenance dose is affected by body size and renal function

(continued)

TABLE 3.4
(continued)

Drug Class	Agent	Dosing and Comments
Pressor agents	Phenylephrine (Neo-Synephrine)	For severe refractory hypotension Bolus • 0.04–0.1 mg IV, can be repeated in 10 min if needed Infusion • Mix 20 mg in 500 mL of D5W or NS (40 mcg/mL) • Infuse 100–180 mcg/min until blood pressure stabilizes • Reduce to 40–60 mcg/min adjusted to maintain desired blood pressure
	Metaraminol (Aramine)	For severe refractory hypotension • Loading dose: 0.5–1 mg, IV push • Infusion: 15 mg (1.5 mL) in 500 mL normal saline; adjust to maintain desired blood pressure • Indirect-acting sympathomimetic amine—mixed alpha and beta, action delayed by 5 min
	Norepinephrine (Levophed)	For severe refractory hypotension • 4 mg in 250 mL of D5W to yield 4 mcg/mL • Initial dose 0.5–1 mcg/min (usual range 0.5–30 mcg/min)
	Vasopressin	Doses for cardiac arrest (option to epinephrine) • 40 U IV push × 1 • Wait 10 minutes before initiating epinephrine protocol For refractory hypotension • 20 U in 250 mL D5W • Infuse at 0.01–0.10 U/min
Vasodilator Systemic arterial	Nitroglycerin	IV infusion: • IV bolus: 12.5–25 mcg • Infuse at 10–20 mcg/min • Titrate to effect Intracoronary (for vasospasm—do not use for no-reflow!) • Dilute to 100–200 mcg/mL • Administer 100 mcg through guiding catheter or selectively into distal coronary • Repeat as needed
	Nitroprusside (Sodium nitroprusside)	IV infusion: • Mix 50 mg in 250 mL D5W • Begin at 0.10 mcg/min titrated to improve blood pressure (up to 10 mcg/min) • Do not administer in same IV line as alkaline solutions
	ACE inhibitors: Enalapril (IV: Enalaprilat)	• IV: 1.25 mg IV initial dose over 5 min • Repeat dose: 1.25–5.0 mg IV every 6 hr • IV ACE inhibitors not approved in STEMI
Coronary	Nitroglycerin	For epicardial vasodilation or treatment of coronary spasm • Dilute to 200 mcg/mL • Administer 100–200 mcg intracoronary • Note: Nitroglycerine is primarily an epicardial vasodilator, and should not be used in situations like no-reflow where small vessel (arteriolar) dilation is required—see below
	Adenosine	For measurement of fractional flow reserve (FFR) • Dilute to 10 mcg/mL • For RCA 18–24 mcg through guiding catheter or selectively into distal coronary • For LCA 24–36 mcg through guiding catheter or selectively into distal coronary • Alternatively, 140–180 mcg/kg per min peripheral intravenous infusion for 3 min For reversal of no-reflow • 100 mcg selective into distal involved vessel

(continued)

TABLE 3.4
(continued)

Drug Class	Agent	Dosing and Comments
	Nitroprusside (Sodium nitroprusside)	For reversal of no-reflow • Dilute to 100 mcg/mL (in non-heparinized saline) • Administer 100 mcg through guiding catheter or selectively into distal coronary • Repeat as needed
	Nicardipine	For reversal of no-reflow • Dilute to 100–200 mcg/mL • Administer 200 mcg selectively into involved coronary
	Diltiazem	For reversal of no-reflow • Dilute to 0.25–1 mg/mL • Administer 1 mg through guiding catheter or selectively into distal coronary • Repeat as needed up to total of 2.5 mg
	Verapamil	For reversal of no-reflow • Dilute to 100 mcg/mL • Administer 100–200 mcg through guiding catheter or selectively into distal coronary • Repeat as needed • Monitor for bradycardia in the right and circumflex coronary
Pulmonary arteriolar	Epoprostenol (Flolan)	IV infusion for pulmonary hypertension • Start at 2 ng/kg/min • Increase by 2 ng/kg per min every 15 minutes until reduction in pulmonary resistance of dose-limiting toxicity (nausea, headache, hypotension)

Additional Abbreviations: FFR, fractional flow reserve; VT, ventricular tachycardia; VEA, ventricular ectopic activity; ASA, American Society Anesthesia; CHF, congestive heart failure; LCA, left coronary artery; RCA, right coronary artery
Prepared in Conjunction with Peg Angel, RN.

and local tradition, so the doses and contraindications for all drugs should be confirmed from a primary source before administration (Table 3.4).

REFERENCES

1. Wyman RM, Safian RD, Portway V, et al. Current complications of diagnostic and therapeutic cardiac catheterization. *J Am Coll Cardiol* 1988;12:1400.
2. Chandrasekar B, Doucet S, Bilodeau L, et al. Complications of cardiac catheterization in the current era: a single-center experience. *Cathet Cardiovasc Interv* 2001;52:289–295.
3. Braunwald E, Swan HJC, Gorlin R, McIntosh HD. Cooperative study on cardiac catheterization. *Circulation* 1968;37(suppl 3):1.
4. Kennedy JW. Complications associated with cardiac catheterization and angiography. *Cathet Cardiovasc Diagn* 1982;8:5.
5. Johnson LW, et al. Coronary angiography 1984–1987: a report of the registry of the Society for Cardiac Angiography and Interventions, I: results and complications. *Cathet Cardiovasc Diagn* 1989;17:5.
6. Lozner E, Johnson LW, Johnson S, et al. Coronary arteriography 1984–1987: a report of the registry of the Society for Cardiac Angiography and Interventions, II: an analysis of 218 deaths related to coronary angiography. *Cathet Cardiovasc Diagn* 1989;17:11.
7. Noto TJ, Johnson LW, Krone R, et al. Cardiac catheterization 1990: a report of the registry of the Society for Cardiac Angiography and Interventions. *Cathet Cardiovasc Diagn* 1991;24:75.
8. Laskey W, Boyle J, Johnson LW, and the Registry Committee of the Society for Cardiac Angiography & Intervention. Multivariable model for prediction of risk of significant complication during diagnostic cardiac catheterization. *Cathet Cardiovasc Diagn* 1993; 30:185.
9. Bourassa MG, Noble J. Complication rate of coronary arteriography. A review of 5250 cases studied by percutaneous femoral technique. *Circulation* 1976;53:106.
10. Boehrer JD, Lange RA, Willard JE, Hillis LD. Markedly increased periprocedure mortality of cardiac catheterization in patients with severe narrowing of the left main coronary artery. *Am J Cardiol* 1992;70:1388.
11. Folland ED, Oprian C, Giacomini J, et al. Complications of cardiac catheterization and angiography in patients with valvular heart disease. *Cathet Cardiovasc Diagn* 1989;17:15.
12. Meine TJ, Harrison JK. Should we cross the valve: the risk of retrograde catheterization of the left ventricle in patients with aortic stenosis. *Am Heart J* 2004;148:41–42.
13. Gobel FL, Steward WJ, Campeau L, et al. Safety of coronary angiography in clinically stable patients following coronary bypass surgery. *Cathet Cardiovasc Diagn* 1998;45:376.
14. Vitiello R, McCrindle BW, Nykanen D, Freedom RM, Benson LN. Complications associated with pediatric cardiac catheterization. *J Am Coll Cardiol* 1998;32:1433.
15. Dorros G, Cowley MJ, Simpson J, et al. Percutaneous transluminal coronary angioplasty. Report of complications from the National Heart, Lung, and Blood Institute PTCA registry. *Circulation* 1983;67:723.
16. Detre K, Holubkov R, Kelsey S, et al. Percutaneous transluminal angioplasty in the 1985–1986 and 1977–1981. The National Heart, Lung and Blood Institute registry. *N Engl J Med* 1988; 318:265.
17. Shaw RE, et al. Development of a risk adjustment mortality model using the American College of Cardiology-National Cardiovascular Data Registry (ACC-NCDR) experience: 1998–2000. *J Am Coll Cardiol* 2002;39:1104–1112.

18. Cutlip DE, et al. Risk assessment for percutaneous coronary intervention: our version of the weather report? *J Am Coll Cardiol* 2003;42:1986–1989.

19. Singh M, et al. Correlates of procedural complications and a simple integer risk score for percutaneous coronary intervention. *J Am Coll Cardiol* 2002;40:387–393.

20. Queshi MA, et al. Simplified scoring system for predicting mortality after percutaneous coronary intervention. *J Am Coll Cardiol* 2003;42:1890–1895.

21. Davis K, Kennedy JW, Kemp HG Jr., et al. Complications of coronary arteriography from the Collaborative Study of Coronary Artery Surgery (CASS). *Circulation* 1979;59:1105.

22. Judkins MP, Gander MP. Prevention of complications of coronary arteriography. *Circulation* 1974;49:599.

23. Alpert JS, et al. Myocardial infarction redefined—a consensus document of The Joint European Society of Cardiology/ American College of Cardiology Committee for the redefinition of myocardial infarction. *J Am Coll Cardiol* 2000;36: 959–969.

24. Kini A, et al. Incidence and mechanism of creatine kinase-MB enzyme elevation after coronary intervention with different devices. *Cathet Cardiovasc Interv* 1999;48:123–129.

25. Jeremias A, et al. Nonischemic chest pain induced by coronary interventions: a prospective study comparing coronary angioplasty and stent implantation. *Circulation* 1998;98:2656.

26. Stone GW, et al. Differential impact on survival of electrocardiographic Q-wave versus enzymatic myocardial infarction after percutaneous intervention: a device-specific analysis of 7147 patients. *Circulation* 2001;104:642–647.

27. Abdelmeguid AE, Topol EJ. The myth of the myocardial "infarctlet" during percutaneous coronary revascularization procedures. *Circulation* 1996;94:3369.

28. Mehran R, et al. Atherosclerotic plaque burden and CK-MB enzyme elevation after coronary intervention – an IVUS study of 2256 patients. *Circulation* 2000;101:604–610.

29. Reeder GS. Elevation of creatine kinase, MB fraction after elective coronary intervention: a valid surrogate end point of poor late outcome? *J Am Coll Cardiol* 1999;34:670.

30. Adams DF, Fraser DB, Abrams HL. The complications of coronary arteriography. *Circulation* 1973;48:609.

31. Sandoval AE, Laufer N. Thromboembolic stroke complicating coronary intervention – acute evaluation and management in the cardiac catheterization laboratory. *Cathet Cardiovasc Diagn* 1998;44:412.

32. Fuchs S, et al. Stroke complicating percutaneous coronary intervention – incidence, predictors, and prognostic implications. *Circulation* 2002;106:86–91.

33. Eggebrecht H, al. Potential embolization by atherosclerotic debris dislodged from aortic wall during cardiac catheterization - histological and clinical findings in 7,621 patients. *Catheter Cardiovasc Interv* 2000;49:389–394.

34. Bladin CF, et al. Transcranial doppler detection of microemboli during percutaneous transluminal coronary angioplasty. *Stroke* 1998;29:2367–2370.

35. Omran H, et al. Silent and apparent cerebral embolism after retrograde catheterisation of the aortic valve in valvular stenosis: a prospective, randomised study. *Lancet* 2003;361: 1241–1246.

36. Blanco VR, et al. Retinal cholesterol emboli during diagnostic cardiac catheterization. *Catheter Cardiovasc Interv* 2000;51: 323–325.

37. Fukumoto Y, et al. The incidence and risk factors of cholesterol embolization syndrome, a complication of cardiac catheterization: a prospective study. *J Am Coll Cardiol* 2003;42:211–216.

38. Rocha P, Mulot R, Lacombe P, et al. Brain magnetic resonance imaging before and after percutaneous mitral balloon commissurotomy. *Am J Cardiol* 1994;74:955.

39. Welton DE, Young JB, Raizner AE, et al. Value and safety of cardiac catheterization during active infective endocarditis. *Am J Cardiol* 1979;44:1306.

40. Green GS, McKinnon CM, Rosch J, Judkins MP. Complications of selective percutaneous transfemoral coronary arteriography and their prevention. *Circulation* 1972;45:552.

41. Samal AK, White CJ. Percutaneous management of access site complications. *Catheter Cardiovasc Interv* 2002;57:12–23.

42. Shammas RL, Reeves WC, Mehta PM. Deep venous thrombosis and pulmonary embolism following cardiac catheterization. *Cathet Cardiovasc Diagn* 1993;30:223.

43. Gowda S, Bollis AM, Haikal AM, Salem BI. Incidence of new focal pulmonary emboli after routine cardiac catheterization comparing the brachial to the femoral approach. *Cathet Cardiovasc Diagn* 1984:10:157.

44. Skillman JJ, Kim D, Baim DS. Vascular complications of percutaneous femoral cardiac interventions. *Arch Surg* 1988;123:1207.

45. Butler R, Webster MW. Meralgia paresthetica: an unusual complication of cardiac catheterization via the femoral artery. *Catheter Cardiovasc Interv.* 2002;56:69–71.

46. Witz M, et al. Retroperitoneal haematoma: a serious vascular complication of cardiac catheterisation. *Eur J Vasc Endovasc Surg* 1999;18:364–365.

47. Mak GYK, Daly B, Chan W, et al. Percutaneous treatment of post catheterization massive retroperitoneal hemorrhage. *Cathet Cardiovasc Diagn* 1993;29:40.

47a. Farouque HM, Tremmel JA, Raissi Shabari F, et al. Risk factors for the development of retroperitoneal hematoma after percutaneous coronary intervention in the era of glycoprotein IIb/IIIa inhibitors and vascular closure devices. *J Am Coll Cardiol* 2005;45:363–8.

48. Sheikh KH, Adams DB, McCann R, et al. Utility of color flow imaging for identification of femoral arterial complications of cardiac catheterization. *Am Heart J* 1989;117:623.

49. Taylor BS. Thrombin injection versus compression of femoral artery pseudoaneurysms. *J Vasc Surg* 1999;30:1052–1059.

50. Samal AK. Treatment of femoral arterial pseudoaneurysms with percutaneous thrombin injection. *Cathet Cardiovasc Interven* 2001;53:259–263.

51. Kent KC, McArdle CR, Kennedy B, et al. A prospective study of the clinical outcome of femoral pseudoaneurysms and arteriovenous fistulas induced by arterial puncture. *J Vasc Surg* 1993; 17:125.

52. Kim D, Orron DE, Skillman JJ, et al. Role of superficial femoral artery puncture in the development of pseudoaneurysm and arteriovenous fistula complicating percutaneous transfemoral cardiac catheterization. *Cathet Cardiovasc Diagn* 1002;25:91.

53. Smith SM, Galland RB. Late presentation of femoral artery complications following percutaneous cannulation for cardiac angiography or angioplasty. *J Cardiovasc Surg* 1992;33:437.

54. Kelm M, et al. Incidence and clinical outcome of iatrogenic femoral arteriovenous fistulas: implications for risk stratification and treatment. *J Am Coll Cardiol* 2002;40:291–297.

55. Moscucci M, et al. Peripheral vascular complications of directional coronary atherectomy and stenting—predictors, management, and outcome. *Am J Cardiol* 1994;74:448.

56. Koreny M, et al. Arterial puncture closure devices compared with standard manual compression after cardiac catheterization: systematic review and meta-analysis. *JAMA* 2004;291:350–357.

57. Kiemeneij F, et al. A randomized comparison of percutaneous transluminal coronary angioplasty by the radial, brachial and femoral approaches – the Access Study. *J Am Coll Cardiol.* 1997;29:1269.

58. Bashore TM, et al. American College of Cardiology/Society for Cardiac Angiography and Interventions Clinical Expert Consensus Document on cardiac catheterization laboratory standards. *J Am Coll Cardiol* 2001;37:2170–2214.

59. Advanced cardiovascular life support. Section 1: introduction to ACLS 2000: overview of recommended changes in ACLS from the guidelines 2000 conference. *Circulation* 2000;102(suppl 1): 1–370.

60. Sprung CL, Pozen RG, Rozanski JJ, et al: advanced ventricular arrhythmias during bedside pulmonary artery catheterizations. *Am J Med* 1982;72:203.

61. Arrowood JA, Mullan DF, Kline RA, Engel TR, Kowey PR. Ventricular fibrillation during coronary angiography: the precatheterization QT interval. *J Electrocardiol* 1987;20:255.

62. Kowey PR, Marinchak RA, Rials JJ, Filert RA. Intravenous amiodarone. *J Am Coll Cardiol* 1997;29:1190.

63. Greenberg ML, Kelley TA, Lerman BB, et al. Atrial pacing for conversion of atrial flutter. *Am J Cardiol* 51986;8:95.

64. Kirshenbaum JM, Kloner RF, McGowan N, Antman EM. Use of an ultrashort-acting beta-receptor blocker (esmolol) in patients

with acute myocardial ischemia and relative contraindications to beta-blockage therapy. *J Am Coll Cardiol* 1988;12:773.

65. Murray KT. Ibutilide. *Circulation* 1998;97:493.

66. Weissler AM, Warren JV. Vasodepressor syncope. *Am Heart J* 1959;57:786.

67. Landau C, Lange RA, Glamann DB, Willard JE, Hillis LD. Vasovagal reactions in the cardiac catheterization laboratory. *Am J Cardiol* 1993;73:95.

68. Gupta PK, Haft JI. Complete heart block complicating cardiac catheterization. *Chest* 1972;61:185.

69. Sprung CL, Elser B, Schein RM, et al. Risk of right bundle branch block and complete heart block during pulmonary artery catheterization. *Crit Care Med* 1989;17:1.

70. Friedrich SP, Berman AD, Baim DS, Diver DJ. Myocardial perforation in the cardiac catheterization laboratory—incidence, presentation, diagnosis, and management. *Cathet Cardiovasc Diagn* 1994;32:99.

71. Tsang TM, Freeman WK, Barnes ME, Reeder GS, Packer DL, Seward JB. Rescue echocardiographically guided pericardiocentesis for cardiac perforation complicating catheter-based procedures – the Mayo Clinic experience. *J Am Coll Cardiol* 1998;32:1345.

72. Saffitz JE, Rose TE, Oaks JB, et al. Coronary artery rupture during coronary angioplasty. *Am J Cardiol*. 1983;51:902.

73. Ellis SG, Ajluni S, Arnold AZ, et al. Increased coronary perforation in the new device era—incidence, classification, management, and outcome. *Circulation* 1994;90:2725.

74. Fejka M, Simon R. Dixon SR, Safian RD, et al. Diagnosis, management, and clinical outcome of cardiac tamponade complicating percutaneous coronary intervention. *Am J Card* 2002;90: 1183–1186.

75. Awadallla H, et al. Catheter-induced dissection of the left main coronary with and without extension into the aortic root: a report of two cases and review of the literature. *J Interven Cardiol* 2004;17:253–257.

76. Foote GA, Schabel SI, Hodges M. Pulmonary complications of the flowdirected balloon-tipped catheter. *N Engl J Med* 1974; 290:927.

77. Heupler FA, Heisler M, Keys TF, et al. Infection prevention guidelines for cardiac catheterization laboratories. *Cathet Cardiovasc Diagn* 1992;25:260.

78. Ramsdale D, et al. Bacteremia following complex percutaneous coronary intervention. *J Invas Cardiol* 2004;16:632.

79. Wiener RS, Ong LS. Local infection after percutaneous transluminal coronary angioplasty: relationship to early repuncture of ipsilateral femoral artery. *Cathet Caridovasc Diagn* 1989;16:180.

80. McCready RA, Siderys H, Pittman JN, et al. Septic complications after cardiac catheterization and percutaneous transluminal coronary angioplasty. *J Vasc Surg* 1991;14:170.

80a. Polard GA, Jacobson RM. Prevention of Hepatitis B Vaccine. *N Engl J Med* 2004;351:2832–8.

81. Beltrami EM, et al. Risk and management of blood-borne infections in health care workers. *Clinical Microbiol Rev* 2000;13: 385–407.

82. Reyes MP, Ganguly S, Fowler M, et al. Pyrogenic reactions after inadvertent infusion of endotoxin during cardiac catheterizations. *Ann Intern Med* 1980;93:32.

83. Feldman T, Moss J, Teplinsky K, Carroll JD. Cardiac catheterization in the patient with a history of allergy to local anesthetics. *Cathet Cardiovasc Diagn* 1990;20:165.

84. Wittbrodt ET, Spinler SA. Prevention of anaphylactoid reactions in high-risk patients receiving radiographic contrast media. *Ann Pharmacother* 1994;28:236.

85. Bertrand ME, et al. Influence of a nonionic, iso-osmolar contrast medium (iodixanol) versus an ionic, low-osmolar contrast medium (ioxaglate) on major adverse cardiac events in patients undergoing percutaneous transluminal coronary angioplasty: a multicenter, randomized, double-blind study. Visipaque in Percutaneous Transluminal Coronary Angioplasty VIP Trial Investigators. *Circulation* 2000;101:131–136.

86. Schrader R, et al. A randomized trial comparing the impact of a nonionic (Iomeprol) versus an ionic (Ioxaglate) low osmolar contrast medium on abrupt vessel closure and ischemic complications after coronary angioplasty. *J Am Coll Cardiol* 1999;33: 395–402.

87. Freed KS, et al. Breakthrough adverse reactions to low-osmolar contrast media after steroid premedication. *Am J Roentgenol* 2001;176:1389–1392.

88. Goss, JE, Chambers CE, Heupler FA, et al. Systematic anaphylactoid reactions to iodinated contrast media during cardiac catheterization procedures—guidelines for prevention, diagnosis, and treatment. *Cathet Cardiovasc Diagn* 1995;34:99.

89. Stewart WJ, McSweeney SM, Kellet MA, Faxon DB, Ryan TJ. Increased risk of severe protamine reactions in NPH insulin dependent diabetics undergoing cardiac catheterization. *Circulation* 1984;70:788.

90. Brieger DB, Mak KH, Kottke-Marchant K, Topol EJ. Heparin-induced thrombocytopenia. *J Am Coll Cardiol* 1998;31:1449.

91. Walenga JM, et al. Heparin-induced thrombocytopenia, paradoxical thromboembolism, and other adverse effects of heparin-type therapy. *Hematol Oncol Clin North Am* 2003;17: 259–282.

91a. Jang IK, Hursting MJ. When heparins promote thrombosis–review of heparin–induced thrombocytopenia. *Circulation* 2005;111: 2671–83.

92. Tommaso CL. Contrast-induced nephrotoxicity in patients undergoing cardiac catheterization. *Cathet Cardiovasc Diagn* 1994;31:316.

93. McCullough PA, et al. Acute renal failure after coronary intervention: incidence, risk factors, and relationship to mortality. *Am J Med* 1997;103:368–375.

94. Steinberg EP, Moore RD, Powe NR, et al. Safety and cost effectiveness of high-osmolality as compared with low-osmolality contrast material in patients undergoing cardiac angiography. *N Engl J Med* 1992;326:425.

95. Rudnick MR, Goldfarb S, Wexler L, et al. Nephrotoxicity of ionic and non-ionic contrast media in 1196 patients: a randomized trial (the Iohexol Cooperative Study). *Kidney Int* 1995;47:254.

96. Aspelin P, Aubry P, Fransson SG, et al. Nephrotoxic effects in high-risk patients undergoing angiography. *N Engl J Med* 2003;348:491–499.

97. Solomon R, Werner C, Mann D, et al. Effects of saline, mannitol, and furosemide on acute decreases in renal function induced by radiocontrast agents. *N Engl J Med* 1994;331:1416.

98. Merten GJ, et al. Prevention of contrast-induced nephropathy with sodium bicarbonate: a randomized controlled trial. *JAMA* 2004;291:2328–2334.

99. Marenzi G, et al. The prevention of radiocontrast-agent-induced nephropathy by hemofiltration. *N Engl J Med* 2003;349: 1333–1340.

100. Tepel M, et al. Prevention of radiographic-contrast-agent-induced reductions in renal function by acetylcysteine. *N Engl J Med* 2000;343:180–184.

101. Briguori C, et al. Acetylcysteine and contrast agent-associated nephrotoxicity. *J Am Coll Cardiol* 2002;40:298–303.

102. Birck R, et al. Acetylcysteine for prevention of contrast nephropathy: meta-analysis. *Lancet* 362:598–603.

103. Abizaid AS, et al. Effects of dopamine and aminophylline on contrast-induced acute renal failure after coronary angioplasty in patients with preexisting renal insufficiency. *Am J Cardiol* 1999;83:260–263.

104. Tumlin JA, et al. Fenoldopam mesylate blocks reductions in renal plasma flow after radiocontrast dye infusion: a pilot trial in the prevention of contrast nephropathy. *Am Heart J* 2002; 143:894–903.

105. Stone GW, et al. Fenoldopam mesylate for the prevention of contrast-induced nephropathy: a randomized controlled trial. *JAMA* 2003;290:2284–2291.

106. Rosman HS, et al. Cholesterol embolization—clinical findings and implications. *J Am Coll Cardiol* 1990;15:1296.

107. Amar D, et al. Should all patients undergoing cardiac catheterization or percutaneous transluminal coronary angioplasty receive oxygen? *Chest* 1994;105:727.

108. Lipp H, O'Donoghue K, Resnekov L. Intracardiac knotting of a flow-directed balloon-tipped catheter. *N Engl J Med* 1972; 284:220.

109. Kober G, Hilgermann R. Catheter entrapment in a Bjork-Shiley prosthesis in aortic position. *Cathet Cardiovasc Diagn* 1987; 13:262.

110. Hartzler GO, et al. Retained percutaneous transluminal coronary angioplasty equipment components and their management. *Am J Cardiol* 1987;60:1260.

111. Grabenwoeger F, Bardach G, Dock W, et al. Percutaneous extraction of centrally embolized foreign bodies: a report of 16 cases. *Br J Radiol* 1988;61:1014.

112. Braunwald E, et al. ACC/AHA guideline update for the management of patients with unstable angina and non-ST-segment elevation myocardial infarction. *Circulation* 2002;106: 1893–1900.

113. Antman EM, et al. ACC/AHA guidelines for the management of patients with ST-elevation myocardial infarction—executive summary. *Circulation* 2004;110:588–6364.

114. Popma J, et al. Antithrombotic therapy during percutaneous coronary intervention: the Seventh ACCP Consensus Conference on Antithrombotic and Thrombolytic Therapy. *Chest* 2004; 126:576S–599S.

115. Awtry EH, Loscalzo J. Aspirin. *Circulation* 2000;101:1206–1218.

116. Patrono C, et al. Platelet-active drugs: the relationships among dose, effectiveness, and side effects. *Chest* 1998;114:470S–488S.

117. Peters R, et al. Effects of aspirin dose when used alone or in combination with clopidogrel in patients with acute coronary syndromes: observations from the Clopidogrel in Unstable angina to prevent Recurrent Events (CURE) study. *Circulation* 2003; 108:1682–1687.

118. Antithrombotic Trialists' Collaboration. Collaborative meta-analysis of randomised trials of antiplatelet therapy for prevention of death, myocardial infarction, and stroke in high risk patients. *BMJ* 2002;324:71–86.

119. Schwartz L, et al. Aspirin and dipyridamole in the prevention of restenosis after percutaneous transluminal coronary angioplasty. *N Engl J Med* 1988;318:1714–1719.

120. Lembo N, et al. Effect of pretreatment with aspirin versus aspirin plus dipyridamole on frequency and type of acute complications of percutaneous transluminal coronary angioplasty. *Am J Cardiol* 1990;65:422–426.

121. Leon MB, et al. A clinical trial comparing three antithrombotic-drug regimens after coronary-artery stenting. Stent Anticoagulation Restenosis Study Investigators. *N Engl J Med* 1998;339:1665–1671.

122. Howard PA. Aspirin resistance. *Ann Pharmacother* 2002;36: 1620–1624.

123. Bhatt DL. Aspirin resistance: more than just a laboratory curiosity. *J Am Coll Cardiol* 2004;43:1127–1129.

124. Kurth T, et al. Inhibition of clinical benefits of aspirin on first myocardial infarction by nonsteroidal antiinflammatory drugs. *Circulation* 2003;108:1191–1195.

125. Eikelboom JW, et al. Aspirin-resistant thromboxane biosynthesis and the risk of myocardial infarction, stroke, or cardiovascular death in patients at high risk for cardiovascular events. *Circulation* 2002;105:1650–1655.

126. Grotemeyer KH, et al. Two-year follow-up of aspirin responder and aspirin non responder. A pilot-study including 180 post-stroke patients. *Thromb Res* 1993;71:397–403.

127. Mueller MR, et al. Variable platelet response to low-dose ASA and the risk of limb deterioration in patients submitted to peripheral arterial angioplasty. *Thromb Haemost* 1997;78:1003–1007.

128. Grundmann K, et al. Aspirin non-responder status in patients with recurrent cerebral ischemic attacks. *J Neurol* 2003;250:63–66.

129. Gum PA, et al. A prospective, blinded determination of the natural history of aspirin resistance among stable patients with cardiovascular disease. *J Am Coll Cardiol* 2003;41:961–965.

130. Wang J, et al. Incidence of aspirin nonresponsiveness using the Ultegra Rapid Platelet Function Assay-ASA. *Am J Cardiol* 2003;92:1492–1494.

131. Chen WH, et al. Aspirin resistance is associated with a high incidence of myonecrosis after non-urgent percutaneous coronary intervention despite clopidogrel pretreatment. *J Am Coll Cardiol* 2004;43:1122–1126.

132. Wong J, et al. Rapid oral challenge-desensitization for patients with aspirin-related urticaria-angioedema. *J Allergy Clin Immunol* 2000;105:997–1001.

133. Andre P, et al. P2Y12 regulates platelet adhesion/activation, thrombus growth, and thrombus stability in injured arteries. *J Clin Invest* 2003;112:398–406.

134. Herbert J, et al. The antiaggregating and antithrombotic activity of clopidogrel is potentiated by aspirin in several experimental models in the rabbit. *Thromb Haemost* 1998;80:512–518.

135. Gachet C. ADP receptors of platelets and their inhibition. *Thromb Haemost* 2001;86:222–232.

136. Weber AA, et al. Recovery of platelet function after discontinuation of clopidogrel treatment in healthy volunteers. *Br J Clin Pharmacol* 2001;52:333–336.

137. Mehta SR, et al. Effects of pretreatment with clopidogrel and aspirin followed by long-term therapy in patients undergoing percutaneous coronary intervention: the PCI-CURE study. *Lancet* 2001;358:527–533.

138. Steinhubl SR, et al. Early and sustained dual oral antiplatelet therapy following percutaneous coronary intervention: a randomized controlled trial. *JAMA* 2002;288:2411–2420.

139. Chan AW, et al. Triple antiplatelet therapy during percutaneous coronary intervention is associated with improved outcomes including one-year survival: results from the Do Tirofiban and ReoProGive Similar Efficacy Outcome Trial (TARGET). *J Am Coll Cardiol* 2003;42:1188–1195.

140. Schomig A, et al. A randomized comparison of antiplatelet and anticoagulant therapy after the placement of coronary-artery stents. *N Engl J Med* 1996;334:1084–1089.

141. Budaj A, et al. Benefit of clopidogrel in patients with acute coronary syndromes without ST-segment elevation in various risk groups. *Circulation* 2002;106:1622–1626.

142. Yusuf S, et al. Effects of clopidogrel in addition to aspirin in patients with acute coronary syndromes without ST-segment elevation. *N Engl J Med* 2001;345:494–502.

143. Wilson S, et al. Clinical outcome of patients undergoing non-cardiac surgery in the two months following coronary stenting. *J Am Coll Cardiol* 2003;42:234–240.

144. Taniuchi M, et al. Randomized comparison of ticlopidine and clopidogrel after intracoronary stent implantation in a broad patient population. *Circulation* 2001;104:539–543.

145. Muller C, et al. A randomized comparison of clopidogrel and aspirin versus ticlopidine and aspirin after the placement of coronary-artery stents. *Circulation* 2000;101:590–593.

146. Mueller C, et al. A randomized comparison of clopidogrel and aspirin versus ticlopidine and aspirin after the placement of coronary artery stents. *J Am Coll Cardiol* 2003;41:969–973.

147. Bertrand ME, et al. Double-blind study of the safety of clopidogrel with and without a loading dose in combination with aspirin compared with ticlopidine in combination with aspirin after coronary stenting: the clopidogrel aspirin stent international cooperative study (CLASSICS). *Circulation* 2000;102: 624–629.

148. Nguyen TA, Diodati JG, Pharand C. Resistance to clopidogrel–a review of the evidence. *J Am Coll Cardiol* 2005;45:1157–64.

149. Matetzky S, et al. Clopidogrel resistance is associated with increased risk of recurrent atherothrombotic events in patients with acute myocardial infarction. *Circulation* 2004;09:3171–3175.

150. Bowers J, Ferguson J. The use of activated clotting times to monitor heparin therapy during and after interventional procedures. *Clin Cardiol* 1994;17:357–361.

151. Dougherty K, et al. Activated clotting times and activated partial thromboplastin times in patients undergoing coronary angioplasty who receive bolus doses of heparin. *Cathet Cardiovasc Diagn* 1992;26:260–263.

152. Ferguson J, et al. Relation between procedural activated clotting time and outcome after percutaneous transluminal coronary angioplasty. *J Am Coll Cardiol* 1994;23:1061–1065.

153. Narins CR, et al. Relation between activated clotting time during angioplasty and abrupt closure. *Circulation* 1996;93: 667–671.

154. Chew D, et al. Defining the optimal activated clotting time during percutaneous coronary intervention: aggregate results from 6 randomized, controlled trials. *Circulation* 2001;103:961–966.

155. Ellis S, et al. Effect of 18- to 24-hour heparin administration for prevention of restenosis after uncomplicated coronary angioplasty. *Am Heart J* 1989;117:777–782.

156. Weitz JI. Low-molecular-weight heparins. *N Engl J Med* 1997;337:688–698.

157. Invasive compared with non-invasive treatment in unstable coronary-artery disease: FRISC II prospective randomised multicentre study. FRagmin and Fast Revascularisation during InStability in Coronary artery disease Investigators. *Lancet* 1999;354:708–715.

158. Bhatt DL, et al. Safety of concomitant therapy with eptifibatide and enoxaparin in patients undergoing percutaneous coronary

intervention: results of the Coronary Revascularization Using Integrilin and Single bolus Enoxaparin Study. *J Am Coll Cardiol* 2003;41:20–25.

159. Goodman SG, et al. Randomized evaluation of the safety and efficacy of enoxaparin versus unfractionated heparin in high-risk patients with non-ST-segment elevation acute coronary syndromes receiving the glycoprotein IIb/IIIa inhibitor eptifibatide. *Circulation* 2003;107:238–244.

160. Kereiakes DJ, et al. Low-molecular-weight heparin therapy for non-ST-elevation acute coronary syndromes and during percutaneous coronary intervention: an expert consensus. *Am Heart J* 2002;144:615–624.

161. Moliterno D, et al. A novel point-of-care enoxaparin monitor for use during percutaneous coronary intervention. Results of the Evaluating Enoxaparin Clotting Times (ELECT) Study. *J Am Coll Cardiol* 2003;42:1132–1139.

162. Neumann FJ, et al. Evaluation of prolonged antithrombotic pretreatment ("cooling-off" strategy) before intervention in patients with unstable coronary syndromes: a randomized controlled trial. *JAMA* 2003;290:1593–1599.

163. Lincoff A, et al. Bivalirudin with planned or provisional abciximab versus low-dose heparin and abciximab during percutaneous coronary revascularization: results of the Comparison of Abciximab Complications with Hirulog for Ischemic Events Trial (CACHET). *Am Heart J* 2002;143:847–853.

164. Lincoff AM, et al. Bivalirudin and provisional glycoprotein IIb/IIIa blockade compared with heparin and planned glycoprotein IIb/IIIa blockade during percutaneous coronary intervention: REPLACE-2 randomized trial. *JAMA* 2003;289: 853–863.

165. Bittl J, et al. Bivalirudin versus heparin during coronary angioplasty for unstable or postinfarction angina: final report reanalysis of the Bivalirudin Angioplasty Study. *Am Heart J* 2001; 142:952–959.

166. Coller BS. 1985. A new murine monoclonal antibody reports an activation-dependent change in the conformation and/or microenvironment of the platelet glycoprotein IIb/IIIa complex. *J Clin Invest* 1985;76:101–108.

167. Topol EJ, et al. Platelet GPIIb-IIIa blockers. *Lancet* 1999;353: 227–231.

168. Kleiman NS, et al. Differential inhibition of platelet aggregation induced by adenosine diphosphate or a thrombin receptor-activating peptide in patients treated with bolus chimeric 7E3 Fab: implications for inhibition of the internal pool of GPIIb/IIIa receptors. *J Am Coll Cardiol* 1995;26:1665–1671.

169. Mascelli MA, et al. Pharmacodynamic profile of short-term abciximab treatment demonstrates prolonged platelet inhibition with gradual recovery from GP IIb/IIIa receptor blockade. *Circulation* 1998;97:1680–1688.

170. Scarborough RM, et al. Barbourin. A GPIIb-IIIa-specific integrin antagonist from the venom of Sistrurus m. barbouri. *J Biol Chem* 1991;266:9359–9362.

171. Kleiman NS. Pharmacokinetics and pharmacodynamics of glycoprotein IIb-IIIa inhibitors. *Am Heart J* 1999;138:263–275.

172. Li D, et al. Tirofiban, a Non-Peptide Inhibitor of the Platelet Glycoprotein IIb/IIIa Receptor. New York: Marcel Dekker, 1971:355–365.

173. Coller BS. Platelet GPIIb/IIIa antagonists: the first anti-integrin receptor therapeutics. *J Clin Invest* 1997;99:1467–1471.

174. Kereiakes DJ, et al. Time course, magnitude, and consistency of platelet inhibition by abciximab, tirofiban, or eptifibatide in patients with unstable angina pectoris undergoing percutaneous coronary intervention. *Am J Cardiol* 1999;84:391–395.

175. Simon DI, et al. A comparative study of light transmission aggregometry and automated bedside platelet function assays in patients undergoing percutaneous coronary intervention and receiving abciximab, eptifibatide, or tirofiban. *Catheter Cardiovasc Interv* 2001;52:425–432.

176. Kabbani S, et al. Suboptimal early inhibition of platelets by treatment with tirofiban and implications for coronary interventions. *Am J Cardiol* 2002;89:647–650.

177. Topol EJ, et al. Comparison of two platelet glycoprotein IIb/IIIa inhibitors, tirofiban and abciximab, for the prevention of ischemic events with percutaneous coronary revascularization. *N Engl J Med* 2001;344:1888–1894.

178. Valgimigli M, et al. The additive value of tirofiban administered with the high-dose bolus in the prevention of ischemic complications during high-risk coronary angioplasty: the ADVANCE Trial. *J Am Coll Cardiol* 2004;44:14–194.

179. The EPIC Investigators. Use of a monoclonal antibody directed against the platelet glycoprotein IIb/IIIa receptor in high-risk coronary angioplasty. *N Engl J Med* 1994;330:956–961.

180. The EPISTENT Investigators. Randomised placebo-controlled and balloon-angioplasty-controlled trial to assess safety of coronary stenting with use of platelet glycoprotein-IIb/IIIa blockade. The EPISTENT Investigators. Evaluation of Platelet IIb/IIIa Inhibitor for Stenting. *Lancet* 1998;352:87–92.

181. ESPRIT Investigators. Novel dosing regimen of eptifibatide in planned coronary stent implantation (ESPRIT): a randomised, placebo-controlled trial. *Lancet* 2000;356:2037–2044.

182. Topol EJ, et al. Outcomes at 1 year and economic implications of platelet glycoprotein IIb/IIIa blockade in patients undergoing coronary stenting: results from a multicentre randomised trial. EPISTENT Investigators. Evaluation of Platelet IIb/IIIa Inhibitor for Stenting. *Lancet* 1999;354:2019–2024.

183. O'Shea J, et al. Platelet glycoprotein IIb/IIIa integrin blockade with eptifibatide in coronary stent intervention: the ESPRIT trial: a randomized controlled trial. *JAMA* 2001;285:2468–2473.

184. Labinaz M, et al. Comparison of one-year outcomes following coronary artery stenting in diabetic versus nondiabetic patients (from the Enhanced Suppression of the Platelet IIb/IIIa Receptor With Integrilin Therapy [ESPRIT] Trial). *Am J Cardiol* 2002;90: 585–590.

185. Randomised placebo-controlled trial of abciximab before and during coronary intervention in refractory unstable angina: the CAPTURE Study. *Lancet* 1997;349:1429–1435.

186. Inhibition of the platelet glycoprotein IIb/IIIa receptor with tirofiban in unstable angina and non-Q-wave myocardial infarction. Platelet Receptor Inhibition in Ischemic Syndrome Management in Patients Limited by Unstable Signs and Symptoms (PRISM-PLUS) Study Investigators. *N Engl J Med* 1998;338:1488–1497.

187. Montalescot G, et al. Platelet glycoprotein IIb/IIIa inhibition with coronary stenting for acute myocardial infarction. *N Engl J Med* 2001;344:1895–1903.

188. Brener SJ, et al. Randomized, placebo-controlled trial of platelet glycoprotein IIb/IIIa blockade with primary angioplasty for acute myocardial infarction. ReoPro and Primary PTCA Organization and Randomized Trial (RAPPORT) Investigators. *Circulation* 1998;98:734–741.

189. Stone GW, et al. Comparison of angioplasty with stenting, with or without abciximab, in acute myocardial infarction. *N Engl J Med* 2002;346:957–966.

190. Ellis SG, et al. Facilitated percutaneous coronary intervention versus primary percutaneous coronary intervention: design and rationale of the Facilitated Intervention with Enhanced Reperfusion Speed to Stop Events (FINESSE) trial. *Am Heart J* 2004;147:E16.

191. Karvouni E, et al. Intravenous glycoprotein IIb/IIIa receptor antagonists reduce mortality after percutaneous coronary interventions. *J Am Coll Cardiol* 2003;41:26–32.

192. Dasgupta H, et al. Thrombocytopenia complicating treatment with intravenous glycoprotein IIb/IIIa receptor inhibitors: a pooled analysis. *Am Heart J* 2000;140:206–211.

193. Berkowitz SD, et al. Acute profound thrombocytopenia after C7E3 Fab (abciximab) therapy. *Circulation* 1997;95:809–813.

194. Merlini PA, et al. Thrombocytopenia caused by abciximab or tirofiban and its association with clinical outcome in patients undergoing coronary stenting. *Circulation* 2004;109: 2203–2206.

Basic Techniques

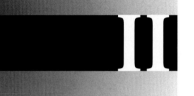

Percutaneous Approach, Including Trans-septal and Apical Puncture

Donald S. Baim   Daniel I. Simon

In contrast with the brachial cutdown technique (see Chapter 5), the *percutaneous* approach to left and right heart catheterization uses needle puncture to achieve vascular access (1) and thus obviates the need for surgical isolation of the vessel during either the insertion or the subsequent withdrawal of the cardiac catheter. Once the needle has been positioned within the vessel lumen, a flexible guidewire is advanced through the needle and well into the vessel being accessed (2). This guidewire remains in an intravascular position as the needle is withdrawn to allow direct insertion of a dilator and an end-hole catheter, or more commonly the introduction of an appropriately sized sheath that is equipped with a back-bleed valve and a side-arm port. The desired catheters can then be placed through the sheath and into the vasculature (3,4). This modification reduces patient discomfort and eliminates repetitive local arterial trauma during catheter exchanges, although it does increase the size of the puncture slightly since the outer diameter of the sheath is 1F size (0.33 mm), larger than the corresponding bare catheter. At the termination of the percutaneous catheterization procedure, the catheters and introducing sheaths are withdrawn, and bleeding from the puncture sites is controlled by the application of direct pressure or the use of one of several vascular closure devices (see below).

Because of its speed and simplicity, percutaneous entry via the femoral approach has become the dominant approach to cardiac catheterization. More than 85% of the procedures contained in the 1990 registry of the Society for Cardiac Angiography and Intervention (SCA&I) were performed via this route (5). With appropriate skill and knowledge of regional anatomy, moreover, the same percutaneous techniques used for femoral artery and vein cannulation can be adapted to allow catheter insertion from a variety of other entry sites. Venous catheterization can thus be performed via the internal jugular, subclavian, or median antecubital vein, whereas arterial catheterization can be performed via the brachial, axillary, or radial arteries, or even the lumbar aorta.

CATHETERIZATION VIA THE FEMORAL ARTERY AND VEIN

Patient Preparation

After palpation of the femoral arterial pulse within the inguinal skin crease, a safety razor is used to shave an area approximately 10 cm in diameter surrounding this point. Although most catheterizations can be performed quickly and easily from a single groin, we have found it expedient to prepare both groins routinely. The right groin is generally used, since it is more easily accessed by the operator standing on that side of the table. If difficulties in catheter advancement force a switch to the other groin once the procedure has begun, however, having the left groin already prepared saves time and inconvenience. The shaved areas are scrubbed with a povidone-iodine/detergent mixture and then painted with povidone-iodine solution. The latter is blotted dry using a sterile towel, and the patient is draped from clavicles to below the feet, leaving only the sterile prepared groin areas exposed. Most laboratories now use disposable paper drapes with adhesive-bordered apertures for this purpose, frequently packaged together with other disposable supplies (syringes, needles, bowls, and so on) in a custom kit available from any of several vendors.

Selection of Puncture Site

The adjacent femoral artery and vein (Fig. 4.1A and B) are the most commonly used vessels for percutaneous diagnostic cardiac catheterization (5). It is important to puncture these vessels at the correct level (1 or 2 cm below the inguinal ligament) to facilitate vessel entry and effective compression to minimize local vascular complications. Although some operators rely on the location of the inguinal skin crease to position the skin nicks through which puncture will be attempted (see below), we prefer locating the skin nicks in reference to the inguinal *ligament* (which runs from the anterior superior iliac spine to the pubic tubercle)—the position of the skin crease itself can be misleading in obese patients. More recently, we have begun to confirm the appropriate localization of the skin nick by fluoroscopy, which should show the nick to overlie the inferior border of the femoral head (6; Fig. 4.1C and D). Making the skin nicks at this level increases the chance that needle puncture will take place in the common femoral segment (overlying the middle of the femoral head) rather than either too high (above the inguinal ligament) or too low (in the superficial femoral or profunda branches of the common femoral artery). The femoral artery should be easily palpable over a several-centimeter span above and below the skin nick site. The femoral vein will lie approximately one fingerbreadth medial to the artery along a parallel course.

Most difficulties in entering the femoral artery and vein—and most vascular complications—arise as the result of inadequate identification of these landmarks prior to attempted vessel puncture. Puncture of the artery at or above the inguinal ligament makes catheter advancement difficult and predisposes to inadequate compression, hematoma formation, and/or retroperitoneal bleeding following catheter removal (see Chapter 3). Puncture of the artery >3 cm below the inguinal ligament increases the chance that the femoral artery will have divided into its profunda and superficial femoral branches. Puncture in the crotch between these two branches fails to enter the arterial lumen, whereas puncture of either one of the branches increases the risk of false aneurysm formation or thrombotic occlusion owing to smaller vessel caliber. Because the superficial femoral artery frequently overlies the femoral vein, low venous punctures may pass inadvertently through the superficial femoral artery, leading to excessive bleeding and possible arteriovenous fistula formation (6; see Chapter 3).

Local Anesthesia

Adequate local anesthesia is essential for a successful catheterization. Inadequate anesthesia leads to poor patient cooperation and makes the time in the catheterization laboratory unpleasant for both patient and operator. Once the inguinal ligament and femoral artery have been identified, the femoral artery is palpated along its course using the three middle fingers of the left hand, with the uppermost finger positioned just below the inguinal ligament. Without moving the left hand, a linear intradermal wheal of 1 or 2% lidocaine is raised slowly by tangential insertion of a 25- or 27-gauge needle along a course overlying both the femoral artery and vein at the desired level of entry.

With the left hand remaining in place, transverse skin punctures are made over the femoral artery and vein, using the tip of a no. 11 scalpel blade. The smaller needle is then replaced by a 22-gauge 1½-in needle, which is used to infiltrate the deeper tissues along the intended trajectory for arterial and venous entry. As this needle is advanced, small additional volumes of lidocaine are infiltrated by slow injection. Each incremental infiltration should be preceded by aspiration so that intravascular boluses can be avoided. To avoid unnecessary injury to the femoral artery, we sometimes intentionally infiltrate medially and laterally to the pulse and infiltrate deeply only through the venous nick. If the anesthetic track passes through the artery, infiltration should be suspended until the tip of the needle has passed out of the back wall of the vessel and then continued to the full length of the needle or to the point where the needle tip contacts the periosteum. Approximately 10 to 15 mL 1% Xylocaine administered in this fashion usually provides adequate local anesthesia. The patient should be warned that he or she may experience some burning as the anesthetic is injected, but that the medication will prevent any subsequent sharp sensations.

Once local anesthesia has been achieved, the small skin nicks can be enlarged and deepened, using the tips of a curved mosquito forceps. This procedure decreases the resistance that is encountered during subsequent advancement of the needle and subsequent vascular sheath and increases the likelihood that any vascular bleeding will become manifest as oozing through the puncture rather than hidden in the formation of a deep hematoma.

Femoral Vein Puncture

If right heart catheterization is to be performed, or secure venous access is desired (for administration of fluids and medications or rapid placement of a temporary pacing catheter), the femoral venous puncture is usually performed prior to arterial puncture. With the left hand palpating the femoral artery along its course below the inguinal ligament, the needle is introduced through the more medial skin nick.

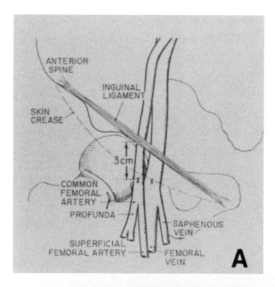
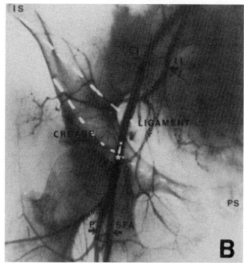
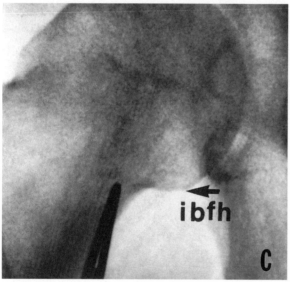
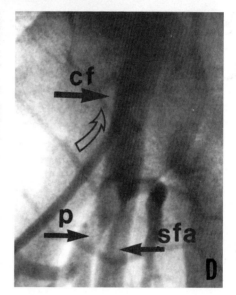

Figure 4.1   Regional anatomy relevant to percutaneous femoral arterial and venous catheterization: **A.** Schematic diagram showing the right femoral artery and vein coursing underneath the inguinal ligament, which runs from the anterior superior iliac spine to the pubic tubercle. The arterial skin nick (indicated by X) should be placed approximately 3 cm below the ligament and directly over the femoral arterial pulsation, and the venous skin nick should be placed at the same level but approximately one fingerbreadth more medial. Although this level corresponds roughly to the skin crease in most patients, anatomic localization relative to the inguinal ligament provides a more constant landmark (see text for details). **B.** Corresponding radiographic anatomy as seen during abdominal aortography. **C.** Fluoroscopic localization of skin nick (marked by clamp tip) to the inferior border of the femoral head (ibfh). **D.** Catheter (*open arrow*) inserted via this skin nick has entered the common femoral artery (cf), safely above its bifurcation into the superficial femoral (sfa) and profunda branches. (For further details, see Kim D, Orron DE, Skillman JJ, et al. Role of superficial femoral artery puncture in the development of pseudoaneurysm and arteriovenous fistula complicating percutaneous transfemoral cardiac catheterization. *Cathet Cardiovasc Diagn* 1992;25:91.)

Classically, the 18-gauge thin-walled Seldinger needle was used; this needle consists of a blunt, tapered external cannula through which a sharp solid obturator projects (Fig. 4.2). The needle should be grasped so that the index and middle fingers lie below the lateral flanges of the needle and the thumb rests on the top of the solid obturator as the needle is advanced along the sagittal plane angled approximately 45° cephalad. Although this needle can

occasionally be advanced up to its hub, the tip of the needle will usually stop more superficially as it encounters the periosteum of the underlying pelvic bones. The periosteum is well innervated and may be quite tender if the initial lidocaine infiltration failed to reach this level. Accordingly, forceful contact with the periosteum is neither necessary nor desirable. If the patient experiences significant discomfort, some operators will remove the

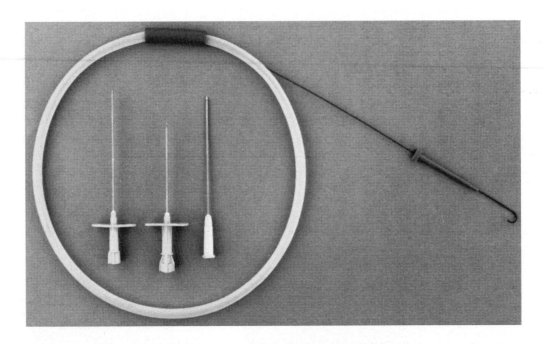

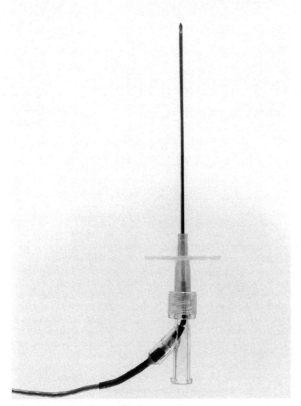

Figure 4.2   Percutaneous needles and guide wire. **Top.** A Seldinger needle (left) with its sharp solid obturator in place, a Potts-Cournand needle (center), which differs in that its obturator is hollow and therefore allows the operator to see blood flashback as the artery is punctured, and an 18-gauge thin-wall needle (right) used for internal jugular vein puncture and now frequently also for arterial entry. These percutaneous needles are surrounded by an 0.038-inch, 145-cm J guidewire. **Bottom.** A Doppler-guided SmartNeedle.

obturator from the Seldinger needle and infiltrate additional lidocaine into the deep tissues through the outer cannula. At this point, the Seldinger needle should have transfixed the femoral vein. The obturator is removed, and a 10-mL syringe is attached to the hub of the cannula. The syringe and cannula are then depressed so that the syringe lies closer to the anterior surface of the thigh (Fig. 4.3) and the needle is more parallel (rather than perpendicular) to

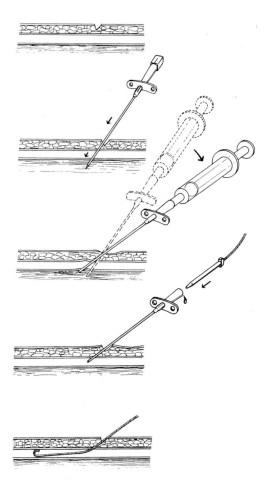

Figure 4.3 Seldinger technique for venous puncture. A skin nick has been created overlying the desired vein, which is punctured through and through by a Seldinger needle with its solid obturator in place. In the center illustration, the obturator is removed and the needle cannula is attached to a syringe. Depression of the syringe toward the surface of the skin tents the vessel slightly and facilitates axial alignment of the cannula at the moment that slow withdrawal brings the tip of the cannula back into the vessel lumen. This is recognized by the sudden ability to withdraw venous blood freely into the syringe, which is then removed from the needle cannula to permit advancement of the J guidewire (shown here with a plastic straightener in place). Once the guidewire has been advanced safely into the vessel, the needle cannula can be removed.

the vein. Gentle suction is applied to the syringe, and the whole assembly is slowly withdrawn toward the skin surface. In doing so, it is helpful to control the needle with both the left hand (which also rests on the patient's leg for support) and the right hand (which also controls the aspirating syringe). As the tip of the cannula is withdrawn into the lumen, venous blood will flow freely into the syringe.

We and most laboratories, however, have now switched from the Seldinger needle in favor of an 18-gauge single-wall puncture needle that has a sharpened tip and lacks the inner obturator. Placement of a fluid-filled syringe on the needle's hub allows direct front-wall entry of the vein without the need to first exit the back wall and then pull back. Otherwise, the technique used is identical after entry of the venous lumen has been achieved.

With the left hand stabilizing the needle, the right hand is used to remove the syringe and to advance a 0.035- or 0.038-inch J guidewire into the hub of the needle. The wire tip may be straightened by hyperextension of the wire shaft in the right hand or by leaving the tip of the wire within the plastic introducer supplied by the manufacturer. The wire should slide through the needle and 30 cm into the vessel with no perceptible resistance. Fluoroscopy should then show the tip of the guidewire just to the left (patient's right) of the spine.

If difficulty is encountered in advancing the guidewire, it should never be overcome by the application of force. Fluoroscopy may simply reveal that the tip of the wire has lodged in a small lumbar branch; it can be drawn back slightly and redirected or gently prolapsed up the iliac vein. When resistance to advancement is encountered at or just beyond the tip of the needle, however, even greater care is required. This resistance may simply be caused by apposition of the tip of the needle to the back wall of the vein, which can be corrected by further depression of the needle hub, with or without slight withdrawal of the needle shaft. If this maneuver fails to allow free advancement of the wire, however, the wire should be removed, and the syringe should be reattached to the needle hub to ensure that free flow of venous blood is still present before additional wire manipulation is attempted—the wire should not be reintroduced unless free flow is obtained. If it is necessary to withdraw the wire, this should always be done gently, since it is theoretically possible for the wire to snag on the tip of the needle. Were this to occur, the needle and wire should be removed as a unit. If the wire still cannot be advanced after these maneuvers, the needle should be withdrawn and the puncture site should be compressed for 1 to 3 minutes. The anatomic landmarks should be reconfirmed and puncture reattempted. In some cases, puncturing the vein during a Valsalva maneuver may help by distending the femoral vein and making clean puncture more likely.

After the wire has freely entered the vein, the needle is removed, leaving the wire well within the vein and secured at the skin entry site by the left hand. The protruding wire is wiped with a moistened gauze pad, and its free end is threaded into the lumen of a sheath and dilator combination adequate to accept the intended right-sided heart catheter. All current sheaths are equipped with a back-bleed valve and side-arm connector (Fig. 4.4) to control bleeding around the catheter shaft and to provide a means of administering drugs or extra intravenous fluids during the right-sided heart catheterization. The operator must make sure that he or she has control of the proximal end of the guidewire and that it is held in a fixed position as the sheath and dilator are introduced through the skin. Insertion is eased if the sheath and dilator are rotated as a unit while they are advanced progressively through the soft tissues. If excessive resistance is encountered, it may be necessary to remove the dilator from the sheath and to

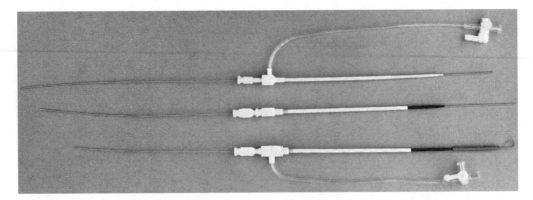

Figure 4.4 Vascular sheaths. **Center.** An original sheath and dilator assembly (USCI "888"). In contrast to the original design, modern arteriovenous introducers are equipped with back-bleed valves and side-arm attachment. **Top.** A Cordis sheath. **Bottom.** A USCI Hemaquet. Each device is inserted over a conventional guidewire as a unit, following which the inner Teflon dilator is removed to permit catheter introduction. The sidearm sheaths also permit fluid infusion and an additional site for pressure monitoring with the catheter in place.

introduce the dilator alone before attempting to introduce the combination. If inspection shows that initial attempts have created significant burring at the end of the sheath, a new sheath should be obtained.

Once the sheath is in place, the wire and dilator are removed, and the sheath is flushed by withdrawal of blood and injection of heparinized saline solution. In our laboratory we usually infuse the sidearm of the venous sheath from a 1-liter bag of normal saline solution, connected via a sterile length of intravenous extension tubing, to maintain sheath patency and provide a carrier for drug administration by the nurse. Although drug administration can also take place via a peripheral intravenous line, the side arm of the sheath avoids any concerns about how quickly volume can be administered or whether infiltration of the peripheral line might jeopardize drug delivery in an emergency. Even if right heart catheterization is not planned, the femoral sheath makes it easy to place a right heart catheter or a temporary transvenous pacemaker lead if hemodynamic instability or bradyarrhythmia ensue.

Catheterizing the Right Heart from the Femoral Vein

A right (as well as a left) heart catheterization is needed to obtain a full profile of the hemodynamic state. Only the right heart catheterization can provide data regarding mean left heart filling pressure (the pulmonary capillary wedge, rather than just the post–A wave left ventricular end diastolic pressure), detect pulmonary arterial hypertension, measure the cardiac output, and detect left-to-right intracardiac shunts. Leaving the right heart catheter in the pulmonary artery during a complex interventional procedure also gives an ongoing measure of changes in the hemodynamic state as fluid and contrast loading take place, various medications (nitrates, diuretics, and so on) are given, and as episodes of ischemia develop and are treated.

For these reasons, it was once common to perform a right heart catheterization in *every* patient who came to the cardiac catheterization laboratory. In contrast, the 1990 SCA&I survey showed that the practice was to perform right heart catheterization in only 28% of procedures (5). The use of right heart catheterization has fallen further after several standard-setting and regulatory agencies ruled that a left heart catheterization alone is adequate for most patients undergoing evaluation for coronary artery disease. The time (<5 minutes), added expense (<$100), and added risk (<1/10,000) of right heart catheterization are small, but so is the added information. So we now skip the right heart catheterization in patients with a primary diagnosis of coronary artery disease, unless they have symptoms of congestive heart failure, noninvasive evidence of depressed left ventricular function or associated valvular disease, or recent myocardial infarction. In such patients, however, we still believe that the quantitation of overall hemodynamic function provided by right heart catheterization justifies performance of this low-risk adjunctive part of the overall catheterization evaluation.

If right heart catheterization *is* to be performed, the desired right heart catheter (Fig. 4.5) is flushed, attached to the venous manifold, introduced into the sheath, and advanced up the inferior vena cava. Although conventional woven Dacron (Goodale-Lubin or Cournand) catheters provide excellent torque control, their inherent stiffness makes them poorly suited for routine use in a training laboratory. It is considerably safer to use 7F balloon flotation catheters to exploit their ease of passage, low risk of injury to the right-sided heart chambers, and (with a suitably equipped catheter) their ability to perform thermodilution measurements of cardiac output. Unfortunately, such soft catheters with smaller internal diameters tend to have poor frequency response (see Chap. 7), may not adequately transmit the torque required for easy catheterization of the right-sided heart from the femoral approach, and accept only 0.021-inch guidewires. To bridge this gap,

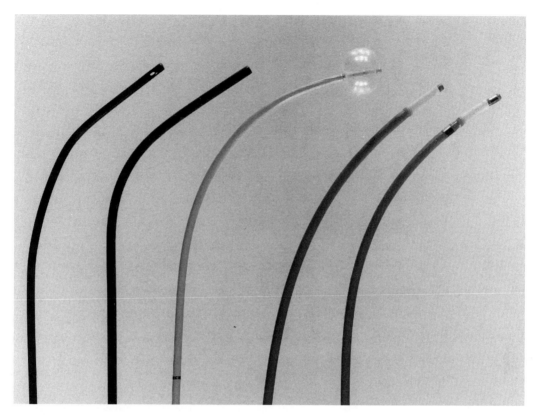

Figure 4.5 Right-sided heart catheters used from the femoral approach. **Left.** Woven Dacron Goodale-Lubin, Cournand catheters. **Center.** Swan-Ganz catheter. **Right.** Newer balloon catheters, including the PWP pressure measurement catheter and the Baim-Turi catheter with bipolar pacing electrodes (USCI).

stiffer, balloon-tipped catheters (PWP monitoring catheter, Medtronic) have been developed that combine the safety of the Swan-Ganz catheter with the catheter control and frequency response previously found only in the woven Dacron catheters. The larger lumen diameter also allows the passage of conventional 0.035- and 0.038-inch diameter guidewires when necessary.

Deviation of the catheter tip from its paraspinous position during advancement from the leg suggests entry into a renal or hepatic vein, which can be corrected by slight withdrawal and rotation of the catheter. Once the catheter is above the diaphragm and within the right atrium, it is rotated counterclockwise to face the lateral wall of the right atrium (Fig. 4.6). Additional counterclockwise rotation and gentle advancement allow passage of the catheter tip into the superior vena cava, which is contiguous with the posterolateral wall of the right atrium. In contrast, anterior orientation of the catheter tip at this point may result in its entrapment in the right atrial appendage and inability to reach the superior vena cava. If passage to the superior vena cava is difficult, the tip of the catheter can be withdrawn to the inferior vena cava, where a 0.035-inch J guidewire can be introduced to traverse the straight-line path from the inferior to the superior vena cava along the back wall of the right atrium. Once in position, a baseline superior vena caval blood sample is obtained for measurement of oxygen saturation and comparison with the subsequently measured pulmonary arterial blood O_2 saturation to screen for unsuspected left-to-right shunts. The catheter is then flushed with heparinized saline solution and withdrawn to the right atrium for pressure measurement.

To advance a catheter from the femoral vein to the pulmonary artery, the tip of the catheter is positioned in the lower portion of the right atrium, directed toward its lateral border. If a balloon flotation catheter is being used, the balloon is inflated at this point. Clockwise rotation is applied, which causes the catheter tip to sweep the anterior and anteromedial wall of the right atrium, along which the tricuspid valve is located (Fig. 4.6). As the catheter tip passes over the tricuspid orifice, slight advancement causes it to enter the right ventricle, where pressure is again recorded. If the right atrium is enlarged, greater curvature of the catheter may be necessary, i.e., a large J loop. Such a loop may be formed by bending the tip of the catheter against the lateral right atrial wall or by engaging in the ostium of the hepatic vein (just below the diaphragm). This larger loop can then be rotated clockwise in the atrium as described above, causing the tip of the catheter to enter the right ventricle. Right ventricular pressure is then recorded.

Simple advancement of the catheter in the right ventricle causes the tip to move toward the apex of that chamber

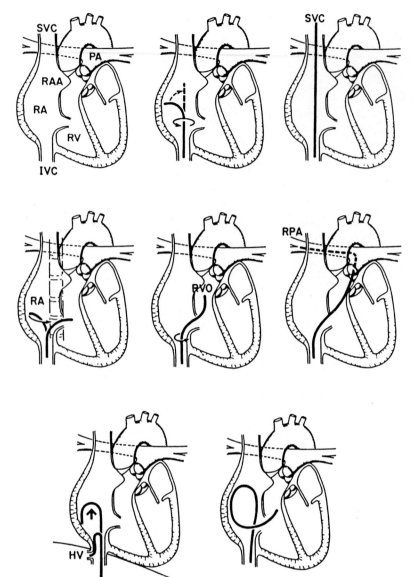

Figure 4.6 Right heart catheterization from the femoral vein, shown in cartoon form. **Top row.** The right heart catheter is initially placed in the right atrium (RA) aimed at the lateral atrial wall. Counterclockwise rotation aims the catheter posteriorly and allows advancement into the superior vena cava (SVC). Although not evident in the figure, clockwise catheter rotation into an anterior orientation would lead to advancement into the right atrial appendage (RAA), precluding SVC catheterization. **Center row.** The catheter is then withdrawn back into the right atrium and aimed laterally. Clockwise rotation causes the catheter tip to sweep anteromedially and cross the tricuspid valve. With the catheter tip in a horizontal orientation just beyond the spine, it is positioned below the right ventricular outflow tract (RVO). Additional clockwise rotation causes the catheter to point straight up, allowing for advancement into the main pulmonary artery and from there into the right pulmonary artery (RPA). **Bottom row.** Two maneuvers useful in catheterization of a dilated right heart. A larger loop with a downward-directed tip may be required to reach the tricuspid valve and can be formed by catching the catheter tip in the hepatic vein (HV) and advancing the catheter quickly into the right atrium. The reverse loop technique (bottom right) gives the catheter tip an upward direction, aimed toward the outflow tract.

and usually does not result in catheterization of the pulmonary artery. To achieve this latter end, the catheter must be withdrawn slightly so that its tip lies horizontally and just to the right (patient's left) of the spine. In this position, clockwise rotation causes the tip of the catheter to point upward (and slightly posteriorly) in the direction of the right ventricular outflow tract (Fig. 4.6). The catheter should be advanced only when it is in this orientation to minimize the risk of ventricular arrhythmias or injury to the right ventricle. Advancement may be facilitated if performed as the patient takes a deep breath.

If these maneuvers fail to achieve access to the pulmonary artery owing to enlargement of the right atrial and ventricular chambers, the catheter may be withdrawn to the right atrium and formed into a large reverse loop, which allows the tip of the catheter to cross the tricuspid valve in an upward orientation (similar to that when right heart catheterization is performed from above), which makes it more likely to enter the outflow tract (Fig. 4.6,

bottom right). When manipulated appropriately, the catheter tip should cross the pulmonic valve and advance to a wedge position without difficulty. Having the patient take a deep breath and cough during advancement is often of assistance in achieving a wedge position. Alternatively, a small amount of air may be released from the balloon to decrease its size and facilitate wedging in a smaller, more distal branch of the pulmonary artery. Catheters advanced from the leg are more likely to seek the left pulmonary artery, whereas catheters advanced from above tend to seek the right pulmonary artery as they make a continuous counterclockwise curve through the right heart chambers. If needed, either pulmonary artery can be catheterized by appropriate manipulation or careful introduction of a curved J guidewire, but extending guidewires into the thin-walled pulmonary arteries should be avoided unless absolutely necessary.

Following measurement of the wedge pressure, the balloon (if a balloon-tip catheter is being used) is deflated and the catheter is withdrawn into the more proximal left or right pulmonary artery. There, pulmonary arterial pressure is measured and another blood sample for measurement of oxygen saturation is obtained. If a more simultaneous "snapshot" of the hemodynamic state is desired, these entry pressures can be re-recorded during a right-sided heart pull-back. For practical reasons, we now tend to re-record only the wedge pressure (simultaneous with the left ventricular pressure) and pulmonary artery pressure, coincident with the measurement of the cardiac output. When baseline hemodynamics are abnormal, we commonly leave the right heart catheter in the proximal pulmonary artery for the duration of the case to allow continuous monitoring of the pulmonary artery diastolic pressure as an index of volume status and ischemic left ventricular dysfunction.

Attempts to perform right heart catheterization occasionally result in entry into other structures. If a woven Dacron catheter is advanced in the right atrium with a posteromedial orientation, it may cross a patent foramen ovale and enter the left atrium. This is sometimes hard to detect by catheter position alone because the catheter appearance in the left atrium or ventricle may be indistinguishable (in the anteroposterior view) from its course during usual right heart catheterization. It can, however, be recognized by a change to a left atrial pressure waveform, position of the catheter tip across the spine and frequently out into the left lung field (i.e., into a pulmonary vein, Fig. 4.7A and B), and the ability to withdraw fully oxygenated blood from the catheter tip. Although more unusual, a woven Dacron catheter can also enter the ostium of the coronary sinus, located inferiorly and posteriorly to the tricuspid orifice. There will be continued presence of a right atrial waveform, but blood sampling will disclose far lower oxygen saturation (20 to 30%) than was present in the superior vena cava. In the right anterior oblique projection, the catheter will be seen to remain in the atrioventricular groove rather than passing rightward into the ventricle. Anatomic abnormalities can also be suspected when the catheter takes an unusual position or course during attempted right heart catheterization. Figure 4.7C, D, and E depict the appearance of the right-sided heart catheter course in three such congenital abnormalities (persistent left superior vena cava, patent ductus arteriosus, and anomalous pulmonary venous return). *The most important points about these side trips off the beaten path to the right ventricle are that the operator should recognize that the tip of the catheter is not in the right ventricle (i.e., one should not attempt to get to the pulmonary artery) and should decide where the catheter is (by pressure monitoring, saturation analysis, or hand injection of a small amount of contrast agent) before withdrawing the catheter to the right atrium and proceeding with the right heart catheterization.*

In patients with elevated right heart pressures or prior placement of an inferior vena caval filter or umbrella, those undergoing specialized procedures (endomyocardial biopsy, coronary sinus catheterization), or those in whom prolonged postprocedural monitoring with a balloon flotation catheter is desired, the *right internal jugular vein* offers an excellent alternative to the femoral vein. The technique for jugular puncture is described in Chapter 20, and the method of advancing the right-sided heart catheter to the pulmonary artery is identical to that described for the brachial approach in Chapter 5. On occasion, percutaneous right heart catheterization is performed from the subclavian or median basilic vein, using a similar technique.

Femoral Artery Puncture

The common femoral artery is punctured by inserting the Seldinger or single-wall puncture needle through the more lateral skin nick. Again, the needle is inserted at approximately 45° along the axis of the femoral artery as palpated by the three middle fingers of the left hand. The experienced operator may feel the transmitted pulsations as the tip of the needle contacts the wall of the femoral artery.

With the Seldinger needle, it is customary to advance the needle completely through the artery until the periosteum is encountered. The obturator is then removed, and the hub of the needle is depressed slightly toward the anterior surface of the thigh. Arterial pressure makes it unnecessary to attach a syringe to the cannula, so that both hands can be used to stabilize the needle as it is slowly withdrawn. When the needle comes back into the lumen of the femoral artery, as evidenced by vigorous pulsatile flow of arterial blood, a 0.035- or 0.038-inch J guidewire should then be advanced carefully into the needle.

If a single-wall puncture is desired, the operator may prefer a Potts-Cournand needle (Fig. 4.2), in which the obturator has a small lumen that transmits a flashback of arterial blood as the vessel is entered, or the same 18-gauge single-wall puncture needle described for venous entry. When the femoral pulse is difficult to palpate or numerous needle insertions have been fruitless, it may be easiest to use the 18-gauge SmartNeedle (Escalon Vascular Access, New Berlin, WI; see Fig. 4.2, bottom panel). The obturator of this device contains a Doppler crystal that picks up pulsatile arterial or more continuous venous flow, and thereby helps aim the needle tip toward the center of the desired vascular lumen.

Whichever needle is used to enter the arterial lumen, the guidewire introduced through the needle should move freely up the aorta (located to the right [patient's left] side of the spine on fluoroscopy) up to the level of the diaphragm. When difficulty in advancing the guidewire is encountered at or just beyond the tip of the needle and is not corrected by slight depression or slight withdrawal of the needle, the guidewire should be withdrawn to ensure that vigorous arterial flow is still present before any further wire manipulation is attempted. If flow is not brisk or if the wire still cannot be advanced, the needle should be

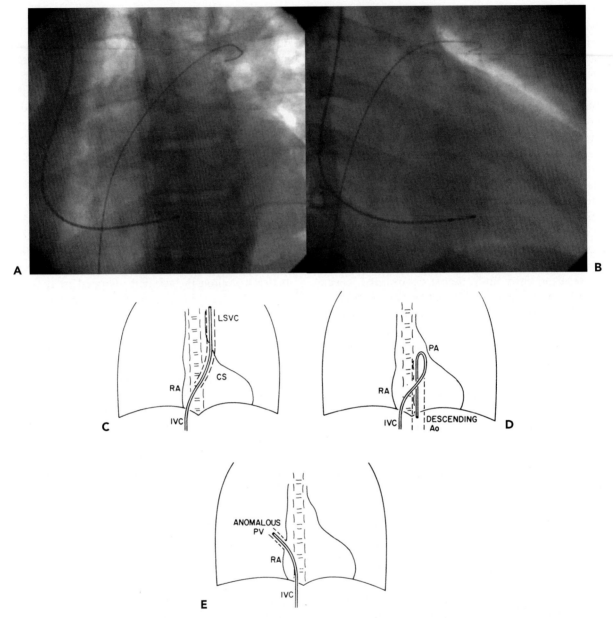

Figure 4.7 Alternative paths occasionally encountered while attempting to advance the right heart catheter from right atrium to ventricle. **A and B.** A J-tipped guidewire has crossed a patent foramen ovale into the left atrium and left upper pulmonary vein; the right anterior oblique view confirms that the guidewire has remained on the atrial side of the atrioventricular plane and thus could not be in the pulmonary artery. **C.** The course of a catheter passed from the femoral vein to the inferior vena cava (IVC), right atrium (RA), coronary sinus (CS), and up into an anomalous left superior vena cava (LSVC). **D.** The catheter crossing from the pulmonary artery (PA) to the descending aorta (Ao) by way of a patent ductus arteriosus. **E.** The catheter entering an anomalous pulmonary vein that drains into the right atrium.

removed and the groin should be compressed for 5 minutes. The operator should verify the correctness of the anatomic landmarks and attempt repuncture of the femoral artery. If the second attempt is still unsuccessful in allowing wire advancement, a third attempt on the same vessel is unwise, and an alternative access site should generally be selected.

If wire motion is initially free, but resistance is encountered after several centimeters (particularly if the patient complains of any discomfort during wire advancement), extensive iliac disease or subintimal wire position are distinct possibilities. The wire should be pulled back slightly under fluoroscopic control, and the needle should be removed as the left hand is used to stabilize the wire and control arterial bleeding. After the wire is wiped with a moist gauze pad, a small (4F or 5F) dilator can be cautiously introduced to a point just below where wire movement became difficult. The wire is then withdrawn from the dilator, blood is aspirated to ensure free flow, and a small bolus of low osmolar contrast medium is then injected gently under fluoroscopic monitoring. This should disclose the anatomic reason for difficult wire advancement—generally iliac tortuosity, stenosis, or dissection. Problems advancing the wire above the aortic bifurcation may also suggest the presence of an abdominal aortic aneurysm (7). Either can usually be overcome by use of a floppy steerable (Wholey wire, Malinckrodt, Hazelwood, MO) or hydrophilic (Glidewire, Terumo) guidewire, carefully reintroduced through the dilator in an attempt to reach the descending aorta, using extreme care to avoid perforation, dissection, or dislodgment of atherothrombotic debris (Fig. 4.8A). In an era when the obstructing lesion can be quickly and effectively treated by angioplasty or stent placement (see Chapter 27), iliac stenosis is no longer a firm indication to abandon trans-femoral left heart catheterization!

If contrast injection through the small dilator reveals that subintimal wire passage has occurred or that the ipsilateral iliac artery is occluded, retrograde left heart catheterization should be relocated to the other femoral artery, the brachial or radial artery. Patients with retrograde dissection should be observed for signs of progressive dissection or arterial compromise, both of which are fortunately rare with retrograde guidewire dissections.

In an aging population with diffuse atherosclerotic disease, the question of performing left heart catheterization via a prosthetic (e.g., aortobifemoral) graft arises frequently (8,9). This is not an ideal approach because the graft wall is tough (making sheath insertion difficult), such grafts may contain diffuse atherosclerotic or thrombotic debris, and graft closure or serious graft infection may occur. The graft should be identified as a separate structure from the adjacent native femoral artery and punctured using a front-wall approach. Even if the graft hood is punctured correctly, the guidewire may pass through the anastomosis and into the native femoral artery rather than proximally up the graft (8). In that event, contrast injections through a small dilator in a RAO projection (right leg) will disclose the problem. Partial withdrawal of the dilator and the use of special steerable guidewires may then allow the wire to be redirected into the graft lumen and thereby reach the descending aorta (Fig. 4.8B). A vascular introducing sheath should always be used to avoid excessive friction during catheter movement or excessive traction on catheter tips during withdrawal, but serial dilators may be needed to facilitate sheath passage through the tough graft wall. This approach via a vascular graft can thus be used with care, particularly when other alternatives (e.g., brachial, axillary, or radial artery) are themselves less than desirable. Some operators choose to administer prophylactic antibiotics (Kefzol 1 gm every 8 hours for 24 hours) when achieving vascular access via a prosthetic graft.

Catheterizing the Left Heart from the Femoral Artery

Once the guidewire has been advanced to the level of the diaphragm and the needle has been removed, the operator's left hand is used to stabilize the wire and control arterial bleeding while the wire is wiped with a moistened gauze pad to remove any adherent blood. If the catheter is to be introduced directly into the artery, the soft tissues are predilated by brief introduction of a Teflon arterial dilator one F size smaller than the intended catheter before insertion into the left heart catheter itself. Essentially all left heart catheterizations from the femoral approach, however, are now performed using an appropriate-sized vascular sheath (e.g., a 6F sheath for a 6F catheter) that is equipped with a back-bleed valve and side-arm tubing as described above. The 15-cm-long sheath is commonly used for diagnostic catheterization, but can reach only the midiliac. In the presence of severe tortuosity, it may be preferable to use the 23-cm-long sheath designed for interventional procedures, which is sufficiently long to enter the distal aorta above the bifurcation. This helps improve the torque responsiveness of diagnostic catheters under those circumstances.

The chosen sheath is introduced over the guidewire (the proximal end of which is held in a straightened, fixed position) with a rotational motion, following which the guidewire and dilator are removed and the sheath is aspirated, flushed, and connected to a pressurized flush system (Intraflo II [30 mL/hour], Abbot Critical Care, North Chicago, IL) to avoid clot formation in the sheath. Alternatively, this side arm can be connected to a manifold for monitoring arterial pressure at a separate site (e.g., during passage of a pigtail catheter across a stenotic aortic valve). This sheath should be power flushed immediately after each catheter is introduced or withdrawn by briefly activating the Intraflo device.

In the classic approach as described above, the guidewire was removed once the sheath had been inserted. This required that the desired left heart catheter be flushed and loaded with a 145-cm J guidewire before its nose was introduced into the back-bleed valve of the sheath. The soft end of the guidewire was then advanced carefully through the catheter, out the end of the sheath, and to the level of the diaphragm before the catheter itself was advanced. One concern, however, is that readvancement of the guidewire out the end of the sheath can cause vascular injury in the presence of severe iliac tortuosity or disease. We therefore adopted a modified technique in which a short exchange length (175 cm) Newton J (Cook, Inc.) is placed through the access needle, and its tip is left at the level of the diaphragm as the dilator is removed from the sheath, the sheath is flushed, and the left heart catheter is inserted over the wire and through the sheath lumen. This obviates the need to renegotiate complex iliofemoral anatomy with the guidewire.

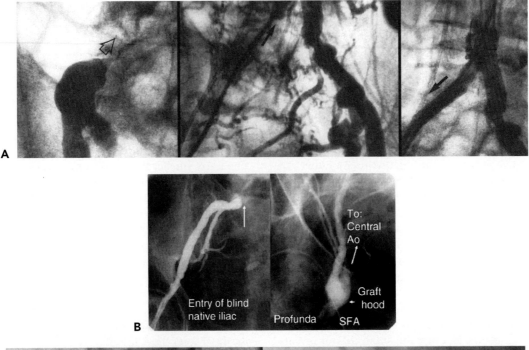

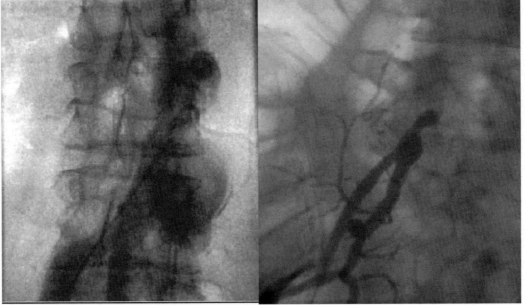

Figure 4.8   A. Entry of the right femoral artery was straightforward, but guidewire advancement stopped in the iliac system. **Left.** Contrast injection through a 5F dilator shows severe iliac stenosis with extensive cross-pelvic collaterals. This was crossed with a Terumo Glidewire to allow completion of the diagnostic angiography and a right coronary artery angioplasty (not shown). **Center.** Injection in the abdominal aorta shows the proximal extent of the iliac stenosis. **Right.** Iliac stenosis then dilated and treated by placement of a Palmaz-Schatz iliac stent, with restored antegrade iliac flow. **B.** Retrograde left heart catheterization in a patient with previous aortic-bifemoral grafting. **Left.** Entry of the graft hood has resulted in passage of the wire into the blind native iliac. **Right.** In a RAO projection, the more anterior pathway to the central aorta (Ao) via the graft can be seen overlying the native iliac, with the bifurcation of the common femoral artery into the profunda and superficial femoral artery (SFA) just below. **C.** Difficult wire passage led to placement of a 5F dilator and hand injection of contrast, showing distal aortic aneurysm (negotiated with Wholey wire). **D.** In another patient, hand injection through a 5F dilator showed occlusion of both iliac arteries (only the right is shown here) leading to conversion to the percutaneous radial approach for completion of the procedure.

Once the catheter has been advanced to the desired level (either above the diaphragm or into the ascending aorta), the guidewire is removed so that the catheter can be connected to the arterial manifold and double-flushed (withdrawal and discarding of 10 mL of blood, followed by injection of heparinized saline solution). All subsequent left heart catheters are then introduced by reinserting this wire to the level of the diaphragm (allowing one catheter to be removed and the second to be reintroduced safely), rather than withdrawing the first catheter completely and then inserting the second catheter and wire through the sheath de novo. Of course, if the left heart catheterization is being performed without the aid of a sheath, the operator must leave the tip of the wire in the abdominal aorta during the removal of the first catheter and the introduction of a second catheter to retain access to the vessel. These over-the-wire catheter exchanges are facilitated by extending the back end of the wire straight down the patient's leg and holding it fixed there to ensure that the wire remains in constant position within the aorta as the newer catheter is advanced.

A Word About Heparin

As described in Chapter 3, early catheterizations from the femoral artery had a higher incidence of major complications than catheterization from the brachial artery. One difference was that brachial catheterization used systemic heparinization to avoid thrombosis in the smaller diameter brachial artery. When systemic heparinization was adopted in femoral procedures, the rates of complications became equivalent, and it became standard practice to achieve full intravenous heparinization (5,000 U) immediately after the left-sided sheath was inserted. Lesser amounts of heparin (2,500 to 3,000) were used, particularly in smaller patients, and additional heparin (up to a total of 50 to 70 U per kg) was given if the procedure went on to a coronary intervention. This type of higher heparin dosing is routinely monitored by an activated clotting time (ACT) machine in the cardiac catheterization laboratory, and titrated to an ACT of roughly 300 seconds (10). If it is planned to use an intravenous IIb/IIIa receptor blocker, lower levels of heparin anticoagulation (ACT 250 to 275) may be desired to prevent excessive bleeding risk.

Although the use of heparin is mandatory for interventional or prolonged diagnostic procedures, most laboratories have abandoned the use of systemic heparinization for simple diagnostic catheterizations, where the complications are extremely low with or without heparin (11). For this issue to be decided scientifically, more than 100,000 patients would have to be randomized to undergo diagnostic catheterization with versus without systemic heparinization. Absent such trial data, we now withhold systemic heparinization for simple procedures, although we still feel that systemic anticoagulation is appropriate for more prolonged or complex diagnostic catheterizations,

cases where a guide wire will be required to cross a stenotic aortic valve, and (absolutely) for all percutaneous coronary interventions.

If systemic heparinization is used, its effects must be reversed at the termination of the left heart catheterization and associated angiography. This was previously accomplished by the administration of protamine (1 mL equals 10 mg of protamine for every 1,000 IU of heparin; 12). The operator should be watchful for potential adverse reactions to protamine, characterized by hypotension and vascular collapse, as discussed in Chapter 3. Protamine reactions appear to be more common in insulin-dependent diabetics and patients with previous protamine exposure, who are more likely to have elevated levels of IgG or IgE antiprotamine antibodies (13). With the decreasing use of heparin during diagnostic catheterization and the increasing use of vascular closure devices, protamine is now rarely used to reverse heparin.

Catheter Selection

The initial left heart catheter in most cases is a pigtail catheter with end- and multiple side-holes (Fig. 4.9). This catheter usually can be flushed in the descending aorta and then advanced to the ascending aorta without difficulty. If left ventricular and femoral arterial (sheath side-arm) pressures are being monitored (as in catheterization to evaluate aortic stenosis), the rough equality of central aortic and femoral arterial pressure should be confirmed at this time (Fig. 4.10; 3,4,14). The systolic peak in the femoral waveform may be slightly delayed and accentuated compared with the ascending aortic pressure trace, but the diastolic and mean pressures should be virtually identical. A greater

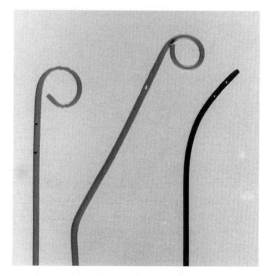

Figure 4.9 Left heart catheters used from the femoral approach. **Left to right.** Pigtail, 145° angled pigtail, and Teflon Gensini catheter (no longer in common use). All three catheters have an end hole to allow placement over a guide wire and multiple side holes to minimize the tendency for catheter whipping or intramyocardial injection during power injection of contrast.

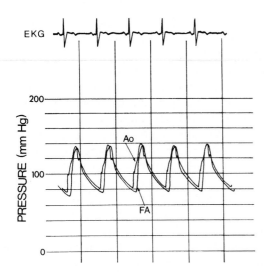

Figure 4.10 Central aortic pressure (Ao) measured through a 7.3F pigtail catheter (Cook) and femoral artery (FA) pressure measured from the side arm of an 8F arterial sheath (Cordis). Only minimal damping of the femoral artery pressure is seen, blunting its systolic overshoot, which frequently exceeds central aortic systolic pressure (see Chapter 7). With larger (8F) catheters, more damping may occur in the side-arm pressure.

difference in mean pressure between the catheter and the sheath may be seen in a patient with a small or extensively diseased iliac artery, which may require the use of a longer sheath, as described above. For the highest pressure fidelity, the sheath size should be one F size larger than the intended left heart catheter (e.g., a 5F pigtail advanced though a 6F sheath). Alternatively, catheters can be advanced from separate arterial entry sites to record left ventricular and ascending aortic pressure; a specially designed pigtail with a separate end-hole lumen and side-hole lumen may be used to perform such pressure recordings (15), or only a pullback pressure recording from left ventricle to ascending aorta can be analyzed.

Crossing the Aortic Valve

After measurement of the ascending aortic pressure, the pigtail catheter is then advanced across the aortic valve and into the left ventricle. If the aortic valve is normal and the pigtail is oriented correctly, it will usually cross the valve directly. In many cases, however, it may be necessary to advance the pigtail down into one of the sinuses of Valsalva to form a secondary loop (Fig. 4.11). As the catheter is withdrawn slowly, this loop will open to span the full diameter of the aorta, at which point a very subtle further withdrawal will often cause the pigtail to fall across the valve.

If significant aortic stenosis is present, the pigtail must be advanced across the valve with the aid of a straight 0.038-inch guidewire. Approximately 6 cm of the guidewire is advanced beyond the end of the pigtail catheter, and the catheter is withdrawn slightly until the tip of the

guidewire is leading (Fig. 4.11). The position of the tip of the guidewire within the aortic root can then be controlled by rotation of the pigtail catheter and adjustment of the amount of wire that protrudes; less wire protruding directs the wire tip more toward the left coronary ostium, whereas more wire protruding directs the wire more toward the right coronary ostium. With the wire tip positioned so that it is directed toward the aortic orifice, the tip of the wire usually quivers in the systolic jet. Wire and catheter are then advanced as a unit until the wire crosses into the left ventricle. If the wire buckles in the sinus of Valsalva instead of crossing the valve, the catheter–wire system is withdrawn slightly and readvanced with or without subtle change in the length of protruding wire or the orientation of the pigtail catheter. Alternatively, some operators prefer to leave the pigtail catheter fixed and move the guidewire independently in attempts to cross stenotic aortic valves. In either case, the wire should be withdrawn and cleaned and the catheter should be double-flushed vigorously every 3 minutes despite systemic heparinization. If promising wire positions are not obtained, the process should be repeated using a different catheter: an angled pigtail or left Amplatz catheter if the aortic root is dilated or a Judkins right coronary catheter if the aortic root is unusually narrow (16). Other catheters have been proposed for this purpose (17), but we have found these standard catheters to suffice in virtually all cases.

When the tip of the guidewire is across the aortic valve, additional wire should be inserted before any attempt is made to advance the catheter itself. Otherwise the catheter may be diverted into a sinus of Valsalva, causing the wire to flip out of the left ventricle. The straight wire should be advanced carefully, since there is a potential (admittedly small in the hypertrophic left ventricle of a patient with aortic stenosis) to perforate the left ventricular wall if the guide wire is advanced farther when it has become trapped in an endocardial surface feature. Once the catheter is in the left ventricle, the wire is immediately withdrawn and the catheter is aspirated vigorously, flushed, and hooked up for pressure monitoring, so that a gradient can be measured even if the catheter is rapidly ejected from the left ventricle or must be withdrawn because of arrhythmias. When using a left Amplatz catheter to cross a stenotic valve, however, we prefer to cross the valve with a full exchange length (260-cm) guidewire. Once the tip of this wire has entered the left ventricle, it is left in position as the Amplatz catheter is removed, and a conventional pigtail catheter is substituted before an attempt is made to measure left ventricular (LV) pressure.

The same approach applies to retrograde catheterization across a porcine aortic valve prosthesis, although it is more common to use a J-tip guidewire to help avoid the area between the support struts and the aortic wall. Ball valves (Starr-Edwards) can be crossed retrograde with this approach, but use of a small (4F or 5F) catheter will minimize the amount of aortic regurgitation resulting from

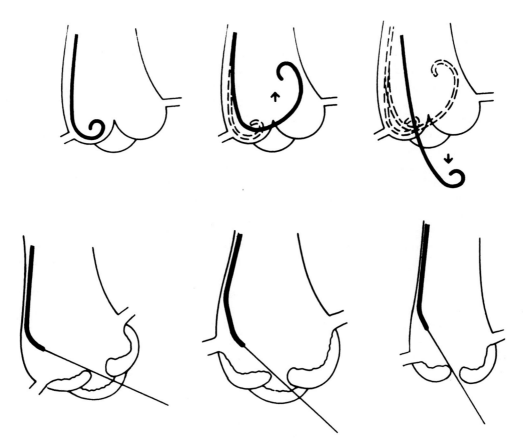

Figure 4.11 Crossing the aortic valve with a pigtail catheter. **Top left.** Although a correctly oriented pigtail catheter will frequently cross a normal aortic valve directly, it may also come to rest in the right or noncoronary sinus of Valsalva. **Top center.** Further advancement of the catheter enlarges the loop to span the aortic root and positions the catheter. **Top right.** Slow withdrawal causes the catheter to sweep across the aortic orifice and fall into the left ventricle. **Bottom left.** To cross a stenotic aortic valve, the pigtail catheter must be led by a segment of straight guidewire. Increasing the length of protruding guidewire straightens the catheter curve and causes the wire to point more toward the right coronary ostium; reducing the length of protruding wire restores the catheter curve and causes the wire to point more toward the left coronary ostium. Once the correct length of wire and the correct rotational orientation of the pigtail catheter have been found, repeated advancement and withdrawal of both the catheter and guidewire as a unit will allow the wire to cross the valve. **Bottom center.** In a dilated aortic root, an angled pigtail provides more favorable wire positions. **Bottom right.** In a small aortic root, a Judkins right coronary catheter may be preferable.

catheter interference with diastolic ball seating. Tilting disc valves (Bjork-Shiley, St. Jude, Carbomedics), however, should not be crossed retrograde because of the potential for producing torrential aortic regurgitation, catheter entrapment, or even disc dislodgement if the catheter passes across the smaller (minor) orifice. Although safe passage through the major orifice may be possible under careful fluoroscopic control (18), we still prefer a trans-septal or even apical puncture approach (see below) when it is necessary to enter the left ventricle in a patient who has a tilting disc valve in the aortic position.

Control of the Puncture Site Following Sheath Removal

Originally, standard groin management required the effect of heparin to wear off or be reversed by protamine to an

ACT <160 seconds before the arterial catheter and sheath were removed and manual pressure applied. Manual pressure method is best applied using three fingers of the left hand that are positioned sequentially up the femoral artery beginning at the skin puncture. With the fingers in this position, there should be no ongoing bleeding into the soft tissues or through the skin puncture, and it should be possible to apply sufficient pressure to obliterate the pedal pulses and then release just enough pressure to allow them to barely return. Pressure is then gradually reduced over the next 10 to 15 minutes, at the end of which time pressure is removed completely. The venous sheath is usually removed 5 minutes after compression of the arterial puncture has begun, with gentle pressure applied over the venous puncture using the right hand. To avoid tying up the catheterization laboratory during this period, patients were usually taken to a special holding room in the catheterization laboratory or back to their hospital beds before the sheaths were removed. If such relocation is to be performed prior to sheath removal, it is important that the sheaths are secured in place (suture, or at least tape) to prevent them being pulled out during transport.

When procedures are performed using larger arterial sheaths or with thrombolytic agents or IIb/IIIa receptor blockers, more prolonged (30- to 45-minute) compression is typically required. To avoid fatigue of the operator or other laboratory personnel performing compression, we typically use a mechanical device (Compressar [Applied Vascular Dynamics, Portland, OR] or FemoStop [Radi Medical, Wilmington, MA]) to apply similar local pressure. These devices can be equally or even more effective in prolonged holds (19), but manual compression may be preferred for removal of smaller (6F) sheaths or in patients with peripheral vascular disease or prior peripheral grafting surgery where occlusive compression or flow restriction might cause arterial occlusion. In every case, however, it should be emphasized that a trained person must be in attendance throughout the compression to ensure that the device is providing adequate control of puncture site bleeding and is not compromising distal perfusion.

After compression has been completed, the puncture site and surrounding area are then inspected for hematoma formation and active oozing, and the quality of the distal pulse is assessed before application of a bandage. The patient is usually kept at bed rest with the leg straight for 4 to 6 hours following percutaneous femoral catheterization (20), with a sandbag in place over the puncture site for the first few hours after catheter removal. In patients at higher risk for rebleeding (those with hypertension, obesity, or aortic regurgitation), application of a pressure bandage in addition to the sandbag may be of value. Elevation of the head and chest to 30 to 45° by the electrical or manual bed control, without muscular effort by the patient, will greatly increase the patient's comfort and will not increase the risk of local bleeding. The only reason to insist that the patient lie completely flat is if there is significant orthostatic hypotension. Before ambulation and again before discharge, the puncture site should be reinspected for recurrent bleeding, hematoma formation, development of a bruit suggestive of pseudoaneurysm or A-V fistula formation, or loss of distal pulses.

Puncture Closure Devices

The technique described above relies on manual or mechanical pressure for initial control of arterial bleeding and then on local hemostasis for ongoing plugging of the arterial puncture site. The potential for ongoing bleeding (with formation of hematoma, false aneurysm, or arteriovenous fistula) has already been described in Chapter 2 and tends to be more common with interventional procedures that require larger sheath size or more aggressive antithrombotic therapy. This has prompted the development of a variety of new devices that seek to provide more positive closure of the arterial puncture site (Fig. 4.12; 21). These devices allow sheath removal in the catheterization laboratory in even a fully anticoagulated patient and shorten the time to hemostasis and ambulation.

The simplest devices are the VasoSeal (Datascope, Paramus, NJ) and Sure Stat (Sub-Q, San Clemente, CA), which apply a collagen or other resorbing hemostatic plug in the skin track apposed to the outer wall of the femoral artery. In randomized trials, the VasoSeal device shortened the time to hemostasis (from 17 to 4 minutes) and ambulation (from 19 to 13 hours) without clear benefit in terms of hematoma formation or the need for vascular surgery compared with manual compression. In diagnostic catheterization, it can also accelerate the time to ambulation to 1 to 2 hours (22).

Next in complexity is the AngioSeal hemostatic puncture closure device (Sherwood, Davis & Geck), which positions a rectangular absorbable "anchor" made of absorbable suture material against the inside wall of the artery and uses an attached suture to winch a small collagen plug down against the outside of the artery (23). In a randomized trial of mostly diagnostic procedures (24), the AngioSeal reduced the time to hemostasis (from 15.3 to 2.6 minutes) and ambulation (from 4 to 6 hours to 1 hour) compared with manual compression, with a modest decrease in hematoma formation.

The Duet device (25) differs in that it uses a liquid procoagulant mixture (thrombin and collagen) that is injected into the soft-tissue tract leading from the outside of the artery to the skin. A compliant balloon on a wire is first positioned and inflated within the artery, pulled into contact with the end of the sheath that was used for the catheterization, and then pulled back against the inside of the puncture site to tamponade bleeding. The sheath is then withdrawn roughly 1 cm farther so that its end lies outside the vessel lumen, and the sheath side arm is used to inject the procoagulant into the soft-tissue tract leading to the outside of the artery. The Matrix VSG system (Access Closure, Inc, Mountain View, CA) differs in the use of a two-component gel that solidifies in the skin tract and adheres to the outside of the artery, but whose dilution sensitivity prevents gelation if inadvertently injected into the arterial lumen.

Although each of these devices depends greatly on the procoagulant properties of its collagen component, the approach of Prostar (Abbott Vascular, Redwood City, CA) relies on the use of a sheathlike device to perform suture-mediated closure of the arterial puncture site. This device has undergone several design improvements to improve the ease of delivery, but it still relies on the passage of fine nitinol needles through the margins of the arterial puncture and out through the skin tunnel, where they can be tied to

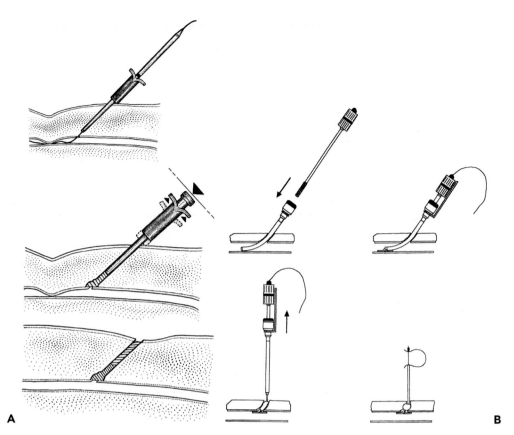

A   B

Figure 4.12 Schematic diagrams of various new devices for the closure of femoral arterial punctures. **A.** The VasoSeal. **B.** The AngioSeal (Kensey-Nash) device. **C.** The Prostar suture device. **D.** The Duet device. (See text for details.)

provide surgical hemostasis (26). It shortens the time from the end of the procedure to hemostasis (19 minutes versus 243 minutes) and ambulation (106 minutes for diagnostic and 232 minutes for interventional procedures versus 4 to 6 hours and 6 to 12 hours, respectively), with a comparably low incidence of major complications (27). Other suturing devices have been released by SuperStitch (Sutura, Fountain Valley CA) and X-site (Datascope). A similar effect can be achieved using external metallic clips (EVS, Angiolink, Taunton, MA, or Integrated Vascular Systems Clip, Abbott, Sunnyvale, CA). The external application of focused ultrasound to thermally seal the puncture site (TheraSeal) is currently being explored by Therus (Seattle WA).

Given this array of new devices, groin closure devices are now being used in most cases in some laboratories, whereas others under less pressure to provide early ambulation and same-day discharge restrict them to patients with an increased risk of bleeding with manual compression or other conditions (back pain, trouble voiding) that make prolonged bed rest undesirable. As these devices continue to evolve and the demand for early ambulation offsets the moderate cost ($100 to $300) of a closure device, they may ultimately replace prolonged local man-

ual or mechanical pressure in the control of postprocedural bleeding from the femoral artery. The conversion to puncture-sealing devices will be accelerated if they can consistently reduce the 1 to 2% incidence of hemorrhagic complications at the arterial puncture site, which constitute one of the most common morbidities associated with catheterization from this route. Of course, the success of these puncture-sealing approaches rests on the premise that a single, accurate, front-wall puncture of the common femoral artery has been performed and that favorable conditions prevail within the vessel and the surrounding soft tissue. Each also requires a modest level of skill and training on the part of the operator and the realization that difficulties encountered in performing a clean closure, once the sheath has been removed and wire access has been given up, may increase rather than decrease the incidence of complications requiring vascular surgery, deep infection, or transfusion. A meta-analysis of groin closure devices (28) suggests that early generations of these devices may have slightly increased complications such as pseudoaneurysm or infection compared with manual or mechanical compression, but they are now used with good results in most femoral catheterizations.

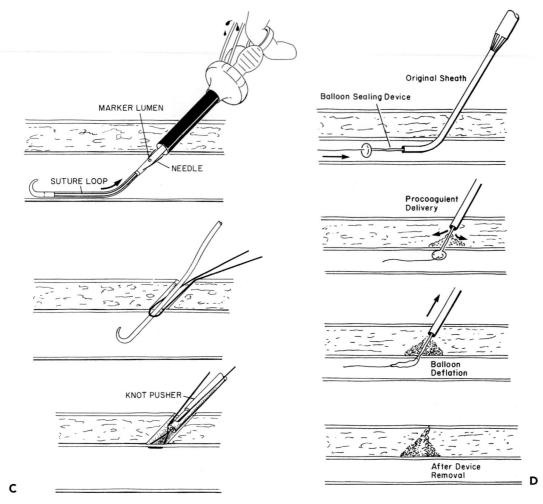

Figure 4.12 (continued)

In an era of increasingly sophisticated catheter-based therapies, it seems likely that an effective device for definitive closure of the femoral artery puncture site will replace the 50-year-old practice of pressing on the puncture site until the bleeding stops!

Contraindications to Femoral Approach to Left Heart Catheterization

As discussed in Chapter 1, the choice of catheterization approach (femoral or brachial) is usually a function of operator, institution, and patient preference. Because of technical ease, however, data from the 1990 Society for Cardiac Angiography and Intervention registry show that 83% of diagnostic (and 96% of interventional) catheterizations are performed via the femoral approach (5). In patients with peripheral vascular disease (femoral bruits or diminished lower extremity pulses), abdominal aortic aneurysm, marked iliac tortuosity, prior femoral arterial graft surgery, or gross obesity, however, catheter insertion and manipulation may present technical challenges even for experienced operators. Recognition of these relative

contraindications may favor the use of the percutaneous axillary, brachial, radial, or even translumbar aortic approaches (see below). Each laboratory should thus have one or more operators skilled in these alternative percutaneous routes, particularly if no operators skilled in the brachial cutdown approach (see Chapter 5) are available.

Beyond the limitations of access to the central arterial circulation, one important parameter in the selection of a percutaneous access site is the ability to obtain hemostasis after catheter removal. In the femoral arterial entry technique, this is usually obtained easily after removal of a percutaneous arterial catheter, but patients with a wide pulse pressure (e.g., severe aortic incompetence or systemic hypertension), gross obesity, or ongoing anticoagulation have more problems with bleeding after femoral catheterization than do patients without these factors, particularly if a groin closure device is not used. The vascular complications of percutaneous retrograde arterial catheterization are usually not life threatening (29–32) and have already been discussed in Chapter 3. In the final analysis, however, there are relatively few patients who absolutely cannot be catheterized from the femoral approach.

ALTERNATIVE SITES FOR LEFT HEART CATHETERIZATION

The techniques described above for percutaneous insertion of a femoral catheter also can be used successfully from the axillary, brachial, or radial arteries, or even the lumbar aorta, with the use of an introducing sheath. In certain cases, access to the left heart may be gained by trans-septal puncture from the right atrium to the left atrium, or even by direct percutaneous entry via the left ventricular apex. Although these other access sites may use needle puncture, guidewire advancement, and sheath insertion skills similar to those outlined above for the femoral approach, the operator wishing to use one of the alternative percutaneous routes must master the local anatomy, details of maximal allowable catheter size, limitations on catheter selection, techniques for achieving postprocedural hemostasis, and the range of complications that may ensue from bleeding or thrombosis at that anatomic location. Individuals interested in mastering one or more of these approaches are referred to the growing body of literature.

Percutaneous Entry of the Axillary or Brachial Arteries

Axillary puncture has long been used as an alternative to femoral entry by the vascular radiologist (33). The patient's hand is brought behind his or her head to expose the axillary fossa, in which the artery can be felt to course. Using local anesthesia and needle puncture and guidewire techniques like those described above, the axillary artery is entered over the head of the humerus. The left axillary artery is generally preferred to allow use of preformed Judkins catheters and avoid the brachiocephalic trunk. Effective control of the puncture site after catheter removal is critical, since accumulation of even modest amounts of hematoma around the artery can cause nerve compression (34).

The *brachial* artery is, of course, readily approached by surgical cutdown (see Chap. 5) but may also be approached using percutaneous (needle and guidewire) techniques (35). The antecubital fossa is prepared and anesthetized as for the cutdown approach. A 21-gauge arterial needle, a special 0.021-inch heavy-duty guidewire, and a 5F or 6F sheath (MicroPuncture set, Cook) can be used to gain access, after which traditional percutaneous catheter techniques are used. Working from the right brachial artery, Amplatz coronary curves are preferred (see Chapter 11). At the end of the procedure, the sheath is removed and the area is compressed manually. Alternatively, proximal occlusion can be obtained by inflation of a blood pressure cuff while a gauze pad and a clear intravenous infusion pressure bag is inflated to above systolic pressure over the puncture site (36). Pressure is then released gradually over 20 to 25 minutes. Comparisons of this percutaneous brachial technique to brachial cutdown show a shorter procedure time (without the need for dissection or repair) and no increase in complications, although surgical repair may be needed occasionally (37). This represents a viable approach for outpatient catheterization or an excellent alternative for access in a patient with difficult femoral or iliac anatomy when a Sones-trained angiographer is not available.

Percutaneous Entry of the Radial Artery

The radial artery was previously viewed as a site for placement of monitoring lines in the coronary care unit, rather than an access route for cardiac catheterization. Largely through the efforts of champions like Kiemeneij (38), however, this has now been adapted to the performance of diagnostic angiography and many types of percutaneous coronary intervention (including stent placement; 38–41). The transradial approach is particularly advantageous for patients with peripheral vascular disease or morbid obesity. Although transradial procedures currently account for fewer than 10% of all coronary diagnostic and interventional procedures in the United States, this percentage is higher in Europe and East Asia and is expected to grow.

Access site bleeding complications are exceedingly rare, and hospital length of stay is significantly shortened, offering better outcomes at lower cost (42–44). Transradial access is preferred by most patients because of reduced periprocedural discomfort, faster time to ambulation, and improved postprocedural quality of life (43). In comparison with femoral and brachial artery approaches, transradial access has a number of advantages. The radial artery is superficial, is easily compressible, and there are no major nerves or veins in its vicinity, reducing the risk of neuropathies or arteriovenous fistulae (45). Limitations of transradial access include significant operator learning curve and smaller artery size, sometimes restricting interventional device options. The availability of hydrophilically coated sheaths and large-bore 6F and 7F guiding catheters, however, provides virtually complete device flexibility for complex procedures involving, for example, bifurcation treatment, vascular brachytherapy, rotational atherectomy, embolic protection, or rheolytic thrombectomy.

Because postprocedural occlusion of the radial artery occurs in up to 3% of transradial procedures, assessment of palmar arch patency must be addressed prior to the procedure (Fig. 4.13). Most operators use a modification of the Allen test, first developed by Hovagim and coworkers (46) and validated by Dr. Gerard Barbeau in >1,000 patients. This approach simply places a pulse oximeter probe on the thumb while compressing the radial and ulnar arteries. The presence of an arterial waveform (even if with reduced amplitude or delayed appearance) and hemoglobin saturation >90% (Barbeau grades A, B, and C) confirms the adequacy of palmar arch blood flow (Fig. 4.14).

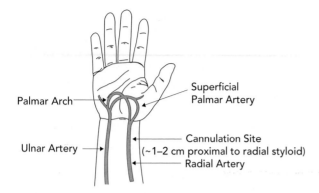

Figure 4.13 Radial artery anatomy, collateral circulation, and cannulation site. The preferred radial artery cannulation site is approximately 1 to 2 cm proximal to the radial styloid.

Although more challenging than routine transfemoral access, success rates for achieving transradial access are typically above 95% (3,6). For cannulation of the radial artery during the learning-phase, we recommend placing the arm in an abducted position with extension of the wrist. Successful cannulation is then followed by adduction of the arm to allow for body positioning and room setup identical to transfemoral cases. Experienced operators often access the radial artery in an adducted position without need for subsequent repositioning.

The right arm is preferred owing to several considerations. First, cardiothoracic surgeons prefer to harvest the left radial artery as a conduit for CABG, and conduit arteries should be avoided because routine catheterization is associated with intimal thickening by intravascular ultrasound. Second, access via the left arm requires marked adduction of the arm to retain routine room setup and allow positioning of the operator and cath lab team to the right of the patient. However, it should be noted that in post-CABG patients, left internal mammary angiography is most easily accomplished via the left radial artery.

The preferred radial artery cannulation site is approximately 1 to 2 cm proximal to the radial styloid. Access of the radial artery over the flexor retinaculum should be avoided. Local anesthesia with Xylocaine is used sparingly (skin infiltration only) to minimize radial artery manipulation and spasm. We recommend cannulation of the radial artery with a micropuncture needle (21 gauge, 4 cm long) that allows for placement of a 0.018-inch guidewire (MicroPuncture Set, Cook Incorporated, Bloomington, IN; Table 4.1). The guidewire should be advanced with great care. Resistance to passage is associated with subintimal passage or radial artery tortuosity, and further advancement can lead to dissection or perforation. Faced with resistance to wire advancement, placement of a short small-bore plastic introducer over the wire can be used for angiography of the distal portion of the radial artery. Once fully advanced, this guidewire allows for the placement of a long 5F hydrophilic sheath (23 cm) with a tapered introducer. Anticoagulation (typically 2,500 to 5,000 U heparin intravenously) is administered immediately after sheath insertion, and many operators also administer a cocktail of vasodilators (nitroglycerine 100 to 200 μg, verapamil 1.25 to 2.5 mg) via the sheath to reduce radial artery spasm. The use of hydrophilic sheaths, however, has resulted in a dramatic reduction in radial artery spasm that can in turn lead to significant discomfort during catheter manipulation or sheath removal.

Diagnostic angiography via the radial artery approach requires some modifications from routine transfemoral angiography. Diagnostic catheters (usually 5F) are advanced into the aortic root over a 0.035-inch 1-mm J wire. If passage of the J wire into the ascending aorta is difficult owing to subclavian artery tortuosity, having the patient take a deep inspiration helps avoid the descending aorta, as does counterclockwise catheter rotation. Catheter selection depends on the site of radial access. Standard diagnostic catheters (i.e., JL4, JR4) may be used via the left radial artery approach for most cases, but catheterization from the right radial artery requires either alternative shapes (Kimny [trade name for the catheter shape developed by Dr. Kiemeneij], Barbeau, AL1, AL2) or different Judkins catheter shapes. In general, engagement of the left main via the right radial artery requires smaller catheters (e.g., JL3.5 compared with JL4, XB3 compared with XB3.5) compared

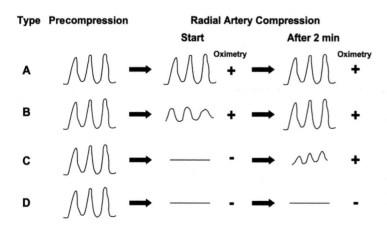

Figure 4.14 Modified Allen test to assess palmar arch patency. Palmar arch patency is addressed prior to the procedure using a modified Allen test first developed by Hovagim (see reference 46) and validated by Dr. Gerard Barbeau (Hospital Laval, Quebec City, Quebec, Canada). A pulse oximeter probe is placed on the thumb while the radial artery is compressed. The presence of an arterial waveform (even if with reduced amplitude or delayed appearance) and hemoglobin saturation >90% (Barbeau Grades A, B, and C) confirm the adequacy of palmar arch blood flow (kindly provided by Dr. Gerard Barbeau).

TABLE 4.1

TRANSRADIAL EQUIPMENT

Xylocaine needle 25 gauge
Radial access kit
  Cook
  Scimed
  Cordis/Johnson & Johnson
  Mayo Healthcare
1-mm 0.35-inch J wire
Diagnostic angiography (4F, 5F)
  Kimny
  Barbeau
  JL3.0, JL3.5, JR4
  AL1.0, AL2.0
Guiding catheters (5F, 6F, 7F, 8F)
  XB 3.0, 3.5
  EBU 3.0, 3.5
  Barbeau
  Kimny
  JL3.0, 3.5, JR4
  Muta left
  Muta right
  Radial
  Mann internal mammary
  MAC 3.0, 3.5, 4.0
Radial artery compression devices
  Hemo Band, Hemo Band Corp., Portland, OR
  TR band, Terumo
  Adapty, Nichiban Co., Japan
  Rad Stat, IEP Group, Inc., Raleigh, NC
  RadiStop, Radi Medical Systems AB, Uppsala, Sweden

with those used for femoral or left radial procedures. Engagement of the coronary ostia may be facilitated by leaving the guidewire within the catheter to enhance torquability. Use of a smaller injecting syringe (i.e., 8 mL rather than 12 mL) or a power injector may optimize angiography with 4F and 5F catheters. To limit exchanges, some operators prefer using a single catheter (e.g., AL1, AL2, Kimny, Barbeau) for both left and right coronary angiography. Catheter exchanges should always be performed with a guidewire remaining in the ascending aorta.

Coronary intervention via transradial access requires only minor modifications relative to the femoral approach, but guiding catheter selection and lack of support are frequent sources of frustration during the learning phase. More than 90% of PCIs performed transradially at Brigham and Women's Hospital are performed with either XB/EBU 3.0 or 3.5, JR4, or hockey stick guides. Many alternative shapes are available for radial interventions, including among others, MAC, Kimny, Barbeau, Muta left, Muta right, radial, and Mann internal mammary. Intervention with 5F and 6F guiding catheters requires periodic deep catheter engagement for stent deployment (see Chapter 22). In larger male patients, it may be possible to use 7F or 8F guiding catheters—a long (23-cm) sheath should be used in these cases—but they should be introduced gradually and delicately. Sheath

changes should be performed with meticulous attention to hemostasis since compartment syndrome is a known and serious complication of even brief forearm bleeding. Antithrombotic therapy for transradial PCI is administered as per usual protocol for transfemoral procedures. Technical tips for diagnostic and interventional transradial procedures are reviewed by Barbeau (47).

Radial Sheaths are removed immediately after diagnostic angiography or coronary intervention in the cardiac catheterization laboratory. Since the radial artery is superficial and easily compressible and since transradial procedures are associated with only rare bleeding complications, ACT is not used to guide sheath removal in radial procedures. A compression strap (Hemo Band, Hemo Band Corp., Portland, OR; TR band, Terumo; Adapty, Nichiban Co., Japan) or device (Rad Stat, IEP Group, Inc., Raleigh, NC; RadiStop, Radi Medical Systems AB, Uppsala, Sweden) is placed directly over the radial artery puncture site and occlusive pressure is applied for approximately 90 minutes for diagnostic procedures and approximately 180 minutes for interventional procedures. Venous engorgement and paresthesias are not uncommon during compression. Care must be taken to avoid compression of the ulnar artery, which may be monitored using the modified Allen test with the pulse oximeter probe. In the absence of lingering sedation, immediate ambulation is permissible following transradial catheterization.

Major complications with transradial access are rare (41, 47a). The most common complication is radial artery occlusion, which has been documented by serial ultrasound studies in approximately 3% of patients. Occlusion is rarely associated with clinical symptoms as long as the Allen test showed patency of the palmar arch. Forearm hematomas require careful management to prevent progression to compartment syndrome. Placement of a second compression device proximal to the first is occasionally helpful in optimizing hemostasis. We have also seen two cases in which the radial artery adhered to the sheath so tenaciously that a segment of artery was transected and removed with the sheath, requiring immediate compression and vascular surgical repair! Access site infections and sterile abscesses, likely secondary to hydrophilic coating, have been reported (48). Repuncturing of the same radial artery in the days, weeks, or months following initial puncture is routine, although patency of the palmar arch should be ensured before each procedure. This is usually preferable to the use of both radial arteries over time, leaving one pristine for potential future use as a bypass conduit.

Institution of a transradial catheterization program requires a team approach within the cardiac catheterization laboratory and hospital wards. Preprocedural evaluation includes bilateral upper extremity blood pressure determination and a modified Allen test. Procedural modifications require additional equipment with the cardiac catheterization laboratory inventory. Postprocedural care requires meticulous attention to the radial artery compression device.

Lumbar Aortic Puncture

Percutaneous puncture of the lumbar aorta is a technique that has been used by radiologists to study patients with extensive peripheral vascular disease since the early 1980s and was then adapted to the performance of coronary angiography (49). More recently, this approach has even been used for coronary stent placement (50), although the fact that the procedure must be done with the patient prone complicates angiographic views and limits resuscitative efforts. The inability to apply direct pressure over the arterial entry site (the posterior wall of the aorta) also limits aggressive anticoagulation. Because of these negative factors, direct aortic puncture should be considered a last resort for vascular entry.

Trans-septal Puncture

With refinements and improvements in techniques for retrograde left heart catheterization, the use of trans-septal puncture for access to the left atrium and left ventricle (51,52) had become an infrequent procedure in most adult cardiac catheterization laboratories (53). In these laboratories, trans-septal puncture was reserved for situations in which direct left atrial pressure recording was desired (pulmonary venous disease), in which it was important to distinguish true idiopathic hypertrophic subaortic stenosis (IHSS) from catheter entrapment, or in which retrograde

left-sided heart catheterization had failed (e.g., owing to severe peripheral arterial disease or aortic stenosis) or was dangerous owing to the presence of a certain type of mechanical prosthetic valve (e.g., Bjork-Shiley or St. Jude valves). The infrequency with which the procedure was performed made it difficult for most laboratories to maintain operator expertise and to train cardiovascular fellows in trans-septal puncture and thus gave the procedure an aura of danger and intrigue. With the advent of percutaneous mitral valvuloplasty and antegrade aortic valvuloplasty using the Inoue balloon (54; Chapter 25), as well as the availability of improved equipment, trans-septal catheterization has again become a relatively common procedure (55).

The goal of trans-septal catheterization is to cross from the right atrium to the left atrium through the fossa ovalis. In approximately 10% of patients, this maneuver is performed inadvertently during right heart catheterization with a woven Dacron catheter because of the presence of a probe-patent foramen ovale, but in the remainder, mechanical puncture of this area with a needle and catheter combination is required to enter the left atrium. Although puncture of the fossa ovalis itself is quite safe, the danger of the trans-septal approach lies in the possibility that the needle and catheter will puncture an adjacent structure (i.e., the posterior wall of the right atrium, the coronary sinus, or the aortic root). To minimize this risk, the operator must have a detailed familiarity with the regional anatomy of the atrial septum (Fig. 4.15). As viewed from the feet with the patient lying supine, the plane of the atrial septum runs from 1 o'clock to 7 o'clock. The fossa ovalis is posterior and

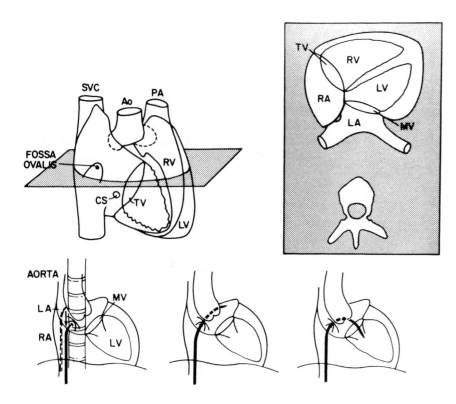

Figure 4.15 Regional anatomy for transseptal puncture. **Top left.** The position of the fossa ovalis is shown relative to the superior vena cava (SVC), aortic root (Ao), coronary sinus (CS), and tricuspid valve (TV). **Top right.** A cross section through the fossa (looking up from the feet) demonstrating the posteromedial direction of the interatrial septum (*bold line*) and the proximity of the lateral free wall of the right atrium. **Bottom row.** The appearance of the trans-septal catheter as it is withdrawn from the SVC in a posteromedial orientation. As the catheter tip slides over the aortic root (**bottom left,** *dotted position*) it appears to move rightward onto the spine. Slight further withdrawal leads to more rightward movement into the fossa (*solid position*). **Bottom center.** Puncture of the fossa with advancement of the catheter into the left atrium. **Bottom right.** Advancement into the left ventricle with the aid of a curved tip occluder. (Redrawn from Ross J Jr. Considerations regarding the technique for transseptal left heart catheterization. *Circulation* 1996;34:391.)

caudal to the aortic root and anterior to the free wall of the right atrium. The fossa ovalis is located superiorly and posteriorly to the ostium of the coronary sinus and well posterior of the tricuspid annulus and right atrial appendage. The fossa ovalis itself is approximately 2 cm in diameter and is bounded superiorly by a ridge—the limbus.

This anatomy can be distorted somewhat by the presence of aortic or mitral valve disease (56). In aortic stenosis, the plane of the septum becomes more vertical and the fossa may be located slightly more anteriorly. In mitral stenosis, the intra-atrial septum becomes flatter with a more horizontal orientation and the fossa tends to lie lower. Combined with the fact that the septum (and fossa) may then bulge into the right atrium, this makes detailed familiarity with the anatomy even more important when trans-septal catheterization is attempted in patients with advanced valvular heart disease. Several algorithms using fluoroscopic landmarks determined by right and left atrial angiography, or the position of a pigtail catheter in posterior (noncoronary) aortic sinus of Valsalva, have been developed to aid localization of the best site for trans-septal puncture (57,58; Fig. 4.16). Alternatively, intraprocedural transthoracic (59), transesophageal (60), or intracardiac (61–63) ultrasound may aid in identifying the optimal location for puncture of the intra-atrial septum (Fig. 4.17).

Classically, trans-septal catheterization is performed only from the right femoral vein, although the technique for a transjugular approach has also been described (63a). For the femoral approach we use a 70-cm curved Brockenbrough needle (USCI, Billerica, MA), which tapers from 18 gauge to 21 gauge at the tip (Fig. 4.18). The needle is introduced via a matching Brockenbrough catheter or 8F Mullins sheath and dilator combination (64; USCI) that has been inserted to the superior vena cava over a flexible 0.032-inch, 145-cm J guidewire. Once the wire has been removed and the catheter has been flushed, the Brockenbrough needle is advanced through the catheter, with an obturator (Bing stylet) protruding slightly beyond the tip of the needle to avoid abrasion or puncture of the catheter wall during needle advancement. As the needle and its stylet are advanced through the catheter, the patient may experience a slight pressure sensation owing to distortion of the venous structures by the rigid needle. During needle advancement, it is thus essential to allow the needle and its direction indicator to rotate freely so that it may follow the curves of the catheter and venous structures; the hub of the needle should never be grasped and rotated at this point. The progress of the needle tip should be monitored fluoroscopically, looking for any sign of perforation of the catheter by the needle. The stylet is then removed at the diaphragm, and the needle hub is connected to a pressure manifold, using a stopcock with a short length of tubing, and is carefully flushed. The needle is then advanced to lie just inside the tip of the catheter or sheath,

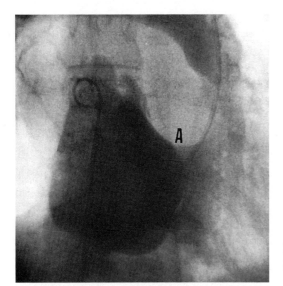 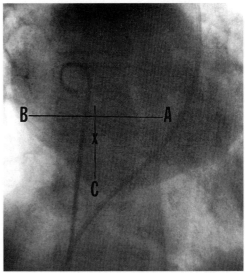

Figure 4.16 Fluoroscopic landmarks for localizing the fossa ovalis. **Left.** As described by Inoue, right atrial injection can be used to locate the upper corner of the tricuspid valve (*point A*), which is marked on the TV monitor. **Right.** Continued filming during the levophase fills the left atrium. A horizontal line is drawn from point A to the back wall of the left atrium, defining point B. That line is divided in half, and a vertical line is dropped to the floor of the left atrium, defining point C. The location of the fossa (X) is along this vertical line, approximately one vertebral body height above point C. When the borders of the left atrium are visible fluoroscopically, the position of a pigtail catheter in the noncoronary sinus of Valsalva can be substituted for point A, allowing localization of the ideal puncture site without contrast injection. A similar localization scheme (not shown) has been proposed in the 40° RAO projection by Croft and associates (reference 57), using the aortic pigtail and the posterior border of the left atrium. Puncture is made 1 to 3 cm below the midpoint of a line connecting the posterior wall of the aorta to the back wall of the left atrium.

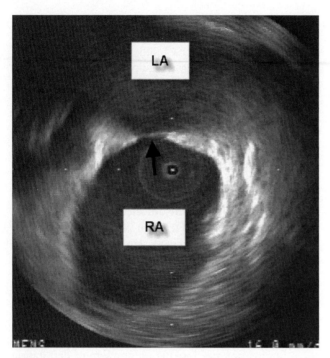

Figure 4.17 Intracardiac echo from within the right atrium (catheter at the center of the grid) shows the thin foramen ovale (arrow) and the left atrium clearly. Images during positioning of the trans-septal needle (not shown) show clear tenting of the foramen by the needle and reduce the uncertainty regarding correct puncture position.

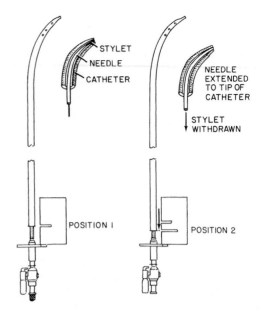

Figure 4.19 The Brockenbrough system with the needle and stylet inserted into the catheter. Ruler measurement of the distance from the catheter hub to the needle flange is shown with the tip of the stylet at the tip of the catheter (position 1) and with the stylet withdrawn and the needle tip extended to the tip of the catheter (position 2). (Redrawn from Ross J Jr. Considerations regarding the technique for trans-septal left heart catheterization. *Circulation* 1966;34:391.)

as indicated by measurements made by comparing the distance between the needle flange and the catheter hub to similar measurements made with a sterile ruler before insertion (Fig. 4.19). Alternatively, current high-quality fluoroscopy can be used to visually monitor advancement of the needle to the catheter tip.

The superior vena caval pressure should then be recorded through the needle, with the needle rotated so that the direc-

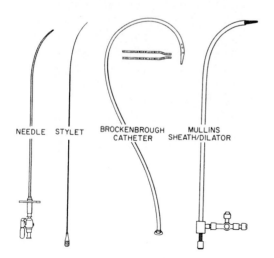

Figure 4.18 Equipment for trans-septal puncture. The Brockenbrough needle **(far left)** and Bing stylet **(left)** can be used in conjunction with the traditional Brockenbrough catheter **(center)** and Mullins sheath/dilator system **(right)**.

tion indicator points anteriorly. Under continuous fluoroscopic and pressure monitoring, the needle and catheter are then held in constant relationship as they are withdrawn slowly, using both hands. The direction indicator is firmly controlled with the right hand and used to rotate the needle clockwise during this withdrawal from the superior vena cava until the arrow is oriented posteromedially (4 o'clock when looking from below). As the tip of the catheter enters the right atrium, it moves slightly rightward (toward the patient's left). The needle and catheter are maintained in their posteromedial orientation, and they continue to be withdrawn slowly. As the catheter tip slips over the bulge of the ascending aorta, it again moves rightward to overlie the vertebrae in the anterior projection. Further slow withdrawal maintaining the 4 o'clock orientation will be associated with a third rightward movement as the catheter tip "snaps" into the fossa ovalis. This is confirmed by the fact that advancement will cause the catheter tip to flex slightly (rather than move back up the atrial septum) if its tip is lodged in the fossa. Clear fluoroscopic evidence of fossa engagement is thus essential to successful trans-septal puncture.

If the foramen is patent, the catheter may actually cross into the left atrium spontaneously at this point, as indicated by a change in atrial pressure waveform and the ability to withdraw oxygenated blood from the needle. Otherwise, the catheter is advanced slightly to flex its tip against the limbus at the superior portion of the foramen ovale. Once the operator is satisfied with this position, she or he advances the Brockenbrough needle smartly so that its point emerges from the tip of the catheter and perforates the atrial septum. Successful entry into the left atrium should be confirmed by both the recording of a left atrial pressure waveform and the withdrawal of oxygenated blood or the demonstration of the typical fluoroscopic appearance of the left atrium during a contrast puff through the needle. Once the operator is confident that the needle tip is across the interatrial septum, the needle and catheter are advanced as a unit a short distance into the left atrium, taking care to control their motion so that the protruding needle does not injure left atrial structures. When the catheter is across the atrial septum, the needle is withdrawn and the catheter is double-flushed vigorously and connected to a manifold for pressure recording.

The main risk during trans-septal catheterization is inadvertent puncture of adjacent structures (the aortic root, coronary sinus, or posterior free wall of the right atrium) rather than the fossa ovalis. As long as the patient is not anticoagulated and perforation is limited to the 21-gauge tip of the Brockenbrough needle (i.e., perforation is recognized and the catheter itself is not advanced), this is usually benign. However, if the 8F catheter itself is advanced into the pericardium or aortic root, potentially fatal complications may occur, underscoring the need for the operator to monitor closely the location of the trans-septal apparatus by fluoroscopic, pressure, and oxygen saturation at each stage of the procedure. Damped pressure waveform during attempted septal puncture may indicate puncture into the pericardium or simply incomplete penetration of a thickened interatrial septum. Injection of a small amount of contrast through the needle can be useful in this case by staining the atrial septum and allowing confirmation of an appropriate position in the left anterior oblique (LAO) and RAO projection before more forceful needle advancement is attempted. If the initial attempt at trans-septal puncture is unsuccessful, the operator may wish to repeat the catheter positioning procedure by removing the trans-septal needle from the catheter, withdrawing the catheter slightly, and reinserting the 0.032-inch guidewire into the superior vena cava. In general, one should never attempt to reposition the catheter–needle combination in the superior vena cava in any other way, since perforation of the right atrium or atrial appendage is a distinct possibility during such maneuvers.

Once the catheter is safely in the left atrium, additional manipulation may be required to enter the left ventricle. If the tip of the catheter has entered an inferior pulmonary vein (as evident by its projection outside the posterior heart border in the right anterior oblique projection), the left ventricle can be approached by torquing the catheter 180° in a counterclockwise direction so that its tip moves anteriorly as it is withdrawn slightly. As the catheter tip moves anteriorly and downward, further advancement will usually allow it to cross the mitral valve and enter the left ventricle. If not, it may be necessary to insert a curved tip occluder into the catheter through an O-ring side-arm adapter to tighten the tip curve and facilitate advancement

into the ventricle. By converting the Brockenbrough catheter from an end- and side-hole device to a side-hole-only device, the tip occluder also minimizes the chance for left ventricular staining and perforation during contrast ventriculography. However, contrast angiography at 8 to 10 mL/second for 40 to 50 mL total injection (as with the Sones catheter) can usually be accomplished safely without a tip occluder, if desired. Following the completion of hemodynamic and angiographic evaluation, the Brockenbrough catheter is withdrawn in the usual manner during continuous pressure recording.

The technique for trans-septal catheterization using the Mullins sheath (64) is similar, except that care must be taken to advance both the dilator and the 8F sheath into the left atrium without injuring the opposite left atrial wall. Slight counterclockwise rotation and repeated puffs of contrast to define location of the catheter tip may be helpful in this regard. Once the sheath is secure in the left atrium, the needle and dilator are withdrawn and the sheath is flushed carefully. Either a specially curved pigtail catheter (in patients with a normal mitral valve) or a CO_2-inflated balloon flotation catheter (in patients with mitral stenosis) may then be inserted through the sheath and passed into the left ventricle. The current Mullins sheath designs have a side-arm connection and back-bleed valve, allowing ongoing measurement of left atrial pressure around the left ventricular catheter. Another recent modification is the use of radiofrequency ablation rather than the Brockenbrough needle to pass through the atrial septum (65).

Complications of trans-septal catheterization are generally infrequent (needle tip perforation <%, tamponade <1%, and death <0.5%) in experienced hands. This is supported by experience in 1,279 cases from the Massachusetts General Hospital (66), 597 cases from Los Angeles (56), and 500 cases from Taiwan (58). The excellent results in these large series indicate that the technique for trans-septal puncture has not been lost (or may even have improved) since its first wave of popularity in the 1960s and 1970s! Because serious complications can occur and are significantly more common early in an operator's experience or in high-risk patients, however, performance of this procedure should be limited to a few operators at each site who can do enough annual procedures to perfect their technique. This is particularly true in patients with distorted anatomy owing to congenital heart disease, marked left or right atrial enlargement, significant chest or spine deformity, inability to lie flat, ongoing anticoagulation, or left atrial thrombus/tumor, in whom the technique should generally be avoided.

Apical Left Ventricular Puncture

Historically, a variety of direct puncture techniques were used to enter the cardiac chambers before the introduction of percutaneous left and right heart catheterization. These techniques included transbronchial (67) and transthoracic (68) approaches to the left atrium, the suprasternal puncture

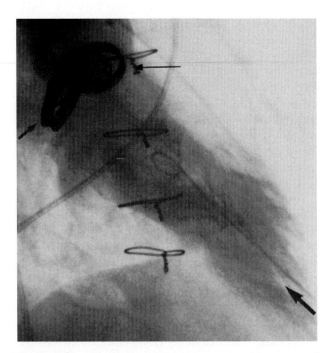

Figure 4.20 Apical left ventricular puncture. In this patient with Björk-Shiley aortic and mitral valve prostheses (*arrow, upper left*), percutaneous puncture of the left ventricular apex was performed to allow left ventricular pressure measurement and contrast ventriculography using a 4F angiographic pigtail catheter shown entering the LV apex (*arrow, lower right*). This catheter was advanced into the left ventricle over an 0.035-inch guide wire, following apical puncture with an 18-gauge thin-wall needle (see text for details).

technique of Radner (69), and apical left ventricular puncture (70,71). Of these, only the last has survived, albeit as an infrequent (roughly one per year in our laboratory) way to measure left ventricular pressure in a patient where retrograde and trans-septal catheterization of the LV are precluded by the presence of mechanical aortic and mitral prostheses.

The site of the apical impulse is located by palpation and confirmed by fluoroscopy of a hemostatic clamp placed at the intended puncture site. Alternatively, the true left ventricular apex can be located using echocardiography (72) and may be found to lie significantly more lateral than the palpated apical impulse in patients with right ventricular enlargement. After liberal local anesthesia, an 18-gauge needle (like that used for internal jugular puncture) is introduced at the apex and directed along the long axis of the left ventricle. This is accomplished by aiming the needle tip roughly toward the back of the right shoulder. Contact with the left ventricular wall can usually be felt as a distinct impulse (and the onset of ventricular premature beats). Sharp advancement of the needle at this point will cause its tip to enter the left ventricular cavity, with pulsatile ejection of blood.

In the technique of Semple (71), an outer Teflon catheter was then advanced over the puncture needle and into the left ventricle (sometimes out through the aortic

valve, as well). We, however, have preferred the technique in which a 0.035-inch 65-cm-long J guidewire is advanced through the needle and into the left ventricle under fluoroscopic guidance. This allows the advancement of a 4F dilator followed by a 4F pigtail catheter to allow pressure measurement and/or left ventricular angiography (Fig. 4.20).

One series describes excellent results of apical puncture in 102 patients (73), whereas a recent series from the Massachusetts General Hospital describes excellent results in 38 patients (74). A variation of apical puncture is a subxiphoid approach through the right ventricle and septum into the left ventricle (75). Major complications (tamponade or pneumothorax) occur in roughly 3% of patients, although tamponade is very rare in postoperative patients (who have adhesive pericardium). Other complications of apical puncture can include hemothorax, intramyocardial injection, and ventricular fibrillation, as well as pleuritic chest discomfort (approximately 10%) and reflex hypotension owing to vagal stimulation (approximately 5%). *We thus reserve this technique for patients in whom it is essential to enter the left ventricle and in whom neither retrograde nor anterograde (trans-septal) entry of the left ventricle is feasible.*

REFERENCES

1. Seldinger SI. Catheter replacement of the needle in percutaneous arteriography, a new technique. *Acta Radiol* 1953;39:368.
2. Judkins MP, Kidd HJ, Frische LH, Dotter CT. Lumen-following safety J-guide for catheterization of tortuous vessels. *Radiology* 1967;88:1127.
3. Barry WH, Levin DC, Green LH, et al. Left heart catheterization and angiography via the percutaneous femoral approach using an arterial sheath. *Cathet Cardiovasc Diagn* 1979;5:401.
4. Hillis LD: Percutaneous left heart catheterization and coronary arteriography using a femoral artery sheath. *Cathet Cardiovasc Diagn* 1979;5:393.
5. Noto TJ, Johnson LW, Krone R, et al. Cardiac catheterization 1990: a report of the registry of the Society for Cardiac Angiography and Interventions. *Cathet Cardiovasc Diagn* 1991;24:75.
6. Kim D, Orron DE, Skillman JJ, et al. Role of superficial femoral artery puncture in the development of pseudoaneurysm and arteriovenous fistula complicating percutaneous transfemoral cardiac catheterization. *Cathet Cardiovasc Diagn* 1992;25:91.
7. Ernst CB. Abdominal aortic aneurysm. *N Engl J Med* 1993;328:1167.
8. Smith DC, Willis WH. Transfemoral coronary arteriography via a prosthetic aortic bifurcation graft. *Cathet Cardiovasc Diagn* 1988;14:121.
9. Lesnefsky EJ, Carrea EP, Groves BM. Safety of cardiac catheterization via peripheral vascular grafts. *Cathet Cardiovasc Diagn* 1993;29:113.
10. Ferguson JJ, Dougherty KG, Gaos CM, Bush HD, Marsh KC, Leachman DR. Relationship between procedural activated clotting time and outcome after percutaneous transluminal coronary angioplasty. *J Am Coll Cardiol* 1994;23:1061.
11. Pepine CJ. ACC/AHA guidelines for cardiac catheterization and cardiac catheterization laboratories. *J Am Coll Cardiol* 1991;18:1149.
12. Dehmer GJ, Haagen D, Malloy CR, et al. Anticoagulation with heparin during cardiac catheterization and its reversal by protamine. *Cathet Cardiovasc Diagn* 1987;13:16.
13. Weiss ME, Nyhan D, Peng ZK, et al. Association of protamine IgE and IgG antibodies with life-threatening reactions to intravenous protamine. *N Engl J Med* 1989;320:886.

14. Krueger SK, Orme EC, King CS, Barry WH. Accurate determination of the transaortic valve gradient using simultaneous left ventricular and femoral artery pressures. *Cathet Cardiovasc Diagn* 1990; 16:202.

15. Jayne JE, Catherwood E, Niles NW, Friedman BJ. Double-lumen catheter assessment of aortic stenosis—comparison with separate catheter techniques. *Cathet Cardiovasc Diagn* 1993;29:157.

16. Harrison JK, Davidson CJ, Phillips HR, et al. A rapid, effective technique for retrograde crossing of valvular aortic stenosis using standard coronary catheters. *Cathet Cardiovasc Diagn* 1990;21:51.

17. Feldman T, Carroll JD, Chiu YC. An improved catheter design for crossing stenosed aortic valves. *Cathet Cardiovasc Diagn* 1989; 16:279.

18. MacDonald RG, Feldman RL, Pepine CJ. Retrograde catheterization of the left ventricle through tilting disc valves using a modified catheter system. *Am J Cardiol* 1984;54:1373.

19. Pracyk JB, Wall TC, Longabaugh P, et al. A randomized trial of vascular hemostasis techniques to reduce femoral vascular complications after coronary intervention. *Am J Cardiol* 1998;81:970.

20. Lau KW, Tan A, Kob TH, et al. Early ambulation following diagnostic 7-French cardiac catheterization—a prospective randomized trial. *Cathet Cardiovasc Diagn* 1993;28:34.

21. Hoffer EK, Bloch RD. Percutaneous arterial closure devices. *J Vasc Interv Radiol* 2003;14:865–885.

22. Brachmann J, Ansah M, Kosinski E, Schuler G. Improved clinical effectiveness with a collagen vascular hemostasis device for shortened immobilization time following diagnostic angiography and percutaneous transluminal coronary angioplasty. *Am J Cardiol* 1998;81:1502.

23. Aker UT, Kensey KR, Heuser RR, et al. Immediate arterial hemostasis after cardiac catheterization—initial experience with a new puncture closure device. *Cathet Cardiovasc Diagn* 1994;31:228.

24. Kussmaul WG, Buchbinder M , Whitlow P, et al. Rapid arterial hemostasis after cardiac catheterization and percutaneous transluminal angioplasty—results of a randomized trial of a novel homeostatic device. *J Am Coll Cardiol* 1995;25:1685.

25. Silber S, Gershony G, Schoen N, et al. A novel vascular sealing device for closure of percutaneous arterial access sites. *Am J Cardiol* 1999;83:1248.

26. Carere RG, Webb JG, et al. Initial experience with Prostar, a new device for percutaneous suture-mediated closure of the arterial puncture site. *Cathet Cardiovasc Diagn* 1996;37:367.

27. Baim DS, Knopf WD, Hinohara T, et al. Suture-mediated closure of the femoral access site after cardiac catheterization – results of the Suture To Ambulate aNd Discharge (STAND I and STAND II) trials. *Am J Cardiol* 2000;85:864–869.

28. Koreny M, et al. Arterial puncture closure devices compared with standard manual compression after cardiac catheterization – systematic review and meta-analysis. *JAMA* 2004;291:350–357.

29. Skillman JJ, Kim D, Baim DS. Vascular complications of percutaneous femoral cardiac interventions—incidence and operative repair. *Arch Surg* 1988;123:1207.

30. Mills JL, Wiedeman JE, Robison JG, Hallet JW. Minimizing mortality and morbidity from iatrogenic arterial injuries—the need for early recognition and prompt repair. *J Vasc Surg* 1986;4:22.

31. Kent KC, McArdle CR, Kennedy B, et al. A prospective study of the clinical outcome of femoral pseudoaneurysms and arteriovenous fistulas induced by arterial puncture. *J Vasc Surg* 1993; 17:125.

32. Lumsden AB, Miller JM, Kosinski AS, et al. A prospective evaluation of surgically treated groin complications following percutaneous cardiac procedures. *Am Surg* 1994;60:132.

33. Valeix B, Labrunie P, Jahjah F, et al. Selective coronary arteriography by percutaneous transaxillary approach. *Cathet Cardiovasc Diagn* 1984;10:403.

34. Molnar W, Paul DJ. Complication of axillary arteriotomies – analysis of 1762 consecutive studies. *Radiology* 1972;104;269.

35. Fergusson DJG, Kamada RO. Percutaneous entry of the brachial artery for left heart catheterization using a sheath: further experience. *Cathet Cardiovasc Diagn* 1986;12:209.

36. Cardenas JAR, Yellayi S, Schatz RA, Franklin M. A new method for brachial artery hemostasis following coronary angiography. *J Invas Cardiol* 1994;6:285.

37. Cohen M, Rentrop P, Cohen BM, Holt J. Safety and efficacy of percutaneous entry of the brachial artery versus cutdown arteriotomy for left-sided cardiac catheterization. *Am J Cardiol* 1986; 57:682.

38. Kiemeneij F, Laarman GJ, de Melker E. Transradial artery coronary angioplasty. *Am Heart J* 1995;129:1–7.

39. Campeau L. Percutaneous radial artery approach for coronary angiography. *Cathet Cardiovasc Diagn* 1989;16:39.

40. Mann T, Cubeddu G, Schneider J, et al. Right radial access for PTCA: a prospective study demonstrates reduced complications and hospital charges. *J Invas Cardiol* 1996;8:30–35.

41. Kiemeneij F, Laarman GJ, Odekerken D, Slagbloom T, Wieken R. A randomized comparison of percutaneous transluminal coronary angioplasty by the radial, brachial and femoral approaches – the access study. *J Am Coll Cardiol* 1997;29:1269.

42. Cohen DJ. Outpatient transradial coronary stenting: implications for cost-effectiveness. *J Invasive Cardiol* 1996;8(suppl D):36D–39D.

43. Cooper CJ, El-Shiekh RA, Cohen DJ, et al. Effects of transradial access on quality of life and cost of cardiac catheterization: a randomized comparison. *Am Heart J* 1999;138:430–436.

44. Mann T, Cowper PA, Peterson ED, et al. Transradial coronary stenting: comparison with femoral access closed with an arterial suture device. *Catheter Cardiovasc Interv* 2000;49:150–156.

45. Rihal CS, Holmes DR, Jr. Transradial cardiac catheterization: is femoral access obsolete? *Am Heart J* 1999;138:392–393.

46. Hovagim AR, Katz RI, Poppers PJ. Pulse oximetry for evaluation of radial and ulnar arterial blood flow. *J Cardiothorac Anesth* 1989;3:27–30.

47. Barbeau GR. Radial loop and extreme vessel tortuosity in the transradial approach: advantage of hydrophilic-coated guidewires and catheters. *Catheter Cardiovasc Interv* 2003;59: 442–450.

47a. Bazemore E, Mann JT. Problems and complications of the transradial approach for coronary interventions: a review. *J Invas Cardiol* 2005;17:156–159.

48. Kozak M, Adams DR, Ioffreda MD, et al. Sterile inflammation associated with transradial catheterization and hydrophilic sheaths. *Catheter Cardiovasc Interv* 2003;59:207–213.

49. Nath PH, Soto B, Holt JH, Satler LF. Selective coronary angiography by translumbar aortic puncture. *Am J Cardiol* 1983;52; 425.

50. Henry GA, et al. Placement of an intracoronary stent via translumbar puncture. *Cathet Cardiovasc Diagn* 1999;46;340.

51. Ross J Jr: Considerations regarding the technique for transseptal left heart catheterization. *Circulation* 1966;34:391.

52. Brockenbrough EC, Braunwald E. A new technique for left ventricular angiocardiography and transseptal left heart catheterization. *Am J Cardiol* 1960;6:1062.

53. Schoonmaker FW, Vijay NK, Jantz RD. Left atrial and ventricular transseptal catheterization review: losing skills? *Cathet Cardiovasc Diagn* 1987;13:233.

54. Eisenhauer AC, Hadjipetrou P, Piemonte TC. Balloon aortic valvuloplasty revisited: the role of the inoue balloon and transseptal antegrade approach. *Catheter Cardiovasc Interv* 2000; 50:484–491.

55. O'Keefe JH, Vlietstra RE, Hanley PC, et al. Revival of the transseptal approach for catheterization of the left atrium and ventricle. *Mayo Clin Proc* 1985;60:790.

56. Clugston R, Lau FYK, Ruiz C. Transseptal catheterization update 1992. *Cathet Cardiovasc Diagn* 1992;26:266.

57. Croft CH, Lipscomb K. Modified technique of transseptal left heart catheterization. *J Am Coll Cardiol* 1985;5:904.

58. Hung JS. Atrial puncture technique in percutaneous transvenous mitral commissurotomy, mitral valvuloplasty using the Inoue balloon catheter technique. *Cathet Cardiovasc Diagn* 1992; 26:275.

59. Kronzon I, Glassman E, Cohen M, et al. Use of two-dimensional echocardiography during transseptal cardiac catheterization. *J Am Coll Cardiol* 1984;4:425.

60. Ballal RS, Mahan EF 3rd, Nanda NC, et al. Utility of transesophageal echocardiography in interatrial septal puncture during percutaneous mitral balloon commissurotomy. *Am J Cardiol* 1990;66:230.

61. Hung JS, Fu M, Yeh KH, et al. Usefulness of intracardiac echocardiography in transseptal puncture during percutaneous transvenous mitral commissurotomy. *Am J Cardiol* 1993;72:853.

62. Szili-Torok T, Kimman G, Theuns D, et al. Transseptal left heart catheterisation guided by intracardiac echocardiography. *Heart* 2001;86:E11.

63. Hanaoka T, Suyama K, Taguchi A, et al. Shifting of puncture site in the fossa ovalis during radiofrequency catheter ablation: intracardiac echocardiography-guided transseptal left heart catheterization. *Jpn Heart J* 2003;44:673–680.

63a. Joseph G, Chandy S, George P, et al. Evaluation of a simplified transseptal mitral valvuloplasty technique using over-the-wire single balloons and complementary femoral and jugular venous approaches to 1,407 consecutive patients. *J Invas Cardiol* 2005; 17:132–138.

64. Mullins CE. Transseptal left heart catheterization: experience with a new technique in 520 pediatric and adult patients. *Ped Cardiol* 1983;4:239.

65. Justino H, Benson LN, Nykanen DG. Transcatheter creation of an atrial septal defect using radiofrequency perforation. *Catheter Cardiovasc Interv* 2001;54:83–87.

66. Roelke M, Smith AJC, Palacios IF. The technique and safety of transseptal left heart catheterization—the Massachusetts General Hospital experience with 1279 procedures. *Cathet Cardiovasc Diagn* 1994;32:332.

67. Morrow AG, Braunwald E, Lanenbaum HL. Transbronchial left heart catheterization: modified technique and its physiologic evaluation. *Surg Forum* 1958;8:390.

68. Bjork VD. Direct pressure measurement in the left atrium, the left ventricle and the aorta. *Acta Chir Scand* 1954;107:466.

69. Radner S. Extended suprasternal puncture technique. *Acta Med Scand* 1955;151:223.

70. Brock R, Milstein BB, Ross DN. Percutaneous left ventricular puncture in the assessment of aortic stenosis. *Thorax* 1956;11:163.

71. Semple T, McGuiness JB, Gardner H. Left heart catheterization by direct ventricular puncture. *Brit Heart J* 1968;30:402.

72. Vignola PA, Swaye PS, Gosselin AJ. Safe transthoracic left ventricular puncture performed with echocardiographic guidance. *Cathet Cardiovasc Diagn* 1980;6:317.

73. Morgan JM, Gray HH, Gelder C, et al. Left heart catheterization by direct ventricular puncture: withstanding the test of time. *Cathet Cardiovasc Diagn* 1989;16:87.

74. Walters DL, Sanchez PL, Rodriguez-Alemparte M, et al. Transthoracic left ventricular puncture for the assessment of patients with aortic and mitral valve prostheses: the Massachusetts General Hospital experience, 1989–2000. *Catheter Cardiovasc Interv* 2003;58:539–544.

75. Zuguchi M, Shindoh C, Chida K, et al. Safety and clinical benefits of transsubxiphoidal left ventricular puncture. *Catheter Cardiovasc Interv* 2002;55:58–65.

Brachial Cutdown Approach

5

Ronald P. Caputo[a]   *William Grossman*

Although once the dominant technical approach to cardiac catheterization and angiography, the brachial cutdown (or Sones) approach has decreased progressively in popularity over the past 30 years as the percutaneous femoral, brachial, and radial approaches described in Chapter 4 have risen to dominance. The brachial cutdown approach is now used in only a few (<10%) cardiac catheterization procedures, and the skills required for brachial arterial and venous cutdown and vascular repair are rapidly vanishing among the invasive cardiology community. Because this approach may still be of value in occasional patients, this chapter will summarize the technique as a guide for those learning to perform it, or as a refresher for those previously trained in the brachial approach who need to use this technique in a particular patient. The brachial cutdown approach, however, should *not* be used by an inexperienced operator unless backed up by a vascular surgeon or a cardiologist with expertise in this technique.

INDICATIONS

The brachial approach may be indicated for patients with (1) severe peripheral vascular disease, making upper extremity vascular access preferable; (2) urgent or emergent cardiac catheterization with an increased risk for bleeding (owing to chronic oral anticoagulation or recent thrombolytic therapy); (3) a need for early ambulation or mobility (outpatient procedures, severe back pain, and so on). Many of these situations can also be addressed by percutaneous radial artery catheterization (see Chapter 4), but the

brachial cutdown approach can provide the following additional advantages: (1) the ability to perform concomitant *right* heart catheterization in patients with suspected or known valvular heart disease, congestive heart failure, intracardiac shunts, and so on; (2) reliable arterial access with 7 French or greater catheter sizes; and (3) venous access to allow for foreign body retrieval (from the superior and inferior vena cava, right ventricle, or pulmonary artery).

Relative contraindications to brachial artery cutdown are few. They include absence of a brachial pulse, presence of an arteriovenous fistula, overlying soft tissue infection, severe ipsilateral axillary or subclavian vascular disease, and inability to extend the arm at the elbow or supinate the hand.

PREPROCEDURE EVALUATION

Proper preprocedure patient evaluation is critical for a successful brachial catheterization. Inspection and identification of the antecubital folds, biceps tendon, and medial and lateral epicondyles of the humerus takes only a few seconds but is essential. This inspection should be performed with the patient's arm extended and the hand supinated to assess for the ability to position the arm properly for the procedure. The general location for arterial cutdown will be approximated 2 to 3 cm above the antecubital skin folds, slightly superior to the level of the humeral epicondyles, and medial to the biceps tendon. A cutdown below this level is not recommended because the artery subsequently courses under the biceps tendons and bifurcates. A cutdown performed above this level is feasible, but may be awkward owing to the medial course of the artery.

[a] The contributions of Alessandro Giambartolomei and Paolo Esente to this chapter in the prior edition are gratefully acknowledged.

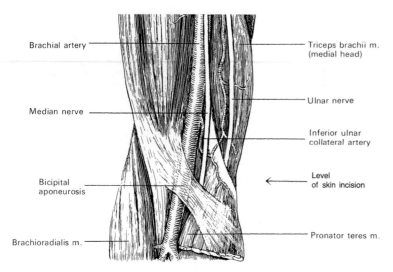

Brachial artery

Median nerve

Bicipital
aponeurosis

Brachioradialis m.

Triceps brachii m.
(medial head)

Ulnar nerve

Inferior ulnar
collateral artery

Level
of skin incision

Pronator teres m.

Figure 5.1 Anatomy of antecubital fossa illustrating course of the brachial artery. The artery is best sought at or slightly above the antecubital skin crease, medial to the bicipital aponeurosis. Care must be taken not to disturb the median nerve, which usually lies medial to the brachial artery. (From Clemente, C. *Gray's Anatomy of the Human Body*, 30th American ed. Philadelphia: Lea & Febiger, 1985.)

The brachial pulses should be carefully palpated bilaterally. A weak unilateral pulse usually indicates proximal vascular occlusive disease. Auscultation should be performed over the brachial, axillary, and subclavian areas to assess for bruits. A diminished pulse and/or bruits should lead the operator to anticipate proximal vascular occlusive disease and plan accordingly with consideration for a contralateral procedure, femoral access, or the use of soft and steerable guidewires. If a prior cutdown has been performed, the brachial pulse should be assessed 1 to 2 cm from the scar (to avoid the need to dissect through scar tissue with potential adhesions to the pervious arteriotomy site), with the new cutdown preferably performed proximally to the previous one.

INCISION, ISOLATION OF VESSELS, AND CATHETER INSERTION

With the direct brachial approach, a single cutdown is made in the right antecubital fossa, through which both

the brachial artery and vein can be isolated and used to perform left and right heart catheterization, respectively. With the arm fully extended flat on the armboard and the hand supinated, the brachial artery (Fig. 5.1) is identified by palpation and local anesthesia is induced in the overlying soft tissues using 1 to 2% lidocaine. This is first injected intradermally through a short 25- or 27-gauge needle to raise a bleb and then deeper using a long (1 1/2-inch) 22-gauge needle to infiltrate the subcutaneous, deep fascial, and periosteal tissues. Liberal amounts of 2% lidocaine are injected, 5 to 15 mL initially. During the course of the procedure, an additional four 4-mL aliquots of lidocaine may be applied topically within the incision. If anesthesia is achieved properly, the catheter insertion site ought to be virtually painless throughout the procedure.

Prior to starting the procedure, the proper instruments should be on hand, including the following: a no. 15 blade with handle, a no. 11 blade without a handle (or with a short handle) for improved control during arteriotomy, two or three curved hemostats, two straight hemostats, one self-retaining retractor, two soft tissue retractors, one small

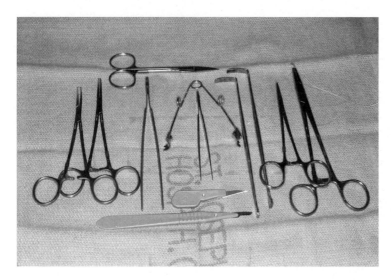

Figure 5.2 Instruments used for brachial cutdown: two Halstead curved 5-inch mosquito hemostats, one Halstead straight mosquito 5-inch hemostat, one thumb dressing 6-inch forceps without teeth, one straight iris forceps without teeth, one short-handled scalpel (no. 11 blade), one long-handled scalpel (no. 15 blade), one Grieshaber wire self-retaining retractor, two Davis double-end soft tissue retractors, one straight 4-inch iris scissors, and one Halsey 5-inch needle holder. All except scalpels are from Pilling Instruments, Washington, PA.

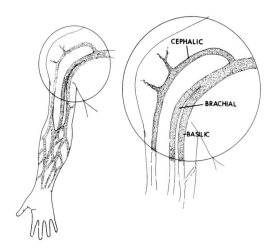

Figure 5.3 Venous anatomy of the arm. Brachial and basilic veins are medial to the cephalic vein within the antecubital fossa. Note that the brachial and basilic veins continue directly into the axillary and subclavian system, whereas the cephalic system frequently joins the subclavian vein at a right angle. Passage of a catheter from the cephalic system to the right atrium may thus be quite difficult; the medial veins provide the straightest pathway.

scissors, one needle holder, one toothless forceps, one small forceps, two segments of umbilical tape or vascular loops, 6.0 Prolene suture on a 3/8-inch needle, 3–0 absorbable suture with a curved needle, silk or chromic ties, and a vein lifter. These items are sufficient for almost all cases (Fig. 5.2).

A transverse incision is made with a no. 15 surgical blade just proximal to (i.e., approximately 2 cm above) the flexor crease. If right and left heart catheterization is contemplated, the incision is wide and made over the palpable brachial artery; if a right heart study alone is planned, the incision is narrow and made directly over a previously identified medial vein. Even large veins of the lateral antecubital fossae usually drain into the cephalic system, through which it may be difficult to navigate the catheter into the right atrium, whereas the medial veins drain into

either the basilic or brachial venous systems (which join the axillary vein by direct continuation and thus provide the easiest routes to the superior vena cava and right atrium [Fig. 5.3]).

The operator performs blunt dissection through the subcutaneous fat with a curved hemostat, simultaneously performing lateral retraction, while the assistant retracts medially. As the handheld retractors are applied to the lateral ends of the incision, the self-retaining retractor is applied superoinferiorly. This provides optimal exposure, particularly when substantial amounts of adipose tissue are present. After the fascia overlying the brachial artery is exposed, the artery is palpated again and blunt dissection through the fascia is then performed immediately overlying or *lateral* to the artery. This further decreases the chance for median nerve injury. When the artery is partially exposed, dissection is continued to separate the artery from adjacent veins and other structures.

At this point, the artery is easily recognized by its pulsation and characteristic silvery-white color. Veins, in contrast, are nonpulsatile, much darker in color, and usually of smaller caliber. The median nerve is yellowish with a slightly corrugated surface, and should not be further manipulated! A few patients have an accessory brachial artery, which is smaller and usually not suitable for catheterization. This vessel has a more superficial course and generally is not surrounded by veins, but deeper palpation will often reveal the location of the true brachial artery. The tissues are separated by blunt dissection with a curved Kelly forceps, and an appropriate vein is brought to the surface, separated from adjacent nerves and fascia, and tagged proximally and distally with a loop of 3–0 or 4–0 silk suture material. The brachial artery is similarly brought to the surface with a curved Kelly forceps, isolated from adjacent nerves, veins, and fascia, and tagged proximally and distally with moistened umbilical tape or silicone elastomer surgical tape (Retract-o-tape, Med-Pro Division, Quest Medical, Dallas, TX; Fig. 5.4).

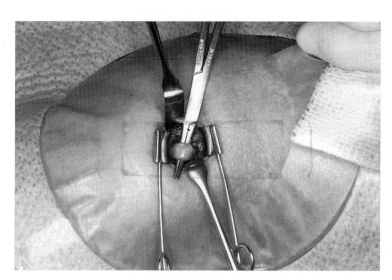

Figure 5.4 Isolation of the brachial artery. The incision is held open superoinferiorly by the self-retractor and laterally by the manual retractors while a curved hemostat is manipulated underneath the artery.

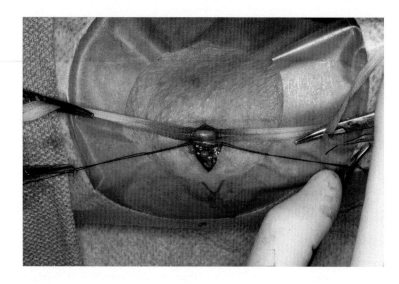

Figure 5.5 Isolating and securing the brachial artery and adjacent vein. The brachial artery is secured superiorly and inferiorly with moistened umbilical tapes fixed with curved hemostats. The isolated segment of vein is secured in similar fashion with 4–0 suture.

After isolating the brachial artery and basilic or brachial vein, an appropriate right heart catheter is selected and flushed. A 1- to 2-mm longitudinal incision is made in the vein with a no. 11 blade, and the catheter is introduced with the aid of either curved tissue forceps or a small plastic catheter introducer. Alternatively, the vein may be placed over a bridge formed by straight forceps to enable better control and to diminish oozing during passage of the catheter. Once the catheter has been introduced and passed a short distance, blood is aspirated, and the catheter is again flushed with heparinized solution. The catheter may then be connected either directly or by means of flexible plastic tubing to the side port of a manifold with an appropriate pressure transducer (see Chapter 7).

After passage of the right heart catheter (discussed below), the brachial artery is cleaned and positioned by applying gentle pressure on the hemostats or umbilical tapes using thumb and index finger to stretch the artery longitudinally (Fig. 5.5). This maneuver is critical because it allows for arterial positioning, stabilization, and (with

adequate tension) excellent hemostatic control. Most operators incise it transversely by making a small (2-mm) nick in its anterior surface with a no. 11 surgical blade. Others favor a *longitudinal* arteriotomy with the no. 11 surgical blade held at a 30° angle to the artery and the sharp edge facing upward (toward the ceiling) to minimize risk of injury to the posterior wall. The longitudinal direction requires a more cautious repair to avoid narrowing the lumen.

An appropriately selected left heart catheter (see the following section) is flushed. Tapered tip catheters, such as the Sones or multipurpose, can be inserted without a sheath (Fig. 5.6), but a sheath may be preferable when multiple catheter exchanges are planned or when catheters with a nontapered tip, such as guiding catheters for percutaneous coronary interventions, are used. To minimize the risk for arterial dissection during insertion of a relatively rigid arterial sheath, it should be introduced over a wire and carefully aspirated and flushed after insertion.

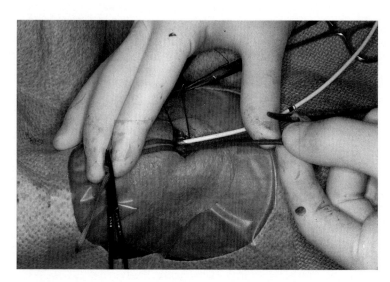

Figure 5.6 Insertion of an 8F Sones I catheter (Cordis Corp., Miami, FL) into the brachial artery during gentle retraction exerted by the thumb and index finger on umbilical tapes to control bleeding. A 7F balloon-tipped Swan-Ganz catheter has already been placed into the adjacent vein.

Many laboratories administer heparin solution (e.g., 50 units per kg) to help prevent thromboembolic events to the hand. This can be given into the distal brachial artery, central aorta, or intravenously.

Catheter Selection

Right Heart Catheters

When right heart catheterization is being performed only for measurement of right atrial, right ventricular, pulmonary artery, and pulmonary capillary wedge pressures, any of the end-hole catheters is adequate. Classic woven Dacron right heart catheters (e.g., Goodale-Lubin and Cournand, Fig. 5.7) have now been replaced by flow-directed balloon flotation catheters. Passage of the right heart catheter may occasionally produce transient right bundle branch block. Should this occur in a patient with pre-existing left bundle branch block, bilateral or complete heart block will develop and may require emergency ventricular pacing. If right-sided angiography is planned, a closed-end catheter with multiple side holes can be used (see Chapter 13).

Left Heart Catheters

When the direct brachial approach is used, potential catheters include both open-end and closed-end multiple-

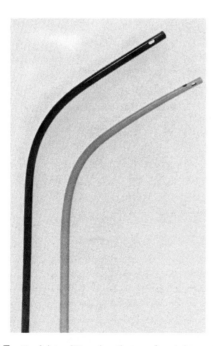

Figure 5.7 Useful traditional catheters for right and left heart catheterization. **Left.** The Goodale-Lubin catheter has an end-hole and two side-holes and is ideal for right heart catheterization, including measurement of pulmonary capillary wedge pressure. **Right.** The polyurethane Sones catheter tapers to a 5F tip with an end-hole and four side-holes; it is useful for coronary angiography and for left ventriculography (at low flow rates).

side-hole designs (used for left ventricular pressure measurement and angiography). The classic Sones B or a multipurpose catheter can also be used for most coronary and left ventriculographic purposes, although they tend to recoil at injection rates greater than 8 mL/second and have to be positioned carefully within the left ventricle to avoid myocardial staining. Pigtail catheters (7 or 8 French) should be used whenever contrast flows greater than 10 mL/second are needed.

Coronary angiography can usually be completed with the Sones catheter. Alternatively, Castillo 1, 2, or 3 type curves are available (Cordis Corp, Miami, FL) and are very useful for angiography of coronary artery bypass grafts, coronary engagement in patients with large aortic roots, and in situations where more forceful torque must be applied (see below). The Sones A type curve is also useful for patients with a high takeoff of the left coronary artery. Multipurpose type I and type II catheters have applications generally similar to the Sones. From the right brachial approach, the femoral mammary catheter is adequate for angiography of the right internal mammary artery, whereas the brachial mammary catheter is required for angiography of the left internal mammary (see below).

ADVANCING THE RIGHT HEART CATHETER

Both right and left heart catheters should be advanced as soon as possible after introduction into the vascular system, because letting them sit in the bloodstream at body temperature may result in loss of catheter stiffness and also diminishes catheter control. The right heart catheter is advanced under fluoroscopic control to the superior vena cava. If a balloon-tip catheter is used, advancement is generally straightforward. The description below applies to use of a nonballoon woven Dacron catheter and is presented because the technique may be useful for maneuvering other stiff catheters through the right heart.

If there is difficulty entering the superior vena cava, it is sometimes helpful to try the following maneuvers: Have the patient take a deep breath; raise the right arm and shoulder toward the head (ask the patient to shrug his or her right shoulder); turn the patient's head to the extreme left; remove the patient's pillow. On occasion, a guidewire may be helpful in passing from the subclavian vein into the superior vena cava. Arterial or venous spasm may develop and inhibit catheter movement. It may resolve if the catheter is withdrawn by a distance of 10 to 20 cm, and the same cocktail of intravenous nitroglycerine and diltiazem may be administered as used in radial artery catheterization. However, *intravenous* papaverine (30 to 60 mg) is often more efficacious (note, it should never be given intra-arterially because of intense local pain). Persisting in attempts to advance or manipulate the catheter in the presence of spasm produces pain, vagal reactions, and hypotension, and may convert a minor problem into a large one.

When the catheter tip has been advanced to the superior vena cava (SVC), the operator should draw a blood sample for oximetry. If the SVC blood oxygen saturation is substantially lower than the pulmonary artery oxygen saturation, a full oximetry run should be done (Chapter 9). To pass from the right atrium to right ventricle and pulmonary artery with a nonballoon catheter, a J loop technique should be tried first. The catheter is advanced so that its tip catches on the lateral right atrial wall and the catheter looks like the letter J on fluoroscopy (Fig. 5.8). Next, the catheter is rotated counterclockwise so that the tip of the J sweeps the anterior right atrial wall (thus avoid-

ing the coronary sinus, whose ostium lies posterior to the tricuspid valve) and jumps across the tricuspid valve into the right ventricle. Because the catheter usually still retains its J curve, its tip will now be pointing toward the right ventricular outflow tract and can easily be advanced into the pulmonary artery. Right ventricular pressure may be recorded during the transit or subsequently during the catheter pullback. It should never, however, be advanced against resistance, since perforation of the right ventricular outflow tract can occur.

The catheter is then advanced to the "wedge" position by having the patient take a deep breath and hold it while the catheter is advanced until its tip will go no farther and ceases to pulsate with the heart. Having the patient cough

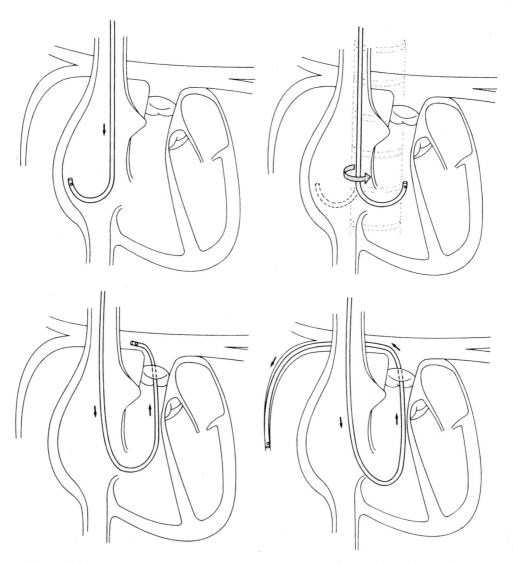

Figure 5.8 Advancing the right heart catheter. In navigating from right atrium to pulmonary artery, the J loop technique should be tried first. **Top left.** The catheter is advanced so that its tip catches on the lateral right atrial wall and forms the letter J. **Top right.** It is then rotated counterclockwise so that the catheter tip sweeps the anterior right atrial wall (thus avoiding the coronary sinus) and jumps across the tricuspid valve into the right ventricle. **Bottom left.** The catheter tip, pointing toward the right ventricular outflow tract, can be easily advanced into the pulmonary artery. **Bottom right.** The patient takes a deep breath, and the catheter is advanced to the "wedge" position (see text).

at this time will frequently advance the catheter tip into a true wedge position. The pressure waveform is examined, and if it has the appearance of a true wedge pressure, it is recorded. If there is any doubt that a true wedge position has been achieved, blood is sampled from the catheter. The pressure is confirmed as a true wedge pressure only if blood that is completely ($\geq$95) saturated with oxygen can be aspirated gently from the catheter (1). In patients who are hypoxemic, a wedge blood oxygen saturation of 90% or more may be accepted, especially if the oxygen saturation of pulmonary artery blood is much lower (e.g., $\leq$70). When mitral stenosis is not expected to be present, the wedge pressure may be confirmed simply by observing its typical waveform and its match against the simultaneously recorded left ventricular diastolic pressure. After measuring (and possibly confirming) the wedge pressure, the right heart catheter is withdrawn into the pulmonary artery.

If a Swan-Ganz catheter is used to obtain pulmonary capillary wedge pressure, it is often necessary to aspirate and discard the 5 to 15 mL of pulmonary artery blood that lie between the balloon and the pulmonary capillary bed before bright red pulmonary capillary blood can be sampled.

ADVANCING THE LEFT HEART CATHETER

After the right heart catheter has been advanced to the pulmonary artery or wedge position, an appropriately selected left heart catheter is inserted into the brachial artery as described previously. This catheter is then advanced into the ascending aorta just above the aortic valve. Although the Sones and multipurpose shapes can sometimes be advanced gently without a guidewire, advancement over a J-tipped guidewire is safer in the presence of subclavian disease or tortuosity. Passage may be aided by deep and held inspiration while lifting the chin and rotating the head leftward and over the left shoulder, but severe tortuosity may then impair catheter control once the aortic root has been reached.

Once the catheter is in the ascending aorta, central aortic pressure is measured and recorded. The catheter is then advanced across the aortic valve into the left ventricle by probing the valve with small to-and-fro excursions while gradually rotating the catheter through 360° so that the catheter tip moves up and down on the aortic valve over its entire plane. The soft-tipped Cordis polyurethane Sones catheter may be advanced directly (tip first) into the left ventricle, or it may be prolapsed across the aortic valve, loop first, as illustrated in Fig. 5.9. In severe aortic stenosis, the Sones catheter usually crosses tip first, but can be aided by insertion of a 0.035-inch straight guidewire (see Chapter 4). Success in crossing a tight aortic valve sometimes depends on the combination of experience, luck, and sheer determination.

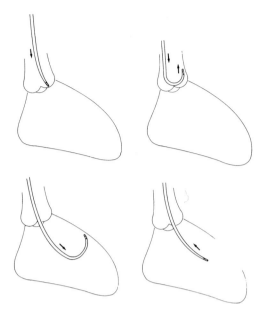

Figure 5.9 Technique for retrograde catheterization of the left ventricle using the Sones catheter. The catheter is advanced **(top left)** to touch the aortic valve. Further advancement usually produces a loop **(top right)** in the ascending aorta, which prolapses readily **(bottom left)** into the left ventricle. The catheter is then withdrawn **(bottom right)** to eliminate the loop and obtain a proper axial orientation for left ventriculography.

Once in the left ventricle, the full baseline hemodynamic measurements are made, including simultaneous pulmonary capillary wedge and left ventricular pressure recording. If a right heart catheterization was not performed, a special-purpose left heart catheter developed by Dr. Earl Shirey can be used for retrograde catheterization of the left atrium from the left ventricle. It can be prolapsed loop first into the left ventricle so that its tip faces the aortic and mitral valves (Fig. 5.10) rather than the left ventricular apex.

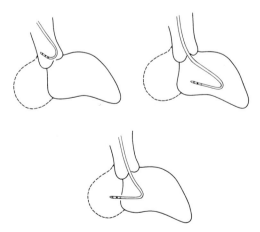

Figure 5.10 Retrograde catheterization of the left atrium using the Shirey catheter. It can be prolapsed loop-first into the left ventricle **(top left)** so that its tip faces the aortic and mitral valves **(top right)** rather than the left ventricular apex. Withdrawal of the redundant loop frequently guides the catheter tip into the left atrium **(bottom)**.

Withdrawal of the redundant loop frequently guides the catheter tip into the left atrium.

After completion of hemodynamic and cardiac output measurements (Chapter 8), most cardiac catheterization procedures today proceed to left ventriculography and coronary angiography. The details of these techniques as applied to both brachial and femoral approaches will be discussed in Chapters 11 and 12, but some special brachial techniques are described below.

SPECIAL TECHNIQUES

Coronary Bypass Grafts

Aortocoronary vein grafts have a high takeoff compared with coronary arteries; therefore, a longer-curve Sones or multipurpose catheter (such as a Sones A or MP 2) is preferable. Engagement techniques are similar to those used with native coronary arteries. When proximal vessel tortuosity limits maneuverability, when the aorta is dilated, and when the graft ostia are outside their usual locations, a preshaped catheter such as the Castillo or Amplatz type 2 or 3 curve is preferable.

Internal Mammary Arteries

The mammary arteries usually originate from the subclavian arteries with inferior takeoffs opposite to the origin of the vertebral arteries. Although the internal mammary artery is best engaged from an ipsilateral brachial approach using preformed femoral catheters, it is usually possible to engage the left mammary from the right brachial approach using one of two techniques. An Amplatz catheter (generally an AR 2 or AL 0.75) can be advanced to the aortic arch and engaged into the left subclavian artery through clockwise rotation. An exchange length wire is passed through this catheter into the subclavian artery and used to exchange the Amplatz for a femoral mammary catheter.

Anomalous Coronary Takeoff

Preshaped catheters with Castillo or Amplatz curves are preferable for anomalous origins not easily reached with the Sones or multipurpose curves. Some catheter recommendations for specific situations include the following:

1. Right coronary artery with inferior takeoff or horizontal heart—AR 2, Castillo 1
2. Right coronary artery with anterior takeoff—Castillo 1 or 2
3. Left coronary artery with a high takeoff—Castillo 3, Sones A, MP 1
4. Left circumflex coronary originating from the right coronary—AR 2, Castillo 1, if the Sones catheter overshoots the origin of the circumflex that is very proximal or is immediately adjacent to the right coronary ostium

5. Right coronary artery with anomalous takeoff from the left sinus of Valsalva or left coronary artery arising from the right sinus of Valsalva—Castillo 2 or 3 to "scan" the aortic wall seeking the ostium

Percutaneous Coronary Interventions

A sheath should always be inserted into the brachial artery for these procedures, as guiding catheters are nontapered and difficult to insert without causing arterial trauma. The sheath can be secured to the skin with a suture or by wrapping the umbilical tape loops around the hub. This helps to stabilize the sheath during catheter manipulations. Guiding catheters must always be inserted over a wire because of their reduced flexibility and sharp edges. The 6F or 7F catheter sizes are often useful for PTCA and stenting (see Chapters 22 and 24). Because of the size of the brachial artery, 8F catheters may be used for rotational atherectomy, kissing balloons, large profile stents, or when extra support is needed. Visual assessment of brachial artery size will allow the operator to assess its suitability for the 10F catheter often required for directional coronary atherectomy.

The following guiding catheter shapes are suggested for the brachial approach.

Right Coronary. The secondary curve of guiding catheters advanced from the right brachial position necessarily lies against the left wall of the aorta yielding superior backup support when compared with catheters advanced from the femoral position. Therefore, we often prefer the right brachial approach in cases of severe right coronary tortuosity, calcification, and so on. The hockey stick design is usually optimal; however, in patients with a small aorta, an AR 2 may be needed. When deep seating of the catheter is required, the AL 0.75 type 1 or 2 curve is useful.

Left Coronary. Amplatz shapes AL 0.75 through AL 3 are excellent, especially when engaging a left main coronary with a superior takeoff or when approaching a left anterior descending coronary with superior angulation. Other useful curves include the JCL or Q, Voda or XB, and Kimny (6 French). From the left brachial approach, standard femoral guiding catheter shapes can be used.

Bypass Grafts. Amplatz 1, 2, and 3, hockey stick and multipurpose shapes are usually adequate.

REPAIR OF VESSELS AND AFTERCARE

After the completion of diagnostic studies, the left heart catheter is removed and the brachial arteriotomy is repaired. Repair may be done in many ways (purse string, interrupted, continuous sutures). Prior to initiation arterial repair release, pressure on the proximal loop is released

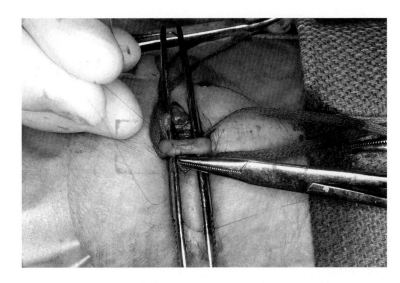

Figure 5.11 Suture repair of the brachial arteriotomy. The artery is stabilized by placing a large forceps underneath in transverse orientation. A stay suture has been placed above the superior margin of the longitudinal incision. Lock-stitch running sutures will be placed beyond the inferior margin of the incision to close the arteriotomy.

briefly to allow generous antegrade bleeding and flush out thrombi that may have formed around the catheter. The proximal bleeding is then controlled, and pressure on the distal umbilical tape is released to allow for retrograde (collateral-fed) bleeding to ensure patency of the distal artery. If there is brisk back-bleeding, no further maneuvers are indicated and arterial closure can commence. If no back-bleeding is present, the area overlying the radial and distal brachial artery should be manually "milked" or massaged in distal to proximal fashion to dislodge and remove any thromboemboli. If there is still no retrograde flow, a Sones or multipurpose catheter can be inserted distally through the arteriotomy, carefully advanced until resistance is met, and then slowly withdrawn while gentle suction is applied to its lumen with a syringe. If these maneuvers fail to restore back-bleeding, a Fogarty embolectomy procedure is then warranted. Dr. Grossman has traditionally favored routine use of a Fogarty arterial embolectomy catheter (Arterial embolectomy catheter; 3F, 40 cm, Shiley Laboratories, Irvine, CA) is used (11).

A common approach to arteriotomy repair calls for stabilization of the vessel by applying pressure with the umbilical tapes or placing a large forceps transversely beneath the artery. A stay suture is placed approximately 1 mm above the proximal end of the arteriotomy, and a continuous lock-stitch is created with sutures evenly spaced at 0.5-mm intervals (Fig. 5.11). The lock-stitch is closed with a second stay suture located 1 to 2 mm distal to the incision (Fig. 5.12). Minor bleeding around the sutures can often be controlled with gentle manual pressure and/or temporary application of a small Gelfoam pad. Once the assistant has confirmed the presence of an adequate radial pulse, the skin and subcutaneous tissues are closed using absorbable suture material and the subcutaneous technique. Two or three 1/4-inch Steri-strips are then applied in transverse fashion across the incision. A small Telfa pad coated with an antibacterial ointment is applied directly over the site and covered with a small stack of 4 × 4 gauze pads that are then wrapped in firm fashion with a 3-inch-wide Ace bandage.

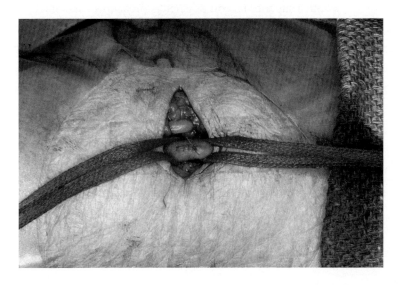

Figure 5.12 Completed repair of a brachial arteriotomy.

Dr. Grossman has favored administration of 10 to 15 mL of a concentrated solution of heparinized saline (3,000 IU of heparin in 30 mL normal saline) into the proximal and distal artery through the Sones catheter, locking this into the vessel by application of a vascular bulldog-type clamp (DeBakey peripheral vascular bulldog clamps with 45 to 60° angled jaws, V. Mueller, Chicago, IL) as far above and below the arteriotomy as possible (Fig. 5.13). He then placed a stay suture at each end of the arteriotomy and closed it with a continuous or running stitch of fine non-wettable suture material such as 6–0 Tevdek (Tevdek, Deknatel Company, Queens Village, NY). The stay suture at one end of the incision is the start of the running stitch, and the stitch is completed by tying to the other stay suture. The advantage of a continuous suture is that it tightens as the artery expands after the clamps are removed.

After suturing the artery, he removed the distal bulldog clamp first and then massaged the forearm gently from the wrist toward the elbow to milk out any air within the lumen of the artery before releasing the proximal bulldog clamp. The proximal clamp was then removed, and any minor leaks were controlled by direct finger pressure while ensuring that the radial pulse could be palpated. If leaking did not stop within a few minutes of such finger pressure, an additional suture or two was required. In this procedure, if the radial pulse is not palpable and essentially of the same amplitude as before the arteriotomy, the artery may be reopened and a Fogarty catheter again passed proximally and distally. When unsuccessful, prompt consultation should be obtained with an experienced vascular surgeon who usually will be able to identify and correct the problem. After repairing the arteriotomy successfully, the vein used in the right heart catheterization may be tied off or repaired (a purse string repair is usually adequate), followed by flushing the wound with copious quantities of fresh sterile saline solution followed by 10% povidone-iodine

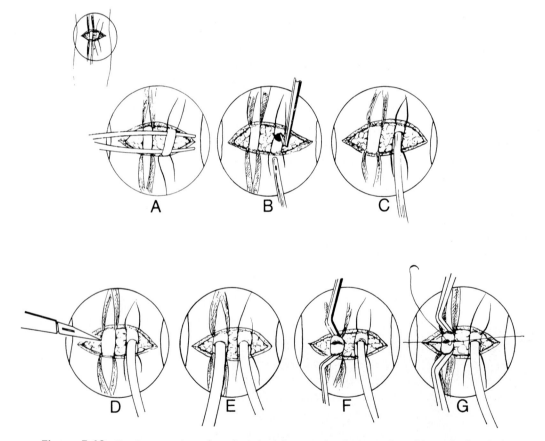

Figure 5.13 Dr. Grossman's preferred method for vessel isolation and repair. **A.** The brachial artery and vein have been isolated. Both are tagged proximally and distally, the artery with moist umbilical or silicone-elastomer tape, the vein with 3–0 silk. The vein has been placed over a bridge formed by a straight forceps to enable better control. **B.** The vein has been incised with a small scissors, and the catheter is about to be inserted with the aid of a plastic catheter introducer. **C.** Passage of the right heart catheter. **D.** Incision of the brachial artery with a no. 11 surgical blade. The cutting edge of the blade is facing upward, and the point approaches the artery from the side and at an angle of 10 to 20° to the horizontal to avoid perforating the posterior wall. **E.** Passage of the left heart catheter. **F.** In preparation for arterial repair, concentrated heparinized saline solution is locked in the vessel by placing bulldog clamps as far above and below the arteriotomy as possible (see text). **G.** Closure of the arteriotomy by continuous or running stitch. Stay sutures are placed at each end of the arteriotomy (see text).

solution (Pharmadine, Sherwood Pharmaceutical, Mahwah, NJ). The skin is closed using a subcuticular stitch of an absorbable suture (4–0 Dexon Plus, Davis and Geck, Inc., Manati, Puerto Rico, on a cutting needle), thereby avoiding the need for suture removal. Antibiotic ointment is placed on the suture line and covered with a firm dressing (although not so firm that it diminishes the radial pulse).

During the postprocedure period, blood pressure measurements should not be performed on the arm for 24 hours. Distal pulses, sensation, motor function, and local bleeding should be assessed, without unwrapping the Ace bandage. The Ace bandage is first released 2 hours following the procedure to reassess the surgical site and then rewrapped firmly but comfortably for 48 hours. The incision should be kept dry for at least 3 days, with the Steri-Strips removed in one week.

TROUBLESHOOTING

Loss of Radial Pulse

The most frequent causes of an absent or diminished radial pulse following a brachial procedure are the following: thrombosis at the arteriotomy site, embolization to the radial artery, dissection at the arteriotomy site, inappropriate suturing, and spasm. If arterial spasm was not a factor during catheter manipulation, it is unlikely to develop after arteriotomy repair and, therefore, should not be assumed to be responsible for a poor radial pulse. When the radial pulse is absent, the artery should be reisolated and secured with umbilical tapes and curved hemostats. The arteriotomy sutures are then carefully removed and antegrade and retrograde bleeding reassessed. If proximal and distal blood flows are normal, a problem with the initial arterial closure should be suspected (e.g., suturing through the posterior wall of the artery, creation of a significant cross-sectional narrowing of the arterial lumen, and so on). The arteriotomy should then be carefully resutured to avoid such problems.

If blood flow remains diminished from either direction, further massaging or milking of the artery is performed, as described previously, to dislodge and flush out any thrombi. The arteriotomy can be inspected proximally and distally to assess for a dissection flap by inserting a small forceps. If a dissection is evident, the true arterial lumen should be located with the small forceps and a soft tipped catheter (Sones) carefully inserted a short distance to act as a stent to appose all layers of the arterial wall. While the catheter is in place, two or three interrupted sutures are used to bind the layers of the arterial wall together, and the arteriotomy is then repaired. When dissection is not evident, the catheter aspiration maneuver described earlier should be performed before resorting to passage of a no. 3 Fogarty catheter. Following embolectomy, the arteriotomy

is resutured, slightly extending the length and depth of the suture line in order to tack down any intimal disruptions (flaps). If the radial pulse is re-established but diminished, this may be due to arterial spasm. Administration of oral nifedipine (10 mg) or intravenous papaverine (30 mg) is frequently beneficial, but prompt consultation with a vascular surgeon is imperative if a radial pulse is not re-established, particularly if signs of neurovascular compromise are present.

Hand Numbness

Hand numbness may result from impaired circulation or median nerve compromise. If the brachial dressing is not overly tight and the radial pulse is palpable, the cause of numbness is unlikely to be circulatory. Severe median nerve injury during cutdown is usually apparent immediately as the patient experiences a striking and characteristic discomfort (electric shock sensation). The most common cause of later median nerve injury is compression induced by hematoma formation following skin closure. This usually develops gradually over the course of several hours postprocedure and should be evacuated promptly to avoid potentially irreversible damage from long-standing median nerve compression.

REFERENCES

1. Rapaport E, Dexter L. Pulmonary capillary pressure. *Methods Med Res* 1958;7:85.
2. Dexter L, Burwell CS, Haynes FW, Seibel RE. Oxygen content of pulmonary "capillary" blood in unanesthetized human beings. *J Clin Invest* 1946;25:913.
3. Dexter L, et al. Studies of congenital heart disease, II: the pressure and oxygen content of blood in the right auricle, right ventricle and pulmonary artery in control patients, with observations on the oxygen saturation and source of pulmonary "capillary" blood. *J Clin Invest* 1947;26:554.
4. Hellens HK, Haynes FW, Dexter L. Pulmonary "capillary" pressure in man. *J Appl Physiol* 1949;2:24.
5. Werko L, Varnauskas E, Eliasch H, et al. Further evidence that the pulmonary capillary venous pressure pulse in man reflects cyclic changes in the left atrium. *Circ Res* 1953;1:337.
6. Connolly DC, Kirklin JW, Wood EH. The relationship between pulmonary artery wedge pressure and left atrial pressure in man. *Circ Res* 1954;2:434.
7. Batson GA, Chandrasekhar KP, Payas Y, Rickards DF. Measurement of pulmonary wedge pressure by the flow directed Swan-Ganz catheter. *Cardiovasc Res* 1972;6:748.
8. Schoenfeld MH, Palacios IF, Hutter AM, Jacoby SS, Block PC. Underestimation of prosthetic mitral valve areas: role of transseptal catheterization in avoiding unnecessary repeat mitral valve surgery. *J Am Coll Cardiol* 1985;5:1387.
9. Hosenpud JD, McAnulty JH, Morton MJ. Overestimation of mitral valve gradients obtained by phasic pulmonary capillary wedge pressure. *Cathet Cardiovasc Diagn* 1983;9:283.
10. Lange RA, Moore DM Jr, Cigarroa RG, Hillis LD. Use of pulmonary capillary wedge pressure to assess severity of mitral stenosis: is true left atrial pressure needed in this condition? *J Am Coll Cardiol* 1989;13:825.
11. Baker LD, Leshin SJ, Mathur VS, Messer JV. Routine Fogarty thrombectomy in arterial catheterization. *N Engl J Med* 1968;279:1203.

6

Diagnostic Catheterization in Childhood and Adult Congenital Heart Disease

Michael J. Landzberg, MD   *James E. Lock, MD*

Although congenital heart disease is generally the province of pediatric cardiologists or adult cardiologists with additional training in congenital heart disease, previously unrecognized or surgically corrected congenital defects are sometimes encountered in the course of adult cardiac catheterization. In addition, some defects such as patent foramen ovale are common, have been implicated in the causation of stroke owing to paradoxic embolization, and may become a target for catheter-based intervention based on the several closure devices now in clinical trials. Although this field cannot be covered comprehensively in a text such as this one, this chapter on diagnostic techniques, Chapter 27 on interventional techniques, and Chapter 33 on profiles in congenital heart disease should offer a basic overview of the current range of diagnostic and therapeutic procedures and access to some of the key current literature. Anyone wishing further training in this field is urged to partner with experienced pediatric or adult congenital cardiologists in the institution or region.

Like other areas of valvular heart disease and ventricular function, progressive advances in noninvasive anatomic and physiologic imaging modalities have provided generally accurate pictures of congenital heart disease. However, precise catheter-based definition of anatomy and physiology remains invaluable in the primary and adjunctive management of many pediatric and older patients with congenital heart disease. In particular, catheterization in this challenging patient group improves the definition of:

1. The varying and sometimes unique anatomy and associated physiologic consequences of natural (unoperated) and postoperated defects (Table 6.1)
2. The inter-relationship and codependency of the pulmonary (ventricle/vasculature/parenchymal) and the systemic circulation in these defects
3. The correlation between anatomic defects and physiologic function
4. Precise angiographic resolution of small (<2 to 3 mm) or tortuous structures, and accurate definition of multiple entry or exit sites or connections (1)
5. The increasing interaction of congenital defects with premature acquired disease (hypertension, reduced left ventricular compliance, neuro-hormonal responses (2)

In past decades, most patients with congenital heart disease presented with one of several classes of "simple" anatomy or physiology. These included *obstructions* (pulmonary/aortic stenosis [PS/AS], aortic coarctation [CoA]), and *intravascular shunts* (atrial/ventricular septal defects [ASD/VSD], patent ductus arteriosus [PDA]). At present, most surviving patients have increasingly complex

TABLE 6.1

CONFOUNDING PHYSIOLOGIC ABNORMALITIES IN PATIENTS WITH CONGENITAL HEART DISEASE

Abnormalities in atrial, or preventricular, transport
Alterations in pulmonary blood flow (quantity, pulsatility, resistance)
Variations in pulmonary capacitance (conduit vessels)
Shunt-, obstruction-, or impedance-related changes in ventricular loading conditions
Myocardial-pericardial interaction
Abnormalities of electrical conduction

anatomy and physiology (3), in part owing to the fact that >60% of adult congenital heart disease (ACHD) patients have had at least one surgery in childhood (approximately half with a reoperation during adulthood). A complete review of every aspect of each individual's "natural" and prior operated history (Table 6.2), with particular attention to the specifics of each intervention, is required prior to embarking on any catheter-based investigation (Table 6.3). This should be coupled with a full understanding of potential anatomic and physiologic variations and sequelae, as well as preparation for selecting and performing an addi-

tional intervention, as needed. As in patients with acquired heart disease, a detailed preprocedural investigational plan, with attention to adequately trained support staff, available equipment, trained operators, and adequate pre procedural and postprocedural monitoring, is required.

GENERAL PRINCIPLES IN THE CATHETERIZATION OF PATIENTS WITH CONGENITAL HEART DISEASE

Vascular Access/Vessel and Chamber Entry

Although usually femoral or jugular arterial and venous access can be used in larger children and adults (see Chapter 4), special access routes are usually required in neonates and infants. Options for vascular access vary depending on body habitus, vessel patency, and the area to be accessed. Patient size, chamber dilation, and vessel distortion present additional technical challenges, which can usually be overcome by an experienced operator.

Umbilical Vessels

Umbilical vessels have decreasing patency over the first 72 postnatal hours, but their use allows sparing of other vessels.

TABLE 6.2

TYPICAL CATEGORIZATION OF SURGICAL REPAIRS[a]

Name	Typical Lesion Application	Surgical Connection	
Glenn (classic)	Single ventricle/TA	SVC to (right) pulmonary artery	End to end
(bidirectional)	Single ventricle/TA	SVC to R/MPA	End to side
Fontan (atriopulmonary)	Single ventricle/TA	Atrial appendage to RV or PA	
(cavopulmonary)		IVC-SVC intracardiac or extracardiac baffle to PAs	
Waterston	TOF/DORV/pulmonary atresia	Ascending aorta to RPA	Side to side
Pott	TOF/DORV/pulmonary atresia	Descending aorta to LPA	Side to side
Blalock-Taussig (classic)	TOF/DORV/pulmonary atresia	Subclavian artery to branch PA	End to side
(modified)	TOF/DORV/pulmonary atresia	Conduit from subclavian artery to branch PA	Side to side
Mustard/Senning (atrial switch)	TGA	Baffle directing SVC-IVC flow to subpulmonary LV, pulmonary venous flow to subsystemic RV	End to end
Arterial switch	TGA	Translocation of more-posterior MPA to anterior supra-LV position, more-anterior aorta to posterior supra-PA position, coronary arterial reimplantation	
Rastelli	TGA/TOF	Conduit between subpulmonary ventricle and PA	
Norwood	HLHS	Translocation of proximal MPA to supra-LV position, end-to-side anastomosis of distal MPA to aorta, modified Blalock-Taussig shunt	
Double switch	TGA	Atrial switch plus arterial switch	

[a] All patients have variations mandating detailed review of operative reporting. DORV, double-outlet right ventricle; HLHS, hypoplastic left heart syndrome; IVC, inferior vena cava; LPA, left pulmonary artery; LV, left ventricle; MPA, main pulmonary artery; PA, pulmonary artery; RPA, right pulmonary artery; RV, right ventricle; SVC, superior vena cava; TA, tricuspid atresia; TGA, transposition of the great arteries (L, left, D, right); TOF, tetralogy of Fallot.

TABLE 6.3

TYPICAL INDICATIONS FOR DIAGNOSTIC CATHETERIZATIONS, PREFERRED IMAGING MODALITIES, AND INTERVENTIONS

Typical Lesion(s)	Diagnostic Cath Typical Indications	Preferred Imaging Modalities	Cath Indication: Interventional
ASD secundum	No: useful for PVR when PHT suspect → ASD test occlusion; PHT vasodilator testing; HD-based management of RV and LV dysfunction	TEE/ICE	ASD closure
PFO	No	TEE/ICE	PFO closure when indicated
ASD sinus venosus	Debated: higher incidence PHT: useful for PVR when PHT suspect; see above	MRI	
ASD primum	No	TEE	
AV canal defect	No: with increasing age, increased risk of PHT → check PVR; see above	TEE	
TAPVR	Debated: PVR, PV anatomy and rule out stenoses	Cath/MRI	
VSD (membranous)	No; uncommon need to assess PVR	TTE/MRI	Investigational closure
VSD (multiple muscular)	No; HD-based management of ventricular dysfunction, when indicated	TTE/MRI	VSD closure
Ao stenosis/regurgitation: subvalvar/supravalvar	Debated: Hemodynamic changes remain the standard for intervention in children and young adults with valvar AS Supravalvar AS: useful to define relationship to CA origins AR: demonstration of fistulous connections when indicated	TTE/TEE/MRI	AS: valve dilations
Aortic coarctation	No: Hemodynamic changes remain the standard for intervention in children and adults	MRI	Dilation/stent
PDA	No: PA pressure when PHT suspect → PDA test occlusion	TTE/MRI	PDA closure
Valvar PS	No: HD-based management of RV failure when appropriate	TTE/MRI	Valve dilation
Peripheral PS	No: HD-based management of RV failure or PHT when appropriate	Nuclear scintigraphy/MRI	PA dilation/stent
TOF preop	No: Anatomy when CAs, VSDs, Ao-PA collaterals cannot be sufficiently imaged otherwise	TTE/MRI	Close muscular VSDs
TOF postop	Assess for residual shunts; HD-based management of RV or LV dysfunction; PHT therapy	TTE/MRI	Close residual shunts /VSDs; PA or conduit dilation/stent
TOF pulmonary atresia	Yes: define PA anatomy and hemodynamics	MRI	Close Ao-PA connections; dilate/stent stenoses
Pulmonary atresia/intact septum	In children: define coronary anatomy; in adults: define CA anatomy or HD-based management of ventricular dysfunction, as indicated		
TGA-D preop	No	TTE	Atrial septostomy
TGA-D postop atrial switch	Assessment of residual shunting; HD-based management of systemic ventricular dysfunction or PHT	MRI	Shunt closure
TGA-D VSD/PS; truncus; DORV postop	No; HD-based management of systemic ventricular dysfunction or PHT	MRI	Shunt closure; conduit dilation/stent
TGA-D postop arterial switch	Assessment of PA stenoses, coronary arterial stenoses	MRI; IVUS	CA dilation/stent
TGA-L	HD-based management of systemic ventricular dysfunction	MRI	
Single ventricle preop	Yes: hemodynamics/PVR	TTE/MRI	Close collaterals, PA dilation/stent
Single ventricle post Fontan	Yes: HD-based management of load and ventricular function	MRI	Conduit and PA dilation/stent; close collaterals

Ao, aorta; AR, aortic regurgitation; AS, aortic stenosis; ASD, atrial septal defect; AV, atrioventricular; CA, coronary artery; DORV, double-outlet right ventricle; HD, hemodynamics; ICE, intracardiac echocardiography; IVUS, intravascular ultrasonography; LV, left ventricle; MRI, magnetic resonance imaging; PA, pulmonary artery; PFO, patent foramen ovale; PHT, pulmonary hypertension; PS, pulmonary stenosis; PV, pulmonary valve; PVR, pulmonary vascular resistance; RV, right ventricle; TAPVR, total anomalous pulmonary venous return; TEE, transesophageal echocardiography; TGA, transposition of the great arteries (L, left; D, right); TOF, tetralogy of Fallot; TTE, transthoracic echocardiography; VSD, ventricular septal defect.

Vascular access via the umbilical vein (5 French umbilical catheter entry) directs the catheter position posteriorly in the right atrium, which assists balloon atrial septostomy but adds considerable difficulty to achieving stable access to the right ventricle (RV) and pulmonary artery (PA). Given the nearly 180° turns involved in catheter passage (umbilical vein [UV] → portal vein → ductus venosus → inferior vena cava → right atrium), concomitant angiographic delineation of the course during entry is suggested. Hand-administered contrast injection to demonstrate ductus patency, combined with use of either a tip-deflecting or torque-controlled wire, permits posterior advancement of the catheter, avoidance of intubation of the liver, and successful passage of the catheter to the inferior vena cava (IVC), where it can be exchanged for a long access sheath after angiographic corroboration. Likewise, the additional curve required to pass a catheter from the umbilical artery (patent for up to 7 to 10 days postnatally) may decrease the success of retrograde catheter passage to the systemic ventricle, although this maneuver is frequently successful.

Hepatic Vein

Direct hepatic vein entry can be considered when the femoral veins are impassable (2). A Chiba needle is passed between the mid and anterior axillary line, near the costal margin between the diaphragm and the inferior liver edge. The needle is typically advanced using ultrasound guidance, passing posteriorly and cephalad toward the intrahepatic IVC or just caudal to the IVC-right atrial (RA) junction, to within a few centimeters of the right border of the spine. When contrast injection confirms entry into a large central hepatic vein, a sheath and dilator are advanced over a guidewire to the RA. Large sheath entry and trans-septal passage can be performed without complication via this route using the following technique: At end procedure, a catheter one French size smaller than the entry catheter is exchanged, and this sheath is withdrawn, with hand injection of contrast until the tip of the sheath is seen to be out of the vessel and within the liver parenchymal tract. This tract is then filled with either coils or Gelfoam. Subsequent pain at the entry site is expected for an ensuing 24 hours owing to peritoneal irritation.

Even after vessel access, catheter passage into the desired chambers may require particular knowledge and experience. Appropriate catheter positioning may be facilitated by use of torque-controllable, extendible, tip-deflecting, stiff or extra-stiff, 0.035-inch and 0.038-inch guidewires, as well as by increased use of shaped catheters designed for peripheral or coronary use.

Superior Vena Cava

Entry to the superior vena cava (SVC) is easiest via advancement of a straight wire or catheter in from the IVC (soft catheters tend to advance anteriorly toward the atrial appendage, away from the SVC). A straight catheter may be gently advanced with a soft counterclockwise rolling to ensure freedom of the catheter tip. Foreshortening of the catheter tip in the anteroposterior (AP) projection typically marks successful posterior angulation, permitting advancement of the free catheter tip to the SVC.

On occasion, interruption of the IVC, with azygous continuation, may complicate catheter passage, markedly elongating the catheter course. Multiple curves along the catheter course make further posterior or trans-septal passage extremely difficult from this access.

Passage to the RV may be complicated when (1) the RA is excessively large, (2) the tricuspid valve or RV is diminutive, (3) marked tricuspid valve regurgitation is present, (4) pulmonary atresia is present. Entry can be facilitated either by advancement of a preformed catheter with curvature aimed toward the tricuspid valve (TV) or with a soft-tipped catheter into which may be introduced the preformed bend on the stiff end of a wire or a tip-deflecting wire—*always leaving the wire within the catheter rather than allowing it to protrude into the vasculature.* The guidewire–soft catheter technique allows for adjustment of entry angle and length of curvature by balancing the distance of the guidewire tip from the catheter end prior to catheter advancement over the guidewire. Particular care must be taken with this approach so that the catheter tip is moving freely prior to further manipulation or balloon tip inflation.

Intubation of a normally positioned RV outflow/main pulmonary artery may be difficult when the RV is particularly dilated or the TV is regurgitant. Passage via an internal jugular or subclavian vein approach may increase stability and aid in anterior angulation to and through the RV outflow tract. A multipurpose or similarly precurved soft-tipped catheter can be turned gently in clockwise fashion, either with concomitant contrast injection or use of a torque-controlled wire. Similarly, a soft balloon end-hole catheter can be stiffened at its distal end either with a sharp S-shaped bend to the stiff end of a 0.035-inch guidewire or with a tip-deflecting wire to facilitate passage to the RV outflow tract.

Passage of a catheter from the femoral vein through the RV outflow typically is directed toward a normally positioned, posteriorly directed left pulmonary artery (LPA). When the PAs are in altered positions, or are dilated, shaping the stiff end of a guidewire with a compound clockwise or counterclockwise loop and advancing it to the end of a soft catheter may help direct the catheter to the right or to the left PA, respectively. Such compound curves may prove extremely useful in individual circumstances, transforming basic shaped catheters into individualized, custom-fitted entry devices—for example, use of a similar, tight S-shaped compound guidewire curve can assist in directing a catheter from the proximal branch right pulmonary artery (RPA) to the upper lobe vessel. Similarly, a preshaped catheter can be used with contrast injection or a torque-controlled guidewire to assist entry of a branch PA. Intubation of a dilated or angulated branch RPA may be particularly difficult from a femoral approach, and we have found that retraction of a left Judkins coronary catheter from the left pulmonary artery into the main pulmonary artery and angulation toward the right can facilitate RPA entry.

Subpulmonary Left Ventricle

When the pulmonary arteries are posteriorly directed (TGA), entry via the subpulmonary left ventricle (LV) is generally performed with a soft-tipped, balloon end-hole catheter placed in the LV apex. After ensuring that the catheter tip is free, a tip-deflecting wire is placed within the catheter, proximal to its tip, and is deflected with sufficient traction to guide the catheter tip in a posterior direction, away from the ventricular apex, and toward the base of the heart. A slight retraction of both catheter and guidewire, as a unit, is typically performed, allowing alignment with the LV outflow. The guidewire is held firmly, acting as a fulcrum from which the catheter is extruded, away from the ventricular apex and into the LV outflow.

Left Atrial

Left atrial entry via a transseptal approach can be accomplished on retraction from the SVC with gentle counterclockwise rotation of a leftward-facing catheter or with clockwise advancement from a similarly leftward-facing catheter positioned near the tricuspid valve (see Chapter 4). Biplane fluoroscopic assessment facilitates safe trans-septal passage, although many centers are making increasing use of intracardiac echocardiographic guidance. Typical AP location of the atrial septum is frequently just rightward of the center of the spine. Posterior clockwise catheter rotation from this position will facilitate passage into the pulmonary veins, which may be probed with use of a torque-controlled guidewire. Lower pulmonary vein entry is frequently facilitated by use of a tight, near 180° C-shaped compound curve to the stiff end of a guidewire placed within the entry catheter, directing it to the vessel orifice. Left pulmonary venous entry is typical on crossing the atrial septum, although the atrial appendage may also be entered. Considerable catheter retraction and further posterior redirection outside of the appendage typically facilitates prompt left pulmonary venous entry. The right-sided pulmonary veins typically require further posterior clockwise rotation until the catheter tip appears on AP projection to be to the right of the spine, and then subsequent catheter advancement.

Shunt

Shunt entry is typically facilitated by precise pre-entry knowledge (MRI angiography) of the shunt location. High-volume shunts (Waterston/Pott/alternative central aorta to PA) may be entered via transiently inflated, balloon-tipped flotation catheters, or with preformed individually adjusted catheters (e.g., Judkins right coronary catheter modified by cutting its distal tip), or via tip-deflecting or torque-controlled wires. A preformed Cobra catheter or a modified pigtail (individually cut to approximately 180° may facilitate torque-controlled wire passage from the subclavian artery through a Blalock-Taussig shunt.

Ductus Arteriosus

The ductus arteriosus was one of the original congenital defects intubated during early catheterization attempts. The ductus, when present, can be intubated relatively easily from either an anterograde venous or retrograde arterial approach. From the descending aorta, a preshaped catheter (Cobra, right Judkins, or multipurpose in children; left Judkins in adult) can direct a soft-tipped torque-controlled guidewire across the ductus. From a venous approach, stationing of a multipurpose catheter within the MPA angled slightly leftward to the MPA-LPA junction allows similar passage of a soft-tipped straight or torque-controlled guidewire across the ductus into the descending aorta.

Pressure Measurement and Oximetry

Pressure and systolic or diastolic gradient measurements require stability of loading conditions and contractility, as well as precise localization of the catheter tip. Improved atrioventricular compliance in youth contributes to lower "normal" values of filling pressures in children (RA ≤3 to 5 mm, PCW/LA ≤5 to 8 mm (5). Localization of pressure gradients can be facilitated by pressure transduction through manufactured or modified (cut) side-hole pigtail catheters equipped with a Touhey-Borst Y-arm adapter so that pressure can be measured continuously as the catheter is retracted over a stable guidewire. Alternatively, a double-lumen end-hole catheter may accomplish this goal of near-simultaneous pressure measurements.

Oximetry remains the gold standard for shunt detection (see Chapter 9). Error range of modern high-fidelity oximeters remains approximately ±3%. This, combined with flow-sampling and venous mixing errors, leads to a required oximetric saturation difference of between 4 and 9% to be assured of the presence of left to right shunting (6). These errors must be taken into account when assessing the accuracy of shunt and resistance calculations (Table 6.4, Fig. 6.1). Common correctable errors in assessing oximetric values include the following:

1. Use of IVC sampling as measure of mixed venous saturation. Especially in the fetus, but also at other ages, hepatic, renal (and ductus venosus) flow may not mix completely within the IVC, giving inaccurate reflection of flow due to streaming effects.

2. Use of wedged samples that do not reflect the sampled chamber or vessel, but rather, are partially contaminated by values from proximal or distal chambers.

3. Mistaking elevated SVC saturation as normal rather than as an indicator of a shunt directly into the SVC from anomalous pulmonary veins or regurgitation from the RA in the presence of atrial level shunting.

4. Focusing on a particular degree of shunting without noting overall flows. For example, in a patient with a secundum atrial septal defect (ASD), SVC oxygen (O_2) saturation 50%, pulmonary artery O_2 saturation 80%, aortic O_2 saturation of 100%, hemoglobin (Hgb) 14, and pulmonary flow/systemic flow (Qp/Qs) ratio of 2.6, correction of atrial shunting does not necessarily correct low systemic flow (Qs equals 1.3 L/minute per m^2), which may require additional investigation.

5. Averaging pulmonary vein saturations in the presence of pulmonary venous desaturation. Segmental pulmonary blood flow is never uniform or sufficiently predictable to allow for estimation without direct measurement. Hence, in the setting of nonuniform pulmonary venous saturations (all pulmonary veins should be sampled for maximal accuracy), the relative contribution of each pulmonary segment to total pulmonary blood flow must be known to calculate pulmonary vascular resistance. If supplemental oxygen corrects desaturation and re-establishes uniformity of venous sampling, improved estimation of pulmonary vascular resistance (PVR) can be made. However, disparities in dissolved oxygen (at $pO_2 > 100$) and hence total blood oxygen content among the pulmonary veins may still contribute to inaccuracy.

TABLE 6.4

COMMONLY USED FORMULAS FOR SHUNT AND RESISTANCE CALCULATIONS[a]

Qp	$\dfrac{VO_2}{(PV\ sat - PA\ sat)(Hgb)(1.36)(10)}$
Qs	$\dfrac{VO_2}{(Ao\ sat - SVC\ sat)(Hgb)(1.36)(10)}$
Qp/Qs	$\dfrac{(Ao\ sat - SVC\ sat)}{(PV\ sat - PA\ sat)}$
Qp effective (Qs effective)	$\dfrac{VO_2}{(PV\ sat - SVC\ sat)(Hgb)(1.36)(10)}$
Q Left → Right	$(Qp - Qp\ effective)$
Q Right → Left	$(Qs - Qs\ effective)$
% Left → Right = 1 − (Qp effective/Qp)	$\dfrac{(PA\ sat - SVC\ sat)}{(PV\ sat - SVC\ sat)}$
% Right → Left = 1 − (Qs effective/Qs)	$\dfrac{(PV\ sat - Ao\ sat)}{(PV\ sat - SVC\ sat)}$
PVR	$\dfrac{(mean\ PA\ pressure - LA\ pressure)}{Qp}$
PVR of multiple lung segments	$\dfrac{1}{R_{Total}} = \dfrac{1}{R_{segment\ 1}} + \dfrac{1}{R_{segment\ 2}} + \cdots\cdots\cdots$ $= \dfrac{Flow_{segment\ 1}}{(pressure\ (PA_1 - PV_1))} + \cdots\cdots\cdots$ pressure

[a]See also Chapter 9.
Q, flow; p, pulmonary; s, systemic; PVR, pulmonary vascular resistance; VO_2, oxygen consumption; R, resistance; PV, pulmonary vein; PA, pulmonary artery; Hgb, hemoglobin (gm/dL); Ao, aorta; SVC, superior vena cava.

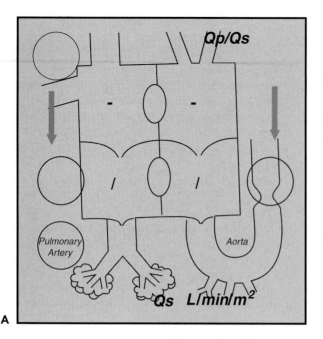
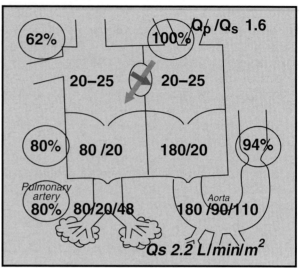

Q_p	$\dfrac{VO_2}{(PV\ sat - PA\ sat)(Hgb)(1.36)(10)}$	$\dfrac{125}{(1-0.80)(13)(1.36)(10)}$	3.6 L/min/m^2
Q_s	$\dfrac{VO_2}{(Ao\ sat - SVC\ sat)(Hgb)(1.36)(10)}$	$\dfrac{125}{(0.94-0.62)(13)(1.36)(10)}$	2.2 L/min/m^2
Q_p/Q_s	$\dfrac{(Ao\ sat - SVC\ sat)}{(PV\ sat - PA\ sat)}$	$\dfrac{(0.94-0.62)}{(1-0.80)}$	1.6 L/min/m^2
Q_p effective (Q_s effective)	$\dfrac{VO_2}{(PV\ sat - SVC\ sat)(Hgb)(1.36)(10)}$	$\dfrac{125}{(1-0.62)(13)(1.36)(10)}$	1.9 L/min/m^2
Q Left $\rightarrow$ Right	$(Q_p - Q_p$ effective$)$	$\dfrac{3.6-1.9}{}$	1.7 L/min/m^2
Q Right $\rightarrow$ Left	$(Q_s - Q_s$ effective$)$	$\dfrac{2.2-1.9}{}$	0.3 L/min/m^2
% Left $\rightarrow$ Right = $1-(Q_p$ effective$/Q_p)$	$\dfrac{(PA\ sat - SVC\ sat)}{(PV\ sat - SVC\ sat)}$	$\dfrac{(.8-.62)}{(1-0.62)}$	0.47 = 47%
% Right $\rightarrow$ Left = $1-(Q_s$ effective$/Q_s)$	$\dfrac{(PV\ sat - Ao\ sat)}{(PV\ sat - SVC\ sat)}$	$\dfrac{(1-0.94)}{(1-0.62)}$	0.16 = 16%
PVR	$\dfrac{(mean\ PA\ pressure - LA\ pressure)}{Q_p}$	$\dfrac{(48-23)}{3.6}$	6.9 Wood units

Figure 6.1 **A.** Commonly used box diagram for displaying hemodynamic and oximetric data. Open circles surround oximetric percent at a given location, whereas pressures are recorded directly where they were measured. Anatomic variants are drawn in yellow circles, with shunt or blood flow direction shown by arrows and color. **B and table.** Hemodynamic and oximetric (including shunt) calculations and measures noted for a patient with atrial level bidirectional shunting.

Furthermore, certain additional facts regarding oximetry and measure of vascular flow and resistance in patients with congenital heart disease should be recognized:

1. Shunt detection is *enhanced* in the presence of low systemic venous saturation.

2. Total PVR is lowered by recruitment of any additional conduit for flow, regardless of resistance of that vessel.

3. Pulmonary vascular resistance is typically flow dependent. Typical recruitment of additional zones of pulmonary blood flow at greater pulmonary blood flow allow for decrease in overall resistance. Hence,

surgical elimination of shunt flow to the lungs may not, in fact, lead to decrease in pulmonary pressures (as would be expected if pulmonary blood flow decreased and PVR remained constant), but rather, may remain elevated due to offsetting reduction in Qp and elevation in PVR.

4. When multiple sources of pulmonary blood flow with differing oxygen saturations (e.g., Qp effective from a systemic venous shunt along with ineffective systemic arterial flow from an aorta-pulmonary shunt) exist in given lung segments or to the entire lung, segmental or total Qp cannot be directly measured. Isolation of each source of flow, temporary occlusion of all but one source, and measurement of pulmonary blood flow (mean PA and PV pressures, PA and PV saturations) from that single source to the lung segment/s in question can allow calculation of PVR, albeit in a lower flow (worst case scenario of PVR).

5. Acute vasoreactivity to vasodilatory agents (inhaled nitric oxide, intravenous prostacyclin, intravenous adenosine, intravenous endothelin antagonists), used to estimate PVR for assistance in planning modern medical or surgical strategies typically increases Qp and hence lowers PVR compared with the free-living environments. PVR measured in such fashion may be sufficiently low to permit acute convalescence from cardiopulmonary surgery, but longer-term postoperative care of such patients may require additional, longer-term pulmonary vasomodulatory therapy (5,6).

6. Measurement of vascular pressures and resistance may be affected by recent trauma (vascular intervention) or contrast administration. Optimally, key aspects of hemodynamic assessment are performed prior to significant contrast exposure or intervention. Likewise, hemodynamics obtained after such exposure may be worst case and may improve with time.

Angiography

Few human structures are perfectly symmetrical, so viewing vessels, chambers, and their connections requires multiple (typically orthogonal) views that minimize overlap and foreshortening of critical areas (Table 6.5). Optimally, biplane or multiplane imagery is used to decrease radiation and contrast exposure. Recording of individualized angiographic angles and views enhances the accuracy of later comparisons.

Contrast administration is typically limited to a dose per injection that is tolerated by the affected ventricle (e.g., segmental or subsegmental PA injections are preferable to larger branch or MPA injections in patients with elevated

---

TABLE 6.5
TYPICAL ANGIOGRAPHIC PROJECTIONS AND LESIONS BEST IMAGED

Projection	Degrees	Vessel/Chamber Imaged	Lesion(s)
Long axial oblique	70° LAO, 30° cranial	LV	Membranous VSD, conotruncal VSD, LVOT obstruction
Hepatoclavicular	45° LAO, 45° cranial	LV	AV canal defect, midmuscular VSD
		Four chambers	LV-RA connections
Lateral	90°	RV/branch PAs	PS/PPS/TGA/DORV
		Descending aorta	Coarctation/PDA
LAO	60–70° LAO	Aorta	Coarctation/aortic valve disease
LAO-cranial	15° LAO, 30° cranial	MPA-branch origins	TOF/PA stenoses
Steep LAO-cranial	60° LAO, 15° cranial	Atrial septum	ASD, PFO
AP-cranial	0° LAO, 30° cranial	RV/conduits	TOF/PS/DORV
AP-caudal	0° LAO, 45° caudal	Ascending aorta/ coronary artery origins	TGA/DORV/ anomalous CA origins
AP	0°	RV, peripheral PAs	TGA/DORV/peripheral PS
		Pulmonary veins	Pulmonary vein stenoses/anomalies of origin/connection
RAO	30° RAO	LV	Anterior VSD, mitral valve disease

Ao, aorta; ASD, atrial septal defect; AV, atrioventricular; CA, coronary artery; DORV, double-outlet right ventricle; LAO, left anterior oblique; LV, left ventricle; LVOT, left ventricular outflow tract; PA, pulmonary artery; PDA, patent ductus arteriosus; PFO, patent foramen ovale; (P) PS, (peripheral) pulmonary stenosis; RAO, right anterior oblique; RV, right ventricle; TGA, transposition of the great arteries (L, left; D, right); TOF, tetralogy of Fallot; VSD, ventricular septal defect.

PVR or RV contractile dysfunction), as long as they are sufficient for maximal anatomic documentation. Prior limitation in fluoroscopic equipment required contrast administration of approximately 1 cc/kg given over 1 second to permit complete chamber delineation in infants and young children with normal volume flow, and ≥1.5 cc/kg over 1 second when excessive shunt flow is present (1). With modern angiographic laboratories, enhanced fluoroscopic fidelity appears to have reduced this contrast requirement substantially.

Given that total contrast administration is designed optimally to be ≤5 cc/kg per catheterization, complete angiographic planning should be performed before the procedure, with ability to shift in "midstream" to optimize obtainment of required data with greatest patient safety.

1. Certain angiographic views serve as reasonable starting points for imaging specific sites or lesions, with individualized adjustment. (Table 6.5).
2. Angiography may be performed with greatest fidelity and least contrast exposure when performed in local fashion, typically via a side-hole angiographic catheter placed over a wire (7). The catheter is adjusted to allow the side holes to be at, upstream, or downstream of flow through the region of question to maximize anatomic imaging with minimal contrast.
3. Retrograde imaging via wedge angiography may assist in delineation of otherwise unreachable vessels or chambers. Some patients, as a result of a congenital defect or prior cardiac surgery, have complete occlusion of a proximal pulmonary artery (typically the left). Owing to bronchial arterial collateralization of the more distal portion of the occluded branch PA, however, this vessel may remain patent decades later. Aortic and collateral vessel angiography or MRI may not be able to establish vessel patency or size adequately owing to restricted baseline flow and vessel underfilling. But a balloon-tipped end-hole catheter can be placed into the draining vessel (typically the corresponding pulmonary vein), so that injection of ≤0.3 mL/kg of nonionic contrast agent followed immediately by an equal volume of saline with the balloon inflated in the pulmonary vein can outline parenchymal vessels with back-filling of the mediastinal segment. On occasion, the main and contralateral PA may also fill in, if they are in continuity. It is important to use biplane cineangiography for these injections to accurately identify the degree of proximal extension of the vessel relative to landmarks, such as the bronchus, on that side. (Similar technique may be used for angiography of particular pulmonary venous pathways when vessel access is restricted or difficult. Catheter placement within the feeding pulmonary artery may be followed by biplane balloon inflation angiography.)

SPECIAL CIRCUMSTANCES

Certain circumstances lead to specific diagnostic considerations for individuals affected by congenital heart disease. These are discussed below.

Pregnancy

Increased preload, heart rate, and cardiac output, coupled with varying ventricular contractile function, may exacerbate pre-existing hemodynamic compromise. Catheterization is safe to mother and fetus when limited to those circumstances (usually mitral or ventricular outflow obstruction) where a combined cardiology and high-risk obstetrics team determines that catheter-based diagnostics or interventions are required despite adequate volume and heart rate control. Choice in timing of catheterization may not be feasible, but should be timed to optimize maternal safety while minimizing fetal teratogenicity or mortality risk. Regardless of food intake, the pregnant woman is considered to have a full stomach, and hence is at increased risk of reflux and aspiration. Overall and uterine radiation exposure should be minimized (direct shielding with lead aprons may intensify rather than reduce exposure, and should be avoided; 8). In such circumstances, the unknown long-term teratogenic risks of low-dose radiation exposure to the fetus in modern laboratories is often outweighed by fetal benefit by improving understanding of ramifications of further management strategies or by direct change in hemodynamics. Availability of fetal monitoring and urgent access to the delivery room should be determined by the obstetric staff prior to catheterization. Typical scenarios leading to catheterization during pregnancy might include maternal suspected or known pulmonary vascular disease, suspected coronary arterial abnormalities, pulmonary venous or functional left atrial outflow obstruction, ventricular outflow obstruction, or subpulmonary or subaortic ventricular failure, unresponsive to standard therapy.

Down Syndrome

The adult patient with Down syndrome frequently has increasing medical comorbidity (thyroid disease, upper and lower airway disease, gastrointestinal reflux, aspiration, limited communication skills, and dementia). Despite restricted alimentation, the Down syndrome patient should be considered to have a full stomach and to be at increased aspiration risk. Hemodynamic assessment of pulmonary vascular resistance should take into account alterations in ventilation and increased incidence of pulmonary vascular disease (9,10). Mechanical ventilation to ensure adequate assessment of pulmonary vascular resistance should be used, as necessary.

Pulmonary Ventricular Failure/Pulmonary Vascular Disease

In the adult, the failing right pulmonary ventricle appears to be less forgiving when acutely compromised, and rapid uncorrectable hemodynamic collapse may ensue. Avoidance of large shifts in preload (rapid volume infusion) and afterload (large contrast bolus, embolization) are thus particularly important in this setting. Recent therapeutic advances for patients with acquired or congenital pulmonary vascular disease have markedly improved the potential for increased quantity and improved quality of life. Assessment of pulmonary vascular reactivity as a marker for further surgical or medical therapy has taken an increasingly larger role in the congenital catheterization laboratory. Extreme care should be taken to avoid acute confounding in-laboratory worsening of PVR by excessive sedation-induced hypoventilation, anesthetic-induced negative inotropy, pain, hemorrhage, acidemia, or severe alterations of loading conditions. In-laboratory support with intravenous (prostacyclin) or inhaled (nitric oxide) pulmonary vasodilators or mechanical assist may be required for even basic hemodynamic assessments in such patients. An intensive monitoring environment outside of the catheterization laboratory is needed for optimization and tailoring of longer-term management strategies.

Improvement in device manufacture, safety testing, and operator experience has led to the extension of transcatheter device septal closure to populations with increased risk and less-well-defined criteria for intervention, such as the patient with ASD, RV dysfunction, and/or cyanosis (see below, and Chapter 27). The concept of transcatheter temporary balloon occlusion to mimic the acute physiologic change of defect closure was pioneered by pediatric cardiologists for the management of surgically placed fenestrations in Fontan baffles, establishing criteria to best estimate the long-term cardiopulmonary tolerance of a removal of a pop-off between circulatory systems (11). Extrapolation of these criteria to the older adult with RV dysfunction and cyanosis is unsubstantiated, but serves as a guide for acute testing of physiologic tolerance. Performance of temporary balloon defect occlusion with compliant large balloon catheters and subsequent measure of change in cardiac output and right atrial pressures is recommended in highest-risk patients contemplating catheter-based or surgical ASD closure (12).

Right Ventricular Outflow Enlargement

Use of transannular patch repair, persistence or recurrence of right ventricular outflow obstruction, or elevation of distal pulmonary artery pressure in patients with tetralogy of Fallot may contribute to increased incidence of right ventricular outflow and pulmonary arterial aneurysmal dilation. Criteria for timing of right ventricular outflow reconstruction in this setting remain unknown. Catheterization of such patients may be indicated to define hemodynamics in the setting of changing exercise capacity or worsening arrhythmia, or to define anatomy in the setting of chest pain or cyanosis with either suspected encroachment of pulmonary venous drainage or pulmonary arterial dissection.

Cyanosis

Long-standing effects of hypoxia-mediated secondary erythrocytosis lessen glomerular filtration rate and increase viscosity, raising the risk for contrast-induced acute tubular necrosis and vascular thrombosis (13). Catheterization should be planned appropriately in such patients and may be accompanied by preprocedural organized reduction in red blood cell mass. The congenital patient has an increased risk of developing pulmonary parenchymal and ventilatory cyanosis, but congenital or acquired vascular causes of decreased systemic arterial saturation should be sought vigorously to avoid the long-term ravages of chronic cyanosis and erythrocytosis. Right to left shunting at the level of systemic veins to pulmonary veins, atrial baffle leaks, patent foramen ovale, and pulmonary artery to pulmonary veins should be sought and potentially treated in the catheterization laboratory. Similarly, pulmonary venous desaturation in the setting of pulmonary venous hypertension owing to (a) systolic or diastolic subaortic ventricular failure, (b) AV valve regurgitation, (c) intravascular obstruction or extravascular compression by an enlarging right atrium or pulmonary artery should be explored for potential medical, surgical, or transcatheter intervention.

Systemic Ventricular "Heart Failure"

The inability of the heart and lungs to meet the metabolic demands imposed by the patient with congenital heart disease may have unique anatomic and physiologic etiologies, and widely differing therapies than those used for children or adults with acquired heart disease (Table 6.6). Use of tailored, hemodynamic-based changes in medical therapy, to date, have not been studied in patients with congenital heart disease.

Coronary Artery Disease

Patients may have abnormalities of coronary artery origin (e.g., anomalous coronary sinus origin of either the right or left coronary artery [RCA or LCA], or origin of LCA/RCA from the pulmonary artery: i.e., ALCAPA), passage (intramural, or between the great arteries), and vessel characteristics (such as those seen in ALCAPA, Kawasaki disease, or coronary reimplantation during arterial switch for TGA). Definition of such abnormalities combines knowledge of congenital cardiology with expertise in the use of tools of the adult cardiologist (including intravascular ultrasound,

TABLE 6.6

ETIOLOGIES OF "HEART FAILURE" IN THE CONGENITAL CARDIAC PATIENT

Afterload
Vascular obstruction
Abnormal arterial impedance
   structural
   neurohormonal
   Systemic right/single ventricle
Preload
   Residual/acquired shunts
   Single ventricle
   Valvar/paravalvular regurgitation
   Renal/hepatic disease and volume retention
   Abnormal venous capacitance
Atrial function/fluid conductance
   Fontan, single ventricle/tricuspid atresia, atrial switch: transposition of great arteries
Loss of subpulmonary ventricle function (Fontan)
Loss of native atrioventricular synchrony
   Atrial flutter → fibrillation
   Artificial pacing
   Ventricular ectopy
Abnormal epicardial/intramural coronary artery flow/formation
   Anomalous left coronary artery origin from the pulmonary artery (ALCAPA)
   Transposition of the great arteries, systemic/pulmonary arterial switch
   Coronary artery between great arteries/intramural/single

thrombolysis in myocardial infarction [TIMI] frame count, provocative endothelial function testing), and may ultimately lead to improved understanding of causes, and therapy, for such diseases.

SUMMARY

Hemodynamic evaluation of both young and older patients with congenital heart disease requires accurate planning and coordinated multidisciplinary care, based on an intricate understanding and assessment of:

1. Interactions between circulations (systemic ⇔ pulmonary)
2. Coupling between chambers and circulation (subpulmonary ventricle ⇔ pulmonary arteries, subaortic ventricle ⇔ systemic arteries)
3. Coupling between chambers (right ⇔ left ventricles, atrioventricular transport post atrial switch repair)
4. Electromechanical coupling

All appear to have such a profound effect on functional capacity and survival. With the increasing complexity of children with congenital heart disease and the more common survival of such children into adulthood, the congenital heart disease physician must be prepared to provide expert hemodynamic assessment and an ever-increasing range of medical, surgical, and catheter-based (see Chapter 27) interventions, as appropriate. Future incorporation of physiologic imaging (primary MRI-based imaging for

catheter manipulations, intracardiac echocardiography, intravascular ultrasonography, high-fidelity tonometry) with catheter-based diagnostics for this population is anticipated, but the cardiac catheter is still certain to play an important tool in making these decisions and delivering the requisite therapies.

REFERENCES

1. Chung T, Burrows PE. Angiography of congenital heart disease. In: Lock JE, Keane JF, Perry SB. Diagnostic and Interventional Catheterization in Congenital Heart Disease, 2nd ed. Boston: Kluwer, 2000:73.
2. Fernandes SM, Landzberg MJ. Transitioning the young adult with congenital heart disease for life-long medical care. *Pediatr Clin North Am.* 2004;51:1739–48.
3. Shim D, Lloyd TR, Cho KJ, et al. Transhepatic cardiac catheterization in children. Evaluation of efficacy and safety. *Circulation* 1995;92:1526–1530.
4. Lock JE, Einzig SA, Moller JH. Hemodynamic responses to exercise in normal children. *Am J Cardiol* 1978;41:1278–1284.
5. Freed MD, Miettinen O, Nadas AS. Oximetric detection of intracardiac left-to-right shunts. *Br Heart J* 1979;42:690–694.
6. Fernandes SM, Newburger JW, Lang P, et al. Usefulness of epoprostenol therapy in the severly ill adolescent/adult with Eisenmenger physiology. *Am J Cardiol* 2003;91:632–635.
7. Rosenzweig EB, Kerstein D, Barst RJ. Long term prostacyclin for pulmonary hypertension with associated congenital heart defects. *Circulation* 1999;99:1858–1865.
8. Verma R, Keane JF. Use of cut-off pigtail catheters with intraluminal guide wires in interventional procedures in congenital heart disease. *Cathet Cardiovasc Diag* 1994;33:85.
9. Damilakis J, Theocharopoulus N, Perisnakis K, et al. Conceptus radiation dosea and risk from cardiac catheter ablation procedures. *Circulation* 2001;104:893–897.

10. Jacobs IN, Tegue WG, Bland JW. Pulmonary vascular complications of chronic airway obstructions in children. *Arch Otolaryngol Head Neck Surg* 1997;123:700–704.

11. Freeman SB, Taft LF, Dooley KI, et al. Population-based study of congenital heart defects in Down syndrome. *Am J Med Genet* 1998;80:213–217.

12. Bridges ND, Lock JE, Mayer JE, Burnett J, Castaneda AR. Cardiac catheterization and temporary occlusion of the interatrial communication after the fenestrated Fontan operation. *J Am Coll Cardiol* 1995;25:1712–1717.

13. Landzberg MJ. Catheterization of the adult with congenital heart disease (ACHD): beyond "shooting the coronaries." *J Interv Cardiol* 2001;14:329–337.

14. Flanagan MF, Hourihan M, Keane JF. Incidence of renal dysfunction in adults with cyanotic congenital heart disease. *Am J Cardiol* 1991;68:403–406.

Hemodynamic Principles

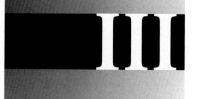

Pressure Measurement

7

William Grossman

The measurement of dynamic blood pressure has been of interest to physiologists and physicians since 1732, when Reverend Stephen Hales measured the blood pressure of a horse by using a vertical glass tube (1). Methodology has advanced impressively since Reverend Hales' day, but with increased technical capability has come greater complexity of instrumentation, so that few physicians today have a firm understanding of the instruments on which they rely.

THE INPUT SIGNAL: WHAT IS A PRESSURE WAVE?

Force is transmitted through a fluid medium as a pressure wave, and an important objective of the cardiac catheterization procedure is to assess accurately the forces and therefore the pressure waves generated by various cardiac chambers. For example, a ventricular pressure wave may be considered a *complex periodic fluctuation in force per unit area*, with one cycle consisting of the time interval from the onset of one systole to the onset of the subsequent systole. The number of times the cycle occurs in 1 second is termed the *fundamental frequency* of cardiac pressure generation. Thus, a fundamental frequency of two corresponds to a heart rate of 120 beats per minute (bpm). Definitions of terms relevant to the theory and practice of pressure measurement are listed in Table 7.1.

Considered as a complex periodic waveform, the pressure wave may be subjected to a type of analysis developed by the French physicist Fourier, whereby any complex wave form may be considered the mathematical summation of a series of simple sine waves of differing amplitude and frequency (Fig. 7.1). Even the most complex waveform can be represented by its own Fourier series, in which the sine wave frequencies are usually expressed as *harmonics*, or multiples of the fundamental frequency. For example, at a heart rate of 120 bpm, the fundamental frequency is 2 cycles per second (Hz) and the first five harmonics are sine waves whose frequencies are 2, 4, 6, 8, and 10 Hz. The practical consequence of this analysis is that, to record pressure accurately, a system must respond with equal amplitude for a given input throughout the range of frequencies contained within the pressure wave. If components in a particular frequency range are either suppressed or exaggerated by the transducer system, the recorded signal will be a grossly distorted version of the original physiologic waveform. For example, the dicrotic notch of the aortic pressure wave contains frequencies above 10 Hz. If the pressure measurement system were unable to respond to frequencies greater than 10 Hz, the notch would be slurred or absent.

PRESSURE MEASURING DEVICES

The manometer used by Starling, Wiggers (2), and others was a modification of that devised by Hürthle (3) in 1898 and is illustrated in Fig. 7.2. A rubber tambour was coupled with a writing lever that recorded change in pressure on a rotating smoked drum. The system had a high inertia and a low elasticity, giving it a narrow range of usefulness. However, consideration of the mechanics of this primitive system helps give a tangible meaning to key concepts applicable to modern pressure measurement devices.

Sensitivity

The sensitivity of such a measurement system may be defined as the ratio of the amplitude of the recorded signal to the amplitude of the input signal. With the Hürthle manometer illustrated in Fig. 7.2, the more rigid the sensing membrane, the lower the sensitivity; conversely,

TABLE 7.1	
DEFINITIONS OF TERMS RELEVANT TO THE THEORY AND PRACTICE OF PRESSURE MEASUREMENT	

Term	Definition
Pressure wave	Complex periodic fluctuation in force per unit area Units: dynes/cm^2: 1 dyne/cm^2 = 1 microbar = 10^{-1} N/M^2 = 7.5×10^{-4} mm Hg mm Hg: 1 mm Hg = 1 Torr = 1/760 atmospheric pressure
Fundamental frequency	Number of times the pressure wave cycles in 1 second
Harmonic	Multiple of the fundamental frequency
Fourier analysis	Resolution of any complex periodic wave into a series of single sine waves of differing frequency and amplitude
Sensitivity of pressure measurement system	Ratio of the amplitude of the recorded signal to the amplitude of the input signal
Frequency response of pressure measurement system	Ratio of output amplitude to input amplitude over a range of frequencies of the input pressure wave
Natural frequency	Frequency at which the pressure measurement system oscillates or responds when shock- excited; also, the frequency of an input pressure wave at which the ratio of output/input amplitude of an undamaged system is maximal. Units: cycles/sec, Hz
Damping	Dissipation of the energy of oscillation of a pressure measurement system owing to friction. Units: damping coefficient, D (see text)
Optimal damping	Damping that progressively blunts the increase in output/input ratio that occurs with increasing frequency of pressure wave input. Optimal damping can maintain frequency response flat (output/input ratio = 1) to 88% of the natural frequency of the system
Strain gauge	Variable-resistance transducer in which the strain (ΔL/L) on a series of wires is determined by the pressure on the transducer's diaphragm. Over a wide range, electrical resistance (R) of the wire is directly proportional to ΔL/L
Wheatstone bridge	Arrangement of electrical connections in a strain gauge such that pressure-induced changes in resistance result in proportional changes in voltage across the bridge
Balancing a transducer	Interpolating a variable resistance across the output of a Wheatstone bridge/strain gauge transducer so that atmospheric pressure at the zero level (e.g., midchest) induces an arbitrary voltage output on the monitor/recording device (i.e., a voltage that positions the transducer output on the oscilloscopic pressure baseline)

the more flaccid the membrane, the higher the sensitivity. This general principle applies to manometers currently in use.

Frequency Response

A second crucial property of any pressure measurement system is its frequency response. The frequency response of a pressure measurement system may be defined as the ratio of output amplitude to input amplitude over a range of frequencies of the input pressure wave. To measure pressure accurately, the frequency response (amplitude ratio) must be constant over a broad range of frequency variation. Otherwise, the amplitude of major frequency components of the pressure waveform may be attenuated while minor components are amplified, so that the recorded waveform becomes a distorted caricature of the physiologic event. Referring again to the Hürthle manometer in Fig. 7.2, the range of good frequency response is improved by stiffening the membrane, and it is narrowed

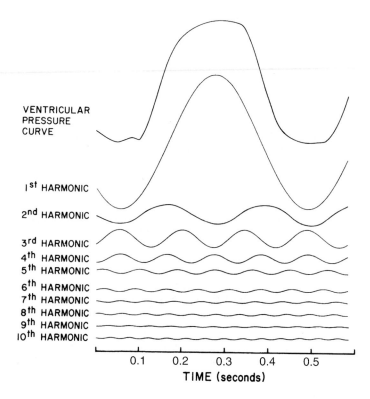

VENTRICULAR
PRESSURE
CURVE

1st HARMONIC

2nd HARMONIC

3rd HARMONIC
4th HARMONIC
5th HARMONIC
6th HARMONIC
7th HARMONIC
8th HARMONIC
9th HARMONIC
10th HARMONIC

0.1   0.2   0.3   0.4   0.5
TIME (seconds)

Figure 7.1   Resolution of a normal ventricular pressure curve (*top*) into its first 10 harmonics by Fourier analysis. If components in a particular frequency range (e.g., the third harmonic, which in this case is 7 Hz) were either suppressed or exaggerated by the transducer system, the recorded signal would be a grossly distorted version of the original physiologic signal. (Adapted from Wiggers CJ. *The Pressure Pulses in the Cardiovascular System.* London: Longmans, Green, 1928:1.)

by making the membrane more flaccid, because the flaccid membrane cannot respond well to higher frequencies. Thus, *frequency response* and *sensitivity* are related reciprocally, and one can be obtained only by sacrificing the other.

Natural Frequency and Damping

A third important concept is the *natural frequency* of a sensing membrane and how it determines the degree of damping required for optimal recording. If the sensing membrane were to be shock-excited (like a gong) in the absence of friction, it would oscillate for an indefinite period in simple harmonic motion. The frequency of this motion would be the natural frequency of the system. Any means of dissipating the energy of this oscillation, such as friction, is called *damping*. The dynamic response characteristics of such a system are determined largely by the natural frequency and the degree of damping that the system possesses (4).

The significance of the natural frequency and the importance of proper damping are illustrated in Fig. 7.3. The amplitude of an output signal tends to be augmented as the frequency of the input signal approaches the natural frequency of the sensing membrane. The physical counterpart of this augmentation is that the sensing membrane of the pressure transducer vibrates with increasing energy and violence. The same mechanism underlies the fracture of a crystal glass when an opera singer vocalizes the appropriate

input frequency. Damping dissipates the energy of the oscillating sensing membrane, and optimal damping dissipates the energy gradually, thereby maintaining the frequency response curve nearly flat (constant output/input ratio) as it approaches the region of the pressure measurement system's natural frequency.

As an analogy to further help the reader understand the significance of damping, consider the simple case of a weight suspended from a spring. If the weight is displaced and then released, the stretched spring recoils

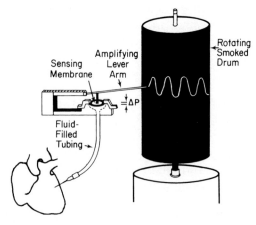

Figure 7.2   Schematic illustration of the Hürthle manometer. A rubber tambour serves as the sensing membrane and is coupled with an amplifying lever arm that records changes in pressure (ΔP) on a rotating smoked drum. Pressure is transmitted from the heart (*lower left corner*) to the sensing membrane by fluid-filled tubing.

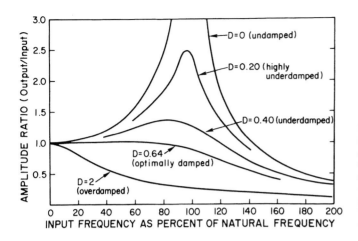

Figure 7.3 Frequency response curves of a pressure measurement system, illustrating the importance of optimal damping. The amplitude of an input signal tends to be augmented as the frequency of that signal approaches the natural frequency of the sensing membrane. Optimal damping dissipates the energy of the oscillating sensing membrane gradually and thereby maintains a nearly flat natural frequency curve (constant output/input ratio) as it approaches the region of the pressure measurement system's natural frequency (see text). D, damping coefficient.

so that the weight moves past its original position and then oscillates up and down. In the absence of frictional forces (damping), the oscillation would continue indefinitely at a frequency determined by the stiffness of the spring and an amplitude determined by the mass of the weight. In practice there is always some damping, and this has two effects: The amplitude of the oscillations gradually diminishes, and the frequency of oscillation is reduced. This second important consequence of damping—reduction of the natural frequency of a system—is not widely appreciated. If we continue with our analogy, imagine that the spring and its weight are suspended in a jar of syrup or honey; the spring will clearly vibrate with lesser amplitude of vibration and lesser frequency than before. The effect of the viscous medium is to further damp the oscillations. If the medium's viscosity is high enough, it prevents any overshoot or oscillation: The weight returns to its original position regardless of its initial displacement. Further damping at this point simply slows the return of the weight to its equilibrium position, thereby depressing the frequency response characteristics of the system. Therefore, damping helps to prevent overshoot artifacts resulting from resonance of the system, but at the cost of diminished frequency response.

WHAT FREQUENCY RESPONSE IS DESIRABLE?

Wiggers (2) suggested that the shortest significant vibrations contained within physiologic pressure waves have one-tenth the period of the entire pressure curve—that is, the essential physiologic information is contained within the first 10 harmonics of the pressure wave's Fourier series. At a heart rate of 120 bpm, the fundamental frequency is 2 Hz and the tenth harmonic is 20 Hz. Therefore, a pressure measurement system with a frequency response range that is flat to 20 Hz should be adequate in such a circum-

stance, and support for this hypothesis has come from experimental work comparing high frequency-response systems with conventional catheter systems (5).

The useful frequency response range of commonly used pressure measurement systems is usually <20 Hz unless special care is taken. Wood and colleagues (6) and Gleason and Braunwald (7) found that frequency response was flat to <10 Hz with small-bore (6F) catheters attached to standard strain gauge manometers.

To ensure a high frequency-response range, the pressure measurement system must be set up in such a way that it has the highest possible *natural frequency* as well as *optimal damping*. The natural frequency is directly proportional to the lumen radius of the catheter system. It is inversely proportional to the length of the catheter and associated tubing and to the square root of the catheter and tubing compliance and the density of fluid filling the system. The highest natural frequency is obtained by using a short, wide-bore, stiff catheter connected to its transducer without intervening tubing or stopcocks and filled with a low-density liquid from which small air bubbles, which increase compliance, have been excluded (e.g., boiled saline solution). Such a system is impractical for routine use, but deviation from it occurs only at a significant sacrifice.

If such a system is constructed, it will be found to be grossly underdamped (Fig. 7.3). Accordingly, it is important to introduce damping into the system to keep the frequency response flat as the frequency of the input signal approaches the natural frequency of the pressure measurement system. With optimal damping, the frequency response can be maintained flat (±5%) to within 88% of the natural frequency, according to Fry (4), although it is unusual to achieve >50% in most laboratories. Damping may be introduced by interposing a damping needle between the catheter and manometer (6) and gradually shortening it until optimal damping is obtained; by filling the manometer or tubing with a viscous medium, such as Renografin (a radiographic contrast agent); or by any of several other methods.

EVALUATION OF FREQUENCY RESPONSE CHARACTERISTICS

Ideally, the frequency response characteristics of a pressure measurement system should be evaluated using a sine wave pressure generator to construct curves similar to those seen in Fig. 7.3. By altering the characteristics of the system discussed in the previous section, a reasonable compromise between frequency response, damping, and practicality can be achieved for each laboratory. Such a sine wave pressure generator is commercially available (Millar Instruments, Houston, TX). An example of the use of this device in estimating frequency response of a pressure measurement system is provided in Fig. 7.4.

Another method, which does not require the use of such a pressure waveform generator, is described here. This technique may be used for measuring the dynamic response characteristics of a pressure measurement system.

The catheter to be studied is connected by means of a three-way stopcock with or without intervening tubing to one arm of a strain gauge transducer (Fig. 7.5). The transducer used should be of the low-volume-displacement type (small chamber capacity) to enhance frequency response. The tip of the catheter is snugly projected through a hole in a no. 6 rubber stopper, which is tightly inserted into the cut-off barrel of a 60-mL plastic syringe. The syringe plunger is removed, and the barrel is fixed in a vertical position, pointing downward, so that the catheter enters from below. The

manometer and catheter are filled with saline solution, care being taken to avoid even small air bubbles, and the catheter is flushed until the catheter tip and holes are submerged in approximately 30 mL of saline solution. The plunger is slowly inserted into the syringe, producing an upward deflection of the pressure trace on the oscilloscope of the recording apparatus. When the trace comes to rest at the top of the oscilloscope, the recorder is turned on at rapid paper speed and the plunger is suddenly withdrawn. This method, modified from Hansen (8), produces shock-excitation vibrations of the type seen in Fig. 7.6. The mathematical foundation for analysis of such a shock excitation has been described by Wiggers (2) and Fry (4) and may be summarized as follows.

The frequency of the after-vibrations produced by shock excitation is the damped natural frequency of the system. This is obtained by measuring the time, t, between two successive vibrations and obtaining the damped natural frequency, N_D as $1/t$. In the example in Fig. 7.6, $N_D = 1/0.04 = 25$ Hz. Next, the damping coefficient, D, is calculated as a function of the ratio by which successive single vibrations decrease. In Fig. 7.6, this may be calculated from the ratio of x_2 to x_1, the percent overshoot:

$$D = \sqrt{\ln^2 (x_2/x_1)/[\pi^2 + \ln^2 (x_2/x_1)]} \qquad (7.1)$$

where $\ln(x_2/x_1)$ is the natural logarithm of the percent overshoot. In our example, $x_2/x_1 = 0.093$, $\ln(x_2/x_1) =$

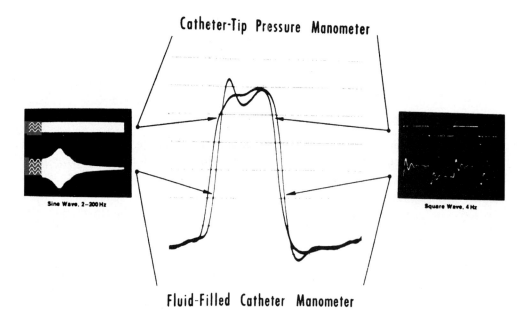

Figure 7.4 Left ventricular pressure **(center)** measured with a fluid-filled standard catheter and micromanometer (catheter-tip pressure manometer) in a patient undergoing cardiac catheterization. **Left and right.** In vitro frequency response for micromanometer (*upper*) and fluid-filled (*lower*) systems. The left panel recordings were obtained by continuously increasing the input frequency of a sine wave pressure waveform from 2 to 200 Hz. The fluid-filled system resonated (natural frequency) at 37 Hz but was flat (±5%) only to 12 Hz. Therefore its useful range is only to approximately 12 Hz. The right panel shows the response of each system to a square wave pressure input signal. (From Nichols WW, Pepine CJ, Millar HD, et al. Percutaneous left ventricular catheterization with an ultraminiature catheter-tip pressure transducer. *Cardiovasc Res* 1978;12:566, with permission.)

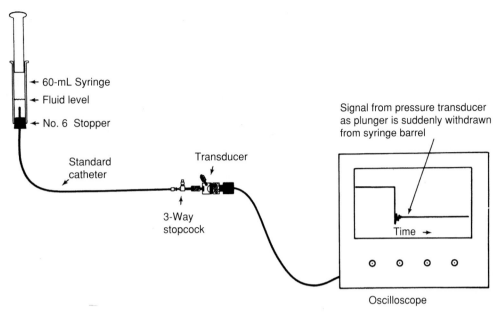

Figure 7.5 Practical evaluation of dynamic response characteristics of a catheter–transducer system. The catheter hub is connected by means of a three-way stopcock to one arm of a low-volume-displacement pressure transducer. The tip of the catheter is snugly projected through a hole in a no. 6 rubber stopper, which is tightly inserted into the cutoff barrel of a 60-mL plastic syringe. The manometer and catheter are filled with saline solution, care being taken to avoid even small air bubbles, and the catheter is flushed until the catheter tip and holes are submerged in approximately 30 mL of saline solution. Next, the plunger is slowly inserted into the syringe, producing an upward deflection of the pressure trace on the oscilloscope of the recording apparatus. When the pressure trace comes to rest at the top of the oscilloscope screen, the recorder is turned on and the plunger is suddenly withdrawn from the syringe barrel. Dynamic response characteristics are then calculated as shown in Fig. 7.6.

−2.379, and D = 0.603. From the damping coefficient D and the damped natural frequency N_D, we may determine the undamped natural frequency N as

$$N = N_D/\sqrt{1 - D^2} \qquad (7.2)$$

A simple practical goal is to try to regulate the damping of an actual pressure measurement system so that its damping coefficient is as close to 0.64 (so-called optimal damping) as possible. At this value, the pressure measurement system shows uniform frequency response ($\pm 5\%$) to about 88% of its natural frequency, according to Fry (2). If such optimal damping is achieved for the system illustrated in Fig. 7.6, its frequency response could be considered flat to 0.88 N, or 27.5 Hz. Improperly damped systems with low natural frequencies (because of small air bubbles or excessively compliant tubing) may achieve uniform frequency response to <10 Hz.

TRANSFORMING PRESSURE WAVES INTO ELECTRICAL SIGNALS: THE ELECTRICAL STRAIN GAUGE

Pressure measurement systems today generally use electrical strain gauges based on the principle of the Wheatstone bridge. In its simplest form, the strain gauge is a variable-resistance transducer whose operation depends on the fact that when an electrical wire is stretched, its resistance to the flow of current increases. As long as the strain remains well below the elastic limit of the wire, there is a wide range within which the increase in resistance is accurately proportional to the increase in length.

Figure 7.7 illustrates how the Wheatstone bridge uses this principle in converting a pressure signal to an electrical signal. In this schematic representation of a pressure transducer, pressure is transmitted through port P and acts on diaphragm D, which is vented to atmospheric pressure on its opposite side. In the illustration, the diaphragm is attached on its undersurface to a plunger, which in turn is attached to four wires, G_1 through G_4, as illustrated. The manner of attachment is such that increased pressure on the diaphragm stretches and therefore increases the electrical resistance of G_1 and G_2 and has the opposite effect on G_3 and G_4. In the Wheatstone bridge, G_1, G_2, G_3, and G_4 are connected electrically as in Fig. 7.8 and are attached to a voltage source, B. If all four resistances are equal, then exactly half the voltage of battery B exists at the junction of G_1 and G_4 and half at the junction of G_2 and G_3; therefore, no current flows between the output terminals. However, when pressure is applied to the diaphragm (Fig. 7.7), the resistances are unbalanced, so that the junction of G_1 and

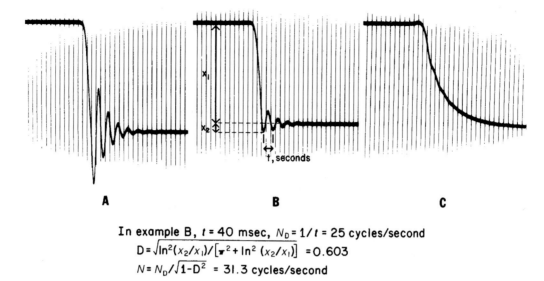

A   B   C

In example B, $t = 40$ msec, $N_D = 1/t = 25$ cycles/second

$$D = \sqrt{\ln^2(x_2/x_1)/[\pi^2 + \ln^2(x_2/x_1)]} = 0.603$$

$$N = N_D/\sqrt{1-D^2} = 31.3 \text{ cycles/second}$$

Figure 7.6 Records of dynamic frequency response characteristics obtained from the system illustrated in Fig. 7.5. **A, B,** and **C.** Progressive increases in damping produced by introducing increasing amounts of a viscous radiographic contrast agent (Renografin-76) into the catheter–transducer system. The catheter was 80 cm long, and its diameter was 8F. **A.** Underdamped. **B.** Almost optimally damped. **C.** Overdamped. The percent overshoot (x_2/x_1) is used in the calculation of the damping coefficient, **D.** The undamped natural frequency, N, is calculated from D and the damped natural frequency, N_D. Time lines are 20 milliseconds. Using the curves shown in Fig. 7.3 for various values of D, the frequency response of the system in **B** can probably be considered flat ($\pm 5\%$) to 0.88 N, or 27.5 Hz.

G_4 becomes negative, and a current flows across the output terminals.

Because movement of the diaphragm (D) in Fig. 7.7 is necessary to produce current flow in the Wheatstone bridge, a certain volume of fluid must actually move through the catheter and connecting tubing to produce a recorded pressure. Therefore, the use of a low-volume-displacement transducer with a small chamber volume improves the frequency-response characteristics of the system.

Balancing a transducer is simply a process whereby a variable resistance (the R balance of most amplifiers) is

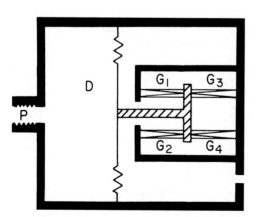

Figure 7.7 Schematic representation of a strain gauge pressure transducer. Pressure is transmitted through port P and acts on diaphragm D, which is vented to atmospheric pressure on its opposite side. Pressure causes the diaphragm to stretch, in turn stretching and therefore increasing the resistance of wires G_1 and G_2, while having the opposite effect on wires G_3 and G_4. The wires are electrically connected as shown in Fig. 7.8.

interpolated into the circuit (Fig. 7.8) so that at an arbitrary baseline pressure, the voltage across the output terminal, can be reduced to zero. Some amplifiers use an alternating current (AC) signal in place of the DC current source shown in Fig. 7.8. When these carrier current amplifiers are used, a variable capacitor (the C balance) must be used in addition to the variable resistor to balance the bridge.

PRACTICAL PRESSURE TRANSDUCER SYSTEM FOR THE CATHETERIZATION LABORATORY

Incorporating all the principles discussed so far in this chapter, many laboratories have settled on a practical system in which a fluid-filled catheter is attached by means of a manifold to a small-volume-displacement strain gauge type pressure transducer (Fig. 7.9).

The system illustrated is used for pressure measurement from the right side of the heart and for arterial monitor lines. The system used for left-sided heart pressure measurement is more complex because it also incorporates ports for radiographic contrast administration and blood discard, as well as a syringe for coronary angiography (see also Chapter 11). Virtually all catheterization laboratories use relatively inexpensive, sterile, disposable pressure transducers in which a tiny integrated circuit on a thin silicon diaphragm serves as the sensing element. Fluid pressure is transmitted to this element through a gel medium, bending the circuit and altering the resistance of resistors in the silicon diaphragm. The

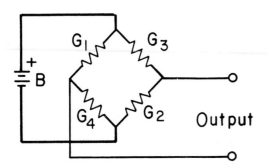

Figure 7.8 Strain gauge connection of the Wheatstone bridge. In this arrangement, if all resistances are equal, then exactly half the voltage of battery B exists at the junction of G_1 and G_4 and half at the junction of G_2 and G_3; therefore, no current will flow between the output terminals. However, when pressure is applied to the diaphragm (see Fig. 7.7), the resistances are unbalanced, so that the junction of G_1 and G_4 becomes negative and a current flows across the output terminals.

circuit delivers an electrical output proportional to the pressure being applied, as discussed previously.

To the first side arm of the manifold (Fig. 7.9), a fluid-filled connecting tube is attached, the distal end of which is adjusted to the zero reference level (see above). The second side arm is connected by a fluid-filled tube to a pressurized flush bag containing heparinized saline solution. The cardiac catheter is connected directly to the front of the manifold through a built-in rotating adapter. By turning the stopcock attached to the flush solution, the operator can flush the catheter intermittently (e.g., every 3 minutes) to clear blood. Turning this stopcock the other way permits filling and flushing of the zero line or the pressure transducer. With this system, a frequency response that is flat ($\pm 5\%$) up to 20 Hz can be achieved routinely. If a reusable (rather than disposable) transducer is employed, it may be sterilized with gas or Cidex between uses.

The establishment of a zero reference is an important practical undertaking that must be accomplished as a part of each catheterization procedure. Midchest level is used widely as zero reference, because fluoroscopic visualization in a lateral projection confirms that the left ventricle and aorta are generally located midway between the sternum and the table top when the patient is supine. However, the validity of choosing the midchest level for zero reference has been challenged in an excellent study by Courtois et al. (9). They carefully examined the influence of hydrostatic forces (caused by the effects of gravity) and concluded that intracardiac pressures should be referenced to an external fluid-filled transducer aligned with the uppermost blood level in the chamber where pressure is being measured. In practical terms, for measurement of left ventricular and aortic pressure, the zero level should be positioned approximately 5 cm below the left sternal border at the fourth left intercostal space (LICS). This eliminates the gravitational/hydrostatic effect of a column of blood above the catheter tip and within the ventricular chamber. Although the right ventricle and left atrium are at different levels in the chest than the left ventricle, Courtois et al. (9) calculated that the error introduced by use of a point 5 cm below the fourth LICS, at the left sternal border, is approximately ± 0.8 mm Hg for chambers other than the left ventricle.

If a decision has been made to use the midchest level for zero reference, each case should begin with measurement of the patient's anteroposterior (AP) thoracic diameter at the level of the angle of Louis. This is done with the use of a large square chest caliper (Picker Instruments), as illustrated in Fig. 7.10. The patient then lies supine on the catheterization table and is draped and otherwise prepared for catheterization (a 12-lead electrocardiogram is recorded, skin sites are shaved and cleansed), and the zero level is established on an adjustable pole attached to the side of the table. This is accomplished with the use of a yardstick to which a carpenter's level has been taped. One end of the yardstick is placed on the patient's sternum at the angle of Louis and the other end against the adjustable metal pole. As illustrated in Fig. 7.10, the metal pole has a centimeter-ruled tape attached to it, allowing identification of the level

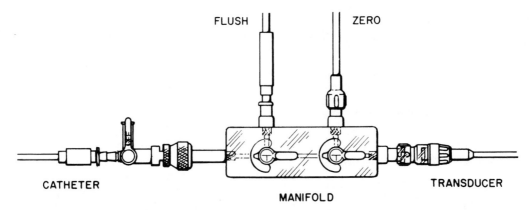

Figure 7.9 A practical system for pressure measurement with excellent frequency response. The catheter is connected by a stopcock to a manifold, which is connected at its other end to a small-volume fluid-filled pressure transducer. The manifold's two sidearms are connected by fluid-filled tubing to a zero-pressure reference level and to a pressurized flush solution.

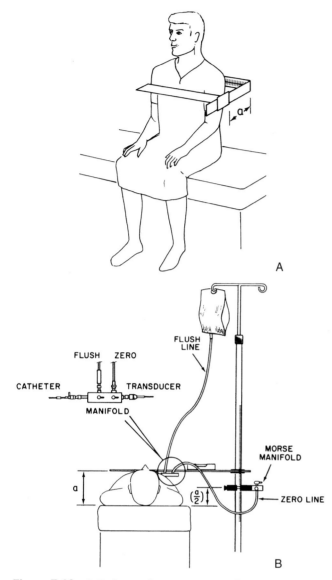

Figure 7.10 **A.** Technique for measurement of a patient's antero-posterior diameter (a), using a metal chest caliper. **B.** Establishment of zero level. (See text for detailed explanation.)

the Morse manifold, 100 mm Hg pressure being transmitted through the fluid-filled zero line to all pressure transducers to be used in a particular case (e.g., left heart, right heart, arterial monitor). Otherwise, the free port of the Morse manifold is left open to air, in communication with the individual zero lines of the various left and right heart manifold systems by way of the series of stopcocks that constitute the Morse manifold, thus referencing all the transducer systems to a common zero level.

PHYSIOLOGIC CHARACTERISTICS OF PRESSURE WAVEFORMS

Reflected Waves

Recognizing the appearance of normal pressure waveforms is a prerequisite to identifying abnormalities that characterize certain cardiovascular disorders. As shown in Fig. 7.11, *forward* pressure and flow waves, as seen in the central aorta, are intrinsically identical in shape and timing. The pressure wave is modified by summation with a *reflected* pressure wave ($P_{backward}$), and the resultant *measured* central aortic pressure wave shows a steady increase throughout ejection (10,11). The flow wave is also modified by summation with a reflected flow wave ($F_{backward}$), but because flow is directional, $F_{backward}$ reduces the magnitude of flow in late ejection, giving the characteristic $F_{measured}$ as is seen with aortic flowmeters or Doppler signals.

The reflections for pressure occur from many sites within the arterial tree, but the major effective reflection site in humans appears to be the region of the terminal abdominal aorta (11). As seen in Fig. 7.12, ascending aortic pressure is increased substantially within one beat after bilateral occlusion of the femoral arteries by external manual compression. High-speed recordings (Fig. 7.12, right) show that the major part of the increase in pressure occurs late in systole, consistent with an increase in the magnitude of the reflected pressure.

Various factors influence the magnitude of reflected waves (Table 7.2). Pressure reflections are diminished during the strain phase of the Valsalva maneuver (10), with the result that pressure and flow waveforms become similar in appearance (Fig. 7.13). After release of the Valsalva strain, reflected waves return and are exaggerated. Therefore, the commonly noted late-peaking appearance of central aortic and left ventricular pressure tracings in humans (Fig. 7.14), referred to as the type A waveform pattern (10), is a result of strong pressure reflections in late systole. In addition to the Valsalva maneuver, pressure reflections are diminished during hypovolemia, hypotension, and in response to a variety of vasodilator agents (Table 7.2). In these circumstances, the left ventricular and central aortic pressure waves exhibit a type C pattern (Fig. 7.14). However, vasoconstriction and hypertension may be expected to accentuate the normal type A waveform. Because the contribution

of midchest (one half of the patient's AP diameter below the angle of Louis). Alternatively, the yardstick with its level can be used to identify the position on the metal pole that is 5 cm below the left sternal border at the fourth LICS. With this technique, a Morse manifold (NAMIC, Medical Products Division, Hudson Falls, NY) or similar device that can be moved up and down the metal pole is set at either the midchest level or 5 cm down from the fourth LICS; one end of the zero line (clear polyethylene tubing) is connected to the manifold, and the other end is connected to the pressure measurement manifold (Fig. 7.9). The zero line, manifold, and pressure transducer are next filled with saline from the flush line so that the pressure transducer can be connected directly with the zero line by the turn of a stopcock on the pressure manifold. The pressure transducers are calibrated by means of a mercury manometer attached to a free port on

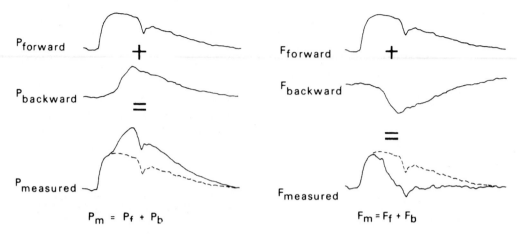

$P_m = P_f + P_b$ $F_m = F_f + F_b$

Figure 7.11   Central aortic pressure (P) and flow (F) measured in a patient during cardiac catheterization. Computer-derived forward and backward pressure and flow components are shown individually: Their sum results in the measured waves. (See text for discussion.) (From Murgo JP, Westerhof N, Giolma JP, et al. Manipulation of ascending aortic pressure and flow wave reflections with Valsalva maneuver: relationship to input impedance. *Circulation* 1981;63:122, with permission.)

of reflections to the arterial pressure waveform should move earlier in systole the closer one gets to the source of the reflections, it is not surprising that the pressure peaks earlier as the catheter is withdrawn from the central aorta to the periphery (Fig. 7.15).

Reflected waves can be of substantial magnitude and are increased in the patient with heart failure (12). Laskey and Kussmaul (12) showed that reflected pressure waves were increased in amplitude in 17 patients with heart failure secondary to idiopathic dilated cardiomyopathy, often producing an exaggerated dicrotic wave. The magnitude of these reflections did not decrease consistently during exer-

cise, as is characteristic of the normal circulation. Infusion of sodium nitroprusside intravenously markedly reduced the magnitude of the reflected pressure waves and delayed their timing; both these changes were deemed beneficial with regard to left ventricular systolic load (12).

Wedge Pressures

A physiologic aspect of pressure measurement that has been of interest for many years is the concept of the "wedge pressure." Broadly stated, a wedge pressure is obtained when an end-hole catheter is positioned in a designated

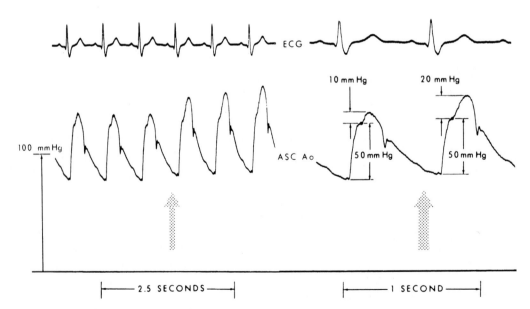

Figure 7.12   Ascending aortic (ASC Ao) pressure waveform in a patient before and after bilateral occlusion of the femoral arteries by external manual compression (*left arrow*). On the right, high-speed recordings show that the major portion of the increase in pressure results from augmentation of the late (reflected) wave. ECG, electrocardiogram. (From Murgo JP, Westerhof N, Giolma JP, et al. Aortic input impedance in normal man: relationship to pressure wave forms. *Circulation* 1980; 62:105, with permission.)

TABLE 7.2
FACTORS THAT INFLUENCE THE MAGNITUDE OF REFLECTED WAVES

Factors that augment pressure wave reflections
    Vasoconstriction
    Heart failure
    Hypertension
    Aortic or iliofemoral obstruction
    Valsalva maneuver—after release

Factors that diminish pressure wave reflections
    Vasodilation
        Physiologic (e.g., fever)
        Pharmacologic (e.g., nitroglycerin, nitroprusside)
    Hypovolemia
    Hypotension
    Valsalva maneuver—strain phase

blood vessel with its open end-hole facing a capillary bed, with no connecting vessels conducting flow into or away from the designated blood vessel between the catheter tip and the capillary bed. *A true wedge pressure can be measured only in the absence of flow.* In the absence of flow, pressure equilibrates across the capillary bed so that the catheter tip pressure is equal to that on the other side of the capillary bed. If minimal damping occurs between the catheter tip and the opposite side of the capillary bed—that is, if there is a large, relatively dilated capillary bed, if the precapillary arterioles and postcapillary venules are not constricted, and if there is no other source of obstruction, such as the presence of microthrombi–phasic as well as mean pressure may be transmitted to the wedged catheter. Thus, an end-hole catheter wedged in a hepatic vein may be used to measure portal venous pressure; a catheter wedged in a distal pulmonary artery measures pulmonary venous pressure; and if it is wedged in a pulmonary vein. It measures pulmonary artery pressure. The details involved in measurement of pulmonary artery wedge pressure, commonly termed *pulmonary capillary wedge pressure,* are discussed in Chapter 5. Properly performed, this determination accurately measures pulmonary venous pressure. In the absence of cor triatriatum or obstruction to pulmonary venous outflow, the pulmonary venous and left atrial pressures are equal, so that pulmonary artery wedge pressure may be used as a substitute for left atrial pressure. Issues of damping and time delay need to be considered when using this pressure to assess a transmitral gradient in a patient with mitral stenosis or prosthetic valve obstruction. These issues have been addressed by Lange et al. (13).

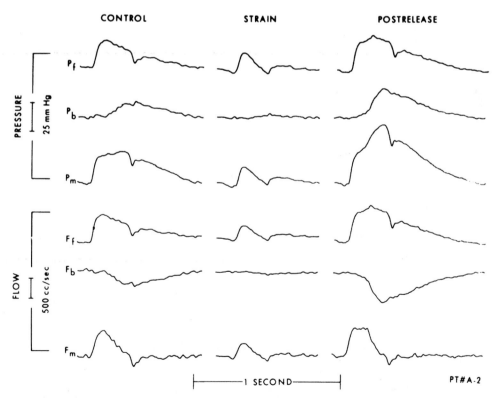

Figure 7.13 Measurements of central aortic pressure (P_m) and flow (F_m) in a patient performing Valsalva maneuver during cardiac catheterization. Control, Valsalva strain, and post–Valsalva release tracings are shown. P_m is the sum of forward (P_f) and backward or reflected (P_b) pressure waves; F_m is the sum of F_f and F_b. (See text for discussion.) (From Murgo JP, Westerhof N, Giolma JP, et al. Manipulation of ascending aortic pressure and flow wave reflections with Valsalva maneuver: relationship to input impedance. *Circulation* 1981;63:122, with permission.)

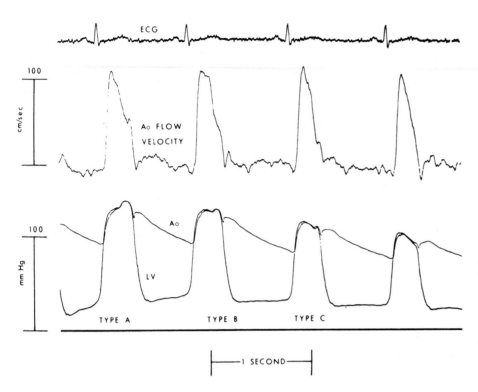

Figure 7.14 Left ventricular (LV) and central aortic (Ao) pressure and aortic flow velocity tracings in a patient at the initiation of the strain phase of a Valsalva maneuver. (See text for details.) (From Murgo JP, Westerhof N, Giolma JP, et al. Manipulation of ascending aortic pressure and flow wave reflections with Valsalva maneuver: relationship to input impedance. *Circulation* 1981;63: 122, with permission.)

SOURCES OF ERROR AND ARTIFACT

Even when every effort has been made to design a pressure measurement system with high sensitivity, uniform frequency response, and optimal damping, distortions and inaccuracies in the pressure waveform may occur. Some common sources of error and artifact in clinical pressure measurement include deterioration in frequency response, catheter whip artifact, end pressure artifact, catheter impact artifact, systolic pressure amplification in the periphery, and errors in zero level, balancing, and calibration.

Deterioration in Frequency Response

Although frequency response may be high and damping optimal during setup of the transducers, substantial deteriora-

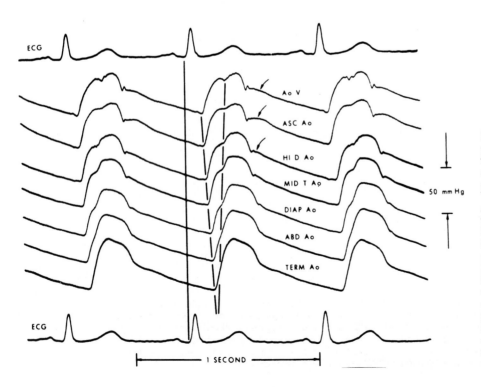

Figure 7.15 Pressure waveforms in a patient undergoing cardiac catheterization, as a function of distance from the aortic valve (Ao V). Ao, aorta; ASC, ascending; Hi D, high descending; MID T, midthoracic; DIAP, diaphragmatic; ABD, abdominal; TERM, just above aortic bifurcation; ECG, electrocardiogram. First vertical line marks onset of primary (forward) pressure wave, which occurs progressively later after the QRS complex with increasing distance from the aortic valve. Second vertical line marks onset of secondary pressure rise associated with the backward or reflected pressure wave. See text for discussion. (From Murgo JP, Westerhof N, Giolma JP, et al. Aortic input impedance in normal man: relationship to pressure wave forms. *Circulation* 1980;62:105, with permission.)

tion in the characteristics can develop during the course of a catheterization study. Air bubbles may be introduced into the catheters, stopcocks, or tubing, or dissolved air may come out of the saline solution used to fill the transducer (just as dissolved air may come out of solution in a glass of water allowed to stand unperturbed for a few hours). Even the smallest air bubbles have a drastic effect on pressure measurement because they cause excessive damping and lower the natural frequency (by serving as an added compliance). When the natural frequency of the pressure measurement system falls, high-frequency components of the pressure waveform (such as those that occur with intraventricular pressure rise and fall) may set the system in oscillation, producing the ventricular pressure overshoot commonly seen in early systole and diastole (Figs. 7.4 and 7.16). Flushing out the catheter, manifold, and transducer dispels these small air bubbles and restores the frequency response of the pressure measurement system.

Catheter Whip Artifact

Motion of the tip of the catheter within the heart and great vessels accelerates the fluid contained within the catheter. Such catheter whip artifacts may produce superimposed waves of ±10 mm Hg. Catheter whip artifacts are particularly common in tracings from the pulmonary arteries and are difficult to avoid.

End Pressure Artifact

Flowing blood has a kinetic energy by virtue of its motion, and when this flow suddenly comes to a halt, the kinetic energy is converted in part into pressure. Therefore, an end-hole catheter pointing upstream (e.g., radial or femoral arterial pressure monitoring line) records a pressure that is artifactually elevated by the converted kinetic energy. This added pressure may range from 2 to 10 mm Hg.

Catheter Impact Artifact

Catheter impact artifact is similar but not identical to catheter whip artifact. When a fluid-filled catheter is hit (e.g.,

by valves in the act of opening or closing or by the walls of the ventricular chambers), a pressure transient is created. Any frequency component of this transient that coincides with the natural frequency of the catheter–manometer system causes a superimposed oscillation on the recorded pressure wave. Catheter impact artifacts are common with pigtail catheters in the left ventricular chamber, where the terminal pigtail may be hit by the mitral valve leaflets as they open in early diastole.

Systolic Pressure Amplification in the Periphery

When radial, brachial, or femoral arterial pressures are measured and used to represent aortic pressure, it must be remembered that peak systolic pressure in these arteries may be considerably higher (e.g., by 20 to 50 mm Hg) than peak systolic pressure in the central aorta (Fig. 7.17), although mean arterial pressure will be the same or slightly lower. There has been debate concerning the mechanism of this amplification of systolic pressure. McDonald (5) and Murgo (10,11) presented convincing evidence that the change in waveform of arterial pressure as it travels away from the heart is largely a consequence of reflected waves. These waves, presumably reflected from the aortic bifurcation, arterial branch points, and small peripheral vessels, reinforce the peak and trough of the antegrade pressure waveform, causing amplification of the peak systolic and pulse pressures (Fig. 7.17). This phenomenon may mask and distort pressure gradients across the aortic valve or left ventricular outflow tract. Use of a double-lumen catheter (e.g., double-lumen pigtail) allows measurement of left ventricular and central aortic pressures simultaneously, thus avoiding this problem. Another method is the transseptal technique with a second catheter in the central aorta (see Chapter 4). Finally, special attention to performing careful pullback tracings may also help the operator to avoid this particular error.

The operator should record central aortic pressure together with peripheral arterial pressure routinely, immediately before entering the left ventricle during retrograde

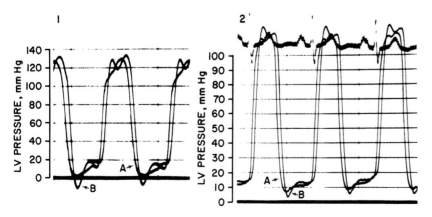

Figure 7.16 Left ventricular (LV) pressure signals as recorded with a micromanometer and with a system using long, fluid-filled tubing and several interposed stopcocks between the pressure transducer and the 7F NIH catheter. The micromanometer tracing is labeled A, and the fluid-filled catheter tracing is labeled B. Note both the early diastolic and the early ejection phase overshoots recorded with the fluid-filled catheter, indicating a poor frequency response, especially in the graph on the left.

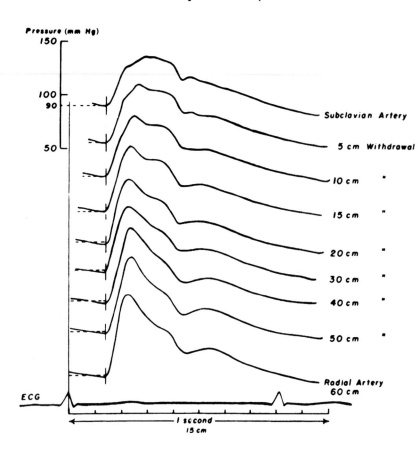

Figure 7.17 Transformation of arterial pressure waveform with transmission to the periphery in a healthy 30-year-old man. Onsets of pressures are aligned for comparison. As the pulse wave moves peripherally, the upstroke steepens and increases in magnitude, giving the pressure a spiky appearance. The horizontal line intersecting onset of each pulse contour is a calibration reference of 90 mm Hg. (From Marshall, HW, et al. Physiologic consequences of congenital heart disease. In: Hamilton WF, Dow P, eds. *Handbook of Physiology: section 2. Circulation*, vol. 1. Washington DC: American Physiologic Society, 1962:417.)

left heart catheterization. If this tracing shows a reverse gradient (peak systolic pressure in periphery higher than in central aorta), the amount of this pressure difference must be considered when subsequent comparisons of left ventricular and systemic arterial pressure are made for the detection of aortic or subaortic stenosis. The peripheral arterial systolic pressure may commonly appear to be 20 mm Hg higher than the left ventricular systolic pressure as a result of this phenomenon. This pressure amplification in the periphery is particularly marked in the radial artery (Fig. 7.17), especially if there is also some end pressure artifact, and may mask the presence of aortic stenosis. If any doubt exists concerning the presence of a true pressure gradient, either a double-lumen left heart catheter or a second central aortic catheter should be introduced to measure accurately the gradient across the aortic valve.

Errors in Zero Level, Balancing, or Calibration

Error in the quantitation of pressures because of improper zero reference is common. As mentioned earlier, in many laboratories the zero reference point is taken at the mid-chest with the patient supine, although some laboratories use a point 10 cm vertically up from the back or 5 cm vertically down from the sternal angle. All manometers must be zeroed at the same point (Fig. 7.10), and the zero reference point should be changed if the patient's position is

changed during the course of the study (e.g., if pillows are placed to prop up the patient). Transducers should be calibrated before each period of use: Electrical calibration signals and calibration factors can usually be relied on as a substitute for mercury calibration, but they should be confirmed regularly against a standard mercury reference. Linearity of response should be checked by using mercury inputs of 25, 50, and 100 mm Hg. If possible, all transducers should be exposed to the calibrating system simultaneously to avoid false gradients caused by unequal amplification of the same pressure signal. In the system described here (Fig. 7.10), a bubble in the zero-reference line can result in a false zero level; therefore, in tracking down an unexpected pressure gradient, flushing of the zero line is an important initial step. If the unexpected gradient persists, catheter attachments should be switched between the two involved manifolds. An artifactual gradient reverses direction, whereas a true gradient persists after this maneuver.

MICROMANOMETERS

To reduce the mass and inertia of the pressure measurement system, improve the frequency response characteristics, and decrease artifacts associated with overdamping and catheter whip, miniaturized transducers have been developed that fit on the distal tip of standard catheters and therefore may be used as intracardiac manometers (Figs. 7.4 and 7.16). Several models are commercially available, but many still have major technical shortcomings, such as fragility, electrical drift problems, temperature sensitivity, and inability to withstand the usual catheter sterilization techniques. Particularly reliable catheter-tip manometers are made by Millar Instruments. Available modifications of this catheter have multiple side holes and therefore permit angiography and high-fidelity pressure measurement through the same catheter. A modification of this catheter has a pigtail tip. The catheter may be subjected to gas sterilization (ethylene oxide) along with other catheters and instruments, and it may be calibrated externally at room temperature because its response characteristics are not appreciably affected by temperature changes over a wide range. In addition, modifications are available with electromagnetic flow velocity sensors and other special capabilities for research applications. Some laboratories have used a disposable high-fidelity transducer catheter and have shown that the pressures measured with these catheters are superior in waveform and accuracy to those measured with standard techniques (14).

For accurate measurement of the rate of ventricular pressure rise (dP/dt) and other parameters of myocardial performance occurring during the first 40 to 50 microseconds of ventricular systole, high frequency-response characteristics are necessary. Although there is some debate on this subject (15), micromanometer-tipped catheters are generally required in patient studies when myocardial mechanics are being examined. Gersh et al. (16) published a careful study on the physical criteria for measurement of left ventricular pressure and its first derivative. They showed that pressure measurement flat to ±5% of the first 20 harmonics of the left ventricular pressure curve is required for accurate reproduction of the amplitude of maximal dP/dt. In their study, accuracy to six harmonics led to a 20% underestimation of peak dP/dt. At a heart rate of 80 bpm, the fundamental frequency is 80/60, or 1.33 Hz, and the 20th harmonic is 26.7 Hz. As seen in Fig. 7.6, this may be possible to achieve with a short, wide-bore catheter attached directly to the pressure transducer, with optimal damping. If the heart rate increases to 100 bpm, however, the 20th harmonic becomes 100/60 × 20, or 33.3 Hz, which exceeds the capacity for even this optimal fluid-filled system. Therefore, to minimize the chance of error, micromanometer catheters should be used exclusively when dP/dt is being measured. Examples of pressure recordings taken with and without micromanometer-tipped catheters may be seen in Figs. 7.4 and 7.16.

REFERENCES

1. Hales S. In: Willius FA, Keys TE, eds. *Classics in Cardiology.* New York: Dover, 1961:131.
2. Wiggers CJ. *The Pressure Pulses in the Cardiovascular System.* London: Longmans, Green, 1928:1.
3. Hürthle K. Beiträge zur Hämodynamik. *Arch Ges Physiol* 1898; 72:566.
4. Fry DL. Physiologic recording by modern instruments with particular reference to pressure recording. *Physiol Rev* 1960;40:753.
5. McDonald DA. *Blood Flow in Arteries,* 2nd ed. Baltimore: Williams & Wilkins, 1974.
6. Wood EH, Leusen IR, Warner HR, et al. Measurement of pressures in man by cardiac catheters. *Circ Res* 1954;2:294.
7. Gleason WL, Braunwald E. Studies on the first derivative of the ventricular pressure pulse in man. *J Clin Invest* 1962;41:80.
8. Hansen AT. Pressure measurement in the human organism. *Acta Physiol Scand* 1949;19(suppl 68):87.
9. Courtois M, Fattal PG, Kovacs SJ, et al. Anatomically and physiologically based reference level of measurement of intracardiac pressures. *Circulation* 1995;92:1994.
10. Murgo JP, Westerhof N, Giolma JP, et al. Manipulation of ascending aortic pressure and flow wave reflections with Valsalva maneuver: relationship to input impedance. *Circulation* 1981;63:122.
11. Murgo JP, Westerhof N, Giolma JP, et al. Aortic input impedance in normal man: relationship to pressure wave forms. *Circulation* 1980;62:105.
12. Laskey WK, Kussmaul WG. Arterial wave reflection in heart failure. *Circulation* 1987;75:711.
13. Lange RA, Moore DM Jr, Cigarroa RG, et al. Use of pulmonary capillary wedge pressure to assess severity of mitral stenosis: is true left atrial pressure needed in this condition? *J Am Coll Cardiol* 1989;13:825.
14. Cha SD, Roman CF, Maranhao V. Clinical trial of the disposable transducer catheter. *Cathet Cardiovasc Diagn* 1988;14:63.
15. Falsetti HL, Mates RE, Greene DG, et al. V_{max} as an index of contractile state in man. *Circulation* 1971;43:467.
16. Gersh BJ, Hahn CEW, Prys-Roberts C. Physical criteria for measurement of left ventricular pressure and its first derivative. *Cardiovasc Res* 1971;5:32.

Blood Flow Measurement: Cardiac Output and Vascular Resistance

8

William Grossman

The maintenance of blood flow commensurate with the metabolic needs of the body is a fundamental requirement of human life. In the absence of major disease of the vascular tree (e.g., arterial obstruction), the maintenance of appropriate blood flow to the body depends largely on the heart's ability to pump blood in the forward direction. The quantity of blood delivered to the systemic circulation per unit time is termed the *cardiac output*, generally expressed in liters per minute.

ARTERIOVENOUS DIFFERENCE AND EXTRACTION RESERVE

Because the extraction of nutrients by metabolizing tissues is a function not only of the rate of delivery of those nutrients (the cardiac output) but also of the ability of each tissue to extract those nutrients from the circulation, tissue viability can be maintained despite a fall in cardiac output as long as there is increased extraction of required nutrients. The extraction of a given nutrient (or of any substance) from the circulation by a particular tissue is expressed as the *arteriovenous difference* across that tissue, and the factor by which the arteriovenous difference can increase at constant flow (owing to changes in metabolic demand) may be termed the *extraction reserve*. For example, arterial blood in humans is normally 95% saturated with oxygen; that is, if 1 L of blood has the capacity to carry approximately 200 mL of oxygen when fully saturated, arterial blood will usually be found to contain 190 mL of

oxygen per liter (190/200 = 95%). Venous blood returning from the body normally has an average oxygen saturation of 75%; that is, mixed venous blood generally contains 150 mL of oxygen per liter of blood (150/200 = 75%). Thus the normal arteriovenous difference for oxygen is 40 mL/L (190 mL/L − 150 mL/L).

The normal extraction reserve for oxygen is 3, which means that under extreme metabolic demand, the body's tissues can extract up to 120 mL of oxygen (3 × 40 mL) from each liter of blood delivered (1). Thus if arterial saturation remains constant at 95%, full use of the extraction reserve will result in a mixed venous oxygen content of 70 mL/L (190 mL/L − 120 mL/L) or a mixed venous oxygen saturation of 35% (70/200 = 35%). This is essentially the value found for mixed venous (i.e., pulmonary artery) oxygen saturation in normal men studied at maximal exercise. The relation between cardiac output and arteriovenous O_2 difference is illustrated in Fig. 8.1.

Lower Limit of Cardiac Output

The value of 3 for the oxygen extraction reserve predicts that in progressive cardiac decompensation, meeting the basal oxygen requirements of the body demands that oxygen extraction increases as cardiac output falls until the arteriovenous oxygen difference has tripled and cardiac output has fallen to one-third of its normal value (Fig. 8.1). Because the extraction reserve has now been used fully, further reduction of cardiac output will result in tissue hypoxia, anaerobic metabolism, acidosis, and eventually, circulatory collapse.

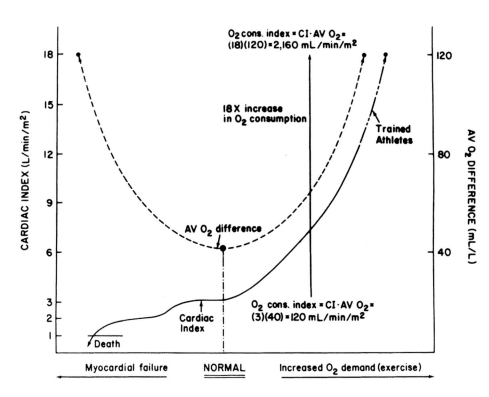

Figure 8.1 Relationship between arteriovenous oxygen (AV O$_2$) difference (*broken line*) and cardiac index (*solid curve*) in normal subjects at rest (**center**) and during exercise (**right**), and in the patient with progressively worsening myocardial failure (**left**). (See text for discussion.)

This prediction appears to be quite accurate; clinical investigators have observed for many years that a fall in resting cardiac output to below one-third of normal (i.e., a cardiac index of ≤ 1.0 L/minute per m^2) is incompatible with life.

Upper Limit of Cardiac Output

Several studies have indicated that the largest increase in cardiac output that can be achieved by a trained athlete at maximal exercise is 600% of the resting output. If a normal 70-kg man has a cardiac output of 5 L/minute or 3.0 L/minute per m^2, his maximal cardiac output might be as high as 30 L/minute (18 L/minute per m^2). Because cardiac output increases approximately 600 mL for each 100-mL increase in oxygen requirements of the body, an increase in cardiac output of 25 L/minute with maximal exercise would suggest an increase in total-body oxygen requirements of 4,167 mL/minute, which is approximately an 18-fold increase over the normal resting value of 250 mL/minute. The 18-fold increase in total-body oxygen requirements is met by the combined sixfold increase in oxygen delivery (i.e., cardiac output) and threefold increase in oxygen extraction (extraction reserve). These relations are illustrated in Fig. 8.1.

Factors Influencing Cardiac Output in Normal Subjects

The range of the "normal" cardiac output is difficult to define with precision because it is influenced by several variables. Obviously, body size is important, and the ranges of normal values for cardiac output of 2-year-old children, 10-year-old children, and 50-year-old men are so different that they show only minimal overlap. For this reason, normalization of the cardiac output for differing body size is considered fundamental by all students of this subject, although there is disagreement about the best way to accomplish this normalization. Because cardiac output seems to be predominantly a function of the body's oxygen consumption or metabolic rate (1,2) and because metabolic rate was thought to correlate best with body surface area (3,4), it has become customary to express cardiac output in terms of the cardiac index ([liters/minute]/[body surface area, m^2]). Body surface area is not measured directly, but is instead calculated from one of the experimentally developed formulas, such as that of Dubois (4).

$$\text{Body surface area (m}^2) = 0.007184 \times$$
$$\text{weight}^{0.425} \text{ (kg)} \times \text{height}^{0.725} \text{ (cm)} \qquad (8.1)$$

Despite the shortcomings and weaknesses of this approach to normalization of the cardiac output (1,5), the method has gained nearly universal acceptance by clinicians over the past 40 years and will be used throughout this book. A chart to aid calculation of body surface area (if weight and height are known) appears in Fig. 8.2.

Although expression of cardiac output as the cardiac index greatly narrows the range of normal values among our groups of 2-year-old children, 10-year-old children, and 50-year-old men, it does not completely abolish the differences in these ranges. In fact, the normal cardiac output appears to vary with age, steadily decreasing from approximately 4.5 L/minute per m^2 at age 7 years to 2.5 L/minute per m^2 at age 70 years (1,6). This is not surpris-

BSA

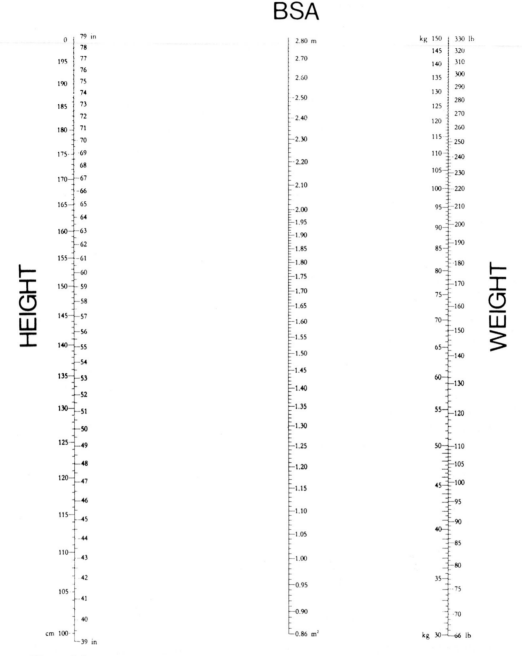

Figure 8.2 Nomogram for calculation of body surface area given the weight and height of the patient. From the formula of Dubois (4).

ing, because it is well known that the body's metabolic rate is affected greatly by age, being highest in childhood and progressively diminishing to old age.

In addition to age, cardiac output is affected by posture, decreasing approximately 10% when a person rises from a lying to a sitting position and approximately 20% when a person rises (or is tilted) from a lying to a standing position. Also, body temperature, anxiety, environmental heat and humidity, and a host of other factors influence the normal resting cardiac output (1), and these must be considered in interpreting any value of cardiac output measured in the clinical setting.

Techniques for Determination of Cardiac Output

Of the numerous techniques devised over the years to measure cardiac output, two have won general acceptance in cardiac catheterization laboratories: the Fick oxygen technique and the indicator dilution technique. Both techniques are similar in that they are based on the theoretical principle enunciated by Adolph Fick (7) in 1870. The principle, which was never actually applied by Fick, states that the total uptake or release of any substance by an organ is the product of blood flow to the organ and the arteriovenous

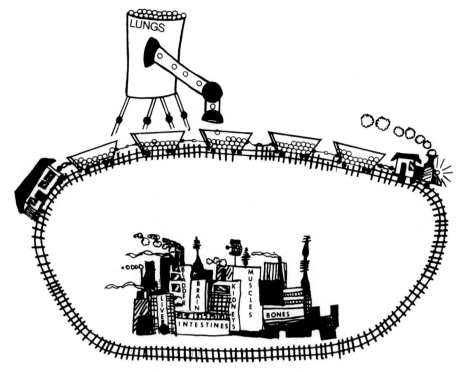

Figure 8.3 Illustration of Fick's principle. A train, representing the circulation, passes by a hopper (the lungs) that delivers marbles (oxygen) to the train's boxcars at a rate of 20 marbles per minute. Because the boxcars each contain 16 marbles before and 20 marbles after passing under the hopper, each boxcar is picking up 4 marbles and must be taking only 0.20 minute to pass under the hopper, since it would pick up 20 marbles in each full minute under the hopper. If each boxcar takes only 0.20 minute to pass by the hopper, the train is moving at a speed sufficient to deliver 5 boxcars per minute to any point down the line. This could have been calculated as

Train's speed (boxcars/minute) = marble delivery rate (marbles/minute)/"AV" marble difference (marble/minute)

= (20 marbles/minute)/(4 marbles/boxcar)

= 5 boxcars/minute

If one boxcar is 1 L of blood and each marble is 10 mL of oxygen, then we have an arteriovenous oxygen difference of 40 mL/L, an O_2 consumption of 200 mL/minute, and a cardiac output of 5 L/minute. (Illustration kindly provided by Jennifer Grossman, age 11.)

concentration difference of the substance. For the lungs, the substance released to the blood is oxygen, and the pulmonary blood flow can be determined by knowing the arteriovenous difference of oxygen across the lungs and the oxygen consumption per minute.

Fick's principle is illustrated in Fig. 8.3. In this figure, a train is passing by a hopper that is delivering marbles to the boxcars at a rate of 20 marbles per minute. If the boxcars each contain 16 marbles before passing under the hopper and 20 marbles after passing under the hopper, each boxcar is picking up four marbles and must be taking only 0.20 minute to pass under the hopper, because it would pick up 20 marbles in each full minute under the hopper. If each boxcar takes 0.20 minute to pass by the hopper, the train is moving at a speed sufficient to deliver five boxcars per minute to any point down the line. This could have been calculated as shown in Fig. 8.3:

Train's speed (boxcars/minute)

= marble delivery rate (marbles/minute)

÷ "AV" marble difference (marbles/boxcar)

= (20 marbles/minute)/(4 marbles/boxcar)

= 5 boxcars/minute

If one boxcar is 1 L of blood and each marble is 10 mL of oxygen, then we have an arteriovenous O_2 difference of 40 mL/L, an oxygen consumption of 200 mL/minute, and a cardiac output of 5 L/minute.

Fick Oxygen Method

In the Fick oxygen method, pulmonary blood flow should be determined ideally by measuring the arteriovenous difference of oxygen across the lungs and the rate of oxygen uptake by blood from the lungs. If there is no intracardiac shunt and pulmonary blood flow is equal to systemic blood flow, the Fick oxygen method also measures systemic blood flow. Thus, *cardiac output equals oxygen consumption divided by arteriovenous oxygen difference.*

In actual practice, the rate at which oxygen is taken up from the lungs by blood is not measured, but rather the uptake of oxygen from room air by the lungs is measured, because in a steady state these two measurements are equal. Furthermore, arteriovenous oxygen difference across the lungs is not measured directly. Generally, pulmonary arterial blood (true mixed venous blood) is sampled, but pulmonary venous blood is not sampled. Instead, left ventricular or systemic arterial blood is sampled and assumed to have an oxygen content representative of mixed pulmonary venous blood. Actually, because of bronchial venous and thebesian venous drainage, the oxygen content of systemic arterial blood is commonly 2 to 5 mL/L of blood lower than pulmonary venous blood as it leaves the alveoli.

Oxygen Consumption

Two different methods for measurement of oxygen consumption are widely used today: the polarographic method and the paramagnetic method. The older Douglas bag method is rarely used, and interested readers are referred to earlier editions of this book for details.

Oxygen consumption may be measured using the metabolic rate meter (MRM), made by Waters Instruments (Rochester, MN), or the Deltatrac II, made by SensorMedics (Yerba Linda, CA). The MRM instrument contains a polarographic oxygen sensor cell (gold and silver/silver chloride electrodes), a hood or face mask, and a blower of variable

speed connected to a servo control loop with the oxygen sensor (Fig. 8.4). This device is convenient and accurate and represents a significant advance over the older, standard procedure of collecting expired air for 3 minutes in a Douglas bag and measuring volume (Tissot spirometer) and oxygen content. The principle of operation for the MRM involves using a variable-speed blower to maintain a unidirectional flow of air from the room through the hood and via a connecting hose to the polarographic oxygen-sensing cell. As illustrated in Fig. 8.4, room air enters the hood at a rate $\dot{V}_R$ (mL/minute), which is determined by the blower's discharge rate $\dot{V}_M$ (mL/minute), as well as the patient's ventilatory rate ($\dot{V}_i$, inhaled air in mL/minute; $\dot{V}_E$, exhaled air). The blower speed $\dot{V}_M$ is controlled by a servo loop designed to maintain the oxygen content of air flowing past the polarographic cell constant at a predetermined value. In a steady state, the average value of $\dot{V}_M$ together with the oxygen content of room air and of air flowing past the polarographic cell can be used to calculate the patient's oxygen consumption, as follows:

The patient's oxygen consumption $\dot{V}O_2$ is given by

$$\dot{V}_{O_2} = (F_RO_2 \cdot \dot{V}_R) - (F_MO_2 \cdot \dot{V}_M) \tag{8.2}$$

where F_RO_2 and F_MO_2 are the fractional contents of oxygen in room air and in air flowing past the polarographic cell, respectively.

As can be seen from Fig. 8.4,

$$\dot{V}_M = \dot{V}_R - \dot{V}_i + \dot{V}_E \tag{8.3}$$

which can be rewritten as

$$\dot{V}_R = \dot{V}_M + \dot{V}_i - \dot{V}_E \tag{8.4}$$

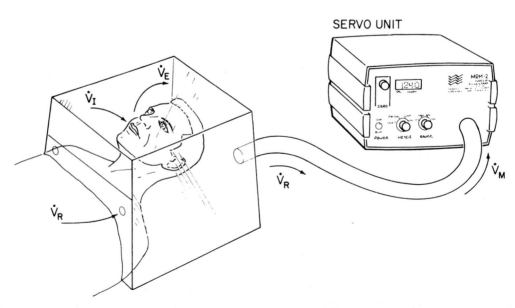

Figure 8.4 Measurement of O$_2$ consumption by a polarographic cell technique using the Waters Instruments metabolic rate meter (MRM). A transparent hood fits snugly over the patient's head, resting on a pillow. Air enters the hood through holes in a plastic sheet at a flow rate of $\dot{V}_R$. The patient's inspiratory ($\dot{V}_I$) and expiratory ($\dot{V}_E$) flow rates subtract and add to $\dot{V}_R$ to yield $\dot{V}_M$, the flow rate leaving the hood and entering the servo unit. A blower motor in the servo unit adjusts $\dot{V}_M$ to keep the O$_2$ sensed by a polarographic cell constant. (See text for details.)

Substituting this in Eq. (8.2) gives

$$V_{O_2} = F_R O_2(\dot{V}_M + \dot{V}_i - \dot{V}_E) - F_M O_2 \cdot \dot{V}_M \quad (8.5)$$

$$= F_R O_2(\dot{V}_M) - F_M O_2(\dot{V}_M) + F_R O_2(\dot{V}_i) - F_R O_2(\dot{V}_E)$$

$$= \dot{V}_M(F_R O_2 - F_M O_2) + F_R O_2(\dot{V}_i - \dot{V}_E)$$

Because the fractional content of oxygen in room air $(F_R O_2)$ is 0.209, oxygen consumption is given by

$$\dot{V}_{O_2} = \dot{V}_M(0.209 - F_M O_2) + 0.209(\dot{V}_i - \dot{V}_E) \quad (8.6)$$

Thus in a steady state (where $\dot{V}_i - \dot{V}_E$ is constant), oxygen consumption can be determined by measuring the volume rate of air moved by the blower motor $(\dot{V}_M)$ and the fractional oxygen content of air moving past the polarographic sensor. In the MRM, a servo-controlled system adjusts $\dot{V}_M$ to keep $F_M O_2$ at a constant predetermined value. In practice, $F_M O_2$ is set at 0.199 so that Eq. (8.6) becomes

$$\dot{V}_{O_2} = \dot{V}_M(0.209 - 0.199) + 0.209(\dot{V}_i - \dot{V}_E) \quad (8.7)$$

$$\dot{V}_{O_2} = 0.01 \dot{V}_M + 0.209(\dot{V}_i - \dot{V}_E).$$

For practical purposes, the respiratory quotient (RQ) is assumed to be 1.0; accordingly, $\dot{V}_i = \dot{V}_E$ and $\dot{V}_{O_2} = 0.01 \dot{V}_M$. If the RQ is actually 0.9 (e.g., the patient releases 0.9 L of CO_2 for each liter of O_2 consumed), the error in $\dot{V}_{O_2}$ resulting from the assumption of an RQ of 1.0 is 1.6%, and if RQ is 0.8, the error is 3.2%. The MRM O_2 consumption monitor has a calibrated blower motor in addition to the servo-control polarographic sensor and gives a readout of oxygen consumption in liters per minute by digital scale (MRM-2) or by meter and paper (MRM-1). The MRM-2 model is calibrated to be highly accurate in the oxygen consumption range from 10 to 1,000 mL O_2/minute and is thus best suited for measurement of resting O_2 consumption in the catheterization laboratory. The MRM-1 model, which is calibrated in the range of 150 to 5,000 mL O_2/minute, is best suited for exercise studies.

The SensorMedics Deltatrac II differs from the Waters Instruments MRM device in several aspects. First, it is more sophisticated than the MRM and directly measures the fractional content of oxygen as well as the concentration of carbon dioxide in expired flow, and thus calculates the RQ of each patient. The SensorMedics device is calibrated prior to each period of use with a cylinder containing a test gas of 95% oxygen and 5% carbon dioxide. The SensorMedics device uses a constant flow rate $\dot{V}_M$ leaving the canopy or hood and entering the metabolic monitor unit. The sensors in this unit measure oxygen (paramagnetic sensor) and carbon dioxide (infrared sensor), and the unit adjusts for temperature and the partial pressure of water vapor, expressing O_2 consumption and CO_2 production at standard temperature and pressure and dry (STPD; dry gas at 0°C and 760 mm Hg).

Both the Waters Instruments and SensorMedics devices are relatively easy to use, although a fair amount of attention to detail is required to obtain reproducible readings consistently. A study by Lange et al. (8), however, found that values of oxygen consumption measured by metabolic rate meter (MRM-2, Waters Instruments, Rochester, MN) were significantly lower than those measured using the standard Douglas bag technique, mentioned previously.

Arteriovenous Oxygen Difference

The arteriovenous oxygen difference across the lungs must be measured to calculate cardiac output by Fick's principle, and this can be accomplished by the following method. From appropriately positioned catheters, systemic arterial and mixed venous (pulmonary arterial) blood samples are obtained during the period when O_2 consumption is being measured. The samples are drawn into heparinized syringes and capped quickly. If the patient has received heparin systemically, the syringes for collection of these blood samples need not be heparinized. If the samples will be analyzed immediately by oximetry, plastic syringes may be used. O_2 may diffuse through the walls of plastic syringes, however, and glass syringes are considered preferable by some if there will be a delay in oximetric analysis of the blood. In a test in my laboratory, no appreciable increase in O_2 saturation of venous blood could be detected over 2 hours. (A capped plastic 15-mL syringe filled with venous blood sitting at room temperature was sampled every 15 minutes for oximetry.) The samples should be drawn simultaneously and as close to the midpoint of the oxygen consumption determination as possible. Care must be taken to avoid contamination of the blood samples with air bubbles.

Oxygen content (in milliliters of oxygen per liter of blood) can be determined by a variety of methods, the most classic of which (and the one that serves as a standard for all others) is the manometric technique of Van Slyke and Neill (9). The major drawback of the Van Slyke and Neill technique is that 15 to 30 minutes are required to run a single blood sample. The different devices for oximetry measurement have been studied and compared by Shepherd and McMahan (9). The older Van Slyke methodology is rarely used today, and the Lex-O_2-Con fuel cell technique is no longer available. Devices in widespread use today are of the co-oximeter class and either hemolyze the blood sample (by ultrasonic or chemical techniques) or use whole blood; both types of co-oximeter depend on spectrophotometric measurement of the percent oxygen saturation of hemoglobin. Several devices in use today have been demonstrated to be accurate (9), including the Radiometer OSM2 and AVOXimeter 1000 (A-Vox Systems, San Antonio, TX) devices. Using these devices, oximetry of heparinized blood samples is simple and quick and measures the percentage of hemoglobin present as oxyhemoglobin. This percentage, multiplied by the theoretical oxygen-carrying capacity of the patient's blood, yields the

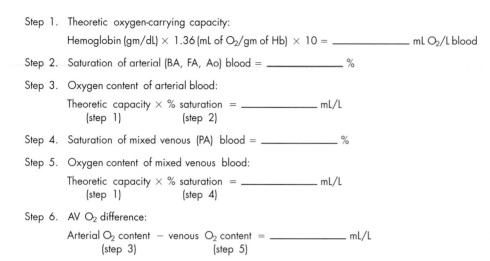

Step 1. Theoretic oxygen-carrying capacity:

Hemoglobin (gm/dL) × 1.36 (mL of O_2/gm of Hb) × 10 = _____ mL O_2/L blood

Step 2. Saturation of arterial (BA, FA, Ao) blood = _____ %

Step 3. Oxygen content of arterial blood:

Theoretic capacity × % saturation = _____ mL/L
　　　(step 1)　　　　　　(step 2)

Step 4. Saturation of mixed venous (PA) blood = _____ %

Step 5. Oxygen content of mixed venous blood:

Theoretic capacity × % saturation = _____ mL/L
　　　(step 1)　　　　　　(step 4)

Step 6. AV O_2 difference:

Arterial O_2 content − venous O_2 content = _____ mL/L
　　(step 3)　　　　　　(step 5)

Figure 8.5 Calculation of oxygen content and AV oxygen difference when using the reflectance oximetry method.

calculated oxygen content of that sample (Fig. 8.5). A formula for approximating the theoretical oxygen-carrying capacity in humans is

Hemoglobin (g/dL)

× 1.36 (mL O_2/g of hemoglobin)　　　　(8.8)

× 10 = theoretical O_2

= carrying capacity (mL O_2/liter of blood)

In several textbooks the constant is given as 1.34, but studies on crystalline human hemoglobin suggest that the correct number may be 1.36 (10,11). Whatever its correct value, the formula is only an approximation. The steps of Fig. 8.5 may be used to calculate oxygen content of blood samples and arteriovenous oxygen difference when the spectrophotometric oximeter method is used. Oxygen contents of arterial and mixed venous blood samples are calculated as the percentage of oxyhemoglobin saturation of these samples multiplied by the oxygen-carrying capacity (steps 2 to 5, Fig. 8.5). The arteriovenous oxygen difference (step 3 minus step 5, Fig. 8.5) may then be divided into the oxygen consumption to yield the cardiac output. Current oximeters, such as the AVOXimeter 1000, illuminate a very small sample of heparinized blood (volume, 50 mL) with light of multiple wavelengths and record the optical density of each transmitted wavelength. This approach allows estimation of total hemoglobin concentration as well as the concentrations of various components: oxyhemoglobin, methemoglobin, and carboxyhemoglobin. This permits instantaneous calculation of oxygen content, which is displayed on the oximeter's liquid crystal display (LCD) screen. This value can then be entered directly in steps 3, 5, and 6 of Fig. 8.5.

Arterial blood may be taken from a systemic artery, the left ventricle, the left atrium, or the pulmonary veins. Theoretically, pulmonary venous blood is preferable to peripheral arterial blood for the arteriovenous oxygen differ-

ence calculations. However, except in the presence of a right-to-left intracardiac shunt, pulmonary venous oxygen content may be approximated by systemic arterial oxygen content, ignoring the small amount of venous admixture resulting from bronchial and thebesian venous drainage. If arterial desaturation (e.g., arterial blood oxygen saturation <95%) is present, a central right-to-left shunt should be excluded before accepting systemic arterial oxygen content as representative of pulmonary venous blood. Techniques for detecting and quantifying such shunts are described in Chapter 9.

The most reliable site for obtaining mixed venous blood is the pulmonary artery. Because of streaming and incomplete mixing, using blood from more proximal sites such as the right atrium or vena cavae as representative of mixed venous blood is much less accurate (12,13). Right ventricular blood is closer to true mixed venous blood and may be substituted for pulmonary arterial blood if necessary.

Sources of Error

The techniques described for cardiac output measurement by application of Fick's principle assume that a steady state exists (i.e., that the cardiac output and oxygen consumption are constant during the period of measurement). Therefore strict quiet, calm, and decorum must be maintained in the cardiac catheterization laboratory during this time to encourage the achievement of a steady state condition. Potential errors in the determination of cardiac output by the Fick oxygen technique may come from a number of sources.

The spectrophotometric determination of blood oxygen saturation may introduce inaccuracies related to carboxyhemoglobin or other abnormal hemoglobins, as discussed previously. This method also may be inaccurate if indocyanine green dye is present in the circulation, although the newer oximeters are not affected by this problem. Reflectance oximetry, as performed on whole blood, is accurate in the range of blood oxygen saturations from 45 to 98%, but may not be reliable when blood O_2 saturation is <40%, as is the case in pulmonary artery blood from patients with very low cardiac output or during strenuous exercise.

Improper collection of the mixed venous blood sample (e.g., air bubbles) is a common source of error. Partial contamination of pulmonary arterial blood with pulmonary capillary wedge blood may result in a falsely high mixed venous oxygen content. If the mixed venous blood sample is taken from the right atrium, inferior vena cava, coronary sinus, or similar sites, a falsely low or high value for arteriovenous difference may result. Also, care must be taken not to dilute the blood sample with too much heparinized saline solution.

The average error in determining oxygen consumption has been estimated to be approximately 6% (13). The error for arteriovenous oxygen difference has been estimated at 5% (14,15). Narrow arteriovenous oxygen differences are more prone to introduce error than wide arteriovenous oxygen differences. Thus the Fick oxygen method is most accurate in patients with low cardiac output, in whom the arteriovenous oxygen difference is wide. The total error in determination of the cardiac output by the Fick oxygen method has been established to be about 10% (16).

Does oxygen consumption actually need to be measured? To avoid the technical difficulties and expense associated with measurement of oxygen consumption, some laboratories assume that O_2 consumption can be predicted from the body surface area, with or without a correction for age and sex. Thus, some laboratories assume that resting O_2 consumption is 125 mL/m^2, or 110 mL/m^2 for older patients. The validity of such an assumption has been addressed in a study from the University of Texas at Dallas (17). Cardiac output was determined by the indicator dilution technique, and O_2 consumption was calculated by dividing cardiac output by arteriovenous oxygen difference, which was measured directly. In the 108 patients studied, the O_2 consumption index averaged 126 ± 26 mL/minute per m^2 (mean ± standard deviation), but there was wide variability as indicated by the standard deviation, and the authors concluded that O_2 consumption varies greatly among adults at the time of cardiac catheterization. In another study from Bristol Royal Infirmary in the United Kingdom (18), direct measurement of O_2 consumption was compared with assumed values in 80 patients (aged 38 to 78 years). Large discrepancies were evident, with more than half the values differing by more than ±10% and several by ±25% or more. Thus, assumed values for O_2 consumption are likely to introduce considerable error.

Indicator Dilution Methods

The indicator dilution method is merely a specific application of Fick's general principle. In the Fick oxygen method,

the indicator is oxygen, the site of injection is the lungs, and the injection procedure is that of continuous infusion. Stewart (19) was the first to use the so-called indicator dilution method for measuring cardiac output; he used the continuous-infusion technique and reported his first studies in 1897.

There are two general types of indicator dilution methods: the continuous-infusion method and the single-injection method. The single-injection method is the most widely used and is discussed here in detail. The fundamental requirements for this method include the following:

A bolus of nontoxic indicator substance is injected; the substance mixes completely with blood, and its concentration can be measured accurately.

The indicator substance is neither added to nor subtracted from the blood during passage between injection and sampling sites.

Most of the indicator must pass the site of sampling before recirculation begins.

The indicator substance must go through a portion of the central circulation where all the blood of the body becomes mixed.

For the single-injection method, theoretical considerations may be summarized as follows: An injection of a specified amount of an indicator, I, into a proximal vessel or chamber (e.g., the vena cava or right atrium for the thermodilution method and the pulmonary artery for the indocyanine green dye method) is followed by continuous measurement of the indicator concentration C in blood as a function of time, t, at a point downstream from the injection (e.g., pulmonary artery for thermodilution technique and radial or femoral artery for the indocyanine green dye method). Because all the injection indicator I must pass the downstream measurement site,

$$I = \dot{Q} \int_0^\infty C(t)\,dt \qquad (8.9)$$

where $\dot{Q}$ is the volume flow (in milliliters per minute) between the sites of injection and measurement. Thus $\dot{Q}$ (which is the cardiac output in the methods to be described) may be calculated as

$$\dot{Q} = \frac{I}{\displaystyle\int_0^\infty C(t)\,dt} \qquad (8.10)$$

Numerous indicators have been used successfully, and the history of this subject is reviewed thoroughly by Guyton et al. (1). Indocyanine green previously had enjoyed long-standing acceptance in clinical practice but is rarely used today for routine measurement of cardiac output. Accordingly, it will not be discussed here and the interested reader is referred to previous editions of this textbook. We will only discuss thermodilution (in which "cold" is the indicator), which is now the dominant technique.

Thermodilution Method

A thermal indicator method for measuring cardiac output was first introduced by Fegler (20) in 1954 but was not applied to the clinical situation until the work of Branthwaite and Bradley (21) and Ganz et al. (22,23). In the initial report by Ganz et al. (22), two thermistors were used: one in the superior vena cava at the site at which the cold dextrose solution was injected into the bloodstream and a second downstream thermistor in the pulmonary artery. These two thermistors allowed accurate measurement of the temperature of the injectate T_I as well as the temperature of blood T_B downstream from the injectate. Using the basic indicator dilution equation, the cardiac output by thermodilution CO_{TD} in milliliters is given as

$$CO_{TD} = \frac{V_I(T_B - T_I)(S_I \cdot C_I / S_B \cdot C_B)60(\text{sec/min})}{\int_0^\infty \Delta T_B(t)\,dt} \quad (8.11)$$

where V_I = volume of injectate (mL) and S_B, S_I, C_B, and C_I are the specific gravity and specific heat of blood and injectate, respectively. When 5% dextrose is used as an indicator, $S_I \cdot C_I / S_B \cdot C_B = 1.08$. Most commercially available thermodilution systems use a single thermistor only, placed at the downstream site, and assume that the temperature of the injectate (measured in a bowl before injection) increased by a predictable amount (catheter warming) during injection. The calculated cardiac output by the thermodilution equation is multiplied by an empirical correction factor (0.825) to correct for the catheter warming (23). However, a recent report (24) has demonstrated that improved accuracy and precision can be obtained with the thermodilution technique when cardiac output is measured using a dual-thermistor catheter system. These investigators used a specialized dual-thermistor right heart catheter, constructed with a second thermistor positioned to measure temperature at the point where the injectate exits the catheter in the right atrium. This takes into account any warming of the injectate that may take place as it travels from the injectate syringe to the point of exit from the catheter in the right atrium. This technique provided substantially less measurement variability and better agreement with simultaneously measured Fick cardiac output (the latter determined using a 5-minute Douglas bag collection of expired air and paired blood samples from pulmonary and femoral arteries).

The thermodilution method for measuring cardiac output has several advantages over the indocyanine green dye method, and these include the following:

1. It does not require withdrawal of blood.
2. It does not require an arterial puncture.
3. An inert and inexpensive indicator is used.
4. There is virtually no recirculation, making computer analysis of the primary curve simple.

Sources of Error

1. The method is unreliable in the presence of significant tricuspid regurgitation.
2. The baseline temperature of blood in the pulmonary artery usually shows distinct fluctuations associated with respiratory and cardiac cycles. If these fluctuations are large, they may approach the magnitude of the temperature change produced by the cold indicator injection.
3. Loss of injected indicator (cold) between injection and measuring sites (vena cava and pulmonary artery) is not usually a problem, but in low-flow, low-output states, loss of indicator may occur because of warming of blood by the walls of the cardiac chambers and surrounding tissues. This concern is supported by the study of van Grondelle et al. (25), who found that thermodilution cardiac output measurements overestimated cardiac output consistently in patients with low output (<3.5 L/minute), and this overestimation was greatest, averaging 35%, in patients whose cardiac outputs were <2.5 L/minute. This is what might be expected from the equation for calculation of cardiac output by thermodilution, since the change in pulmonary artery blood temperature (ΔT_B) will be reduced if cold is lost by warming of the injectate during slow passage through the vena cava, right atrium, and right ventricle. Because ΔT_B is the denominator in the equation for cardiac output calculation, reduction in ΔT_B will result in a rise in calculated cardiac output.
4. The empirical correction factor of 0.825 may be inadequate to correct for deviations in true injectate temperature from the temperature of the injectate bowl or reservoir owing to warming in the syringe by the hand of the individual injecting the dextrose solution from the syringe or by catheter warming.

In general, indicator dilution cardiac output determinations have an error of 5 to 10% when performed carefully. The values obtained correlate well with those calculated by the Fick oxygen method.

Clinical Measurement of Vascular Resistance

Poiseuille's Law

The French physician Jean Léonard Marie Poiseuille (1799–1869) made many important contributions to the study of hemodynamics. At age 18, he introduced the mercury manometer for the measurement of blood pressure, a technical innovation that continues in use to this day. In 1846, he formulated a series of equations describing the flow of fluids through cylindrical tubes. Although Poiseuille was interested in blood flow, he substituted simpler liquids in his measurements of flow through rigid glass tubes. His discoveries, later modified by others, are expressed in what is regarded as Poiseuille's law (26), which may be stated as follows:

$$Q = \frac{\pi\,(P_i - P_o)\,r^4}{8\eta l} \qquad (8.12)$$

where Q is volume flow; $P_i - P_o$ is inflow pressure − outflow pressure; r is the radius of the tube; l is the length of the tube; and η is the viscosity of the fluid.

This relationship applies in the specific circumstance of steady state laminar flow of a homogeneous fluid through a rigid tube. Under these conditions, flow, Q, varies directly as the pressure difference, $P_i - P_o$, and the fourth power of the tube's radius, r. It varies inversely as the length, l, of the tube and the viscosity, η, of the fluid.

Hydraulic resistance, R, is defined by analogy to Ohm's law as the ratio of mean pressure drop, ΔP, to flow, Q, across the vascular circuit. The various factors contributing to vascular resistance can be illustrated by rearranging Poiseuille's law as follows:

$$R = \frac{P_i - P_o}{Q} = \frac{8\eta l}{\pi r^4} \qquad (8.13)$$

It is apparent from this equation that, in the condition of steady laminar flow of a homogeneous fluid through a rigid cylindrical tube, resistance to flow depends only on the dimensions of the tube and the viscosity of the fluid. In particular, the resistance is remarkably sensitive to changes in the radius of the tube, varying inversely with its fourth power.

Vascular Resistance and Pressure–Flow Relationships

The applicability of laws derived from steady state fluid mechanics in assessing vascular resistance is somewhat ambiguous because blood flow is pulsatile, blood is a non-homogeneous fluid, and the vascular bed is a nonlinear, elastic, frequency-dependent system. In such a system, resistance varies continuously with pressure and flow and is influenced by many factors, such as inertia, reflected waves, and the phase angle between pulse and flow wave velocities (26–28).

To assess both vessel caliber and elasticity, the resistive and compliant characteristics of the vascular system, the concept of *vascular impedance* has been used (27). Vascular impedance has been defined as the instantaneous ratio of pulsatile pressure to pulsatile flow (28,29). Because impedance may not be the same for all frequencies, its calculation requires resolution of the harmonic components of both pressure and flow pulsations. The *impedance modulus* so calculated is then expressed as a spectrum of impedance versus frequency. Although measurement of impedance is important in research studies, it is rarely included in routine diagnostic cardiac catheterization, and the reader is referred elsewhere (26) for a full discussion.

As a consequence of the foregoing considerations and the many active and passive factors that influence pressure and flow in blood vessels, the concept of vascular resistance in its pure physical sense is limited in application. In the context of the clinical and physiologic setting, however, pulmonary and systemic vascular resistances calculated from hemodynamic measurements made during cardiac catheterization have acquired empiric pathophysiologic meaning and are often important factors in clinical decision making.

Estimation of Vascular Resistance in the Clinical Situation

Calculations of vascular resistance are usually applied to both the pulmonary and systemic circulations. Although many authors refer to systemic or pulmonary arteriolar resistance, I prefer the term *vascular resistance* because it is less committal concerning the anatomic site of the resistance. As has been mentioned, arteriolar tone is only one determinant of vascular resistance to blood flow. To estimate pulmonary and systemic vascular resistances quantitatively, knowledge of both the driving pressure across the pulmonary and systemic vascular beds and the respective blood flow through them is required.

The formulas generally used are:

A. Systemic vascular resistance $= \dfrac{\overline{Ao} - \overline{RA}}{Q_s}$

B. Total pulmonary resistance $= \dfrac{\overline{PA}}{Q_p}$ $\qquad$ (8.14, A–C)

C. Pulmonary vascular resistance $= \dfrac{\overline{PA} - \overline{LA}}{Q_p}$

where $\overline{Ao}$ is mean systemic arterial pressure, $\overline{RA}$ is mean right atrial pressure, $\overline{PA}$ is mean pulmonary arterial pressure, $\overline{LA}$ is mean left atrial pressure, Q_s is systemic blood flow, and Q_p is pulmonary blood flow.

In many laboratories, the mean pulmonary capillary wedge pressure is used as an approximation of mean left atrial pressure. This should cause no problem because there is ample evidence that pulmonary capillary wedge pressure, properly obtained, closely approximates the level of left atrial pressure (30–32). The flows are volume flows (as opposed to velocity flows) and are expressed in liters per minute, and pressures are expressed in millimeters of mercury (mm Hg). These equations yield resistance in arbitrary resistance units (R units) expressed in mm Hg per liter per minute, also called *hybrid resistance units* (HRUs). These HRUs are sometimes referred to as Wood units because they were first introduced by Dr. Paul Wood. They may be converted to metric resistance units expressed in dynes-sec-cm^{-5} by use of the conversion factor 80. In this system, resistance is expressed as:

Resistance =

$$\frac{\Delta P(\text{mm Hg}) \times 1{,}332 \text{ dynes/cm}^2/\text{mm Hg}}{Q_s \text{ or } Q_p (\text{L/min}) \times 1{,}000 \text{ mL/L} \div 60 \text{ sec/min}}$$

$$= \frac{\Delta P}{Q_s \text{ or } Q_p} \times 80 = \text{dynes-sec-cm}^{-5} \qquad (8.15)$$

There is no particular advantage to either system, since both express precisely the same ratio. Most pediatric cardiologists use hybrid resistance units, whereas cardiologists with adult practices generally use metric units.

In pediatric practice, it is conventional to normalize vascular resistances for body surface area (BSA), thus giving a resistance index. Although this is not commonly done in adult cardiac catheterization laboratories, the practice makes sense because normal cardiac output and therefore vascular resistance may be substantially different in a 260-lb man and a 110-lb woman. The normalized resistance, however, is not obtained by dividing resistance (as calculated in Eq. 8.14) by body surface area. Rather, normalized resistance is calculated by substituting the blood flow index for blood flow in the resistance formula. Thus systemic vascular resistance index (SVRI) is calculated as

$$\text{SVRI} = \frac{(\overline{Ao} - \overline{RA})\,80}{\text{CI}} \qquad (8.16)$$

where CI is the cardiac (or systemic blood flow) index. Therefore, SVRI equals SVR multiplied by BSA.

Cardiac output, usually measured by either the Fick or the thermodilution method, is used as mean blood flow. It is important to realize that in conditions of intracardiac shunts or shunts between the pulmonary and systemic circulations, pulmonary blood flow and systemic flow may not be equal, and the respective flow through each circuit must be measured and used in the appropriate resistance calculation. Normal values for vascular resistance in adults are given in Table 8.1.

Clinical Use of Vascular Resistance

As can be deduced from the Poiseuille equation, changes in systemic or pulmonary vascular resistance may result theoretically from one of three mechanisms. Because changes in length of the vascular beds are uncommon after growth has been completed, changes in vascular resistance reflect either altered viscosity of blood or a change in cross-sectional area (radius) of the vascular bed.

There is ample evidence that changes in blood viscosity alter measured vascular resistances. Nihill (33) has shown that an approximate doubling of pulmonary vascular resistance occurs with increases in hematocrit from 43 to 64%. Similarly, low values for measured vascular resistance are commonly seen in patients with severe chronic anemia, although the low vascular resistance in such cases probably represents more than a viscosity effect alone.

With regard to changes in cross-sectional area of the pulmonary or systemic vascular bed, such changes do not invariably imply altered arteriolar tone. In the normal systemic circulation, mean aortic pressure may be 100 mm Hg, whereas right atrial pressure is only 5 mm Hg. Although the greatest part of this pressure drop occurs at the arteriolar level (approximately 60%), about 15% occurs in the capillaries, 15% in small veins, and 10% in the arterial system proximal to the arterioles (27). Thus although systemic vascular resistance is dominated by the caliber of the arterioles, the other components of the systemic vascular bed are by no means negligible. For example, Read and coworkers (34) studied systemic vascular resistance in dogs with constant (pump-controlled) cardiac output and found that a rise in venous pressure consistently caused a fall in resistance. The magnitude of the fall was proportional to the increment in venous pressure rise and was about 20% for an increase in venous pressure of 20 mm Hg. Other studies show no change in resistance when arterial pressure is so manipulated (in the absence of baroreceptor control). These findings have been interpreted by McDonald (28) to suggest that the decline in systemic vascular resistance with increased venous pressure results from dilation of small venous channels, whereas systemic arterioles do not distend passively with increased pressure. Therefore, measurement of vascular resistance is not a precise tool for assessing the dynamics of individual sections of the vascular bed, and the term *vascular resistance* should not be used as synonymous with arteriolar resistance.

TABLE 8.1

NORMAL VALUES FOR VASCULAR RESISTANCE

Systemic vascular resistance	$1{,}170 \pm 270$ dynes-sec-cm^{-5}
Systemic vascular resistance index	$2{,}130 \pm 450$ dynes-sec-cm$^{-5} \cdot$ M^2
Pulmonary vascular resistance	67 ± 30 dynes-sec-cm^{-5}
Pulmonary vascular resistance index	123 ± 54 dynes-sec-cm$^{-5} \cdot$ M^2

Values are expressed as mean $\pm$ standard deviation and are derived from 37 subjects without demonstrable cardiovascular disease (17 males, 20 females, age 47 ± 9 years) who underwent diagnostic cardiac catheterization at the Peter Bent Brigham Hospital between July 1, 1975, and June 30, 1978.

Systemic Vascular Resistance

The minute-to-minute control of vascular resistance, at least in the systemic bed, is an amalgam of autonomic nervous system influences and local metabolic factors. Hypotension or reduced cardiac output generally triggers increased systemic resistance by means of the baroreceptors, α-adrenergic neural pathways, and release of humoral vasoconstrictor hormones, but these influences may be opposed by metabolic factors if the hypotension or low cardiac output results in decreased tissue perfusion with local hypoxia and acidosis. This latter circumstance is commonly seen in congestive heart failure or shock.

Knowledge of changes in systemic vascular resistance is also important in evaluating the hemodynamic response to stress tests, such as dynamic or isometric exercise (35). In this regard, there is ample evidence that normally, the systemic vascular resistance falls in response to dynamic exercise, but pulmonary vascular resistance is unchanged (at least with supine bicycle exercise). Transient elevations in systemic vascular resistance have been provoked by infusions of vasopressor drugs to evaluate the left ventricular response to a sudden increase in afterload (36).

Low systemic vascular resistance may be seen in conditions in which blood flow is abnormally high, such as may occur in patients with arteriovenous fistula, severe anemia, and other high-output states. It is important to realize that in these circumstances there may well be regional differences in vascular resistance (e.g., very low in the arteriovenous fistula but normal or increased in other vascular beds), and calculations based on mean pressure and flow in the entire systemic circulation must be interpreted with caution.

Total Pulmonary Resistance

Calculated as the ratio of mean pulmonary artery pressure to pulmonary blood flow, total pulmonary resistance expresses the resistance to flow in transporting a volume of blood from the pulmonary artery to the left ventricle in diastole, neglecting left ventricular diastolic pressure. This relationship is obviously influenced by alterations in left atrial pressure and will not consistently provide useful information about the condition of the pulmonary vasculature. Although widely used 25 years ago, this parameter is less commonly used today and in general should be used primarily in the patient where measurement of left atrial or pulmonary capillary wedge pressure is not possible.

Pulmonary Vascular Resistance

Sometimes (inappropriately) called pulmonary arteriolar resistance, pulmonary vascular resistance expresses the pressure drop across the major pulmonary vessels, the precapillary arterioles, and the pulmonary capillary bed and is more precise in assessing the presence and degree of pulmonary vascular disease than is total pulmonary resistance. Simple calculation of pulmonary vascular resistance provides general information about the pulmonary circulation, but this must be interpreted in the context of the clinical situation and other hemodynamic data obtained during cardiac catheterization. The pulmonary vasculature is a dynamic system and is subject to many mechanical, neural, and biochemical influences.

Measured pulmonary vascular resistance may be *increased* by hypoxia, hypercapnia, increased sympathetic tone, polycythemia, local release of serotonin, mechanical obstruction by multiple pulmonary emboli, precapillary pulmonary edema, or lung compression (pleural effusion, increased intrathoracic pressure via respirator). Pulmonary vascular resistance may be *decreased* by oxygen, adenosine, isoproterenol, α-antagonists such as phentolamine or tolazoline, inhaled nitric oxide, prostacyclin infusions, and high doses of calcium channel blockers. These vasodilators may be used to test for fixed, irreversible pulmonary hypertension. A practical approach used in many laboratories to test for responsiveness and determine therapeutic dosage uses intravenous epoprostenol (Flolan, Glaxo Wellcome, Research Triangle Park, NC), starting at 2 ng/kg per minute and increasing by increments of 2 ng/kg per minute every 15 minutes until dose-limiting pharmacologic effects (such as nausea, headache, or hypotension) are seen.

The tolazoline test for fixed pulmonary hypertension is rarely performed at present, and the interested reader is referred to earlier editions of this textbook for details as to its use. *Oxygen inhalation* may be of value in assessing pulmonary vascular reactivity. Patients with high pulmonary vascular resistance (i.e., $\geq$600 dynes-sec-cm^{-5}) in association with a central shunt (e.g., ventricular septal defect) should be given 100% oxygen by face mask before concluding that the changes are fixed. Older patients with a combination of left heart failure and chronic obstructive lung disease may have considerable pulmonary vasoconstriction owing to alveolar hypoventilation and its resultant hypoxia. Inhalation of 100% oxygen in such cases may result in a dramatic fall in pulmonary arterial pressure and vascular resistance.

Most studies demonstrating the usefulness of tolazoline or oxygen inhalation in the assessment of pulmonary vascular disease associated with central shunts were carried out in patients living at high altitudes. The usefulness of such assessment in patients living at sea level is less certain.

PULMONARY VASCULAR DISEASE IN PATIENTS WITH CONGENITAL CENTRAL SHUNTS

The decision as to whether a patient with congenital heart disease would profit from corrective surgery often hinges on the calculated pulmonary vascular resistance. Although each case must be evaluated on its own characteristics, many criteria for operability have been proposed (37,38). It has been suggested that the ratio between pulmonary vascular resistance and systemic vascular resistance (resistance ratio, PVR/SVR) be used as a criterion for operability in dealing with congenital heart disease (37). Normally, this ratio is ≤0.25. Values of 0.25 to 0.50 indicate moderate pulmonary vascular disease, and values greater than 0.75 indicate severe pulmonary vascular disease. When the PVR/SVR resistance ratio equals 1.0 or more, surgical correction of the congenital defect is considered contraindicated because of the severity of the pulmonary vascular disease.

The resistance ratio has the value of factoring in miscellaneous neural, hormonal, and blood viscosity influences that may be affecting both pulmonary and systemic vascular beds and that may be primarily related to the patient's immediate clinical status more than to intrinsic pulmonary vascular changes. Many patients with left ventricular failure and low systemic output (from any cause) have associated high systemic and pulmonary vascular resistance, but the resistance ratio will be normal in the absence of intrinsic vascular pathology.

We have reported (37) three patients with congenital heart disease (two with atrial septal defect and one with patent ductus arteriosus) having cyanosis and pulmonary arterial hypertension at nearly systemic levels. Each of our patients (37) had PVR/SVR ratios of <0.50 and net left-to-right shunts, despite severe pulmonary hypertension (e.g., pulmonary artery pressure 110/55 mm Hg). Each patient had progressive improvement in pulmonary vascular resistance toward normal following operative closure of the shunts. These cases illustrate the importance of increased blood viscosity associated with the polycythemia of cyanosis (hematocrits in the 56 to 66% range), which may contribute substantially to the measured increase in pulmonary and systemic vascular resistances. As mentioned earlier, studies in dogs showed that calculated pulmonary vascular resistance doubled when hematocrit was raised from 43 to 64%. Accordingly, elimination of severe cyanosis with return of hematocrit to normal may lead to a 50% reduction in pulmonary vascular resistance. This influence of viscosity, as well as the generalized vasoconstriction often seen in patients with advanced cardiac disease, will be factored out by the ratio of PVR/SVR.

In his classic description of the Eisenmenger syndrome, Wood pointed out that attempted surgical repair of the shunt defect was a major source of death in these patients (38). He stated that in patients with pulmonary blood flow of <1.75 times systemic flow or with total pulmonary vascular resistance >12 Wood or hybrid units (960 dynes-sec-cm^{-5}), ordinary surgical repair of the defect should not be attempted. Others have suggested similar criteria for special instances or conditions. In my opinion, surgical repair should be limited to patients in whom the net shunt is left to right and the pulmonary vascular resistance is less than systemic vascular resistance, preferably with a resistance ratio of <0.50.

PULMONARY VASCULAR DISEASE IN PATIENTS WITH MITRAL STENOSIS

Marked elevations in pulmonary vascular resistance may also be seen in acquired heart disease, notably in mitral stenosis. The effect of mitral valve replacement in patients with mitral stenosis and/or regurgitation associated with pulmonary hypertension has been evaluated (39,40). Most patients experience significant reduction in pulmonary vascular resistance following successful repair of the mitral valve lesion. Although some degree of pulmonary hypertension may persist postoperatively, significant palliative benefit usually occurs, and the decision regarding surgery must be made in light of information regarding left and right ventricular function as well as the degree of pulmonary hypertension.

Currently, percutaneous balloon mitral valvuloplasty is used widely as an alternative to surgery for treating patients with advanced mitral stenosis. The procedure results in an immediate improvement in mitral valve area and in pulmonary hypertension. Its effects on pulmonary vascular resistance have been studied in a cohort of 14 patients with critical mitral stenosis and severe pulmonary hypertension (41). Balloon mitral valvuloplasty resulted in an immediate improvement in mitral valve area (0.7 ± 0.2 cm^2 to 1.6 ± 0.7 cm^2, $P <$ .01), mean left atrial pressure (26 ± 6 mm Hg to 15 ± 5 mm Hg, $P <$ .01), mean pulmonary artery pressure (51 ± 17 mm Hg to 40 ± 14 mm Hg), and pulmonary vascular resistance (630 ± 570 dynes-sec-cm^{-5} to 447 ± 324 dynes-sec-cm^{-5}, $P <$ .01). At an average of 7 months follow-up, repeat catheterization showed that pulmonary vascular resistance had declined further and now averaged 280 ± 183 dynes-sec-cm^{-5}. Of note, two patients who showed substantial restenosis to mitral valve areas of less than 1.0 cm^2 exhibited a return of pulmonary vascular resistance to prevalvuloplasty values (41). The decline in pulmonary vascular resistance after balloon valvuloplasty is not offset by the bronchopulmonary stresses associated with thoracotomy and general anesthesia, making mitral balloon valvuloplasty appealing as either an alternative to surgery or a preparatory procedure before surgery in patients with mitral stenosis and advanced pulmonary hypertension.

ASSESSMENT OF VASODILATOR DRUGS

Cardiac catheterization provides an ideal opportunity for assessing the potential response of a patient to a change in medical regimen, particularly with regard to vasodilator drugs. In recent years, vasodilator drugs have assumed a major role in the treatment of patients with congestive heart failure. There is, however, great variability among currently used vasodilator agents, and the relative effects of a particular drug on resistance and capacitance vessels is of major importance in predicting its hemodynamic effects (42). This problem may become complex when a particular drug may have different effects, depending on the level of resting tone in resistance and capacitance beds. For example, nitrate preparations are well known to influence venous capacitance; this influence is presumably responsible (at least in part) for the fact that ventricular filling pressures and pulmonary congestion are consistently improved when nitrate therapy is given to patients with congestive heart failure. Despite this consistent effect on preload, the effect of nitrates on forward cardiac output has been variable (43–45), and studies have reported decreases, increases, or mixed effects on cardiac output in normal subjects and in patients with heart failure.

Goldberg and colleagues (46) studied 15 patients with chronic congestive heart failure who were given an oral nitrate (erythrityl tetranitrate) at the time of cardiac catheterization to identify predictors of nitrate effect on cardiac output. There were significant reductions in right atrial, pulmonary capillary wedge, and mean arterial pressure in nearly all patients. Augmentation in cardiac output by ≥10% occurred in eight patients (thereby defined as responders), but no change or decline occurred in seven patients (nonresponders). The level of peripheral vasoconstriction, as reflected by resting systemic vascular resistance, was significantly higher for the responders than for the nonresponders (2,602 ± 251 versus 1,744 ± 193 dynes-sec-cm^{-5}, $P < .02$). Furthermore, a significant reduction in systemic vascular resistance occurred only in responders, and the decline was a linear function of resting resistance (Fig. 8.6).

Thus, although reductions in arterial pressure and left and right ventricular filling pressures are a constant result of nitrate therapy, significant augmentation in forward cardiac output is likely only in patients with the most intense resting peripheral vasoconstriction. The design of a catheterization protocol in a patient with congestive heart failure can include assessment of vasodilator therapy based on these principles. For example, if the resting cardiac output is low and if right and left ventricular filling pressures as well as systemic vascular resistance are high, a long-acting nitrate or a balanced agent (e.g., sodium nitroprusside or an angiotensin-converting enzyme inhibitor) might be expected to be particularly beneficial and can be tested while the catheters are still in place. On the other hand, if the output is low and resistance is high but filling pressures are near normal, a nitrate might not help because the lowered resistance may be offset by the fall of the already normal preload, with the result being no increase in output. In such a patient, a selective lowering of resistance would be desirable, and hydralazine could be tested before removing the catheters. If the cardiac output is low but resistance is normal, neither a nitrate nor a converting enzyme inhibitor

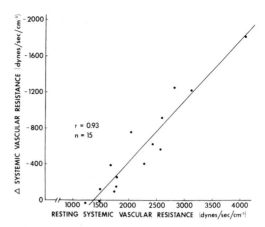

Figure 8.6   The change (Δ) in systemic vascular resistance following administration of erythrityl tetranitrate plotted as a function of resting systemic vascular resistance in 15 patients with congestive heart failure. Patients with the greatest degree of vasoconstriction at rest demonstrated the greatest fall in resistance in response to the nitrate. (From Goldberg et al. Nitrate therapy of heart failure in valvular heart disease. *Am J Med* 1978;65:161, with permission.)

is likely to increase output and should be tested only if filling pressures are high and symptoms of congestion are a prominent part of the clinical picture. In such patients, the combination of an inotropic agent and a nitrate may be particularly helpful and could be tested at the time of catheterization. Finally, if the output is low but filling pressures and systemic vascular resistance are normal, vasodilator drugs will probably do more harm than good, and a therapeutic trial of preload elevation (administration of colloid) with or without an inotropic agent could be tested during the catheterization.

These examples are presented merely to illustrate the principle of using cardiac catheterization parameters (i.e., resistances, flows, and filling pressures) to design a therapeutic regimen and then, while the catheters are still in place, put it to the test. We have found this most useful with regard to the patient with heart failure, and cardiac catheterization in such patients should include full right and left heart catheterization with measurement of cardiac output, left and right heart pressures, and systemic and pulmonary vascular resistances.

REFERENCES

1. Guyton AC, Jones EC, Coleman TG. *Circulatory Physiology: Cardiac Output and Its Regulation.* Philadelphia: WB Saunders, 1973:4.
2. Dexter L, et al. Effect of exercise on circulatory dynamics of normal individuals. *J Appl Physiol* 1951;3:439.
3. Berkson J, Boothby WB. Studies of metabolism of normal individuals: comparison of estimation of basal metabolism from linear formula and surface area. *Am J Physiol* 1936;116:485.
4. Dubois EF. *Basal Metabolism in Health and Disease.* Philadelphia: Lea & Febiger, 1936.
5. Holt JP, Rhode EA, Kines H. Ventricular volumes and body weight in mammals. *Am J Physiol* 1968;215:704.
6. Brandfonbrener M, Landowne M, Shock NW. Changes in cardiac output with age. *Circulation* 1955;12:556.

7. Fick A. Uber die Messung des Blutquantums in den Herzventrikeln. *Sitz der Physik-Med ges Wurtzberg* 1870:16.

8. Lange RA, Dehmer GJ, Wells PJ, et al. Limitations of the metabolic rate meter for measuring oxygen consumption and cardiac output. *Am J Cardiol* 1989;64:783.

9. Shepherd AP, McMahan CA. Role of oximeter error in the diagnosis of shunts. *Cathet Cardiovasc Diagn* 1996;37:435.

10. Bernhard FW, Skeggs L. The iron content of crystalline human hemoglobin. *J Biol Chem* 1943;147:19.

11. Diem K, ed. *Documenta Geigy-Scientific Tables*, 6th ed. Ardsley, NY: Geigy Pharmaceuticals, 1962:578.

12. Dexter L, et al. Studies of congenital heart disease, II: the pressure and oxygen content of blood in the right auricle, right ventricle, and pulmonary artery in control patients. *J Clin Invest* 1947;26:554.

13. Barratt-Boyes BG, Wood EH. The oxygen saturation of blood in the venae cavae, right heart chambers, and pulmonary vessels of healthy subjects. *J Lab Clin Med* 1957;50:93.

14. Selzer A, Sudrann RB. Reliability of the determination of cardiac output in man by means of the Fick principle. *Circ Res* 1958;6:485.

15. Thomassen B. Cardiac output in normal subjects under standard conditions: the repeatability of measurements by the Fick method. *Scan J Clin Lab Invest* 1957;9:365.

16. Visscher MB, Johnson JA. The Fick principle: analysis of potential errors in the conventional application. *J Appl Physiol* 1953;5:635.

17. Dehmer GJ, Firth BG, Hillis LD. Oxygen consumption in adult patients during cardiac catheterization. *Clin Cardiol* 1982;5:436.

18. Kendrick AH, West J, Papouchado M, Rozkovec A. Direct Fick cardiac output: are assumed values of oxygen consumption acceptable? *Eur Heart J* 1988;9:337.

19. Stewart GN. Researches on the circulation time and on the influences which affect it, IV: the output of the heart. *J Physiol* 1897; 22:159.

20. Fegler G. Measurement of cardiac output in anesthetized animals by a thermodilution method. *Q J Exp Physiol* 1954;39:153.

21. Branthwaite MA, Bradley RD. Measurement of cardiac output by thermodilution in man. *J Appl Physiol* 1968;24:434.

22. Ganz W, et al. A new technique for measurement of cardiac output by thermodilution in man. *Am J Cardiol* 1971;27:392.

23. Forrester JS, et al. Thermodilution cardiac output determination with single flow-directed catheter. *Am Heart J* 1972;83:396.

24. Lehmann KG, Platt MS. Improved accuracy and precision of thermodilution cardiac output measurement using a dual thermistor catheter system. *J Am Coll Cardiol* 1999;33:883.

25. van Grondelle AV, Ditchey RV, Groves BM, et al. Thermodilution method overestimates low cardiac output in humans. *Am J Physiol* 1983;245:H690.

26. Milnor WR. *Hemodynamics*, 2nd ed. Baltimore: Williams & Wilkins, 1989.

27. O'Rourke MF. *Arterial function in health and disease*. Edinburgh: Churchill Livingstone, 1982.

28. McDonald DA. *Blood flow in arteries*, 2nd ed. Baltimore: Williams & Wilkins, 1974.

29. Murgo JP, Westerhof N, Giolma JP, Altobelli SA. Aortic input impedance in normal man: relationship to pressure wave forms. *Circulation* 1980;62:105.

30. Connolly DC, Kirklin JW, Wood CH. The relationship between pulmonary artery pressure and left atrial pressure in man. *Circ Res* 1954;2:434.

31. Rapaport E, Dexter L. Pulmonary capillary pressure. *Methods Med Res* 1958;7:85.

32. Lange RA, Moore DM Jr, Cigarroa RG, Hillis LD. Use of pulmonary capillary wedge pressure to assess severity of mitral stenosis: is true left atrial pressure needed in this condition? *J Am Coll Cardiol* 1989;13:825.

33. Nihill MR, McNamara DG, Vick RL. The effects of increased blood viscosity on pulmonary vascular resistance. *Am Heart J* 1976; 92:65.

34. Read RC, Kuida H, Johnson JA. Venous pressure and total peripheral resistance in the dog. *Am J Physiol* 1958;192:609.

35. Grossman W, et al. Changes in inotropic state of the left ventricle during isometric exercise. *Br Heart J* 1973;35:697.

36. Ross J Jr, Braunwald E. The study of left ventricular function in man by increasing resistance to ventricular ejection with angiotensin. *Circulation* 1964;29:739.

37. DiSesa VJ, Cohn LH, Grossman W. Management of adults with congenital bidirectional shunts, cyanosis, and pulmonary vascular obstruction: successful operative repair in 3 patients. *Am J Cardiol* 1983;51:1495.

38. Wood P. The Eisenmenger syndrome or pulmonary hypertension with reversal central shunt. *Br Med J* 1958;2:701.

39. Braunwald E, Braunwald NS, Ross J Jr, Morrow AG. Effects of mitral-valve replacement on the pulmonary vascular dynamics of patients with pulmonary hypertension. *N Engl J Med* 1965; 273:509.

40. Dalen JE, et al. Early reduction of pulmonary vascular resistance after mitral valve replacement. *N Engl J Med* 1967;277:387.

41. Levine MJ, Weinstein JS, Diver DJ, et al. Progressive improvement in pulmonary vascular resistance following percutaneous mitral valvuloplasty. *Circulation* 1989;79:1061.

42. Braunwald E, Colucci WS. Vasodilator therapy of heart failure: Has the promissory note been paid? *N Engl J Med* 1984;310:459.

43. Ferrer MI, et al. Some effects of nitroglycerin upon the splanchnic, pulmonary and systemic circulations. *Circulation* 1966;33:357.

44. Williams JF, Glick G, Braunwald E. Studies on cardiac dimensions in intact unanesthetized man, V: effects of nitroglycerin. *Circulation* 1965;32:767.

45. Gold HK, Leinbach RC, Sanders CA. Use of sublingual nitroglycerin in congestive failure following acute myocardial infarction. *Circulation* 1972;46:389.

46. Goldberg S, Mann T, Grossman W. Nitrate therapy of heart failure in valvular heart disease: importance of resting level of peripheral vascular resistance in determining cardiac output response. *Am J Med* 1978;65:161.

Shunt Detection and Quantification

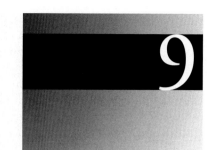

William Grossman

Detection, localization, and quantification of intracardiac shunts are an integral part of the hemodynamic evaluation of patients with congenital heart disease. In most cases, an intracardiac shunt is suspected on the basis of the clinical evaluation of the patient before catheterization. There are several circumstances, however, in which data obtained at catheterization should alert the cardiologist to look for a shunt that had not been suspected previously:

1. Unexplained arterial desaturation should immediately raise the suspicion of a right-to-left intracardiac shunt, which may then be assessed by the methods to be discussed. Most commonly, arterial desaturation (i.e., arterial blood oxygen saturation <95%) detected at the time of cardiac catheterization represents alveolar hypoventilation. The causes for this alveolar hypoventilation and its associated physiologic right-to-left shunt include (a) excessive sedation from the premedication, (b) chronic obstructive lung disease or other pulmonary parenchymal disease, and (c) pulmonary congestion/edema secondary to the patient's cardiac disease. Alveolar hypoventilation associated with each of these problems is exacerbated by the supine position of the patient during the catheterization procedure. Helping the patient to assume a more upright posture (head-up tilt or propping the patient up with a large wedge if tilt mechanism is not available) and encouraging the patient to take deep breaths and to cough will correct or substantially ameliorate arterial hypoxemia in most cases. If arterial desaturation persists, oxygen should be administered by face mask for both therapeutic and diagnostic purposes. If full arterial blood oxygen saturation cannot be achieved by face-mask administration of oxygen (it is best in this regard to use a rebreathing mask that fits snugly), a right-to-left shunt is presumed to be present, and its anatomic site and magnitude should be determined using the methods described later in this chapter.

2. Conversely, when the oxygen content of blood in the pulmonary artery is unexpectedly high (i.e., if the pulmonary artery [PA] blood oxygen saturation is >80%), the possibility of a left-to-right intracardiac shunt should be considered. It is for these two reasons that arterial and pulmonary artery saturation should be measured routinely *during* cardiac catheterization.

3. When the data obtained at cardiac catheterization do not confirm the presence of a suspected lesion, one should consider the presence of an intracardiac shunt. For example, if left ventricular cineangiography fails to reveal mitral regurgitation in a patient in whom this was judged to be the cause of a systolic murmur, it is prudent to look for evidence of a ventricular septal defect (VSD) with left-to-right shunting.

DETECTION OF LEFT-TO-RIGHT INTRACARDIAC SHUNTS

Many techniques are available for the detection, localization, and quantification of left-to-right intracardiac shunts. The techniques vary in their sensitivity, in the type of indicator they use, and in the equipment needed to sense and read out the presence of the indicator.

Measurement of Blood Oxygen Saturation and Content in the Right Heart (Oximetry Run)

In the oximetry run, a basic technique for detecting and quantifying left-to-right shunts, the oxygen content or percent saturation is measured in blood samples drawn sequentially from the pulmonary artery, right ventricle (RV), right atrium (RA), superior vena cava (SVC), and inferior vena cava (IVC). A left-to-right shunt may be detected and localized if a significant step-up in blood oxygen saturation or content is found in one of the right heart chambers. A *significant step-up* is defined as an increase in blood oxygen content or saturation that exceeds the normal variability that might be observed if multiple samples were drawn from that cardiac chamber.

The technique of the oximetry run is based on the pioneering studies of Dexter and his associates in 1947 (1). They found that multiple samples drawn from the right atrium could vary in oxygen content by as much as 2 volumes percent (vol%).[a] This variability has been attributed to the fact that the right atrium receives its blood from three sources of varying oxygen content: the superior vena cava, the inferior vena cava, and the coronary sinus. The maximal normal variation within the right ventricle was found to be 1 vol%. Because of more adequate mixing, a maximal variation within the pulmonary artery of only 0.5 vol% was found by Dexter. Thus, using the Dexter criteria, a significant step-up is present at the atrial level when the highest oxygen content in blood samples drawn from the right atrium exceeds the highest content in the venae cavae by 2 vol%. Similarly, a significant step-up at the ventricular level is present if the highest right ventricular sample is 1 vol% higher than the highest right atrial sample, and a significant step-up at the level of the pulmonary artery is present if the pulmonary artery oxygen content is more than 0.5 vol% greater than the highest right ventricular sample.

Dexter's study described normal variability and gave criteria for a significant oxygen step-up only for measurement of blood oxygen content. This in part reflects the methodology available to him, because spectrophotometric oximetry was not used widely at that time. In recent years, nearly all cardiac catheterization laboratories (especially those primarily involved in pediatric catheterization) have moved toward the measurement of percentage oxygen saturation by spectrophotometric oximetry as the routine method for oximetric analysis of blood samples. Oxygen content may then be calculated from knowledge of percentage saturation, the patient's blood hemoglobin concentration, and an assumed constant relationship for oxygen-carrying capacity of hemoglobin, as discussed in Chapter 8 (1.36 mL O_2/g hemoglobin). When oxygen content is derived in this manner, rather than by measurement by the Van Slyke or other direct oximetric technique, the value is no more accurate (and probably less so because of the potential presence of carboxyhemoglobin or hemoglobin variants with O_2 capacity other than 1.36) than the percentage oxygen saturation values from which it is calculated.

To clarify this situation, Antman and coworkers studied prospectively the normal variation of both oxygen content and oxygen saturation of blood in the right heart chambers (2). The study population consisted of patients without intracardiac shunts who were undergoing diagnostic cardiac catheterization for evaluation of coronary artery disease, valvular heart disease, cardiomyopathy, or possible pulmonary embolism. Each patient had a complete right heart oximetry run (see later discussion) with sampling of multiple sites in each chamber. Oxygen content was measured directly by an electrochemical fuel-cell method (Lex-O_2-Con, Lexington Instruments, Lexington, MA), a method that had been validated previously against the Van Slyke method. Oxygen saturation was calculated as blood oxygen content divided by oxygen-carrying capacity. The relationship between oxygen content and oxygen saturation obviously depends on the hemoglobin concentration of the patient's blood (e.g., 75% oxygen saturation of pulmonary artery blood will be associated with a substantially lower oxygen content in an anemic patient than in one with normal hemoglobin concentration). Also, systemic blood flow may be an important determinant of oxygen variability in the right heart chambers because high systemic flow tends to equalize the differences across various tissue beds.

In the context of these considerations, I have listed criteria in Table 9.1 for a significant step-up in right heart oxygen content and percentage oxygen saturation associated with various types of left-to-right shunt, based on the study of Antman and coworkers (2) and other investigators (1,3,4). As can be seen from the bottom line ("Any level") of Table 9.1, the simplest way to screen for a left-to-right shunt is to sample SVC and PA blood and measure the difference, if any, in percentage O2 saturation. We recommend obtaining blood samples from SVC and PA routinely at the time of right heart catheterization and determining their O_2 saturation by reflectance oximetry. If the ΔO_2 saturation between these samples is $\geq 8\%$, a left-to-right shunt may be present at atrial, ventricular, or great vessel level, and a full oximetry run should be done.

Oximetry Run

The blood samples needed to localize a step-up in the right heart are obtained by performing what is called an oximetry run. The samples needed and the order in which we recommend they be obtained follow.

Obtain a 2-mL sample from each of the following locations:

1. Left and/or right pulmonary artery
2. Main pulmonary artery[b]
3. Right ventricle, outflow tract[b]
4. Right ventricle, mid[c]
5. Right ventricle, tricuspid valve or apex[b,c]

---

[a] 1 vol% = 1 mL O_2/100 mL blood, or 10 mL O_2/L of blood.

[b] Confirm location by pressure measurement.
[c] If frequent extrasystoles occur, do not persist. Obtain samples from three different locations in right ventricle and right atrium.

TABLE 9.1

DETECTION OF LEFT-TO-RIGHT SHUNT BY OXIMETRY

Level of Shunt	Criteria for Significant Step-Up				Approximate Minimal Q_p/Q_s Required for Detection (Assuming SBFI = 3L/min/M²)	Possible Causes of Step-Up
	Mean of Distal Chamber Samples	Mean of Proximal Chamber Samples	Highest Value in Proximal Chamber	Highest Value in Distal Chamber		
	O_2 %sat	O_2 vol%	O_2 %sat	O_2 vol%		
Atrial (SVC/IVC to RA)	≥7	≥1.3	≥11	≥2.0	1.5–1.9	Atrial septal defect; partial anomalous pulmonary venous drainage; ruptured sinus of Valsalva; VSD with TR; coronary fistula to RA
Ventricular (RA to RV)	≥5	≥1.0	≥10	≥1.7	1.3–1.5	VSD; PDA with PR; primum ASD; coronary fistula to RV
Great Vessel (RV to PA)	≥5	≥1.0	≥5	≥1.0	≥1.3	PDA; aorta-pulmonic window; aberrant coronary artery origin
Any level (SVC to PA)	≥7	≥1.3	≥8	≥1.5	≥1.5	All the above

SVC and IVC, superior and inferior vena cavae; RA, right atrium; RV, right ventricle; PA, pulmonary artery; VSD, ventricular septal defect; TR, tricuspid regurgitation; PDA, patent ductus arteriosus; PR, pulmonic regurgitation; ASD, atrial septal defect; SBFI, systemic blood flow index; Q_p/Q_s, pulmonary to systemic flow ratio.

6. Right atrium, low or near tricuspid valve
7. Right atrium, mid
8. Right atrium, high
9. Superior vena cava, low (near junction with right atrium)
10. Superior vena cava, high (near junction with innominate vein)
11. Inferior vena cava, high (just at or below diaphragm)
12. Inferior vena cava, low (at L4–L5)
13. Left ventricle
14. Aorta (distal to insertion of ductus)

In performing the oximetry run, an end-hole catheter (e.g., Swan-Ganz balloon flotation catheter) or one with side holes close to its tip (e.g., a Goodale-Lubin catheter) is positioned in the right or left pulmonary artery. Cardiac output is measured by the Fick method. As soon as the determination of oxygen consumption is completed, the operator begins to obtain 2-mL blood samples from each of the locations indicated. This is done under fluoroscopic control, with catheter tip position further confirmed by pressure measurement at the sites noted. The entire procedure should take less than 7 minutes. If a sample cannot be obtained from a specific site because of ventricular premature beats, that site should be skipped until the rest of the run has been completed.

Oxygen saturation and/or content in each of the samples is determined as discussed previously, and the presence and localization of a significant step-up are determined by applying the criteria listed in Table 9.1.

An alternative method for performing the oximetry run is to withdraw a fiberoptic catheter from the pulmonary artery through the right heart chambers and the inferior and superior venae cavae. This permits a continuous readout of oxygen saturation that allows detection of a step-up in oxygen content.

If the oximetry run reveals that a significant step-up is present, the pulmonary blood flow, systemic blood flow, and magnitude of left-to-right and right-to-left shunts may be calculated according to the following formulas.

Calculation of Pulmonary Blood Flow (Q_p)

Pulmonary blood flow is calculated by the same formula used in the standard Fick equation:

$$\frac{Q_p}{(\text{L/min})} = \frac{O_2 \text{ consumption (mL/min)}}{\begin{bmatrix} PV\ O_2 \\ \text{content} \\ \text{(mL/L)} \end{bmatrix} - \begin{bmatrix} PA\ O_2 \\ \text{content} \\ \text{(mL/L)} \end{bmatrix}} \quad (9.1)$$

If a pulmonary vein (PV) has not been entered, systemic arterial oxygen content may be used in the preceding formula, if systemic arterial oxygen saturation is ≥95%. If systemic oxygen saturation is <95%, one must determine whether a right-to-left intracardiac shunt is present. If there is an intracardiac right-to-left shunt, an assumed value for pulmonary venous oxygen content of 98% oxygen capacity should be used in calculating pulmonary blood flow. If arterial desaturation is present and is not owing to a right-to-left intracardiac shunt, the observed systemic arterial oxygen saturation should be used to calculate pulmonary blood flow.

Example

Let us suppose that a patient is found to have an atrial septal defect with a left-to-right shunt clearly detected by oximetry run. Furthermore, the catheter crosses the defect and a pulmonary vein is entered, from which a blood sample shows O_2 saturation of 98%. Let us further suppose, however, that systemic arterial blood saturation is 90% and that this is owing to chronic pulmonary disease. After ruling out a right-to-left shunt (e.g., inhalation of 100% oxygen, indocyanine green dye injection in inferior vena cava, echocardiogram-bubble study), should we use 98% or 90% for pulmonary venous blood O_2 saturation in the calculation of Q_p? As indicated earlier, because arterial desaturation is not caused by a right-to-left intracardiac shunt, the observed systemic arterial O_2 saturation (90%) should be used because this summates all the pulmonary veins draining both lungs, not just the one with 98% O_2 saturation.

Calculation of Systemic Blood Flow (Q_s)

Use the following equation for systemic blood flow:

$$\frac{Q_s}{(L/min)} = \frac{O_2 \text{ consumption (mL/min)}}{\left[\begin{array}{c} SA\ O_2 \\ content \\ (mL/L) \end{array}\right] - \left[\begin{array}{c} MV\ O_2 \\ content \\ (mL/L) \end{array}\right]} \quad (9.2)$$

The key to the measurement of systemic blood flow in the presence of an intracardiac shunt is that the mixed venous oxygen content must be measured in the chamber immediately proximal to the shunt, as shown in Table 9.2.

The formula generally used by cardiologists who treat adults for the calculation of venous content in the presence of an atrial septal defect (ASD) was derived by Flamm and coworkers (5). They found that systemic blood flow calculated from mixed venous oxygen content as determined from the formula listed in Table 9.2 most closely approximates systemic blood flow as measured by left ventricular to brachial artery (BA) dye curves in patients with atrial septal defect studied at rest. It should be noted that Flamm's formula weights blood returning from the superior vena cava more heavily than might be expected on the basis of relative flows in the superior and inferior cavae. The success of this empirical weighting of the relatively desaturated superior vena cava blood (O_2 saturation is almost always less in blood from the superior as opposed to the inferior vena cava) probably reflects the fact that the third contributor to mixed venous blood—desaturated coronary sinus blood—is not sampled during the oximetry run and therefore cannot be included directly in the formula. The formula (3 SVC O_2 + 1 IVC O_2)/4 was validated by Flamm and associates for mixed venous oxygen content at rest (5). Thus in 18 patients without shunt, this value agreed closely with pulmonary artery blood oxygen content at rest. During supine bicycle exercise, however, a different relationship was found to apply, in which mixed venous (pulmonary artery) oxygen content in patients without shunts was best approximated as (1 SVC O_2 + 2 IVC O_2)/3. This formula was then used for patients with atrial septal defect during exercise, and it reliably predicted systemic blood flow measured by left ventricular to brachial artery dye-dilution curve. Therefore, for patients with left-to-right shunt at the atrial level, the formula in Table 9.2 should be used only for calculation of resting mixed venous O_2 content.

Obviously, calculations from the formula in Table 9.2 would be little changed in many cases by ignoring inferior vena cava blood altogether, and this is done in some laboratories (especially those involved in pediatric catheterization). Flamm and associates, however, examined the effects of assuming that superior vena cava O_2 content equaled mixed venous O_2 content and concluded that this was somewhat less accurate (both in the 18 subjects without shunt and in the 9 patients with atrial septal defect and left-to-right shunt) than the formula given in Table 9.2 (5).

TABLE 9.2

CALCULATION OF SYSTEMIC BLOOD FLOW IN THE PRESENCE OF LEFT-TO-RIGHT SHUNT

Location of shunt as determined by site of O_2 step-up	Mixed venous sample to use in calculating systemic blood flow
1. Pulmonary artery (e.g., patent ductus arteriosus)	Right ventricle, average of samples obtained during oximetry run
2. Right ventricle (e.g., ventricular septal defect)	Right atrium, average of all samples during oximetry run
3. Right atrium (e.g., atrial septal defect)	3(SVC O_2 content) + 1(IVC O_2 content)

Calculation of Left-to-Right Shunt

If there is no evidence of an associated right-to-left shunt, the left-to-right shunt is calculated by

$$L \to R \text{ shunt} = Q_p - Q_s \qquad (9.3)$$
$$\text{(measured in L/min)}$$

Examples of Left-to-Right Shunt Detection and Quantification

Some examples of oximetry runs are presented to illustrate interpretation.

Atrial Septal Defect

In the example seen in Fig. 9.1, there is a step-up in oxygen saturation in the mid–right atrium. The average or mean value for the vena caval samples in this patient is calculated as $[3(\text{SVC}) + 1(\text{IVC})] \div 4$. SVC is the average of SVC samples (i.e., 67.5% in this example), and IVC is the value for the IVC sample taken at the level of the diaphragm only (i.e., 73%). Thus the vena caval mean O_2 saturation for the patient in Fig. 9.1 is $[3(67.5) + 1(73)] \div 4 = 69\%$. The right atrial mean O_2 saturation for this patient is $(74 + 84 + 79) \div 3 = 79\%$. The 10% step-up in mean O_2 saturation from vena cava to right atrium is higher than the 7% value listed in Table 9.1 as a criterion for a significant step-up at the atrial level. Note that for this example, the highest-to-highest approach (highest right atrial O_2 saturation to highest vena caval O_2 saturation) would barely meet criteria for a significant step-up, because of the high value for IVC saturation (73%)

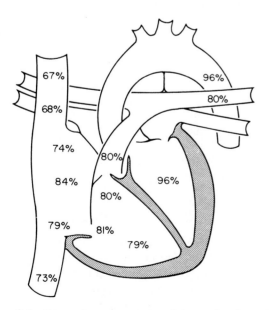

Figure 9.1 Schematic representation of the results of an oximetry run in a patient with a small to moderate atrial septal defect. Values represent percentage O_2 saturation of blood at multiple locations. (See text for details.)

compared with SVC saturation. Thus for the detection of a significant step-up at the atrial level using the highest-to-highest approach, it is best to use the highest RA and SVC samples. In this case, the result would be $(84\% - 68\%) = 16\%$, which is clearly above the 11% value listed in Table 9.1 for detection of a significant step-up. Also, the screening samples that we recommend for all right heart catheterizations (single sample from SVC and PA) would have strongly indicated a shunt at some level in the right heart, since ΔO_2 saturation from SVC to PA is 12 to 13%, well above the 8% value for a significant step-up.

To calculate pulmonary and systemic blood flows for the example given in Fig. 9.1, we need to know O_2 consumption and blood O_2 capacity. If the patient's O_2 consumption determined by the methods described in Chapter 8 is 240 mL O_2/minute and the blood hemoglobin concentration is 14 g%, pulmonary and systemic blood flows may be calculated as follows:

$$Q_p = \frac{O_2 \text{ consumption (mL/min)}}{\left[\begin{array}{c} \text{PV } O_2 \\ \text{content} \\ \text{(mL/L)} \end{array}\right] - \left[\begin{array}{c} \text{PA } O_2 \\ \text{content} \\ \text{(mL/L)} \end{array}\right]} \qquad (9.4)$$

PV O_2 content was not measured, but left ventricular (LV) and arterial blood O_2 saturation was 96% (effectively ruling out a right-to-left shunt), and therefore it may be assumed that PV blood O_2 saturation was 96%. As described in Chapter 8, oxygen content for PV blood is calculated as follows:

$$0.96 \left(\frac{14 \text{ g Hgb}}{100 \text{ mL blood}} \right) \times \left(\frac{1.36 \text{ mL } O_2}{\text{g Hgb}} \right)$$

$$= 18.3 \text{ mL } O_2/100 \text{ mL blood} \qquad (9.5)$$
$$= 183 \text{ mL } O_2/\text{liter}$$

Similarly, PA O_2 content is calculated as

$$0.80(14)1.36 \times 10 = 152 \text{ mL } O_2/\text{liter} \qquad (9.6)$$

Therefore,

$$Q_p = \frac{240 \text{ mL } O_2/\text{min}}{[183 - 152] \text{ mL } O_2/\text{L}} \qquad (9.7)$$
$$= 7.74 \text{ L/min}$$

Systemic blood flow for the patient in Fig. 9.1 is calculated as

$$Q_s = \frac{240 \text{ mL } O_2/\text{min}}{\left[\begin{array}{c} \text{systemic} \\ \text{arterial} \\ O_2 \text{ content} \end{array}\right] - \left[\begin{array}{c} \text{mixed} \\ \text{venous} \\ O_2 \text{ content} \end{array}\right]} \qquad (9.8)$$

$$= \frac{240}{(0.96 - 0.69)14(1.36)10}$$

$$= 4.7 \text{ L/min}$$

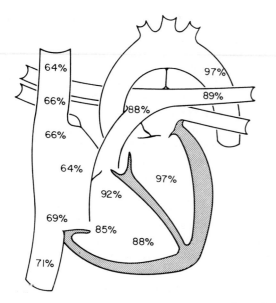

Figure 9.2 Findings from an oximetry run performed in a patient with a large ventricular septal defect. (See text for details.)

For this calculation, mixed venous O_2 saturation was derived from the formula given in Table 9.2 as 69%. Thus the ratio of Q_p/Q_s in this example is 7.74/4.7 = 1.65, and the magnitude of the left-to-right shunt is 7.7 − 4.7 = 3 L/min. This patient has a small to moderate atrial septal defect.

Ventricular Septal Defect

Figure 9.2 shows another example of findings in an oximetry run. In this case, the patient has a large O_2 step-up in the right ventricle, indicating the presence of a ventricular septal defect. If O_2 consumption is 260 mL/minute and hemoglobin is 15 g%, then

$$Q_p = \frac{260}{(0.97 - 0.885)15(1.36)10} = 15 \text{ L/minute}$$

$$Q_s = \frac{260}{(0.97 - 0.66)15(1.36)10} = 4.1 \text{ L/minute} \quad (9.9)$$

$$Q_p/Q_s = 15/4.1 = 3.7$$

$$L \rightarrow \text{shunt} = 15 - 4.1 = 10.9 \text{ L/minute}$$

In this case, the O_2 saturation of mixed venous blood is calculated by averaging the right atrial O_2 saturations because the right atrium is the chamber immediately proximal to the O_2 step-up.

Flow Ratio

The ratio Q_p/Q_s gives important physiologic information about the magnitude of a left-to-right shunt. In addition, because it factors out other variables (e.g., O_2 consumption), the ratio can be calculated from knowledge of blood

O_2 saturation alone. A Q_p/Q_s ratio of <1.5 signifies a small left-to-right shunt and is often felt to argue against operative correction, particularly if the patient has an otherwise uncomplicated atrial or ventricular septal defect. A ratio of ≥2.0 indicates a large left-to-right shunt and is generally considered sufficient evidence to recommend surgical repair of the defect, to prevent late pulmonary vascular disease as well as other complications of prolonged circulatory overload. Flow ratios between 1.5 and 2.0 are obviously intermediate in magnitude; surgical correction is generally recommended if operative risk is low. A flow ratio of less than 1.0 indicates a net right-to-left shunt and is often a sign of the presence of irreversible pulmonary vascular disease.

A *simplified formula* for calculation of flow ratio can be derived by combining the equations for systemic and pulmonary blood flow to obtain

$$\frac{Q_p}{Q_s} = \frac{(SA\ O_2 - MV\ O_2)}{(PV\ O_2 - PA\ O_2)} \quad (9.10)$$

where SA O_2, MV O_2, PV O_2, and PA O_2 are systemic arterial, mixed venous, pulmonary venous, and pulmonary arterial blood oxygen saturations, respectively. For the patient illustrated in Fig. 9.1,

$$Q_p/Q_s = (96\% - 69\%)/(96\% - 80\%) = 1.69.$$

Calculation of Bidirectional Shunts

A simplified approach to the calculation of simultaneous right-to-left and left-to-right (also known as bidirectional) shunts makes use of a hypothetic quantity known as the *effective blood flow*, the flow that would exist in the absence of any left-to-right or right-to-left shunting:

$$Q_{eff} = \frac{O_2 \text{ consumption (mL/min)}}{\begin{bmatrix} PV\ O_2 \\ \text{content} \\ (mL/L) \end{bmatrix} - \begin{bmatrix} MV\ O_2 \\ \text{content} \\ (mL/L) \end{bmatrix}} \quad (9.11)$$

The approximate left-to-right shunt then equals $Q_p − Q_{eff}$, and the approximate right-to-left shunt equals $Q_s − Q_{eff}$. Actually, this effective blood flow approach is an approximation of the significantly more complex formula shown in Eq. (9.12)(b).

Limitations of Oximetry Method

There are several limitations and potential sources of error in the calculations of blood flow using the data obtained from an oximetry run. A primary source of error may be the absence of a steady state during the collection of blood samples. That is, if the oximetry run is prolonged because of technical difficulties, if the patient is agitated, or if arrhythmias occur during the oximetry run, the data may not be consistent.

TABLE 9.3

EXPECTED VALUE OF O_2 CONTENT (VOLUMES PERCENT) FOR VARIOUS LEVELS OF O_2 STEP-UP AND BLOOD HEMOGLOBIN CONCENTRATION[a]

Increase in O_2 saturation (%)	Hemoglobin Concentration (vol%)		
	(g/100 mL)		
	10	**12**	**15**
5	0.68	0.82	1.02
10	1.36	1.63	2.04
15	2.04	2.45	3.06
20	2.72	3.26	4.08

[a] Modified from Antman EM, Marsh JD, Green LH, Grossman W. Blood oxygen measurements in the assessment of intracardiac left to right shunts: a critical appraisal of methodology. *Am J Cardiol* 1980;46:265, with permission.

TABLE 9.4

GUIDELINES FOR OPTIMUM USE OF OXIMETRIC METHOD FOR SHUNT DETECTION AND QUANTIFICATION[a]

1. Blood samples at multiple sites should be obtained rapidly.
2. Blood O_2 saturation data rather than O_2 content data are preferable to identify the presence and location of a shunt.
3. Comparison of the mean of all values obtained in the respective chambers is preferable to comparison of highest values in each chamber.
4. Because of the important influence of systemic blood flow on shunt detection, exercise should be used in equivocal cases where a low systemic blood flow is present at rest.

[a] Based on the data of Antman EM, Marsh JD, Green LH, Grossman W. Blood oxygen measurements in the assessment of intracardiac left to right shunts: a critical appraisal of methodology. *Am J Cardiol* 1980;46:265.

An important limitation of the oxygen step-up method for detecting intracardiac shunts is that it lacks sensitivity. Most shunts of a magnitude that would lead to a recommendation for surgical closure of a ventricular septal defect or patent ductus arteriosus are detected by this method. Small shunts, however, are not consistently detected by this technique.

As pointed out by Antman and coworkers (2), the normal variability of blood oxygen saturation in the right heart chambers is strongly influenced by the magnitude of systemic blood flow. High levels of systemic flow tend to equalize the arterial and venous oxygen values across a given vascular bed. Therefore, elevated systemic blood flow will cause the mixed venous oxygen saturation to be higher than normal, and interchamber variability owing to streaming will be blunted. Even a small increase in right heart oxygen saturation under such conditions might indicate the presence of a significant left-to-right shunt; larger increases would indicate voluminous left-to-right shunting of blood. For a patient with a systemic blood flow index of 3.0 L/minute per M^2, minimum shunt sizes that could be detected reliably by oximetry are listed in Table 9.1.

Fundamental to the oximetric method of shunt detection is the fact that left-to-right shunting across an intracardiac defect will cause an increase in blood O_2 saturation in the chamber receiving the shunt proportional to the magnitude of the shunt. The increase in blood O_2 content in the chamber receiving the shunt, however, depends not only on the magnitude of the shunt but also on the O_2-carrying capacity of the blood (i.e., the hemoglobin concentration). As reported by Antman and colleagues (2), the influence of blood hemoglobin concentration may be important when blood O_2 content (rather than O_2 saturation) is used to detect a shunt (Table 9.3).

Thus, the same shunt giving the same blood O_2 saturation step-up would give markedly different blood O_2 content step-ups if the blood hemoglobin concentration varied significantly. Accordingly, when evaluating oximetric data for shunt detection, it is more precise to exclude the potential influence of blood O_2-carrying capacity and use only O_2 saturation data. This is especially true in pediatric cases (4) where the normal blood O_2-carrying capacity may vary from 20 to 28 vol% in the neonate to 12 to 16 vol% in infancy. To minimize errors and maximize the physiologic strengths of the oximetry method for shunt detection and quantification, the guidelines listed in Table 9.4 should be followed.

Other Indicators

Many more sensitive techniques are available to detect smaller left-to-right shunts (7–19). These include indocyanine green dye curves, radionuclide techniques, contrast angiography, and echocardiographic methods. Some of these methods (e.g., green dye) were discussed extensively in previous editions of this textbook, and the interested

$$L \rightarrow R = \frac{Q_p \, (MV \, O_2 \text{ content} - PA \, O_2 \text{ content})}{(MV \, O_2 \text{ content} - PV^e \, O_2 \text{ content})}$$

$$R \rightarrow L = \frac{Q_p \, (PV^e \, O_2 \text{ content} - SA \, O_2 \text{ content})(PA \, O_2 \text{ content} - PV^e \, O_2 \text{ content})}{(SA \, O_2 \text{ content} - MV \, O_2 \text{ content}) \times (MV \, O_2 \text{ content} - PV^e \, O_2 \text{ content})}$$

(9.12)

[e] If pulmonary vein is not entered, use 98% $\times$ O_2 capacity.

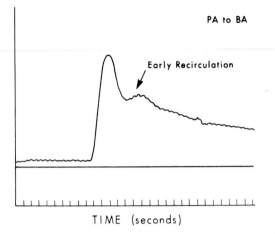

PA to BA

Early Recirculation

TIME (seconds)

Figure 9.3 Left-to-right shunt. This indicator dilution curve, performed by injecting indocyanine green into the pulmonary artery with sampling in the brachial artery, demonstrates early recirculation on the downslope, indicating a left-to-right shunt. Injection was at time zero. This technique does not localize the site of the left-to-right shunt.

reader is referred there for details. For discussion of other predominantly non–catheter-based methods (e.g., echo, radionuclide) the reader is referred to textbooks devoted to those techniques. We will give only one example here of one of the older methods.

Early Recirculation of an Indicator

Standard indicator dilution curves, performed by injection of indocyanine green into the pulmonary artery with sampling in a systemic artery, are rarely done today, and most laboratories are not even equipped to do them. In the presence of a left-to-right shunt, however, a green dye curve produced by this technique will demonstrate early recirculation on the downslope of the dye curve (7; Fig. 9.3).

This technique can detect left-to-right shunts too small to be detected by the oxygen step-up method (8). Thus if there is no evidence of a left-to-right shunt by this method, there is no need to perform an oximetry run. The studies of Castillo and coworkers (9) suggest that left-to-right shunts as small as 25% of the systemic output can be detected by standard pulmonary artery to systemic artery dye curves.

Although a simple pulmonary to systemic artery indocyanine green dye curve may detect the presence of a shunt, it does not localize it. That is, a pulmonary artery to systemic artery dye curve will show evidence of early recirculation in the presence of a left-to-right shunt owing to an atrial septal defect, ventricular septal defect, or patent ductus arteriosus.

Angiography

Selective angiography is effective in visualizing and localizing the site of left-to-right shunts. Angiographic demonstration of anatomy has become a routine part of the preoperative evaluation of patients with congenital or acquired shunts and is useful in localizing the anatomic site of the shunt. Actually, the use of angiography in this fashion should be considered an indicator-dilution method, with the radiographic contrast agent being the indicator and the cinefluoroscopy unit serving as the densitometer.

In general, assessment of the patient with a left-to-right shunt virtually always includes a left ventriculogram. If this is performed in the left anterior oblique projection with cranial angulation (or done as a biplane study with both left and right anterior oblique views), excellent visualization of the interventricular septum, sinuses of Valsalva, and ascending and descending thoracic aorta will allow diagnosis and localization of essentially all the causes of left-to-right shunt other than atrial septal defect and anomalous pulmonary venous return.

Complicated lesions (e.g., endocardial cushion defects, coronary artery/right heart fistulas, ruptured aneurysms at the sinus of Valsalva) commonly require angiographic delineation before surgical intervention can be undertaken. Angiography also helps to assess the "routine" cases more completely. For instance, does the patient with secundum atrial septal defect have associated left ventricular dysfunction or mitral valve prolapse? Does the patient with ventricular septal defect have associated aortic regurgitation (caused by prolapse of the medial aortic leaflet) or infundibular pulmonic stenosis?

Angiography, however, cannot replace the important physiologic measurements that allow quantitation of flow and vascular resistance. Without quantitative evaluation of pulmonary and systemic flows (Q_p and Q_s) and their associated resistances (PVR and SVR), appropriate decisions regarding patient management cannot be made, nor can prognosis be assessed.

DETECTION OF RIGHT-TO-LEFT INTRACARDIAC SHUNTS

The primary indication for the use of techniques to detect and localize right-to-left intracardiac shunts is the presence of cyanosis or, more commonly, arterial hypoxemia. The presence of arterial hypoxemia raises two specific questions: first, is the observed hypoxemia owing to an intracardiac shunt, or is it owing to a ventilation/perfusion imbalance secondary to a variety of forms of intrinsic pulmonary disease? This problem is particularly important in patients with coexistent congenital heart disease and pulmonary disease. Second, if hypoxemia is caused by an intracardiac shunt, what is its site and what is its magnitude?

Attempts to measure right-to-left shunts in patients with cyanotic heart disease date back at least to 1941 (20–23). Prinzmetal (20), in a series of ingenious experiments, expanded the earlier observation of Benenson and Hitzig that ether injected intravenously in patients with cyanotic heart disease will cause a prickly, burning sensation of the face (18). This sensation is caused by the entrance of ether into the systemic circulation of patients with right-to-left shunts. In normal subjects without right-to-left shunts, the ether is eliminated by the lungs and thus does not reach the systemic circulation. Prinzmetal then measured the time necessary for an intravenous injection of a dilute solution of saccharin to be tasted. This time is equal to the transit time from a peripheral vein through the lungs, through the left heart, and then to the systemic circulation. By increasing the concentration of the saccharin, he found that a second, much shorter appearance time occurred in patients with cyanotic heart disease because of the presence of a right-to-left shunt bypassing the pulmonary circulation. He then estimated the percent right-to-left shunt by the following formula:

$$\% \, R \rightarrow L \, Shunt = \frac{A}{A + C} \qquad (9.13)$$

where A is the smallest concentration of saccharin to be tasted by way of the long circuit and C is the smallest concentration of saccharin to be tasted by the short circuit. Our current methods of documenting and quantitating right-to-left shunts may not be as ingenious and certainly are not as sweet, but they are nonetheless effective.

Angiography

With appropriate techniques, angiography may be used to demonstrate right-to-left intracardiac shunts. This method is particularly important in detecting right-to-left shunting owing to a pulmonary arteriovenous fistula. In this circumstance, the shunt cannot be detected by indicator dilution curves on the basis of a shortened appearance time. That is, the difference in transit time when the pulmonary capillaries are bypassed is not perceptible by standard indicator

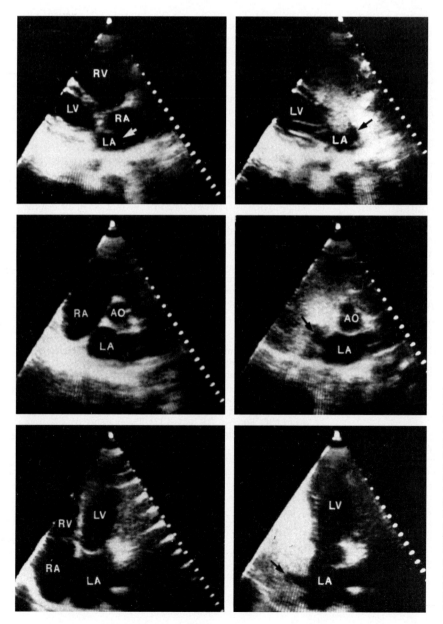

Figure 9.4 Two-dimensional echo showing right ventricular (RV) inflow tract **(top),** short axis views at the base **(middle)** (AO = aorta), and four-chamber apical view **(bottom)** in a patient with an atrial septal defect (ASD) shown at cardiac catheterization to be associated with a Q_p/Q_s of 3.0. **Left views.** The anatomy before echo contrast injection. Following an intravenous injection of agitated saline solution **(right views),** a negative contrast effect *(black arrows)* is seen within the right atrium (RA), compatible with entry of unopacified blood from the left atrium (LA) across the ASD into the RA. The ASD is visualized *(white arrow)* as an area of septal dropout. (Reproduced from Come PC, Riley M. Contrast echocardiography. In: Come PC, ed. *Diagnostic cardiology: noninvasive imaging techniques.* Philadelphia: JB Lippincott, 1984:294, with permission.)

dilution techniques. Although angiography may localize right-to-left shunts, it does not permit quantification.

Oximetry

The site of right-to-left shunts may be localized if blood samples can be obtained from a pulmonary vein, the left atrium, left ventricle, and aorta. The pulmonary venous blood of patients with arterial hypoxemia caused by an intracardiac right-to-left shunt is fully saturated with oxygen. Therefore, the site of a right-to-left shunt may be localized by noting which left heart chamber is the first to show desaturation (i.e., a step-down in oxygen concentration). Thus if left atrial blood oxygen saturation is normal but desaturation is present in the left ventricle and in the systemic circulation, the right-to-left shunt is across a ventricular septal defect. The only disadvantage of this technique is that a pulmonary vein and the left atrium must be entered. This is not as easy in adults as it is in infants, in whom the left atrium may be entered routinely by way of the foramen ovale.

Echocardiographic methods have proved sensitive for the detection and localization of left-to-right and right-to-left shunts. The so-called echocardiographic contrast or "bubble study" using agitated saline solution with microbubbles or some of the newer specifically designed echo contrast agents can detect small shunts, and the use of two-dimensional echocardiographic techniques can usually localize the site of the shunt to the atrial or ventricular septum. Combined echocardiographic and cardiac catheterization studies allow injection of the echo contrast agent into the right or left heart chambers sequentially, thus permitting localization of the shunt and determination as to whether it is unidirectional or bidirectional. Echo-Doppler techniques can also be used to detect and localize intracardiac shunts. In this regard, color Doppler echocardiography is particularly useful in detecting and localizing small intracardiac shunts without the need for injection of an echo contrast agent. An example of the use of echo-contrast technique for the detection of an atrial septal defect with left-to-right shunting is shown in Fig. 9.4.

REFERENCES

1. Dexter L, et al. Studies of congenital heart disease, II: the pressure and oxygen content of blood in the right auricle, right ventricle, and pulmonary artery in control patients, with observations on the oxygen saturation and source of pulmonary capillary blood. *J Clin Invest* 1947;26:554.
2. Antman EM, Marsh JD, Green LH, Grossman W. Blood oxygen measurements in the assessment of intracardiac left to right shunts: a critical appraisal of methodology. *Am J Cardiol* 1980; 46:265.
3. Barratt-Boyes BF, Wood EH. The oxygen saturation of blood in the vena cavae, right heart chambers, and pulmonary vessels of healthy subjects. *J Lab Clin Med* 1957;50:93.
4. Freed MD, Miettinen OS, Nadas AS. Oximetric determination of intracardiac left to right shunts. *Br Heart J* 1979;42:690.
5. Flamm MD, Cohn KE, Hancock EW. Measurement of systemic cardiac output at rest and exercise in patients with atrial septal defect. *Am J Cardiol* 1969;23:258.
6. Dexter L, et al. Studies of congenital heart disease, I: technique of venous catheterization as a diagnostic procedure. *J Clin Invest* 1947;26:547.
7. Swan HJC, Wood EH. Localization of cardiac defects by dye-dilution curves recorded after injection of T-1824 at multiple sites in the heart and great vessels during cardiac catheterization. *Proc Staff Meet Mayo Clin* 1953;28:95.
8. Hyman AL, et al. A comparative study of the detection of cardiovascular shunts by oxygen analysis and indicator dilution methods. *Ann Intern Med* 1962;56:535.
9. Castillo CA, Kyle JC, Gilson WE, Rowe GG. Simulated shunt curves. *Am J Cardiol* 1966;17:691.
10. Braunwald E, Tannenbaum HL, Morrow AG. Localization of left-to-right cardiac shunts by dye-dilution curves following injection into the left side of the heart and into the aorta. *Am J Med* 1958;24:203.
11. Long RTL, Braunwald E, Morrow AG. Intracardiac injection of radioactive krypton: clinical applications of new methods for characterization of circulatory shunts. *Circulation* 1960;21:1126.
12. Levy AM, Monroe RG, Hugenholtz PG, Nadas AS. Clinical use of ascorbic acid as an indicator of right-to-left shunt. *Br Heart J* 1967;29:22.
13. Hugenholtz PG, et al. The clinical usefulness of hydrogen gas as an indicator of left-to-right shunts. *Circulation* 1963;28:542.
14. Amplatz K, et al. The Freon test: a new sensitive technique for the detection of small cardiac shunts. *Circulation* 1969;39:551.
15. Singleton RT, Dembo DH, Scherlis L. Krypton-85 in the detection of intracardiac left-to-right shunts. *Circulation* 1965;32:134.
16. Morrow AG, Sanders RJ, Braunwald E. The nitrous oxide test: an improved method for the detection of left-to-right shunts. *Circulation* 1958;17:284.
17. Long RT, Waldhausen JA, Cornell WP, Sanders RJ. Detection of right-to-left circulatory shunts: a new method utilizing injections of krypton-85. *Proc Soc Exp Biol Med* 1959;102:456.
18. Benenson W, Hitzig LWM. Diagnosis of venous arterial shunt by ether circulation time method. *Proc Soc Exp Biol Med* 1938;38: 256.
19. Parker JA, Treves S. Radionuclide detection, localization, and quantitation of intracardiac shunts and shunts between the great arteries. *Prog Cardiovasc Dis* 1977;20:121.
20. Prinzmetal M. Calculation of the venous arterial shunt in congenital heart disease. *J Clin Invest* 1941;20:705.
21. Swan HJC, Zapata-Diaz J, Wood EH. Dye dilution curves in cyanotic congenital heart disease. *Circulation* 1953;8:70.
22. Swan HJC, Burchell HB, Wood EH. The presence of venoarterial shunts in patients with interatrial communications. *Circulation* 1954;10:705.
23. Banas JS, et al. A simple technique for detecting small defects of the atrial septum. *Am J Cardiol* 1971;28:467.

Calculation of Stenotic Valve Orifice Area

10

Blase A. Carabello   *William Grossman*

The normal cardiac valve offers little resistance to blood flow. As valvular stenosis develops, there is progressively more resistance to flow, causing a pressure drop (pressure gradient) across the valve. At any stenotic orifice size, greater flow across the orifice yields a greater pressure gradient. Using two fundamental hydraulic formulas, Dr. Richard Gorlin and his father developed a formula for the calculation of cardiac valvular orifices from flow and pressure-gradient data (1). Today, this formula is usually calculated by computerized pressure monitoring systems, but it is still valuable to understand its derivation and characteristics.

GORLIN FORMULA

The first hydraulic formula that the Gorlins used was based on Torricelli's law, which describes flow across a round orifice:

$$F = AVC_C \tag{10.1}$$

where F is flow rate, A is orifice area, V is velocity of flow, and C_c is the coefficient of orifice contraction. The constant C_c compensates for the physical phenomenon that, except for a perfect orifice, the area of a stream flowing through an orifice will be less than the true area of the orifice.

Rearranging the terms,

$$A = \frac{F}{VC_C} \tag{10.2}$$

The second hydraulic principle used in the derivation of the Gorlin formula relates pressure gradient and velocity of flow according to Torricelli's law:

$$V^2 = (C_v)^2 \cdot 2gh \quad \text{or} \quad V = (C_v)\sqrt{2gh} \tag{10.3}$$

where V is velocity of flow; C_v is the coefficient of velocity, correcting for energy loss as pressure energy is converted to kinetic or velocity energy; h is the pressure gradient in cm H_2O, and g is the gravitational constant (980 cm/sec^2) for converting cm H_2O to units of pressure.

Combining the two equations,

$$A = \frac{F}{C_v\sqrt{2gh} \cdot C_C} = \frac{F}{C_V C_C \sqrt{2 \cdot 980 \cdot h}}$$
$$= \frac{F}{(C)(44.3)\sqrt{h}} \tag{10.4}$$

where C is an empirical constant accounting for C_V and C_C, the expression of h in mm Hg (rather than cm H_2O), and correcting the calculated valve area to the actual valve area measured at surgery or autopsy.

It is obvious that antegrade flow across the mitral and tricuspid valves occurs only in diastole, whereas that across the aortic and pulmonic valves occurs only in systole. Accordingly, the flow, F, for Eq. (10.4) is the total cardiac output expressed in terms of the seconds per minute during which there is actually forward flow across the valve. For the mitral and tricuspid valves, this is calculated by multiplying the diastolic filling period (seconds per beat) by the heart rate (beats per minute [bpm]), yielding the number of seconds per minute during which there is diastolic flow. The cardiac output in milliliters per minute (or cm^3/minute) is then divided by the seconds per minute during which there is flow, yielding diastolic flow in cubic centimeters per second. For the aortic and pulmonic valves, the systolic ejection period is substituted for the diastolic filling period. The manner in which the diastolic filling period and systolic ejection period are measured is shown in Fig. 10.1. The diastolic filling period begins at mitral valve opening and continues until end-diastole. The systolic ejection period begins with aortic valve opening and proceeds to the dicrotic notch or other evidence of aortic valve closure.

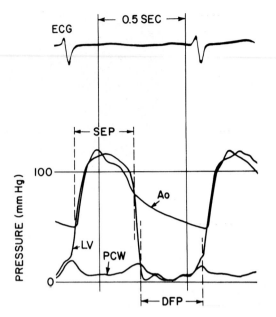

Figure 10.1 Left ventricular (LV), aortic (Ao), and pulmonary capillary wedge (PCW) pressure tracings from a patient without valvular heart disease, illustrating the definition and measurement of diastolic filling period (DFP) and systolic ejection period (SEP). See text for discussion.

Thus the final equation for the calculation of valve orifice area A (in cm^2) is

$$A = \frac{CO/(DFP \text{ or } SEP)(HR)}{44.3\text{C}\sqrt{\Delta P}} \qquad (10.5)$$

where CO is cardiac output (cm^3/minute), DFP is diastolic filling period (seconds/beat), SEP is systolic ejection period (seconds/beat), HR is heart rate (beats/minute), C is an empirical constant, and P is the pressure gradient. The DFP is measured directly from left ventricular versus pulmonary capillary wedge or left atrial pressure tracings as shown in Fig. 10.1.

An empirical constant of 0.7 (later adjusted to 0.85) was derived by comparing calculated and actual mitral valve areas (1,2). Using this constant, the maximum deviation of the calculated valve area from the measured valve area was 0.2 cm^2. The empirical constant for the aortic tricuspid and pulmonic valve was never derived. The constant for these valves has been assumed to be 1.0 (i.e., 1.0 × 44.3 = 44.3) because of lack of data comparing actual with calculated valve areas for those valves. Nonetheless, the Gorlin formula remains the gold standard for assessing the severity of stenotic cardiac valves.

MITRAL VALVE AREA

By rearranging the terms of Eq. (10.5), one sees that for the mitral valve,

$$\Delta P = \left[\frac{CO/(HR)(DFP)}{(MVA)(44.3)(0.85)}\right]^2 \qquad (10.6)$$

where ΔP is mean transmitral pressure gradient and MVA is mitral valve area. Thus, by doubling cardiac output one will quadruple the gradient across the valve, if heart rate and diastolic filling period remain constant. The normal mitral orifice in an adult has a cross-sectional area of 4.0 to 5.0 cm^2 when the mitral valve is completely open in diastole. Considerable reduction in this orifice area can occur without symptomatic limitation, but when the area is 1.0 cm^2 or less, a substantial resting gradient will be present across the mitral valve, and any demand for increased cardiac output will be met by increases in left atrial and pulmonary capillary pressure that lead to pulmonary congestion and edema.

Figure 10.2 demonstrates that a cardiac output of 5 L/minute can be maintained with only a minimal mitral diastolic gradient as the mitral orifice area contracts from its normal 4.0 to 5.0 cm^2 to a moderately stenotic area of 2.0 cm^2. After that, the gradient rises so that, at an orifice area of 1.0 cm^2, a resting gradient of 8 to 10 mm Hg is required to maintain cardiac output at 5 L/minute with a normal resting heart rate of 72 bpm (Fig. 10.2A). Note that even at this level of cardiac output, substantial increases in gradient may occur in response to tachycardia (Fig. 10.2B,C), which reduces the total time per minute available for diastolic filling. Thus, 1.0 cm^2 is generally viewed as the critical mitral valve area because only small increases in cardiac output lead to pulmonary congestion and severe dyspnea. However, some allowance, needs to be made for the patient's size in assessing critical valve area. Larger patients need greater flows than smaller patients need to maintain tissue perfusion, and they also have higher gradients because of greater cardiac output for any given valve orifice area. Thus 1.2 cm^2 could be a critical mitral valve area for a larger patient. Currently, no uniform agreement exists on indexing critical valve area to body size.

Example of Valve Area Calculation in Mitral Stenosis

Figure 10.3 shows pulmonary capillary wedge (PCW) and left ventricular (LV) pressure tracings in a 40-year-old woman with rheumatic heart disease and severe mitral stenosis. This woman also had hypertension and significant elevation of her LV diastolic pressure. The valve orifice area is calculated with the aid of a form reproduced as Table 10.1. In this patient, five beats were chosen from the recordings taken closest in time to the Fick cardiac output determination. Planimetry of the area between PCW and LV pressure tracings (Fig. 10.3) was done for these five beats, and these areas were divided by the length of the diastolic filling periods for each beat, giving an average gradient deflection in millimeters. The mean gradient in millimeters of mercury (Table 10.1, part B) was calculated as the average gradient deflection in millimeters multiplied by the scale factor (mm Hg/mm deflection). In this

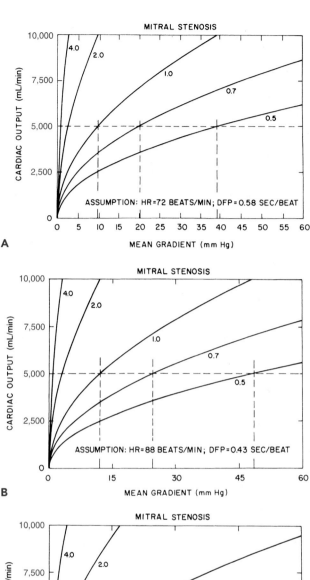

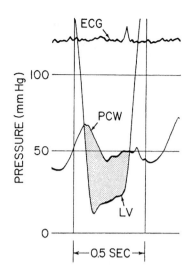

Figure 10.3 Pulmonary capillary wedge (PCW) and left ventricular (LV) pressure tracings in a 40-year-old woman with severe mitral stenosis. This woman also had systemic arterial hypertension and significant elevation of her LV diastolic pressure. See text for discussion.

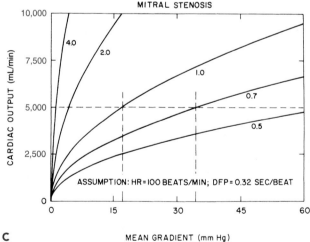

Figure 10.2 Relationships between cardiac output and mean diastolic pressure gradient in patients with mitral stenosis, calculated using Eq. 10.6, derived from the Gorlin formula. Curves represent orifice areas of 4.0, 2.0, 1.0, 0.7, and 0.5 cm². **A–C.** Flow-gradient relations at differing heart rates and diastolic filling periods (see text for discussion). (Courtesy of Dr. James J. Ferguson III.)

case, the mean gradient was 30 mm Hg. Next, the average diastolic filling period was calculated (Table 10.1, part C) using the average measured length between initial PCW-LV

crossover in early diastole and end-diastole (peak of the R wave by ECG). This average length in millimeters is divided by the paper speed (mm/second) to give the average diastolic filling period, which in this case was 0.40 sec. Heart rate and cardiac output (Table 10.1, parts D and E) are recorded, ideally from data collected simultaneously with the recording of the PCW-LV pressure gradient. Heart rate was 80 bpm and cardiac output was 4,680 cm³/minute in the case illustrated in Fig. 10.3. Note that cardiac output must be expressed in cubic centimeters per minute if valve area is expressed in square centimeters of cross-sectional area.

Entering these values in the formula given in Table 10.1, part F, and using a constant of $0.85(44.3) = 37.7$ for the mitral valve, we get

Mitral orifice area =

$$\frac{(4,680\,\text{cm}^3/\text{min})/(80\,\text{beats/min})(0.40\,\text{sec/beat})}{37.7\sqrt{30\,\text{mm Hg}}}$$

$$= 0.71\ \text{cm}^2 \qquad (10.7)$$

Because the accuracy of the method to hundredths of a square centimeter has not been demonstrated, the resulting valve area is rounded off and expressed as 0.7 cm².

Pitfalls

Pulmonary Capillary Wedge Tracing

In most cases, PCW pressure is substituted for left atrial pressure under the assumption that a properly confirmed wedge pressure accurately reflects left atrial pressure. Nishimura et al. (3) found that transmitral gradient was overestimated by 3.3 to 3.5 mm Hg when a Swan-Ganz

TABLE 10.1

VALVE ORIFICE AREA DETERMINATION

Patient _____ Age _____ Unit number _____ Date _____

A. Complex no.	Area of gradient (mm²)	/	Length of diastolic or systolic period (mm)	=	Average gradient (deflection, mm)
1.	_____	/	_____	=	_____
2.	_____	/	_____	=	_____
3.	_____	/	_____	=	_____
4.	_____	/	_____	=	_____
5.	_____	/	_____	=	_____

B. Mean gradient = Average gradient (mm deflection) × scale factor (mm Hg/mm deflection)

= _____ × _____ = _____ mm Hg

C. Average diastolic or systolic period = average length (mm)/paper speed (mm/sec)

= _____ / _____ = _____ sec/beat

D. Heart rate = _____ beat/min

E. Cardiac output (Fick or indicator dilution) = _____ mL/min

F. Valve area = $\dfrac{\text{cardiac output/(heart rate} \times \text{avg. diastolic or systolic period)}}{\text{valve constant}^a \times \sqrt{\text{mean gradient}}}$

$$= \frac{\underline{\hspace{2cm}}/(\underline{\hspace{2cm}} \times \underline{\hspace{2cm}})}{\underline{\hspace{2cm}} \times \sqrt{\quad}} = \underline{\hspace{2cm}} \text{ cm}^2$$

G. Valve area index = valve area body surface area = _____ cm²/m²

[a] Valve constants: for mitral valve use 37.7; for aortic, tricuspid, and pulmonic valves use 44.3.

catheter was used to measure wedge pressure compared with actual left atrial pressure. However, these "wedge" pressures were not confirmed as true wedge pressures, using the techniques described in Chapter 4. Conversely, Lange et al. (4) measured left atrial pressure directly (trans-septal) and compared it with oximetrically confirmed wedge pressure obtained using a stiff woven Dacron catheter. In this study, overestimation of true left atrial pressure was only 1.7 ± 0.6 mm Hg. Thus we and others believe that the weight of evidence (5) and our own experience support the use of the PCW pressure as a satisfactory substitution for left atrial pressure, except in some patients with pulmonary veno-occlusive disease or cor triatriatum. Failure to wedge the catheter properly may, however, cause one to compare a damped pulmonary artery pressure with the LV pressure, yielding a falsely high gradient. To ensure that the right heart catheter is properly wedged, one should verify that

1. The mean wedge pressure is lower than the mean pulmonary artery pressure
2. Blood withdrawn from the wedged catheter is ≥95% saturated with oxygen, or at least equal in saturation to arterial blood.

Alignment Mismatch

Alignment of the PCW and LV pressure tracings does not match alignment of simultaneous left atrial and LV tracings because there is a time delay in the transmission of the left atrial pressure signal back through the pulmonary venous and capillary beds. The resulting pressure mismatch is small when PCW pressure is measured in the distal pulmonary arteries using a 7F or 8F Cournand or Goodale-Lubin catheter, but may be larger when wedge pressure is measured more proximally in the pulmonary arterial tree using a balloon-tipped flow-directed catheter. As illustrated in Fig. 5.8, the A and V waves in an optimally damped PCW tracing are delayed typically by 50 to 70 milliseconds compared with a simultaneous left atrial pressure tracing. Thus, ideally, the wedge pressure should be realigned with the LV pressure (using tracing paper) by shifting it leftward by 50 to 70 milliseconds.

The V wave, which is normally present in the left atrium (where it represents pulmonary venous return), peaks immediately before the downstroke of the LV pressure tracing. With a wedge pressure measured distally using a 7F Goodale-Lubin catheter (Fig. 10.3), the peak of the V wave is bisected by the rapid downstroke of LV pressure decline. Realignment of a wedge tracing so that the V wave peak is bisected by (or slightly to the left of) the downstroke of LV pressure is a practical method for achieving more physiologic realignment.

Calibration Errors

Failure to calibrate pressure transducers properly and adjust them to the same zero reference point may yield an erroneous gradient. A quick way to check the validity of an unsuspected transmitral pressure gradient is to switch left and right heart catheters to opposite transducers, which if calibrated correctly yield the same gradient.

Cardiac Output Determination

Cardiac output must be determined accurately using the techniques described in Chapter 8. The cardiac output used in valve area calculation should be the value measured simultaneously with the gradient determination. The measurement used in the valve area formula is usually the forward cardiac output determined by the Fick method or the thermodilution method. If mitral valvular regurgitation exists, the gradient across the valve will reflect not only net forward flow but forward plus regurgitant or total transmitral diastolic flow. Thus using only net forward flow to calculate the valve orifice area will *underestimate* the actual anatomic valve area in cases where regurgitation coexists with stenosis. It is worth noting that many patients with mitral stenosis have coexistent tricuspid regurgitation. As indicated in Chapter 8, tricuspid regurgitation may cause the thermodilution technique of measuring cardiac output to be inaccurate.

Early Diastasis

Even when left atrial and LV pressures equalize (diastasis) before the end of diastole, there will generally still be flow through the mitral valve after the point of diastasis. The diastolic filling period to be used in valve area calculation should include all of nonisovolumic diastole, not just the period during which a gradient is present.

AORTIC VALVE AREA

An aortic valve area of 0.7 cm^2 or less is generally considered severe enough to account for the symptoms of angina, syncope, or heart failure in a patient with aortic stenosis. Because the development of symptoms in patients with aortic stenosis portends an abrupt worsening of prognosis, this valve area is termed *critical*. However, it must be pointed out that no unique critical valve area has been established and that an aortic valve area as large as 1.0 cm^2 can cause symptoms and thus be critical, especially in a large individual. Conversely, smaller calculated valve orifice areas in a totally asymptomatic patient may not be critical. Figure 10.4 illustrates the relationship between cardiac output and aortic pressure gradient over a range of values for aortic valve area at three values for heart rate and systolic ejection period. For the aortic valve, Eq. (10.4) can be rearranged as

$$\Delta P = \left[\frac{CO/(HR)(SEP)}{44.3 AVA} \right]^2 \qquad (10.8)$$

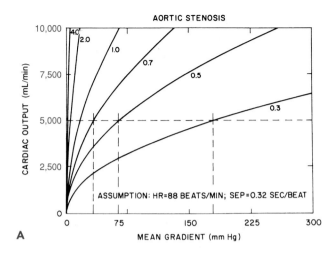

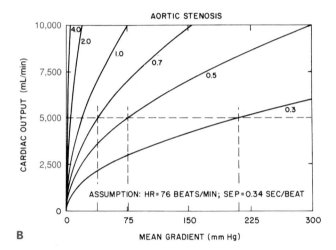

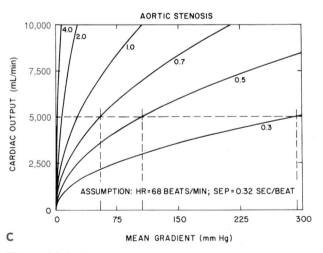

Figure 10.4 Relationships between cardiac output and mean aortic systolic pressure gradient in patients with aortic stenosis, calculated using Eq. 10.7, derived from the Gorlin formula. Curves represent orifice areas of 4.0, 2.0, 1.0, 0.7, 0.5, and 0.3 cm^2. **A–C.** Flow-gradient relations at differing heart rates and systolic ejection periods. (Courtesy of Dr. James J. Ferguson III.)

As can be seen in Fig. 10.4A, at a normal resting cardiac output of 5.0 L/minute, an aortic orifice area of 0.7 cm^2 will result in a gradient of approximately 33 mm Hg across the aortic valve. Doubling of the cardiac output, as might occur with exercise, would increase the gradient by a factor of 4 to 132 mm Hg if the systolic time per minute did not change. This increase in gradient would require a peak LV pressure in excess of 250 mm Hg to maintain a central aortic pressure of 120 mm Hg. Such a major increase in LV pressure obviously increases myocardial oxygen demand and limits ejection performance. These factors contribute to the symptoms of angina and congestive heart failure, respectively (6,7). The limitations in cardiac output imposed by high afterload may contribute to hypotension when peripheral vasodilation occurs during muscular exercise.

Actually, the systolic time per minute does not remain constant during the increase in cardiac output associated with exercise. As heart rate increases during exercise, the systolic ejection period tends to become shorter, but the tendency is counteracted by both increased venous return and systemic arteriolar vasodilation, factors that normally help to maintain LV stroke volume constant (or even allow it to increase) during exercise. Thus, the heart rate is increasing but the systolic ejection period is diminishing only slightly so that their product (systolic ejection time per minute) increases. This is the counterpart of the decreased diastolic filling time per minute during exercise discussed earlier. Examining Eq. (10.8), it can be seen that the increase in cardiac output will be partially offset by the increase in (HR)(SEP) so that the gradient will not quadruple with a doubling of cardiac output during exercise.

Figure 10.4B and C show that with decreasing heart rate, the gradient *increases* in aortic stenosis for any value of cardiac output. This is opposite to the effect of heart rate in mitral stenosis and reflects the *opposite effects* of heart rate on systolic and diastolic time per minute. Viewed another way, as the heart rate slows in aortic stenosis, the stroke volume increases if cardiac output remains constant. Thus the flow per beat across the aortic valve increases and so does the pressure gradient.

As with mitral stenosis, some allowance must be made for body size in defining a critical valve area in patients with aortic stenosis; larger patients who require higher output may become symptomatic at somewhat larger valve areas. Thus, a very large man with a body surface area of 2.4 m^2 and a cardiac index of 3.0 L/minute per m^2 would have a cardiac output of 7,200 mL/min. At a heart rate of 68 bpm (Fig. 10.4C), this man might have a 50-mm Hg aortic valve gradient with an orifice area of 0.9 to 1.0 cm^2. Thus, for him, this might be a critical valve area.

Example

Figure 10.5 demonstrates simultaneous pressure tracings from the left ventricle (LV) and right femoral artery (RFA) in a patient with exertional syncope. Because the pulse wave takes a finite period of time to travel from the left ventricle to the femoral artery, the femoral artery tracing is somewhat delayed (Fig. 10.5A). Figure 10.5B shows the LV and RFA tracings realigned to correct for the delay in transmission time. This is accomplished by using tracing paper and aligning the arterial upstroke to coincide with the LV upstroke. After such alignment, the mean pressure gradient can now be obtained by planimetry, and the orifice area can be calculated using the form given in Table 10.1. For this example, the average aortic pressure gradient is 40 mm Hg, the systolic ejection period is 0.33 sec, the heart rate is 74 bpm, and the cardiac output is 5,000 mL/min. Using these values together with an aortic valve constant of (1)(44.3) = 44.3 in the equation in Table 10.1 gives

Aortic valve area =

$$\frac{(5{,}000\,\text{cm}^3/\text{min})/(74\,\text{beats}/\text{min})(0.33\,\text{sec}/\text{beat})}{44.3\sqrt{40\,\text{mm Hg}}}$$

$$= 0.7\,\text{cm}^2 \qquad (10.9)$$

As discussed in Chapter 7, peripheral arterial pressure waveforms are distorted in ways other than time delay. These distortions include systolic amplification and spreading out (widening) of the pressure waveform. To assess possible errors introduced by the use of peripheral arterial pressure as a substitute for ascending aortic pressure, Folland et al. (8) compared the LV-ascending aortic (LV-Ao) mean gradient in 26 patients with aortic stenosis with the LV-femoral artery (LV-FA) systolic gradient, with and without

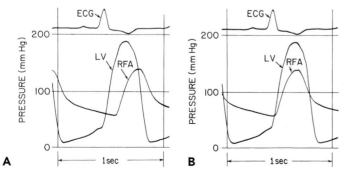

Figure 10.5 Left ventricular (LV) and right femoral artery (RFA) pressure tracings in a patient who presented with exertional syncope owing to aortic stenosis. **A.** The tracings actually recorded, demonstrating the significant time delay for the pressure waveform to reach the RFA. **B.** Realignment using tracing paper. (See text for discussion.)

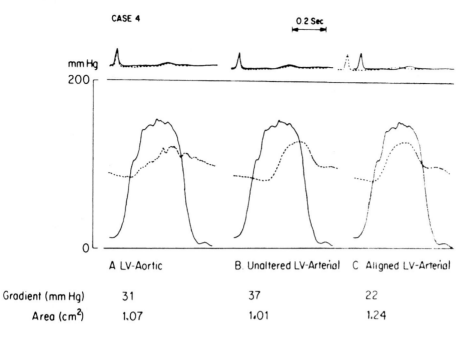

CASE 4

0.2 Sec

	A LV-Aortic	B. Unaltered LV-Arterial	C. Aligned LV-Arterial
Gradient (mm Hg)	31	37	22
Area (cm²)	1.07	1.01	1.24

Figure 10.6 Pressure gradients in aortic stenosis. **A.** The left ventricular (LV)–central aortic gradient. **B.** LV-femoral artery gradient without alignment. **C.** LV-femoral artery gradient with alignment obtained by moving the femoral artery tracing leftward so that its upstroke coincides with the LV pressure upstroke. (Reproduced with permission from Folland ED, Parisi AF, Carbone C. Is peripheral arterial pressure a satisfactory substitute for ascending aortic pressure when measuring aortic valve gradients? *J Am Coll Cardiol* 1984;4:1207.)

realignment (Fig. 10.6). Without realignment, the LV-FA gradient overestimated the LV-Ao gradient by about 9 mm Hg. In contrast, aligned LV-FA gradients underestimated the LV-Ao gradient by about 10 mm Hg, possibly because peak systolic arterial pressure is higher in peripheral arterial pressure tracings than in central aortic tracings so that the planimetered gradient is smaller when using LV-FA. Without realignment, this effect is offset by the fact that much of the arterial systolic waveform is outside and to the right of the LV pressure tracing (Fig. 10.6). A second error

in gradient measurement can occur if the LV catheter is placed in the LV outflow tract (9). As shown in Fig. 10.7, a gradient usually exists between the body of the left ventricle and outflow tract, produced as blood accelerates when it enters this relatively narrow portion of the left ventricle. A catheter tip placed in the LV outflow tract will measure a typical LV pressure tracing, but can underestimate the true LV-aorta gradient by 30 mm Hg.

Assey et al. (10) measured the transaortic valve gradients in 15 patients from eight different combinations of catheter

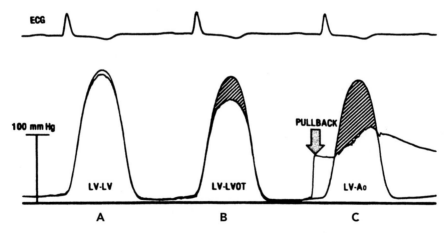

Figure 10.7 **A.** Pressure tracings recorded from two catheters placed within the body of the left ventricular (LV) chamber. Tracings are nearly identical. **B.** Pressures recorded by two catheters, one placed in the body of the left ventricular chamber and the other placed in the left ventricular outflow tract (LVOT), proximal to the aortic valve (AO). Both catheters record characteristic left ventricular pressure tracings; however, there is a substantial pressure gradient between the body of the left ventricle and the outflow tract. This is not owing to anatomic subvalvular stenosis but rather to acceleration of blood as it enters the relatively narrow outflow tract. **C.** Pressures recorded from the catheter in the body of the left ventricle and from a second catheter in the proximal aorta. These tracings demonstrate the gradient across the aortic valve and outflow tract. (Reproduced from Pasipoularides A. Clinical assessment of ventricular ejection dynamics with and without outflow obstruction. *J Am Coll Cardiol* 1990;15:859, with permission.)

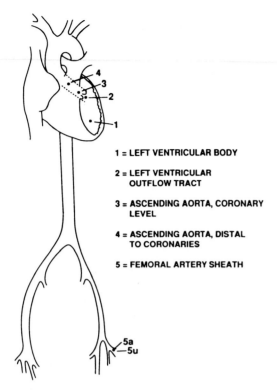

1 = LEFT VENTRICULAR BODY

2 = LEFT VENTRICULAR
    OUTFLOW TRACT

3 = ASCENDING AORTA, CORONARY
    LEVEL

4 = ASCENDING AORTA, DISTAL
    TO CORONARIES

5 = FEMORAL ARTERY SHEATH

Figure 10.8 Two sites for recording left ventricular pressure (1 and 2) and three sites for recording distal pressure (3, 4, and 5) are shown. Site 5u represents the actual femoral artery pressure tracing, which is unaligned with the left ventricular pressure tracing. Site 5a represents the recording obtained from the femoral artery, which is then manually aligned to match the left ventricular pressure tracing in time. The following are the potential recording sites for obtaining the transaortic valve pressure gradient in aortic stenosis: 1–3, 1–4, 1–5a, 1–5u, 2–3, 2–4, 2–5a, and 2–5u. Gradients recorded at these different sites may vary widely in any given patient. (Reproduced with permission from Assey ME, Zile MR, Usher BW, Karavan MP, Carabello BA. Effect of catheter positioning on the variability of measured gradient in aortic stenosis. *Cathet Cardiovasc Diagn* 1993;30:287.)

locations using the schema shown in Fig. 10.8. The average mean gradient recorded between positions 1 and 3 was the greatest, whereas the gradient between positions 1 and 5 using the alignment technique produced the smallest value.

In some patients, the differences in gradient among the different measurement sites were as much as 45 mm Hg. In calculating aortic valve area, the gradient between sites 1 and 3, which records gradient before pressure recovery, is probably the most accurate reflection of the pressure drop across the valve. When the aortic catheter is placed at a more distal site, it records the effect of pressure recovery, which reduces gradient as blood flow again becomes laminar. The more proximal aortic position is probably the ideal location for measuring the gradient for the valve area calculation; the more distal positions may better reflect the actual overload on the myocardium. When the transvalvular gradient recorded from positions 1 and 5a in Fig. 10.8 is larger than 60 mm Hg, these differences are of little clinical importance. When a small transvalvular gradient is present in conjunction with a low cardiac output, however, the differences between aligned and unaligned tracings and between gradients recorded at different catheter locations may affect the decision about whether to replace the valve. In such instances, we recommend that the problem be obviated by placing a second catheter in the proximal ascending aorta without need for alignment (8; Fig. 10.6A). As an alternative, the difference between peak central aortic and peripheral arterial pressure is added to the planimetered gradient measured during the Fick output determination. This compensates for the fact that the planimetered gradient with realignment (Fig. 10.6C) underestimates the true gradient (Fig. 10.6A). The most accurate approach, however, involves the use of a second catheter positioned in the ascending aorta, as discussed earlier.

Another approach to increasing the accuracy of transaortic valve gradient measurement using simultaneous LV and femoral artery pressures has been introduced by Krueger et al. (11) at the University of Utah. As seen in Fig. 10.9, the mean LV systolic pressure during interval A and the mean femoral artery systolic pressure during interval B are determined by planimetry. Their difference was nearly identical to the gradient measured by planimetry of simultaneous LV and central aortic pressures and was more accurate than other techniques commonly used (11).

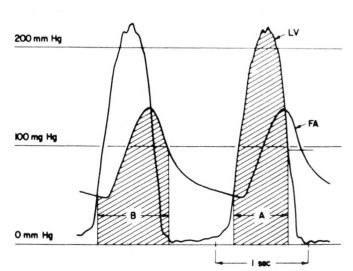

Figure 10.9 Simultaneous recordings of left ventricular (LV) and femoral artery (FA) pressures in a patient with aortic stenosis. The mean LV systolic pressure during interval A and the mean FA systolic pressure during interval B are determined by planimetry, and the systolic LV-aortic gradient is estimated as the difference between these mean pressures. (Reproduced with permission from Krueger SK, Orme EC, King CS, Barry WH. Accurate determination of the transaortic valve gradient using simultaneous left ventricular and femoral artery pressures. *Cathet Cardiovasc Diagn* 1989;16:202.)

If a second catheter is not used to obtain simultaneous LV and peripheral pressures, the gradient may be obtained by recording LV pressure and superimposing it on the aortic pressure obtained immediately after the LV catheter is pulled back into the aorta.

Pitfalls

Transducer Calibration

As with calculation of mitral valve area, attention to cardiac output determination and transducer calibration is critical. Assurance that proper transducer calibration has been accomplished can be obtained by comparing the left heart catheter pressure with the peripheral arterial catheter pressure before insertion of the left heart catheter into the left ventricle. Because in the absence of peripheral stenosis mean arterial pressure will be the same throughout the arterial tree, the mean pressures recorded by both catheters should be identical, confirming identical transducer calibration. Further gradient verification is made by comparing the LV pressure with aortic pressure obtained by the left heart catheter during catheter pullback. In this case, both LV and aortic pressures are recorded by the same catheter and transducer, eliminating the second transducer as a source of error.

Pullback Hemodynamics

When the aortic valve area is diminished to 0.6 cm^2 or less, a 7F or 8F catheter placed retrograde across the valve takes up a significant amount of the residual orifice area, and the catheter may actually increase the severity of stenosis. Conversely, removal of the catheter reduces the severity of stenosis. We have observed that a peripheral pressure rise occurs in severe aortic stenosis when the LV catheter is removed from the aortic valve orifice (12). In our experience, an augmentation in peripheral systolic pressure of more than 5 mm Hg at the time of LV catheter pullback indicates that significant aortic stenosis is present. This sign is present in >80% of patients with an aortic valve area of 0.5 cm^2 or less, a point that is discussed further in Chapter 29.

AREA OF TRICUSPID AND PULMONIC VALVES

Because of the rarity of tricuspid and pulmonic stenosis in adults, no general agreement exists as to what constitutes a critical orifice area for these valves. In general, a mean gradient of 5 mm Hg across the tricuspid valve is sufficient to cause symptoms of systemic venous hypertension. Gradients across the pulmonic valve of <50 mm Hg are usually well tolerated, but gradients of >100 mm Hg indicate a need for surgical correction. Between 50 and 100 mm Hg, decisions regarding surgical correction depend on the clinical features in each case.

ALTERNATIVES TO THE GORLIN FORMULA

A simplified valve formula for the calculation of stenotic cardiac valve areas was proposed by Hakki et al. (13) and tested in 100 consecutive patients with either aortic or mitral stenosis. The simplified formula is

$$\text{Valve area} = \frac{\text{cardiac output (liters/min)}}{\sqrt{\text{pressure gradient}}} \quad (10.10)$$

and is based on their observation that the product of heart rate, SEP or DFP, and the Gorlin formula constant was nearly the same for all patients whose hemodynamics were measured in the resting state, and the value of this product was close to 1.0. For the examples given earlier in this chapter, the simplified formula works reasonably well. Thus for the patient with mitral stenosis (Fig. 10.3) with a cardiac output of 4,680 mL/minute and a mitral diastolic gradient of 30 mm Hg, mitral valve area is 4.68 divided by the square root of 30, or 0.85 cm^2 using the simplified formula as opposed to the value of 0.71 cm^2 calculated using the Gorlin formula. For the patient with aortic stenosis whose tracings are shown in Fig. 10.5 (cardiac output 5 L/minute, aortic gradient 40 mm Hg), the aortic valve area by the simplified formula is 5 divided by the square root of 40, or 0.79 cm^2 as opposed to 0.73 cm^2 by the Gorlin formula. Because the percentage of time per minute spent in diastole or systole changes substantially at higher heart rates, the simplified formula may be less useful in the presence of substantial tachycardia. This point, however, has not been tested adequately.

ASSESSMENT OF AORTIC STENOSIS IN PATIENTS WITH LOW CARDIAC OUTPUT

In the patient with a forward cardiac output of 3 L/min, a mean transvalvular gradient of 20 mm Hg will yield a calculated valve area of 0.7 cm^2, indicating critical aortic stenosis. However, not all such patients actually have severe aortic stenosis. Valve calculations made using the Gorlin formula are flow dependent. That is, as cardiac output increases, calculated area increases, and as cardiac output decreases, calculated area decreases (14,15). Two potential mechanisms exist by which calculated valve orifice area increases with cardiac output: (a) Increased flow through the stenotic aortic valve in conjunction with increased LV pressure physically opens the valve to a greater orifice area, and thus the valve orifice really is wider during increased flow, and (b) inaccuracies in the Gorlin formula cause the calculated area (but not necessarily the actual orifice area) to be flow dependent. The Gorlins themselves noted that they had no data from which to calculate an empirical constant for the aortic valve (1). Indeed, such a constant has never been calculated but has been assumed to be 1.0 by the cardiologic community. The issue remains in doubt, but in all probability both explanations are correct in part.

On one hand, Tardif and coworkers have shown that two-dimensional transesophageal echocardiographic imaging of the stenotic aortic valve has failed to demonstrate true change in valve orifice areas when increased flow caused calculated area to increase (16). These data suggest that the relationship between calculated area and flow dependence resides within the calculation rather than in representing a true change in area. However, it remains unclear whether the echocardiographic method used is sensitive enough to detect tiny (0.2 to 0.4 cm^2) changes in actual valve area. On the other hand, Voelker and colleagues working in vitro concluded that changes in calculated orifice area with changes in flow were probably owing to actual changes in valve area (17). Flow dependence of calculated valve orifice area appears less in bicuspid than in tricuspid valves (18), but is greater at lower than at higher flows (19).

These problems in assessing stenosis severity have substantial clinical importance. Consider a patient with reduced cardiac output and low LV ejection fraction who has both cardiomyopathy and mild aortic stenosis. Despite a calculated valve area of 0.7 cm^2, such a patient will probably not benefit from aortic valve replacement because aortic stenosis was not the cause of the LV dysfunction. On the other hand, although patients with low aortic valve gradients are generally at higher risk for perioperative death associated with aortic valve replacement (7,20), Brogan et al. (21) have demonstrated that some patients with low gradients may improve substantially following surgery. It is likely that such patients have truly severe aortic stenosis, which is the cause of their hemodynamic decompensation; in these patients, correcting the aortic stenosis is beneficial.

Preliminary data from three studies suggest that cautious hemodynamic manipulation in the catheterization laboratory can distinguish between these two different clinical entities (22–25). In patients with mild aortic stenosis, an infusion of nitroprusside or dobutamine increases forward output substantially, but may actually decrease the transvalvular gradient. In such cases, the calculated aortic valve area increases dramatically and is no longer within the critical range. On the other hand, in patients with truly severe aortic stenosis, infusion of nitroprusside widens the transvalvular gradient and increases the calculated aortic valve area only slightly, if at all. The results of nitroprusside infusion in a patient with mild aortic stenosis are demonstrated in Table 10.2 (24). The patient's initial calculated valve orifice area was 0.6 cm^2, which would indicate a need for surgery. However, following nitroprusside infusion, the gradient actually fell and calculated valve area increased. The patient improved on chronic vasodilator therapy, usually contraindicated in aortic stenosis unless the disease is mild. It must be emphasized that infusion of nitroprusside in patients with aortic stenosis must be performed with great caution, because if true aortic stenosis is present, hypotension may result. If it is known that the patient has normal coronary arteries, dobutamine, which produces similar changes in cardiac output, can be infused instead of nitroprusside. However, dobutamine infusion may be dangerous in patients who also have coronary disease, in whom it may precipitate ischemia.

VALVE RESISTANCE

Valve resistance is simply the mean aortic valve gradient divided by the cardiac output per second of systolic flow. It has the advantage of being calculated from two directly obtained pieces of data (output and gradient) and requires no discharge coefficient (26). A simplified formula for calculating aortic valve resistance is

$$\frac{\left(\begin{array}{c}\text{Mean}\\\text{gradient}\end{array}\right)\left(\begin{array}{c}\text{Systolic ejection}\\\text{period}\end{array}\right)\left(\begin{array}{c}\text{Heart}\\\text{rate}\end{array}\right) \times 1.33}{\text{Cardiac output (liters/min)}}$$

$$(10.11)$$

Valve resistance has been shown by Cannon et al. (22) to help separate patients with severe aortic stenosis from those patients who had similarly small calculated aortic valve areas, but who were subsequently demonstrated to have mild disease. Resistance appears less flow dependent than valve area (22,26). Resistance is unlikely to supplant the Gorlin formula in assessing stenosis severity, but may be an important adjunct to it in patients with low cardiac output.

Currently, we recommend cautious hemodynamic manipulation with dobutamine or nitroprusside for patients with a cardiac output of <4.5 L/minute who have a transvalvular gradient of <40 mm Hg and a valve resistance of <275 dyn·sec·cm^{-5}. If patients respond by substantially increasing the measured gradient, they probably have truly severe aortic stenosis and may benefit from aortic valve

---

TABLE 10.2

NITROPRUSSIDE INFUSION IN A PATIENT WITH MILD AORTIC STENOSIS

	Baseline	Nitroprusside (0.5 µg/kg/min)
Cardiac output (liters/min)	3.0	4.5
Left ventricular pressure (mm Hg)	130/30	120/20
Aortic pressure (mm Hg)	90/60	90/50
Aortic valve area (cm^2)	0.6	1.0
Valve resistance (dyn·sec·cm^{-5})	200	160

From Carabello BA, Ballard WL, Gazes PC. Patient 65. *Cardiology Pearls*. Philadelphia: Hanley & Belfus, 1994:142.

replacement. However, if cardiac output increases substantially but gradient increases only slightly or actually declines, the aortic stenosis is mild and the patient is unlikely to benefit from aortic valve replacement.

ACKNOWLEDGMENT

We would like to express our appreciation to Dr. James J. Ferguson III, who supplied Figs. 10.2 and 10.4, constructed by him from computer simulation.

REFERENCES

1. Gorlin R, Gorlin G. Hydraulic formula for calculation of area of stenotic mitral valve, other cardiac valves and central circulatory shunts. *Am Heart J* 1951;41:1.
2. Cohen MV, Gorlin R. Modified orifice equation for the calculation of mitral valve area. *Am Heart J* 1972;84:839.
3. Nishimura RA, Rihal CS, Tajik AJ, Holmes DR Jr. Accurate measurement of the transmitral gradient in patients with mitral stenosis: a simultaneous catheterization and Doppler echocardiographic study. *J Am Coll Cardiol* 1994;24:152.
4. Lange RA, Moore DM, Cigarroa RG, Hillis LD. Use of pulmonary capillary wedge pressure to assess severity of mitral stenosis: is true left atrial pressure needed in this condition? *J Am Coll Cardiol* 1989;13:825.
5. Alpert JS. The lessons of history as reflected in the pulmonary capillary wedge pressure. *J Am Coll Cardiol* 1989;13:830.
6. Strauer BE, Burger SB. Systolic stress, coronary hemodynamics and metabolic reserve in experimental and clinical cardiac hypertrophy. *Basic Res Cardiol* 1980;75:234.
7. Carabello BA, et al. Hemodynamic determinants of prognosis of aortic valve replacement in critical aortic stenosis and advanced congestive heart failure. *Circulation* 1980;62:42.
8. Folland ED, Parisi AF, Carbone C. Is peripheral arterial pressure a satisfactory substitute for ascending aortic pressure when measuring aortic valve gradients? *J Am Coll Cardiol* 1984;4:1207.
9. Pasipoularides A. Clinical assessment of ventricular ejection dynamics with and without outflow obstruction. *J Am Coll Cardiol* 1990;15:859.
10. Assey ME, Zile MR, Usher BW, Karavan MP, Carabello BA. Effect of catheter positioning on the variability of measured gradient in aortic stenosis. *Cathet Cardiovasc Diagn* 1993;30:287.
11. Krueger SK, Orme EC, King CS, Barry WH. Accurate determination of the transaortic valve gradient using simultaneous left ventricular and femoral artery pressures. *Cathet Cardiovasc Diagn* 1989;16: 202.
12. Carabello BA, Barry WH, Grossman W. Changes in arterial pressure during left heart pullback in patients with aortic stenosis: a sign of severe aortic stenosis. *Am J Cardiol* 1979;44:424.
13. Hakki AH, et al. A simplified valve formula for the calculation of stenotic cardiac valve areas. *Circulation* 1981;63:1050.
14. Burwash IG, Thomas DD, Sadahiro M, et al. Dependence of Gorlin formula and continuity equation valve areas on transvalvular volume flow rate in valvular aortic stenosis. *Circulation* 1994;39:827.
15. Carabello BA. Advances in the hemodynamic assessment of stenotic cardiac valves. *J Am Coll Cardiol* 1987;10:912.
16. Tardif JC, Rodrigues AG, Hardy JF, et al. Simultaneous determination of aortic valve area by the Gorlin formula and by transesophageal echocardiography under different transvalvular flow conditions: evidence that anatomic aortic valve area does not change with variations in flow in aortic stenosis. *J Am Coll Cardiol* 1997;29:1296.
17. Voelker W, Reul H, Nienhaus G, et al. Comparison of valvular resistance, stroke work loss and Gorlin valve area for quantification of aortic stenosis: an *in vitro* study in a pulsatile aortic flow model. *Circulation* 1995;91:1196.
18. Shively BK, Charlton GA, Crawford MH, Chaney RK. Flow dependence of valve area in aortic stenosis: relation to valve morphology. *J Am Coll Cardiol* 1998;31:654.
19. Marcus R, Bednarz J, Abruzzo J, et al. Mechanism underlying flow-dependency of valve orifice area determined by the Gorlin formula in patients with aortic valve obstruction. *Circulation* 1993;88 (suppl I):I-103(abstr).
20. Lund O. Preoperative risk evaluation and stratification of long-term survival after valve replacement for aortic stenosis: reasons for earlier operative intervention. *Circulation* 1990;82:124.
21. Brogan WC III, Grayburn PA, Lange RA, Hillis LD. Prognosis after valve replacement in patients with severe aortic stenosis and a low transvalvular pressure gradient. *J Am Coll Cardiol* 1993;21:1657.
22. Cannon JD Jr, Zile MR, Crawford FA Jr, Carabello BA. Aortic valve resistance as an adjunct to the Gorlin formula in assessing the severity of aortic stenosis in symptomatic patients. *J Am Coll Cardiol* 1992;20:1517.
23. Casale PN, Palacios IF, Abascal VM, et al. Effects of dobutamine on Gorlin and continuity equation valve areas and valve resistance in valvular aortic stenosis. *Am J Cardiol* 1992;70:1175.
24. DeFilippi CR, Willett DL, Brickner ME, et al. Usefulness of dobutamine echocardiography in distinguishing severe from nonsevere valvular aortic stenosis in patients with depressed left ventricular function and low transvalvular gradients. *Am J Cardiol* 1995;75:191.
25. Carabello BA, Ballard WL, Gazes PC. *Cardiology Pearls.* Philadelphia: Hanley & Belfus, 1994:142.
26. Ford LE, Feldman T, Chiu YC, Carroll JD. Hemodynamic resistance as a measure of functional impairment in aortic valvular stenosis. *Circ Res* 1990;66:1.

Angiographic Techniques

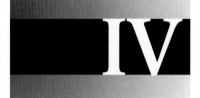

Coronary Angiography

11

Donald S. Baim[a]

Diagnostic coronary angiography (also called coronary arteriography) is now the principal component of cardiac catheterization, with an estimated 2,000,000 procedures (roughly 800 per 100,000 population) performed each year in the United States (1,2). The goal is to examine the entire coronary tree (both native vessels as well as any surgically constructed bypass grafts) while recording details of the coronary anatomy that include the following: the pattern of arterial distribution, anatomic or functional pathology (atherosclerosis, thrombosis, congenital anomalies, or focal coronary spasm), and the presence of intercoronary and intracoronary collateral connections. The procedure is typically performed in 30 minutes or less, under local anesthesia, on an outpatient basis, with a procedure-related major complication rate (death, stroke, myocardial infarction, see Chapter 3) of <0.1%. By performing a series of intracoronary contrast injections in carefully chosen angulated views using current high-resolution x-ray imaging (see Chapter 2), it is possible to define all portions of the coronary arterial circulation down to vessels as small as 0.3 mm, free of any artifacts owing to vessel overlap or foreshortening.

There is currently no other imaging technique that gives as detailed a view of the coronary circulation, although noninvasive techniques such as magnetic resonance angiography (MRA) and multidetector and electron-beam computed tomography (MDCT, EBCT) have improved their resolution and emerged as effective screening tests for coronary artery disease in the proximal coronary arteries, coronary anomalies, and patency of surgical bypass grafts (3,4). But for patients with compelling ischemic symptoms, what begins as a diagnostic procedure can quickly shift to a definitive therapy (percutaneous coronary intervention or PCI, see Chapters 22–24) performed through

the same access site. Even so, coronary angiography is limited to examination of only the coronary lumen and not the endothelial surface, plaque content, vessel wall, or (except indirectly) coronary flow physiology. When those features are in question, coronary angiography may be supplemented by intravascular ultrasound, optical computerized tomography, angioscopy, or intracoronary pressure and flow measurements (see Chapters 18 and 19). Despite these limitations, selective coronary angiography still remains the clinical gold standard for evaluating coronary anatomy. The performance of high-quality coronary angiography to safely define each and every coronary stenosis in an optimal view is an important measure of an operator's skill in cardiac catheterization and is the foundation on which the ability to perform successful coronary intervention is based.

CURRENT INDICATIONS

The various current indications for coronary angiography are summarized comprehensively in the most recent set of AHA/ACC guidelines on coronary angiography (2), available online at http://www.acc.org/clinical/topic/topic.htm. Although the details of these indications continue to evolve as new applications of catheter-based therapy are developed, they are still best summarized by the principle stated by F. Mason Sones—coronary arteriography is indicated when a problem is encountered whose resolution may be aided by the objective demonstration of the coronary anatomy, provided competent personnel and adequate facilities are available and the potential risks are acceptable to the patient and physician.

The most frequent indication is the further evaluation of patients in whom the diagnosis of coronary atherosclerosis is almost certain and in whom anatomic correction by means of coronary bypass surgery or PCI is contemplated. Angiographic evaluation of coronary anatomy in

[a] The contribution of William Grossman to this chapter in prior editions is gratefully acknowledged.

such patients provides the crucial information needed to select the most appropriate treatment strategy—catheter intervention (see Chapters 22–24), bypass surgery, or medical therapy. Included in this category are patients with stable angina pectoris refractory to medical therapy.

Even asymptomatic patients with noninvasive evidence of myocardial ischemia also benefit from revascularization and are thus candidates for coronary angiography (5). In patients with unstable angina (new onset, progressive, or rest pain), intensive drug therapy (beta-blocker, calcium channel blocker, nitrate, heparin, aspirin, clopidogrel or a platelet glycoprotein IIb/IIIa receptor blocker) may be temporizing, but more than two thirds of such patients will come to angiography within 6 weeks of presentation anyway owing to ongoing clinical symptoms or a positive exercise test (6,7). In most cases, therefore, such patients are brought to early coronary angiography, with same-procedure PCI if their anatomy is suitable. Patients with acute myocardial infarction routinely undergo immediate coronary angiography followed by same-procedure primary angioplasty (8). However, the role of routine post-MI coronary angiography in the asymptomatic postinfarct patient who was managed medically or with thrombolysis has not been established (9). The most recent AHA/ACC guidelines for the role of coronary angiography in stable angina, unstable angina, and acute myocardial infarction are available on the Internet at www.acc.org/clinical/topic/topic.htm.

A second group of indications for coronary angiography consists of patients in whom the presence or absence of coronary artery disease is unclear (2). This includes patients with troublesome chest pain syndromes but ambiguous noninvasive test results, patients with unexplained heart failure or ventricular arrhythmias, survivors of out-of-hospital cardiac arrest (10), patients with suspected or proven variant angina (11), and patients with risk factors for coronary artery disease who are being evaluated for major abdominal, thoracic, or vascular surgery (12). This category also includes patients scheduled for correction of congenital or valvular pathology. Patients with congenital defects such as tetralogy of Fallot frequently have anomalies of coronary distribution that may lead to surgical complications if unrecognized (13), whereas patients older than age 45 years with valvular disease may have advanced coronary atherosclerosis without clinical symptoms. Although younger patients with valvular disease are commonly operated on without prior coronary angiograms, given the extraordinary low risk of diagnostic catheterization and the potential benefit of knowing the coronary anatomy, most surgical center personnel believe it is best to perform a preoperative diagnostic catheterization to identify (and then correct) significant coronary lesions, to provide the best and safest outcome during concurrent valve replacement (14).

Finally, coronary angiography is frequently performed when a patient develops recurrent angina after coronary intervention (to detect and treat restenosis, see Chapter 22) or after bypass surgery (to detect vein graft failure, which might require catheter intervention or reoperation). Routine follow-up angiography 6 months after catheter intervention is not indicated clinically, but may play an important role in the research evaluation of new technologies or drug therapies targeted at reducing restenosis (15).

HISTORY AND GENERAL ISSUES

The initial attempts to perform coronary angiography used nonselective injections of contrast medium into the aortic root to opacify both the left and right coronary arteries simultaneously as the angiographic images were recorded on serial conventional sheet films (16). To improve contrast delivery into the coronary ostia, some early investigators used transient circulatory arrest induced by the administration of acetylcholine or by elevation of intrabronchial pressure, followed by occlusion of the ascending aorta by gas-filled balloon and injection of the contrast bolus. Although nonselective aortic root injection is still used occasionally today to evaluate ostial lesions, anomalous coronary ostia, or coronary bypass grafts, intentional circulatory arrest is no longer practiced, and earlier nonselective techniques have largely been replaced by selective injection into each coronary ostium using specially designed catheters advanced from any of several arterial access points.

In most patients, successful coronary angiography can be performed by either the brachial cutdown or the percutaneous approach (from the femoral, brachial, or radial artery), leaving the choice of access site up to physician and patient. Data from the Society for Cardiac Angiography and Intervention in 1990 (17) show the percutaneous femoral approach was used in 83% of cases, with further increase in that percentage over the subsequent years. The brachial cutdown approach (Chapter 5) has decreased, but the percutaneous radial approach (Chapter 4) entry may offer a selective advantage in patients with severe peripheral vascular disease or known abdominal aortic aneurysm. It also allows immediate postprocedure ambulation. Regardless of the approach, however, it is important for the catheterization team to meet the patient before the actual procedure to evaluate the best access site, to gain an appreciation of the clinical questions that need to be answered by coronary angiography, to uncover any history of adverse reaction to medications or organic iodine compounds, and to explain the procedure and its risks in detail.

Coronary angiography was traditionally performed with hospitalization on the night after the procedure and sometimes the night prior to the scheduled procedure as well. In contrast, most patients now come in on the morning of their scheduled procedure, with no oral intake (except for medications and limited quantities of clear liquid) for 6 to 8 hours before catheterization. A preprocedure workup has usually been done on an outpatient basis some days before. A mild sedative premedication (such as diazepam, 5 to 10 mg orally) may be given prior to the procedure, or intravenous conscious sedation may be administered as needed during the procedure itself. Outpatient coronary angiography for low- to moderate-risk patients began in the 1990s (2,18–21), and continues as the dominant practice. However, patients who have undergone a coronary intervention, those with major comorbidities (e.g., heart failure, valve disease, renal insufficiency, peripheral vascular disease), those who live more than a 1-hour drive from the cardiac catheterization facility, or those who have sustained a procedural complication are expected to stay overnight in the hospital following a diagnostic coronary angiogram. If the angiogram shows significant disease and PCI is appropriate, this may be done during the same procedure followed by an overnight hospital stay. Patients needing revascularization but not found to be suitable for PCI at the time of coronary angiography may go for a bypass surgical operation within 24 to 48 hours or may be discharged home to return for surgery, depending on clinical acuity and availability of surgical time. At least 2 hours of bed rest is required after a percutaneous femoral procedure unless a puncture sealing device is used (see Chapter 4) to allow earlier ambulation and discharge.

THE FEMORAL APPROACH

As described in Chapter 4, the femoral approach to left heart catheterization involves insertion of the catheter either directly over a guidewire or through an introducing sheath. Systemic anticoagulation (heparin, 3,000 to 5,000 units at the time of sheath introduction) is used in some laboratories (2), although others now omit heparin in brief diagnostic procedures. A series of preformed catheters are used, starting with a pigtail catheter for left ventriculography followed by separate catheters (either Judkins or Amplatz shapes) for cannulation of the left and right coronary arteries and any surgical bypass grafts. Coronary catheters are available in 5F, 6F, 7F, or 8F end-hole designs that may taper further near the tip. They may be constructed of either polyethylene (Cook Inc, Bloomington, IN) or polyurethane (Cordis, Miami, FL; and USCI, Billerica, MA) and contain either steel braid, nylon, or other reinforcing materials (Kevlar, carbon fiber) within the catheter wall to provide the excellent torque control needed for coronary cannulation. Current catheters may have a soft distal tip to minimize the risk of arterial dissection. In the 1970s, 8F catheters predominated because they provided excellent torque control and permitted rapid contrast delivery. In the 1980s, improvements in the design of 7F catheters allowed for a lumen diameter comparable to that in standard 8F catheters, making them the standard in most laboratories. Smaller (6F and even 5F) coronary angiographic catheters are now available that use technology similar to that used in guiding catheters to provide thinner catheter walls and larger lumens (6F lumens up to

0.064 inches), exceeding the lumen size once available in 8F diagnostic catheters (22). We now use such 6F catheters for all of our routine diagnostic procedures. Some of the catheters used for native coronary injection via the femoral or brachial approach are shown in Fig. 11.1.

Insertion and Flushing of the Coronary Catheter

The desired catheter is inserted into the femoral sheath and advanced to the level of the left mainstem bronchus over the guidewire. Alternatively, some operators prefer to advance the tip of the coronary angiography catheter around the arch and into the ascending aorta before the guidewire is removed. Although this may reduce snagging of the catheter tip on aortic wall plaques and irregularities, it places greater emphasis on the precision of initial catheter flushing. After removal of the guidewire, the catheter is attached to a specially designed manifold system that permits the maintenance of a closed system during pressure monitoring, catheter flushing, and contrast agent administration (Fig. 11.2). The catheter is immediately double-flushed—blood is withdrawn and discarded, after which heparinized saline flush is injected through the catheter lumen. Difficulty in blood withdrawal suggests apposition of the catheter tip to the aortic wall, which can be rectified by slight withdrawal or rotation of

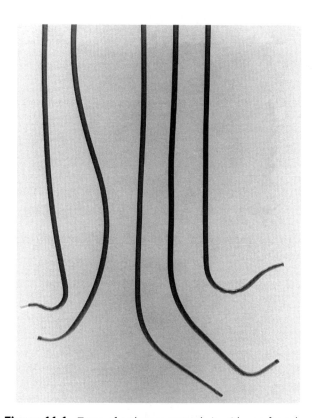

Figure 11.1 Types of catheters currently in wide use for selective native coronary angiography. **Left to right.** Amplatz right, Judkins right, Sones, Judkins left, and Amplatz left.

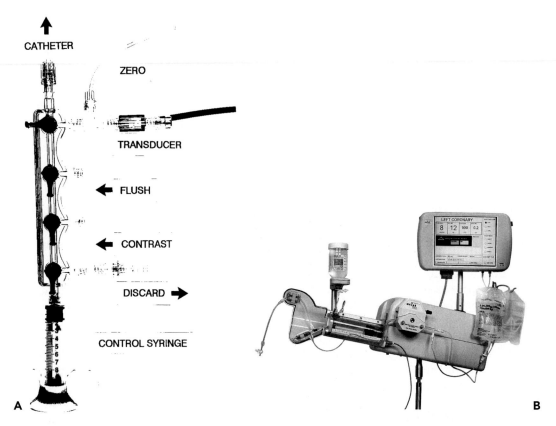

Figure 11.2 **A.** Four-port coronary manifold. This manifold provides a closed system with which blood can be withdrawn from the catheter and discarded. The catheter can be filled with either flush solution or contrast medium, and the catheter pressure can be observed, all under the control of a series of stopcocks. The fourth port is connected to an empty plastic bag and is used as a discard port (for blood from the double flush, air bubbles) so that the syringe need not be disconnected from the manifold at any time during the procedure. Attachment of the transducer directly to the manifold allows optimum pressure waveform fidelity (see Chap. 9), and the fluid-filled reference line allows zeroing of the transducer to midchest level. **B.** The Bracco-Squibb Acist device consists of a contrast filled power injector, controlled by a sterile pneumatic actuator to deliver contrast in amounts and rates up to the limits preprogrammed on the digital panel. A power flushing system and a pressure transducer are also included, duplicating many of the functions of the traditional four-port manifold.

the catheter until free blood aspiration is possible. The lumen of the introducing sheath should also be flushed immediately before and after each catheter insertion and every 5 minutes thereafter to prevent the encroachment of blood into the sheath. Alternatively, the side arm of the sheath may be connected to a 30 mL/hour continuous flow regulator (Intraflo II).

Once the catheter has been flushed with saline solution, tip pressure should be displayed on the physiologic monitor at all times (except during actual contrast injections). Recording this baseline pressure before contrast administration serves as an important baseline reference point. Next, the catheter lumen should be gently filled with contrast agent under fluoroscopic visualization, avoiding selective contrast administration into small branches such as the lumbar arteries if filling is performed in the descending aorta. Filling with contrast results in slight attenuation of high-frequency components in the aortic pressure waveform, whose new shape should be carefully

noted. Any subsequent alteration in that waveform during coronary angiography (see damping and ventricularization, below) may signify an ostial coronary stenosis or an unfavorable catheter position within the coronary artery. Once these measures are completed, the coronary angiographic catheter is advanced into the aortic root in preparation for selective engagement of the desired coronary ostium.

Damping and Ventricularization of the Pressure Waveform

A fall in overall catheter tip pressure (damping) or a fall in diastolic pressure only (ventricularization, Fig. 11.3) during catheter engagement in a coronary ostium indicates obstruction of the catheter tip or interference with coronary inflow. The catheter tip may have been inserted across a proximal coronary stenosis or may have an adverse catheter lie that places it against the coronary wall. If either

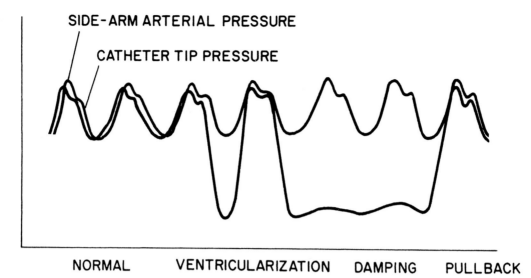

SIDE-ARM ARTERIAL PRESSURE

CATHETER TIP PRESSURE

NORMAL   VENTRICULARIZATION   DAMPING   PULLBACK

Figure 11.3 Pressure tracings as recorded during coronary angiography. Except for its earlier phase and slightly lower systolic pressure, catheter tip pressure should resemble the pressure waveform simultaneously monitored by way of the femoral side-arm sheath or other arterial monitor (e.g., radial artery). In the presence of an ostial stenosis or an unfavorable catheter position against the vessel wall, the waveform shows either ventricularization (in which systolic pressure is preserved but diastolic pressure is reduced) or frank damping (in which both systolic and diastolic pressures are reduced). In either case, the best approach is to withdraw the catheter immediately until the waveform returns to normal and to attempt to define the cause of the problem by nonselective injections in the sinus of Valsalva. Alternatively, a catheter equipped with side holes near the tip may be used to provide ongoing coronary perfusion.

of these phenomena is observed, the catheter should be withdrawn into the aortic root immediately until the operator can analyze the situation further. The catheter may be re-engaged and a cautious small-volume contrast injection made to further clarify the situation. This may disclose a proximal occlusion of the vessel, against which the tip of the coronary catheter is resting, in which case a cine run should be performed to document this finding. The test injection may also indicate ostial stenosis with absent reflux into the aortic root or retention of the injected contrast in the proximal and mid vessel. Lack of reflux indicates that the catheter tip is severely restricting or occluding ostial inflow and mandates that only a gentle injection be performed followed by immediate removal of the catheter at the end of the cine run to restore antegrade flow. Actually, continuing to inject and film as the catheter is removed from the ostium may capture the few frames that show the ostial lesion clearly.

Another approach to evaluating such ostial lesions is to perform a nonselective injection into the sinus of Valsalva in an appropriate view (that displays the ostium of the vessel in question with no overlap by the sinus of Valsalva). Or the standard end-hole diagnostic catheter may be exchanged for an end- and side-hole angioplasty guiding catheter to overcome damping by preserving antegrade flow into the side holes, through the lumen of the catheter, and into the coronary artery, even though the catheter tip may be obstructing entry of blood into the ostium itself (see discussion of cannulation of the right coronary ostium,

below). Vigorous injection despite a damped or ventricularized pressure waveform should be avoided, however, since it predisposes to ventricular fibrillation or dissection of the proximal coronary artery with major ischemic sequelae. Such a dissection is manifest by tracking of contrast down the vessel over the course of the injection and failure of contrast to clear on fluoroscopy after the injection is terminated. Prompt consideration of repair by catheter-based intervention or bypass surgery should be considered if creation of such a dye stain is associated with impeded antegrade coronary flow and signs of myocardial ischemia.

Cannulation of the Left Coronary Ostium

Engagement of the left coronary ostium is usually quite easy with the Judkins technique. As Judkins himself has stated, "No points are earned for coronary catheterization—the catheters know where to go if not thwarted by the operator" (23). If a left Judkins catheter with a 4-cm curve (commonly referred to as a JL4) is simply allowed to remain en face as it is advanced down into the aortic root, it will engage the left coronary ostium without further manipulation in 80 to 90% of patients (Fig. 11.4). Engagement should take place with the arm of the catheter traversing the ascending aorta at an angle of approximately 45°, the tip of the catheter in a more or less horizontal orientation, and with no change in the pressure waveform recorded from the catheter tip.

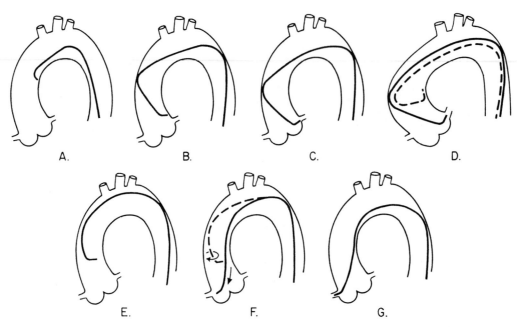

Figure 11.4 Judkins technique for catheterization of the left and right coronary arteries as viewed in the left anterior oblique (LAO) projection. In a patient with a normal-size aortic arch, simple advancement of the JL4 catheter leads to intubation of the left coronary ostium **(A–C)**. In a patient with an enlarged aortic root **(D)**, the arm of the JL4 may be too short, causing the catheter tip to point upward or even flip back into its packaged shape (dotted catheter). A catheter with an appropriately longer arm (a JL5 or JL6) is required. To catheterize the right coronary ostium, the right Judkins catheter is advanced around the aortic arch with its tip directed leftward, as viewed in the LAO projection, until it reaches a position 2 to 3 cm above the level of the left coronary ostium **(E)**. Clockwise rotation causes the catheter tip to drop into the aortic root and point anteriorly **(F)**. Slight further rotation causes the catheter tip to enter the right coronary ostium **(G)**.

In patients with a widened aortic root owing to aortic valve disease or long-standing hypertension, the 4-cm left Judkins curve may be too short to allow successful engagement: The catheter arm may lie nearly horizontally across the aortic root with the tip pointing vertically against the roof of the left main artery, or the catheter may even refold into its packaged shape during advancement into the aortic root (Fig. 11.4D). In this case, a left Judkins catheter with a larger (JL4.5, JL5, or even JL6) curve should be selected. In the long run, changing to a larger catheter under these circumstances may end up saving time compared with trying to make an unsuitable catheter work.

In the occasional patient with a short or narrow aortic root (usually a younger female, particularly if of short stature), even the 4-cm Judkins curve may be too long. When brought down into the aortic root, the catheter arm may lie nearly vertically with the tip pointing downward below the left coronary ostium. The left ostium may still be engaged despite this somewhat unfavorable situation by pushing the catheter down into the left sinus of Valsalva for approximately 10 seconds to tighten the tip angle and then withdrawing the catheter slowly. Having the patient take a deep breath during this maneuver also helps by pulling the heart into a more vertical position to assist in engagement of the left ostium. The most satisfactory approach, however, is to exchange for a JL3.5 catheter with a shorter curve.

On rare occasions, the left coronary ostium lies out of plane (typically high and posterior), as seen in the right anterior oblique (RAO) projection where the ostium is seen to be posterior to the catheter tip. In this case, limited counterclockwise rotation of the left Judkins catheter may help orient the catheter's tip posteriorly and facilitate engagement. Too much rotation of this catheter, however, may result in a refolded catheter that requires guidewire reinsertion to straighten. In that case, it may be helpful to step up to the next larger Judkins curve. Alternately, some operators prefer to switch to a left Amplatz shape (Fig. 11.1; (available in progressively larger curves—1, 2, 3, 4). Amplatz catheters (24) are more tolerant of rotational maneuvering and allow easy engagement of left coronary ostia that lie out of the conventional Judkins plane, as well as subselective engagement of the left anterior descending and circumflex coronary arteries in patients with short left main coronary segments or separate left coronary ostia. The left Amplatz is advanced around the arch oriented toward the left coronary ostium (Fig. 11.5). The tip of the catheter usually comes to rest in the sinus of Valsalva below the coronary ostium. As the catheter is advanced farther, however, the Amplatz shape causes the tip of the catheter to ride up the wall of the sinus until it engages the ostium. At that point,

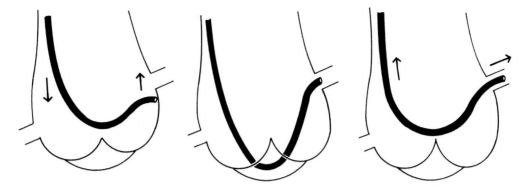

Figure 11.5 Catheterization of the left coronary with an Amplatz catheter. The catheter should be advanced into the ascending aorta with its tip pointing downward so that the terminal catheter configuration resembles a diving duck. As the Amplatz catheter is advanced into the left sinus of Valsalva, its tip initially lies below the left coronary ostium **(left).** Further advancement causes the tip to ride up the aortic wall and enter the ostium **(center).** Slight withdrawal of the catheter causes the tip to seat more deeply in the ostium **(right).**

slight withdrawal of the catheter causes deeper engagement of the coronary ostium, whereas further slight advancement causes paradoxic retraction of the catheter tip.

Cannulation of the Right Coronary Ostium

The Judkins technique for engaging the right coronary ostium requires slightly more catheter manipulation than cannulation of the left coronary ostium (16,23). After being flushed and filled with contrast in the descending aorta (with the catheter tip directed anteriorly to avoid injection into the intercostal arteries), the right Judkins catheter with a 4-cm curve (JR4) is brought around the aortic arch with the tip facing inward until it comes to lie against the right side of the aortic root with its tip aimed toward the left coronary ostium (Fig. 11.4). In a left anterior oblique (LAO) projection, the operator slowly and carefully rotates the catheter clockwise by nearly 180° to engage the right coronary artery. The tip of the right Judkins catheter tends to drop more deeply into the aortic root when the catheter is rotated, as the tertiary curve of the right Judkins shape aligns with the top of the aortic arch. To compensate for this effect, the operator must either begin the rotational maneuver with the tip 2 to 3 cm above the coronary ostium or withdraw the catheter slowly during rotation. Care must be taken to avoid overrotation of the catheter, which tends to cause the catheter tip to engage too deeply into the right coronary artery. To avoid this common technical error, the operator should be prepared to apply a small amount of counterclockwise torque immediately as the tip of the catheter enters the ostium. Catheters with smaller (3.5-cm) or larger (5- or 6-cm) Judkins curves or right Amplatz catheters (AR1 or AR2) may be of value if aortic root configuration and proximal right coronary anatomy make engagement difficult.

Sometimes, the right coronary ostium lies high and anterior above the commissure of the left and right aortic

valve leaflets rather than in the middle of the right sinus. If it has not been possible to engage the right coronary with the approach described above, a nonselective injection should be performed into the right sinus of Valsalva. This will show the high-anterior origin and trigger a change to a left Amplatz (either AL0.75 or AL1) as required to make contact with the aortic wall at that ostium location.

Damping and ventricularization are far more common in the right coronary artery than in the left. The cause may be (a) the generally smaller caliber of the vessel (particularly in nondominant vessels; see below), (b) ostial spasm around the catheter tip, (c) selective engagement of the conus branch, or (d) true ostial stenosis. These problems in right coronary engagement can usually be elucidated by nonselective injections into the right sinus of Valsalva or cautious injections in the damped position with immediate postinjection withdrawal of the catheter. As mentioned above, a 6 or 7F angioplasty guiding catheter with side holes near the tip may be used to allow uninterrupted coronary perfusion between contrast injections, if necessitated by true ostial or proximal right coronary disease.

Cannulation of Saphenous Vein and Free Arterial Grafts

Despite the high initial rate of anginal relief following bypass surgery, 3 to 12% of saphenous vein grafts occlude within the first month. Additional veins occlude between 1 month and 1 year after surgery due to exaggerated neointimal hyperplasia. By far the dominant failure mode of saphenous vein graft failure beyond 1 year, however, is diffuse graft atherosclerosis, which accounts for a 50% graft closure rate by 7 years (25). Free arterial grafts (free radial or free internal mammary) are sometimes used instead of saphenous vein grafts, and these have an intermediate long-term patency between that of saphenous vein grafts and pedicled internal mammary grafts (see next page). An increasing number of patients thus develop recurrent angina after prior bypass surgery owing to vein graft or progressive native vessel disease, and these patients account for more than 20% of the diagnostic procedures in our laboratory.

The proximal anastomosis of a vein graft or free arterial graft is usually placed on the right or left anterior aortic surface, several centimeters above the sinuses of Valsalva. Because many surgeons still resist the practice of placing radiopaque markers on the proximal graft (26), the operator must generally rely on the surgeon's operative report or diagram, as well as knowledge of usual surgical practice in her or his own institution. The operative report always should be obtained before elective angiography on any patient with prior bypass surgery, but is absolutely essential on patients who underwent their operation at another medical center (where local preference may include practices like proximal anastomosis to the right posterior surface of the aorta, see below), or even proximal anastomosis to the descending aorta in patients with aortic root disease. It may thus be quite frustrating to embark on coronary angiography in a patient with prior bypass surgery without a detailed graft map, operative note, or prior detailed catheterization report/films in hand.

Most commonly, grafts to the left coronary arise from the left anterior surface of the aorta, with grafts to the circumflex system usually placed somewhat higher on the aorta than those to the left anterior descending or diagonal branches. Alternatively, some surgeons prefer to route grafts to the circumflex through the transverse sinus behind the heart, in which case the circumflex graft may originate from the posterior surface of the aorta. Grafts to the right coronary (or the distal portions of a dominant circumflex) usually originate from the right anterior surface of the aorta, above and somewhat behind the plane of the native right coronary ostium. We generally use the right Judkins (JR4) or Amplatz (AL1) catheter to engage anterior (i.e., left) coronary grafts. Special left coronary bypass, internal mammary, or hockey stick catheters may be required for left grafts that originate with an upward trajectory (Fig. 11.6). For downward-pointing right coronary grafts, we prefer a soft catheter with no primary curve (a multipurpose, Wexler, or JR3.5 short-tip catheter), which provides better alignment with the proximal portion of the graft and thus better opacification. The Wexler catheter can also be used for grafts originating from the left or posterior surface of the aorta. Since its tip remains in contact with the aortic wall, the shaft of this catheter can be rotated or the tip can be flexed to bring it into alignment with the proximal graft once the ostium has been engaged.

If no markers have been provided, the catheter tip should be oriented against the appropriate aortic wall and slowly advanced and then withdrawn until its tip catches in a graft ostium. The graft is injected in multiple projections that show its origin, shaft, distal anastomosis, and the native vessels beyond the anastomosis. This process must then be repeated until all graft sites have been identified.

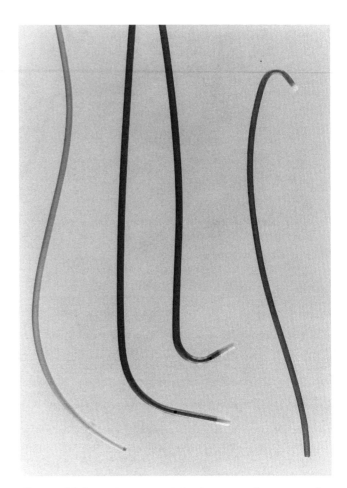

Figure 11.6 Catheters used for bypass graft angiography. Although the right Judkins or Amplatz catheters can be used for many anterior takeoff vein grafts, the catheters shown here may be useful. **Left to right.** Wexler, multipurpose, hockey stick shape, and internal mammary.

Grafts should not be written off as occluded unless a clear stump is demonstrated. If the myocardial territory supplied by a graft assumed to be occluded is still contracting, and there is no evident native or collateral blood supply to that territory, there may be a missed graft—the myocardium cannot function without a visible means of support! In that case, it may be valuable to perform an aortogram in an appropriate view to try to demonstrate flow in and locate the origin of such a missed graft. The emergence of effective therapies for focal lesions in vein grafts has placed a premium on being able to find and fix such diseased grafts before they occlude (Fig. 11.7; see Chapters 23 to 25).

Internal Mammary Cannulation

Based on their superior demonstrated 10-year patency, the pedicled left and right internal mammary arteries (IMAs, also known as internal thoracic arteries [ITAs]) have become the conduits of choice. The proximal end of this graft remains attached to the subclavian artery (supplying

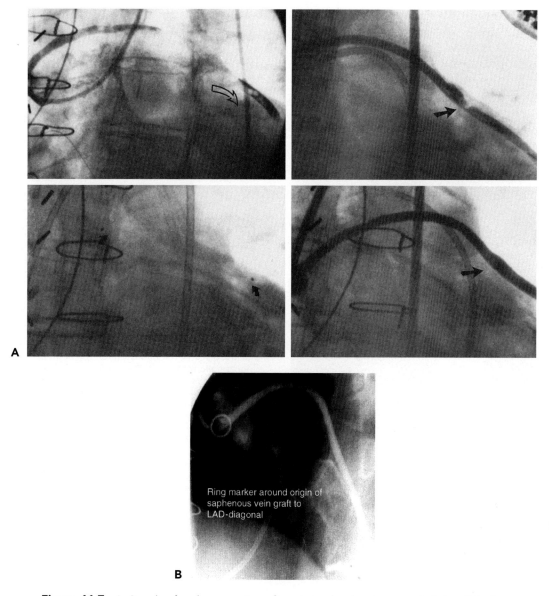

Figure 11.7 **A.** Sample of saphenous vein graft angiography, showing an occluded graft to the circumflex, filled with thrombus **(top left, *open arrow*)**. A drug-infusion catheter (Tracker, Target Therapeutics) was placed **(bottom left, *curved arrow*)** and used to administer Urokinase (50,000 IU/hour) overnight. The following morning **(top right)**, the thrombus had been dissolved, revealing the underlying ulcerated culprit lesion. This was treated with a single Palmaz-Schatz coronary stent **(bottom right),** re-establishing full patency. **B.** Saphenous vein graft with origin localized by ring marker implanted at the time of surgery.

the nutritional needs of the graft itself), as the vessel is freed up from its lower sternal attachments and anastomosed to the target coronary artery (usually the left anterior descending). More than 90% of current elective bypass procedures involve placement of at least one internal mammary graft.

Successful cannulation (27) requires knowledge of the left subclavian and brachiocephalic trunk as well as the right subclavian arteries, as shown in. Fig. 11.8A. It is also important to understand some of the common anatomic variants in the internal mammary artery,

including more proximal origin in the vertical portion of the subclavian, or origin as a common vessel with the thyrocervical trunk.

Although uncommon, these grafts can develop significant lesions, making it important to evaluate such grafts during any postbypass catheterization. In patients with early recurrence of angina (within the first 6 months after surgery), the most common lesion is located at the distal mammary-coronary anastomosis. It is usually due to local intimal hyperplasia rather than atherosclerosis and responds well to balloon angioplasty (see Chapter 22).

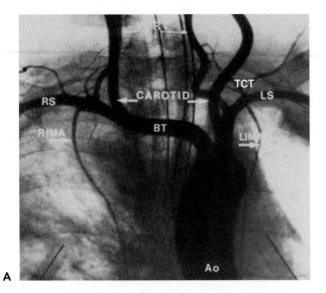

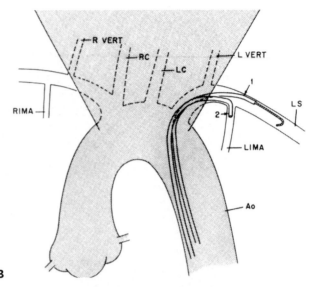

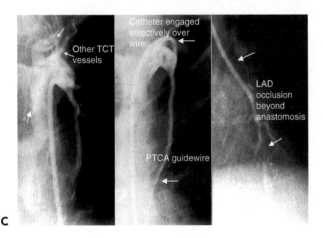

Figure 11.8 Internal mammary angiography. **A.** Aortic arch injection shows the left internal mammary artery (LIMA) originating from the left subclavian (LS), just opposite the thyrocervical trunk (TCT) and distal to the right vertebral artery (VERT). The right internal mammary artery (RIMA) originates from the right subclavian (RS) just distal to the bifurcation of the right carotid from the brachiocephalic trunk (BT). **B.** Schematic diagram shows the corresponding arch vessel origins. Note that the left subclavian originates just inside the patient's leftmost edge of the wedge-shaped shadow cast by the upper-mediastinal structures in the left anterior oblique projection. Catheter manipulation in this projection facilitates advancement of a guidewire into the LS (step 1), facilitating selective cannulation of the LIMA during catheter withdrawal and slight counterclockwise rotation (step 2, see text). **C.** Variant in which internal mammary originates in common with thyrocervical trunk, resulting in poor opacification. An angioplasty guide wire was placed down the internal mammary through the 6F diagnostic catheter and used to advance the tip of the diagnostic catheter selectively down the IMA. From that position, sufficient opacification was obtained to demonstrate occlusion of the distal left anterior descending (LAD) beyond the anastomosis as the cause of the patient's recurrent angina.

Flow-limiting kinks may also be present in the midgraft, and ostial lesions at the origin of the internal mammary from the subclavian may also occur. In patients years postbypass, significant lesions may develop in the native coronary artery beyond the internal mammary touchdown. In addition to establishing the patency of the internal mammary itself, it may also be important to look for large nonligated side branches that may divert flow from the coronary circulation and whose occlusion (in the occasional patient) may be required for angina relief (28). It is also important to look for stenoses in the subclavian artery before the takeoff of the internal mammary that may compromise the inflow to the graft and thereby cause myocardial ischemia (Fig. 11.9). Such lesions may require construction of a carotid-to-subclavian graft, or more commonly stent placement (29) to restore normal flow to the internal mammary and vertebral branches of the subclavian artery (see Chapters 14 and 26).

Although mammary grafts can be studied easily from the ipsilateral brachial approach, we prefer the femoral approach using a soft-tip preformed internal mammary catheter, which resembles a right Judkins catheter except for a tighter primary curve. This used to be a time-consuming (up to 20 minutes for some operators) process, but has been reduced to less than 3 minutes in our laboratory by adoption of a systematic strategy (see Fig. 11.8B; 27). In the LAO projection, cannulation of the left internal mammary artery begins by advancement of this catheter into the aortic arch until it lies just inside the left edge of the wedgelike density formed by the shadow of the upper mediastinum against the lung fields. With 1 to 2 cm of J guidewire protruding from its tip, the mammary catheter is rotated counterclockwise until it falls into the subclavian artery origin. From there, the wire can be advanced well out into the axillary artery. The mammary catheter is then advanced over the wire, into the midsubclavian, where the guidewire is then removed and the catheter is flushed and filled with

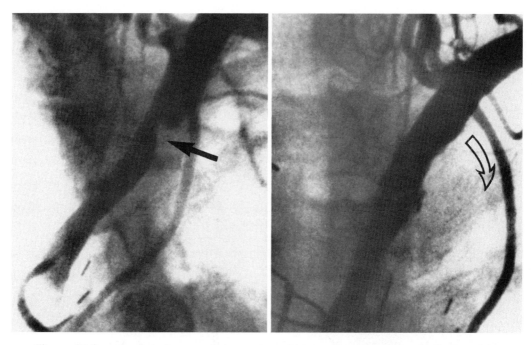

Figure 11.9 Left subclavian stenosis in a patient with recurrent angina in the distribution of the otherwise patent left internal mammary artery **(left)**, treated by stenting **(right)**.

contrast. A low-osmolar contrast agent should be used to avoid causing CNS toxicity by reflux of hyperosmolar ionic contrast up the vertebral arteries. Switching to the straight AP projection, the catheter is rotated counterclockwise slightly (to make the tip point slightly anteriorly) as it is withdrawn slowly until the internal mammary is engaged. Intermittent gentle puffs of contrast will help localize the mammary origin during this withdrawal. Great care should be taken to avoid catheter tip trauma/dissection of the relatively delicate mammary vessel.

If selective cannulation is difficult because of tortuosity or anatomic variations, a variety of superselective or nonselective techniques can be used to permit angiographic evaluation. Nonselective injections into the subclavian will generally allow adequate opacification to see that the internal mammary is open, but generally not to provide detailed information about the distal native vessel. Inflation of a blood pressure cuff on the ipsilateral arm may help reduce runoff through the axillary artery and improve opacification of the internal mammary in cases where selective cannulation is difficult. When selective cannulation proves difficult, we sometimes attach a Y connector to the hub of the diagnostic internal mammary catheter and advance a 0.014 soft-tipped coronary angioplasty guidewire into the mammary to serve as a support for catheter advancement.

Cannulation of the right internal mammary artery may be slightly more difficult because of the need to avoid the right carotid before entering the right subclavian itself. Again in the LAO projection, the upper mediastinal wedge is identified. The mammary catheter with protruding J wire is taken to the right edge of this shadow and rotated coun-

terclockwise until it falls into the brachiocephalic trunk. The wire is then advanced toward the right subclavian artery. Predilection for the wire to advance into the right carotid artery may require removing the guidewire and performing a nonselective contrast injection in the brachiocephalic trunk to identify the origin of the subclavian branch. The RAO-caudal projection often gives the best spatial resolution of the right carotid and right subclavian origins, after which steerable Wholey guidewire (Mallinckrodt) can be used to cannulate the subclavian. Once the wire is firmly out of the subclavian artery, the mammary catheter is advanced as described above. For cannulation of the right internal mammary artery, however, the catheter is rotated slightly clockwise during withdrawal to point its tip anteriorly.

Gastroepiploic Graft Cannulation

Taken together, the left and right internal mammary arteries can be used to revascularize most lesions in the left anterior descending, proximal circumflex, and proximal right coronary arteries. Even with sequential distal anastomoses, however, the fact that there are only two internal mammary arteries means that most revascularization procedures still suffer the long-term limitations associated with the use of saphenous veins. Free segments of radial artery have also been used as bypass conduits, either from the ascending aorta (like a saphenous vein) or from the descending thoracic aorta (30) in some patients undergoing repeat bypass surgery. Although the radial artery may have slight benefit over the saphenous vein, it is prone to

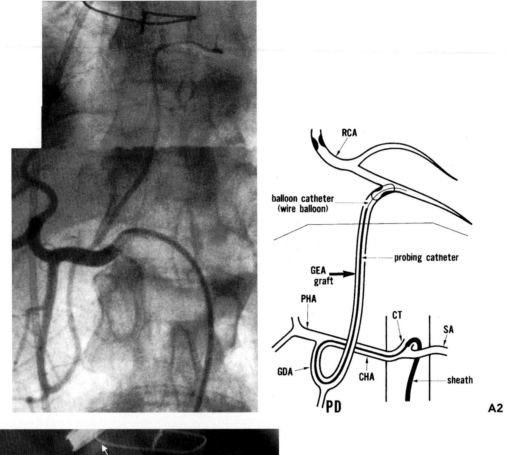

A1   A2

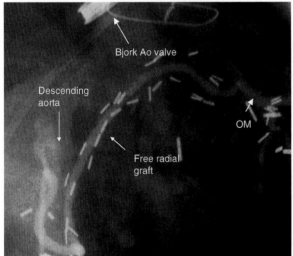

B

Figure 11.10   A. Gastroepiploic graft anatomy. The common hepatic artery (CHA) originates with the splenic artery (SA) from the celiac trunk (CT). The gastroduodenal artery (GDA) originates from the CHA, which then becomes the proper hepatic artery (PHA). The terminal branches of the GDA are the pancreatoduodenal (PD) and the right gastroepiploic artery (GEA), shown here undergoing angioplasty of a lesion at its anastomosis to the right coronary artery (RCA). (Diagram from Ishiki T, et al. Percutaneous angioplasty of stenosed gastroepiploic artery grafts. *J Am Coll Cardiol* 1993,21:727, 1993, with permission.) **B.** Free radial graft from the descending aorta to an obtuse marginal graft, cannulated using a Cobra visceral angiographic catheter. Localization of the graft ostium was aided by the presence of multiple surgical clips used to ligate small side branches of the radial artery at the time of bypass.

spasm in the early postop period, and does not match the long-term patency record of the internal mammary artery (because it does not retain its blood supply and innervation when used as a free graft). The effort to perform all arterial bypass has brought back the right gastroepiploic artery (as an arterial pedicle graft) for anastomosis to the posterior descending or other vessels on the inferior surface of the heart (31,32). The right gastroepiploic normally supplies most of the greater curvature of the stomach, but can be dissected free from that organ and tunneled through the diaphragm to reach the inferior wall of the heart. Angiography of this vessel is possible using standard visceral angiographic catheters (e.g., Cobra) which are designed to enter visceral arteries such as the celiac axis (33). From there, the catheter can be advanced into the common hepatic (as opposed to the splenic) artery and then turned downward into the gastroduodenal artery (Fig. 11.10). A 0.025-inch Glidewire (Terumo) can then be used to cannulate the right gastroepiploic (as opposed to the superior pancreatoduodenal artery) if more selective injection is desired.

THE BRACHIAL OR RADIAL APPROACH

The technique of brachial artery cutdown was the first approach used for selective coronary angiography, as described in Chapter 5. Dr. F. Mason Sones, Jr., designed the original catheter for this approach—a thin-walled radiopaque woven Dacron catheter with a 2.67-mm (8F) shaft diameter (16,34), tapering to 5F external diameter at a point 5 cm from its tip. In addition to the open tip, current models include side holes that are arranged in opposed pairs within 7 mm of the distal end. As Sones stated, this provides a "flexible finger" that may be curved upward into the coronary orifices by pressure of the more rigid shaft against the aortic valve cusps. This enables the Sones catheter to be used for cannulation of both the left and right coronary arteries, as well as entry into the left ventricle for ventriculography. The standard Sones catheter is available in lengths of 80, 100, and 125 cm and 6 to 8F diameters. Most operators now use a different Sones-type coronary catheter constructed of polyurethane and made by Cordis Corporation. This catheter traverses a tortuous subclavian system with much greater facility and smoothness than does the woven Dacron catheter, and its enhanced torque control and reduced coefficient of friction ease engagement of the coronary ostia. See Fig. 11.1 for a variety of preshaped coronary catheters, which are also effective from the brachial approach (35). In general, similar techniques apply for use of standard Judkins and Amplatz shapes from the left brachial or radial arteries, as described above for the femoral approach. From the right brachial or radial arteries, smaller left Judkins curves or special catheter shapes are preferable (see Chapter 4).

When the Sones method is used from the right arm, catheter tip pressure should be monitored continuously once the catheter enters the brachial artery. Further passage of the catheter into the subclavian and brachiocephalic arteries should be accomplished under both pressure monitoring and fluoroscopic visualization. Occasionally, it may be difficult to pass the catheter from the subclavian artery to the aortic arch, but a simple maneuver by the patient—such as a deep inspiration, shrugging the shoulders, or turning the head to the left—often facilitates passage of the catheter into the ascending aorta. If passage of the catheter from the subclavian artery to the ascending aorta is not accomplished immediately and with complete ease, the operator should stop catheter manipulation and use a soft J-tipped 0.035-inch guidewire. Once the catheter is in the ascending aorta, the guidewire is removed and the catheter is aspirated, flushed, and reconnected to the rotating adapter of the manifold, either directly or by a short length of large-bore flexible connecting tubing.

With the Sones technique, selective engagement of the left coronary artery is accomplished as follows. In a left anterior oblique projection, the sinus of Valsalva containing the ostium of the left coronary artery lies to the left, and the sinus containing the ostium of the right coronary artery lies to the right. The noncoronary sinus lies posteriorly. The operator advances the catheter to the aortic valve and then continues to advance the catheter until its tip bends cephalad and points toward the left coronary ostium. When the catheter is properly positioned with its tip bent cephalad, slightly advancing or rotating the catheter usually results in selective engagement of the left coronary ostium, which is verified by a small injection of radiographic contrast agent. Occasionally, a deep breath taken by the patient will facilitate this selective engagement. Our usual approach, illustrated in the upper left panel of Fig. 11.11, involves forming a smooth shallow loop and gradually inching up to the ostium from below. If the distal 2 to 3 mm of the catheter tip bends downward during this inching up process, the tip may enter the left coronary artery, giving a cobra head appearance (see Fig. 11.11, top right) similar to that achieved with the left Amplatz catheter (see Fig. 11.5). For the high takeoff left coronary ostium, the catheter may have the appearance (as in Fig. 11.11, bottom) in which the catheter tip is lying across the ostium at right angles to the course of the left main coronary artery. During contrast injection in this

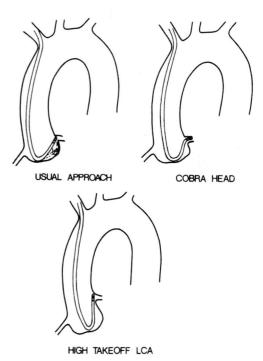

USUAL APPROACH   COBRA HEAD

HIGH TAKEOFF LCA

Figure 11.11 Selective catheterization of the left coronary artery using the Sones catheter. The standard approach involves forming a smooth shallow loop and gradually "inching up" to the ostium from below. If the distal 2 to 3 mm of the catheter tip bends downward during this inching-up process, the tip may enter the left coronary artery, giving a cobra head appearance (upper right). When the left coronary ostium originates high in the left sinus of Valsalva (high takeoff left coronary artery), the catheter may have the appearance seen in the bottom panel, where the tip is lying across the ostium at right angles to the course of the left main coronary artery. During coronary injection in this instance, coronary blood flow usually carries the contrast agent down the vessel, giving good opacification of the entire left coronary artery.

instance, coronary blood flow generally carries the contrast agent down the vessel, giving good opacification of the entire left coronary artery. Once the catheter tip has engaged the coronary ostium and no damping of pressure from the catheter tip is observed, cineangiography may be performed with selective injection of radiopaque material in a variety of views, as described below.

Selective engagement of the right coronary orifice may be accomplished as illustrated in steps 1 to 3 of Fig. 11.12. In the shallow LAO projection, the catheter is curved up toward the left coronary artery (step 1) and clockwise torque is applied. While the operator is gradually applying clockwise torque, a gentle to-and-fro motion of the catheter (the to-and-fro excursions are not more than 5 to 10 mm in length) helps to translate the applied torque to the catheter tip. When the tip starts moving in its clockwise sweep of the anterior wall of the aorta, the operator maintains (but does not increase) a clockwise torque on the catheter and simultaneously pulls the catheter back slightly (step 2, Fig. 11.12) because the right coronary ostium is lower than that of the left coronary artery. At this point, the catheter usually makes an abrupt turn into the right coronary ostium, at which time the operator must release all torque to prevent the catheter tip from continuing its sweep past the ostium. On occasion, the Sones catheter literally leaps into the right coronary artery and will be 4 to 5 cm down its lumen. If this occurs, the catheter should be gently withdrawn until its tip is stable just within the ostium.

Another technique for catheterizing the right coronary artery involves a more direct approach by way of the right coronary cusp. With the catheter in the right sinus, the operator should make a small curve on the tip, directed right-ward. A small dose of contrast material in the right sinus of Valsalva will allow visualization of the right coronary orifice and thus facilitate selective engagement. Occasionally, a deep inspiration by the patient accompanied by gentle advancement of the catheter to the right of the aortic root results in selective engagement of the right coronary artery.

ADVERSE EFFECTS OF CORONARY ANGIOGRAPHY

Once the coronary vessels have been engaged, optimal selective angiography requires transient but nearly complete replacement of blood flow with the radiopaque contrast agent. A wide variety of iodine-containing agents are currently used for coronary angiography and have already been discussed in greater detail in Chapter 2. Older high-osmolar contrast agent had a number of potentially deleterious effects during coronary injection (see Chapters 2 and 3) that include the following: (a) transient (10- to 20-second) hemodynamic depression marked by arterial hypotension and elevation of the left ventricular end diastolic pressure, (b) electrocardiographic effects with T-wave inversion or peaking in the inferior leads (during right and left coronary injection, respectively), sinus slowing or arrest, and prolongation of the PR, QRS, and QT intervals (36,37), (c) significant arrhythmia (asystole or ventricular tachycardia/fibrillation) (38), (d) myocardial ischemia owing to interruption of oxygen delivery or inappropriate arteriolar vasodilatation (coronary "steal"), (e) allergic reaction (39), and (f) cumulative renal toxicity (40). Some (but not all) of these adverse effects are eliminated by use of a low-osmolar contrast agent, albeit at a modest increased expense (41).

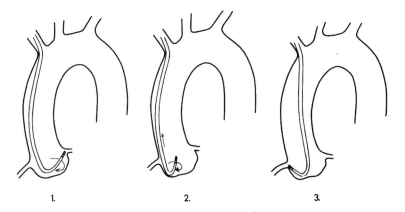

Figure 11.12 Selective catheterization of the right coronary artery using the Sones catheter. In the shallow left anterior oblique (LAO) projection, the catheter is curved upward and to the left **(1)** and clockwise torque is applied. While the operator is gradually applying clockwise torque, a gentle to-and-fro motion of the catheter helps to translate the applied torque to the catheter tip. When the tip starts moving in its clockwise sweep of the anterior wall of the aorta, the operator maintains (but does not increase) a clockwise torque tension on the catheter and simultaneously pulls the catheter back slightly **(2)**, because the right coronary ostium is lower than that of the left coronary artery. At this point, the catheter usually makes an abrupt leap into the right coronary ostium **(3)**, at which time the operator must release all torque to prevent the catheter tip from continuing its sweep and passing by the ostium. See text for details and alternative methods.

Although newer low-osmolar contrast agents have less prominent side effects, patients undergoing coronary angiography should always be monitored continuously in terms of clinical status, surface electrocardiogram, and arterial pressure from the catheter tip. In patients with baseline left ventricular dysfunction or marked ischemic instability, we also like to perform a right heart catheterization, and display pulmonary artery pressure continuously on the same scale as the arterial pressure as an early indicator of procedural problems or progressive decompensation. A significant rise in pulmonary artery mean or diastolic pressure should prompt temporary suspension of angiography and initiation of treatment (e.g., intravenous furosemide, nitroglycerin, nitroprusside) before frank pulmonary edema develops. The venous sheath also provides a ready route for the rapid administration of fluid or medications through its side arm and allows rapid insertion of a temporary pacing electrode if needed. Prophylactic placement of temporary pacing electrodes in patients undergoing coronary angiography is not indicated (42), since most episodes of bradycardia or asystole are brief and are resolved promptly by having the patient give a forceful cough, which elevates central aortic pressure and probably helps wash residual contrast out of the myocardial capillary bed. Similarly, prophylactic drugs are not given routinely to prevent ventricular tachyarrhythmias, although appropriate drugs (lidocaine, amiodarone, atropine, epinephrine, and so on), a defibrillator, and airway management equipment are always kept at the ready and can be brought into play within seconds.

One of the most common adverse effects seen during coronary angiography is the provocation of myocardial ischemia, particularly in patients with unstable angina. In very unstable patients, we modify our usual practice of performing the left ventriculogram before coronary angiography (lest an adverse reaction to the ventriculogram compromise the more crucial coronary study). When myocardial ischemia does occur during coronary angiography, the best course of action is to remove the catheter from the coronary ostium and temporarily suspend injections until angina resolves. If this takes more than 30 seconds, we typically administer nitroglycerin (200 mg bolus, repeated at 30-second intervals up to a total of 1,000 mg) into either the involved coronary artery or the pulmonary artery catheter. If marked arterial hypertension is present and fails to respond to nitroglycerin, we may administer other vasodilators as needed to bring the blood pressure down. In patients with inappropriate tachycardia in the setting of angina and reasonable systolic left ventricular function, intravenous propranolol (1 mg every minute to a total dose of 0.1 to 0.15 mg/kg) or an infusion of a short-acting beta-blocking agent (esmolol) is frequently beneficial. Only rarely (in patients with severe three-vessel and/or left main coronary disease and those whose ischemia is associated with hypotension) is myocardial ischemia severe enough and refractory to the above management program to

prompt placement of an intra-aortic counterpulsation balloon in the contralateral femoral artery before completion of coronary angiography (see Chapter 21). In any patient with prolonged or refractory ischemia during diagnostic coronary angiography, it may be worthwhile to perform limited re-examination of the coronary vessels to determine whether the angiographic procedure has caused a problem (spasm, dissection, thrombosis) that might require immediate treatment with additional vasodilators, coronary intervention, thrombolysis, or emergency bypass surgery.

Severe allergic reactions are uncommon during coronary angiography and are best prevented by 18 to 24 hours of premedication (prednisone 20 to 40 mg and cimetidine 300 mg every 6 hours; 32) and/or use of a nonionic contrast agent in patients with a history of prior allergic reaction to radiographic contrast (41). When a severe unexpected reaction does occur, it usually responds promptly to the intravenous administration of epinephrine (0.1 mg equals 1 mL of the 1:10,000 solution available on most emergency carts, repeated every 2 minutes until the blood pressure and/or wheezing improves). Larger bolus doses of epinephrine are to be avoided, because they may provoke marked tachycardia, hypertension, and arrhythmia.

Renal insufficiency may develop after coronary angiography, particularly in patients who are hypovolemic, who receive large volumes of contrast (more than 3 mL/kg), or who have had prior renal insufficiency, diabetes, or multiple myeloma (33). In these patients, every effort should be made to give adequate hydration preprocedure and postprocedure (see also Chapters 2 and 3). Use of low-osmolar or iso-osmolar contrast agents may be helpful in this situation, but their real benefit remains controversial (41).

INJECTION TECHNIQUE

As mentioned previously, high-quality coronary angiography requires selective injection of radiographic contrast at an adequate rate and volume to transiently replace the blood contained in the involved vessel with slight but continuous reflux into the aortic root. Too timid an injection allows intermittent entry of nonopaque blood into the coronary artery (producing contrast dilution or streaming, which makes interpretation of lesions difficult) and fails to visualize the coronary ostium and proximal coronary branches. However, too vigorous an injection may cause coronary dissection or excessive myocardial blushing, and too prolonged an injection may contribute to increased myocardial depression or bradycardia.

We train our fellows to adjust the rate and duration of manual contrast injection to match the observed filling pattern of the particular vessel being injected. Injection velocity should be built up gradually during the first second until the injection rate is adequate to completely replace antegrade blood flow into the coronary ostium (Fig. 11.13). The associated rate and volume required to

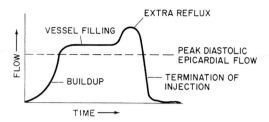

Figure 11.13 Suggested injection pattern for coronary angiography. To appropriately replace antegrade coronary blood flow with contrast medium throughout the cardiac cycle, the operator should build up the velocity of injection over 1 to 2 seconds until no unopacified blood is seen to enter the ostium and there is reflux of contrast medium into the aorta during systole and diastole. This injection is maintained until the entire coronary artery is filled with contrast medium. If the ostium has not been well seen, a brief extra push should be given to cause adequate reflux into the aortic root, and the injection should be terminated. Prolonged held inspiration with some degree of Valsalva maneuver is sometimes used during Sones angiography to reduce coronary flow and make it much easier to replace blood flow during manual contrast injection.

accomplish this goal have been measured (43) and were found to average 7 mL at 2.1 mL/second in the left and 4.8 mL at 1.7 mL/second in the right coronary. In patients with occlusion, much lower rates and volumes are required, and in patients with left ventricular hypertrophy (e.g., aortic stenosis, hypertrophic myopathy) much greater volumes and higher rates of injection may be required.

The injection should be maintained until the entire vessel is opacified. If there is any question about whether the body of the injection has provided adequate reflux to visualize the coronary ostium, an additional burst of contrast (extra reflux) should be given before the injection is terminated. The injection should then be terminated abruptly by turning the manifold stopcock back to monitor pressure, although cine filming should continue until opacification of distal vessels or late-filling branches is complete. The operator should monitor for excessive bradycardia or hypotension, review the video loop, and set up the gantry angles for the next injection. To avoid problems, each injection should begin with a completely full (and bubble-free) injection syringe, held with the handle slightly elevated so that any microbubbles will drift up toward the plunger. The injection syringe should be managed in such a way as to avoid mixtures of blood and contrast, because such mixtures may promote formation of thrombi (particularly when nonionic contrast agents are used).

Although manual contrast injection is the standard technique in coronary angiography, some operators favor use of a power injector (as used in left ventriculography or aortography) to perform coronary injections (44). The injector is preset for a rate to match the involved vessel (2 to 3 mL/second for the right and 3 to 4 mL/second for the left coronary) and activated by a foot switch for a sufficient time to fill the coronary with contrast (generally 2 to 3 seconds). This approach allows a single operator to per-

form injections and move the table and has proved safe in thousands of procedures. A special power injector has also been introduced (Acist, Bracco, Eden Prairie, MN) that can perform such power injections under rate control by finger pressure on a sterile control handle, reverting automatically to pressure monitoring when the injection is terminated. This may be of value when a single operator must perform injections and pan the table during diagnostic coronary angiography.

ANATOMY, ANGIOGRAPHIC VIEWS, AND QUANTITATION OF STENOSIS

Coronary Anatomy

The coronary angiographer must develop a detailed familiarity with normal coronary arterial anatomy and its common variants. For individuals just learning coronary anatomy, the main coronary trunks can be considered to lie in one of two orthogonal planes (Fig. 11.14). The anterior descending and posterior descending coronary arteries lie in the plane of the interventricular septum, whereas the right and circumflex coronary trunks lie in the plane of the atrioventricular valves. In the 60° left anterior oblique (LAO) projection, one is looking down the plane of the interventricular septum, with the plane of the AV valves seen en face; in the 30° right anterior oblique (RAO) projection, one is looking down the plane of the AV valves, with the plane of the interventricular septum seen en face. The major segments and branches have each been assigned a numerical identification in the BARI modification (45) of the CASS nomenclature (Fig. 11.15).

Right-Dominant Circulation

The right coronary artery gives rise to the conus branch (which supplies the right ventricular outflow tract) and one or more acute marginal branches (which supply the free wall of the right ventricle), whether or not the circulation is right dominant. In the 85% of patients who have a right-dominant coronary artery, it goes on to form the AV nodal artery, the posterior descending and the posterolateral left ventricular branches that supply the inferior aspect of the interventricular septum (see Fig. 11.14). The left main trunk branches after a short (but variable) distance into the left anterior descending and the circumflex coronary arteries. The left anterior descending artery gives rise to septal branches that curve down into the interventricular septum, as well as diagonal branches that wrap over the anterolateral free wall of the left ventricle.

Some patients have a twin left anterior descending system, in which one trunk (frequently intramyocardial) supplies the entire septum and the other trunk runs on the surface of the heart supplying all the diagonal branches. The

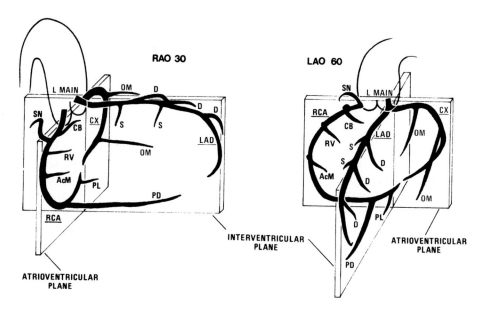

Figure 11.14 Representation of coronary anatomy relative to the interventricular and atrioventricular valve planes. Coronary branches are as indicated—L Main (left main), LAD (left anterior descending), D (diagonal), S (septal), CX (circumflex), OM (obtuse marginal), RCA (right coronary), CB (conus branch), SN (sinus node), AcM (acute marginal), PD (posterior descending), PL (posterolateral left ventricular).

circumflex artery courses clockwise in the AV groove (viewed from the apex) as it gives rise to one or more obtuse marginal branches that supply the lateral free wall of the left ventricle, but does not reach the crux in patients with a right-dominant circulation. In some patients, a large intermedius or ramus medianus branch (neither a diagonal nor a marginal) may originate directly from the left main trunk, bisecting the angle between the left anterior descending and circumflex arteries, to create a trifurcation pattern of the left main coronary artery. Regardless of whether the patient is right or left dominant, the sinus

node originates as a proximal branch of the right coronary in 60% of patients and as a left atrial branch of the circumflex in the remaining 40% of patients.

Left-Dominant Circulation

In 8% of patients, the coronary circulation is left dominant; that is, the posterolateral left ventricular, posterior descending, and AV nodal arteries are all supplied by the terminal portion of the left circumflex coronary artery. In such patients, the right coronary artery is small and supplies only

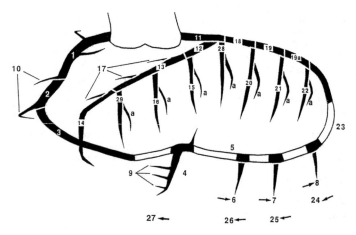

Figure 11.15 The numerical coding system and official names of the coronary segments, as used in the Bypass Angioplasty Revascularization Investigation (BARI) study. Right coronary: 1, proximal; 2, middle; 3, distal; 4, posterior descending; 5, posteroatrioventricular; 6, first posterolateral; 7, second posterolateral; 8, third posterolateral; 9, inferior septals; 10, acute marginals. Left coronary: 11, left main; 12, proximal left anterior descending; 13, middle left anterior descending; 14, distal left anterior descending,;15, first diagonal (a, branch of first diagonal); 16, second diagonal,;17, septals (anterior septals); 18, proximal circumflex; 19, middle circumflex; 19a, distal circumflex; 20, 21, and 22, first, second, and third obtuse marginals; 23, left atrioventricular; 24, 25, and 26, first, second, and third posterolaterals (in left- or balanced-dominant system); 27, left posterior descending (in left-dominant system); 28, ramus (ramus intermedius); 29, third diagonal. (From The BARI Protocol. Protocol for the Bypass Angioplasty Revascularization Investigation. *Circulation* 1991;84:V1, with permission.)

the right atrium and right ventricle. It may be important to visualize, as a potential source of right-to-left collaterals, but the small diameter of a nondominant right coronary artery predisposes it to damping and catheter-induced spasm (see below, which make limited injections advisable.

Balanced-Dominant Circulation

In about 7% of hearts, there is a codominant or balanced system, in which the right coronary artery gives rise to the posterior descending artery and then terminates, and the circumflex artery gives rise to all the posterior left ventricular branches and perhaps also a parallel posterior descending branch that supplies part of the interventricular septum. In some patients, the supply to the inferior wall may be further fractionated among a short posterior descending branch of the right coronary (which supplies the inferobase), branches of the distal circumflex (which supply the midinferior wall), and branches of the acute marginal (which extend to supply the inferoapex).

Anatomic Variants

Although these basic concepts describe the general pattern of the coronary circulation, it must be noted that there is considerable patient-to-patient variability in the size and position of different coronary arterial branches (46). In 1 to 2% of patients, these coronary anatomic features are sufficiently divergent to qualify as coronary anomalies. Every operator must be thoroughly familiar with these anatomic anomalies and continually vigilant for their occurrence, lest failure to recognize an anomaly result in an incomplete and therefore inadequate examination. In a review of 126,595 cases from the Cleveland Clinic (47), the most common of these anomalies was separate ostia of the left anterior descending and left circumflex arteries (0.41%). When separate ostia of the left anterior descending and left circumflex are present, the catheter will generally sit with its tip in the left anterior descending, although there is generally adequate spillover to opacify the circumflex. If not, separate cannulation of the circumflex may be necessary, using the next-larger size left Judkins catheter (e.g., JL5 instead of JL4) or a left Amplatz catheter. A similar situation may exist in the right coronary artery, where the conus branch may have a separate ostium whose separate cannulation may be necessary to demonstrate important collaterals when reflux during the right coronary injection does not provide adequate reflux to opacify the conus.

The next most common anomaly is origin of the circumflex from the right coronary artery or right sinus of Valsalva (0.37%). This should be suspected when the left main is unusually long and a paucity of vessels to the lateral wall is identified. Careful review of the RAO left ventriculogram may show a dot of contrast just behind the aortic valve when the anomalous circumflex runs posterior to the aorta (48). If an anomalous circumflex is not filled

adequately during right coronary injection, it must be cannulated separately (generally with an AL1 catheter). We have seen patients in whom the only coronary lesion was located in such an anomalous circumflex, and failure to identify and opacify this vessel would have led to failure to diagnose and treat the problem.

In another common variant, anomalous vessels (particularly the right coronary artery) may originate unusually high in the aortic root or out of the normal coronary plane (38; Fig. 11.16), making them easier to cannulate using left Amplatz rather than right Judkins catheters. The left coronary may originate from the right sinus of Valsalva (Fig. 11.17), either as a separate ostium (49) or as part of a single coronary (50). Origin of a coronary artery from the noncoronary sinus of Valsalva is rare but has been reported (47,51). The main effect of these coronary anomalies is to test the patience, knowledge, and resourcefulness of the angiographer. Other anomalies, however, may themselves cause myocardial ischemia (even in the absence of atherosclerotic stenosis) and are described later in the section on nonatherosclerotic coronary artery disease.

Angiographic Views

Accurate coronary diagnosis requires coronary injections in multiple views to be sure that all coronary segments are seen clearly without foreshortening or overlap. The angulation of each view is given in two terms. The first term denotes rotation, i.e., the term right anterior oblique (RAO) designates a view where the image intensifier is located over the patient's right anterior chest wall, and left anterior oblique (LAO) designates a view where the image intensifier is located over the patient's left anterior chest wall. The second term denotes skew, i.e., the amount of angulation toward the patient's head (cranial) or foot (caudal). Although the full nomenclature of skew specifies first the source of the beam and then the location of the imaging device (e.g., caudocranial, to denote that the x-ray tube is toward the patient's feet while the image intensifier is located toward the patient's head), in practice this is simplified to give just the location of the imaging device. The term RAO caudocranial is thus stated as RAO-cranial.

When cradle systems were in use in the 1970s, these views were usually limited to different degrees of left or right anterior obliquity in the transverse plane, including the classic 60° LAO and 30° RAO projections (see Fig. 11.14). To allow concurrent cranial angulation of the x-ray beam, cradle systems were then modified by propping the patient's shoulders up on a foam wedge—hence the name *sit-up view*—to provide compound LAO-cranial projection. In the 1980s, cradle systems were abandoned in favor of parallelogram or rigid U-arm systems supported by a rotating pedestal (see Chapter 2) that allow compound beam angulation in any combination of conventional transverse (LAO, RAO) with skew (cranial, caudal) angulation up to

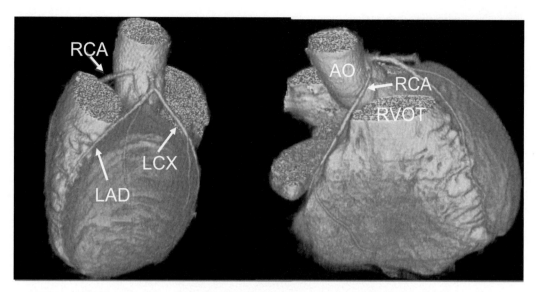

Figure 11.16 Multidetector computed tomographic image of a patient with anomalous origin of the right coronary artery from the left sinus of Valsalva and a course between the aorta and pulmonary artery (RCA, right coronary artery; LAD, left anterior descending; LC, left circumflex; AO, aorta; RVOT, right ventricular outflow tract).

45°. Although these views place increased demands on the generator and increase the scattered radiation, there is no doubt that they have improved our ability to define coronary anatomy (Fig. 11.18; 52–54).

It is not necessary to perform all potential views in a given patient to constitute an adequate study. Rather, a series of screening views should be used as the foundation of the study, adjusted or supplemented by one or more additional views selected to more completely define suspicious areas. This requires the operator to interpret the coronary anatomy as each injection is made or by digital review—it is not acceptable to simply shoot a series of routine views and hope that the study will prove adequate when reviewed later. Although some laboratories rely on a technician to set up shots and pan the table during coronary angiography, I (DB) believe that each operator should know how to do this himself or herself to develop a good understanding of how the choice of gantry angulation influences the projected coronary anatomy. One valuable training tool in this respect is a simple wire model of the coronary anatomy, which is viewed as it is moved into different angles (Fig. 11.19; 55). A computer program that simulates the effect of changing angles on the projected coronary anatomy is provided on the companion DVD-ROM to this text book. Although there is no substitute for this type of hands-on learning, the discussion below is provided as a rough introduction.

Right Anterior Oblique Projections

For historic reasons relating to cradle systems, the screening views used in many laboratories were the straight LAO-RAO angulations. With the availability of more modern gantry systems, it became clear that certain cranial and caudal angulated views offer far better anatomic definition. Thus, we generally avoid the straight 30° RAO projection of the left coronary, because it suffers from overlap and foreshortening of both the left anterior descending and circumflex vessels (see Fig. 11.18). Instead, our initial view of choice is the RAO-caudal projection (0 to 10° RAO and 15 to 20° caudal), since it provides an excellent view of the left main bifurcation, the proximal left anterior descending artery, and the proximal to midcircumflex artery. The second view we perform is a shallow RAO-cranial projection (0 to 10° RAO and 25 to 40° cranial), which provides a superior view of the mid and distal left anterior descending artery, with clear visualization of the origins of the septal and diagonal branches. This shallow RAO cranial view is also quite good for examination of the distal right coronary artery or distal circumflex, since it effectively unstacks the posterior descending and posterolateral branches and projects them without foreshortening. It seldom, however, provides any useful information about the left main or circumflex coronary artery, because it causes them to be overlapped and foreshortened.

Left Anterior Oblique Projections

The conventional 60° LAO projection is limited by overlap and foreshortening of the left coronary artery, although it is very useful in the evaluation of the proximal and midright coronary artery. The LAO-cranial view, created by the addition of 15 to 30° of cranial angulation, elongates the left main and proximal left anterior descending arteries

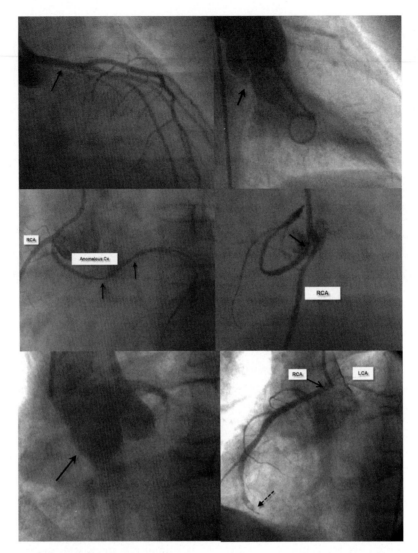

Figure 11.17 Anomalous origin of the circumflex from the right coronary artery. **Top left.** Note the long left main and absence of a circumflex during injection of the left coronary artery. **Top right.** Review of the right anterior oblique (RAO) left ventriculogram shows the telltale dot behind the aortic root, created by an end-on look at the anomalous circumflex coursing behind the aorta. **Center left.** The anomalous circumflex (Cx) originates from the right sinus of Valsalva with severe stenosis (arrows) responsible for the patient's unstable anginal syndrome. **Center right.** The RAO projection shows that the anomalous circumflex (arrow) has a separate ostium immediately posterior to the RCA origin, and then courses behind the aorta to reach the lateral wall of the left ventricle. **Bottom left.** In a different patient with an acute inferior wall myocardial infarction, a right sinus injection was performed after difficulty was encountered engaging the right coronary, and showed no right coronary ostium but faint filling of a vessel crossing the aorta. **Bottom right.** A left Amplatz catheter was used to cannulate the anomalous right coronary ostium originating from the left sinus of Valsalva (slightly anterior to the left coronary artery), revealing the RCA occlusion and thrombus (dotted arrow) responsible for the inferior MI, which then underwent primary angioplasty and stenting.

while projecting the intermedius or first diagonal branch downward off the proximal circumflex. If radiographic penetration in this view is difficult, reducing the LAO angulation to 30 to 40° will usually allow the left anterior descending artery to fall into the lucent wedge between the right hemidiaphragm and the spine. Performing the angiographic run during a sustained maximal inspiration will usually pull the diaphragm down and improve x-ray penetration. The LAO-caudal view (40 to 60° LAO and 10 to

20° caudal) projects the left coronary artery upward from the left main in the appearance of a spider (hence the older term, *spider view*), and usually offers improved visualization of the left main, proximal left anterior descending (LAD), and proximal circumflex arteries. It is particularly valuable in patients whose heart has a horizontal lie, i.e., the origin of the left main artery projects at or below the proximal left anterior descending artery in the standard LAO projection. This view can often be enhanced by film-

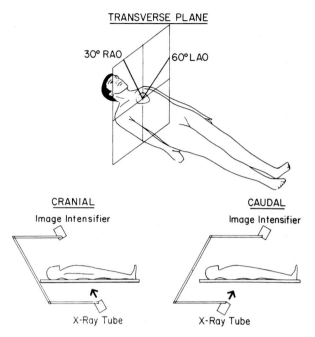

TRANSVERSE PLANE

30° RAO   60° LAO

CRANIAL   CAUDAL
Image Intensifier   Image Intensifier

X-Ray Tube   X-Ray Tube

Figure 11.18 Geometry of angulated views. Conventional coronary angiography was performed previously using angulation only in the transverse plane **(top)**, as demonstrated by the 60° left anterior oblique (LAO) and 30° right anterior oblique (RAO) views. Currently, improved x-ray equipment permits simultaneous cranial or caudal angulation in the sagittal plane. Each view is named based on the location of the image intensifier, rather than the older nomenclature specifying the location of both the x-ray tube and intensifier (i.e., cranial is equivalent to caudocranial).

ing during maximal expiration, which accentuates a horizontal cardiac position and allows a better look from below, although it stresses the radiographic capacity of most older installations.

Posteroanterior and Left Lateral Projections

The straight posteroanterior (PA, or "0-0") and left lateral projections tend to be underused in the era of complex angulation. Because the left main coronary artery curves from a more leftward to an almost anterior direction along its length, the PA projection (sometimes referred to incorrectly as the AP projection) frequently provides the best view of the left main ostium. On the other hand, the shallow RAO-caudal view frequently provides a better look at the more distal left main artery. The left lateral projection is particularly useful in examining the proximal circumflex and the proximal and distal left anterior descending arteries, particularly when combined with slight (10 to 15°) cranial angulation. This projection also provides the best look at the anastomosis of a left internal mammary graft to the middistal left anterior descending and offers an excellent look at the midportion of the right coronary artery, free of the excessive motion seen when this portion of the vessel is viewed in the straight RAO projection. The left lateral projection also has the advantage of allowing easy radiographic penetration in most patients when it is performed with both of the patient's hands posi-

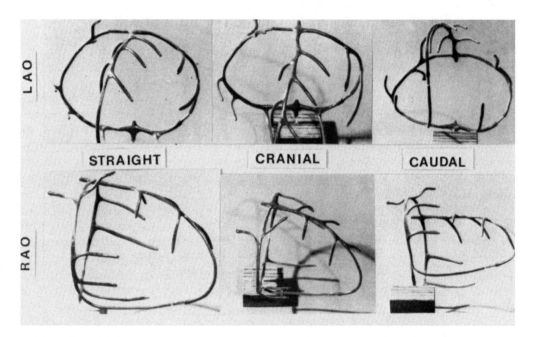

LAO

RAO

STRAIGHT   CRANIAL   CAUDAL

Figure 11.19 Demonstration of angiographic projections using the author's coronary model. LAO and RAO projections are photographed straight (i.e., with no cranial or caudal angulation) as well as with moderate cranial and moderate caudal angulation (see text for details).

tioned behind the head, although it generates the highest degree of backscatter given the proximity of the beam entry point on the patient's right side to the operator.

Over the past several years, operators in our laboratory have adopted a uniform sequence of these views, adjusting the exact angles slightly in each patient as dictated by test puffs of contrast. Beginning with the left coronary artery, these views include the following:

1. RAO-caudal to visualize the left main, proximal LAD, and proximal circumflex
2. RAO-cranial to visualize the mid and distal LAD without overlap of septal or diagonal branches
3. LAO-cranial to visualize the mid and distal LAD in an orthogonal projection
4. LAO-caudal to visualize the left main and proximal circumflex.

One or more supplemental views (PA, lateral-cranial, lateral-caudal) may then be taken to clarify any areas of uncertainty. The right coronary catheter is then placed, after which three screening views are obtained:

1. LAO to visualize the proximal right coronary artery (RCA)
2. RAO-cranial to visualize the posterior descending and posterolateral branches
3. Lateral to visualize the mid-RCA

Lesion Quantification

To quantify a coronary stenosis accurately, it must be seen in profile, free from artifact related to foreshortening or obfuscation by a crossing vessel. Multiple views are important, because many lesions have a markedly eccentric (elliptical rather than round) lumen (56). When seen across its major axis, the width of the lumen may appear nearly normal, but a clue to the presence of a severe degree of narrowing in the other axis may be marked lucency caused by thinning of the contrast column. Any such suspicious lesions must be examined in a variety of other projections to reveal their true severity and to distinguish the lucency caused by eccentric stenosis from a similar lucency that may be seen adjacent to an area of denser contrast (caused by tortuosity or overlapping vessels in the absence of any true abnormality at the site) through a perceptual artifact known as the Mach effect (57).

The ability of coronary angiography to quantify the degree of stenosis at different points in the coronary circulation is fundamentally limited by the fact that it consists of a "lumen-o-gram," in which each stenosis can be evaluated only by comparison to an adjacent reference segment that is presumed to be free of disease. In fact, both intravascular ultrasound (56; see Chapter 19) and pathologic examination (58) show that even segments that appear smooth on angiography may harbor substantial plaque. It is thus important to have a sense of the normal caliber of the major coronary arteries (4.5 ± 0.5 mm for the left

main, 3.7 ± 0.4 mm for the left anterior descending, 3.4 ± 0.5 mm for a nondominant versus 4.2 ± 0.6 mm for a dominant circumflex, and 3.9 ± 0.6 mm for a dominant versus 2.8 ± 0.5 mm for a nondominant right coronary artery (59). By comparing the diameter of a presumably disease-free segment of coronary artery to the size of the diagnostic catheter (6F equals 2 mm), the operator can identify vessels that fall below these normal size ranges and may thus be diffusely diseased.

In addition to the difficulty in finding a disease-free reference segment, a major problem in the interpretation of a coronary angiogram is deciding the severity of any given stenosis. Both animal data (60) and human data (61) show that a stenosis that reduces the lumen diameter by 50% (and hence cross-sectional area by 75%) is hemodynamically significant in that it reduces the normal threefold to fourfold flow reserve of a coronary bed (Fig. 11.20), whereas a 70% diameter stenosis (90% cross-sectional area) eliminates virtually any ability to increase flow above its resting level (see Chapter 18). Stenoses that reduce the lumen diameter by 90%, however, rarely exist without reducing antegrade flow (i.e., TIMI [Thrombolysis in Myocardial Infarction] grade 1 or 2, rather than TIMI grade 3 normal flow).

Instead of the subjective TIMI flow grading system, Gibson et al. (62) have created norms for the number of cine frames (at 30 frames per second [fps]) required for contrast to leave the catheter tip and reach standardized distal landmarks in each coronary artery (the LAD "mustache," the first posterolateral branch of the right coronary). Contrast normally reaches these points in 20 frames for the RCA and 36 frames for the LAD, with TIMI 2 (partial) flow corresponding to more than a doubling of those frame counts. Of course, even more precise data about hemodynamic lesion significance can be determined by performance of flow or pressure gradient measurements, at rest and during arteriolar vasodilation (e.g., after adenosine administration) to calculate the coronary flow or fractional flow reserve (63). Lesions that permit a flow increase of more than twofold, or have a ratio of distal pressure to aortic pressure >0.75 in the setting of peak flow after adenosine injection, are generally considered to be hemodynamically insignificant. Angiographically borderline (40 to 60%) lesions for which there is no clear objective evidence of ischemia (i.e., exercise test, perfusion scan) should thus be interrogated further with intravascular ultrasound or pressure wire measurements before considering intervention (see Chapters 18 and 19).

In clinical practice, however, the degree of lesion stenosis is usually just estimated visually from the coronary angiogram. The operator must thus develop a sense of what constitutes a 50, 70, and 90% diameter stenosis (see Fig. 11.21). Although the process of visually estimating the degree of coronary stenosis may seem straightforward, it is subject to significant operator variability (the standard deviation for repeat estimates is ≤18%: 64) as well as a sys-

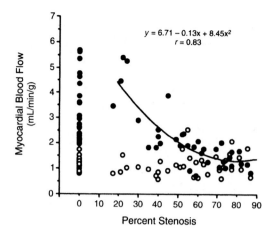

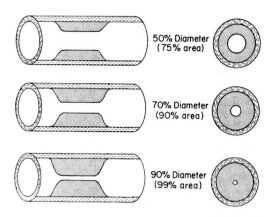

Figure 11.21 Coronary stenoses of 50, 70, and 90% diameter reduction are shown in longitudinal and cross section. The corresponding reductions in cross-sectional area are indicated in parentheses.

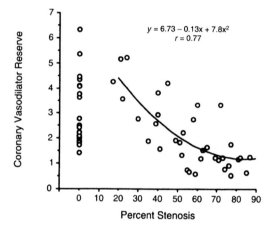

Figure 11.20 Effect of coronary stenosis on myocardial blood flow and coronary vasodilator reserve. **Top.** Resting flow *(open circles)* is well maintained at approximately 1 mL/minute per gram of myocardium throughout the range of evaluated diameter stenosis. The ability to increase flow during vasodilator stimulus *(closed circles)*, however, becomes impaired for stenosis >50% and is virtually abolished >70%. **Bottom.** The vasodilator reserve (dilated flow/resting flow), which has a normal value of 3 to 4 but is reduced with stenosis >50% and falls to 1 at >70%. (From Uren, et al., Relation between myocardial blood flow and the severity of coronary artery stenosis. *N Engl J Med* 1994;330:1782, with permission).

tematic form of "stenosis inflation" that causes operators to estimate a diameter stenosis that is roughly 20% higher than that measured by quantitative coronary angiography (QCA; 65). A stenosis that measures 50% will thus typically be called 70%, whereas a stenosis that measures 70% will be called 90%.

Tools are available to resolve this problem. The simplest is to project the coronary image on a wall-mounted viewing screen and to use inexpensive digital calipers (available from machinist supply houses) to measure the relative diameters of the stenotic and reference segments (66). Percent stenosis then can be calculated as 100 × [1−(stenosis diameter/reference diameter)] to provide a more accurate estimate of stenosis. This technique also reduces the stan-

dard deviation for diameter stenosis to 6 to 8% (64,66). Even greater precision can be obtained by using computer-assisted algorithms to perform automated edge detection on digitally acquired images to measure the coronary lumen with a standard deviation <5% (67,68). The amount of variation in diameter stenosis readings for one study (69) using these different methods concurrently is shown in Fig. 11.22.

The good news is that angiographers who have trained their eye in actual stenosis quantification (by using digital calipers or computer-assisted quantitative coronary angiography) can then actually give visual estimates much closer to true measurements. (70) This would allow angiographers to be more uniform in their visual estimates and move away from reporting physiologically impossible findings like a 95% stenosis with normal distal flow. Until there is a stenosis reading reform, so that those of us who call such lesions accurately (e.g., 70%) will not be accused of intervening on mild lesions, there will be no substitute to seeing the films yourself before making any clinical decisions!

It has also become important to evaluate lesion morphology more accurately from the coronary angiogram. Features such as eccentricity, ulceration, and thrombus may be associated with unstable clinical patterns (71,72), whereas features such as calcification, eccentricity, or thrombus may influence the choice of catheter intervention. Many of these features can be recognized from careful study of high-quality cineangiograms, although angiography is clearly not as sensitive to these features as intravascular ultrasound (73) or angioscopy (for thrombus or dissection; 74). Angiographers may also have trouble predicting the physiologic significance of a coronary lesion, in which case angiography may need to be supplemented by other techniques such as direct flow or distal pressure measurements (63). Finally, the absence of lesions narrowing the coronary lumen by >50% does not necessarily confer immunity from subsequent coronary events, since it is frequently a less severe stenotic lesion that

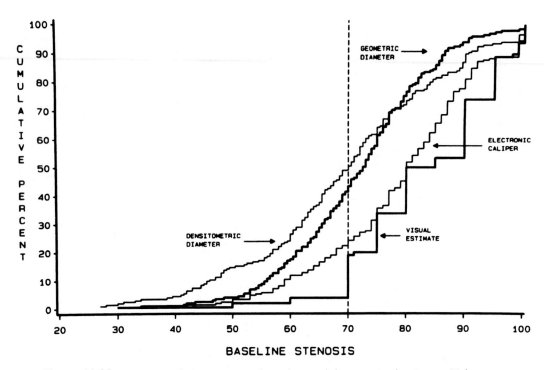

Figure 11.22 In a series of 227 patients with single-vessel disease, visual estimates (right curve, average nearly 90%) were consistently higher than either caliper measurements (average near 80%) or computer-assisted quantitative angiography by either geometric or densitometric techniques (left curves, average near 70% diameter stenosis). (From Folland ED, Vogel RA, Hartigan P, et al. Relation between coronary artery stenosis assessed by visual, caliper, and computer methods and exercise capacity in patients with single-vessel coronary artery disease. *Circulation* 1994;89:2005, with permission).

has the large lipid core and thin fibrous cap that may predispose to subsequent plaque rupture and the resulting coronary thrombosis (75). Despite these recognized limitations in quantification and morphology assessment, contrast coronary angiography remains the clinical standard by which lesions are evaluated and decisions are made regarding the need for (and best mode of providing) revascularization in the patient with ischemic heart disease.

Coronary Collaterals

In reviewing the coronary angiogram, one basic principle is that there should be evident blood supply to all portions of the left ventricle. Previously occluded vessel branches are usually manifest as truncated stumps, but a stump may not be evident if there has been a flush occlusion at the origin of the involved vessel. These occluded or severely stenotic vessels will frequently be seen to fill late in the injection by antegrade (so-called bridging) collaterals or collaterals that originate from the same (intracoronary) or an adjacent (intercoronary) vessel, which are reviewed in an excellent paper by Levin (76) and illustrated in Figs. 11.23 through 11.25. Finally, coronary occlusion may present in some patients simply as an angiographically arid area to which there is no evidence of either antegrade or collateral flow and no evident vascular stump. If such

an area fails to show regional hypokinesis on the left ventriculogram, however, the operator should search carefully for blood supply by way of anomalous vessels or unopacified collaterals (i.e., a separate origin conus branch that was not opacified during the main right coronary injections), because the myocardium cannot continue to function normally with no visible means of support. Functioning collaterals, however, can maintain a coronary wedge pressure that averages nearly 40% of mean aortic pressure (77,78), thereby maintaining myocardial viability in the collateral-fed distribution. Along with other measures of retained or augmentable wall motion, redistributing defects on perfusion imaging, and positron emission tomographic (PET) evidence of ongoing glucose metabolism, the angiographic presence of collateral flow to an area in the distribution of an occluded coronary artery is one of the strongest evidences of ongoing myocardial viability and an important factor in determining the best revascularization strategy.

Although it is uncommon, what appears as a network of collaterals may be the vascular supply to an organized thrombus (in the left ventricle or left atrium) or a cardiac tumor. Those entities should be suspected when filling of an apparent collateral network is seen in the absence of occlusion or severe stenosis of the normal supply to a myocardial territory.

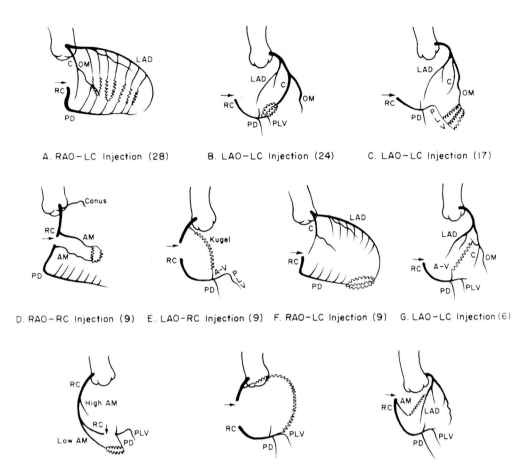

Figure 11.23 Ten collateral pathways observed in patients with right coronary (RC) obstruction (total occlusion or >90% stenosis). LAD, left anterior descending; C, circumflex; OM, obtuse marginal; PD, posterior descending; PLV, posterior left ventricular branch; AM, acute marginal branch of right coronary artery; AV, atrioventricular nodal; LC, left coronary. Numbers in parentheses represent numbers of cases in this series. (From Levin DC. Pathways and functional significance of the coronary collateral circulation. *Circulation* 1974;50:831. By permission of the American Heart Association, Inc.)

NONATHEROSCLEROTIC CORONARY ARTERY DISEASE

Although atherosclerotic stenosis is far and away the most common pathologic process responsible for myocardial ischemia, the angiographer must be aware of various other potential causes. These include certain congenital anomalies of coronary origin (46,79–81)—for example, an anomalous coronary that courses between the aorta and pulmonary artery (Fig. 11.16), in which flow may be compromised by deformation of the ostium or compression of the proximal vessel, potentially even causing sudden death. In patients with such anatomy and objective evidence of ischemia on medical therapy, bypass surgery or stenting of the anomalous segment may be considered (82).

Other abnormalities include coronary fistulae (Fig. 11.26), coronary aneurysms (83,84), and muscle bridges (Fig. 11.27; 85,86). Coronary fistulae, connections mostly from a coronary artery to the right ventricle, right atrium, pulmonary artery, or coronary sinus, are found in roughly 0.1% of patients coming to cardiac catheterization. When they are large (or in the setting of proximal coronary disease), these fistulae may cause chronic volume overload or myocardial ischemia and must be closed, using surgery or newer catheter techniques (embolization coils, covered stents; 87). Smaller, asymptomatic fistulae may close spontaneously, however, and can be managed conservatively (88). Muscle bridges are sections of a coronary artery (almost always the left anterior descending) that run under a strip of left ventricular muscle, which compresses the lumen during ventricular systole despite a normal appearance during diastole (85,86). Similar systolic compression of the first septal branch (saw-toothing) is also seen in many patients with hypertrophic cardiomyopathy (89). When one of these congenital anomalies is present in a patient with ischemic symptoms in whom catheterization has failed to demonstrate the expected finding of coronary atherosclerosis, the angiographer should be able to recognize it

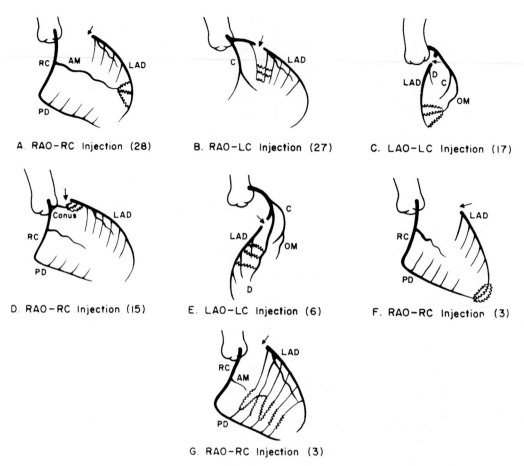

Figure 11.24 Seven collateral pathways observed in patients with left coronary artery obstruction. Abbreviations and format are the same as in Figure 11.23. (From Levin DC: Pathways and functional significance of the coronary collateral circulation. *Circulation* 1974;50:831. By permission of the American Heart Association, Inc.)

as a potential cause of ischemia and recommend additional functional testing with an eye toward surgical or catheter-assisted repair (fistula coil embolization, muscle bridge stent placement).

The coronary arteries may also be affected by medium-vessel vasculitis (90), including polyarteritis nodosa and the mucocutaneous lymph node syndrome (Kawasaki disease). The latter is largely a childhood illness, in which coronary arteritis may lead to aneurysm, stenosis, or thrombosis that was often fatal (usually in the first month of the illness) before the use of high-dose gamma globulin to treat the acute illness. When coronary aneurysms are found in adults, it may thus be difficult to determine if they represent atherosclerotic damage to the vessel wall or the remainders of childhood Kawasaki disease (83). The treatment for the stenotic lesions (bypass or catheter-based intervention), however, are the same regardless of the etiology.

Although not an arteritis, cardiac allograft vasculopathy (91) is one of the most troublesome long-term complications of heart transplantation. The mechanism seems to be an immune-mediated diffuse vascular pro-

liferative response involving distal as well as proximal coronary arteries, with superimposed focal lesions of the proximal vessels. The latter may be amenable to catheter-based revascularization. Patients who have received prior mantle radiation therapy for Hodgkin disease may be at risk for radiation-induced coronary stenosis (92), particularly of the left and right coronary ostia and the proximal left coronary artery, up to 20 years after completing their course of therapy. The pathology is most commonly fibrotic contraction of the vessel wall, rather than intimal proliferation or plaque formation.

Finally, some patients who come to catheterization have no demonstrable coronary abnormality to account for their clinically suspected ischemic heart disease. Although anginalike pain can be seen in patients with noncoronary cardiac abnormality (e.g., mitral valve prolapse, hypertrophic cardiomyopathy, aortic stenosis, myocarditis) or extracardiac conditions (esophageal dysmotility [93], cholecystitis), one must also consider the possibility of epicardial or microvascular coronary vasospastic disease (see below).

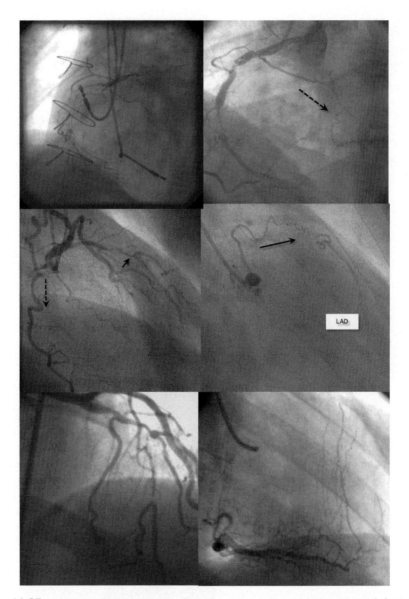

Figure 11.25 Angiographic appearance of some common collateral pathways. **Top left.** Bridging or vasa vasora collaterals in an occluded right coronary artery (RCA). **Top right.** Kugel collateral (sinus node to atrioventricular node, *dotted arrow*) supplying the distal RCA. **Center left.** Full-bore connection (*dotted arrow*) between the distal circumflex and the distal portion of an occluded RCA, in a patient with coexisting left anterior descending (LAD) occlusion (*short arrow*). **Center right.** Classic Vieussens (Raymond de Vieussens, 1641–1715) collateral connecting the conus branch of the RCA to the LAD in the same patient as shown in the previous example. **Bottom left.** Septal-to-septal collateral in severely stenotic LAD. **Bottom right.** Posterior descending septal branches connecting to septal branches of an occluded LAD.

Coronary Vasospasm

Vasospasm of an epicardial coronary artery typically presents as variant (or Prinzmetal) angina in which episodes of rest pain occur despite well-preserved effort tolerance at other times (94). An electrocardiogram recorded during an episode of spontaneous pain usually shows ST elevation in the territory supplied by the vasospastic artery. Absence of a significant coronary lesion in such a patient confirms the diagnosis of variant angina owing to focal coronary spasm (Fig. 11.28). In these patients, coronary angiography is performed mainly to look at the extent of underlying atherosclerosis (95). Provocative maneuvers to initiate spasm were once common to confirm the diagnosis and evaluate drug therapy (96). It is now used mostly when the diagnosis of variant angina is uncertain and a patient with troublesome chest pain fails to manifest sufficient disease to explain its cause.

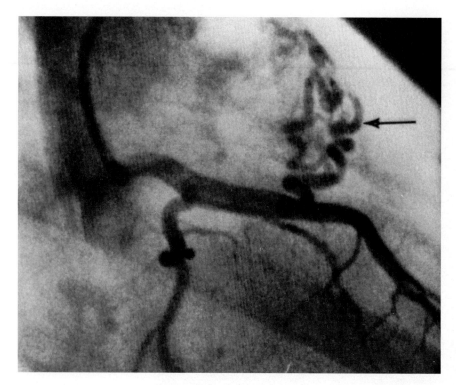

Figure 11.26 Coronary artery fistula (*arrow*) between the midleft anterior descending coronary artery and the pulmonary artery, shown in the right anterior oblique view.

If provocative testing for coronary spasm is contemplated, the patient should be withdrawn from calcium channel blockers for at least 24 hours and long-acting nitrates for at least 12 hours before the study and should not be premedicated with either atropine or sublingual nitroglycerin. Ongoing therapy with any of these agents may render provocative tests falsely negative (96). Although various provocative tests have been used (metha-

choline, epinephrine and propranolol, hyperventilation and tris-buffer, cold pressor), the most commonly used provocative agent has been ergonovine or methylergonovine maleate (Methergine, Sandoz, East Hanover, NJ; 97–99). These agents are stimulants of the α-adrenergic and serotonin receptors in coronary vascular smooth muscle.

Testing for coronary spasm should be performed only after baseline angiographic evaluation of both the left and

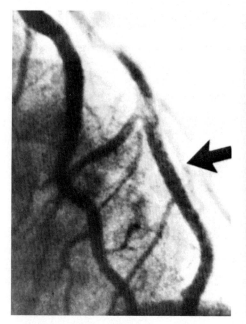 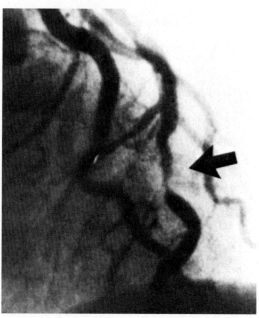

Figure 11.27 Muscle bridge. Moderately severe muscle bridge of the left anterior descending coronary artery (*arrow*) as seen in diastole (**left**) and systole (**right**).

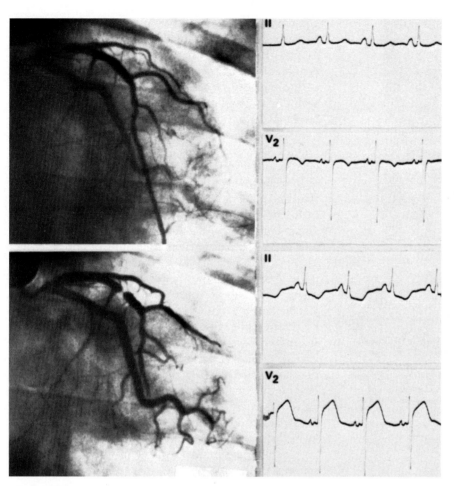

Figure 11.28 True coronary spasm. Intense focal vasospasm of the left anterior descending coronary artery is shown in right anterior oblique projection in a patient with variant angina. Note the absence of a significant underlying atherosclerotic stenosis in the top view, the absence of vasoconstriction of other vessel segments, and the marked ST elevation in the anterior leads during the spontaneous vasospastic episode. (From Baim DS, Harrison DC. Nonatherosclerotic coronary heart disease. In: Hurst JW, ed. *The Heart*, 5th ed. New York: McGraw-Hill, 1985, with permission.)

right coronary arteries. It should not be performed in patients with severe hypertension or severe anatomic cardiac pathology (left ventricular dysfunction, left main or multivessel disease, or aortic stenosis). As an example, our protocol for using methylergonovine calls for a total of 0.4 mg (400 mg equals 2 ampules) to be diluted to a total volume of 8 mL in a 10-mL syringe that is appropriately labeled. The provocative test consists of graded intravenous administration of 1 mL (0.05 mg), 2 mL (0.10 mg), and 5 mL (0.25 mg) of this mixture at 3- to 5-minute intervals. Parenteral nitroglycerin (100 to 200 mg/mL) must be premixed and loaded in a labeled syringe before the testing is begun. It is also advisable to have an intracoronary calcium channel blocker (verapamil 100 μg/mL, diltiazem 250 μg/mL) or nitroprusside (100 μg/mL) close at hand in case nitroglycerin-refractory spasm develops. Temporary pacing and defibrillator equipment should also be available to treat the bradyarrhythmias or tachyarrhythmias that sometimes accompany coronary spasm. At 1 minute before each ergonovine dose, the patient is interrogated about symptoms similar to those of her or his clinical complaint, and a 12-lead electrocardiogram is recorded. After each electrocardiogram, coronary angiography is performed, looking either at both arteries or only at the artery of highest clinical suspicion for vasospasm. In the absence of clinical

symptoms, electrocardiographic changes, or focal coronary vasospasm, the next ergonovine dose is administered, and the cycle is repeated until the total dose of 0.4 mg has been given. The provocative test should be considered positive only if focal spasm (>70% diameter stenosis) occurs and is associated with clinical symptoms and/or electrocardiographic changes. Even if there are no symptoms or electrocardiographic changes, both coronary arteries should be opacified at the end of the provocative test, and any generalized vasoconstrictor effect should be terminated by administration of nitroglycerin to document the resolution of spasm and the extent of underlying atherosclerotic stenosis. Note that coronary artery spasm may occur in two vessels simultaneously (Fig. 11.29), and visualization of only one vessel may fail to adequately assess the magnitude of the vasospastic response.

Some operators have used an intracoronary methylergonovine administration protocol, in which a 4-minute intracoronary infusion (10 μg/minute in the right and 16 μg/min in the left coronary) is administered. Alternatively, discrete doses of 5 to 10 μg may be given into a coronary artery, waiting 3 minutes and imaging before a second dose is given (maximal total dose 50 μg per vessel). These intracoronary protocols may be advantageous in that they produce less systemic effect (hypertension, esophageal

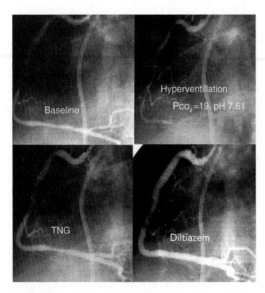

Figure 11.29 A 37-year-old man was admitted with chest pain and ST-segment elevation in the inferior leads. Emergency catheterization was performed for presumed acute myocardial infarction within 30 minutes of presentation **(top left)**, but disclosed a dominant right coronary artery with only mild disease at a time when pain had resolved after nitrate and heparin therapy. Hyperventilation (30 breaths per minute for 5 minutes) was performed with reduction of PCO_2 to 19 mm Hg and elevation of pH to 7.61, resulting in provocation of occlusive focal spasm of the distal right coronary artery with return of chest pain and ST-segment elevation **(top right)**. Relief of vasospasm and marked general dilation of the RCA was produced by intracoronary administration of trinitroglycerin (TNG) 200 μg **(bottom left)** and diltiazem 500 μg **(bottom right)**.

spasm). The other intracoronary provocative test for coronary spasm uses acetylcholine (serial doses of 20-50-100 μg injected into the left coronary, and 20-50-80 μg injected into the right coronary). Some investigators have also used hyperventilation as a provocative test for spasm (100, Figure 11.29). The same caveats regarding ready availability of potent intracoronary vasodilators to treat spasm also apply to any of these prevocational protocols.

Several additional comments about ergonovine are in order. Ergonovine testing should be avoided in patients with severe atherosclerotic stenosis (≥80%), in whom spasm is not required to explain the clinical symptoms. In these patients, however, we frequently do repeat coronary angiography of the stenotic vessel after the intracoronary administration of 200 mg of nitroglycerin to exclude the possibility that spontaneous focal vasospasm is contributing to the appearance of severe atherosclerotic stenosis. Second, the operator should be aware that the positivity rate depends strongly on which patients are studied; the test is almost always positive in patients with known variant angina (if their disorder is active and medications have been withheld) and is positive in approximately one third of patients with clinically suspected variant angina, but it is positive in <5% of patients whose symptoms do not suggest variant angina (99). The Duke group (101) reported

ergonovine testing in 3,447 patients without significant coronary disease or variant angina, with an overall positivity rate of 4% in such patients. There were two independent predictors of a positive test: mild to moderate disease on the angiogram (spasm often takes place at the point of such disease) and a history of smoking, whose presence increased the positivity rate to 10%.

Since finding spasm is so uncommon now that the syndrome is detected clinically in most patients and is treated so effectively by calcium channel blockers, the risk of ergonovine testing to evaluate patients with atypical symptoms and minimal fixed coronary disease is remarkably low. In the Duke study, significant complications occurred in only 11 patients (0.03%), including myocardial infarction in four patients and ventricular tachycardia or fibrillation (VT or VF) in seven patients (101). When provocative testing produces clinical symptoms but no angiographic evidence of vasospasm in either coronary artery, there may still be scintographic evidence of myocardial ischemia due to microvascular spasm. Both multivessel epicardial and microvascular spasm have been implicated in tako-tsubo syndrome where extreme emotional stress is followed by chest pain, ST elevation, and a particular pattern of apical hypokinesis extending beyond the usual single coronary territory. If there are no signs of myocardial ischemia, an alternative diagnosis such as esophageal dysmotility (93), which can also be provoked by methylergonovine, should be considered.

It is also important to distinguish the intense focal spasm seen in patients with variant angina from the normal mild (15 to 20%) diffuse coronary narrowing seen as a pharmacologic response to ergonovine in normal patients (102). True coronary spasm must also be distinguished from spasm induced by mechanical interventions such as rotational atherectomy (see Chapter 28) or catheter-tip spasm (Fig. 11.30). Catheter-tip spasm is most common in the right coronary artery, is not associated with clinical symptoms or electrocardiographic changes, and does not indicate variant angina (103). It should be recognized as such, however, and treated by withdrawal of the catheter, administration of nitroglycerin, and nonselective or cautious repeat selective opacification of the involved vessel to avoid mistaking catheter-tip spasm for an atherosclerotic lesion. Spasm should also be distinguished from a "pleating" artifact that may occur when a curved artery is straightened out by a stiff guidewire (Fig. 11.31), causing folds of the vessel wall to impinge on the lumen. Pleating is refractory to nitroglycerin but resolves immediately when the stiff guidewire is withdrawn (104).

Abnormal Coronary Vasodilator Reserve

Evidence has been accumulating that the patient group with angina and angiographically normal coronary arteries may contain a subgroup of patients who have myocardial ischemia on the basis of abnormal vasodilator reserve. Despite angiographic normality, intravascular

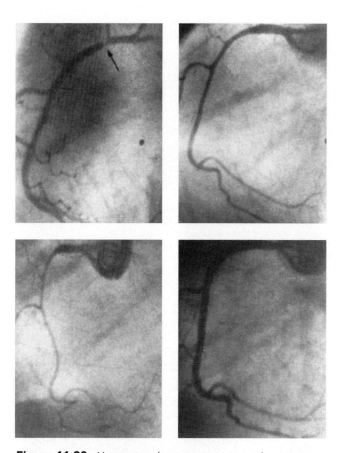

Figure 11.30 Vasomotor changes not representing true coronary spasm. During right coronary catheterization with a Judkins catheter **(top left)**, this patient developed severe catheter-tip spasm. Recatheterization 24 hours later with an Amplatz catheter **(top right)** showed neither catheter-tip spasm nor an atherosclerotic stenosis. Following ergonovine 0.4 mg, marked diffuse coronary narrowing was observed **(bottom left)** without angina or electrocardiographic changes. After the intracoronary administration of nitroglycerin 200 mcg **(bottom right)**, there is marked diffuse vasodilation.

and a unique pattern of apical akinesis (107,108; see also Chapter 12).

MISTAKES IN INTERPRETATION

An inexperienced operator often produces an incomplete or uninterpretable study, especially if she or he is using poor equipment. Such an operator is also likely to misinterpret the angiographic findings, with potentially serious clinical consequences. The following discussion summarizes some of the most common pitfalls that may lead the inexperienced coronary angiographer to mistaken conclusions.

Inadequate Number of Projections

There is no standard number of projections that will always provide complete information. Each major vessel must be viewed in an isolated fashion as it stands apart from other vessels. Usually, the angulated views discussed earlier in this chapter are necessary to visualize clearly the anatomy of the proximal left anterior descending and circumflex arteries.

Inadequate Injection of Contrast Material

The inexperienced operator or assistant has a tendency to hold back on the volume and force of injection into the coronary circulation. This results in inadequate or intermittent, pulsatile opacification of the coronary arterial tree as contrast flow fails short of peak coronary flow during diastole. Because there is inadequate mixing of contrast agent and blood, pockets of nonradiopaque blood in such inadequate injections may even give the appearance of arterial narrowing.

Superselective Injection

It is not uncommon to catheterize the left anterior descending or circumflex coronary artery superselectively, especially when the left main coronary artery is short and its bifurcation is early. To the inexperienced operator, this may give the impression of total occlusion of the nonvisualized vessel (e.g., if only the circumflex artery is opacified, the operator may conclude that the left anterior descending artery is occluded). If adequate filling of the noncannulated vessel cannot be achieved by reflux, selective cannulation of the LAD may be obtained by counterclockwise rotation or use of the next-smaller Judkins catheter (e.g., JL3.5), whereas selection cannulation of the circumflex may be obtained by clockwise rotation or use of the next-larger Judkins catheter (e.g., JL5). With the right coronary artery, superselective injection may occur if the catheter tip is too far down the vessel, leading to failure to visualize the conus and sinus node arteries. Because these are important sources of collateralization

ultrasound examination may show normal vessel wall architecture, intimal thickening, or atheromatous plaque (84). In these patients, coronary blood flow (as described in Chapter 18) may fail to rise normally with pacing tachycardia or exercise, and the coronary vascular resistance is increased abnormally (105). Also, many of these patients show an abnormal rise in left ventricular end diastolic pressure following pacing tachycardia and show less lactate consumption than normal subjects in response to pacing tachycardia (106). A failure of small vessel coronary vasodilation, inappropriate vasoconstriction at the arteriolar level, or functional abnormalities of capillary endothelial cells in releasing endothelium-derived relaxing factor (EDRF) have been postulated to account for these findings. Many patients with so-called syndrome X respond at least partially to treatment with a calcium channel blocker. Disordered small vessel vasoconstriction has also been implicated in the tako-tsubo syndrome where patients with angiographically normal epicardial arteries may present with chest pain, anterior ST elevation,

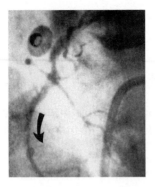
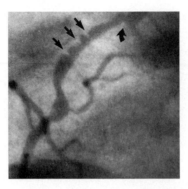
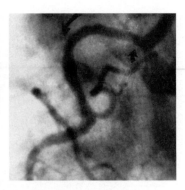

Figure 11.31   Right coronary artery "pleating" artifact. **Left.** Baseline injection shows diffuse disease in this tortuous right coronary artery selected for rotational atherectomy. **Center.** shows straightening of the proximal vessel by the stiff type C wire, creating three areas of infolding of the vessel wall *(arrows)* as well as the appearance of ostial stenosis *(curved arrow)*. Immediately on withdrawal of the guidewire, the artery returned to its baseline curvature and these defects resolved *(arrows)*.

of the left coronary system, important information may be missed (see Fig. 11.13). Adequate injection to give a continuous (nonpulsatile) reflux of contrast agent back into the sinus of Valsalva will help the operator to recognize vessels that originate proximally to the catheter tip and thus avoid the interpretation error of superselective injection.

Selective cannulation of a coronary artery may also fail to detect significant ostial stenosis, particularly if the catheter tip lies beyond the lesion and adequate contrast reflux is not produced. If ostial stenosis is suspected (e.g., if there is partial ventricularization or damping), we have found it helpful to perform a final injection during withdrawal of the catheter from the ostium (Fig. 11.32).

Catheter-Induced Coronary Spasm

Coronary artery spasm may be related to the catheter itself, possibly caused by mechanical irritation and a myogenic reflex (see Fig. 11.30). It is seen most commonly when the right coronary artery is engaged selectively, although it may occur rarely in the left anterior descending artery as well. Although catheter-tip spasm can occur with either the brachial or femoral approach, it is probably more common with the right Judkins catheter, especially if the catheter tip enters the right coronary ostium at an angle and produces tenting of the proximal vessel. If coronary narrowing suggests the occurrence of spasm to the operator, sublingual, intravenous, or intracoronary nitroglycerin should be given and the injection repeated.

Congenital Variants of Coronary Origin and Distribution

This topic has been discussed earlier in this chapter, but it bears re-emphasis. Variation in origin and distribution of the coronary artery branches may confuse the operator and cause him or her to mistakenly diagnose coronary

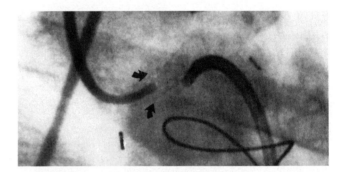
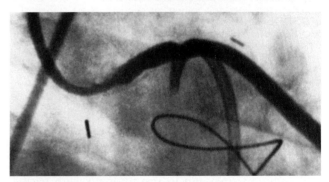
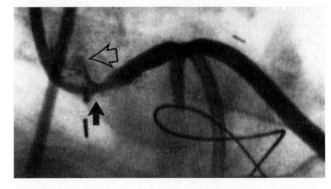

Figure 11.32   Masking of ostial stenosis during superselective cannulation. Ostial stenosis of previously stented vein graft is not apparent with the tip of the catheter well beyond the stenosis **(top and center).** Continued injection during catheter withdrawal **(bottom)** causes reflux into the aorta *(solid arrow)* and clearly shows significant ostial stenosis.

occlusion. For example, a small right coronary artery that terminates in the AV groove well before the crux may be interpreted as an abnormal or occluded artery, whereas it is a normal finding in 7 to 10% of human hearts. Double ostia of the right coronary artery or origin of the circumflex artery from the right coronary artery may be similarly confusing and lead to misdiagnosis.

Myocardial Bridges

As discussed earlier, coronary arteries occasionally dip below the epicardial surface under small strips of myocardium. During systole, the segment of the artery surrounded by myocardium is narrowed and appears as a localized stenosis. These myocardial bridges occur most commonly in the distribution of the left anterior descending artery and its diagonal branches. The key to the recognition of these bridges is that the apparent localized stenosis returns to normal during diastole. Recent studies using the flow wire (see Chapter 18) show clear derangement in phasic flow dynamics in muscle bridge segments and their normalization by stent placement. Although some severe muscle bridges can thus cause true myocardial ischemia under certain circumstances, they are seen in at least 5% of normal angiograms obtained in patients with no evidence of ischemia in the LAD territory.

Total Occlusion

If a coronary artery or branch is totally occluded at its origin, it may not be visualized, and the occlusion may be missed. If the occlusion is flush with the parent vessel, no stump will be seen. Such occlusions are primarily recognized by visualization of the distal segment of the occluded vessel by means of collateral channels or by noting the absence of the usual vascularity seen in a particular portion of the heart.

REFERENCES

1. Bashore TM, et al. American College of Cardiology/Society for Cardiac Angiography and Interventions Clinical Expert Consensus Document on Cardiac Catheterization Laboratory Standards. A Report of the American College of Cardiology Task Force on Clinical Expert Consensus Documents. *J Am Coll Cardiol* 2001; 37:2170–2214.
2. Scanlon PJ, Faxon DP, Audet A, et al. AHA/ACC guidelines for coronary angiography. A report of the ACC/AHA Task force on practice guidelines. *J Am Coll Cardiol* 1999;33:1756.
3. Budoff MJ. Clinical utility of computed tomography and magnetic resonance techniques for noninvasive coronary angiography. *J Am Coll Cardiol* 2003;42:1867–1878.
4. Ropers D, et al. Visualization of coronary artery anomalies and their anatomic course by contrast-enhanced electron beam tomography and three dimensional reconstruction. *Am J Cardiol* 2001;87:193–197.
4a. Martuscelli E, et al. Evaluation of venous and arterial conduit patency by 16-slice spiral computed tomography. Circulation 2004;110:3234–38.
5. Davies RF, Goldberg AD, Forman S, et al. Asymptomatic Cardiac Ischemia Pilot (ACIP) study two-year follow-up: outcomes of patients randomized to initial strategies of medical therapy versus revascularization. *Circulation* 1997;95:2037.
6. The TIMI IIIB Investigators. Effects of tissue plasminogen activator and a comparison of early invasive and conservative strategies in unstable angina and non-Q wave myocardial infarction—results of the TIMI IIIB trial (Thrombolysis in Myocardial Ischemia). *Circulation* 1994;89:1545.
7. Miltenberg AJM, et al. Incidence and follow-up of Braunwald subgroups in unstable angina pectoris. *J Am Coll Cardiol* 1995; 25:1286.
8. Ryan TJ, Anderson JL, Antman EM, et al. ACC/AHA guidelines for the management of patients with acute myocardial infarction: executive summary. *Circulation* 1996;94:2341.
9. The TIMI Study Group. Comparison of invasive and conservative strategies after treatment with intravenous tissue plasminogen activator in acute myocardial infarction. *N Engl J Med* 1989;320: 618.
10. Spaulding CM, Joly L, Rosenberg A, et al. Immediate coronary angiography in survivors of out-of-hospital cardiac arrest. *N Engl J Med* 1997;336:1629.
11. Panza JA, Laurienzo JM, Curiel RV, et al. Investigation of the mechanism of chest pain in patients with angiographically normal coronary arteries using transesophageal dobutamine stress echocardiography. *J Am Coll Cardiol* 1997;29:293.
12. Eagle KA, et al. Guidelines for perioperative cardiovascular evaluation for noncardiac surgery (report of the ACC/AHA Task Force on Practice Guidelines). *J Am Coll Cardiol* 1996; 27:910.
13. Neufeld NH, Blieden LC. Coronary artery disease in children. *Prog Cardiol* 1975;4:119.
14. Roberts WC. No cardiac catheterization before cardiac valve replacement—a mistake. *Am Heart J* 1982;103:930.
15. Baim DS, Kuntz RE. Appropriate uses of angiographic follow-up in the evaluation of new technologies for coronary intervention. Circulation 1994;90:2560.
16. Conti CR. Coronary arteriography. *Circulation* 1977;55:227.
17. Noto TJ, Johnson LW, Krone R, et al. Cardiac catheterization 1990: a report of the registry of the Society for Cardiac Angiography and Interventions. *Cathet Cardiovasc Diagn* 1991;24:75.
18. Fierens E. Outpatient coronary arteriography. *Cathet Cardiovasc Diagn* 1984;10:27.
19. Maher PR, Young C, Magnusson PT. Efficacy and safety of outpatient cardiac catheterization. *Cathet Cardiovasc Diagn* 1987;13:304.
20. Lee JC, et al. Feasibility and cost-saving potential of outpatient cardiac catheterization. *J Am Coll Cardiol* 1990;15:378.
21. Talley JD. The cost of performing diagnostic cardiac catheterization. *J Intervent Cardiol* 1994;7:273.
22. Kohli RS, Vetrovec GW, Lewis SA, Cole S. Study of the performance of 5 French and 7 French catheters in coronary angiography: a functional comparison. *Cathet Cardiovasc Diagn* 1989;18:131.
23. Judkins MP. Selective coronary arteriography, a percutaneous transfemoral technique. *Radiology* 1967;89:815.
24. Amplatz K, Formanek G, Stanger P, Wilson W. Mechanics of selective coronary artery catheterization via femoral approach. *Radiology* 1967;89:1040.
25. Fitzgibbon GM, Kafka HP, Leach AJ, Keon WJ, Hooper DG, Burton JR. Coronary bypass graft fate and patient outcome: angiographic follow-up of 5,065 grafts related to survival and reoperation in 1,388 patients during 25 years. *J Am Coll Cardiol* 1996;28:616.
26. Eisenhauer TL, Collier E, Cambier PA. Beneficial impact of aorto-coronary graft markers on post-operative angiography. *Cathet Cardiovasc Diagn* 1997;40:249.
27. Kuntz RE, Baim DS. Internal mammary angiography: A review of technical issues and newer methods. *Cathet Cardiovasc Diagn* 1990;20:10–16.
28. Ayres RW, et al. Transcatheter embolization of an internal mammary artery bypass sidebranch causing coronary steal syndrome. *Cathet Cardiovasc Diagn* 1994;31:301.
29. Breal JA, et al. Coronary-subclavian steal—an unusual cause of angina pectoris after successful internal mammary artery bypass grafting. *Cathet Cardiovac Diagn* 1991;24:274.
30. Bilazarian SD, Shemin RJ, Mills RM. Catheterization of coroanry artery bypass graft from the descending aorta. *Cathet Cardiovasc Diagn* 1990;21:103.

31. Mills NL, Everson CT. Right gastroepiploic artery: a third arterial conduit for coronary artery bypass. *Ann Thorac Surg* 1989;47:706.

32. Suma H, et al. The right gastroepiploic artery graft—clinical and angiographic mid-term results in 200 patients. *J Thorac Cardiovasc Surg* 1993;105:615.

33. Tanimoto Y, et al. Angiography of right gastroepiploic artery for coronary artery bypass graft. *Cathet Cardiovasc Diagn* 1989;16:35.

34. Sones FM, Shirey EK. Cine coronary arteriography. *Mod Concepts Cardiovasc Dis* 1962;31:735.

35. Schoonmaker FW, King SB. Coronary arteriography by the single catheter percutaneous femoral technique, experience in 6,800 cases. *Circulation* 1974;50:735.

36. Ovitt T, et al. Electrocardiographic changes in selective coronary arteriography: the importance of ions. *Radiology* 1972;102:705.

37. Tragardh B, Bove AA, Lynch PR. Mechanism of production of cardiac conduction abnormalities due to coronary arteriography in dogs. *Invest Radiol* 1976;11:563.

38. Paulin S, Adams DF. Increased ventricular fibrillation during coronary arteriography with a new contrast medium preparation. *Radiology* 1971;101:45.

39. Lasser EC, et al. Pretreatment with corticosteroids to alleviate reactions to intravenous contrast material. *N Engl J Med* 1987;317:845.

40. Parfrey PS, et al. Contrast material-induced renal failure in patients with diabetes mellitus, renal insufficiency, or both. *N Engl J Med* 1989;329:143.

41. Ritchie JL, et al. Use of nonionic or low osmolar contrast agents in cardiovascular procedures (ACC Position Statement). *J Am Coll Cardiol* 1993;21:269.

42. Harvey JR, et al. Use of balloon flotation pacing catheters for prophylactic temporary pacing during diagnostic and therapeutic catheterization procedures. *Am J Cardiol* 1988;62:941.

43. Dodge JT, Nykiel M, Altmann J, Hobkirk Km, Brennan M, Gibson CM. Coronary artery injection technique: a quantitative in vivo investigation using modern catheters. *Cathet Cardiovasc Diagn* 1998;44:34.

44. Ireland MA, et al. Safety and convenience of a mechanical injector pump for coronary angiography. *Cathet Cardiovasc Diagn* 1989;16:199.

45. The BARI protocol. Protocol for the Bypass Angioplasty Revascularization Investigation. *Circulation* 1991;84:V1.

46. Angelini P, Villason S, Chan AV, Diez JG. Normal and anmomalous coronary arteries in humans. In: Angelini P, ed. Coronary artery anomalies—a comprehensive approach. Philadelphia: Lippincott Williams & Wilkins, 1999.

47. Yamanaka O, Hobbs RE. Coronary artery anomalies in 126,595 patients undergoing coronary arteriography. *Cathet Cardiovasc Diagn* 1990;21:28.

48. Serota H, et al. Rapid identification of the course of anomalous coronary arteries in adults—the "dot and eye" method. *Am J Cardiol* 1990;65:891.

49. Ishikawa T, Brandt PWT. Anomalous origin of the left main coronary artery from the right aortic sinus—angiographic definition of anomalous course. *Am J Cardiol* 1985;55:770.

50. Shirani J, Roberts WC. Solitary coronary ostium in the aorta in the absence of other major congenital cardiovascular abnormalities. *J Am Coll Cardiol* 1993;21:137.

51. Cohen DJ, Kim D, Baim DS. Origin of the left main coronary artery from the "non-coronary" sinus of Valsalva. *Cathet Cardiovasc Diagn* 1991;22:190.

52. Aldridge HE. A decade or more of cranial and caudal angled projections in coronary arteriography—another look. *Cathet Cardiovasc Diagn* 1984;10:539.

53. Elliott LP, et al. Advantage of the cranial-right anterior oblique view in diagnosing mid left anterior descending and distal right coronary artery disease. *Am J Cardiol* 1981;48:754.

54. Grover M, Slutsky R, Higgins C, Atwood JE. Terminology and anatomy of angulated coronary arteriography. *Clin Cardiol* 1984; 7:37.

55. Taylor CR, Wilde P. An easily constructed model of the coronary arteries. *Am J Radiol* 1984;142:389.

56. Mintz GS, Popma JJ, Pichard AD, et al. Limitations of angiography in the assessment of plaque distribution in coronary artery disease: a systematic study of target lesion eccentricity in 1446 lesions. *Circulation* 1996;93:924.

57. Randall PA Mach bands in cine coronary arteriography. *Radiology* 1978;129:65.

58. Arnett EN, et al. Coronary artery narrowing in coronary heart disease: comparison of cineangiographic and necropsy findings. *Ann Intern Med* 1979;91:350.

59. Dodge JT, Brown BG, Bolson EL, Dodge HT. Lumen diameter of normal human coronary arteries—influence of age, sex, anatomic variation, and left ventricular hypertrophy or dilation. *Circulation* 1992;86:232.

60. Gould KL, et al. Physiologic basis for assessing critical coronary stenosis—instantaneous flow response and regional distribution during coronary hyperemia as measures of flow reserve. *Am J Cardiol* 1974;33:87.

61. Uren NG, et al. Relation between myocardial blood flow and the severity of coronary artery stenosis. *N Engl J Med* 1994; 330:1782.

62. Gibson CM, Cannon CP, Daley WL, et al. TIMI frame count: a quantitative method of assessing coronary artery flow. *Circulation* 1996;93:879.

63. Pijls NHJ, de Bruyne B, Peels K, et al. Measurement of fractional flow reserve to assess the functional severity of coronary-artery stenoses. *N Engl J Med* 1996;334:1703.

64. Gibson CM, Safian RD. Limitations of cineangiography—impact of new technologies for image processing and quantitation. *Trends Cardiovasc Med* 1992;2:156.

65. Stadius ML, Alderman EL. Coronary artery revascularization—critical need for and consequences of objective angiographic assessment of lesion severity. *Circulation* 1990;82:2231.

66. Scoblionko DP, et al. A new digital electronic caliper for measurement of coronary arterial stenosis—comparison with visual estimates and computer-assisted measurements. *Am J Cardiol* 1984; 53:689.

67. Gronenshild E, Jannsen J, Tijdent F. CAAS II—a second generation system for off-line and on-line quantitative coronary angiography. *Cathetet Cardiovasc Diagn* 1994;33:61.

68. Escaned J, Baptiwsta J, DiMario C, et al. Significance of automated stenosis detection during quantitative angiography: insights gained from intracoronary ultrasound imaging. *Circulation* 1996; 94:966.

69. Folland ED, Vogel RA, Hartigan P, et al. Relation between coronary artery stenosis assessed by visual, caliper, and computer methods and exercise capacity in patients with single-vessel coronary artery disease. *Circulation* 1994;89:2005.

70. Danchin N, Foley D, Serruys PW. Visual versus quantitative assessment of the severity of coronary artery stenoses—can the angiographer's eye be reeducated? *Am Heart J* 1993;126:594.

71. Ambrose JA, Hjemdahl-Monsen CE. Angiographic anatomy and mechanisms of myocardial ischemia in unstable angina. *J Am Coll Cardiol* 1987;9:1397.

72. Dangas G, Mehran R, Wallenstein S, et al. Correlation of angiographic morphology and clinical presentation in unstable angina. *J Am Coll Cardiol* 1997;29:519.

73. Mintz GS, Pichard AD, Popma JJ, et al. Determinants and correlates of lesion calcium in coronary artery disease: a clinical, angiographic and intravascular ultrasound study. *J Am Coll Cardiol* 1997;29:268.

74. Waxman S, Sassower MA, Mittleman MA, et al. Angioscopic predictors of early adverse outcome after coronary angioplasty in patients with unstable angina and non-Q-wave myocardial infarction. *Circulation* 1996;93:2106.

75. Fishbein MC, Siegel RJ. How big are coronary atherosclerotic plaques that rupture? *Circulation* 1996;94:2662.

76. Levin DC. Pathways and functional significance of the coronary collateral circulation. *Circulation* 1974;50:831.

77. Piek JJ, van Liebergen RAM, Koch KT, Peters TJG, David GK. Clinical, angiographic and hemodynamic predictors of recruitable collateral flow during balloon angioplasty of coronary occlusion. *J Am Coll Cardiol* 1997;29:275.

78. Seiler C, Fleisch M, Garachemani A, Meier B. Coronary collateral quantitation in patients with coronary artery disease using intravascular flow velocity or pressure measurements. *J Am Coll Cardiol* 1998;32:1272.

79. Levin DC, Fellows KE, Abrams HL. Hemodynamically significant primary anomalies of the coronary arteries. Angiographic aspects. *Circulation* 1978;58:25.

80. Click RL, et al. Anomalous coronary arteries: location, degree of atherosclerosis and effect on survival—a report from the Coronary Artery Surgery Study. *J Am Coll Cardiol* 1989;13:531.

81. Liberthson RR. Sudden death from cardiac causes in children and young adults. *N Engl J Med* 1996;334:1039.

82. Doorey AJ, et al. Six-month success of intracoronary stenting for anomalous coronary arteries associated with myocardial ischemia. *Am J Cardiol* 1000;86:580–582.

83. Newburger JW, et al. Diagnosis, treatment, and long-term management of Kawasaki Disease. *Circulation* 2004;110: 2747–71.

84. Papadakis MC, et al. Frequency of coronary artery ectasia in patients undergoing surgery for ascending aprtic aneurysms. *Am J Cardiol* 2004;94:1433–35.

85. Ge J, Erbel R, Rupprecht HJ, et al. Comparison of intravascular ultrasound and angiography in the assesssment of myocardial bridging. *Circulation* 1994;89:1725.

86. Klues HG, Schwarz ER, vom Dahl J, et al. Disturbed intracoronary hemodynamics in myocardial bridging: early normalization by intracoronary stent placement. *Circulation* 1997; 96:2905.

87. Dorros G, Thota V, Ramireddy K, Joseph G. Catheter-based techniques for closure of coronary fistulae. *Cathet Cardiovasc Diagn* 1999;46:143.

88. Sherwood MC, Rockenmacher S, Colan SD, Geva T. Prognostic significance of clinically silent coronary artery fistulas. *Am J Cardiol* 1999;83:407.

89. Yetman AT, McCrindle BW, MacDonald C, Freedom RM, Gow R. Myocardial bridging in children with hypertrophic cardiomyopathy—a risk factor for sudden death. *N Engl J Med* 1998; 339:1201.

90. Jennette JC, Falk RJ. Small-vessel vasculitits. *N Engl J Med* 1997; 337:1512.

91. Weis M, von Scheidt W. Cardiac allograft vasculopathy: a review. *Circulation* 1997;96:2069.

92. Om A, Ellaham S, Vetrovec GW. Radiation-induced coronary artery disease. *Am Heart J* 1992;124:1598.

93. Cohen S. Motor disorders of the esophagus. *N Engl J Med* 1979; 301:183.

94. Maseri A, Chierchia S. Coronary artery spasm: demonstration, definition, diagnosis, and consequences. *Prog Cardiovasc Dis* 1982;25:169.

95. Mark DB, et al. Clinical characteristics and long-term survival of patients with variant angina. *Circulation* 1984;69:880.

96. Waters DD, Theroux P, Szlachcic J, Dauwe F. Provocative testing with ergonovine to assess the efficacy of treatment with nifedipine, diltiazem and verapamil in variant angina. *Am J Cardiol* 1981;48:123.

97. Heupler FA, et al. Ergonovine maleate provocative test for coronary arterial spasm. *Am J Cardiol* 1978;41:631.

98. Sueda S, Kohno H, Fukuda H, et al. Frequency of provoked coronary spasms in patients undergoing coronary arteriography using a spasm provocation test via intracoronary administration of ergonovine. *Angiology* 2004;55:403–411.

99. Raizner AE, et al. Provocation of coronary artery spasm by the cold pressor test. *Circulation* 1980;62:925.

99. Sueda S, Kohno H, Fukuda H, et al. Induction of coronary artery spasm by two pharmacological agents: comparison between intracoronary injection of acetylcholine and ergonovine. *Coron Artery Dis* 2003;14:451–457.

100. Nakao K, Ohgushi M, Yoshimura M, et al. Hyperventilation as a specific test for diagnosis of coronary artery spasm. *Am J Cardiol* 1997;80:545.

101. Harding MB, Leithe ME, Mark DB, et al. Ergonovine maleate testing during cardiac catheterization—a 10 year perspective in 3,447 patients without significant coronary artery disease or Prinzmetal's variant angina. *J Am Coll Cardiol* 1992;20:107.

102. Cipriano PR, et al. The effects of ergonovine maleate on coronary arterial size. *Circulation* 1979;59:82.

103. Friedman AC, Spindola-Franco H, Nivatpumin T. Coronary spasm: Prinzmetal's variant angina vs. catheter-induced spasm; refractory spasm vs. fixed stenosis. *Am J Radiol* 1979;132:897.

104. Hays JT, Stein B, Raizner AE. The crumpled coronary artery—an enigma of arteriopathic pseudopathology and its potential for misinterpretation. *Cathet Cardiovasc Diagn* 1994;31:293.

105. Cannon RO III, Watson RM, Rosing DR, Epstein SE. Angina caused by reduced vasodilator reserve of the small coronary arteries. *J Am Coll Cardiol* 1983;1:1359–1373.

106. Cannon RO III, et al. Left ventricular dysfunction in patients with angina pectoris, normal epicardial coronary arteries, and abnormal vasodilator reserve. *Circulation* 1985;72:218–226.

107. Kurisu S, Sato H, Kawagoe T, et al. Tako-tsubo-like left ventricular dysfunction with ST-segment elevation: a novel cardiac syndrome mimicking acute myocardial infarction. *Am Heart J* 2002;143:448–455.

108. Sun H, Mohri M, Shimokawa H, et al. Coronary microvascular spasm causes myocardial ischemia in patients with vasospastic angina. *J Am Coll Cardiol* 2002;39:847–851.

Cardiac Ventriculography

12

Donald S. Baim[a]

Cardiac ventriculography is used to define the anatomy and function of the ventricles and related structures in patients with congenital, valvular, coronary, and myopathic heart disease (1–5). Specifically, left ventriculography may provide valuable information about global and segmental left ventricular function, mitral valvular regurgitation, and the presence, location, and severity of a number of other abnormalities such as ventricular septal defect, hypertrophic cardiomyopathy, or left ventricular mural thrombus. As a result, left ventriculography is often included as part of the routine diagnostic cardiac catheterization protocol in a patient being evaluated for coronary artery disease, aortic or mitral valvular disease, unexplained left ventricular failure, or congenital heart disease. Similarly, right ventriculography may provide information about global and segmental right ventricular function and can be especially helpful in patients with congenital heart disease, although right ventriculography is rarely performed in the adult cardiac catheterization laboratory.

INJECTION CATHETERS

To achieve adequate opacification of the left or right ventricle, it is necessary to deliver a relatively large amount of contrast material in a relatively short time. In adults, this is best done using a 6F, 7F, or 8F catheter with multiple side holes to allow rapid delivery of contrast material with the catheter remaining in a stable position in the midventricle to reduce the chance of arrhythmia. Catheters that have

only an end hole (such as the Cournand or multipurpose) are not well suited for left ventriculography, since the contrast jet out of the single end hole can cause the catheter to recoil during contrast delivery, potentially causing ventricular ectopic beats, inadequate ventricular opacification, and myocardial staining or even perforation.

Pigtail Catheter

The pigtail catheter (developed by Judkins) has several advantages over an end-hole-only design for left and right ventriculography (Fig. 12.1). Its end hole permits its insertion over a J-tipped guidewire so that the pigtail catheter can be advanced safely to the left ventricle from any arterial access site (see Chapter 4), even in the patient with brachiocephalic or iliac arterial tortuosity. The loop shape keeps the end hole away from direct contact with the endocardium, while multiple side holes on the several centimeters of catheter shaft proximal to the pigtail loop provide numerous simultaneous exit paths for contrast material. These offsetting jet directions help stabilize the catheter within the left ventricle during contrast injection and reduce the magnitude of catheter recoil. This virtually eliminates the possibility of endocardial staining, since the end hole usually is not positioned adjacent to ventricular trabeculae, and substantially reduces the occurrence of ventricular ectopic beats.

The pigtail usually passes easily across a normal aortic valve, either directly or by prolapsing across the valve leaflets. Passage across a stenotic aortic valve usually requires use of a straight leading guidewire (see Chapter 4). In patients with porcine aortic valve prosthesis, the pigtail generally passes across the bioprosthesis even more easily than straight catheters such as the multipurpose, since the pigtail

---

[a] David Hillis was a coauthor on this chapter in previous editions, and some of his contributed text remains in the current chapter.

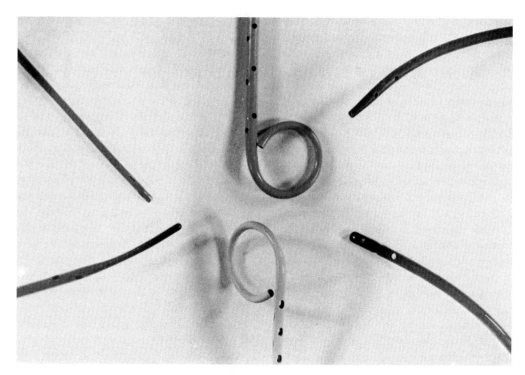

Figure 12.1 Examples of ventriculographic catheters (clockwise from the top): pigtail, 8F (Cook); Gensini, 7F; NIH, 8F; pigtail, 8F (Cordis); Lehman ventriculographic, 8F; Sones, 7.5F tapering to a 5.5F tip (see text for details).

configuration seems to prevent the catheter from sliding down into the lateral sinuses outside the support struts. Pigtail catheters can also be passed retrograde across a ball valve prosthesis (Starr-Edwards), but the resulting interference of the catheter shaft with seating of the ball during diastole may cause significant aortic regurgitation. Only the smallest-diameter (e.g., 4 F) catheter should be used for this purpose, dwell time across the valve should be kept to a minimum, and the patients should be monitored carefully for hemodynamic deterioration until the catheter is withdrawn from the left ventricle. Of course, no catheter should ever be passed across a tilting disc aortic valve prosthesis (Bjork-Shiley, Medtronic-Hall, or St. Jude) because of the risk that the catheter will be entrapped were it to pass through the smaller (minor) orifice of the valve.

The original Judkins pigtail design had a straight shaft leading up to the pigtail end. It was thus designed to sit directly under the aortic valve, and just in front of mitral inflow, relying on that inflow to distribute contrast to the apex of the left ventricle. In routine practice, this has been replaced by angled pigtail catheters, which have a 145 to 155° shaft angle at its distal end (just proximal to the side holes). This angle mimics that between the aortic root and the long axis of the left ventricle and helps the catheter achieve a central position within the left ventricle. This alignment may be improved further if the heart is pulled into a somewhat more vertical orientation by having the

patient take and maintain a deep breath during the left ventriculographic injection. Some authors have suggested that catheter manipulation and overall image quality are better with the angled than with the straight pigtail (6), but adequate ventriculography can be achieved with either shape.

Other Left Ventriculographic Catheters

The Sones catheter is used widely for left ventriculography when catheterization is performed from the brachial approach, although some operators prefer to use a pigtail catheter as described above. The polyurethane Sones catheter (80-cm Cordis SON-II, Sones Technique, Cordis Corporation, Miami, FL) is particularly suitable for left ventriculography because it has four side holes in addition to its end hole. The catheter comes in 6F, 7F, and 8F sizes and tapers to a smaller external diameter near its tip. The catheter will accept a 0.035-inch guidewire, which can be useful in crossing a severely stenotic aortic valve. Techniques for traversing a tortuous subclavian artery system and entering the left ventricle with the Sones catheter are discussed in Chapter 5. For left ventriculography, the Sones catheter should be positioned in an axial orientation (parallel to the ventricular long axis), with its tip midway between the aortic valve and left ventricular apex. Low injection rates (see below) usually minimize the extent and forcefulness of catheter recoil. Catheter recoil may still occur, however, with induction of multiple ventricular extrasystoles and potential danger of endocardial staining. Accordingly, the operator should hold the catheter during injection and be prepared to withdraw it if significant recoil develops.

The NIH and Eppendorf catheters have multiple side holes and no end hole (Fig. 12.1). They are easily inserted through an arteriotomy (by the brachial approach) or percutaneously through a femoral arterial sheath. The Cordis NIH (polyurethane) and Cook NIH Torcon blue (polyethylene) catheters are relatively soft and unlikely to cause dissection or perforation. The NIH and Eppendorf can be gently prolapsed across the aortic valve, but of course cannot be aided by a leading guidewire because of the lack of an end hole. The Lehman ventriculographic catheter has a tapered closed tip that extends beyond multiple side holes (Fig. 12.1). The tapered tip may assist the operator in manipulating the catheter through tortuous arteries and across a stenotic aortic valve. Once in the left ventricle, the tip lessens the likelihood of endocardial staining, but may increase the chance of ventricular ectopy during the injection of contrast material.

INJECTION SITE

The adequate opacification of either ventricle is accomplished only if a large amount of contrast material is delivered in a short time. Although satisfactory opacification of the left ventricle can sometimes be achieved by the injection of contrast material into the left atrium, this requires a transseptal catheterization, does not allow an evaluation of mitral valvular incompetence, and may obscure the basal portion of the left ventricle and the aortic valve. Similarly, the left ventricle may be opacified by aortography in patients with significant aortic regurgitation, and the right ventricle may be opacified by injecting contrast material into the venae cavae or right atrium. The best approach to ventriculography in the adult, however, is via injection of contrast material directly into the ventricular chamber in question.

In the left ventricle, the optimal catheter position is the midcavity, provided that ventricular ectopy is not a problem (Fig. 12.2). Such a midcavitary position ensures (a) adequate delivery of contrast material to the chamber's body and apex; (b) lack of interference with mitral valvular function, thus producing factitious mitral regurgitation; and (c) positioning of the holes through which the contrast material is injected

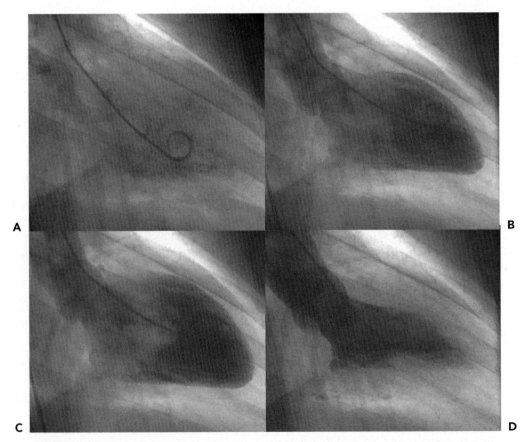

Figure 12.2 An example of midcavitary catheter position for 30° right anterior oblique left ventriculography using an angled pigtail catheter. **A.** Just before the injection of contrast material. **B.** At the end of rapid filling. **C.** At end-diastole (post A wave). **D.** End-systole.

away from ventricular trabeculae (a possible cause of endo-cardial staining). In some patients, however, the midcavitary position induces repetitive ventricular ectopy. In that case, the tip of the catheter is best repositioned so that it lies in the left ventricular inflow tract immediately in front of the posterior leaflet of the mitral valve (Fig. 12.3). This position is usually free of ventricular ectopy, but may produce mitral regurgitation if the catheter is too close to the mitral valve. In occasional patients with vigorous ventricular contraction, no stable midventricular position can be found for the catheter. The pigtail catheter can then be advanced into continuous contact with the left ventricular apex (assuming that there is no evidence of apical aneurysm of mural thrombus) to allow measurement of left ventricular pressure during stable rhythm and left ventriculography with the rate of contrast injection reduced to 10 mL/seconds (see below).

When the pigtail catheter is rotated in the left ventricle, it may pass under chordae. This can be suspected if the catheter shaft passes close to the inferior wall or exhibits an abrupt kink and can be confirmed if the loop of the pigtail opens up as the catheter is withdrawn back to the left ventricular outflow tract. Because the side holes on the catheter shaft are held in close proximity to the myocardial wall by the chordae, this position increases the risk of myocardial staining and should be corrected before ventriculography is performed. If repositioning the catheter would be difficult (as in a patient whose stenotic aortic valve has just been crossed) and ventriculography is required, a reduced injection rate should be used as described above for the Sones catheter.

In the right ventricle (Fig. 12.4), the optimal catheter position is the midcavity, provided that repetitive ventricular ectopy does not occur. If ectopy is uncontrollable, the catheter may be positioned in the outflow tract, just below the pulmonic valve. Even here, however, repetitive ventricular ectopy may present a difficult problem. In our experience, right ventriculography is often accompanied by frequent ventricular premature beats regardless of catheter position.

INJECTION RATE AND VOLUME

The rapid delivery of an adequate amount of contrast material requires the use of a power injector. Flow injectors (most commonly, the device manufactured by Medrad) allow one to select both the volume and the rate of delivery of contrast material. Sufficient pressure to deliver the selected volume of injectate in a selected time is automatically developed, although a maximal pressure limit of roughly 1,000 psi is set to minimize the risk of catheter burst. Of course, this high pressure is not actually delivered to the catheter tip, but is dissipated by frictional losses in the shaft of the catheter. Some injectors permit synchronization of the injection of contrast material with the R wave of the electrocardiogram, so that a set flow rate

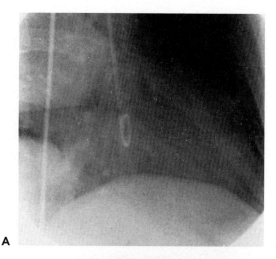

A

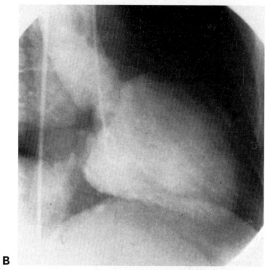

B

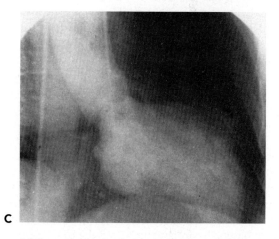

C

Figure 12.3 An example of a pigtail catheter positioned in the left ventricular inflow tract for 30° right anterior oblique left ventriculography. **A.** Before the introduction of contrast material. **B.** At end-diastole. **C.** End-systole. Note that this patient has a large anteroapical aneurysm with dyskinesis during systole.

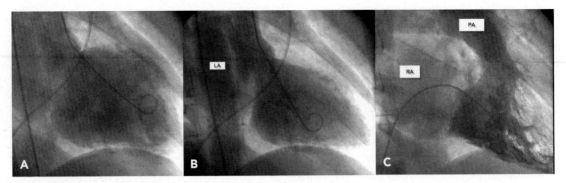

Figure 12.4   Mitral and tricuspid regurgitation. End-diastolic **(A)** and end-systolic **(B)** frames from a left ventriculogram performed in the 30° RAO projection in a patient with normal coronaries and presumptive AIDS cardiomyopathy, showing enlarged end-diastolic and end-systolic volumes, reduced ejection fraction of 38%, and 2+ mitral regurgitation. Note dye to the enlarged left atrial volume; the contrast density method underestimated the severity of regurgitation, shown to be moderately severe by a regurgitant fraction of 36% and transesophageal echo. End-systolic **(C)** frame from a right ventriculogram in the same patient performed in the 30° RAO projection showing 2+ tricuspid regurgitation (LA, left atrium; RA, right atrium; PA, pulmonary artery).

is delivered in each of several successive diastolic intervals (7). Although this technique has been said to lessen the incidence of ventricular ectopic beats and to minimize the volume of contrast material required for adequate ventricular opacification, our impression is that it offers no clear advantage over nonsynchronized methods.

Cine left ventriculography is accomplished using an injection rate and volume that depend on (a) the type and size of catheter, (b) the size of the ventricular chamber to be opacified, (c) the approximate ventricular stroke volume, and (d) the preventriculography hemodynamics. Different operators use different catheters and different injection parameters for left ventricular injection. In most cases performed with pigtail catheters, these parameters are 30 to 36 mL injected at 10 to 12 mL/second (i.e., a 3-second-long injection). Somewhat higher volume and rate may be used in patients with a high cardiac output or large ventricular chamber, and somewhat smaller volumes and rates may be used in smaller or irritable ventricles. When an end-hole (e.g., Sones or multipurpose) catheter is used for left ventriculography, the rate of injection of contrast material should not exceed 7 to 10 mL/second to minimize the chance of recoil and staining.

In the patient with hemodynamic evidence of severe left ventricular dysfunction (mean pulmonary capillary wedge pressure >25 mm Hg), left ventriculography should be performed using a low-osmolar contrast agent. These contrast agents have substantially improved the safety of left ventriculography in patients with depressed myocardial function, severe coronary artery disease, and/or aortic stenosis, as discussed in Chapter 2 (8–11). Even so, if filling pressures are markedly elevated, left ventriculography should be performed only once it has been reduced by the administration of intravenous nitroglycerin or sodium nitroprusside. With current radiographic equipment (12), low-osmolar contrast agents, and techniques using smaller amounts of contrast

material, it is a rare patient who cannot undergo left ventriculography safely. But failure to take a severely elevated preventriculography pulmonary capillary wedge pressure seriously can lead to disastrous consequences, including intractable pulmonary edema and even death. In any patient with increased risk (LV dysfunction, mural thrombus, renal insufficiency), one should always ask whether noninvasive means of assessing left ventricular function (see below) might not be preferable to contrast ventriculography.

Before performing a power injection of contrast material, one should take appropriate precautions in filling and firing the power injector to prevent air embolism. The injection syringe is made of siliconized plastic so that the contrast medium and any air may be easily seen. This syringe is usually loaded from a contrast bottle through a short U-shaped straw while the syringe barrel is pointed upward. With the injector still in the vertical position, 30-inch-long sterile roentgenography tubing is connected to the syringe, and all air is expelled from the syringe and tubing by holding the load switch in the forward position as the operator taps the syringe and its Luer-Lok connector to discharge all air bubbles. Alternatively, some laboratories fill the injector by connecting the sterile roentgenography tubing to the coronary manifold, drawing contrast from that supply (generally a slower process, more prone to bubble formation).

Only after all of the bubbles have been expelled in the nose-up position should the injector head be inverted. A fluid-to-fluid connection is accomplished by touching the meniscus of blood spurting from the hub of the catheter to the meniscus of contrast exiting the roentgenography tubing as the technician slowly advances the syringe plunger of the injector manually. When the connection is made, the injector operator stops advancing and begins retracting the plunger until the interface between contrast material and blood can be seen in the roentgenography tubing and verified to be free of air bubbles. Prior to the left ventriculographic run, a test injection of a small amount of contrast material is often performed under fluoroscopic visualization to enable the physician to assess catheter and patient position and confirm that ventricular ectopy does not occur. If the catheter is repositioned, another test injection is recommended before the definitive injection.

Prior to performing the angiogram, the physician should look closely at the injector syringe to confirm that it is filled with contrast medium, free of air, and oriented in the desired nose-down direction. He or she should grasp the catheter at its hub so that the catheter can be pulled back instantaneously if ventricular extrasystoles, myocardial staining, or other untoward events develop during injection. The technician or other individual firing the injector should be prepared to abort the injection on command from the physician operator in the event of an untoward occurrence. If extrasystoles develop, we withdraw the ventriculographic catheter a distance of approximately 2 to 3 cm slightly after the first extrasystole, which usually results in a quiet position for the remainder of the 3- to 4-second contrast injection.

Instructions to the patient regarding respiration during contrast ventriculography vary from laboratory to laboratory. Previously, imaging systems were often inadequate to give good definition of the left ventricular silhouette unless ventriculography was performed during deep inspiration to move the diaphragm out of the radiographic field. With modern imaging systems, excellent definition of the ventricular silhouette can be achieved without performing ventriculography during held deep inspiration. Left ven-

triculography done during normal quiet breathing allows physiologic interpretation of left ventricular volumes, angiographic stroke volume, and calculated left ventricular regurgitant fraction in cases of valvular regurgitation.

FILMING PROJECTION AND TECHNIQUE

Projections should be used that provide maximal delineation of the structure of interest and minimal overlapping of other structures. The 30° right anterior oblique (RAO) projection eliminates overlap of the left ventricle and the vertebral column, allows one to assess anterior, apical, and inferior segmental wall motion, and places the mitral valve in profile to provide a reliable assessment of the presence and severity of mitral regurgitation. The 60° left anterior oblique (LAO) view allows one to assess ventricular septal integrity and motion, lateral and posterior segmental function, and aortic valvular anatomy. To prevent the foreshortening of the left ventricle and visualize the entire length of the interventricular septum in profile, 15 to 20° cranial angulation should be added to the 60° LAO view, and the angiogram should be performed during a sustained deep inspiration to minimize obstruction by the diaphragm. This view visualizes a ventricular septal defect and the associated left-to-right shunting, or the septal bulge and systolic anterior motion in hypertrophic obstructive cardiomyopathy, or isolated lateral wall motion abnormalities (Figs. 12.5 and 12.6). For routine left or right ventricu-

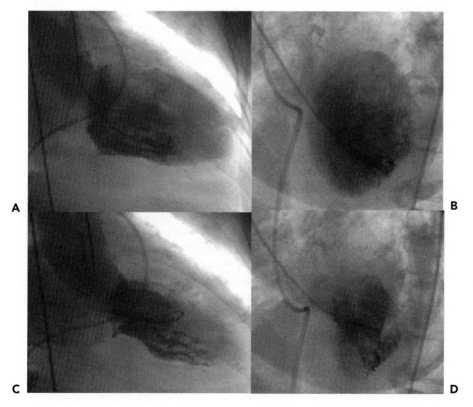

Figure 12.5 Biplane left ventriculogram in a patient with an acute lateral wall myocardial infarction owing to occlusion of the circumflex coronary artery. **A.** End-diastolic frame in the 30° RAO projection. **B.** End-diastolic frame in the 60° LAO, 15° cranial projection. **C.** End-systolic frame in the RAO projection showing midinferior wall hypokinesis and 3+ mitral regurgitation. **D.** End-systolic frame in the LAO projection showing akinesis of the lateral wall.

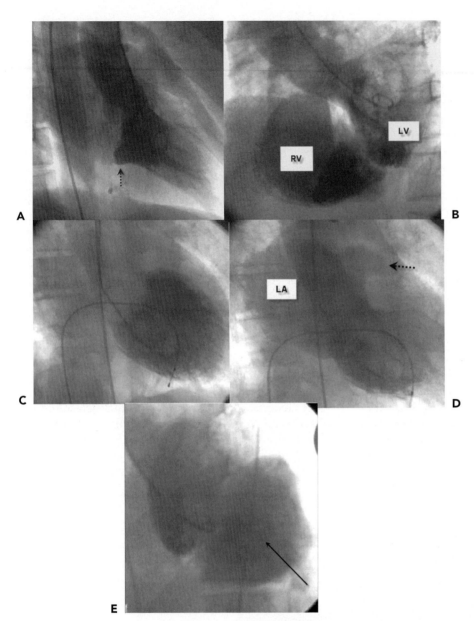

Figure 12.6 Various other pathology seen on left ventriculography. **A.** Mitral valve prolapse, with prolapse of a thickened posterior leaflet behind the fornix *(dotted arrow)* and mitral regurgitation in the RAO projection. **B.** Ventricular septal defect 3 days post inferior myocardial infarction owing to single-vessel right coronary occlusion, with contrast crossing from left to right ventricles in the LAO-cranial projection. **C and D.** Papillary muscle rupture 5 days post inferior myocardial infarction (diastolic and systolic frame respectively, showing dense contrast filling the left atrium and left atrial appendage *(arrow)*. **E.** Pseudoaneurysm (contained myocardial rupture, *arrow*) seen several weeks following a lateral wall myocardial infarction owing to single-vessel circumflex marginal disease.

lography, 30 frames per second using the 9-inch field of view allows the best temporal and spatial imaging, but many laboratories now use 15 frames per second for both ventriculography and coronary angiography to reduce radiation exposure (see Chapter 2).

If both RAO and LAO ventriculograms are indicated in a single-plane room, this requires two separate injections. If available, biplane ventriculography is thus preferable to single-plane ventriculography because it allows one to obtain more information at essentially no additional risk to the patient. In the patient with coronary artery disease, biplane left ventriculography provides more information on the location and severity of segmental wall motion abnormalities than does single plane ventriculography; in the patient with congenital heart disease biplane right ventriculography allows one to assess accurately the anatomy of the right ventricular outflow tract, the pulmonic valve, and the proximal

portions of the pulmonary artery. But biplane ventriculography has several disadvantages, including (a) the increased expense of biplane cineangiographic equipment; (b) the reduced quality of cineangiographic imaging in each plane owing to radiation scatter caused by the opposite plane; (c) the additional time required to position the biplane equipment appropriately, especially when the brachial approach is used; and (d) the additional radiation exposure to personnel in the room. In reality, most laboratories have only one biplane laboratory in their imaging suite, so that almost all left ventriculograms are done single plane.

ANALYSIS OF THE VENTRICULOGRAM

The left ventriculogram is analyzed both qualitatively and quantitatively on a normal sinus beat that follows a previous normal sinus beat in which the ventricle is well opacified. Evaluation of ectopic or postectopic beats will give a false impression of ventricular function. Overall ventricular dysfunction is described as hyperdynamic (>70 %), normal (50 to 69 %), mildly hypokinetic (35 to 49%), moderately hypokinetic (20 to 24%), or severely hypokinetic (<20%). Regional wall motion can be graded qualitatively as normal, hypokinetic, akinetic, or dyskinetic for each of the segments seen in the right anterior oblique projection (anterolateral, apical, inferior, posterobasal segments) and the left anterior oblique projection (basal septal, apical septal, apical lateral, basal lateral segments). Quantitative evaluation involves measurement of ejection fraction (the percent of end-diastolic volume that is ejected during systole), the absolute end-diastolic and end-systolic volumes (using the area-length method), and chord-by-chord local shortening (see Chapters 16 and 17).

The degree of mitral regurgitation can be estimated (on a scale of 1+ to 4+) by examining any systolic leakage of contrast from the left ventricle back into the left atrium and the opacification of the left atrium relative to the left ventricle, in the right anterior oblique projection (see Chapter 28) (Figure 12.6). In patients with a markedly enlarged left atrium from chronic mitral regurgitation, however, the dilution of the regurgitant contrast jet within this larger left atrial volume may lead to underestimation of regurgitation severity by the atrial density scale (Figure 12.4). A more quantitative method involves a comparison of the angiographic stroke volume (end-diastolic volume minus end-systolic volume) with the forward stroke volume (cardiac output divided by heart rate). These should be equal absent significant left-sided valvular regurgitation, but in patients with mitral (or aortic) regurgitation the angiographic stroke volume will be larger than the forward stroke volume (by an amount equal to the regurgitant volume). The severity of the regurgitant lesion can then be estimated by calculating the regurgitant fraction (the regurgitant volume, divided angiographic stroke volume), which indicates the percent of the volume ejected during each systole goes backwards into the left atrium rather than forwards into the aorta. Mild (1+) mitral regurgitation is usually associated with a regurgitant fraction <30%, moderate (2+) with a regurgitant fraction 30 to 39%, moderately severe (3+) with a regurgitant fraction 40 to 49%, and severe mitral regurgitation with a regurgitant fraction >50% (13).

INTERVENTION VENTRICULOGRAPHY

Permanent segmental dysfunction of the left ventricular wall can be caused by frank infarction, but reversible segmental dysfunction can also be caused by ischemia. This can be transient with brief ischemia (Fig. 12.7) more prolonged with stunning following a longer period of ischemia, or chronic with hibernation owing to sustained moderate ischemia, as with a collateralized chronic total occlusion

(14). Several angiographic techniques have been described to help determine if an asynergic segment of the left ventricle is infarcted or just ischemic. Segments whose abnormal wall motion is caused by ischemia generally show improvement in systolic motion, whereas segments whose abnormal wall motion is owing to infarction fail to improve, using these techniques.

For example, left ventricular segmental wall motion can be improved substantially by the administration of catecholamines (15). Two left ventriculograms are performed—the first in the resting (baseline) state, the second during a steady state infusion of epinephrine (1 to 4 mg/minute) or dobutamine (10 to 15 μg/kg per minute). Alternatively, left ventricular segmental wall dysfunction often can be improved by administration of nitroglycerin (16), either by improving collateral blood flow, reducing myocardial oxygen consumption to match available supply, or simply reducing the afterload against which the left ventricle must eject. Left ventricular segmental wall motion can be influenced by postextrasystolic potentiation (17) when a single ventricular premature beat is introduced during left ventriculography and is followed by a potentiated beat. Segmental wall motion during one of the preceding sinus beats is compared with that of the postextrasystolic beat and improvement on the potentiated beat compared with the preceding sinus beat suggests ischemia rather than infarction. It is probably unwise, however, to attempt to induce the ventricular extrasystole by manipulating the left ventriculographic catheter during the injection of contrast material since such manipulation may cause endocardial staining. Segments whose wall motion improves with intervention generally maintain this level of improvement after successful surgical revascularization; in contrast, segments in which contractile function is not influenced are generally not improved by revascularization. Other invasive (i.e., electromechanical mapping, see below) or noninvasive techniques for assessing myocardial viability (delayed thallium, PET, MRI) are more direct, however.

Other types of intervention ventriculography may be of use in the patient with chronic left ventricular volume overload caused by aortic or mitral regurgitation. In the patient with aortic regurgitation and well-preserved left ventricular function, angiotensin in a dose sufficient to increase left ventricular systolic pressure by 20 to 50 mm Hg causes no change in left ventricular ejection fraction (18). But if aortic regurgitation has caused a loss of left ventricular contractile reserve, a similar amount of angiotensin causes a fall in left ventricular ejection fraction of >0.10. Thus, left ventriculography during afterload stress may provide additional information about left ventricular functional capability. Alternatively, intervention ventriculography using sodium nitroprusside may be used in patients with mitral regurgitation, aortic regurgitation, or dilated cardiomyopathy to assess the potential benefit in hemodynamics and ventricular performance during chronic vasodilator therapy.

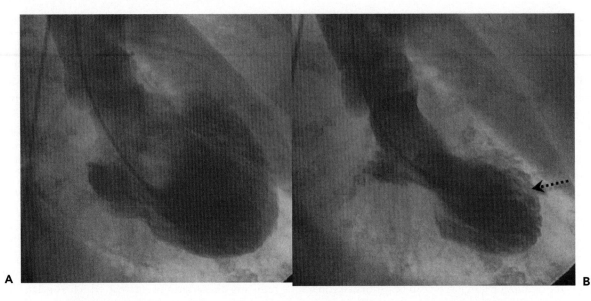

Figure 12.7 Tako-tsubo heart. A 71-year-old woman under extreme emotional stress presented with anterior ST-segment elevation, elevated creatine phosphokinase isoenzymes, and diffuse akinesis of the left ventricular apex (including both anterior and inferior aspects), resembling the shape of a Japanese octopus trap (tako-tsubo; narrow neck and round bottom), despite angiographically normal coronary arteries. Within 3 weeks, left ventricular function had returned to near normal. The mechanism is believed to be intense sympathetic arteriolar vasoconstriction involving the apical myocardium. (Case provided by Alan Yeung, M.D., Stanford University. See also Wittstein IS, et al, Neurohumoral features of myocardial stunning due to sudden emotional stress, *N Engl J Med* 2005; 352:539–548)

COMPLICATIONS AND HAZARDS

Although complications of cardiac catheterization and angiography are discussed in detail in Chapter 3, certain specific points relevant to ventriculography are presented here.

Arrhythmias

Ventricular extrasystoles occur frequently during ventriculography and are usually caused by mechanical stimulation of the ventricular endocardium by the catheter or a jet of contrast agent. Such extrasystoles can usually be eliminated or at least minimized by repositioning the catheter. Although short runs of ventricular tachycardia occur during an occasional ventriculogram, they almost always cease promptly when the catheter is removed from the ventricle. Rarely, the ventricular tachycardia caused by ventriculography is sustained even after catheter removal. It should be treated quickly with a bolus of intravenous lidocaine and, if necessary, direct current countershock. Ventricular fibrillation has been reported to be induced by an improperly grounded power injector (19).

Intramyocardial Injection (Endocardial Staining)

The deposition of contrast material within the endocardium and myocardium is usually caused by improper positioning of the ventriculographic catheter so that it passes under one of the papillary muscles or so that a side hole lies firmly against the endocardium. Although a small endocardial stain usually causes no problem, a large stain may lead to medically refractory ventricular tachyarrhythmias, including ventricular tachycardia or fibrillation. Rarely, the power injection of contrast material causes myocardial perforation, with the resultant leakage of blood and contrast material into the pericardial space and the development of cardiac tamponade. This must be treated by emergency pericardiocentesis and immediate consultation obtained from a cardiothoracic surgeon (see Chapter 32).

Fascicular Block

Because of the proximity of the anterior fascicle of the left bundle to the left ventricular outflow tract, transient left anterior fascicular block may occur during retrograde left heart catheterization. In the patient with underlying right bundle branch block and left posterior fascicular block, complete heart block may occur as the catheter is advanced into the left ventricle (20). Although temporary pacing is usually required, catheter-induced fascicular block usually resolves within 12 to 24 hours. Transient complete left bundle branch block is an extremely rare complication of retrograde left heart catheterization (21).

Embolism

The inadvertent injection of air or thrombus probably poses the greatest risk associated with ventriculography.

The risk of air embolization should be avoidable by good technique in filling the injector and confirming a bubble-free hookup as described above. The presence of thrombi on or within the ventriculographic catheter is minimized by frequent flushing of the catheter with a solution containing heparin when the ventriculographic catheter is first introduced and just prior to hooking up for the ventriculogram. If there is a suspicion (from noninvasive testing) of a thrombus in the left ventricular apex, great care should be taken to position the ventriculographic catheter in the left ventricular inflow tract, avoiding the apical portion completely, or avoided completely by relying on the noninvasive evaluation. Partially organized thrombi may also be dislodged from the left ventricular wall by the catheter tip or the force of a power injection. Accordingly, the ventricular angiographic catheter should not be advanced to the left ventricular apex except under exceptional circumstances (e.g., suspicion of idiopathic hypertrophic subaortic stenosis).

Complications of Contrast Material

For 20 to 30 seconds after ventriculography with a high-osmolar agent, the patient will experience a hot flash owing to the powerful vasodilation caused by the contrast material as it distributes throughout the arterial tree (see Chapter 2). Transient nausea and vomiting may also occur in 20 to 30% of patients. With current low-osmolar contrast agents, these complications are uncommon. With earlier ionic contrast agents, ventriculography produced a modest fall in systemic arterial pressure, a reflex increase in heart rate, and a transient depression of left ventricular contractility that resolved within 1 to 2 minutes.

ALTERNATIVES TO CONTRAST VENTRICULOGRAPHY

Echocardiographic Visualization of the Left Ventricle

Two-dimensional echocardiography may be used as an alternative to contrast ventriculography to assess global and regional left ventricular performance. Echocardiography is noninvasive, does not require exposure to radiation, and does not add to the contrast load of coronary angiography in patients at high risk for contrast-induced renal dysfunction. In a few subjects, echocardiography may fail to provide adequate images owing to extreme obesity or an increased anteroposterior chest dimension unless a transesophageal study is performed. In most patients, however, adequate images of the left ventricle can be acquired in multiple short- and long-axis planes to evaluate segmental and global left ventricular function as well as the degree of mitral regurgitation. Two-dimensional echocardiographic imaging also allows determination of left ventricular volumes using a

modification of Simpson's rule based on analysis of orthogonal long-axis views. The left ventricular volumes provided by echocardiography tend to be somewhat small, and the estimates of mitral regurgitation tend to be somewhat higher than those obtained with contrast ventriculography (13,22). Because two-dimensional echocardiography can be used to determine left ventricular wall thickness, it is an excellent method for quantitating left ventricular mass.

Magnetic Resonance Imaging (MRI) Ventriculography

MRI is another reliable alternative for measuring ventricular dimensions and evaluating regional wall motion. MRI images are acquired in a gated fashion throughout the cardiac cycle, and end-diastolic and end-systolic frames are identified. Because MRI images can be presented in any planes, a detailed assessment of regional wall motion can be accomplished in almost all subjects regardless of body shape or size. Left ventricular volumes are calculated using Simpson's rule (i.e., volume equals Σ area times slice thickness) in serial short-axis slices through the ventricle or from a single long-axis loop by applying the area-length method (as with contrast ventriculography). In general, MRI provides estimates of left ventricular volumes that are similar to those obtained with contrast ventriculography (23,24). As with two-dimensional echocardiography, MRI provides an accurate quantitation of left ventricular wall thickness, mass, perfusion, pericardial thickness, and partial information on valve function (Fig. 12.8; 25).

Electromechanical Mapping

Originally developed for electrophysiology, the Biosense electromechanical mapping catheter uses tip sensors to measure the relative strength of electromagnetic fields emitted by three coils positioned under the patient support, and thereby to calculate the exact position of the catheter tip in three dimensions (26,27). When the catheter is placed in contact with the left ventricular endocardium, the unipolar electrogram can be recorded from multiple locations within the left ventricle. Recording the motion of the catheter over the cardiac cycle allows calculation of cardiac volumes (including those at end-diastole and end-systole), local wall motion, and wall shortening. Areas of myocardial infarction show poor local shortening with low unipolar voltage. In contrast, areas with severe ischemia show reduced local shortening with retained unipolar voltage. Although more time consuming than contrast ventriculography, electromechanical mapping may provide more detailed assessment of ventricular function, the potential for recovery after revascularization (28), and a highly accurate way to deliver local therapies (direct myocardial revascularization, local drug injection, myocardial replacement therapy) to ischemic areas of the left ventricle.

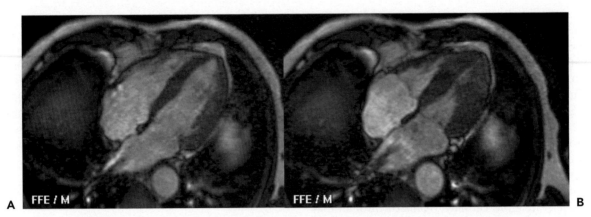

Figure 12.8   Frames from a magnetic resonance (MR) ventriculogram in end-diastole **(A)** and end-systole **(B)** in a patient with aortic stenosis, left ventricular hypertrophy, and preserved ejection fraction. MR and echo assessments of ventricular function should be used liberally in lieu of contrast ventriculography in patients with hemodynamic instability, mural thrombus, or limited contrast tolerance.

Electrical Conductance Catheter

If a multielectrode catheter is positioned along the long axis of the left ventricle (from the aortic valve to the apex) and current is passed between the proximal and distal-most electrodes, the voltage difference between pairs of interposed electrodes will reflect the local conductance and thus the regional blood volume (Fig. 12.9; see also Chapter 16). In actuality, this needs to be corrected for the parallel conductance of the surrounding myocardium by subtracting a correction volume determined by comparing the conductance-calculated stroke volume to the actual stroke volume. A second correction factor to the slope of the relationship between calculated conductance and actual volume is determined by monitoring the signal as 5 mL of

10% saline is injected into the pulmonary artery and passes through the left ventricle. The main application of conductance volume measurements includes monitoring of instantaneous pressure–volume loops in response to various drugs or interventions, and the recording of serial pressure–volume loops during balloon occlusion of the inferior vena cava allows a clinical definition of the end-systolic pressure–volume relationship as a measure of left ventricular function (29). This technique can also be used in the right ventricle or aorta to measure serial volume changes and compares favorably with echocardiographic, magnetic resonance, or nuclear methods (30). An FDA-approved catheter and system for ventricular conductance measurements are available from CD Leycom, Zoetermeer, NL (see www.cardiodynamics.nl).

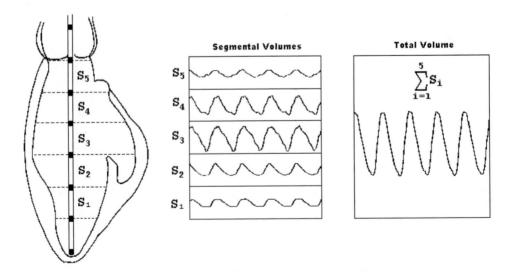

Figure 12.9   A left ventricular conductance (or impedance) catheter is shown in position along the left ventricular long axis, with calculated segmental volumes between each intervening electrode pair summed to provide the total instantaneous ventricular volume.

REFERENCES

1. Hildner FJ, et al. New principles for optimum left ventriculography. *Cathet Cardiovasc Diagn* 1986;12:266.
2. Grossman W. Assessment of regional myocardial function. *J Am Coll Cardiol* 1986;7:327.
3. Herman MV, Gorlin R. Implication of left ventricular asynergy. *Am J Cardiol* 1969;23:538.
4. Bruschke AVG, Proudfit WL, Sones FM Jr. Progress study of 590 consecutive nonsurgical cases of coronary disease followed 5–9 years, II: ventriculographic and other correlations. *Circulation* 1973;47:1154.
5. Rackley CE, Hood WP Jr. Quantitative angiographic evaluation and pathophysiologic mechanisms in valvular heart disease. *Prog Cardiovasc Dis* 1973;15:427.
6. Lehmann KG, Yang JC, Doria RJ, et al. Catheter optimization during contrast ventriculography: a prospective randomized trial. *Am Heart J* 1992;123:1273.
7. Schad N, et al. The intermittent phased injection of contrast material into the heart. *Am J Roentgenol* 1968;104:464.
8. Bourdillon PD, et al. Effects of a new nonionic and a conventional ionic contrast agent on coronary sinus ionized calcium and left ventricular hemodynamics. *J Am Coll Cardiol* 1985;6:845.
9. Salem DN, Konstam MA, Isner JM, Bonin JD. Comparison of the electrocardiographic and hemodynamic response to ionic and nonionic radiocontrast media during left ventriculography: a randomized double-blind study. *Am Heart J* 1986;111:533.
10. Benotti JR. The comparative effects of ionic versus nonionic agents in cardiac catheterization. *Invest Radiol* 1988;23(suppl 2):5366.
11. Wisneski JA, Gertz EW, Dahlgren M, Muslin A. Comparison of low osmolality ionic (ioxaglate) versus nonionic (iopamidol) contrast media in cardiac angiography. *Am J Cardiol* 1989;63:489.
12. Mancini GB, et al. Quantitative assessment of global and regional left ventricular function with low-contrast dose digital subtraction ventriculography. *Chest* 1985;87:598.
13. Dujardin KS, Enriques-Sarano M, Bailey KR, Nishimura RA, Seward JB, Tajik AJ. Grading of mitral regurgitation by quantitative Doppler echocardiography: calibration by left ventricular angiography in routine clinical practice. *Circulation* 1997;96:3409.
14. Kurisu S, Sato H, Kawagoe T, et al. Tako-tsubo-like left ventricular dysfunction with ST-segment elevation: a novel cardiac syndrome mimicking acute myocardial infarction. *Am Heart J* 2002;143:448–455.
15. Horn HR, et al. Augmentation of left ventricular contraction pattern in coronary artery disease by an inotropic catecholamine: the epinephrine ventriculogram. *Circulation* 1974;49:1063.
16. Helfant RH, et al. Nitroglycerin to unmask reversible asynergy: correlation with post coronary bypass ventriculography. *Circulation* 1974;50:108.
17. Dyke SH, Cohn PF, Gorlin R, Sonnenblick EH. Detection of residual myocardial function in coronary artery disease using postextrasystolic potentiation. *Circulation* 1974;50:694.
18. Bolen JL, et al. Evaluation of left ventricular function in patients with aortic regurgitation using afterload stress. *Circulation* 1976;53:132.
19. Rowe GG, Zarnstorff WC. Ventricular fibrillation during selective angiography. *JAMA* 1965;192:947.
20. McBride W, Hillis LD, Lange RA. Complete heart block during retrograde left-sided cardiac catheterization. *Am J Cardiol* 1989;63:375.
21. Shammas NW, Lee JK, Daubert JP, Pomerantz RM. Complete heart block complicating retrograde left ventricular catheterization: case report and review. *Cathet Cardiovasc Diagn* 1994;31:122.
22. Schiller NB, Shah PM, Crawford M, et al. Recommendations for quantitation of the left ventricle by two-dimensional echocardiography. *J Am Soc Echo* 1989;2:358.
23. Cranney GB, Lotan CS, Dean L, Baxley W, Bouchard A, Pohost GM. Left ventricular volume measurement using cardiac axis nuclear magnetic resonance imaging: validation by calibrated ventricular angiography. *Circulation* 1990;82:154.
24. Yang PC, Kerr AB, Liu AC, et al. New real-time interactive cardiac magnetic resonance imaging system complements echocardiography. *J Am Coll Cardiol* 1998;32:2049.
25. Woods T, Grist T, Rahko P. Leaking left ventricular pseudoaneurysm. *Circulation* 1999;100:329.
26. Gepstein L, Hayam G, Sshpun S, Ben-Haim SA. Hemodynamic evaluation of the heart with a non-fluoroscopic electromechanical mapping technique. *Circulation* 1997;96:3672.
27. Gepstein L, Goldin A, Lessick J, et al. Electromechanical characterization of chronic myocardial infarction in the canine coronary occlusion model. *Circulation* 1998;98:2055.
28. Samady H, et al. Electromechanical mapping identifies improvement in function and retention of contractile reserve after revascularization in ischemic cardiomyopathy. *Circulation* 2004;110:2410–2416.
29. Tulner SA, et al. Perioperative assessment of left ventricular function by pressure-volume loops using the conductance catheter method. *Anesth Analg* 2003;97:950–957.
30. White PA, Redington AN. Right ventricular volume measurement: can conductance do it better? *Physiol Meas* 2000;21:R23–R41.

PULMONARY ANGIOGRAPHY

13

Nils Kucher, M.D.   *Samuel Z. Goldhaber, M.D.*[a]

Although right heart catheterization was first described in 1929 (1), angiographic visualization of the pulmonary arteries was not performed until 1938 (2). Pulmonary angiography was performed initially using a nonselective technique (by intravenous injection of contrast material), to avoid venous cutdown, catheter manipulation, and fluoroscopy. Selective pulmonary arteriography recorded on serial cut films was then introduced by Sasahara and colleagues in 1964 (3). The basic objective remains visualization of the lumen of the main and branch pulmonary arteries, and current practice reflects advances in catheter design, the development of rapid digital imaging equipment, and the availability of safer radiographic contrast agents (see also Chapter 2).

Pulmonary angiography remains the gold standard technique for diagnosing pulmonary embolism and is also indicated for evaluating a variety of congenital and acquired diseases, such as pulmonary arteriovenous malformation, pulmonary artery stenosis and aneurysm, pulmonary vein stenosis, anomalous pulmonary venous return, pulmonary artery neoplasm, inflammation, and hemorrhage. Although the frequency of diagnostic pulmonary angiography has declined over the past decade as contemporary noninvasive imaging techniques, including multislice computed tomography (CT) and magnetic resonance (MR) imaging, have reached competitive diagnostic accuracy for diseases involving the pulmonary vasculature, there has been a recent resurgence as various catheter interventions on the pulmonary circulation, including balloon angioplasty with or without stent placement, mechanical

embolectomy, embolization, or foreign body retrieval, have been introduced (4). Although this procedure still remains largely the province of radiologists in many centers, invasive cardiologists should thus have a basic understanding of its technical aspects.

ANATOMY

The main pulmonary artery arises from the conus of the right ventricle, first anterior and then left of the aorta. It progresses 4 to 5 cm in a posteromedial direction before it bifurcates into the right and left pulmonary arteries.

The right pulmonary artery courses horizontally in the mediastinum, passing anterior to the right mainstem bronchus and posterior to the ascending aorta and superior vena cava. The right upper lobe branch (truncus anterior) arises within the mediastinum before reaching the right hilum and divides further into the three segmental upper lobe arteries (Fig. 13.1). The remainder of the right pulmonary artery continues as pars interlobaris until the origin of the middle lobe and upper lobe segmental arteries. From this point, the artery continues as pars basalis and gives rise to four segmental arteries of the lower lobe.

The smaller left pulmonary artery is a direct posterior continuation of the main pulmonary artery, crossing over the left mainstem bronchus before passing posterior to the bronchus as the pars superior. Thus, the proximal portion of the left pulmonary artery is foreshortened in a frontal view and is best seen in a left anterior oblique or lateral view. There is no large upper lobe branch, but a variable number of small segmental arteries supplying the left upper lobe originate from the outer aspect of the pars

[a] Drs. Lorraine K. Skibo and Lewis Wexler were authors of this chapter in the prior editions.

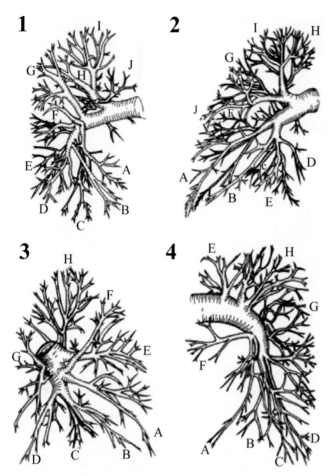

Figure 13.1 Segmental pulmonary arterial anatomy. Right lung, right anterior oblique view **(1)** and left anterior oblique view **(2)**. A, right middle lobe medial segmental artery; B, right lower lobe anterior basal segmental artery; C, right lower lobe lateral basal segmental artery; D, right lower lobe posterior basal segmental artery; E, right lower lobe medial basal segmental artery; F, right middle lobe lateral segmental artery; G, right lower lobe superior segmental artery; H, right upper lobe posterior segmental artery; I, right apical segmental artery; J, right upper lobe anterior segmental artery. Left lung, right anterior oblique view **(3)** and left anterior oblique view **(4)**. A, lingula, inferior segmental artery; B, left lower lobe anteromedial basal segmental artery; C, left lower lobe lateral basal segmental artery; D, left lower lobe posterior basal segmental artery; E, left upper lobe anterior segmental artery; F, lingula, superior segmental artery; G, left lower lobe superior segmental artery; H, left upper lobe apical-posterior segmental artery. (Reprinted with permission from Kandarpa K, ed. *Handbook of Cardiovascular and Interventional Radiology*, Little Brown and Company, 1988)

superior. The pars interlobaris and basalis give rise to two lingular and four lower lobe segmental arteries.

Within the lung, the vessels branch in either a bifurcational (two branches of similar size) or collateral (one small branch at a 30 to 80° angle, and a larger branch of similar size as the parent) pattern. The lobar and segmental branching is remarkably variable, and there are many supernumerary branches that outnumber conventional branches and penetrate the lung directly (5). Each segmental artery supplies a pulmonary perfusion segment

(Fig. 13.2), as resolved on conventional nuclear pulmonary scans.

The segmental pulmonary veins are variable within the lung parenchyma. Ultimately, however, they form a superior and an inferior vein on each side before they enter the left atrium. The left veins, however, may merge to form a common vein within the pericardium (5).

PROCEDURE

Hemodynamic Measurements

Patients who need pulmonary angiography are often acutely ill and may require continuous blood pressure measurements and electrocardiographic monitoring. Sinus bradycardia or heart block may occur as vascular access is gained. Complete heart block during right heart catheterization can also occur owing to impact of the right bundle branch in patients with underlying left bundle branch block, necessitating temporary pacing. Transient supraventricular and ventricular arrhythmias are also common during catheter advancement through the right heart chambers, and sustained tachyarrhythmias with hemodynamic impairment may necessitate electrical cardioversion.

An important part of the procedure is formal hemodynamic measurements (both pressures and oxygen saturation) during catheter advancement. The coronary sinus is occasionally entered while trying to access the right ventricular outflow tract (particularly from subclavian, jugular, or brachial access route). To minimize the risk of perforation, catheter advancement should be halted if a right atrial pressure wave form continues to be present as the catheter is advanced across the spine into what should fluoroscopically be the right ventricle. Catheter position in the coronary sinus may be confirmed or excluded by using a right anterior oblique or left lateral view, withdrawal of desaturated blood (saturation approximately 20%), or a gentle contrast injection through the catheter. Damping of the pressure in the main pulmonary artery may indicate the presence of massive pulmonary embolism (PE), with the catheter holes embedded in the embolus. In that situation, a hand injection of contrast can confirm the diagnosis.

The formal hemodynamics prior to angiography (Table 13.1) may also suggest the presence of congestive heart failure, valvular disease, intracardiac shunts, pulmonary hypertension, or pericardial disease. Severe hemodynamic embarrassment may also require modification of the angiographic procedure, including catheter selection and placement, injection rates, and image recording modes. In particular, complications of pulmonary angiography are more common in patients with pulmonary hypertension (particularly in the presence of right ventricular dysfunction) mandating special precautions such as supplemental oxygen,

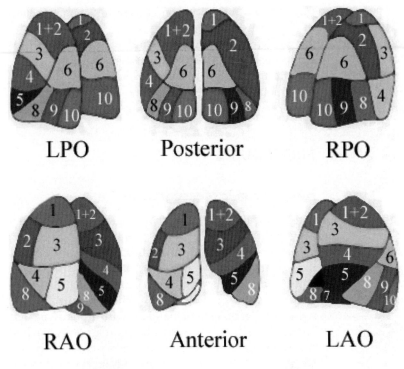

LPO   Posterior   RPO

RAO   Anterior   LAO

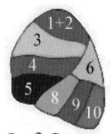

Right Lateral   Left Lateral

Figure 13.2 Pulmonary artery perfusion segments. **Top.** Left posterior oblique (LPO), posterior, and right posterior oblique (RPO) views. **Center.** Right anterior oblique (RAO), anterior, and left anterior oblique (LAO) views. **Bottom.** Right and left lateral views. Left lung, upper lobe: S1+2, apical posterior; S3, anterior; S4, superior lingular; S5, inferior lingular. Left lung, lower lobe: S6, superior; S8, anterior medial basal; S9, lateral basal; S10, posterior basal. Right lung, upper lobe: S1, apical; S2, posterior; S3, anterior. Right lung, middle lobe: S4, lateral; S5, medial. Right lung, lower lobe: S6, superior; S7, medial basal; S8, anterior basal; S9, lateral basal; S10, posterior basal.

TABLE 13.1

HEMODYNAMIC MEASUREMENTS (NORMAL RANGES)

Right atrial pressure, mm Hg	Mean	8–10
	A wave	2–10
	V wave	2–10
Right ventricular pressure, mm Hg	Systolic	15–30
	End-diastolic	0–8
Pulmonary artery pressure, mm Hg	Mean	10–20
	Systolic	15–30
	End-diastolic	3–12
Pulmonary capillary wedge pressure, mm Hg	Mean	5–12
	A wave	3–15
	V wave	3–12
Arteriovenous oxygen difference, mL/L		30–50
Cardiac output, L/min		4.0–8.0
Cardiac index, L/min per m^2		2.6–4.6
Pulmonary vascular resistance,* Wood units		0.7–1.1

* Mean pulmonary artery pressure − pulmonary capillary wedge pressure)/cardiac output.

reduced amounts of contrast agent, or superselective rather than mainstream pulmonary artery injections (6).

Venous Access

The right common femoral vein is the preferred venous access site, because it provides a relatively straight course to the inferior vena cava and right heart. In patients with suspected proximal deep vein thrombosis, ultrasound examination may be considered prior to vascular entry. In some patients, vascular access via the left femoral vein is precluded owing to an abrupt angle of the left iliac vein with the inferior vena cava. To minimize the risk of dislodging thrombi during catheter advancement (7), manual injection of 10 to 15 mL of contrast into the femoral vein may help to exclude massive iliac or caval vein thrombosis prior to advancing the catheter to the right heart.

Upper extremity venous access may be used in patients with proximal lower extremity deep vein thrombosis, inferior vena cava thrombosis, or groin infection. The right

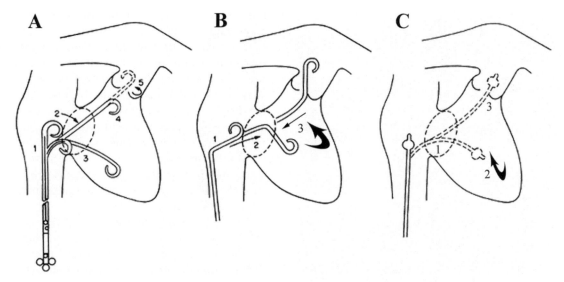

Figure 13.3 Techniques for pulmonary artery catheterization. **A.** Straight body pigtail catheter and tip-deflecting wire. The pigtail catheter is placed in the right atrium (1). The wire is deflected to point toward the right ventricle (2). The wire is fixed, and the catheter is advanced over it into the right ventricle (3). The tip deflection is released (4). Counterclockwise rotation of the catheter swings the pigtail anteriorly (5). Simultaneous advancement of the catheter places it into the main pulmonary artery. Advancing the catheter farther usually takes it into the left main pulmonary artery. The tip-deflecting wire is used to direct the catheter downward and to the right for right main pulmonary artery catheterization. **B.** Grollman pulmonary artery catheter. The pigtail catheter is placed in the right atrium (1). The anteromedial portion of the right atrium is probed to facilitate catheter entry into the right ventricle (2). The catheter is then slightly withdrawn and rotated counterclockwise to allow entry into the right ventricular outflow tract and main pulmonary artery (3). **C.** Balloon-tipped catheter. The balloon is inflated under fluoroscopic guidance in the common iliac vein, and the catheter is advanced under observation into the right atrium (1). The catheter is then rotated anteromedially to facilitate direct entry into the right ventricle (2). As soon the tricuspid valve is passed, documented by a right ventricular pressure waveform, the catheter is rotated to point the balloon tip cranially toward the right ventricular outflow tract before advancing it farther (3). Deep inspiration of the patient may facilitate flow-directed entry of the balloon tip from the outflow tract into the main pulmonary artery, with a preference to enter the left pulmonary artery.

heart may be approached easily with a balloon-directed catheter when gaining vascular access via the internal jugular vein (8; Chapter 4). The basilic vein at the antecubital fossa can also provide adequate access, but the cephalic vein is not suitable since it enters the axillary vein at an abrupt angle.

Catheterization Techniques

Most catheters used for diagnostic pulmonary angiography are between 5F and 7F to provide a lumen that will accommodate contrast injection rates of 20 to 25 mL/second. A 4F nylon pulmonary catheter allows flow rates of 20 mL/second at 1,050 psi (9) and may reduce access site complications. Recognizing that there are many techniques for selectively catheterizing the right and left pulmonary arteries, we describe three common approaches in Fig. 13.3. The presence of a properly placed inferior vena caval filter does not necessarily preclude a transfemoral approach. Safe transfilter angiography has been reported by passing straight or J-tipped guidewires followed by catheters through stainless steel Greenfield, Vena-Tech, and Bird's

Nest filters (10). It is important to insert and withdraw catheters only while they are straightened over a wire to minimize the likelihood of the catheter hooking onto the filter. During interventional procedures that involve multiple catheter exchanges, a long sheath may be placed with its leading tip beyond the filter.

Catheters for pulmonary arteriography are of two basic designs. The pigtail type catheters have multiple side holes whereas the curled catheter tip allows safe passage through the right heart. The pulmonary pigtail should be tighter than that used in the left heart (i.e., <1 cm in diameter) to permit use of the same catheter for subselective injections. All pigtail catheters must be removed from the pulmonary arteries only after straightening with a floppy-tip guidewire under fluoroscopic observation, since the catheter tip may otherwise engage a papillary muscle, chordae tendineae, or tricuspid valve leaflet during withdrawal. In contrast, the balloon-tipped catheters are assisted by blood flow through the right heart chambers and into the pulmonary arteries. Side holes in the catheter shaft then allow power injection in the main branches while the catheter end-hole makes balloon occlusion angiography possible with the

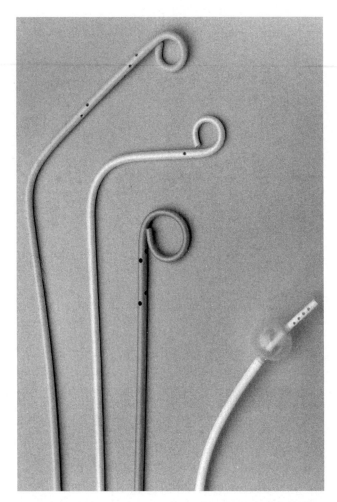

Figure 13.4 Catheters for pulmonary angiography. **Left to right.** Nyman, Grollman, and straight pigtail catheters (Eppendorf type), and the balloon occlusion catheter with side holes distal to the balloon (Berman type).

same catheter (Fig. 13.4). Balloon catheters are first deflated and can then be removed without fluoroscopy.

The most common pigtail catheter is the Grollman pulmonary artery catheter (Cook Inc., Bloomington, IN). This 6.7F polyethylene catheter has a 90° reversed secondary curve 3 cm proximal to the pigtail (Fig. 13.4; 11). It can be advanced easily into virtually any segmental artery with a low risk of the pigtail getting caught in the trabeculated right ventricle. If the catheter tip becomes stuck in the right ventricular outflow tract, having the patient take a deep breath may help straighten the soft catheter shaft and allow passage into the main pulmonary artery. If this maneuver is not successful, use of a soft-tipped J guidewire may facilitate catheter entry into the main pulmonary artery, but care with extruding any wire in the right ventricle is in order to avoid perforation. In challenging cases, the pulmonary artery can be catheterized using a conventional large-lumen balloon flotation catheter, with placement of an exchange-length J-tipped guidewire in

the pulmonary artery, and subsequent advancement of the angiographic pigtail over that wire.

In patients with right atrial enlargement, the right ventricle may be difficult to probe with the standard Grollman catheter because the distal end of the catheter may be too short to allow direct passage. In this case, the 90° angle of the distal tip may be increased by introducing a manually bent proximal end of a guidewire (12). The van Aman catheter is a 7F polyurethane modified Grollman catheter with a 90° reversed secondary curve 6 cm (rather than 3 cm) proximal to the pigtail and has been successfully used for pulmonary artery catheterization in patients with right heart enlargement (13).

The 7F Berman balloon catheter (Critikon Inc., Tampa, FL) has no end-hole, can therefore not be used with a guidewire, and requires introduction through a venous sheath. From the jugular or brachial approach, the catheter follows a continuous curve through the outflow tract and into the right pulmonary artery. The right pulmonary artery may be catheterized from below by using a reverse curve in which the Berman catheter is curved against the lateral right atrial wall before crossing the tricuspid valve, so that it enters the right ventricle pointing up as though it were coming from above. This approach is particularly helpful in the presence of tricuspid regurgitation, since the right atrial catheter loop provides more backup when advancing the catheter than seen with direct transit of the tricuspid valve from below. Catheterization of the left pulmonary artery is frequently more difficult, and may require the use of deflection guidewires into the angiographic catheter if standard attempts at catheter manipulation are unsuccessful.

Preferred catheters for the brachial approach include a 5F nonreversed Grollman catheter or a 5F multiple-bend pigtail catheter (Cordis Corp., Miami, FL; 14,15). Direct catheter entry into the right ventricle may be difficult using the brachial approach. Looping the catheter around the right atrial free wall, counterclockwise rotation, and gentle retraction are necessary to probe the right ventricle.

Contrast Agents and Injection Rates

Low-osmolar contrast agents with an iodine concentration of at least 300 μg/L are recommended for pulmonary angiography (see Chapter 2). The reduction in cough reflex, flushing, hypotension, and nausea with these nonionic agents promotes motion-free image acquisition (16).

In vitro activation of platelets has been reported with the low-osmolar agents iohexol and iopamidol (17). One study found increased plasma levels of plasminogen activator inhibitor-1 in patients following pulmonary angiography with iohexol and increased thrombin-antithrombin III complexes with iohexol and ioxaglate (18). Newer isosmolar nonionic agents have not been tested in patients undergoing pulmonary angiography, but the isosmolar nonionic dimer iodixanol appears to reduce major

TABLE 13.2

SUGGESTED CONTRAST INJECTION RATES (INJECTED OVER 2 SECONDS)

Injection Site	Cut Film	DSA
Right atrium pulmonary mainstem	40–50 mL	30–40 mL
Right/left main pulmonary artery	30–40 mL	20–30 mL
Lobar pulmonary arteries	20–30 mL	20 mL
Segmental pulmonary arteries	10–15 mL	5–10 mL

DSA, digital subtraction angiography.

adverse cardiovascular events compared with low-osmolar ionic contrast in patients with acute coronary syndromes who undergo percutaneous coronary intervention (19). Compared with iohexol, iodixanol also reduced contrast nephropathy in patients undergoing coronary or aortofemoral angiography (20).

The contrast injection rate is determined by the rate of blood flow in the selected vessel, pulmonary artery pressure, imaging modes, and the catheter used for angiography. Less contrast is necessary for digital imaging techniques to obtain adequate diagnostic-quality opacification of segmental and subsegmental arteries (Table 13.2). As smaller vessels are selected for the injection site, the rate and volume are decreased accordingly. Contrast injection should be performed using an automated injector system at a pressure of 600 psi (42 kg/cm^2). For balloon occlusion angiography of segmental vessels, a hand injection of 5 to 10 mL is used. In the presence of pulmonary hypertension, the amount of contrast should be reduced to minimize the adverse hemodynamic impact that may be seen with full contrast injection under those circumstances (21).

Imaging Modes

Digital techniques have virtually replaced conventional cut films. Hagspiel et al. (22) found digital subtraction angiography (DSA) with selective pulmonary arterial injections equivalent to conventional cut-film angiography in diagnostic performance and image quality. In 80 patients, DSA allowed more accurate detection of pulmonary emboli with better interobserver agreement than conventional cut film (23). In 54 patients with suspected PE but a negative digital angiogram, none suffered a thromboembolic event after a mean of 12 months (24).

The major advantage of DSA over cut film is that less contrast agent is required to obtain high-resolution images. This is particularly important for evaluation of patients with pulmonary hypertension and renal insufficiency. Other advantages include rapid image acquisition and flexible display format. Images can be viewed individually or in cine format on the monitor, in either their subtracted or unsubtracted mode. Masks can be selected image by image and

their pixels shifted to best match the anatomy. In addition, DSA may even allow satisfactory opacification of pulmonary arteries when contrast is injected into the superior vena cava or right atrium. The major disadvantage of DSA is the requirement for motionless image acquisition. This may be especially difficult in the evaluation of patients with severe cardiopulmonary symptoms, who may not be able to hold their breath during image acquisition. Mask shifting helps minimizing cardiac motion artifacts but is less helpful in reducing respiratory motion artifacts. But although serial cut film still has greater spatial resolution than cineradiography or DSA, there is no evidence that DSA is inferior to serial cut film in the detection of subsegmental PE.

Filming rates are based on the normal transit of contrast through the lung. Injected contrast reaches the capillaries in 2 to 3 seconds while the left atrium fills in 4 to 6 seconds (25). With cut film, a total of 12 images are usually obtained: 3 per second in 3 seconds, and 1 per second for an additional 6 seconds. With digital systems, a full second of mask images are obtained before injection (about one cardiac cycle), with ongoing acquisition at six images per second. Higher rates may be used in uncooperative patients, in large individuals, or in situations where high flow is expected (for example in pulmonary arteriovenous malformations). Slower acquisition rates are recommended for patients with low cardiac output.

A minimum of two radiographic series are required for each lung to exclude pulmonary embolism. The two standard views are the frontal and 45° ipsilateral posterior oblique view. These views have been validated for pulmonary embolism in a large clinical trial (26). If it is available, *biplane* filming is preferred over monoplane filming to reduce the total amount of contrast. Although the lateral is the true orthogonal view to the frontal projection, it is not desirable for most cases of pulmonary angiography, since even selective right or left injections frequently cause reflux into the opposite lung that may confuse interpretation. If a sufficient amount of contrast (40 to 50 mL) is injected and prolonged filming is carried out, the lateral and oblique views may also be used to evaluate left ventricular size and function as well as the anatomy of the ascending aorta or proximal coronary arteries.

Complications and Contraindications

Major complications can be defined as those that are life threatening or require intervention or intensive monitoring. Minor complications can be defined as those that regress spontaneously without long-term morbidity, even if patients require prolonged monitoring. The complications seen during the Prospective Investigation of Pulmonary Embolism Diagnosis (PIOPED; 26) study were tabulated according to these definitions (Table 13.3). Of note, the study involved injecting high-osmolar ionic contrast through pigtail catheters with images recorded on cut film.

TABLE 13.3

COMPLICATIONS OF PULMONARY ANGIOGRAPHY IN THE PIOPED STUDY (N = 1,111)

Major		
Death	5	(0.5%)
CPR, ventilation	4	(0.4%)
Renal failure (dialysis)	3	(0.3%)
Hematoma (2-unit transfusion)	2	(0.2%)
Total	14	(1.3%)
Minor		
Respiratory distress	4	(0.4%)
Renal dysfunction	10	(0.9%)
Angina	2	(0.2%)
Hypotension	2	(0.2%)
Pulmonary congestion	4	(0.4%)
Urticaria, itching, or periorbital edema	16	(1.4%)
Hematoma	9	(0.81%)
Arrhythmia	6	(0.54%)
Subintimal contrast (dissection)	4	(0.4%)
Narcotic overdose	1	(0.1%)
Nausea and vomiting	1	(0.1%)
Right bundle branch block	1	(0.1%)
Total	60	(5.4%)

From Baum S, ed. *Abrams Angiography*. Boston: Little, Brown and Co, 1997.

Three of the five deaths reported by Stein and colleagues may have been owing to severe baseline cardiopulmonary compromise rather than catheterization or angiography (26). In one study, three deaths occurred in the presence of a right ventricular end-diastolic pressure >20 mm Hg (7).

Unlike previous large series, no myocardial perforations occurred in PIOPED, attributed to the exclusive use of pigtail type rather than straight catheters, such as the Eppendorf. Renal failure and insufficiency occurred in the PIOPED group in 0.3% and 1.0%, respectively, more often in elderly patients (26).

There are no absolute contraindications to pulmonary angiography, although risk clearly increases with severe pulmonary hypertension, allergy to iodine contrast, renal insufficiency, left bundle branch block, or severe congestive heart failure (21). With the use of nonionic, low-osmolar contrast and prophylactic oxygen administration, these risks may be reduced (27). In patients with a history of anaphylactoid reaction to intravenous contrast, we advise use of preprocedural corticosteroids and nonionic low-osmolar contrast agents.

PULMONARY EMBOLISM

The annual incidence of venous thromboembolism—deep vein thrombosis and pulmonary embolism (PE)—exceeds 1 per 1,000 (28). The main cause of early death is acute right ventricular failure, although most deaths beyond 30 days are owing to underlying disease (e.g., cancer, congestive heart failure, or chronic lung disease; 29). The overall 3-month mortality is approximately 15% (30).

Diagnosis

PE may not be suspected, because it can mimic a wide spectrum of medical diseases. Common differential diagnoses are thus chronic lung disease, congestive heart failure, pneumonia, acute myocardial infarction, aortic dissection, pericarditis, cancer, pneumothorax, musculoskeletal pain, and anxiety states. The most common symptoms include dyspnea, chest pain, cough, and hemoptysis. Pleuritic pain is most often present in patients with segmental PE. The presence of syncope and severe painless dyspnea usually indicate a hemodynamically significant PE, particularly when accompanied by tachycardia and tachypnea. Clinical signs of right ventricular dysfunction may include distended neck veins, an accentuated pulmonic component of the second heart sound, or a right ventricular heave. Occasionally, the murmur of tricuspid regurgitation may be present.

Assessment of the *clinical pretest probability* helps improve the diagnostic accuracy of any test in patients with suspected PE. Wells and coworkers (31) have prospectively tested a bedside assessment to estimate this probability based on signs or symptoms of deep vein thrombosis (DVT) (3 score points), no alternative diagnosis is more likely than PE (3 score points), a heart rate >100 beats per minute (1.5 score points), immobilization or surgery within 4 weeks (1.5 score points), a history of DVT or PE (1.5 score points), hemoptysis (1.0 score points), and cancer (1.0 score point). A score ≤4.0 using this schema makes the presence of PE unlikely.

Nonimaging Tests

Electrocardiography

The ECG will exclude acute ST-segment elevation myocardial infarction and may help establish the diagnosis of PE in the presence of a classic S1Q3T3 pattern, incomplete or complete right bundle branch block, right axis deviation, or clockwise rotation in the precordial leads. The Qr pattern in V1 and inverted T waves in the anterior precordial leads indicate hemodynamically significant PE with an increased risk for adverse clinical events (32).

D-Dimer

D-dimer is a specific proteolytic degradation product of cross-linked fibrin via endogenous fibrinolysis. In a pulmonary angiography study, a plasma D-dimer of <500 ng/m (performed with quantitative enzyme-linked immunosorbent assay [ELISA]) had a >90% negative predictive value for excluding PE (33). In another study, the negative predictive value was 99.6%, whereas in an overview the ELISA D-dimer test had a sensitivity of 94%, suggesting that fewer imaging studies may be required in patients with negative D-dimer measurements (34). The specificity of the D-dimer test, however, was only 45% in outpatients with suspected PE (35). Owing to this very low specificity, the D-dimer measurement is not very useful in hospitalized patients with suspected PE, being best suited for the Emergency Department or office setting.

Arterial Blood Gas Analysis

Arterial blood gases (36) and alveolar-arterial oxygen gradients (37) are not helpful in differentiating patients with confirmed or excluded PE by pulmonary angiography. Therefore, arterial blood gases should not be obtained as a screening test, absent respiratory compromise.

Noninvasive Imaging Tests

Ventilation Perfusion Scanning

Lung scanning has been the principal imaging test for suspected PE. However, an increasing number of hospitals obtain lung scans only in patients with allergy to radiographic contrast agents, severe renal insufficiency, or pregnancy. Normal and high-probability lung scans are themselves diagnostic. However, most patients with suspected PE have ventilation perfusion scan results that are nondiagnostic (low or intermediate or indeterminate probability scans). The diagnostic accuracy may be improved when scans are interpreted in conjunction with clinical pretest probability (38), but additional imaging studies are usually required.

Contrast-Enhanced Chest Computed Tomography

Chest CT has virtually replaced lung scanning as the initial imaging test for PE (39). The latest generation of multidetector CT scanners (Fig. 13.5) permits image acquisition of the entire chest with 1-mm resolution and a single breath hold of less than 10 seconds, enabling accurate imaging of the complete pulmonary vasculature. At the same time, the deep veins can be examined for proximal DVT by obtaining additional images from the pelvic and femoropopliteal region. Chest CT also helps detect alternative diagnoses, such as aortic dissection, pneumonia, or pericardial tamponade. Compared with first-generation single-slice scanners, the sensitivity of multirow detector CT increases from about 70% to >90% (40,41). The ongoing PIOPED II study compares various imaging strategies, including lung scanning, venous ultrasound, digital subtraction pulmonary angiography,

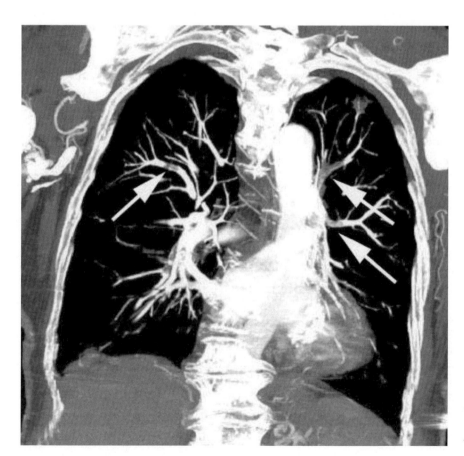

Figure 13.5 Contrast enhanced multirow (16-slice) detector chest CT in a patient with acute pulmonary embolism. In the coronal reconstructed view, multiple segmental emboli can be visualized (*arrows*). (Figure kindly provided by Joseph Schoepf, MD, Department of Radiology, Brigham and Women's Hospital, Boston, MA.)

and contrast venography against multirow detector chest CT (42).

In patients with confirmed PE, chest CT may also provide prognostic information in the presence of right ventricular enlargement if identified in a reconstructed CT four-chamber view. In a study of 63 patients with PE, a ratio of right to left ventricular dimension >0.9 identified patients at risk for adverse clinical events (43).

Gadolinium-Enhanced Magnetic Resonance Angiography

MR imaging avoids ionizing radiation or iodinated contrast agents and also allows assessment of left and right ventricular function and size, potentially important for risk stratification. Under specialized study circumstances, MR may be nearly as sensitive and specific as pulmonary angiography for PE (44). Limitations include restricted spatial resolution for evaluation of peripheral pulmonary arteries, limited round-the-clock availability, prolonged examination time, and difficulties monitoring severely ill patients in the scanner.

Venous Ultrasonography

Compression ultrasound of the deep veins is noninvasive and accurate in diagnosing symptomatic proximal DVT. If it confirms DVT in patients with symptoms suggestive of PE, the diagnosis can be made without further workup. However, more than half of the PE patients have no ultrasound evidence of DVT because the entire clot has already embolized to the lungs. Therefore, patients suspected of PE who have no evidence of DVT still require further investigation for PE.

Contrast Venography

Conventional venography is highly accurate for proximal and distal DVT but may provoke phlebitis or hypersensitivity reactions. Although contrast venography is the gold standard for DVT diagnosis, it is rarely performed in patients with suspected PE. Venography is required for catheter-directed thrombolysis, catheter embolectomy, percutaneous angioplasty, or insertion of an inferior vena caval filter.

Echocardiography

Transthoracic echocardiography has emerged as an important tool for risk stratification of patients with acute PE. The presence of right ventricular dysfunction on the echocardiogram is an independent predictor of early death (30), but echocardiography cannot be recommended to diagnose or exclude PE routinely because it is normal in about half of the patients with confirmed PE (45). However, bedside echocardiography facilitates discrimination of patients suspected of having either PE or cardiogenic shock. Potentially life-saving therapy, including thrombolysis, catheter intervention, or surgical embolectomy, can be initiated based on echocardiographic evidence

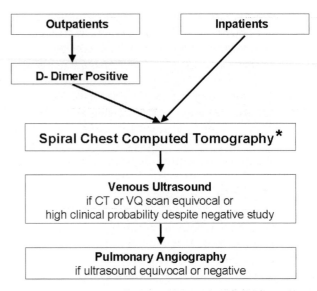

*VQ Scan if contrast allergy, renal insufficiency, or pregnancy

Figure 13.6 Suggested diagnostic strategy for patients with suspected pulmonary embolism without cardiogenic shock. VQ, ventilation perfusion.

of right ventricular dysfunction without necessarily obtaining time-consuming PE imaging tests (46). Transesophageal echocardiography helps visualize clots within the left and right main pulmonary arteries and is an alternative to the transthoracic approach for patients with poor image quality (47).

Overall Diagnostic Strategy

The initial assessment includes clinical pretest probability, physical examination, and an ECG. A plasma ELISA D-dimer should be obtained in all outpatients (Fig. 13.6). If the D-dimer is normal, PE is essentially excluded (48). If D-dimer levels are elevated, we recommend a chest CT as the initial imaging test (Fig. 13.6). In patients with renal insufficiency, pregnancy, or allergy to contrast agents, ventilation perfusion scanning may be used instead of chest CT. If the clinical suspicion remains high after a negative or indeterminate chest CT or lung scan, we recommend obtaining a venous ultrasound study. If the ultrasound study is negative or equivocal, we recommend proceeding to pulmonary angiography. This strategy is safe and only rarely requires pulmonary angiography (48).

Interpretation and Validity of Pulmonary Angiograms

Large cut-film angiographic studies have validated the angiographic criteria for acute PE (26,49,50). Primary angiographic criteria are *persistent central or marginal intraluminal radiolucency* and the *trailing edge of an intraluminal radiolucency obstructive to contrast flow* (Fig. 13.7). Complete obstruction showing abrupt vessel cutoff with a concave

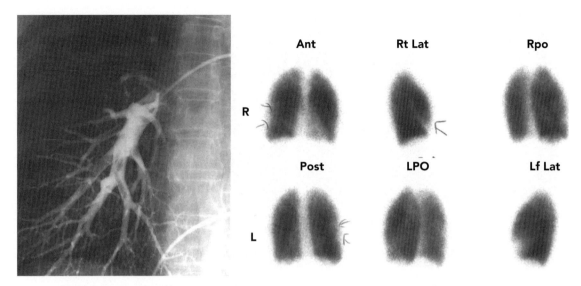

Figure 13.7 Primary evidence of acute pulmonary embolism. Selective cut-film angiogram of the right lower lobe pulmonary artery with multiple intraluminal radiolucencies, almost completely outlined by contrast **(left)**. Corresponding segmental perfusion defects of the right lower lobe **(right)**.

border of the contrast column is also considered primary evidence of acute PE (Fig. 13.8; 48). These criteria have also been validated for DSA (12,13,51). Secondary signs include oligemic or avascular regions, focal prolonged arterial phase, abruptly tapered peripheral vessels, or focal diminished venous flow. The latter signs have not been validated for PE and should be interpreted with caution.

In PIOPED (26), 35% had positive and 61% had negative pulmonary angiograms for PE. Angiography was nondiagnostic in 3% patients and was not completed in 1% because of complications. Two angiographic readers agreed that PE was present or could not be diagnosed with

certainty in 92% of cases. The readers agreed that PE was absent or it could not be excluded with certainty in 82% of cases. Interobserver agreement for cut-film pulmonary angiography decreases with diminishing pulmonary artery caliber. It was 98% for lobar PE, 90% for segmental PE, but only 66% for subsegmental PE. Subsegmental PE was diagnosed in 6% of patients. In another angiographic study, the proportion of patients with subsegmental PE was 30% (52). Interobserver agreement of DSA appears to be superior to cut-film angiography. In 140 patients with suspected PE, the kappa values ranged between 0.28 and 0.59 for cut-film angiography and between 0.66 and 0.89 for DSA (53).

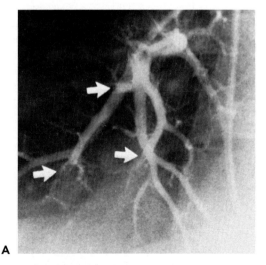

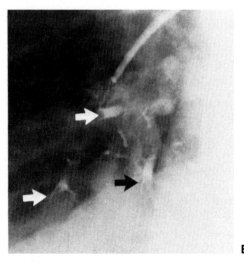

Figure 13.8 A. Right lower lobe balloon occlusion pulmonary cineangiogram demonstrates multiple vessels "cut off" *(arrows)*. **B.** Balloon deflation facilitated distal contrast distribution, with a visible trailing edge of a thrombus *(arrows)*.

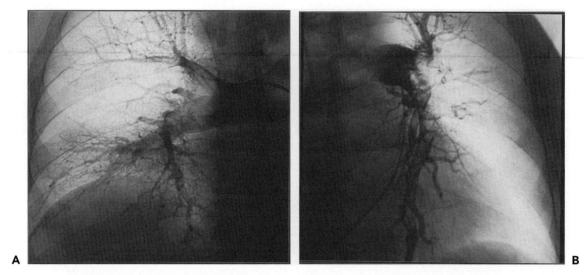

Figure 13.9 Selective cut-film angiograms in a 65-year-old man with recurrent attacks of dyspnea and syncope who presented with preserved systemic arterial pressure and right ventricular dysfunction on the echocardiogram. The angiogram demonstrates extensive intraluminal filling defects in both pulmonary arteries.

Because pulmonary angiography is the diagnostic gold standard for PE, we cannot directly calculate sensitivity, specificity, and predictive values. We estimate sensitivity and specificity as 98% and 95 to 98%, respectively. The validity of pulmonary angiography was assessed with follow-up studies of patients with negative angiograms in whom anticoagulation was withheld. In five studies, 840 patients had at least 3 months of follow-up (39,53–58). Recurrent venous thromboembolism was documented in 1.9% of these patients. Therefore, it is almost always safe to withhold anticoagulants in patients with suspected PE and a negative pulmonary angiogram.

Hemodynamic Characteristics

Many PE patients without cardiopulmonary disease have normal hemodynamics. Systolic right ventricular pressure rarely exceeds 50 mm Hg in patients without pre-existing cardiopulmonary disease (Figs. 13.9, 13.10, and 13.11). Instead, acute increase in right ventricular afterload with a

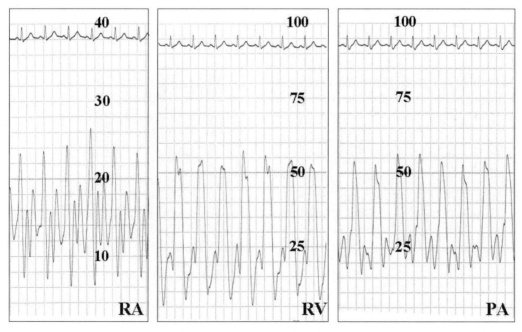

Figure 13.10 Right heart pressure tracings in the patient with acute pulmonary embolism from Fig. 13.9. RA, right atrium; RV, right ventricle; PA, pulmonary artery.

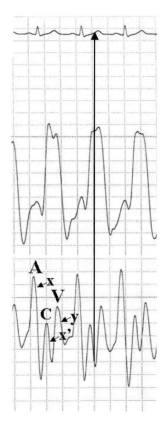

Figure 13.11 Simultaneous right atrial *(lower tracing)* and right ventricular *(upper tracing)* pressure curves from the patient with acute pulmonary embolism from Fig. 13.9. The atrial A wave is most prominent and coincides with the rapid rise in right ventricular diastolic pressure. The C wave is smaller than the V wave and coincides with the rapid rise in systolic right ventricular pressure. The nadir of the prominent right atrial x-descent coincides with systolic peak right ventricular pressure just before the beginning of the T wave *(arrow)*. The nadir of the y-descent coincides with the dip in right ventricular diastolic pressure.

systolic pressure above 50 to 60 mm Hg will result in acute right ventricular dilatation and systolic failure. Patients with recurrent PE may tolerate higher systolic pressure values prior to the development of right ventricular failure. As a result of right ventricular diastolic dysfunction, the right ventricular diastolic pressure approximates pulmonary artery diastolic pressure and typically shows a prominent dip and rapid rise. Right atrial pressure is elevated, with a prominent A wave and steep x descent (59). As right ventricular dilatation and dysfunction evolve, reduced right ventricular output impairs left ventricular filling. Left ventricular distensibility may be further compromised owing to a shift of the interventricular septum toward the left ventricle. Left ventricular cardiac output is decreased, with the systemic arterial waveform showing a sharp upstroke owing to compensatory increase in systemic vascular resistance.

In PE patients, increased myocardial shear stress can be quantified with brain natriuretic peptide levels (60,61); elevated troponin levels indicate myocardial ischemia

and microinfarction (62,63). Myocardial ischemia and microinfarction are probably caused by increased oxygen demand of the failing right ventricle and reduced coronary perfusion as a consequence of a decreased systemic cardiac output.

Catheter Fragmentation and Embolectomy

In patients with massive PE, catheter intervention with or without embolectomy is an alternative to systemic thrombolysis or surgical embolectomy (Figs. 13.12 and 13.13). If the bleeding risk is not increased, catheter intervention may be combined with local or systemic thrombolysis. Most of the devices appear to be effective, safe, and potentially life-saving in the presence of large fresh clots (Table 13.4), but none has been investigated in a controlled clinical trial (64–68). The Greenfield transvenous embolectomy catheter has been available the longest, but it has limited efficacy in the presence of chronic clots and does not address the risk of re-embolization.

OTHER INDICATIONS FOR PULMONARY ANGIOGRAPHY

Pulmonary Hypertension

Chronic Thromboembolic Pulmonary Hypertension

Most patients with chronic thromboembolic pulmonary hypertension have no documented history of DVT or PE nor any identifiable coagulopathy. Dyspnea with exertion and fatigue are the most common complaints. The nonspecific nature of these findings may substantially delay diagnosis. The chest radiograph usually reveals right ventricular enlargement and enlarged main pulmonary arteries. ECG changes are consistent with pulmonary hypertension. Arterial blood gases often reveal resting hypoxemia with a widened A-a gradient. Echocardiography documents pulmonary hypertension and right ventricular dilation and dysfunction. Most patients have a high-probability ventilation perfusion scan. Contrast-enhanced chest CT or MR will usually demonstrate chronic thrombi and may reveal other rare causes of pulmonary hypertension such as mediastinal fibrosis. Chest CT may be helpful to exclude other causes of multiple stenoses and occlusions of pulmonary vessels, such as infection, inflammation, or neoplasm (69).

Right heart catheterization and pulmonary arteriography are performed, both to confirm the diagnosis and to determine operability. In a study of 250 patients with chronic thromboembolic pulmonary hypertension, the characteristic angiographic findings (Table 13.5 and Fig. 13.14) were confirmed surgically (70). In addition to indefinite anticoagulation, pulmonary thromboendarterectomy plus

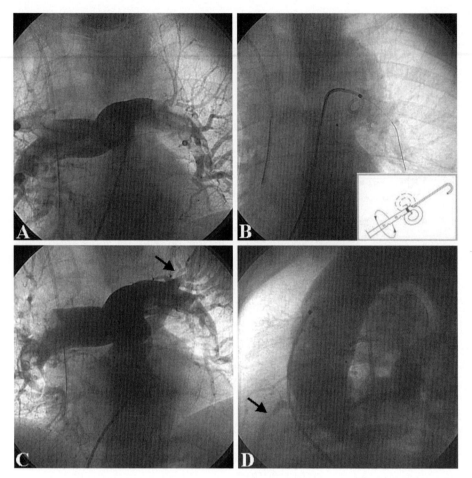

Figure 13.12 Catheter fragmentation in combination with a continuous systemic infusion of 100 mg alteplase over 2 hours in a 64-year-old female with massive pulmonary embolism and cardiogenic shock. **A.** Frontal view demonstrating subtotal filling defects in both main pulmonary arteries. **B.** Catheter thrombus fragmentation in the left pulmonary artery (pars superior) using a pigtail rotational catheter. **C.** Following catheter fragmentation, improved flow in the left upper lobe pulmonary arteries (arrow) was accompanied by a prompt increase in systemic arterial pressure from 70 mm Hg to 95 mm Hg. **D.** Lateral view demonstrating a significant proximal stenosis of the right coronary artery approximately 7 seconds after nonselective injection of 40 mL contrast into the main pulmonary artery (arrow).

inferior vena cava (IVC) filter should be considered in patients with functional class ≥2. The procedure involves a median sternotomy on cardiopulmonary bypass in deep hypothermia with circulatory arrest periods (71). Repeated balloon angioplasty of proximal pulmonary arteries may be considered in patients who are not candidates for surgery (72). Lung transplantation is an option in patients with extensive distal disease.

The presence of downstream pulmonary vascular resistance, defined as a prolonged time from balloon occlusion to the beginning of steady state pulmonary artery occlusion pressure, may identify patients at risk for persistent pulmonary hypertension and poor outcome following pulmonary thromboendarterectomy (73).

Primary Pulmonary Hypertension

Primary pulmonary hypertension (PPH) is a rare disease of unknown etiology, distinguished by characteristic arterial, capillary, and venular lesions (74). The term "primary" is used in the absence of congenital or acquired pulmonary, cardiac, or collagen vascular disease. There is a genetic predisposition in about 10% of patients. The human herpesvirus 8 may play a role in the pathogenesis (75). If this

condition is left untreated, pulmonary artery pressure and pulmonary vascular resistance will increase steadily until the right ventricle fails.

Echocardiography usually first documents the presence of pulmonary hypertension in patients with unexplained dyspnea or fatigue. Chest CT helps exclude secondary forms of pulmonary hypertension. Right heart catheterization is the gold standard for establishing the presence of pulmonary hypertension and is particularly important in excluding pulmonary venous hypertension in the presence of a normal left ventricular filling pressure.

Angiography reveals nonspecific dilatation of the proximal pulmonary arteries with smooth, rapid tapering of distal vessels (Fig. 13.15). A distal corkscrew appearance of the arteries may also be seen (74).

Acute drug challenge with a short-acting, titratable vasodilator during continuous monitoring of the hemodynamic profile is recommended in patients in whom calcium channel blockers are considered (74). Patients in whom a reduction in pulmonary vascular resistance ≥20% is associated with a decrease in mean pulmonary artery pressure ≥20% are considered responders (76). Symptomatic intolerance includes a decrease of >40% in mean systemic arterial pressure, an increase in heart rate >40%, or signs

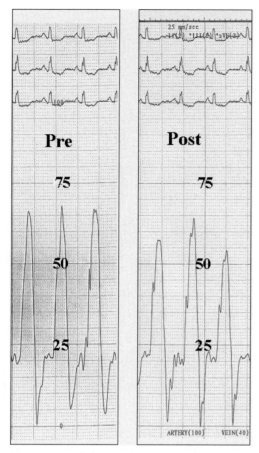

Figure 13.13 Right ventricular pressure curves pre and post catheter fragmentation in the patient from Fig. 13.12. Despite rapid clinical improvement, there was only a mild decrease in right ventricular systolic pressure following catheter fragmentation.

is being considered. An increasing number of vasodilator drugs for chronic use are available to treat PPH (see Chapter 30).

Intravenous epoprostenol (Flolan) is most commonly used to test acute vasodilator response (Table 13.6). The dose is up-titrated until systemic effects (headache, flushing, or nausea) occur. Caution is warranted in patients with coexisting congestive heart failure.

Adenosine is a potent pulmonary vasodilator and has a half-life of <5 seconds. Adverse effects include dyspnea and chest discomfort. It should not be administered in patients on theophylline or with acute asthma.

In contrast to epoprostenol or adenosine, nitric oxide has no inotropic properties and does not increase cardiac output. It is inhaled via a face mask.

Rare Indications

Pulmonary Arteriovenous Malformation (PAVM)

This entity is probably to the result of an embryologic defect in the terminal capillary loop. Polycythemia and reduced arterial PO_2 are manifestations of the extracardiac right-to-left shunt. Most patients with PAVMs are asymptomatic, although dyspnea, cyanosis, digital clubbing, and hemoptysis may be present. Paradoxic emboli via PAVMs can result in cerebrovascular accident or abscess. PAVMs are classified into two types (76). Simple PAVMs are usually a complex branching mass, supplied by one to three subsegmental arteries, all arising from the same segmental artery. Complex PAVMs are supplied by two or more different segmental arteries. Complex PAVMs are more frequent in the right middle lobe or lingula.

The walls of PAVMs are quite thin. Multiple PAVMs are present in one third of cases. From 40 to 65% of PAVMs are associated with hereditary hemorrhagic telangiectasia (Rendu-Osler-Weber syndrome). PAVMs are seen rarely with Fanconi syndrome (pancytopenia, radial deformities, and brown skin pigmentation).

and symptoms leading to discontinuation of drug. Acute drug challenge is also recommended in patients with end-stage congestive heart failure to prove that high pulmonary vascular resistance is not fixed and to ensure eligibility for heart transplantation. However, acute drug challenge is optional in PPH patients in whom bosentan

TABLE 13.4

INTERVENTIONAL DEVICES FOR MASSIVE PULMONARY EMBOLISM

Catheter	Manufacturer	Mechanism of Action
Greenfield catheter	Medi-Tech/Boston Scientific, Watertown, MA	Suction embolectomy
Pigtail catheter	Cook Europe, Bjaerverskov, Denmark	Fragmentation via over-the-wire pigtail rotation
Amplatz device	BARD-Microvena, White Bear Lake, MN	Clot maceration via high-speed impeller rotation
AngioJet	Possis Medical, Minneapolis, MN	Embolectomy via high-pressure saline injection (Venturi effect)
Hydrolyser	Cordis, Warren, NJ	Embolectomy via rheolytic effect
Aspirex	Straub Medical, Wangs, Switzerland	Embolectomy via over-the-wire, high-speed spiral coil rotation

TABLE 13.5

ANGIOGRAPHIC FINDINGS IN CHRONIC THROMBOEMBOLIC PULMONARY HYPERTENSION

Finding	Comment
Pouching	Contrast filling concave pouches in organized thrombus, with delayed opacification or obstruction of the distal artery
Webs/bands	Persistent thin or thick linear radiolucencies in lobar or segmental vessels causing stenosis with or without poststenotic dilatation
Luminal irregularity	Scalloped arterial margins
Vessel tapering	Abrupt narrowing of major pulmonary arteries
Vessel obstruction	Obstruction of lobar arteries, usually at their origin

From Koning R, Cribier A, Gerber L, et al. A new treatment for pulmonary embolism: percutaneous rheolytic thrombectomy. *Circulation* 1997;96:2498–2500.

Screening for PAVMs can be done noninvasively with contrast echocardiography. Spiral chest CT helps establish the diagnosis (Fig. 13.16). When intervention is planned, selective pulmonary angiography is necessary, with frontal and both oblique views of each lung.

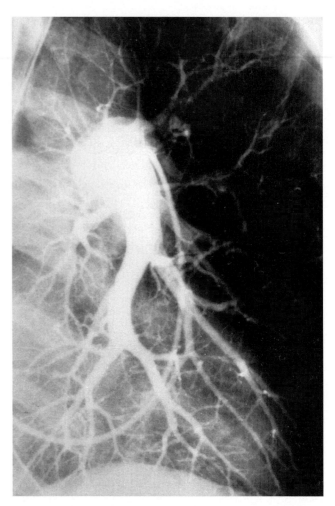

Figure 13.15 Primary pulmonary hypertension. A 45° right anterior oblique view of the left pulmonary angiogram of a 30-year-old male with primary pulmonary hypertension. Note the rapid tapering of segmental vessels.

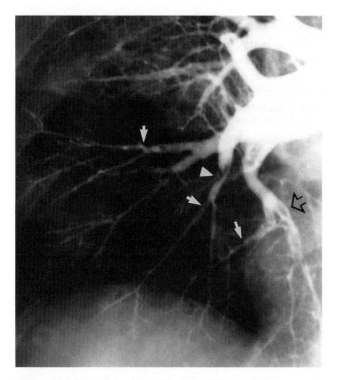

Figure 13.14 Chronic pulmonary thromboembolism. Frontal view of right pulmonary angiogram in a 42-year-old female still dyspneic after an acute pulmonary embolus was documented 6 months earlier and treated. The proximal pulmonary arteries are dilated. The distal vessels taper rapidly and are irregular (*arrows*). Eccentric stenoses are present (*arrowheads*), as are intraluminal webs (*open arrow*).

PAVMs can be percutaneously embolized with detachable balloons or coils (Fig. 13.17; 77). Silicone balloons can be repositioned within the feeding artery prior to final detachment to facilitate precise deployment. With the potential for direct systemic emboli, extreme caution must be exercised, and angiographic technique must be meticulous to avoid air embolism, catheter thrombosis and embolism, or systemic deployment of occlusion devices.

Acquired pulmonary arteriovenous shunts can be secondary to trauma, infection, or hepatogenic angiodysplasia (78). Infection-related shunts are seen in bronchiectasis, invasive aspergillosis, tuberculosis, and schistosomiasis.

Pulmonary Artery or Vein Stenosis

An increasing number of patients with repaired congenital heart disease now survive into adulthood and may present with pulmonary vascular stenoses and occlusions. Most pulmonary arterial and venous stenoses occur in

TABLE 13.6			
DOSE REGIMENS: ACUTE VASODILATOR TESTING			
Drug	**Initial Dose**	**Dose Increments**	**Maximum Dose**
Intravenous epoprostenol	2 ng/kg per minute	2 ng/kg per minute every 15 minutes	16 ng/kg per minute
Intravenous adenosine	50 µg/kg per minute	50 µg/kg per minute every 15 minutes	350 µg/kg per minute
Inhaled nitric oxide	20 ppm	20 ppm every hour	80 ppm

association with congenital cardiac disease such as tetralogy of Fallot, truncus arteriosus, pulmonary valvular stenosis, patent ductus arteriosus, aortic stenosis, ventricular septal defects, or transposition of the great vessels. Pulmonary blood flow is often maintained by surgical shunts or systemic-to-pulmonary collaterals. Isolated stenoses may present following pulmonary artery banding after systemic to pulmonary artery shunts such as Blalock-Taussig, Waterston-Cooley, or Glenn anastomosis. In patients with congenital heart disease, pulmonary angiography may be required to evaluate the indication for reoperation, including assessment of the size of pulmonary vessels and collaterals, or documentation of intracardiac or extracardiac shunt patency.

Stenosis may also be secondary to rubella, chronic infections (such as histoplasmosis), or infestations (such as schistosomiasis). Stenoses are associated with idiopathic hypercalcemia. Lung transplant pulmonary arterial stenoses are not common and carry a poor prognosis (79). Congenital single or multiple stenoses may be present without cardiac anomalies (Fig. 13.18). Angioplasty and stent placement for treatment of pulmonary artery stenoses have

been used primarily for treatment of congenital stenoses (80). Pressure recordings are helpful in establishing hemodynamic significance of pulmonary branch stenoses.

Pulmonary vein stenosis is increasingly seen in patients who undergo radiofrequency ablation of the pulmonary venous ostia for treatment of atrial fibrillation. Balloon angioplasty with or without stent placement has been used successfully to treat symptomatic patients (81).

Pulmonary Artery Aneurysms

Pulmonary artery aneurysms may appear as a perihilar mass on chest radiographs. Spiral chest CT or MR is useful to confirm the diagnosis. Most aneurysms occur centrally, usually secondary to pulmonary hypertension or following surgical correction of congenital heart disease. Degenerative pulmonary aneurysms can be seen in Marfan syndrome. Tuberculosis results in pulmonary artery aneurysms known as Rasmussen aneurysms. Other infectious causes of pulmonary artery aneurysms include syphilis and septic emboli. Rupture of pulmonary artery aneurysms may cause fatal hemorrhage. Multiple pulmonary artery aneurysms

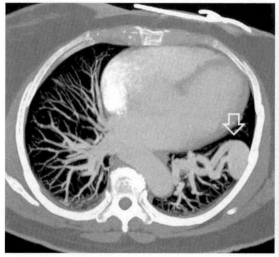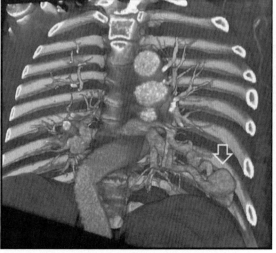

Figure 13.16 Multirow (16-slice) detector chest computed tomogram of a patient with a single large pulmonary arteriovenous malformation *(arrows)*. Axial view **(left)** and reconstructed coronal view **(right)**. (Courtesy of Joseph Schoepf, MD, Department of Radiology, Brigham and Women's Hospital, Boston, MA.

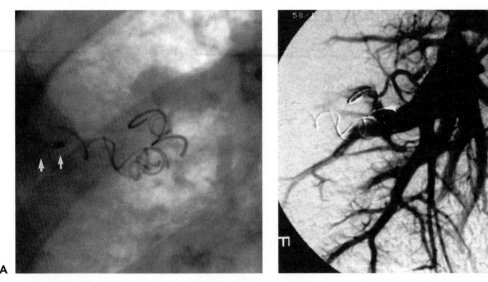

A   B

Figure 13.17 Pulmonary arteriovenous malformation with percutaneous embolization. **A.** Digital image displaying Amplatz spider vascular occlusion device *(arrows)* trailed by multiple coils. **B.** Right pulmonary angiogram confirms occlusion of the fistula.

may be seen in Behçet disease and are associated with poor prognosis (82). Pseudoaneurysms of the pulmonary artery result from penetrating or catheter trauma. Technical and clinical success has been reported for percutaneous embolization of pseudoaneurysms with coils, Gelfoam, and suture material (83).

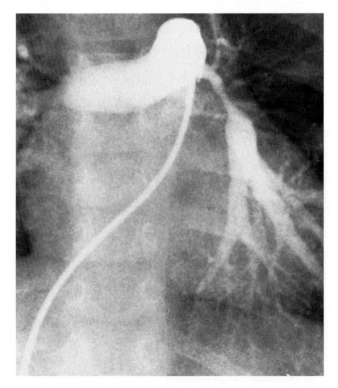

Figure 13.18 Left interlobar pulmonary artery stenosis. Left pulmonary angiogram of isolated pulmonary arterial stenosis in an adolescent male.

Partial Anomalous Pulmonary Vein Return

This entity may be seen in isolation or more often in combination with an atrial septal defect. Anomalous veins commonly enter the right atrium directly. Transesophageal echocardiography is accurate in delineating the cardiac abnormalities. Pulmonary angiography with delayed filming is diagnostic for quantification of the left-to-right shunt. An oxygen saturation run should include a sample from the high superior vena cava to exclude the rare possibility of solitary left anomalous pulmonary vein return (84).

Pulmonary Artery Neoplasms

Leiomyosarcoma of the pulmonary artery is a rare neoplasm. It typically is seen in the main pulmonary artery in relation to the pulmonary valve (Fig. 13.19). The tumor is entirely intraluminal in half the reported cases and spreads along the lumen. Pulmonary angiography with hemodynamic assessment may be required preoperatively (Fig. 13.20). It is important to evaluate the venous phase for any pulmonary venous involvement. Arterial or venous obstruction, encasement, displacement, or rarely intraluminal invasion may be identified.

Inflammation

Inflammatory diseases of the lung manifest a spectrum of findings at pulmonary arteriography. In Takayasu arteritis, the degree of pulmonary involvement correlates with the severity of brachiocephalic disease (85). Findings include stenosis, occlusion, and, rarely, dilatation of pulmonary arteries. CT angiography best demonstrates the wall thickening and enhancement of involved arteries (86). Systemic-to-

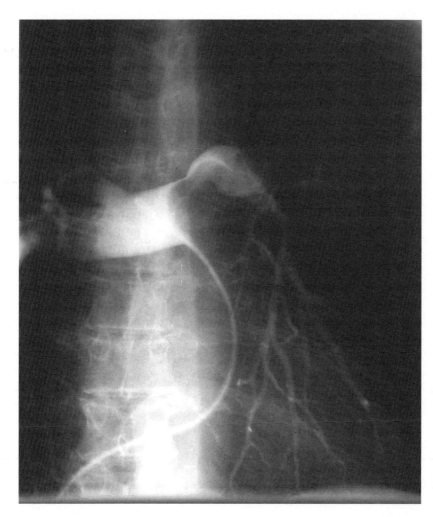

Figure 13.19 Nonselective cut-film pulmonary angiogram in a 62-year-old male with progressive dyspnea and elevated jugular venous pressure. An irregular intraluminal mass (leiomyosarcoma) is seen in the left main pulmonary artery. Severe reduction in distal flow indicates a hemodynamically significant stenosis. (Courtesy of Richard Baum, MD, Department of Radiology, Brigham and Women's Hospital, Boston, MA.)

pulmonary artery communications may exist, with bronchial arteries serving as collaterals to the occluded pulmonary arteries. Behçet disease involves the pulmonary arteries with a nonspecific vasculitis in about 5% of patients. Angiographic findings are predominantly aneurysms, with occlusion noted less frequently. Severe mediastinitis from histoplasmosis can compress and occlude the pulmonary arteries and veins as they traverse the mediastinum. Lymph node involvement can compress adjacent arteries and veins.

Foreign Bodies

The pulmonary arterial system is the final destination for fractured and embolized devices placed in the venous

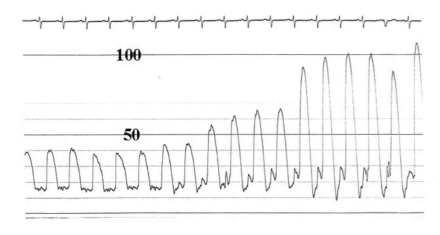

Figure 13.20 Pulmonary artery pressure tracing from the patient in Fig. 13.19. During catheter withdrawal from the left into the main pulmonary artery trunk, hemodynamic significance of the stenosis was confirmed. (Courtesy of Richard Baum, MD, Department of Radiology, Brigham and Women's Hospital, Boston, MA.)

system. In most cases, a hand injection of contrast is helpful to determine the size and orientation of the vessel containing the foreign body. Percutaneous retrieval using a nitinol snare has simplified the approach to foreign body removal. Balloons are well suited to engage lost stents and either to deploy the stent in a safe location or to retrieve it.

REFERENCES

1. Ludwig JW. Heart and coronaries—the pioneering age. In: Rosenbusch G, Oudkerk M, Amman E. *Radiology in Medical Diagnostics—Evolution of X-Ray Applications 1895–1995.* Oxford: Blackwell Science, 1995:213–224.
2. Robb GP, Steinberg I. A practical method of visualization of the chambers of the heart, the pulmonary circulation, and the great blood vessels in man. *J Clin Invest* 1938;17:507.
3. Sasahara AA, Stein M, Simon M, Littmann D. Pulmonary angiography in the diagnosis of thromboembolic disease. *New Engl J Med* 1964;270:1075–1081.
4. Goldhaber SZ. Pulmonary Embolism. *Lancet* 2004;363:1295–1305.
5. Fraser RF, Pare JAP, Pare PD, et al. Diagnosis of diseases of the chest, 3rd ed. Boston: Little, Brown and Co., 1983.
6. Alpert JS, Smith R, Carlson J, et al. Mortality in patients treated for pulmonary embolism. *JAMA* 1976;236:1477–1480.
7. Mills SR, Jackson DC, Older RA, et al. The incidence, etiologies, and avoidance of complications of pulmonary angiography in a large series. *Radiology* 1980;136:295–299.
8. Grollman JH. Pulmonary Arteriography. *Cardiovasc Intervent Radiol* 1992;15:166–170.
9. Koizumi J, Mouri M, Watanabe M, Hiramatsu K. Transbrachial selective pulmonary angiography using a new 4Fr curved pigtail catheter and hydrophilic-coated guidewire. *Cardiovasc Intervent Radiol* 1998;21:347–349.
10. Hansen ME, Geller SC, Yucel EK, et al. Transfemoral venous catheterization through inferior vena caval filters: results in seven cases. *AJR* 1991;157:967–970.
11. Grollman JH, Gyepes MT, Helmer E. Transfemoral selective bilateral pulmonary arteriography with a pulmonary artery-seeking catheter. *Radiology* 1978;96:202–204.
12. Courey WR, de Villsante JM, Waltman AC. A quick, simple method of percutaneous transfemoral arteriography. *Radiology* 1975;113:475–477.
13. Mills CS, van Aman ME. Modified technique for percutaneous transfemoral pulmonary angiography. *Cardiovasc Intervent Radiol* 1986;9:52–53.
14. Grollman JH, Renner JW. Transfemoral pulmonary angiography: update on technique. *Am J Roentgenol* 1981;136:624–626.
15. Tempkin DL, Kadika JE. New catheter design and placement technique for pulmonary arteriography. *Radiology* 1987;163:275–276.
16. Saeed M, Braun SD, Cohan RH, et al. Pulmonary angiography with iopamidol: patient comfort, image quality, and hemodynamics. *Radiology* 1987;165:345–349.
17. Hardeman MR, Konijnenberg A, Sturk A, Reekers JA. Activation of platelets by low-osmolar contrast media: differential effects of ionic and nonionic agents. *Radiology* 1994;192:563–566.
18. Van Beek EJR, Levi M, Reekers JA, et al. Increased plasma levels of PAI-1 after administration of nonionic contrast medium in patients undergoing pulmonary angiography. *Radiology* 1994;193:821–823.
19. Davidson CJ, Laskey WK, Hermiller JB, et al. Randomized trial of contrast media utilization in high-risk PTCA: the COURT trial. *Circulation* 2000;101:2172–2177.
20. Aspelin P, Aubry P, Fransson SG, et al. Nephrotoxic effects in high-risk patients undergoing angiography. *N Engl J Med* 2003;348:491–499.
21. Oudkerk M, van Beek EJR, Reekers JA. Pulmonary angiography: technique, indications and interpretation. In: Oudkerk M, van Beek EJR, ten Cate JW, eds. *Pulmonary Embolism.* Berlin: Blackwell Science, 1999:135–159.
22. Hagspiel KD, Polak JF, Grassi, CJ, et al. Pulmonary embolism: comparison of cut-film and digital pulmonary angiography. *Radiology* 1998;207:139–145.
23. Johnson MS, Stine SB, Shah H, et al. Possible pulmonary embolus: evaluation with digital subtraction versus cut-film angiography—prospective study in 80 patients. *Radiology* 1998;207:131–138.
24. Forauer AR, McLean GK, Wallace LP. Clinical follow-up of patients after a negative digital subtraction pulmonary arteriogram in the evaluation of pulmonary embolism. *J Vasc Interv Radiol* 1998;9:903–908.
25. Baum S, ed. *Abrams Angiography.* Boston: Little, Brown and Co, 1997.
26. Stein PD, Athanasoulis C, Alavi A, et al. Complications and validity of pulmonary angiography in acute pulmonary embolism. *Circulation* 1992;85:462–468.
27. Pitton MB, Duber C, Mayer E, Thelen M. Hemodynamic effects of nonionic contrast bolus injection and oxygen inhalation during pulmonary angiography in patients with chronic major-vessel thromboembolic pulmonary hypertension. *Circulation* 1996;94:2485–2491.
28. Tsai AW, Cushman M, Rosamond WD, Heckbert SR, Polak JF, Folsom AR. Cardiovascular risk factors and venous thromboembolism incidence: the longitudinal investigation of thromboembolism etiology. *Arch Intern Med* 2002;162:1182–1189.
29. Goldhaber SZ, Elliot CG. Acute pulmonary embolism I: epidemiology, pathophysiology, and diagnosis. *Circulation* 2003;108:2726–2729.
30. Goldhaber SZ, Visani L, De Rosa M. Acute pulmonary embolism: clinical outcomes in the International Cooperative Pulmonary Embolism Registry (ICOPER). *Lancet* 1999;353:1386–1389.
31. Wells PS, Anderson DR, Rodger M, et al. Derivation of a simple clinical model to categorize patients' probability of pulmonary embolism: increasing the model's utility with the SimpliRED D-dimer. *Thromb Haemost* 2000;83:416–420.
32. Kucher N, Walpoth N, Wustmann K, Noveanu M, Gertsch M. QR in V1—an ECG sign associated with right ventricular dysfunction and adverse clinical outcome in pulmonary embolism. *Eur Heart J* 2003;24:1113–1119.
33. Goldhaber SZ, Simons GR, Elliott CG, et al. Quantitative plasma D-dimer levels among patients undergoing pulmonary angiography for suspected pulmonary embolism. *JAMA* 1993;270:2819–2822.
34. Dunn KL, Wolf JP, Dorfman DM, et al. Normal D-dimer levels in emergency department patients suspected of acute pulmonary embolism. *J Am Coll Cardiol* 2002;40:1475–1478.
35. Brown MD, Rowe BH, Reeves MJ, et al. The accuracy of the enzyme-linked immunosorbent assay D-dimer test in the diagnosis of pulmonary embolism: a metaanalysis. *Ann Emerg Med* 2002;40:133–144.
36. Stein PD, Goldhaber SZ, Henry JW, Miller AC. Arterial blood gas analysis in the assessment of suspected acute pulmonary embolism. *Chest* 1996;109:78–81.
37. Stein PD, Goldhaber SZ, Henry JW. Alveolar-arterial oxygen gradient in the assessment of acute pulmonary embolism. *Chest* 1995;107:139–143.
38. PIOPED Investigators. Value of the ventilation/perfusion scan in acute pulmonary embolism. Results of the Prospective Investigation of Pulmonary Embolism Diagnosis (PIOPED). *JAMA* 1990;263:2753–2759.
39. Schoepf UJ, Costello P, Goldhaber SZ. Current perspective: Spiral CT for acute pulmonary embolism. *Circulation* 2004;109:2160–2167.
40. Schoepf UJ, Holzknecht N, Helmberger TK, et al. Subsegmental pulmonary emboli: improved detection with thin-collimation multi-detector row spiral CT. *Radiology* 2002;222:483–490.
41. Qanadli SD, Hajjam ME, Mesurolle B, et al. Pulmonary embolism detection: prospective evaluation of dual-section helical CT versus selective pulmonary arteriography in 157 patients. *Radiology* 2000;217:447–455.
42. Gottschalk A, Stein PD, Goodman LR, Sostman HD. Overview of Prospective Investigation of Pulmonary Embolism Diagnosis II. *Semin Nucl Med* 2002;32:173–182.
43. Quiroz R, Kucher N, Kipfmueller F, et al. Right ventricular enlargement on chest computed tomography: prognostic role in acute pulmonary embolism. *Circulation* 2004;109:2401–2404.
44. Oudkerk M, van Beek EJ, Wielopolski P, et al. Comparison of contrast-enhanced magnetic resonance angiography and conventional

pulmonary angiography for the diagnosis of pulmonary embolism: a prospective study. *Lancet* 2002;359:1643–1647.

45. Goldhaber SZ. Echocardiography in the management of pulmonary embolism. *Ann Intern Med* 2002;136:691–700.

46. Kucher N, Windecker S, Meier B, Hess OM. Novel management strategy for patients with suspected pulmonary embolism. *Eur Heart J* 2003;24:366–376.

47. Pruszczyk P, Torbicki A, Kuch-Wocial A, et al. Diagnostic value of transoesophageal echocardiography in suspected haemodynamically significant pulmonary embolism. *Heart* 2001;85:628–634.

48. Musset D, Parent F, Meyer G, et al. Diagnostic strategy for patients with suspected pulmonary embolism: a prospective multicentre outcome study. *Lancet* 2002;360:1914–1920.

49. Dalen JE, Brooks HL, Johnson LW, et al. Pulmonary angiography in acute pulmonary embolism: indications, techniques, and results in 367 patients. *Am Heart J* 1971;81:175–185.

50. Hull RD, Hirsh J, Carter CJ, et al. Pulmonary angiography, ventilation lung scanning, and venography for clinically suspected pulmonary embolism with abnormal perfusion lung scan. *Ann Intern Med* 1983;98:891–899.

51. Sagel SS, Greenspan RH. Nonuniform pulmonary arterial perfusion. *Radiology* 1970;99:541–548.

52. Oser RF, Zuckerman DA, Gutierrez FR, Brink JA. Anatomic distribution of pulmonary emboli at pulmonary angiography: implications for cross-sectional imaging. *Radiology* 1996;199:31–35.

53. Van Beek EJR, Bakker AJ, Reekers JA. Interobserver variability of pulmonary angiography in patients with non-diagnostic lung scan results: conventional versus digital subtraction arteriography. *Radiology* 1996;198:721–724.

54. Cheely R, McCartney WH, Perry JR, et al. The role of noninvasive tests versus pulmonary angiography in the diagnosis of pulmonary embolism. *Am J Med* 198;70:17–22.

55. Van Beek EJ, Reekers JA, Batchelor DA, Brandjes DP, Buller HR. Feasibility, safety and clinical utility of angiography in patients with suspected pulmonary embolism. *Eur Radiol* 1996;6:415–419.

56. Bookstein JJ. Segmental arteriography by pulmonary embolism. *Radiology* 1969;93:1007–1012.

57. Novelline RA, Baltarowich OH, Athanasoulis CA, et al. The clinical course of patients with suspected pulmonary embolism and a negative pulmonary arteriogram. *Radiology* 1978;126:561–567.

58. Henry JW, Relyea B, Stein PD. Continuing risk of thromboemboli among patients with normal pulmonary angiograms. *Chest* 1995; 107:1375–1378.

59. Goldstein JA. Pathophysiology and management of right heart ischemia. *J Am Coll Cardiol* 2002;40:841–853.

60. Kucher N, Printzen G, Goldhaber SZ. Prognostic role of brain natriuretic peptide in acute pulmonary embolism. *Circulation* 2003;107:2545–2547.

61. Kucher N, Printzen G, Doernhoefer T, Windecker S, Meier B, Hess OM. Low pro-brain natriuretic peptide levels predict benign clinical outcome in acute pulmonary embolism. *Circulation* 2003;107:1576–1578.

62. Giannitsis E, Muller-Bardorff M, Kurowski V, et al. Independent prognostic value of cardiac troponin T in patients with confirmed pulmonary embolism. *Circulation* 2000;102:211–217.

63. Konstantinides S, Geibel A, Olschewski M, et al. Importance of cardiac troponins I and T in risk stratification of patients with acute pulmonary embolism. *Circulation* 2002;106:1263–1268.

64. Greenfield LJ, Proctor MC, Williams DM, et al. Long-term experience with transvenous catheter pulmonary embolectomy. *J Vasc Surg* 1993;18:450–458.

65. Schmitz-Rode T, Janssens U, Duda SH, et al. Massive pulmonary embolism: percutaneous emergency treatment by pigtail rotation catheter. *J Am Coll Cardiol* 2000;36:375–380.

66. Uflacker R, Strange C, Vujic I. Massive pulmonary embolism: preliminary results in treatment with the Amplatz thrombectomy device. *J Vasc Interv Radiol* 1996;7:519–528, 1996.

67. Koning R, Cribier A, Gerber L, et al. A new treatment for pulmonary embolism: percutaneous rheolytic thrombectomy. *Circulation* 1997;96:2498–2500.

68. Kucher N, Windecker S, Banz Y, Schmitz-Rode T, Hess O, Meier B. Percutaneous catheter thrombectomy device for acute pulmonary embolism. *Radiology* 2005; in press.

69. Schwickert HC, Schweden F, Schild HH, et al. Pulmonary arteries and lung parenchyma in chronic pulmonary embolism: preoperative and postoperative CT findings. *Radiology* 1994;191:351–357.

70. Auger WR, Fedullo PF, Moser KM, et al. Chronic major-vessel thromboembolic pulmonary artery obstruction: appearance at angiography. *Radiology* 1992;182:393–398.

71. Fedullo PF, Auger WR, Kerr KM, Rubin LJ. Chronic thromboembolic pulmonary hypertension. *N Engl J Med* 2001;345:1465–1472.

72. Feinstein JA, Goldhaber SZ, Lock JE, et al. Balloon pulmonary angioplasty for treatment of chronic thromboembolic pulmonary hypertension. *Circulation* 2001;103:10–13.

73. Kim NHS, Fesler P, Channick RN, et al. Preoperative partitioning of pulmonary vascular resistance correlates with early outcome after thromboendarterectomy for chronic thromboembolic pulmonary hypertension. *Circulation* 2004;109:18–22.

74. Humbert M, Sitbon O, Simonneau G. Treatment of pulmonary arterial hypertension. *N Engl J Med* 2004;351:1425–1436.

75. Cool CD, Rai PR, Yeager ME, et al. Expression of human herpesvirus 8 in primary pulmonary hypertension. *N Engl J Med* 2003;349:1113–1122.

76. Galie N, Ussia G, Passarelli P, at el. Role of pharmacologic tests in the treatment of primary pulmonary hypertension. *Am J Cardiol* 1995;75:55A–62A.

77. White RI, Pollak JS, Wirth JA. Pulmonary arteriovenous malformations: diagnosis and transcatheter embolotherapy. *J Vasc Interv Radiol* 1996;7:787–804.

78. Oh KS, Bender TM, Bowen A, Ledesma-Medina J. Plain radiographic, nuclear medicine and angiographic observations of hepatogenic pulmonary angiodysplasia. *Pediatr Radiol* 1983;13: 111–115.

79. Clark SC, Levine AJ, Hasan A, et al. Vascular complications of lung transplantation. *Ann Thorac Surg* 1996;61:1079–1082.

80. O'Laughlin MP, Slack MC, Grifka RG, et al. Implantation and intermediate-term follow-up of stents in congenital heart disease. *Circulation* 1993;88:605–614.

81. Qureshi AM, Prieto LR, Latson LA, et al. Transcatheter angioplasty for acquired pulmonary vein stenosis after radiofrequency ablation. *Circulation* 2003;108:1336–1342.

82. Numan F, Islak C, Berkmen T, et al. Behcet disease: pulmonary arterial involvement in 15 cases. *Radiology* 1994;192:465–468.

83. Ray CE Jr, Kaufman JA, Geller SC, et al. Embolization of pulmonary catheter-induced pulmonary artery pseudoaneurysms. *Chest* 1996;110:1370–1373.

84. McGaughey MD, Traill TA, Brinker JA. Partial left anomalous pulmonary venous return: a diagnostic dilemma. *Cathet Cardiovasc Diagn* 1986;12:110–115.

85. Yamada I, Shibuya H, Matsubara O. Pulmonary artery disease in Takayasu's arteritis: angiographic findings. *AJR* 1992;159:263–269.

86. Park JH, Chung JW, Im J-G, et al. Takayasu arteritis: evaluation of mural changes in the aorta and pulmonary artery with CT angiography. *Radiology* 1995;196:89–93.

Angiography of the Aorta and Peripheral Arteries

14

Michael R. Jaff   *Briain D. MacNeill*   *Kenneth Rosenfield*[a]

Atherosclerosis is a systemic disease that afflicts millions of patients annually in the United States. Historically, most of the clinical focus has been on its coronary artery manifestations, given their frequency and the potentially grave consequences. Although specialists in vascular medicine and vascular surgery have long recognized that peripheral (i.e., extracardiac) arterial occlusive disease may contribute significantly to morbidity and mortality, it is only recently that invasive and interventional cardiologists have become actively involved in its diagnosis and management. To support that involvement, this chapter includes atherosclerotic manifestations in all major arterial territories. It reviews the natural history, clinical presentation, noninvasive diagnostic modalities, and angiographic techniques used in patients with peripheral vascular disease, including aneurysmal disease of the thoracic and abdominal aorta, and atherosclerotic disease of the extracranial carotid arteries, renal arteries, and lower extremity arteries. Additional information regarding interventional techniques is reviewed in Chapter 26, and representative case profiles are reviewed in Chapter 34.

PERIPHERAL IMAGING TECHNIQUES

Aortography and peripheral angiography have a history as long as that of cardiac catheterization. Shortly after

---

[a] Some of the material in the current chapter was contributed by Robert M. Schainfield, D.O., for the previous edition.

W. Forssmann reported the passage of a catheter from his own arm vein into his right atrium in 1929 (1), dos Santos and colleagues described their experience in performing abdominal aortography by direct needle puncture (2). Seven years later, Nuvoli performed aortography via direct needle puncture of the ascending aorta (3). Fortunately, these direct access techniques have now been virtually replaced by the percutaneous and direct (see Chapters 4 and 5) techniques for catheter introduction, which are the foundation of modern angiography. In the past decade, major improvements have also been made in noninvasive imaging techniques, so that modalities such as duplex ultrasound, computed tomography (CT), and magnetic resonance angiography (MRA) are now frequently the initial investigations for diagnosis and monitoring of peripheral vascular disease. These noninvasive imaging techniques augment traditional techniques of catheter-based angiography, facilitating detection of subclinical disease, strategizing for interventional procedures, and allowing safe and reliable methods for ongoing surveillance.

NONINVASIVE ANGIOGRAPHY

Improvements in imaging techniques and resolution have resulted in widespread clinical application of MRA and CTA. By definition, noninvasive imaging modalities avoid the potential complications of catheter-based angiography.

There are currently three techniques for performing MRA. The first, termed *time-of-flight MRA* (TOF-MRA), was the initial MR-based angiographic application and remains an important method for evaluation of distal runoff vessels (4). It relies on suppression or saturation of the background tissue by rapid sequences of radiofrequency signal to allow detection of high-velocity flowing blood (5). Although its application was met with enthusiasm, it was limited by overestimation and time-consuming imaging protocols (6).

The next MR application applied to peripheral angiography was *phase contrast MRA* (PC-MRA), in which manipulation of the spin states creates a differential signal from flowing blood and background tissue. In the resultant PC-MRA images, the signal of each pixel represents velocity in a given direction (7). An advantage of this technique is that it allows quantification of blood flow volume and velocity. PC-MRA is limited by flow voids arising in regions of flow turbulence, flow-velocity dependence on signal intensity, and the need for gating large arteries.

The third technique, *contrast-enhanced MRA* (CE-MRA), is independent of flow and relies on the intravenous injection of nonnephrotoxic gadolinium-based paramagnetic contrast, which shortens local T1 relaxation time (Fig. 14.1; 8). The application of CE-MRA has been validated for single fields of view, and although it is an excellent method for examining limited fields (e.g., perirenal aorta), it is often insufficient to cover larger vascular beds. As a result, several techniques have been adopted to overcome this limitation, including multistation MRA or moving table MRA. Multistation MRA requires multiple injections, masking the venous and parenchymal signal from the initial injection, and the use of high volumes of contrast (9). Moving table MRA with bolus chasing overcomes some of these limitations by maximizing the data obtained from a single bolus. The rapid transit time from the aorta to the lower limbs is such that venous filling cannot be completely negated (10).

Since its first report in 1992, improvements in CT angiography have resulted in rapid image acquisition and improved image resolution (11). In particular, the development of multidetector CT (MDCT) allows shorter image acquisition time, thinner sections, and improved longitudinal coverage (Fig. 14.2). In general, a scout scan is performed to ensure that the area of interest is covered. A test dose of contrast is required to set the time delay between contrast injection and image acquisition. A total volume of 80 to 100 mL of iodinated contrast is usually required (12). The major disadvantage of CTA is the need for moderate volumes of nephrotoxic contrast, precluding its use in the setting of renal insufficiency.

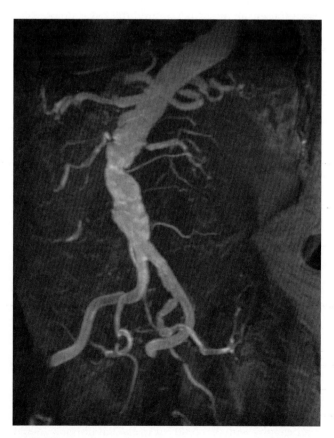

Figure 14.1 Contrast enhanced MRA of the aorta demonstrating aortic tortuosity with evidence of mural thrombus. Both the right and left renal arteries demonstrate high-grade stenoses at their origin.

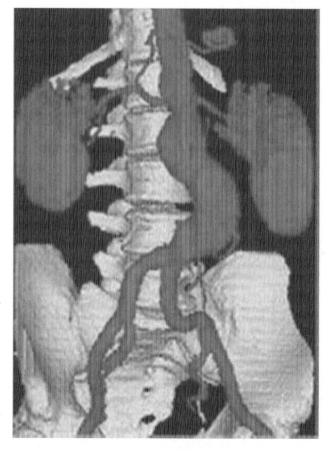

Figure 14.2 Three-dimensional CT angiography of an infrarenal aortic aneurysm, demonstrating the application of novel imaging protocols in current vascular medicine practice.

RADIOGRAPHIC IMAGING

Catheter-based angiography has equally undergone a new level of complexity and sophistication and, at this writing, remains the gold standard for diagnosis of arterial disease. As with cardiac angiography (Chapter 2), the techniques of vascular angiography are predicated on maximizing benefit for the patient while minimizing associated risk. These principles are summarized in the recently updated consensus conference guidelines regarding the clinical competency required for the diagnosis and management of peripheral vascular diseases (13).

Principles of vascular angiography may be divided into general considerations common to all vascular territories and specific considerations relating to individual vascular beds. General considerations include techniques of arterial access, radiographic equipment, catheter design and use, anticoagulation, and contrast selection. Specific principles, discussed in their relevant sections, include the choice of arterial access, catheter selection, optimal angulation, adjunctive methods of evaluation (intravascular ultrasound, translesional pressure gradient measurement, and so on), and classification of angiographic findings.

VASCULAR ACCESS

Although arterial access has been discussed previously (Chapter 4 and 5), its importance in achieving a safe, complication-free procedure cannot be overstated, particularly in patients with known peripheral vascular disease. Deciding on the appropriate site of access for peripheral arteriography is a most important preprocedural decision, analogous to planning a surgical incision. Optimal access reduces the likelihood of complications and shortens the duration of the procedure. The most favorable site of access is determined based on the clinical history, physical examination, and noninvasive studies (e.g., duplex ultrasonography, MRA, or CTA). The most common sites remain the common femoral and brachial arteries. If the femoral pulse is diminished or absent (e.g., owing to occlusion more proximally), one of several methods may be used to facilitate successful entry of the artery (14,15). We strongly recommend confirming the site of femoral access by fluoroscopy in all patients, particularly in those with ambiguous surface landmarks (see Chapter 4). Arterial calcification, which is frequently present in diseased arteries, can also aid as a fluoroscopic target. Ultrasound guidance, and road mapping of a contrast injection performed via a catheter positioned in the distal aorta from the contralateral groin, may also be helpful. For difficult access, a Doppler integrated needle (SmartNeedle) can be used to accurately locate the arterial or venous access site (16).

Although many operators use crossover techniques from the contralateral femoral artery, antegrade puncture of the ipsilateral common femoral artery (CFA) is widely

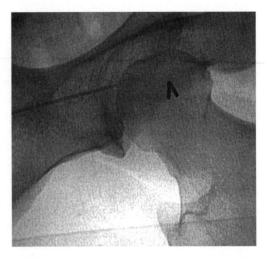

Figure 14.3 Antegrade femoral artery puncture. The skin nick at the top of the femoral head (needle), with ideal entry at the middle of the common femoral artery with angle <45°.

used to approach femoral, popliteal, or infrapopliteal disease. Antegrade access is considered more challenging technically and limits angiography to the ipsilateral leg, but it offers a more stable platform for intervention. The patient's orientation is reversed such that the feet are placed at the head of the gantry, allowing maximal mobility of the image intensifier around the lower limbs. As in retrograde access, the desired site of entry is in the middle of the CFA below the inguinal ligament, but given the different angulation, the skin puncture is made at or above the top of the femoral head (17; Fig. 14.3). A 9-cm needle is frequently required, as compared with the standard 7-cm needle used for retrograde access. A less acute needle angle, generally <45°, facilitates catheter and sheath insertion by avoiding the kinking associated with a steeper-angled entry. Arterial puncture should be performed under fluoroscopic guidance aiming for the mid or upper portion of the femoral head. Aids to antegrade access include arterial calcification or prior studies (angio, CTA, or MRA) that define the bifurcation of the CFA in relation to the femoral head. In cases with a known high CFA bifurcation, the antegrade stick should be modified accordingly.

Having achieved arterial puncture, a 0.035-inch wire is advanced under fluoroscopic guidance into the proximal SFA or PFA. The wires that we recommend include a Wholey wire (which provides a gentle steerable tip) or an angled Glidewire (which gives easy passage into the femoral circulation but must be used with care as it may track subintimally or be skeletonized by the sharp edge of the access needle). We recommend use of a 5F sheath until the site of arteriotomy and procedural requirement has been confirmed. To confirm the site of antegrade access, angiography with 30 to 50° of ipsilateral oblique angulation will define the arteriotomy site in relation to the common femoral bifurcation. Anticoagulation should be administered once the correct position of the access point has been confirmed. Extra care should be taken to remove the antegrade sheath promptly following the procedure to minimize complications. It is our practice to consider reversing anticoagulation to facilitate immediate sheath removal in the catheterization laboratory.

Great care should be exercised in advancing and manipulating catheters and guidewires in the severely diseased peripheral circulation to reduce the chance of embolization related to the traumatic disruption of cholesterol-rich atherosclerotic plaque. This rare but devastating complication of arteriography may lead to livedo reticularis, hypertension, renal failure, stroke, or potentially death (see Chapter 3). Although there are no proven therapies effective in the management of this dreadful complication, prostanoids (e.g., PGE1, PGI2) may serve a palliative role in those cases in which it occurs (18,19).

RADIOLOGIC EQUIPMENT

As in cardiac catheterization, optimal imaging requires a radiographic gantry capable of axial and sagittal orientation with sufficient mobility to allow imaging of all vascular beds. To capture the larger regions of interest (e.g., the entire aortic arch, the pelvic vasculature, or both legs) a large-field (14-inch or 36-cm) image intensifier is recommended. Widespread application of digital imaging has facilitated contrast enhancement and noise reduction, providing superior angiographic results. Digital subtraction angiography (DSA) and road mapping are two techniques commonly used in peripheral angiography and intervention. In DSA, subtraction of a precontrast mask suppresses interfering structures from subsequent projections, thereby

enhancing arterial filling and masking fixed structures (bone, calcifications, soft tissue, and air densities). This allows the use of lower doses of iodinated contrast or use of noniodinated contrast including carbon dioxide or gadolinium (20,21; Fig. 14.4A,B).

Further postprocessing features include reversal, magnification, pixel shifting, picture integration, contour enhancement, image stacking and three-dimensional reconstruction of the subtracted image (22–26). Quantitative analysis (QA) may be used to assess vessel diameters and lengths, degree of luminal narrowing, and blood flow velocity (27). Another useful technique used in DSA is road mapping. This technique is used for selective catheterization and is a useful aid for visualization of a moving catheter. Prior to moving the catheter, a small amount of contrast medium is injected. The image with filled vessels is stored in memory as a mask (a road map along which the catheter is to be moved). This mask is then subtracted from the following fluoroscopic images, which will display both the vessels and the catheter with its tip. Although it is not used in cardiac work (where cardiac motion precludes acquiring as suitable "mask" image), DSA is of great value in peripheral angiography as it reduces contrast volume, procedure time, and radiation exposure.

CATHETERS AND GUIDEWIRES

Just as there are a wide range of cardiac catheters and guidewires, vascular angiography and intervention have a wide range of tools available to meet different anatomic challenges. In addition to standard, thin-walled 18-gauge needles that will accommodate a 0.038-inch wire, micropuncture

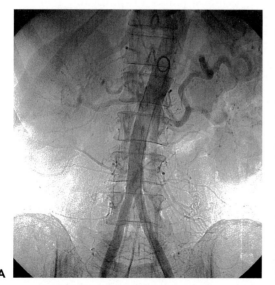
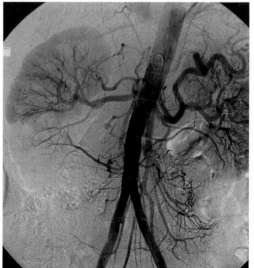

A   **B**

Figure 14.4 **A.** Normal abdominal aortogram using iodinated contrast material obtained by digital imaging technique. **B.** Same imaging data, but with enhancement of contrast-filled vessels obtained by the subtraction of all background densities (bones, soft tissue, gas) as recorded on a mask immediately prior to contrast injection.

(i.e., 21-gauge) needle sets are available that allow conversion to a standard (i.e., 0.035-inch) guidewire in situations with a high risk of bleeding or unsuccessful needle puncture attempts.

Most peripheral guidewires are made of a stainless steel coil surrounding a tapered inner core that runs the length of the wire for additional strength. A central safety wire filament is incorporated to prevent separation were the wire coil ever to fracture. Standard wires vary in diameter from 0.012 to 0.052 inch, with 0.035 and 0.038 being the most commonly used sizes. The length of most standard wires is between 100 and 180 cm; longer exchange-length guidewires (measuring 260 to 300 cm) permit keeping the tip of the wire in a selected position during catheter exchange. Tip configurations include straight or angled tip and J shape. Special features may include the ability to move the wire's inner core to vary the length of the floppy tip, deflect the wire tip, or transmit torque from the shaft to the tip so that it can be steered within the vascular tree. Varying degrees of shaft stiffness (e.g., extra-support wires) allow advancement of stiff devices through tortuous vessels, and low-friction wires with a hydrophilic coating (glide wires) have revolutionized peripheral work and made it possible to perform superselective catheterization and traverse complex stenoses and long occlusions.

Peripheral angiographic catheters are constructed of polyurethane, polyethylene, Teflon, or nylon with a wire braid in the wall of the catheter to impart torque ability. An ideal catheter has good memory, is nonthrombogenic, has sufficient torque control to facilitate rotational positions, can accommodate high-pressure injection, and tracks well (frequently aided by hydrophilic polymer coating). Catheters vary in French size, length, and hole pattern—either a single end hole for selective injections, both end and side holes, or a blocked end with side holes only. For catheters designed to be positioned in the abdominal aorta, 60- to 80-cm lengths are sufficient; in the thoracic or carotid areas, 100- to 120-cm lengths (similar to those of left heart catheters) may be required. The most common diagnostic catheter sizes are 5 to 7 French, although 3 and 4 French systems have gained popularity when brachial and radial arteries are used for access.

Several catheter shapes have been designed, which ultimately determines a specific function (Fig. 14.5). They fall into these general families:

- Straight catheters with multiple side ports that are used for rapid injection into large vessels and for exchange.
- Pigtail or tennis-racket catheters that are used for nonselective angiography in large vessels (i.e., aorta, pulmonary artery, or cardiac chambers). Multiple side holes along the distal shaft allow rapid delivery of contrast without a single forceful jet that could cause catheter whipping or subintimal dissection as might be seen with contrast exiting the end-hole alone.
- Simple curved catheters (i.e., Berenstein, Cobra, Headhunter) that are used for vessel selection.

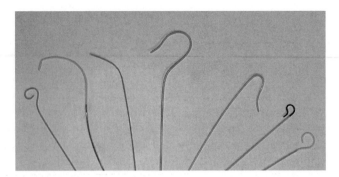

Figure 14.5 Peripheral angiographic catheters. **Left to right.** Pigtail, Cobra, multipurpose, Headhunter, Simmons, SOS-omni, tennis racket.

- Complex reverse-curve catheters (i.e., Simmons, sidewinder, SOS-OMNI) that are used for selective catheterization of certain aortic branches.

CONTRAST AGENTS

The principles of contrast agents are similar for peripheral angiography as for coronary angiography (Chapter 2). In general, high-osmolar contrast materials are avoided as they are associated with increased side effects (nausea, vomiting, light-headedness, local pain during peripheral injection), all of which reduce patient tolerance (28). Low-osmolar or iso-osmolar contrast delivers less osmotic load, resulting in reduced intravascular volume augmentation. Although their use has traditionally been confined to certain high-risk patient groups, they have more recently become standard in all catheterization laboratories.

Contrast-induced nephropathy (CIN, see Chapters 2 and 3) has become one of the most common complications of angiography, accounting for a 14.5% incidence of acute renal failure postangiography, and making it the third most common cause of new onset renal failure in hospitalized patients (29). CIN is particularly prevalent in peripheral angiography; owing to the large volumes of contrast required, the high incidence of comorbidities such as baseline renal dysfunction, diabetes, hypertension, and renal artery atherosclerosis (30). Aggressive prehydration, particularly with isotonic (0.9%) rather than hypotonic (0.45%) saline, reduces CIN, especially in high-risk patients (31). Use of iso-osmolar contrast agents (e.g., iodixanol) similarly decreases the incidence of CIN (32). Attempts to target the final pathway of free radical injury have focused on the use of the antioxidant acetylcysteine. Although the results have been conflicting, there appears to be little disadvantage in its use and possible benefit (33) (34–37). More definitive benefit has recently been published with periprocedural infusion of sodium bicarbonate, resulting in a significant reduction in CIN in what was shown to be a safe, inexpensive, and simple protocol (38).

Preventative methods for CIN have focused on the development of nonnephrotoxic contrast agents. Two such agents have now emerged as alternatives in patients with renal dysfunction or a history of contrast allergy. Carbon dioxide (CO_2) as a contrast agent has been used extensively in many vascular beds (39–44). Its primary advantage is that it obviates any risk of allergic reaction or nephrotoxicity (45). Its application is limited to arteries below the diaphragm to minimize the risk of cerebral embolization, and digital subtraction equipment is required. Another agent, gadolinium (gadopentetate dimeglumine), has traditionally been used with magnetic resonance imaging, but can also be applied to catheter-based imaging (46–48). Like CO_2, it is relatively nontoxic, although the maximal dose is limited to 0.4 mmol/kg (approximately 60 mL; Fig. 14.6A,B).

Beyond these general peripheral imaging techniques, there are a number of important considerations relating to each portion of the arterial tree. In this and subsequent chapters relating to the peripheral circulation (Chapters 26 and 34), we will review the territories in a head-to-foot sequence.

THORACIC AORTA

Anatomy

The aortic valve is composed of three leaflets that form the three sinuses of Valsalva: right, left, and posterior (49). The ascending aorta itself begins just beyond the sinus segment, and courses in a mostly anterior-posterior direction. The diameter of the ascending aorta varies between 2.2 cm

and 3.8 cm in middle-aged adults and increases slightly with advancing age (50). After it passes over the main pulmonary artery and left mainstem bronchus, the aorta gives rise to the brachiocephalic trunk and then courses posteriorly and leftward in front of the trachea. It then gives rise to the remaining arch vessels—the left common carotid, and left subclavian arteries—from its upper surface (Fig. 14.7A).

Distal to the origin of the left subclavian artery, the aorta narrows slightly at the site of the isthmus where the ligamentum arteriosum (the remnant of the fetal ductus arteriosus) tethers the aorta to the left pulmonary artery. Just distally to this point, a fusiform dilatation, called the aortic spindle, may occur. The descending aorta then continues anterior to the spine, with a diameter of approximately 2.5 cm. Vessels deriving from the descending portion of the aorta are nine pairs of posterior intercostal arteries (levels T3 to T11). The first and second posterior intercostal arteries are supplied by the superior intercostal artery, which is a branch of the subclavian artery. At the level of the fourth to sixth thoracic vertebrae, anteriorly directed bronchial arteries come off to supply each lung.

Disorders of the Thoracic Aorta

Aortic Coarctation

Coarctation of the aorta (see also Chapters 27 and 33) occurs in 0.02% to 0.06% of the population and may be associated with bicuspid aortic valve (33% of cases), patent ductus arteriosus, ventricular septal defect (VSD), or Turner syndrome (51). To bypass the resulting bandlike narrowing of the aorta, collateral flow occurs retrograde

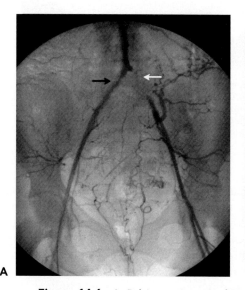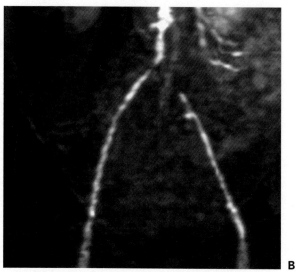

Figure 14.6 **A.** Pelvic arteriogram of 75-year-old female with bilateral hip claudication demonstrating diffuse infrarenal aortic atherosclerosis, right common iliac artery stenosis (black arrow), and left common iliac artery occlusion (white arrow) with external iliac artery reconstitution via collaterals. **B.** Corresponding MRA with two-dimensional gadolinium-enhanced technique that mirrors the DA image.

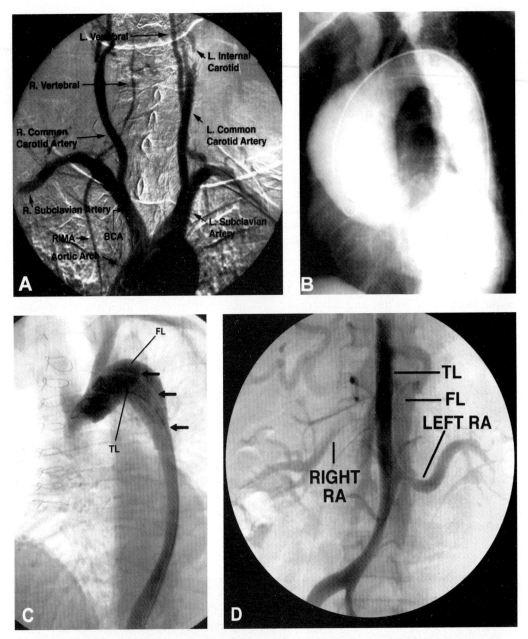

Figure 14.7 **A.** Normal ascending and arch aortogram with great vessels. **B.** Ascending aortic aneurysm owing to cystic medial degeneration. **C.** Stanford type A aortic dissection following aortic valve replacement. The intimal dissection flap *(arrows)* separates the contrast-filled true lumen (TL) from the false lumen (FL) that compromises the TL as it proceeds distally. **D.** The dissection extending into the abdominal aorta with origination of the left renal artery from the FL and TL supplying the right renal artery.

into the posterior intercostal branches of the descending aorta. The resultant enlargement and tortuosity of these intercostal arteries are responsible for the "rib notching" seen on chest radiographs.

The classical findings by aortography or MRA are of a high-grade, discrete narrowing of the aorta at the level of the isthmus, with associated dilatation of the ascending aorta and enlargement of the internal thoracic and the intercostal arteries (52). Aortography assumes a significant role in differentiating the great variety of abnormal patterns,

including complete aortic interruption, hypoplastic aorta and the most common type—a stenosis at the site of the isthmus, distal to the origin of the left subclavian artery. Both AP and lateral (RAO/LAO) aortography should be initially undertaken, with contrast injection performed proximal to the presumed site of coarctation using either large-film or cineangiographic technique. When attempting to traverse the site of narrowing in retrograde fashion, care must be taken to avoid inadvertent perforation of the thin-walled poststenotic segment. Entrance to the prestenotic aorta from the brachial or axillary arteries may thus be preferred.

Patent Ductus Arteriosus

The prevalence of patent ductus arteriosus is 1/5,500 in children younger than 14 years of age (53). Selective aortic angiography is sensitive in demonstrating small shunts and surpasses the sensitivity of right heart catheterization with stepwise oximetry (see also Chapters 9, 27, and 33).

Aortic Aneurysms

Thoracic aortic aneurysms (TAAs) and pseudoaneurysms may have various causes, including those that are degenerative, atherosclerosis-related, or congenital (aneurysms of the Valsalva sinus); other causes include trauma, infection (syphilitic, bacterial), cystic medial degeneration, connective tissue disorders, vasculitic, and chronic dissection. Degenerative aneurysms involving the descending aorta account for approximately 75% of TAAs (54,55). Cystic medial degeneration (as seen in Marfan syndrome) may also result in aneurysms of the ascending aorta (56); Fig. 14.8B). Aneurysms caused by blunt or penetrating trauma often involve the proximal descending thoracic aorta where the mobile arch segment joins the descending segment that is fixed to the spine (57–59). These may present as pseudoaneurysms—contained ruptures that lack intimal and medial components and are contained only by adventitia and periaortic tissue.

The natural history of TAAs is poorly understood as compared with the extensive data available on untreated infrarenal abdominal aortic aneurysms (60). Many patients with thoracic aortic aneurysms are asymptomatic at the time of diagnosis, with the aneurysm incidentally detected during testing for an unrelated disorder. Thoracic aneurysms appear to enlarge at a more rapid rate than abdominal aneurysms (0.42 versus 0.28 cm/year), and aneurysms larger than 5 to 6 cm in diameter enlarge even faster and have a greater likelihood of rupture (60–62). The cumulative five-year risk of rupture is increased fivefold in aneurysms ≥6 cm in diameter. Symptoms tend to develop late in the course of the enlargement of the aorta and are usually related to impingement on adjacent structures. In addition to presenting with catastrophic rupture, patients with TAA may report dyspnea, hoarseness, dysphagia, stridor, and plethora with edema from superior vena cava (SVC) compression. Neck or jaw pain may also be present in patients with aneurysms of the aortic arch. Dilatation of the aortic valve annulus and aortic valve may produce aortic regurgitation and congestive heart failure. Aneurysms of the descending thoracic aorta may produce pleuritic left-sided or interscapular pain, whereas thoracoabdominal aortic aneurysms may induce complaints of abdominal pain and left shoulder discomfort from irritation of the left hemidiaphragm.

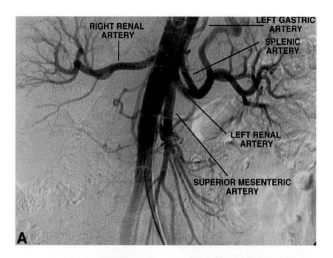

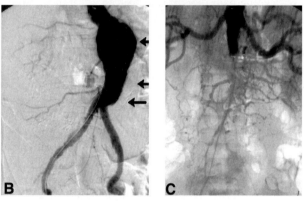

Figure 14.8 **A.** Normal abdominal aortogram in anteroposterior projection. **B.** Aortogram demonstrating an infrarenal abdominal aortic aneurysm (4.7 cm) that underestimates the accurate size owing to the presence of mural thrombus *(arrows)*. **C.** Distal aortic occlusion below the renal arteries.

The primary treatment for TAAs is surgical repair when the diameter >5 to 6 cm or symptoms develop (63). The standard procedure is to use a Dacron graft to replace the diseased segment. In most patients undergoing elective thoracic aorta surgical repair, aortography is required to provide information about the location of the aneurysm and its relationship to major aortic branches in the chest and abdomen. Optimal surgical approaches, as well as operative risks, are best defined by imaging the coronary, brachiocephalic, visceral, and renal arteries during injections. Stent–graft devices have been successfully used as an alternative to surgical grafting for both thoracic and aortic degenerative and post-traumatic descending TAAs (64–66). Early experience has been limited by incomplete aneurysm thrombosis, graft leak, and failure. However, further refinements in the technology may make this modality a viable option in poor surgical candidates.

Aortic Dissection

Aortic dissection is a longitudinal cleavage of the aortic media by a dissecting column of blood (67). An intimal tear allows the passage of blood into the aortic wall, separating the inner and outer layers of the aortic wall and creating a "double-barrel lumen" (68). Men are affected about twice as frequently as women (69). Most patients are between 50 and 70 years of age and have arterial hypertension (70). Other risk factors include cystic medial degeneration (71), Marfan syndrome (72), bicuspid aortic valve, aortic coarctation, blunt trauma (70), pregnancy (73,74), connective tissue disorders (72), and thoracic aorta operative procedures (75). The dissection may extend proximally from its origin to the aortic annulus, or distally to involve the entire length of the aorta and any or all of its major branches, until terminated by an aortic branch or atherosclerotic plaque.

Dissection is usually heralded by the sudden onset of excruciating pain described as tearing, throbbing, lacerating, ripping or burning in the anterior chest, neck or intrascapular region (76). Similar pain may occur with rupture or sudden expansion of a chronic dissection. If the acute dissection results in compression of aortic branches, symptoms and signs of acute myocardial infarction (77,78), stroke or TIA, paraparesis (79), mesenteric ischemia, renal failure (80), paraplegia, and extremity ischemia (81) may result. Most patients with ascending aortic extension who are treated medically die within 3 months, usually from dissection into the pericardium, mediastinum, or pleural cavity.

Once considered the gold standard for diagnosis of aortic dissection, aortography (which has a sensitivity of 80% and specificity of about 95%) has largely been replaced by CT, MRA, and transesophageal echocardiography (TEE; 82). Visualization of an intimal flap is the only direct aortographic sign that is pathognomonic of dissection. This is frequently in association with delayed or sluggish filling of a second lumen, although about 20% of patients with aortic dissection have only one visible aortic channel. The presence of a false lumen may still be suspected, however, if that single channel shows evidence of extrinsic compression by a hematoma in the false lumen. Beyond documenting the dissection, aortography provides information about aortic insufficiency and branch vessel or coronary artery involvement, particularly in cases where CT or MRI findings are equivocal and there is a strong clinical suspicion of aortic dissection (83).

Two classification systems of aortic dissection are widely used. The *DeBakey classification* is based on the anatomical extent of the dissection (71,84). In type I, the tear originates in the ascending aorta and extends distally. Type II dissections are confined to the ascending aorta. In type III, the dissection may be confined to the descending aorta (type IIIa) or extend into the abdominal aorta and iliac arteries (type IIIb). The *Stanford classification* is based solely on the location of the origin of the dissection (85). Type A includes all cases where the ascending aorta is involved, and type B includes those where the ascending aorta is not involved (Fig. 14.7C,D).

When approaching a patient with suspected aortic dissection, the preferred entry point is the femoral artery with the best pulse. An atraumatic diagnostic catheter (e.g., pigtail or tennis racket) with a soft J-tipped guidewire should be advanced under fluoroscopic guidance with frequent test injections. Since the entry to the false lumen is commonly on the greater (outer) curve of the aorta, the catheter may be used to direct the wire toward the inner curve to maximize the chance of remaining in the true lumen. If this is done successfully, structures like the aortic leaflets and coronary arteries will be observed, and it will be possible to enter the left ventricle. It is not uncommon, however, to enter the false lumen during initial catheter advancement. When this becomes apparent on test injections, care should be taken to avoid extending the false lumen, pulling the catheter back and using the techniques discussed above to re-enter the true lumen.

Surgical repair of Stanford type A aortic dissections entails Dacron graft placement of the ascending aorta (86). If the aortic valve is abnormal, it is replaced (87). In contrast, most patients with type B acute aortic dissections can be initially treated with medical therapy, reserving surgical intervention for those with signs of impending rupture (persistent pain and hypotension), ischemia of legs or mesentery, renal failure, paraparesis, or paraplegia (77). In cases of chronic dissection, operative treatment should be considered if the diameter of the descending aorta exceeds 5 to 6 cm or symptoms develop. Endovascular stents and balloon fenestration have been successfully used in treating the ischemic complications associated with aortic dissection (65,88–90).

Vasculitides

Vasculitis, highlighted by inflammation of the vessel wall, has two forms that commonly affect the aorta and its branches. These produce dilation of the proximal aorta, narrowing or occlusion of large aortic branches, or both. Takayasu arteritis is characterized by irregularity of the ascending aorta, narrowing of the descending aorta, obstructions of arch vessels, and aortic insufficiency or dissection (91–93). Therapeutic options include surgical bypass or balloon angioplasty demonstrating adjunctive stenting in patients with end organ ischemia (94,95). Intervention should generally be reserved until acute inflammation has subsided.

Giant cell or temporal arteritis is a vasculitis of large and medium arteries. Angiographic evidence of aortic branch involvement shows long, smooth stenoses alternating with relatively normal segments. The intracranial carotid artery and its branches, or the distal subclavian arteries, are usually involved, with aortic disease relatively uncommon (96).

Connective Tissue Disorders

Several inherited diseases, including Marfan syndrome, Ehlers-Danlos syndrome, and hereditary annuloaortic ectasia, may be responsible for noninflammatory degeneration of the aortic wall. These may lead to aneurysm formation, rupture, or dissection.

Marfan syndrome is a rare autosomal dominant disorder that may affect the aorta, heart, eye, and skeleton. Cardiovascular complications occur in >50% of patients (97,98). Cystic medial degeneration accounts for the resultant changes in aortic root dilation with aortic ectasia, aortic insufficiency, aneurysm formation, or dissection (99). In Marfan syndrome, the aortic dilatation is primarily confined to the aortic root. Asymptomatic aortic dissection may be seen in approximately 10% of patients. Treatment for patients with Marfan syndrome and cystic medial degenerative disease should undergo elective replacement of the ascending aorta and the aortic sinuses when the greatest diameter of the aorta is 5.0 to 5.5 cm (100). The most commonly performed procedure is replacement of the ascending aorta and the aortic valve with a composite graft containing Dacron and a mechanical valve prosthesis. The coronary arteries are reimplanted in the Dacron graft (101).

Ehlers-Danlos syndrome is a rare set of genetic disorders of collagen production. The literature describes more than nine types of this syndrome with features of hyperextensibility of joints and thick skin. Vascular complications include vessel thrombosis, rupture, or embolization from aneurysms (102).

Thoracic Aortography

Arch aortography has historically been used to examine the aorta for aortic valve or root disease; suspected aneurysms or dissections; congenital anomalies such as vascular rings, coarctation, or patent ductus arteriosus; evaluation of vascular injuries associated with blunt or penetrating chest trauma; and for examination of stenoses at the origins of the great vessels. Although TEE, CT, and magnetic resonance arteriography (MRA) have been applied to many of these clinical settings, aortography remains the gold standard for aortic imaging.

Thoracic aortography is usually performed from the femoral approach. In cases of suspected aortic dissection with diminished or absent femoral pulses or a history of catheter-related cholesterol embolization, angiography may also be performed safely via a brachial access. A high-flow multi-side-hole (pigtail) catheter is positioned in the ascending aorta, just above the sinus of Valsalva. Contrast (40 to 60 mL injected at 20 mL/second) is injected using a power injector. For cine imaging, 30 frames per second may be used; for digital imaging four to six frames/second should be used with breath-holding to minimize motion artifact. The left anterior oblique (LAO) projection optimally delineates the aortic arch—in the right anterior oblique (RAO) projection, the ascending and descending aorta are often superimposed and the origin of the great vessels tends to be obscured. Use of digital subtraction angiography (DSA) allows a lower concentration of contrast to be used (20 mL/second for a total of 30 mL at four to six frames/second). The aortogram should be centered and angulated to provide the maximum information for clinical setting. For example, aortography used to evaluate blunt injury should include sufficient imaging of the descending thoracic aorta, whereas aortography for ascending aortic dissection should also enable detection of regurgitation into the left ventricle.

ABDOMINAL AORTA

Anatomy

The abdominal aorta starts at the level of the diaphragm (T12) and proceeds anterior to the spine and to the left of the inferior vena cava until it bifurcates into the common iliac arteries at the level of the fourth lumbar vertebra (49; Figure 14.8A). The normal diameter of the midabdominal aorta varies between 1.50 cm and 2.15 cm, with a slight increase in size with age and male gender (103). Three main branches of the aorta originate from its ventral surface. The first is the celiac artery at the level of T12-L1. The second branch is the superior mesenteric artery (SMA), which takes off about 1 cm caudal to the celiac axis at the L1–L2 level. The third is the inferior mesenteric artery (IMA), which originates at the L3–L4 level and takes off in an anterolateral direction, slightly to the left. The renal arteries originate posterolaterally from the aorta at the level of L1–L2 (just below the SMA). Four pairs of lumbar arteries arise in a posterolateral direction below the main renal arteries.

Clinical Manifestations of Abdominal Aortic Disease

In patients with abdominal aortic aneurysms (AAA), the goals of preoperative imaging are detection, staging, surveillance, and diagnosis of rupture (104,105). Important information in planning a management strategy includes the size and length of the AAA, proximal and distal margins, number, location and patency of renal and mesenteric arteries, presence of lower extremity occlusive disease, and any associated aneurysmal disease (e.g., iliac, hypogastric, femoral, or other intra-abdominal vessels; Fig. 14.6B). The role of abdominal aortography in the preoperative assessment of patients with AAA has diminished with the advent of CT, MRI, and sonography (Fig. 14.7). Preoperative angiography may be useful in the cases of suspected suprarenal or juxtarenal aortic aneurysm involvement, renal or mesenteric artery stenosis, horseshoe kidney, and iliofemoral occlusive disease.

Atherosclerotic occlusive disease, or atherosclerosis obliterans (ASO), may warrant arteriographic examination of the aorta. ASO may result in complete occlusion of the aorta (106; Fig. 14.8C). The cause usually is a chronic thrombotic occlusion superimposed on severe atherosclerosis of the distal aorta and iliac arteries. Leriche syndrome is a chronic aortic occlusion that consists of buttock and thigh claudication, impotence, and the absence of femoral pulses (107). Congenital coarctation syndromes, which include Williams syndrome (108), neurofibromatosis (109), congenital rubella (110), and tuberous sclerosis (111), may also involve the abdominal aorta and its branches. Aortography reveals a smooth tapered proximal and midabdominal aorta with proximal renal artery involvement and narrowing of the superior mesenteric or celiac arteries. Middle aortic syndrome (abdominal aortic coarctation) produces stenoses of the midaorta and its associated major branches (112). Treatment options include surgical bypass or percutaneous transluminal angioplasty with endovascular stenting in certain cases, although experience is limited and the exact role of the latter is controversial (113).

Abdominal Aortography

Abdominal aortography is typically performed from a femoral approach, using a 4 to 6 French multi-side-hole pigtail or an Omni Flush diagnostic catheter. If the femoral pulse is not palpable on either side, alternative options include translumbar, axillary, brachial, or radial approaches. The tip of the catheter should be positioned at the T12 or L1 level, thus placing the side holes adjacent to the first and second lumbar vertebrae. Contrast medium should be injected (30 to 50 mL at a rate of 15 mL/second). At least four frames/second should be obtained when evaluating the mesenteric or renal arteries. When performing arteriography in an aorta with suspected or known aneurysmal disease or severe atherosclerotic involvement, meticulous care should be taken to avoid dislodging mural thrombus or plaque, resulting in distal embolization.

Ideally, two views of the aorta—anteroposterior and lateral—are performed, particularly if the origins of the mesenteric vessels are being evaluated. Assessment of a translesional pressure gradient can also be used to augment angiographic severity of an aortic narrowing. This is most easily performed by measuring the pressure gradient between a 4 or 5F catheter above the lesion and the side port of a long femoral sheath placed at the level of the aortic bifurcation. For aortic lesions, a gradient of 10 mm Hg is considered significant. Further augmentation of the gradient using vasodilators (200 μg of intra-arterial nitroglycerin) delivered into the lower aorta can also be used. Intravascular ultrasound (IVUS) provides additional information, and is a useful adjunct for aortic intervention by providing accurate lesion measurements. Although a 15-MHz transducer provides superior imaging for the aorta, it requires a larger sheath for access (8F). A 30-MHz (2.4F) transducer allows superior far-field imaging compared

with a 40-MHz coronary transducer without the need for up-sizing the arterial sheath.

SUBCLAVIAN AND VERTEBRAL ARTERIES

Anatomy

The brachiocephalic, left common carotid, and left subclavian arteries arise from the aortic arch after it passes over the main pulmonary artery and left main stem bronchus (49). Whereas the right subclavian artery and right common carotid originate as branches of the brachiocephalic trunk (also known as the *innominate* artery), the left common carotid and left subclavian usually originate separately from the aortic arch. An aortic arch variant in which the brachiocephalic and left common carotid artery may have a common origin (i.e., bovine arch), is present in about 10% of the population (114). The major branches of the subclavian artery that deserve special attention are the internal mammary and vertebral arteries; the latter originate from the superior aspect of the vessel (opposite the internal mammary) and proceed into the skull through the cervical transverse processes.

Manifestations of Subclavian Disease

Atherosclerosis of the proximal subclavian artery may manifest clinically as arm claudication, subclavian steal, or (in patients with previous internal mammary grafting) coronary ischemia (115). In classic subclavian steal, stenosis or occlusion of the proximal subclavian artery causes blood from the contralateral vertebral artery to flow antegrade across the basilar system and then retrograde down the ipsilateral vertebral to fill the subclavian artery distal to the lesion (Fig. 14.9A). In rare cases, this may cause cerebral ischemia during upper extremity exercise. In patients who have undergone internal mammary artery bypass grafting to a coronary artery, a proximal subclavian obstruction may cause retrograde flow in the graft during arm exercise and lead to coronary ischemia (coronary-subclavian steal; Fig. 14.9B,C). Stenosis of the vertebral origin is relatively common, particularly at its origin from the subclavian artery; however, cerebral symptoms are unusual, given the dual blood supply (from both vertebrals and from the carotid arteries by way of the posterior communicating artery) unless both vertebrals are diseased.

Subclavian and Vertebral Arteriography

An aortic arch arteriogram with a 5 French pigtail catheter can visualize the origin of the great vessels to evaluate for atherosclerotic occlusive disease. (See "Thoracic Aortography.") The optimum catheter for selective catheterization of the innominate or subclavian artery depends on the configuration of

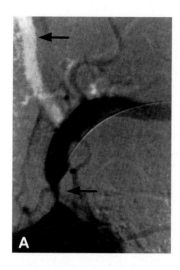

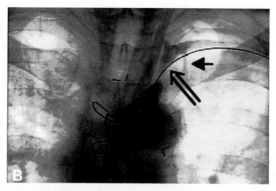

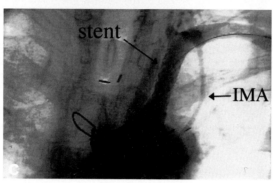

Figure 14.9 **A.** Selective left subclavian arteriogram depicting severe ostial stenosis *(arrow)* and retrograde flow through left vertebral artery *(white).* **B.** Arteriogram of subclavian artery in patient status post CABG with a LIMA graft and a high-grade ostial stenosis *(double arrow)* resulting in poor visualization of the graft *(arrow).* **C.** Following successful stenting of the subclavian artery stenosis and restoration of antegrade flow into the LIMA graft.

the great vessels of the neck. For the simple origin take off, angiography can generally be performed with a 5F Davies, Berenstein, JR4, hockey stick, or VTK catheter. If the arch aortogram demonstrates an elongated arch, a reverse-curve catheter such as a 5F VTK or Simmons may be required. A 30 to 45° LAO projection is useful for selecting each of the branches, with the catheters formed and oriented in the ascending aorta and withdrawn sequentially from innominate to left common carotid to left subclavian. Angiography of the innominate is usually best performed with 30 to 40° of RAO and mild caudal angulation to open out the innominate–subclavian bifurcation. Subclavian and vertebral angiography can generally be performed in the anteroposterior view, with the addition of an oblique view (RAO or LAO) if there is suspicion of an eccentric lesion. The origins of the internal mammary arteries are often clearly defined in the RAO cranial angulation, a point of particular importance in subclavian intervention.

If a proximal vertebral artery stenosis is expected, selective injection of the ipsilateral subclavian artery in the anteroposterior projection is usually diagnostic. Modest angulation may sometimes be necessary. Translesional gradients across innominate or subclavian lesions can be performed with either a 0.014-inch pressure wire or simultaneous pressures measured between a 4 or 5F catheter beyond the lesion and the side port of a long 6F sheath placed in the distal aorta. Augmentation of the gradient with injection of vasodilators into the distal subclavian circulation can be used to simulate exercise and augment the

gradient. A gradient of 15 mm Hg is considered significant for subclavian or innominate stenosis.

CAROTID ARTERIES

Anatomy

The brachiocephalic artery bifurcates into the right subclavian and right common carotid arteries as the first main branch off the aorta. The left common carotid is typically the second main branch of the aorta. Each common carotid runs within a fascial (carotid) sheath, lateral to the vertebrae, and bifurcates into an external and internal carotid artery branch at the fourth cervical vertebrae. Although the internal carotid artery normally has no main branches prior to entering the skull, it forms a tortuous portion known as the carotid siphon within the cavernous and supraclinoid segment, after which it divides into the anterior and posterior cerebral arteries. The external carotid artery has several major branches named for their territory of supply.

Extracranial Carotid Atherosclerosis

Approximately 700,000 strokes occur annually in the United States, of which 25 to 30% are owing to extracranial carotid artery disease. In the Minneapolis-St. Paul, Minnesota, metropolitan area during 1985, there were 1,792 hospital discharges with the diagnosis of acute stroke, representing an event rate of 828/100,000 population in men and 551/100,000 in women (116,117). Patients with carotid disease frequently have severe coronary artery disease. In a population of 506 patients undergoing evaluation for potential carotid revascularization, 16% of patients without clinical clues suggestive of coronary heart disease were found to have severe, surgically correctable coronary artery disease (118). Even patients with asymptomatic carotid artery stenosis have an increased risk of coronary events. In one study of 444 male patients, the 4-year mortality rate was 37%, with 61% of the deaths owing to coronary artery disease. Multivariate analysis shows diabetes mellitus, an abnormal electrocardiogram, and the presence of intermittent claudication to be associated with an increased mortality risk (two or three risk factors revealed annual mortality rates of 11.3% and 13%, respectively). Just the finding of increased carotid intima-media thickness on duplex ultrasonographic predicts a higher risk of myocardial infarction or stroke, as much as 3.87 times that compared to patients with minimal thickness (119,120).

Most patients with extracranial carotid artery disease are identified by the presence of a carotid bruit on physical examination, with no referable symptoms. Estimates of the prevalence of asymptomatic carotid bruits in adults range from 1 % (121) to 2.3 % in patients age 45 to 54 years and 8.2% in patients older than age 75 years (122). Among patients scheduled to undergo other vascular surgical procedures, however, the incidence of cervical bruits ranged from 6% (123) to 16% (124), with a mean prevalence of 10% (125). An asymptomatic carotid bruit carries a 1.5% annual incidence of stroke and a 3-year stroke risk of 2.1% (as demonstrated by the European Carotid Surgery Trialists; 126). Among patients with an asymptomatic bruit and with severe (70 to 99%) carotid stenosis, the 3-year risk of stroke was 5.7% (127).

Absence of a bruit, however, does not imply absence of significant carotid disease. In a substudy of the North American Symptomatic Carotid Endarterectomy Trial (NASCET), 1,268 patients with recent transient cerebral ischemia or nondisabling stroke were examined for the presence of a carotid bruit. Fifty-eight percent of patients had a bruit localized to the ipsilateral carotid artery, 31% had a carotid bruit involving the contralateral vessel, and 24% had bilateral carotid bruits. The sensitivity and specificity of a focal bruit to predict high-grade ipsilateral carotid stenosis was 63% and 61%, respectively. In this patient subgroup, absence of a bruit lowered the pretest 70 to 99% probability of a carotid stenosis from 52% only to 40% (128).

Once established, extracranial carotid artery stenosis progresses in approximately 20 to 40% of cases. In one prospective natural history study of 232 patients with mild (<50%) and moderate (50 to 79%) carotid stenosis followed with annual carotid duplex ultrasonography for a mean of 7 years, 23% demonstrated disease progression.

One half of these patients developed severe stenosis (80 to 99%) or occlusion. Progression to either 80 to 99% stenosis or occlusion was more likely in patients whose initial stenosis was 50 to 79% rather than <50% (129,130). More recent data in 425 asymptomatic patients with 50 to 79% carotid stenosis followed for a mean of 38 months demonstrated progression of stenosis in 17% of 282 arteries with at least two serial carotid duplex examinations. In general, this carried a moderately low incidence of ipsilateral stroke (0.85% at 1 year, 3.6% at 3 years, 5.4% at 5 years; 131), but patients with 80 to 99% carotid stenosis had an annual neurologic event rate of 20.6% (132).

Many carotid lesions are discovered only after the patient begins to experience symptoms, which may vary from transient monocular blindness (amaurosis fugax) to expressive or receptive aphasia, hemiparesis/hemiplegia, and mental status changes. Although these episodic symptoms last minutes to hours and then completely resolve, they are harbingers of recurrent and potentially nonreversible events, and thus warrant urgent evaluation and therapy in an attempt to prevent a catastrophic stroke. The first study in this evaluation is carotid duplex ultrasonography, which provides two-dimensional images of the extracranial carotid arteries and may provide information about plaque morphology (Fig. 14.10A). Color-coded images can detect increased velocities of blood flow, which correlate to greater degrees of stenosis, while Doppler waveforms and velocities can also be measured to evaluate stenosis severity when performed by skilled vascular ultrasonographers.(100; Fig. 14.10B) Once a significant stenosis is identified, contrast or magnetic resonance angiography (MRA) can be performed to corroborate the ultrasound findings (101; Fig. 14.10C). Conversely, if the ultrasound is performed by a reliable vascular laboratory, many surgeons proceed with endarterectomy based on this diagnostic test alone (102). A strategy of duplex ultrasonography followed by CTA yielded sensitivity of 100% and specificity of 84% (133).

Publication of a recent randomized trial comparing carotid endarterectomy to carotid artery stent placement in high-surgical risk patients demonstrated noninferiority of the endovascular procedure, prompting approval of this procedure in the United States (134; Fig. 14.10D). (See Chapters 26 and 34.)

Carotid Arteriography

Carotid arteriography remains the gold standard in assessing the presence and quantitative narrowing of the carotid and intracerebral vasculature. Despite the advances made with noninvasive techniques such as duplex ultrasonography, MRA, and spiral CTA, selective carotid catheterization may be indicated to more accurately delineate the degree of stenosis involving the distal common and internal carotid arteries, extent of disease at the bifurcation, as well as information about the intracranial circulation, including collateral flow patterns.

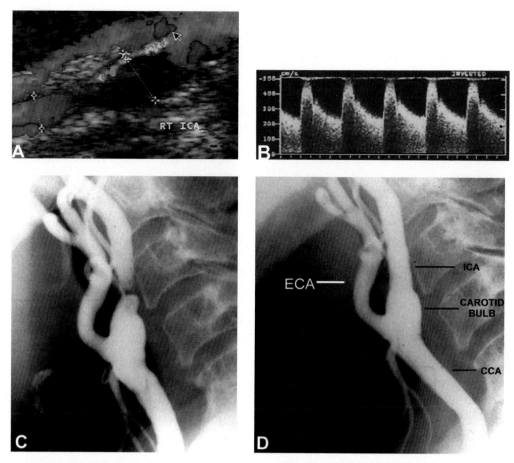

Figure 14.10 **A.** Color duplex image of severely narrowed right ICA. **B.** Corresponding spectral waveform of ICA showing accelerated peak systolic and end-diastolic velocities. **C.** Carotid arteriogram confirming severe stenosis involving the right ICA. **D.** Arteriogram of carotid bifurcation following successful stenting of stenotic right internal carotid artery (ICA).

To completely evaluate cerebral circulation, carotid angiography should be performed in conjunction with arch aortography and selective vertebral angiography. Arch aortography is a crucial first step because it allows characterization of the arch configuration and optimal catheter selection. Anatomical variations of the typical aortic arch include origin of the left common carotid from the innominate (bovine arch) seen in 25%, origin of the left vertebral from the aorta in 3%, or origin of the right subclavian as the distalmost vessel in 1%. For normal arch anatomy, a 5F Davies, Berenstein, or Headhunter catheter can be used. For elongated arch anatomy, a retroflexed catheter such as a VTK or Simmons may be required to selectively engage the greater vessels. Having engaged the carotid ostium, the catheter can be advanced over a 0.035-inch glide wire.

Once the catheter is beyond the aortic arch, careful double-flushing is mandatory to minimize risk of embolization. Injections of diluted low-osmolar contrast are typically performed with digital subtraction at 4 to 6 mL/second for a total of 8 mL in the common carotid

artery (CCA) with DSA at four or six frames/second, and at 3 to 4 mL/second for a total of 5 to 6 mL in the vertebral artery. In general, we begin with lower rates and volumes of contrast in the cerebral circulation and make adjustments as needed for subsequent images. Angiography should be extended into the venous filling phase to rule out any venous abnormality.

Multiple oblique projections are necessary, including anteroposterior, lateral, and oblique views to optimally visualize narrowing at the carotid bifurcation and proximal ICA. The lateral projection is best to visualize the proximal ICA and carotid siphon.

The angiographic views commonly used to delineate the intracerebral course of the internal carotid arteries includes the Town view (AP cranial to bring the petrous ridge over the roof of the orbit) and the straight lateral views. To calculate the percent diameter stenosis, the projection that demonstrates the highest degree of stenosis should be used. Many methods of calculating carotid artery stenosis have been used in previous trials; however, the NASCET methodology is the most widely accepted. It compares the stenotic area with the most normal-appearing artery distal to the stenosis.

RENAL ARTERIES

Anatomy

The renal arteries arise from the lateral aspect of the aorta at the L1–L2 level (49). Accessory renal arteries may occur in 25 to 35% of cases and usually supply the lower pole of the kidney. These may originate anywhere from the suprarenal aorta down to the iliac arteries.

Atherosclerotic Renal Artery Stenosis

Atherosclerotic renal artery stenosis (ARAS) is clearly more common than previously believed, with increasing prevalence in certain patient populations. In one series of 395 arteriograms performed in patients with abdominal aortic aneurysms, aortoiliac atherosclerosis, or infrainguinal atherosclerosis, 33 to 50% had a renal artery stenosis of >50% (135). In 346 patients with aneurysmal or occlusive vascular disease prompting arteriography, 28% had significant ARAS. The presence of coronary artery atherosclerosis is also a marker for ARAS. In a prospective study of 1,302 patients undergoing coronary arteriography, concurrent abdominal aortography demonstrated significant RAS in 15% of patients. The number of coronary arteries involved with atherosclerosis also appears to predict the likelihood of renal artery stenosis in this series. For example, if one coronary artery demonstrated atherosclerosis, the incidence of significant ARAS was 10.7%. If three coronary arteries and the left main trunk were involved with atherosclerosis, the incidence of ARAS was 39.0% (136). Conversely, 58% of patients with ARAS had clinically overt coronary artery disease.

Several clinical clues may suggest the presence of ARAS. Patients who develop diastolic hypertension after 55 years of age, who have exacerbation of previously well-controlled hypertension, who demonstrate refractory hypertension (uncontrolled hypertension despite treatment with three antihypertensive medications of synergistic classes at maximal doses), who develop azotemia after treatment with an angiotensin-converting enzyme inhibitor, or who present with malignant hypertension (severe hypertension and acute myocardial infarction, acute stroke or transient ischemic attack, aortic dissection, acute renal failure) should all be suspected of having renal artery stenosis. A discrepancy in renal size, the physical finding of a systolic and diastolic abdominal bruit with radiation to one or both flank regions, unexplained azotemia, or the presence of diffuse atherosclerosis with hypertension and azotemia without obvious cause must prompt the physician to search for renal artery disease. Up to 24% of patients with ESRD being considered for dialysis in one series had severe

ARAS (137). The 15-year survival of patients committed to end-stage renal disease (ESRD) because of ARAS was 0%, compared with 32% in patients committed to dialysis for other causes such as polycystic kidney disease.

The natural history of ARAS has been studied extensively in many retrospective series, which suggest that approximately 50% of renal artery stenoses progress over time (106). More recent prospective data using duplex ultrasonography to assess renal artery patency demonstrated that 48% of renal arteries whose baseline stenosis was <60% progressed to >60% stenosis after 36 months, compared with only 8% in vessels with no stenosis at baseline (138).

A number of noninvasive diagnostic tests have been used to determine if renal artery stenosis is present. Historically, rapid-sequence intravenous pyelography was used, but this test has now been shown to be inaccurate. Equally inaccurate are plasma renin levels, only elevated in 50 to 80% of patients with RAS (139). Captopril-stimulated nuclear renography is a prominent diagnostic test for patients with suspected renal artery stenosis, with sensitivity and specificity in the range of 90% (140). However, in a recent comparison with clinical clues for the diagnosis of renal artery stenosis, the isotopic renal scan was no better than the clinical prediction rule to predict renal artery stenosis, particularly in the presence of bilateral renal artery stenosis or impaired renal function.

Renal artery duplex ultrasonography can be an excellent test to diagnose renal artery stenosis if performed by a skilled operator. In one prospective series, of 29 patients (58 renal arteries) who underwent contrast arteriography and duplex ultrasonography, sensitivity of the latter was 84%, specificity was 97%, and positive predictive value was 94% for detection of >60% stenosis (141). Using criteria of peak systolic velocity within the renal artery >180 cm/second, duplex scanning was able to discern between normal and diseased renal arteries with sensitivity of 95% and specificity of 90% (142). The ratio of peak systolic velocity (PSV) in the area of renal artery stenosis compared with the PSV within the aorta (renal to aortic ratio, or RAR) of >3.5 predicts the presence of >60% renal artery stenosis with a sensitivity of 92%. In another large prospective series of 102 consecutive patients who underwent both duplex ultrasonography and contrast arteriography within 1 month of each other, 62 of 63 arteries with <60% stenosis, 31 of 32 arteries with 60 to 79% stenosis, and 67 of 69 arteries with 80 to 99% stenosis were correctly identified by duplex ultrasonography. Occluded renal arteries were correctly identified in 22 of 23 cases. The overall sensitivity of duplex ultrasonography was 98%, specificity was 99%, positive predictive value was 99%, and negative predictive value was 97% (143).

Limitations of direct ultrasound visualization of the renal arteries include large body habitus and overlying bowel gas obscuring identification of the renal arteries. Some authors have suggested that renal hilar scanning is easier and as accurate as complete interrogation of the renal arteries (144). However, direct comparison of both techniques has revealed limitations of hilar scanning, including low sensitivity, inability to discriminate between stenosis and occlusion, and inadequate determination of accessory renal arteries. The sensitivity was 67% for hilar scanning, with a specificity of 89 to 99% (145). Given that many patients have both main renal artery disease and intraparenchymal disease, the addition of resistive indices within the parenchyma may help predict which patients will benefit from revascularization (146).

Duplex ultrasonography is an excellent method for determining patency following revascularization (147). Given the proliferation of endovascular therapy (percutaneous angioplasty with stent deployment; 148), duplex ultrasonography is helpful in detecting restenosis.

Magnetic resonance arteriography has demonstrated great promise as a highly accurate noninvasive test for the diagnosis of renal artery stenosis (149,150). Limitations of this technology, predominantly overestimating degrees of stenosis, are decreasing with the addition of intravenous gadolinium, a nonnephrotoxic contrast agent (151), and perhaps with the addition of captopril (152).

Computed tomographic angiography (CTA) has demonstrated efficacy in the diagnosis of renal artery stenosis. When compared with contrast arteriography, the sensitivity of CTA is 92%, with specificity of 95% (153). Recent studies have even suggested the potential use of CTA in determining the patency of renal artery stents (154).

Renal Arteriography

Access for renal angiography is most commonly achieved from the femoral approach. A brachial approach may be advantageous if there is significant infrarenal aortic atheroma or aneurysmal disease or an extreme downward angulation of the renal arteries detected by preprocedural noninvasive testing. The first stage of renal angiography is an abdominal aortogram, allowing identification of ostia of the renal arteries and locating any accessory renal arteries seen in as many as 25% of the population. Frequently, an aortogram will suffice in ruling out significant renal artery stenosis. As with abdominal aortography described above, a 5F multiholed catheter placed at the L1–L2 interspace for a power injection of a total of 30 mL at 15 mL/second using DSA at four frames/second is generally sufficient to provide adequate opacification. If DSA is not available, the concentration of contrast should be increased accordingly, a total of 40 mL at 20 mL/second. In the setting of renal insufficiency, carbon dioxide can be used as a surrogate contrast agent. In this setting a bolus dose of 40 to 50 mL of carbon dioxide delivered by hand injection during breath-holding using DSA (four frames/second) can allow adequate localization of the renal artery origins to allow selective angiography.

Using the abdominal aortogram, or noninvasive imaging, as a guide, the appropriate catheter can be selected for selective renal arteriography. Commonly used catheters include 5F internal mammary, hockey stick, or renal double-curve catheters. For downward angulated renal arteries, a reverse-curve catheter such as an Omni selective catheter may be more appropriate from the femoral approach or a 5F multipurpose catheter from a brachial approach. Contrast should be injected at a rate of 5 mL/second for a total of 5 to 8 mL using DSA at four frames/second. Angiography should include both the arterial phase and the nephrographic phase.

The origin of the renal arteries is variable, necessitating varied angulations to adequately display the renal ostia en face. A useful technique is to modify the LAO/RAO angulation while fluoroscopically watching the catheter until its tip appears maximally opened. Additionally, disease involving renal bifurcations may require cranial or caudal angulation to open out the lesion in its full severity.

If there is evidence of aortic atheroma, either by noninvasive imaging or by aortography, a technique of no-touch angiography is recommended. In this technique a 0.014-inch wire is left in the catheter, sitting in the abdominal aorta to prevent the catheter from dislodging atheroma as its tip is manipulated toward the renal artery.

Occasionally, renal angiography will yield equivocal or indeterminate results, particularly in complex conditions such as fibromuscular dysplasia, Takayasu arteritis, radiation, aneurysms, or vasculitis. In this setting, measurement of a trans-stenotic gradient provides useful information regarding the hemodynamic significance of a stenosis. Pressure measurement is most accurately measured using a 0.014-inch pressure wire, but alternatively can be performed by measuring the differential pressure between a 4F catheter placed beyond the lesion and a 5 or 6F sheath or guide placed in the aorta. Gradients greater than 10 mm Hg mean or 20 mm Hg systolic are considered significant (Fig. 14.11).

Intravascular ultrasound (IVUS) provides a further method of renal artery evaluation for indeterminate lesions. IVUS is particularly useful in guiding or evaluating renal intervention. A standard 40-MHZ IVUS catheter affords sufficient image resolution for most renal sizes while maintaining a low profile.

PELVIC AND LOWER EXTREMITIES

Anatomy

The bifurcation of the abdominal aorta into the common iliac arteries (CIAs) occurs at the level of L4–L5 (49; Fig. 14.12A). The common iliac arteries divide at the lumbosacral junction, with the internal iliac arteries (IIAs) taking off medially and posteriorly, and the external iliac arteries (EIAs) continuing anteriorly and laterally to the

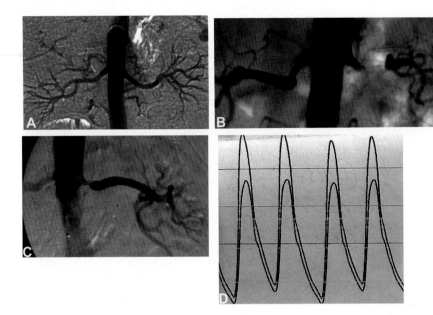

Figure 14.11 **A.** Abdominal aortogram demonstrating normal renal arteries. **B.** Atherosclerosis of the aorta resulting in bilateral renal artery stenosis. **C.** Selective injection of the left renal artery depicting an apparent moderate degree of luminal narrowing. **D.** However, an intra-arterial pressure tracing obtained across the lesion demonstrates a peak systolic and mean gradient of 23 mm Hg and 12 mm Hg respectively, indicating a hemodynamic significant lesion.

groin where they exit the pelvis just posterior to the inguinal ligament to become the common femoral artery. The inferior epigastric artery takes off medially at the junction of the EIA and common femoral artery. The deep iliac circumflex artery takes off laterally and superiorly.

The common femoral artery (CFA) originates at the inguinal ligament and then bifurcates (usually at the lower portion of the femoral head) into the superficial femoral artery (SFA) anteromedially and the deep femoral artery (DFA or "profunda") posterolaterally (Fig. 14.12B). The DFA has two major branches, the lateral circumflex and medial circumflex femoral arteries. The SFA proceeds down the anteromedial thigh and dives deep at the adductor (Hunter) canal, where it becomes the popliteal artery running posterior to the femur. Major popliteal branches include the sural and geniculate (superior, middle, and inferior) arteries around the knee (Fig. 14.12C).

Below the knee, at the border of the popliteus muscle, the popliteal artery divides, with the anterior tibial (AT) artery proceeding laterally and anterior to the tibia toward the foot. As it passes over the ankle onto the dorsum of the foot, it continues as the dorsalis pedis (DP) artery. After the takeoff of the AT, the popliteal continues as the tibioperoneal trunk (TPT), which then bifurcates into the posterior tibial (PT) and peroneal (PER) arteries. The PT courses posteromedially in the calf, whereas the peroneal runs near the fibula between the AT and PT arteries. The peroneal artery then rejoins the PT above the ankle via its posterior division, and the AT via its anterior division (Fig. 14.12D). On the dorsum of the foot, the DP artery has lateral and medial tarsal branches. After the PT artery passes behind the medial malleolus, it divides into medial and lateral plantar arteries. The lateral plantar and distal DP arteries join to form the plantar arch (Fig. 14.12E).

Lower-Extremity Arterial Occlusive Disease

The prevalence of peripheral arterial occlusive disease (PAD) remains difficult to appreciate among the general population. Since a significant segment of the population with PAD has no symptoms of the disorder, true prevalence rates are difficult to ascertain. Patients with asymptomatic PAD are at minimal risk of developing critical limb ischemia that threatens limb survival, with the obvious exception of the patient who suffers acute limb ischemia from an embolic event or trauma. Instead, patients first develop intermittent claudication to some degree before progressing to rest pain, a nonhealing ischemic ulcer, or gangrene.

The United States National Institutes of Health suggests that lower-extremity arterial occlusive disease causes over 60,000 hospitalizations annually, each stay lasting an average of >11 days (155). Manifestations of arteriosclerosis obliterans, namely diminished pedal pulses and carotid bruits, occur with increasing frequency as the population ages. Although intermittent claudication occurs more often in men at any age, physical examination findings of peripheral arterial disease occur with identical frequency in men and women (156). Several investigators have attempted to define the prevalence of PAD using noninvasive testing modalities and symptom questionnaires. In one series of 613 men and women with a mean age of 66 years, using segmental limb blood pressures, Doppler flow velocities, reactive hyperemia, and pulse reappearance times, researchers found an 11.7% incidence of large-vessel PAD (157). Although 11.7% of the population thus had evidence of PAD, only 2.2% of men and 1.7% of women had intermittent claudication. In this same population, however, 20.3% of men and 22.1% of women had

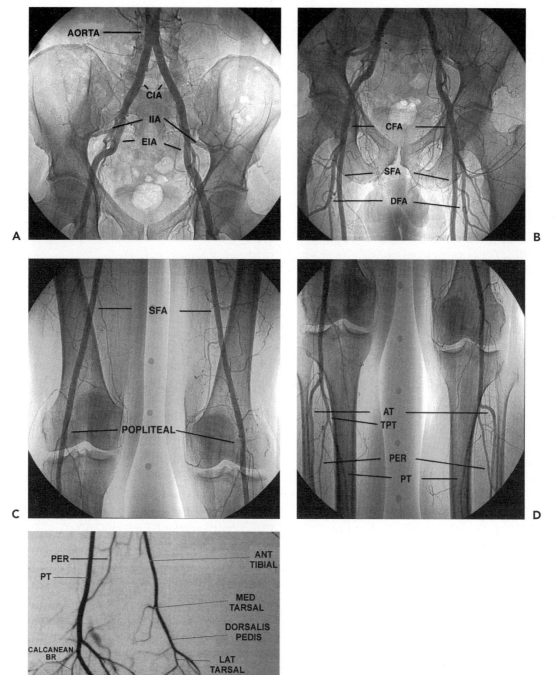

Figure 14.12 Normal pelvic and lower-extremity arteriogram. **A.** The distal abdominal aorta bifurcating into the iliac arteries. **B.** The common femoral artery (CFA) dividing into the deep femoral (DFA) and superficial femoral arteries (SFA). **C.** The SFA traversing the thigh into the popliteal artery as it dives through the adductor (Hunter) canal. **D.** The popliteal artery dividing laterally into the anterior tibial (AT) artery and continuing directly into the tibioperoneal trunk (TPT), which bifurcates into the posterior tibial (PT) and peroneal arteries (PER). **E.** The dorsalis pedis artery (DP) originates from the AT artery beyond the ankle and PT artery, which gives off plantar branches. (CIA, common iliac arteries; IIA, internal iliac arteries; EIA, external iliac arteries.)

abnormalities in the femoral or posterior tibial artery pulse examination.

The currently accepted methods of determining the presence of PAD include an historical review of patient symptoms and atherosclerotic risk factors, physical examination, and the use of noninvasive vascular tests. Unfortunately, the history is often quite unreliable for confirming the diagnosis of PAD, as <50% of patients actually have classic symptoms of intermittent claudication (158).

A simple, accurate, painless, and noninvasive test is the ankle-brachial index (ABI). This test compares the blood pressure obtained with a handheld Doppler in the dorsalis pedis or posterior tibial artery (whichever is higher) to the blood pressure in the higher of the two brachial pressures. Generally, an ABI >0.9 is considered normal, >0.5 to <0.9 reflects mild to moderate PAD, and <0.5 suggests severe arterial occlusive disease.

It is widely accepted that the presence of PAD increases the likelihood of myocardial infarction, stroke, renovascular disease (159), and cardiovascular mortality. The 5-year survival of a patient with intermittent claudication is only 70%, with 75% of these deaths attributable to cardiovascular events (160). Many studies have confirmed the association between cardiovascular morbidity and mortality and an abnormal ABI (161–166). Some have suggested that there is a significant proportion of the population with asymptomatic PAD, and their risk of cardiovascular morbidity and mortality is similar to their symptomatic counterparts. However, it is assumed that because of their lack of symptoms, this risk may not be recognized until an event has occurred.

The risk factors for the development of PAD include hypertension, hypercholesterolemia, tobacco use, and diabetes mellitus. Tobacco use remains the most important modifiable risk factor for PAD. Hughson et al. found that 56% of patients with intermittent claudication were active users of cigarettes and 24% were former smokers (167,168). In addition, active cigarette smoking causes more severe claudication pain and diminished peripheral circulation in comparison with patients who do not smoke, leading to a reduction in the exercise capacity of patients with claudication (169). Finally, the risk of progression of PAD and atherosclerosis in other vascular beds is significantly greater in those patients who continue to smoke as compared with those who stop smoking. In 343 patients with intermittent claudication, only 11% stopped smoking 1 year after the diagnosis. Ischemic rest pain developed in 16% of continued smokers after 7 years, whereas none of the former smokers suffered with rest pain. The incidence of myocardial infarction 10 years after the diagnosis of claudication was 11% in former smokers and 53% in active smokers. Ten-year overall survival rates were 82% in former smokers and 46% in active smokers (170).

Diabetes mellitus and PAD is an ominous combination. Although the prevalence of PAD is higher in the diabetic than in the nondiabetic population, it is the relatively rapid progression to ischemic rest pain and ulceration that portends a poor prognosis for the patients with diabetes. There is a twofold to threefold increase in risk of intermittent claudication in diabetic patients when compared with the nondiabetic population (171). This holds true for both men and women. The severity of PAD is also greater in the diabetic population. In a study of 47 patients with diabetes mellitus, all of whom had intermittent claudication at baseline, in comparison with 224 patients with intermittent claudication but no diabetes, the incidence of ischemic rest pain and/or gangrene after 6 years of follow-up was 40% and 18% respectively (172). The duration of diabetes and the type of diabetes therapy (i.e., diet, oral hypoglycemic agent, and insulin) did not play a role in the incidence or severity of PAD.

Independent predictors of progression of PAD in diabetic patients include a decreased postexercise ankle-brachial index, increased arm systolic blood pressure, and current smoking, demonstrating the additive effects of atherosclerotic risk factors on the natural history of PAD (173). Interestingly, among the risk factors for amputation in patients with diabetes mellitus, neuropathic symptoms and lack of outpatient diabetes education are of importance and must be viewed concomitantly with the location and severity of PAD (174). Unfortunately, there remains no definitive evidence that strict glycemic control can prevent macrovascular complications from diabetes mellitus (175). There are several potential other risk factors for peripheral arterial occlusive disease including Lp(a) (176), hyperhomocysteinemia (177), fibrinogen (178), and C-reactive protein (179). The specific role of each of these factors in the prevention and therapy of peripheral arterial disease remains unclear.

The most common symptom described by patients with peripheral arterial disease is intermittent claudication. Although the description of the symptom may vary among patients from pain to ache to numbness and weakness, there are several distinct characteristics of intermittent claudication. The discomfort is usually brought on by walking and alleviated by rest. The discomfort generally involves muscle groups immediately distal to the arterial segments involved (i.e., superficial femoral artery stenosis causes calf discomfort). The onset of intermittent claudication is quite predictable and occurs at similar distances providing that the speed, incline, and terrain have remained unchanged. Patients generally stop, stand, and wait for 1 to 5 minutes for relief prior to resumption of walking.

Progression to critical limb ischemia is manifest by ischemic pain at rest, generally in the arch of the foot or toes. This occurs with the patient lying supine and is relieved by hanging the foot over the bedside. Paradoxically, patients with ischemic rest pain may note improvement in their pain with walking. Patients may resort to sleeping in a reclining chair to provide a dependent position to the foot. Ischemic ulcerations occur as a result of trauma to toes or areas where bony prominences are exposed. Even minimal trauma, such as an ill-fitting shoe, may result in ulceration. The presence of ischemic rest pain or ulceration warrants a prompt and aggressive strategy for revascularization.

Physical examination must include palpation of all pulses, including the superficial temporal and carotid arteries, the arteries of the upper extremities, and the arteries of the lower extremities. Auscultation for bruits in the region of the cervical carotid arteries, abdomen, flank, and inguinal regions should be routinely performed, and the phase of the cardiac cycle during which the bruit occurs should be noted. Attempts to palpate the abdominal aorta for aneurysmal dilatation should me made. Close inspection of the feet and toes should include a search for ischemic ulceration or tinea infection. Kissing ulcerations between the toes in the web spaces are often subtle and easily missed on examination.

Once the ankle-brachial index has been performed to provide objective evidence of the overall severity of PAD, more specific noninvasive information can be obtained in the vascular laboratory. The addition of segmental limb pressures can aid in localizing stenoses or occlusions. A series of limb pressure cuffs are placed on the thigh (some centers prefer high- and low-thigh cuffs), calf, ankle, transmetatarsal region of the foot, and digit. The ABI is calculated, and then the pressure is sequentially inflated in each cuff to approximately 20 to 30 mm Hg above systolic pressure. Using a continuous wave Doppler probe placed at a pedal vessel, the pressure in the cuff is gradually released, and the pressure at each segment is measured. If a decrease in pressure between two consecutive levels of >30 mm Hg is identified, this suggests arterial occlusive disease of the artery proximal to the cuff. In addition, comparing the two limbs, a 20 to 30 mm Hg discrepancy from one limb to the other at the same cuff level also suggests a significant arterial stenosis or occlusion proximal to the cuff (180).

Pulse volume recordings (PVR) are plethysmographic tracings that detect the changes in the volume of blood flowing through a limb. Using similar equipment as described previously, the cuffs are inflated to 65 mmHg, and a plethysmographic tracing is recorded at various levels (181). The normal PVR is similar to the normal arterial pulse wave tracing and consists of a rapid systolic upstroke and rapid downstroke with a prominent dicrotic notch. With increasing severity of disease, the waveform becomes more attenuated, with a wide downslope, and ultimately, virtually absent waveforms.

Ankle-brachial indices, segmental pressures, and pulse volume recordings are useful objective tests in patients with suspected lower-extremity arterial occlusive disease or limb discomfort without an obvious cause, and as a method of evaluating the success of an intervention, and as a method of follow-up. The tests are inexpensive, painless, reproducible, and relatively easy to perform. The equipment required to perform these examinations is significantly less expensive than modern color-flow duplex ultrasound units.

Native vessel arterial duplex ultrasonography is widely performed. This examination is generally accepted as a method of defining arterial stenoses or occlusions (Fig. 14.13A). The sensitivity of duplex ultrasonography to detect occlusions and stenoses has been reported to be 95% and 92%, with specificities of 99% and 97%, respectively (182). Limitations have included tandem stenosis (183), tibial vessel imaging (184), and difficulty imaging the inflow arteries (185). Using a 5.0- to 7.5-MHz transducer, imaging of the suprainguinal and infrainguinal arteries is performed. The vessels are studied in the sagittal plane, and Doppler velocities are obtained using a 60° Doppler angle. Vessels are classified into one of five categories: normal, 1 to 19% stenosis, 20 to 49% stenosis, 50 to 99% stenosis, and occlusion. The categories are determined by alterations in the Doppler waveform, as well as increasing peak systolic velocities. For a stenosis to be classified as 50 to 99%, for example, the peak systolic velocity must increase by 100% in comparison with the normal segment of artery proximal to the stenosis (186; Fig. 14.13B).

Arterial duplex ultrasonography has been used to guide the interventionist toward appropriate access to a lesion potentially amenable to endovascular therapy (187; Fig. 14.13C). This technology has also been used after endovascular therapy to determine technical success (188) and durability of the procedure (189; Fig. 14.13D). Unfortunately, it appears that duplex ultrasonography soon after balloon angioplasty may overestimate residual stenosis and may limit the use of this technology after endovascular therapy (190).

In patients who have undergone surgical bypass graft revascularization, particularly with saphenous vein, 21 to 33% will develop graft stenosis. Once the graft becomes thrombosed, secondary patency rates are dismal, so detection of a graft stenosis should lead to its repair prior to graft thrombosis—if this is done, an estimated 80% of grafts can be salvaged (191). A well-organized graft surveillance program is thus crucial to preserving patency of bypass grafts. In one series of 170 saphenous vein bypass grafts, 110 stenoses were detected over a 39-month period. In those grafts that underwent surgical revision once a stenosis was detected, the 4-year patency was 88%, whereas in those grafts that did not undergo revision despite the detection of a stenosis, the 4-year patency was 57% (192). The use of an intensive surveillance program has been less beneficial in prosthetic grafts (193).

The procedure for graft surveillance is performed in a similar manner as used in native vessel arterial duplex ultrasonography. The inflow artery to the bypass graft is initially imaged using a 5.0- to 7.5-MHz transducer and a Doppler angle of 60°. Subsequently, the proximal anastomosis,

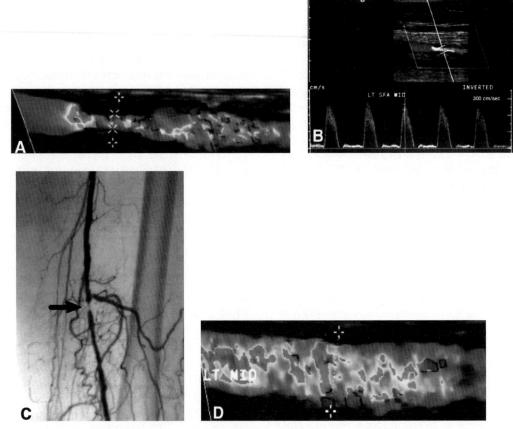

Figure 14.13   A. Severe stenosis of the left superficial femoral artery (SFA) as depicted by color duplex scanning. **B.** Spectral waveform shows an increased peak systolic velocity of 300 cm/second. **C.** Arteriogram confirming a severe SFA stenosis at the corresponding site. **D.** Nine-month follow-up arteriogram demonstrating a widely patent SFA at the site of revascularization with adjunctive pHVEGF165 to accelerate re-endothelialization.

proximal, mid, and distal graft, distal anastomosis, and outflow artery are interrogated. Peak systolic and end-diastolic velocities are obtained at each segment and compared with the segment of graft proximal to the area being studied. If the ratio of the peak systolic velocity within a stenotic segment relative to the normal segment proximal to the stenosis is >2, this suggests 50 to 75% diameter reduction. The addition of end-diastolic velocities >100 cm/second suggest >75 % stenosis (194).

Vein bypass grafts should be studied within 7 days of formation, and then in 1 month, followed by 3-month intervals for the first year. If the graft remains normal after year 1, follow-up surveillance should be done every 6 months thereafter. Ankle pressures and waveforms should be performed at the time of each surveillance study. The development of a stenosis during a surveillance examination should prompt consideration toward arteriography, either with contrast or using magnetic resonance (195).

Magnetic resonance angiography has been promoted as an excellent method of evaluating the anatomy of the lower-extremity arteries. Initially touted as a unique and effective method of identifying angiographically occult runoff arteries that would be suitable as targets for surgical

revascularization (196), investigators have studied the use of MR angiography as the sole imaging modality prior to surgical revascularization (197). Recent comparative trials of MR angiography and standard contrast arteriography have revealed high sensitivity and specificity (97.1 and 99.2%, respectively) for MR angiography in patients suspected of having PAD (198).

CTA has also been studied in PAD as a primary method of diagnosis. Although there is a requirement for the administration of iodinated contrast and significant external beam radiation exposure, images have provided excellent anatomic visualization of the lower-extremity arteries, even in the most acute situations (199). Given the impressive advances in the field of endovascular therapy for PAD with percutaneous transluminal angioplasty, stent deployment, atherectomy, and stent-grafting for aneurysmal and occlusive disease, however, diagnostic arteriography continues to play an important role in the management of patients with PAD.

Pelvic and Lower-Limb Angiography

Although angiography remains the gold standard for evaluation of peripheral vascular disease (PVD), with improved noninvasive imaging, it should be reserved only for patients in whom endovascular or surgical interventions are contemplated. The history, clinical examination, and noninvasive imaging allow a targeted approach to peripheral angiography. Indications for arteriographic study of the upper and lower extremities include ischemia (either exertional or resting) owing to atherosclerosis, embolus, thrombosis, and vasculitis. Other potential causes warranting arteriography are peripheral aneurysms, vascular tumors, trauma, extrinsic compression (e.g., popliteal artery entrapment syndrome, cystic adventitial disease, and vasculitis, collagen vascular disease, and radiation).

Pelvic arteriography can be performed from the femoral or brachial approach. From either access point, a multiholed catheter (pigtail or Omni Flush) can be passed to the level of L4–L5 in the abdominal aorta. Power injection in the AP projection at a rate of 15 mL/second for a total of 30 mL using DSA at four frames/second will define the aortoiliac bifurcation and common iliac arteries. If an iliac artery occlusion is suspected, the catheter should be positioned just below the renal arteries to visualize the lumbar arteries that provide important collaterals into the pelvis (Fig. 14.14).

Selective angiography of the iliac arteries can similarly be achieved via femoral or brachial approaches. From the brachial access, a 5F multipurpose catheter can selectively engage each common iliac. From the ipsilateral femoral artery, iliac angiography can be performed by either retrograde injections through the access sheath or through a straight catheter placed retrograde in the common iliac. The contralateral femoral approach requires engaging the common iliac by unfolding an Omni Flush catheter using a

guidewire and engaging the aorta bifurcation. A 0.035–inch angled glide wire can be manipulated through the catheter into the external iliac and used to anchor the catheter as it is advanced into the common iliac. Alternatively, a 4 or 5F glide catheter could be placed over the glide wire and selective angiography performed through it. Alternatives for engaging the contralateral common iliac include a Cobra, SOS-OMNI, hook, or internal mammary artery catheters.

No consensus has been reached as to which common femoral artery should be punctured—that on the side of the more symptomatic or less symptomatic leg. The advantages of accessing the less symptomatic leg are that groin complications would not interfere with surgical bypass procedures, there is less risk of iliac artery trauma (e.g., dissection or occlusion), and the option remains to then perform an antegrade puncture of the affected leg.

The most favorable angulation for iliac angiography is the contralateral oblique angle, generally 30 to 40°. Hand injections or power injections at 10 mL/second for a total of 10 mL are usually sufficient. Translesional gradients in the iliac vessels are useful guides to the hemodynamic severity of a lesion and also to the success of intervention. A 15-mm Hg gradient is considered significant across an iliac stenosis.

Lower-extremity arteriography is also easily performed using a single femoral access point. The ipsilateral lower limb can be imaged through the common femoral access sheath, while the contralateral lower limb can be imaged using the technique described above for crossing the aortoiliac bifurcation and selective iliac angiography. The optimal view for the common femoral bifurcation is 30 to 45° of ipsilateral oblique angulation, performed with a hand injection of 6 to 8 mL of contrast using DSA at four frames/second. Runoff of the lower limb can then be performed either in sequential stations using DSA or as a single angiographic run. DSA in sequential stations yields improved resolution and facilitates varied angulation for each station. In general, the SFA can be imaged in an anteroposterior view with the addition of an oblique angle if a stenosis is suspected. The popliteal artery, tibeoperoneal trunk, and trifurcation are best imaged in an ipsilateral oblique angle (30°). Infrapopliteal runoff can be performed in either an anteroposterior or an ipsilateral oblique projection. If DSA is used, an image rate of four frames/second is suitable for above the knee and two frames/second for beneath the knee. To optimize the visualization of the tibial or pedal arteries, selective catheter positioning into the superficial femoral artery with the use of vasodilating agents, such as nitroglycerin (100 to 300 μg), papaverine (30 to 60 mg), or tolazoline (12.5 to 25 mg) may enhance digital images (200).

Intra-arterial pressure monitoring may thus be more accurate than multiple angiographic images in assessing the hemodynamic significance of a vascular lesion (201). There exists no consensus as to the threshold that defines a significant gradient. However, a resting peak systolic gradient

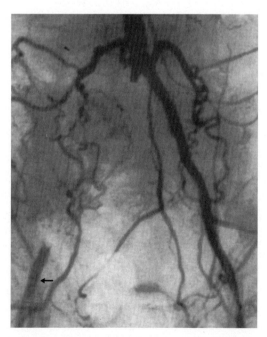

Figure 14.14 Pelvic arteriogram showing right iliac artery occlusion with common femoral artery *(arrow)* reconstitution via collaterals.

of 5 mm Hg or an increase greater than 10 mm Hg after augmentation with a vasodilator (e.g., nitroglycerin) is considered of hemodynamic significance (187). Intravascular ultrasound permits direct planimetry of luminar cross-sectional narrowing, obviating the multiple, oblique views required to unwind and/or eliminate overlap, which may obscure important luminal obstructions (202).

REFERENCES

1. Forssmann W. Die Sondierung des rechten Herzens. *Klin Wochenschr* 1929;1929;8:2085.
2. Dos Santos R, Lama AC, Pereira-Caldas J. Arteriorgafa da aorta e dos vasos abdominalis. *Med* Contempo 1929;47:93.
3. Nuvoli I. Arteriografa dell' aorta ascendente o del ventriculo. *Policlinico (Prat)* 1936;43:227.
4. Cambria RP, Kaufman JA, L'Italien GJ, et al. Magnetic resonance angiography in the management of lower extremity arterial occlusive disease: a prospective study. *J Vasc Surg* 1997;25:380–389.
5. Meaney JF. Magnetic resonance angiography of the peripheral arteries: current status. *Eur Radiol* 2003;13:836–852.
6. McCauley TR, Monib A, Dickey KW, et al. Peripheral vascular occlusive disease: accuracy and reliability of time-of-flight MR angiography. *Radiology* 1994;192:351–357.
7. Steinberg FL, Yucel EK, Dumoulin CL, Souza SP. Peripheral vascular and abdominal application of MR flow imaging techniques. *Magn Reson Med* 1990;14:315–320.
8. Prince MR, Arnoldus C, Frisoli JK. Nephrotoxicity of high-dose gadolinium compared with iodinated contrast. *J Magn Reson Imaging* 1996;6:162–166.
9. Rofsky NM, Johnson G, Adelman MA, Rosen RJ, Krinsky GA, Weinreb JC. Peripheral vascular disease evaluated with reduced-dose gadolinium-enhanced MR angiography. *Radiology* 1997;205:163–169.
10. Kopka L, Vosshenrich R, Rodenwaldt J, Grabbe E. Differences in injection rates on contrast-enhanced breath-hold three-dimensional MR angiography. *AJR Am J Roentgenol* 1998;170:345–348.
11. Napel S, Marks MP, Rubin GD, et al. CT angiography with spiral CT and maximum intensity projection. *Radiology* 1992;185:607–610.
12. Lookstein RA. Impact of CT angiography on endovascular therapy. *Mt Sinai J Med* 2003;70:367–374.
13. Creager MA, Goldstone J, Hirshfeld JW Jr, et al. ACC/ACP/SCAI/SVMB/SVS clinical competence statement on vascular medicine and catheter-based peripheral vascular interventions: a report of the American College of Cardiology/American Heart Association/American College of Physician Task Force on Clinical Competence (ACC/ACP/SCAI/SVMB/SVS Writing Committee to develop a clinical competence statement on peripheral vascular disease). *J Am Coll Cardiol* 2004;44:941–957.
14. Millward SF, Burbridge BE, Luna G. Puncturing the pulseless femoral artery: a simple technique that uses palpation of anatomic landmarks. *J Vasc Intervent Radiol* 1993;4:415–417.
15. Khangure MS, Chow KC, Christensen MA. Accurate and safe puncture of a pulseless femoral artery: an aid in performing iliac artery percutaneous transluminal angioplasty. *Radiology* 1982;144:927–928.
16. Kluge A, Rauber K, Breithecker A, Rau WS, Bachmann G. Puncture of the popliteal artery using a Doppler-equipped (SMART) needle in transpopliteal interventions. *Eur Radiol* 2003;13:1972–1978.
17. Sacks D, Summers TA. Antegrade selective catheterization of femoral vessels with a 4- or 5-F catheter and safety wire. *J Vasc Intervent Radiol* 1991;2:325–326.
18. Hirai M, Nakayama R. Haemodynamic effects of intra-arterial and intravenous administration of prostaglandin E1 in patients with peripheral arterial disease. *Br J Surg* 1986;73:20–23.
19. Gruss JD. Experience with PGE1 in patients with postoperative trashfoot. *Vasa* 1989;28(suppl):57–60.
20. Spinosa DJ, Kaufmann JA, Hartwell GD. Gadolinium chelates in angiography and interventional radiology: a useful alternative to iodinated contrast media for angiography. *Radiology* 2002;223:319–325.
21. Spinosa DJ, Angle JF, Hartwell GD, Hagspiel KD, Leung DA, Matsumoto AH. Gadolinium-based contrast agents in angiography and interventional radiology. *Radiol Clin North Am* 2002;40:693–710.
22. Bosanac Z, Miller RJ, Jain M. Rotational digital subtraction carotid angiography: technique and comparison with static digital subtraction angiography. *Clin Radiol* 1998;53:682–687.
23. Seymour HR, Matson MB, Belli AM, Morgan R, Kyriou J, Patel U. Rotational digital subtraction angiography of the renal arteries: technique and evaluation in the study of native and transplant renal arteries. *Br J Radiol* 2001;74(878):134–141.
24. Unno N, Mitsuoka H, Takei Y, et al. Virtual angioscopy using 3-dimensional rotational digital subtraction angiography for endovascular assessment. *J Endovasc Ther* 2002;9:529–534.
25. Meijering EH, Niessen WJ, Bakker J, et al. Reduction of patient motion artifacts in digital subtraction angiography: evaluation of a fast and fully automatic technique. *Radiology* 2001;219:288–293.
26. Ashleigh RJ, Hufton AP, Razzaq R, MacDiarmaid-Gordon L. A comparison of bolus chasing and static digital subtraction arteriography in peripheral vascular disease. *Br J Radiol* 2000;73:819–824.
27. Kwan ES, Hall A, Enzmann DR. Quantitative analysis of intracranial circulation using rapid-sequence DSA. *AJR Am J Roentgenol* 1986;146:1239–1245.
28. Krouwels MM, Overbosch EH, Guit GL. Iohexol vs. ioxaglate in lower extremity angiography: a comparative randomized double-blind study in 80 patients. *Eur J Radiol* 1996;22:133–135.
29. McCullough PA, Wolyn R, Rocher LL, Levin RN, O'Neill WW. Acute renal failure after coronary intervention: incidence, risk factors, and relationship to mortality. *Am J Med* 1997;103:368–375.
30. Baliga R, Ueda N, Walker PD, Shah SV. Oxidant mechanisms in toxic acute renal failure. *Am J Kidney Dis* 1997;29:465–477.
31. Mueller C, Buerkle G, Buettner HJ, et al. Prevention of contrast media-associated nephropathy: randomized comparison of 2 hydration regimens in 1620 patients undergoing coronary angioplasty. *Arch Intern Med* 2002;162:329–336.
32. Aspelin P, Aubry P, Fransson SG, Strasser R, Willenbrock R, Berg KJ. Nephrotoxic effects in high-risk patients undergoing angiography. *N Engl J Med* 2003;348:491–499.
33. Tepel M, van der Giet M, Schwarzfeld C, Laufer U, Liermann D, Zidek W. Prevention of radiographic-contrast-agent-induced reductions in renal function by acetylcysteine. *N Engl J Med* 2000;343:180–184.
34. Diaz-Sandoval LJ, Kosowsky BD, Losordo DW. Acetylcysteine to prevent angiography-related renal tissue injury (the APART trial). *Am J Cardiol* 2002;89:356–358.
35. Briguori C, Manganelli F, Scarpato P, et al. Acetylcysteine and contrast agent-associated nephrotoxicity. *J Am Coll Cardiol* 2002;40:298–303.
36. Shyu KG, Cheng JJ, Kuan P. Acetylcysteine protects against acute renal damage in patients with abnormal renal function undergoing a coronary procedure. *J Am Coll Cardiol* 2002;40:1383–1388.
37. MacNeill BD, Harding SA, Bazari H, et al. Prophylaxis of contrast-induced nephropathy in patients undergoing coronary angiography. *Cathet Cardiovasc Intervent* 2003;60:458–461.
38. Merten GJ, Burgess WP, Gray LV, et al. Prevention of contrast-induced nephropathy with sodium bicarbonate: a randomized controlled trial. *JAMA* 2004;291:2328–2334.
39. Hawkins IF. Carbon dioxide digital subtraction arteriography. *AJR Am J Roentgenol* 1982;139:19–24.
40. Weaver FA, Pentecost MJ, Yellin AE, Davis S, Finck E, Teitelbaum G. Clinical applications of carbon dioxide/digital subtraction arteriography. *J Vasc Surg* 1991;13:266–272.
41. Kerns SR, Hawkins IF Jr, Sabatelli FW. Current status of carbon dioxide angiography. *Radiol Clin North Am* 1995;33:15–29.

42. Kerns SR, Hawkins IF Jr. Carbon dioxide digital subtraction angiography: expanding applications and technical evolution. *AJR Am J Roentgenol* 1995;164:735–741.

43. Caridi JG, Hawkins IF Jr. CO$_2$ digital subtraction angiography: potential complications and their prevention.[see comment]. *J Vasc Intervent Radiol* 1997;8:383–391.

44. Hawkins IF, Caridi JG. Carbon dioxide (CO$_2$) digital subtraction angiography: 26-year experience at the University of Florida. *Eur Radiol* 1998;8:391–402.

45. Sullivan KL, Bonn J, Shapiro MJ, Gardiner GA. Venography with carbon dioxide as a contrast agent. *Cardiovasc Intervent Radiol* 1995;18:141–145.

46. Prince MR, Yucel EK, Kaufman JA, Harrison DC, Geller SC. Dynamic gadolinium-enhanced three-dimensional abdominal MR arteriography. *J Magn Reson Imaging* 1993;3:877–881.

47. Kaufman JA, Geller SC, Waltman AC. Renal insufficiency: gadopentetate dimeglumine as a radiographic contrast agent during peripheral vascular interventional procedures. *Radiology* 1996;198:579–581.

48. Kaufman JA, Hu S, Geller SC, Waltman AC. Selective angiography of the common carotid artery with gadopentetate dimeglumine in a patient with renal insufficiency. *AJR Am J Roentgenol* 1999;172:1613–1614.

49. Gabella G. Cardiovascular System. In: Williams PL, Bannister LH, Berry MM, eds. *Gray's Anatomy*. New York: Churchill Livingstone, 1995:1505–1546.

50. Aronberg DJ, Glazer HS, Madsen K, Sagel SS. Normal thoracic aortic diameters by computed tomography. *J Comput Assist Tomogr* 1984;8:247–250.

51. Hougen TJ. Congenital anomalies of the aortic arch. In: Lindsay J, ed. *Diseases of the Aorta*. Philadelphia: Lea & Febiger, 1994.

52. Ho VB, Prince MR. Thoracic MR aortography: imaging techniques and strategies. *Radiographics* 1998;18:287–309.

53. Perloff JK. Patent ductus arteriosus. In: *The Clinical Recognition of Congenital Heart Disease*. Philadelphia: WB Saunders, 1994: 510–545.

54. Rizzo RJ, McCarthy WJ, Dixit SN, et al. Collagen types and matrix protein content in human abdominal aortic aneurysms. *J Vasc Surg* 1989;10:365–373.

55. Milewicz DM, Michael K, Fisher N, Coselli JS, Markello T, Biddinger A. Fibrillin-1 (FBN1) mutations in patients with thoracic aortic aneurysms. *Circulation* 1996;94:2708–2711.

56. Kouchoukos NT, Dougenis D. Surgery of the thoracic aorta. *New Engl J Med* 1997;336:1876–1888.

57. Creasy JD, Chiles C, Routh WD, Dyer RB. Overview of traumatic injury of the thoracic aorta. *Radiographics* 1997;17:27–45.

58. Parmley LF, Mattingly TW, Manison WC. Non-penetrating traumatic injury of the thoracic aorta. *Circulation* 1958;17:1086.

59. Cohen AM, Crass JR, Thomas HA, Fisher RG, Jacobs DG. CT evidence for the "osseous pinch" mechanism of traumatic aortic injury. *AJR Am J Roentgenol* 1992;159:271–274.

60. Dapunt OE, Galla JD, Sadeghi AM, et al. The natural history of thoracic aortic aneurysms. *J Thorac Cardiovasc Surg* 1994;107: 1323–1332.

61. Hirose Y, Hamada S, Takamiya M, Imakita S, Naito H, Nishimura T. Aortic aneurysms: growth rates measured with CT. *Radiology* 1992;185:249–252.

62. Cambria RA, Gloviczki P, Stanson AW, et al. Outcome and expansion rate of 57 thoracoabdominal aortic aneurysms managed nonoperatively. *Am J Surg* 1995;17:213–217.

63. Lawrie GM, Earle N, De Bakey ME. Evolution of surgical techniques for aneurysms of the descending thoracic aorta: twenty-nine years experience with 659 patients. *J Card Surg* 1994;9: 648–661.

64. Semba CP, Kato N, Kee ST, et al. Acute rupture of the descending thoracic aorta: repair with use of endovascular stent-grafts. *J Vasc Intervent Radiol* 1997;8:337–342.

65. Dake MD, Miller DC, Semba CP, Mitchell RS, Walker PJ, Liddell RP. Transluminal placement of endovascular stent-grafts for the treatment of descending thoracic aortic aneurysms. *New Engl J Med* 1994;331:1729–1734.

66. Girardi LN, Bush HL Jr. Type B aortic dissection and thoracoabdominal aneurysm formation after endoluminal stent repair of abdominal aortic aneurysm. *J Vasc Surg* 1999;29:936–938.

67. Crawford ES. The diagnosis and management of aortic dissection. *JAMA* 1990;264:2537–2541.

68. DeSanctis RW, Doroghazi RM, Austen WG, Buckley MJ. Aortic dissection. *New Engl J Med* 1987;317:1060–1067.

69. Spittell PC, Spittell JA Jr, Joyce JW, et al. Clinical features and differential diagnosis of aortic dissection: experience with 236 cases (1980 through 1990). *Mayo Clin Proc* 1993;68:642–651.

70. Larson EW, Edwards WD. Risk factors for aortic dissection: a necropsy study of 161 cases. *Am J Cardiol* 1984;53:849–855.

71. DeBakey ME, Henly WS, Cooley DA. Surgical management of dissecting aneurysms of the aorta. *J Thorac Cardiovasc Surg* 1965;49:130.

72. Marsalese DL, Moodie DS, Vacante M, et al. Marfan's syndrome: natural history and long-term follow-up of cardiovascular involvement. *J Am Coll Cardiol* 1989;14:422–428; discussion 429–431.

73. Pumphrey CW, Fay T, Weir I. Aortic dissection during pregnancy. *Br Heart J* 1986;55:106–108.

74. Wahlers T, Laas J, Alken A, Borst HG. Repair of acute type A aortic dissection after cesarean section in the thirty-ninth week of pregnancy. *J Thorac Cardiovasc Surg* 1994;107:314–315.

75. Strichartz SD, Gelabert HA, Moore WS. Retrograde aortic dissection with bilateral renal artery occlusion after repair of infrarenal aortic aneurysm. *J Vasc Surg* 1990;12:56–59.

76. Crawford ES, Svensson LG, Coselli JS, Safi HJ, Hess KR. Aortic dissection and dissecting aortic aneurysms. *Ann Surg* 1988;208: 254–273.

77. Glower DD, Fann JI, Speier RH, et al. Comparison of medical and surgical therapy for uncomplicated descending aortic dissection. *Circulation* 1990;82(suppl IV):IV39–46.

78. Glower DD, Speier RH, White WD, Smith LR, Rankin JS, Wolfe WG. Management and long-term outcome of aortic dissection. *Ann Surg* 1991;214:31–41.

79. Strouse PJ, Shea MJ, Guy GE, Santinga JT. Aortic dissection presenting as spinal cord ischemia with a false-negative aortogram. *Cardiovasc Intervent Radiol* 1990;13:77–82.

80. Cambria RP, Brewster DC, Gertler J, et al. Vascular complications associated with spontaneous aortic dissection. *J Vasc Surg* 1988;7:199–209.

81. Raby N, Giles J, Walters H. Aortic dissection presenting as acute leg ischaemia. *Clin Radiol* 1990;42:116–117.

82. Fradet G, Jamieson WR, Janusz MT, Ling H, Miyagishima RT, Munro AI. Aortic dissection: current expectations and treatment. Experience with 258 patients over 20 years. *Can J Surg* 1990;33: 465–469.

83. Soto B, Harman MA, Ceballos R, Barcia A. Angiographic diagnosis of dissecting aneurysm of the aorta. *Am J Roentgenol Radium Ther Nucl Med* 1972;116:146–154.

84. DeBakey ME, McCollum CH, Crawford ES, et al. Dissection and dissecting aneurysms of the aorta: twenty-year follow-up of five hundred twenty-seven patients treated surgically. *Surgery* 1982; 92:1118–1134.

85. Daily PO, Trueblood HW, Stinson EB, Wuerflein RD, Shumway NE. Management of acute aortic dissections. *Ann Thorac Surg* 1970;10:237–247.

86. Taniguchi K, Nakano S, Matsuda H, et al. Long-term survival and complications after composite graft replacement for ascending aortic aneurysm associated with aortic regurgitation. *Circulation* 1991;84(suppl III):III31–39.

87. Wheat MW Jr. Acute dissection of the aorta. *Cardiovasc Clin* 1981;12:177–196.

88. Walker PJ, Dake MD, Mitchell RS, Miller DC. The use of endovascular techniques for the treatment of complications of aortic dissection. *J Vasc Surg* 1993;18:1042–1051.

89. Slonim SM, Nyman U, Semba CP, Miller DC, Mitchell RS, Dake MD. Aortic dissection: percutaneous management of ischemic complications with endovascular stents and balloon fenestration. *J Vasc Surg* 1996;23:241–251.

90. Slonim SM, Nyman UR, Semba CP, Miller DC, Mitchell RS, Dake MD. True lumen obliteration in complicated aortic dissection: endovascular treatment. *Radiology* 1996;201:161–166.

91. Matsunaga N, Hayashi K, Sakamoto I, Ogawa Y, Matsumoto T. Takayasu arteritis: protean radiologic manifestations and diagnosis. *Radiographics* 1997;17:579–594.

92. Yamato M, Lecky JW, Hiramatsu K, Kohda E. Takayasu arteritis: radiographic and angiographic findings in 59 patients. *Radiology* 1986;161:329–334.

93. Cho YD, Lee KT. Angiographic characteristics of Takayasu arteritis. *Heart Vessels Suppl* 1992;7:97–101.

94. Sharma S, Saxena A, Talwar KK, Kaul U, Mehta SN, Rajani M. Renal artery stenosis caused by nonspecific arteritis (Takayasu disease): results of treatment with percutaneous transluminal angioplasty. *AJR Am J Roentgenol* 1992;158:417–422.

95. Kumar S, Mandalam KR, Rao VR, et al. Percutaneous transluminal angioplasty in nonspecific aortoarteritis (Takayasu's disease): experience of 16 cases. *Cardiovasc Intervent Radiol* 1989;12:321–325.

96. Klein RG, Hunder GG, Stanson AW, Sheps SG. Large artery involvement in giant cell (temporal) arteritis. *Ann Intern Med* 1975;83:806–812.

97. Pyeritz RE. Ehlers-Danlos syndrome. In: Steinberg AG, Bearn AG, Mlfulsky AG, eds. *Genetics of Cardiovascular Disease*. Philadelphia: WB Saunders, 1983.

98. Pyeritz RE, McKusick VA. The Marfan syndrome: diagnosis and management. *New Engl J Med* 1979;300:772–777.

99. McKusick VA. Heritable *Disorders of Connective Tissue*. St Louis, MO: CV Mosby, 1972.

100. Gott VL, Cameron DE, Pyeritz RE, et al. Composite graft repair of Marfan aneurysm of the ascending aorta: results in 150 patients. *J Card Surg* 1994;9:482–489.

101. Coselli JS, LeMaire SA, Buket S. Marfan syndrome: the variability and outcome of operative management. *J Vasc Surg* 1995;21:432–443.

102. Steinberg AG, Bearn AG, Motulsky AGH. Progress in medical genetics. In: *Genetics of Cardiovascular Disease*. Philadelphia: WB Saunders, 1983.

103. Horejs D, Gilbert PM, Burstein S, Vogelzang RL. Normal aortoiliac diameters by CT. *J Comput Assist Tomogr* 1988;12:602–603.

104. Nuno IN, Collins GM, Bardin JA, Bernstein EF. Should aortography be used routinely in the elective management of abdominal aortic aneurysm? *Am J Surg* 1982;144:53–57.

105. Campbell JJ, Bell DD, Gaspar MR. Selective use of arteriography in the assessment of aortic aneurysm repair. *Ann Vasc Surg* 1990;4:419–423.

106. Shepherd J, Cobbe SM, Ford I, Isles et al. Prevention of coronary heart disease with pravastatin in men with hypercholesterolemia. West of Scotland Coronary Prevention Study Group. *New Engl J Med* 1995;333:1301–1307.

107. Leriche R, Morel A. The syndrome of thrombotic obliteration of the aortic bifurcation. *Ann Surg* 1948;127:193.

108. Sumboonnanonda A, Robinson BL, Gedroyc WM, Saxton HM, Reidy JF, Haycock GB. Middle aortic syndrome: clinical and radiological findings. *Arch Dis Child* 1992;67:501–505.

109. Itzchak Y, Katznelson D, Boichis H, Jonas A, Deutsch V. Angiographic features of arterial lesions in neurofibromatosis. *Am J Roentgenol, Radium Ther Nucl Med* 1974;122:643–647.

110. Siassi B, Klyman G, Emmanouilides GC. Hypoplasia of the abdominal aorta associated with the rubella syndrome. *Am J Dis Child* 1970;120:476–479.

111. Flynn PM, Robinson MB, Stapleton FB, Roy S 3rd, Koh G, Tonkin IL. Coarctation of the aorta and renal artery stenosis in tuberous sclerosis. *Pediatr Radiol* 1984;14:337–339.

112. Lewis VD 3rd, Meranze SG, McLean GK, O'Neill JA Jr, Berkowitz HD, Burke DR. The midaortic syndrome: diagnosis and treatment. *Radiology* 1988;167:111–113.

113. Messina LM, Reilly LM, Goldstone J, Ehrenfeld WK, Ferrell LD, Stoney RJ. Middle aortic syndrome. Effectiveness and durability of complex arterial revascularization techniques. *Ann Surg* 1986;204:331–339.

114. Kadir S. Regional anatomy of the thoracic aorta. In: Kadir S, ed. *Atlas of Normal & Variant Angiographic Anatomy*. 1991: WB Saunders, 1991:19.

115. Brown AH. Coronary steal by internal mammary graft with subclavian stenosis. *J Thorac Cardiovasc Surg* 1977;73:690–693.

116. McGovern PG, Pankow JS, Burke GL, et al. Trends in survival of hospitalized stroke patients between 1970 and 1985. The Minnesota Heart Survey. *Stroke* 1993;24:1640–1648.

117. American Heart Association. *2002 Heart and Stroke Statistical Update*. Dallas, TX: American Heart Association, 2001.

118. Hertzer NR, Young JR, Beven EG, et al. Coronary angiography in 506 patients with extracranial cerebrovascular disease. *Arch Intern Med* 1985;145:849–852.

119. O'Leary DH, Polak JF, Kronmal RA, Manolio TA, Burke GL, Wolfson SK Jr. Carotid-artery intima and media thickness as a risk factor for myocardial infarction and stroke in older adults. Cardiovascular Health Study Collaborative Research Group. *New Engl J Med* 1999;340:14–22.

120. Wang TJ, Nam BH, D'Agostino RB, et al. Carotid intima-media thickness is associated with premature parental coronary heart disease: the Framingham Heart Study. *Circulation* 2003;108:572–576.

121. Wadia NH, Monckton G. Intracranial bruits in health and disease. *Brain* 1957;80:492–509.

122. Heyman A, Wilkinson WE, Heyden S, et al. Risk of stroke in asymptomatic persons with cervical arterial bruits: a population study in Evans County, Georgia. *New Engl J Med* 1980;302:838–841.

123. Ivey TD, Strandness E, Williams DB, Langlois Y, Misbach GA, Kruse AP. Management of patients with carotid bruit undergoing cardiopulmonary bypass. *J Thorac Cardiovasc Surg* 1984;87:183–189.

124. Evans WE, Cooperman M. The significance of asymptomatic unilateral carotid bruits in preoperative patients. *Surgery* 1978;83:521–522.

125. Sauve JS, Laupacis A, Ostbye T, Feagan B, Sackett DL. The rational clinical examination. Does this patient have a clinically important carotid bruit? *JAMA* 1993;270:2843–2845.

126. MRC European Carotid Surgery Trial: interim results for symptomatic patients with severe (70–99%) or with mild (0–29%) carotid stenosis. European Carotid Surgery Trialists' Collaborative Group. *Lancet* 1991;337:1235–1243.

127. Risk of stroke in the distribution of an asymptomatic carotid artery. The European Carotid Surgery Trialists Collaborative Group. *Lancet* 1995;345:209–212.

128. Sauve JS, Thorpe KE, Sackett DL, et al. Can bruits distinguish high-grade from moderate symptomatic carotid stenosis? The North American Symptomatic Carotid Endarterectomy Trial. *Ann Intern Med* 1994;120:633–637.

129. Johnson BF, Verlato F, Bergelin RO, Primozich JF, Strandness E Jr. Clinical outcome in patients with mild and moderate carotid artery stenosis. *J Vasc Surg* 1995;21:120–126.

130. Verlato F, Camporese G, Bernardi E, et al. Clinical outcome of patients with internal carotid artery occlusion: a prospective follow-up study. *J Vasc Surg* 2000;32:293–298.

131. Rockman CB, Riles TS, Lamparello PJ, et al. Natural history and management of the asymptomatic, moderately stenotic internal carotid artery. *J Vasc Surg* 1997;25:423–431.

132. Bock RW, Gray-Weale AC, Mock PA, et al. The natural history of asymptomatic carotid artery disease. *J Vasc Surg* 1993;17:160–169.

133. Herzig R, Burval S, Krupka B, Vlachova I, Urbanek K, Mares J. Comparison of ultrasonography, CT angiography, and digital subtraction angiography in severe carotid stenoses. *Eur J Neurol* 2004;11:774–781.

134. Yadav JS, Wholey MH, Kuntz RE, et al. Protected carotid-artery stenting versus endarterectomy in high-risk patients.[see comment]. *New Engl J Med* 2004;351:1493–1501.

135. Olin JW, Melia M, Young JR, Graor RA, Risius B. Prevalence of atherosclerotic renal artery stenosis in patients with atherosclerosis elsewhere. *Am J Med* 1990;88:46–51.

136. Harding MB, Smith LR, Himmelstein SI, et al. Renal artery stenosis: prevalence and associated risk factors in patients undergoing routine cardiac catheterization. *J Am Soc Nephrol* 1992;2:1608–1616.

137. Scoble JE, Maher ER, Hamilton G, Dick R, Sweny P, Moorhead JF. Atherosclerotic renovascular disease causing renal impairment—a case for treatment. *Clin Nephrol* 1989;31:119–122.

138. Zierler RE, Bergelin RO, Isaacson JA, Strandness DE Jr. Natural history of atherosclerotic renal artery stenosis: a prospective study with duplex ultrasonography. *J Vasc Surg* 1994;19:250–257.

139. Brunner HR, Laragh JH, Baer L, et al. Essential hypertension: renin and aldosterone, heart attack and stroke. *New Engl J Med* 1972;286:441–449.

140. Mann SJ, Pickering TG, Sos TA, et al. Captopril renography in the diagnosis of renal artery stenosis: accuracy and limitations. *Am J Med* 1991;90:30–40.

141. Taylor DC, Kettler MD, Moneta GL, et al. Duplex ultrasound scanning in the diagnosis of renal artery stenosis: a prospective evaluation. *J Vasc Surg* 1988;7:363–369.

142. Strandness DE Jr. Duplex imaging for the detection of renal artery stenosis. *Am J Kidney Dis* 1994;24:674–678.

143. Olin JW, Piedmonte MR, Young JR, DeAnna S, Grubb M, Childs MB. The utility of duplex ultrasound scanning of the renal arteries for diagnosing significant renal artery stenosis.[see comment]. *Ann Intern Med* 1995;122:833–838.

144. Nazzal MM, Hoballah JJ, Miller EV, Sharp WJ, Kresowik TF, Corson J. Renal hilar Doppler analysis is of value in the management of patients with renovascular disease. *Am J Surg* 1997;174:164–168.

145. Isaacson JA, Zierler RE, Spittell PC, Strandness DE Jr. Noninvasive screening for renal artery stenosis: comparison of renal artery and renal hilar duplex scanning. *J Vasc Tech* 1995;19:105–110.

146. Cohn EJ Jr, Benjamin ME, Sandager GP, Lilly MP, Killewich LA, Flinn WR. Can intrarenal duplex waveform analysis predict successful renal artery revascularization? *J Vasc Surg* 1998;28:471–480.

147. Eidt JF, Fry RE, Clagett GP, Fisher DF Jr, Alway C, Fry WJ. Postoperative follow-up of renal artery reconstruction with duplex ultrasound. *J Vasc Surg* 1988;8:667–673.

148. Dorros G, Jaff M, Mathiak L, et al. Four-year follow-up of Palmaz-Schatz stent revascularization as treatment for atherosclerotic renal artery stenosis. *Circulation* 1998;98:642–647.

149. Grist TM. Magnetic resonance angiography of renal arterial stenosis. *Coron Artery Dis* 1999;10:151–156.

150. Grist TM. Magnetic resonance angiography of the aorta and arteries. *Magn Reson Imaging Clin North Am* 1993;1:253–269.

151. De Cobelli F, Vanzulli A, Sironi S, et al. Renal artery stenosis: evaluation with breath-hold, three-dimensional, dynamic, gadolinium-enhanced versus three-dimensional, phase-contrast MR angiography. *Radiology* 1997;205:689–695.

152. Grenier N, Trillaud H, Combe C, et al. Diagnosis of renovascular hypertension: feasibility of captopril-sensitized dynamic MR imaging and comparison with captopril scintigraphy. *AJR Am J Roentgenol* 1996;166:835–843.

153. Kaatee R, Beek FJ, de Lange EE. Renal artery stenosis: detection and quantification with spiral CT angiography versus optimized digital subtraction angiography. *Radiology* 1997;205:121–127.

154. Raza SA, Chughtai AR, Wahba M, Cowling MG, Taube D, Wright AR. Multislice CT angiography in renal artery stent evaluation: prospective comparison with intra-arterial digital subtraction angiography. *Cardiovasc Intervent Radiol* 2004;27:9–15.

155. U.S. Department of Heath & Human Services. *Chartbook on Cardiovascular, Lung and Blood Diseases*. Bethesda, MD: NIH, NHLBI, 1994.

156. Abbott RD, Brand FN, Kannel WB. Epidemiology of some peripheral arterial findings in diabetic men and women: experiences from the Framingham Study. *Am J Med* 1990;88:376–381.

157. Criqui MH, Fronek A, Barrett-Connor E, Klauber MR, Gabriel S, Goodman D. The prevalence of peripheral arterial disease in a defined population. *Circulation* 1985;71:510–515.

158. Hiatt WR. Medical treatment of peripheral arterial disease and claudication. *New Engl J Med* 2001;344:1608–1621.

159. Gross CM, Kramer J, Waigand J, Luft FC, Dietz R. Relation between arteriosclerosis in the coronary and renal arteries. *Am J Cardiol* 1997;80:1478–1481.

160. Weitz JI, Byrne J, Clagett GP, et al. Diagnosis and treatment of chronic arterial insufficiency of the lower extremities: a critical review. *Circulation* 1996;94:3026–3049.

161. McKenna M, Wolfson S, Kuller L. The ratio of ankle and arm arterial pressure as an independent predictor of mortality. *Atherosclerosis* 1991;87:119–128.

162. Criqui MH, Langer RD, Fronek A, et al. Mortality over a period of 10 years in patients with peripheral arterial disease. *New Engl J Med* 1992;326:381–386.

163. Newman AB, Siscovick DS, Manolio TA, et al. Ankle-arm index as a marker of atherosclerosis in the Cardiovascular Health Study. Cardiovascular Heart Study (CHS) Collaborative Research Group. *Circulation* 1993;88:837–845.

164. Vogt MT, Cauley JA, Newman AB, Kuller LH, Hulley SB. Decreased ankle/arm blood pressure index and mortality in elderly women. *JAMA* 1993;27:465–469.

165. Kornitzer M, Dramaix M, Sobolski J, Degre S, De Backer G. Ankle/arm pressure index in asymptomatic middle-aged males: an independent predictor of ten-year coronary heart disease mortality. *Angiology* 1995;46:211–219.

166. Leng GC, Fowkes FG, Lee AJ, Dunbar J, Housley E, Ruckley CV. Use of ankle brachial pressure index to predict cardiovascular events and death: a cohort study. *BMJ* 1996;313:1440–1444.

167. Hughson WG, Mann JI, Garrod A. Intermittent claudication: prevalence and risk factors. *BMJ* 1978;1:1379–1381.

168. Hughson WG, Mann JI, Tibbs DJ, Woods HF, Walton I. Intermittent claudication: factors determining outcome. *BMJ* 1978;1:1377–1379.

169. Gardner AW. The effect of cigarette smoking on exercise capacity in patients with intermittent claudication. *Vasc Med* 1996;1:181–186.

170. Jonason T, Bergstrom R. Cessation of smoking in patients with intermittent claudication. Effects on the risk of peripheral vascular complications, myocardial infarction and mortality. *Acta Med Scand* 1987;221:253–260.

171. Brand FN, Abbott RD, Kannel WB. Diabetes, intermittent claudication, and risk of cardiovascular events. The Framingham Study. *Diabetes* 1989;38:504–509.

172. Jonason T, Ringqvist I. Diabetes mellitus and intermittent claudication. Relation between peripheral vascular complications and location of the occlusive atherosclerosis in the legs. *Acta Med Scand* 1985;218:217–221.

173. Palumbo PJ, O'Fallon WM, Osmundson PJ, Zimmerman BR, Langworthy AL, Kazmier FJ. Progression of peripheral occlusive arterial disease in diabetes mellitus. What factors are predictive? *Arch Intern Med* 1991;151:717–721.

174. Reiber GE, Pecoraro RE, Koepsell TD. Risk factors for amputation in patients with diabetes mellitus. A case-control study.[see comment]. *Ann Intern Med* 1992;117:97–105.

175. The Diabetes Control and Complications Trial Research Group. The effect of intensive treatment of diabetes on the development and progression of long-term complications in insulin-dependent diabetes mellitus. *N Engl J Med* 1993;329:977–986.

176. Valentine RJ, Grayburn PA, Vega GL, Grundy SM. Lp(a) lipoprotein is an independent, discriminating risk factor for premature peripheral atherosclerosis among white men. *Arch Intern Med* 1994;154:801–806.

177. Malinow MR, Kang SS, Taylor LM, et al. Prevalence of hyperhomocyst(e)inemia in patients with peripheral arterial occlusive disease. *Circulation* 1989;79:1180–1188.

178. Lowe GD, Fowkes FG, Dawes J, Donnan PT, Lennie SE, Housley E. Blood viscosity, fibrinogen, and activation of coagulation and leukocytes in peripheral arterial disease and the normal population in the Edinburgh Artery Study. *Circulation* 1993;87:1915–1920.

179. Ridker PM, Cushman M, Stampfer MJ, Tracy RP, Hennekens CH. Plasma concentration of C-reactive protein and risk of developing peripheral vascular disease. *Circulation* 1998;97:425–428.

180. Strandness DE Jr. Noninvasive vascular laboratory and vascular imaging. In: Young JR, Olin JW, Bartholomew JR, eds. *Peripheral Vascular Disease.* St Louis, MO: Mosby, 1996:369–374.

181. MacDonald NR. Pulse volume plethysmography. *J Vasc Tech* 1994;18:241–248.

182. Whelan JF, Barry MH, Moir JD. Color flow Doppler ultrasonography: comparison with peripheral arteriography for the investigation of peripheral vascular disease. *J Clin Ultrasound* 1992;20:369–374.

183. Allard L, Cloutier G, Durand LG, Roederer GO, Langlois YE. Limitations of ultrasonic duplex scanning for diagnosing lower limb arterial stenoses in the presence of adjacent segment disease. *J Vasc Surg* 1994;19:650–657.

184. Larch E, Minar E, Ahmadi R, et al. Value of color duplex sonography for evaluation of tibioperoneal arteries in patients with femoropopliteal obstruction: a prospective comparison with anterograde intraarterial digital subtraction angiography. *J Vasc Surg* 1997;25:629–636.

185. Lewis WA, Bray AE, Harrison CL. A comparison of common femoral waveform analysis with aorto-iliac duplex scanning in assessment of aorto-iliac disease. *J Vasc Tech* 1994;18:337–44.

186. Kohler TR, Nance DR, Cramer MM, Vandenburghe N, Strandness DE Jr. Duplex scanning for diagnosis of aortoiliac and femoropopliteal disease: a prospective study. *Circulation* 1987;76:1074–1080.

187. Legemate DA, Teeuwen C, Hoeneveld H, Eikelboom BC. Value of duplex scanning compared with angiography and pressure measurement in the assessment of aortoiliac arterial lesions. *Br J Surg* 1991;78:1003–1008.

188. Silke CM, Grouden MC, Nicholls S. Non-invasive follow-up of peripheral angioplasty: a prospective study. *J Vasc Tech* 1997;21: 23–25.

189. Mewissen MW, Kinney EV, Bandyk DF, et al. The role of duplex scanning versus angiography in predicting outcome after balloon angioplasty in the femoropopliteal artery. *J Vasc Surg* 1992;15:860–865.

190. Sacks D, Robinson ML, Marinelli DL, Perlmutter GS. Evaluation of the peripheral arteries with duplex US after angioplasty. *Radiology* 1990;176:39–44.

191. Bandyk D. Ultrasonic duplex scanning in the evaluation of arterial grafts and dilatations. *Echocardiography* 1987;20:251–264.

192. Mattos MA, van Bemmelen PS, Hodgson KJ, Ramsey DE, Barkmeier LD, Sumner DS. Does correction of stenoses identified with color duplex scanning improve infrainguinal graft patency? J Vasc Surg 1993;17:54–64.

193. Lalak NJ, Hanel KC, Hunt J, Morgan A. Duplex scan surveillance of infrainguinal prosthetic bypass grafts. *J Vasc Surg* 1994;20: 637–641.

194. Bandyk DF. Postoperative surveillance of infrainguinal bypass. *Surg Clin North Am* 1990;70:71–85.

195. Jaff MR, Breger R, Deshur W, Pipia J. Detection of an arterial bypass graft threatening lesion by use of duplex ultrasonography and magnetic resonance angiography in an asymptomatic patient. *Vasc Surg* 1998;32:109–114.

196. Owen RS, Carpenter JP, Baum RA, Perloff LJ, Cope C. Magnetic resonance imaging of angiographically occult runoff vessels in peripheral arterial occlusive disease. *New Engl J Med* 1992;326: 1577–1581.

197. Cambria RP, Yucel EK, Brewster DC, et al. The potential for lower extremity revascularization without contrast arteriography: experience with magnetic resonance angiography. J Vasc Surg 1993; 17:1050–1056.

198. Sueyoshi E, Sakamoto I, Matsuoka Y, et al. Aortoiliac and lower extremity arteries: comparison of three-dimensional dynamic contrast-enhanced subtraction MR angiography and conventional angiography. *Radiology* 1999;210:683–688.

199. Poletti PA, Rosset A, Didier D. Subtraction CT angiography of the lower limbs: a new technique for the evaluation of acute arterial occlusion. *AJR Am J Roentgenol* 2004;183:1445–1448.

200. Cohen MI, Vogelzang RL. A comparison of techniques for improved visualization of the arteries of the distal lower extremity. *AJR Am J Roentgenol* 1986;147(5):1021–1024.

201. Moore WS, Hall AD. Unrecognized aortoiliac stenosis. A physiologic approach to the diagnosis. *Arch Surg* 1971;103:633–638.

202. Isner JM, Rosenfield K. Enough with the fantastic voyage: will IVUS pay in Peoria? *Cathet Cardiovasc Diagn* 1992;26: 192–199.

Evaluation of Cardiac Function

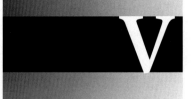

Stress Testing During Cardiac Catheterization: Exercise and Pacing Tachycardia

15

William Grossman[a]

Patients with significant heart disease may have entirely normal hemodynamics when assessed in the resting state during cardiac catheterization. Because most cardiac symptoms are precipitated by exertion or some other stress, however, it also may be important to assess hemodynamic performance during some form of stress such as muscular exercise, pharmacologic intervention (e.g., dobutamine infusion), or pacing-induced tachycardia. Such an evaluation enables the physician to assess the *cardiovascular reserve* and the relationship (if any) between specific symptoms and hemodynamic impairment. Physiologic information so obtained is often valuable in prescribing specific medical therapy, selecting patients for corrective cardiac surgery, and estimating prognosis.

Muscular exercise, both dynamic and isometric, has been studied extensively in the cardiac catheterization laboratory, and the normal hemodynamic responses are reasonably well understood. There are major differences between the hemodynamic responses to dynamic exercise (done either in the supine or the erect position) and the responses to static, isometric exercise, and these two types of exercise are discussed separately.

DYNAMIC EXERCISE

During dynamic exertion, skeletal muscles are actively contracting and developing force that is translated into motion and work. This is accompanied by an increase in both carbon dioxide production and oxygen (O_2) consumption by skeletal muscle, and a corresponding increase in alveolar gas exchange needed to support the higher metabolic rate. In normal sedentary individuals, the level of O_2 consumption during maximal exercise ($\dot{V}_{O_2}$max) can increase about 12-fold in comparison with that during the resting state (1). Age and fitness also modify $\dot{V}_{O_2}$max. During aging, there is a decrease in $\dot{V}_{O_2}$max of about 5% per decade. During athletic training, $\dot{V}_{O_2}$max increases because of both cardiovascular and skeletal muscle adaptation. In marathon runners and Olympic-class athletes, $\dot{V}_{O_2}$max may represent an 18-fold increase in O_2 consumption above the resting state. The increased oxygen requirements of muscular exercise are met by both an increase in the cardiac output and an increased extraction of oxygen from arterial blood by skeletal muscle, which causes widening of the arteriovenous oxygen difference (AV O_2 difference).

The need for the heart to increase cardiac output appropriately for the increase in O_2 consumption resulting from exercise is met by an increase in *heart rate* and an increase in *stroke volume*. The relative contributions of these increases to the rise in cardiac output depend on the type of exercise (supine versus upright), the intensity of exercise, the limitation of diastolic filling at high heart rates, and the response to sympathetic stimulation. Metabolic adaptations of exercising muscle include a switch from use of free fatty acids at rest to an accelerated breakdown of muscle glycogen stores and enhanced uptake of bloodborne glucose, which is supplied by

[a] Some material in this chapter was developed for previous editions by Drs. Beverly Lorell, Mark Feldman, and Raymond McKay.

increased hepatic gluconeogenesis. Because carbohydrate metabolism produces more carbon dioxide than fat metabolism does, the *respiratory quotient* (ratio of carbon dioxide production to O_2 consumption) rises from a resting value of 0.7 to 0.8 toward 1.0. The delivery of bloodborne oxygen and glucose to working skeletal muscle is enhanced in the presence of normal vasculature by a reduction in skeletal muscle vascular resistance mediated by metabolic byproducts and by sympathetically mediated vasoconstriction elsewhere, which causes a redistribution of blood away from the renal and splanchnic beds to exercising muscle.

Exercise depends on the adequacy of pulmonary function to increase oxygen supply. During progressive exercise, there is a linear increase in minute ventilation relative to the increase in O_2 consumption. When the intensity and duration of exercise are such that insufficient oxygen is delivered to exercising muscle, anaerobic metabolism of glucose develops, causing metabolic acidosis and an increase in respiratory quotient to values >1.0; minute ventilation increases out of proportion to O_2 consumption. Beyond this *anaerobic threshold*, the accumulation of hydrogen ions usually causes skeletal muscle weakness, pain, and severe breathlessness, followed by exhaustion and cessation of exercise. It is best to conduct exercise studies in the catheterization laboratory so that the patient reaches a *steady state level of submaximal exercise* below the anaerobic threshold and exercise can be sustained for several minutes. This approach permits estimation of cardiovascular reserve and allows the physician to determine whether the increase in cardiac output is appropriate for the increase in O_2 consumption occurring at that particular level of exercise.

Oxygen Uptake and Cardiac Output

There is a linear relationship between O_2 consumption and increasing workload (Fig. 15.1). Oxygen uptake increases abruptly after initiation of dynamic exercise, reflecting additional work needed to overcome inertia of the legs, and then increases steadily over a few minutes to reach a new steady

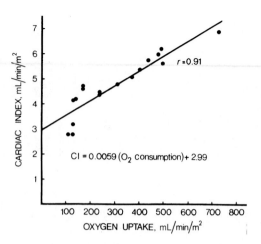

Figure 15.2 The relationship between cardiac output and oxygen consumption (both indexed for body surface area) during supine dynamic exercise of varying intensity in normal subjects, based on the data of Dexter. As can be seen from the regression equation for this relationship, for each increment of 100 mL/minute per m² of oxygen consumption, there is an increase in cardiac output of 0.59 L/minute per m² or 590 mL/minute per m². CI, cardiac index. (Data from Dexter L, et al. Effects of exercise on circulatory dynamics of normal individuals. *J Appl Physiol* 1951;3:439.)

state that is directly related to the intensity or level of exercise (2–4). Simultaneously, the mixed venous blood oxygen saturation decreases to a lower steady level related to the intensity of exercise, producing an increase in the AV O_2 difference.

The cardiac output increases linearly with increasing workload during both supine and upright exercise in normal subjects (2–5). As can be seen from the regression equation for this relationship (Fig. 15.2), for each increment of 100 mL/minute per m² of O_2 consumption during exercise, there is an increase in cardiac output of 590 mL/minute per m².

Exercise Index

The linear relationship between oxygen uptake and cardiac output during exercise, illustrated in Fig. 15.2, may be used to assess whether the cardiac output response measured in an individual patient is appropriate to the level of exercise and increased oxygen uptake. The regression formula is $CI = 0.0059X + 2.99$, where CI is the cardiac index in liters per minute per square meter of body surface area (BSA) and X is the O_2 consumption in mL/minute per m² BSA. This formula may be used to calculate the *predicted cardiac index* for a given level of O_2 consumption (X), and the predicted cardiac index may then be compared with the *measured cardiac index*. Note that this assessment can be performed at any steady state level of exercise and does not depend on achieving any specific target level of exertion. This equation can be used to calculate a predicted cardiac index by measuring O_2 consumption during dynamic exercise. The patient's actual measured cardiac index during exercise is then divided by the predicted cardiac index to determine the deviation from normal:

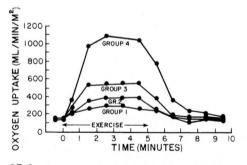

Figure 15.1 Oxygen consumption in normal subjects during exercise. Each group represents a different level of exercise, with the most intense exercise being performed by group 4. Note the prompt increase and establishment of a new steady state in oxygen uptake that is directly related to the intensity of the exercise. (From Donald KW, et al. The effect of exercise on the cardiac output and circulatory dynamics of normal subjects. *Clin Sci* 1955; 14:37, with permission.)

Exercise index =

$$\frac{\text{Measured cardiac index (L/min/m}^2)}{\text{Predicted cardiac index (L/min/m}^2)} \quad (15.1)$$

We have termed this ratio the *exercise index*, since it allows expression of exercise capacity as a percentage of the normal response. An exercise index of 0.8 or higher indicates a normal cardiac output response to exercise.

Exercise Factor

Another way of using this relationship between cardiac output and O_2 consumption involves calculation of the *exercise factor*, which is the increase in cardiac output with exercise divided by the corresponding increase in O_2 consumption:

Exercise factor =

$$\frac{\text{Increase in cardiac output (mL/min)}}{\text{Increase in O}_2 \text{ consumption (mL/min)}} \quad (15.2)$$

A normal exercise factor is an increase of 600 mL/minute in cardiac output per 100 mL/minute increase in O_2 consumption. An exercise factor <6.0 indicates a subnormal response in cardiac output; like an exercise index of <0.8, such a factor suggests some pathologic process limiting the heart's ability to meet the exercise-induced increase in O_2 consumption with an appropriate increase in cardiac output, forcing an excessive reliance on oxygen extraction from arterial blood and widening of the AV O_2 difference.

Systemic and Pulmonary Arterial Pressure and Heart Rate

Systolic arterial pressure and mean arterial pressure also increase linearly in relation to O_2 consumption during dynamic exercise in normal subjects, although the response is somewhat variable (4,6–8). Despite this increase in arterial pressure, systemic vascular resistance decreases substantially during dynamic exercise, indicating that the elevated arterial blood pressure is secondary to increased cardiac output. Patients who are unable to generate an adequate increase in cardiac output during dynamic exercise may also increase their arterial pressure, but in this circumstance systemic vascular resistance does not decline and may actually increase.

The behavior of the pulmonary circulation in response to dynamic exercise is different from that of the systemic circulation in normal individuals. Mean pulmonary artery pressure increases almost proportionally with cardiac output (pulmonary blood flow), so that there is only a slight decrease in pulmonary vascular resistance, in contrast to the normal substantial decrease in resistance of the systemic vasculature.

Heart rate increases consistently during both supine and upright dynamic exercise and tends to increase linearly in relation to O_2 consumption. During dynamic supine exercise in the catheterization laboratory, tachycardia is the predomi-

nant factor in increasing cardiac output. Tachycardia exerts a positive inotropic effect (the so-called treppe phenomenon), but increased sympathetic nervous system activity appears to be the most significant factor leading to enhanced myocardial contractility. In most normal subjects, supine bicycle exercise is accompanied by an increase in ejection fraction and other ejection indices of left ventricular (LV) systolic function with a decrease in LV end-systolic volume.

Several investigators (2,3,6–8) examined the responses of cardiac output, stroke volume, and heart rate to a given intensity of supine exercise in normal subjects and showed that the increase in cardiac output is caused primarily by an increase in heart rate with a negligible contribution by increased stroke volume. During repeat exercise when heart rate is held constant, there is a comparable increase in cardiac output caused by a marked increase in stroke volume (7). When heart rate is artificially increased by electrical pacing in the absence of dynamic exercise, however, cardiac output remains unchanged and a major fall in stroke volume occurs (7), indicating that further cardiovascular adjustments are required for an adequate hemodynamic response to dynamic exercise.

Therefore, to adequately interpret the response to supine exercise in the catheterization laboratory, it is important to recognize that the increase in cardiac output in normal young subjects is caused by a proportionate increase in heart rate. As discussed later, when chronotropic reserve is depressed, an appropriate increase in cardiac output relative to O_2 consumption depends on the capacity to augment LV diastolic filling and end-diastolic fiber tension, leading to an increase in stroke volume by means of the Frank-Starling mechanism.

Upright Versus Supine Exercise

The contributions of heart rate and stroke volume to cardiac output differ in supine and upright bicycle exercise. End-diastolic volumes at rest are near maximum when normal subjects are supine, smaller when they are sitting, and smallest when they are standing (4). When subjects are in the upright position, LV end-diastolic volume, cardiac output, and stroke volume are lower than when they are in the supine position (6,8). During erect bicycle exercise, most normal subjects demonstrate an increase in ejection fraction and reduction in end-systolic volume, some enhancement of LV end-diastolic volume, and an increase in stroke volume as well as heart rate. LV end-diastolic volume and stroke volume tend to increase up to about 50% of peak O_2 consumption and then to plateau or actually decrease at high levels of exercise (4). At high levels of exercise and fast heart rates, recruitment of the Frank-Starling mechanism may be blunted by the effects of tachycardia and limitation of diastolic filling owing to shortening of diastole. At high levels of upright exercise, stroke volume is preserved by a progressive decrease in end-systolic volume and increase in ejection fraction in the presence of a constant or decreased LV end-diastolic volume (4,5).

Caution must be used in interpreting the relative contributions of inotropic reserve and use of the Frank-Starling mechanism in patients studied during dynamic exercise in the catheterization laboratory. The effects of advancing age profoundly alter the exercise response. In healthy subjects, there appear to be no age-related changes in resting cardiac output, ejection fraction, end-systolic volume, or end-diastolic volume (9). With age, there is a reduction in both peak O_2 consumption and cardiac output during exercise. Also, with advancing age there is a reduction in heart rate and contractility response during exercise, so that the increase in cardiac output at any level of exercise is accomplished by significant increases in end-diastolic volume and in stroke volume (9,10). Therefore, as discussed earlier, studies of the effects of dynamic supine bicycle exercise in young adults have generally shown no change or a fall in LV end-diastolic pressure (LVEDP) and volume during exercise. In contrast, studies of older normal subjects or patients with atypical chest pain and normal coronary arteries have generally shown that both dynamic supine and upright bicycle exercise are associated with an increase in LVEDP (8,11), which is consistent with an age-dependent reliance on an increase in preload during exercise. For example, in a group of 10 sedentary men whose average age was 46 years, there was a rise in LVEDP from 8 ± 1 to 16 ± 2 mm Hg during supine bicycle exercise and a rise from 4 ± 1 to 11 ± 1 mm Hg during upright bicycle exercise (8). The diminished heart rate and contractility responses during exercise and resultant increased dependence on the Frank-Starling mechanism with aging may reflect an age-related decrease in responsiveness to β-adrenergic stimulation (12).

There are also gender-related differences in the normal response to exercise. Normal men and women can achieve comparable increases in weight-adjusted peak O_2 consumption, heart rate, and blood pressure. However, normal women generally achieve increases in stroke volume during upright exercise through an increase in end-diastolic volume without an increase in ejection fraction, whereas normal men exhibit a progressive increase in ejection fraction to peak exercise (13).

The interpretation of normal versus abnormal LV systolic performance during dynamic exercise may also be complicated by the effects of chronic β-adrenergic blockade. Studies of the hemodynamic effects of chronic β-adrenergic blockade on graded exercise in hypertensive but otherwise healthy young adults have shown that no impairment of maximal exercise capacity (maximal O_2 consumption) or cardiac output response occurs during chronic β-adrenergic blockade. β-Blockade, however, causes a reduction in heart rate at any level of exercise, and this relative reduction in heart rate is compensated for by both a widening of the AV O_2 difference and an increase in stroke volume, associated with an increased LV end-diastolic volume and a reduced arterial blood pressure (decreased impedance to ejection).

In normal beta-blocked subjects, increases in cardiac output during exercise depend on increasing stroke volume by means of the Frank-Starling mechanism. Therefore, the dynamic exercise response of a patient receiving chronic β-adrenergic blocking therapy may be associated with an inappropriately low increase in cardiac output relative to O_2 consumption, accompanied by excessive widening of the AV O_2 difference with an increased reliance on an increase in LV end-diastolic volume. During dynamic supine exercise in the catheterization laboratory, the finding that an increase in cardiac output depends on an increase in LV end-diastolic volume (and pressure) could be caused by either β-adrenergic blockade per se or intrinsic impairment of LV systolic function. For these reasons, strong consideration should be given to discontinuation of β-adrenergic blocking drugs at least 24 hours before catheterization if analysis of the hemodynamic response to dynamic exercise is planned to assess the adequacy of cardiovascular reserve.

Left Ventricular Diastolic Function

Interpretation of the changes in LV diastolic pressure with exercise depends greatly on an appreciation of the adaptations in diastolic function that occur. In normal subjects, multiple adjustments occur to accommodate an increased transmitral flow into the left ventricle in the face of an abbreviated diastolic filling period and to maintain low pressures throughout diastole. Exercise is associated with a progressive acceleration of isovolumetric relaxation so that enhanced diastolic filling occurs with minimal change in mitral valve opening pressure (14). The exercise-induced enhancement of diastolic relaxation and filling is probably modulated by both β-adrenergic stimulation and increased heart rate.

In normal subjects, there is either no change or a downward shift in the LV diastolic pressure-volume relation during exercise (Fig. 15.3). In the presence of ischemia or cardiac hypertrophy, however, exercise may provoke an upward shift in the LV diastolic pressure-volume relationship so that any level of LV end-diastolic volume is associated with a much higher LVEDP. In such patients, the left ventricle may be regarded as exhibiting increased chamber stiffness (decreased distensibility) during exercise. In patients with coronary artery disease, a transient but striking upward shift in the LV diastolic pressure-volume relation is common during episodes of ischemia (15). Patients with coronary artery disease who develop angina during dynamic exercise in the catheterization laboratory commonly show a marked rise in LVEDP. A careful study of the dynamics of LV diastolic filling during exercise in patients with coronary artery disease has been reported by Carroll et al. (16). These authors studied LV diastolic pressure-volume relations in 34 patients with coronary disease who developed ischemia during exercise and compared the finding with those from 5 patients with minimal cardiovascular disease (control) and 5 patients with an akinetic area at rest from a prior infarction but no active ischemia

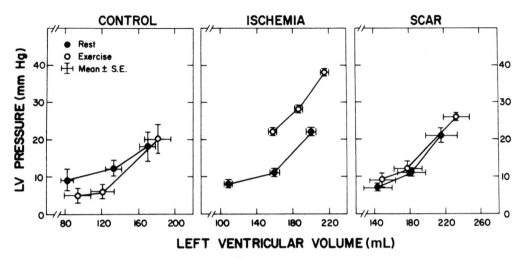

Figure 15.3 Left ventricular (LV) diastolic pressure-volume relations at rest and during exercise in patients without heart disease (control), compared with patients with coronary disease who developed ischemia during exercise (ischemia), and patients with akinetic areas owing to previous infarction but no active ischemia during exercise (scar). Pressure and volume are averaged at three diastolic points: early diastolic pressure nadir, mid-diastole, and end-diastole. The control group had a downward shift of the early diastolic pressure-volume relation, but the ischemia group showed an upward and rightward shift. (From Carroll JD, Hess OM, Hirzel HO, et al. Dynamics of left ventricular filling at rest and during exercise. *Circulation* 1983;68:59, with permission.)

during exercise (scar group). There was an upward shift in the LV diastolic pressure-volume relationship during exercise-induced ischemia, which was not seen in either the scar or the control group (Fig. 15.3). Therefore, interpretation of an exercise-induced rise in LVEDP in patients with coronary artery disease is complex and may be related to both a decrease in LV chamber distensibility and an increase in LV end-diastolic volume secondary to a reduction in ejection fraction (11,16).

The presence of cardiac hypertrophy is frequently characterized by depression of the rates of LV relaxation and diastolic filling at rest, and this depression profoundly impedes LV filling during exercise-induced tachycardia. In patients with conditions such as hypertrophic cardiomyopathy or hypertensive hypertrophic cardiomyopathy, in whom baseline LV end-systolic volumes are small, there is no reserve to further enhance systolic shortening, and abnormal diastolic properties limit the capacity to recruit the Frank-Starling mechanism during exercise. Furthermore, tachycardia may provoke ischemia (owing to impaired coronary vasodilator reserve), accompanied by an upward shift in the diastolic pressure-volume relationship. These findings with exercise-induced tachycardia in patients with coronary disease and/or advanced LV hypertrophy are remarkably similar to the changes in diastolic function seen during angina induced by pacing tachycardia, as described later in this chapter.

Marked abnormalities in LV diastolic function occur with exercise in patients with clinical evidence of heart failure but normal resting systolic function (so-called diastolic heart failure). Kitzman and Sullivan (17) studied seven patients with New York Heart Association (NYHA) class III

or IV heart failure with one or more documented episodes of pulmonary edema and no significant coronary artery disease. All had LV ejection fractions of ≥50%, without echocardiographic evidence of regional wall motion abnormalities or valvular or pericardial disease. Four of these patients were elderly with a medical history remarkable only for chronic hypertension. Most patients had increased LV wall thickness and mass. Patients were studied by symptom-limited upright exercise with simultaneous hemodynamic and radionuclide measurements, and data were compared to those seen in age- and sex-matched healthy volunteers who served as controls. As can be seen in Fig. 15.4, maximum exercise capacity was reduced, and the cardiac output increased primarily as a result of tachycardia, with no change in stroke volume. Figure 15.5 shows that LV ejection fraction was normal at rest and with exercise for both patients and control subjects, but there was a striking rise in pulmonary capillary wedge pressure in those patients with diastolic heart failure, compared with the control subjects. Accordingly, these patients clearly have "pure" diastolic heart failure: Efforts to treat their heart failure by improving systolic function (e.g., digoxin) will not be successful. As seen in Fig. 15.6, diastolic distensibility was markedly decreased with exercise in these patients.

Examples of the Use of Exercise to Evaluate Left Ventricular Failure in the Cardiac Catheterization Laboratory

Examples of the hemodynamic changes that can occur during supine bicycle exercise are shown in Tables 15.1 and

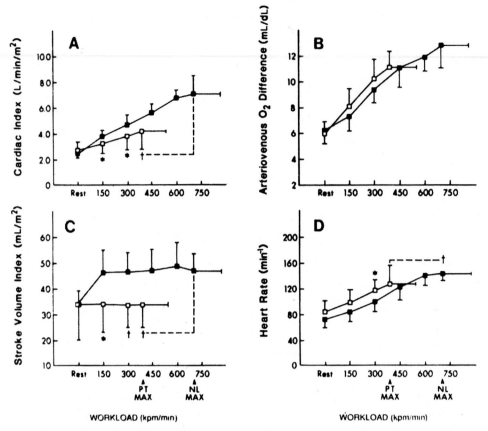

Figure 15.4   Seven patients with heart failure and normal left ventricular systolic function *(open symbols)* compared with 10 age- and gender-matched healthy volunteers *(solid symbols)* who served as controls. All subjects underwent upright bicycle exercise with hemodynamic evaluation. Cardiac output increased for the patients with heart failure as a result of an increase in heart rate, with fixed stroke volume. PT MAX, patient maximum exercise; NL MAX, normal subject maximum exercise. (From Kitzman D, et al. Exercise tolerance in patients with heart failure and preserved left ventricular systolic function: failure of the Frank-Starling mechanism. *J Am Coll Cardiol* 1991;17:1065, with permission.)

15.2. Table 15.1 illustrates the response to 6 minutes of supine bicycle exercise of a 36-year-old woman with an idiopathic dilated cardiomyopathy (ejection fraction, 40%) whose major symptom was exertional dyspnea. Because her ejection fraction was only moderately depressed and her hemodynamic values were almost normal at rest, resting hemodynamic data alone did not clarify whether her cardiovascular reserve was impaired and whether her exertional dyspnea was likely to be cardiac in origin. During exercise, the cardiac index increased appropriately in relation to the increase in O_2 consumption, yielding an exercise index of 1.1 and an exercise factor of 8.5:

$$\frac{\Delta \text{ cardiac index}}{\Delta \; O_2 \text{ consumption}} = \frac{3,300}{387} = 8.5 \qquad (15.3)$$

The increase in cardiac output, however, was accomplished at the cost of a substantial increase in mean pulmonary capillary wedge pressure, which rose from 11 to 27 mm Hg. These data suggest that the patient had some limitation of inotropic reserve and that her ability to increase cardiac output depended heavily on use of the Frank-Starling

mechanism. Therefore, her dyspnea can be considered to be of cardiac origin.

A patient with more severe impairment of cardiovascular reserve is illustrated in Table 15.2, which shows the response to 6 minutes of supine bicycle exercise of a 60-year-old man with idiopathic dilated cardiomyopathy and symptoms of marked fatigue and dyspnea with minimal exertion. His chest radiograph showed cardiomegaly with no evidence of pulmonary edema, and his rest hemodynamics were almost normal. Supine bicycle exercise was associated with a marked rise in both left and right heart filling pressures and a marginal ability to increase cardiac output appropriately in relation to his increase in O_2 consumption. His exercise index was 0.85, with a low exercise factor at 4.9:

$$\frac{\Delta \text{ cardiac index}}{\Delta \; O_2 \text{ consumption}} = \frac{1,700}{341} = 4.9 \qquad (15.4)$$

The cause of exercise intolerance in some patients with LV failure is diminished cardiovascular reserve, so that inadequate oxygen is delivered to working skeletal muscle to meet the demands of aerobic metabolism. Other patients

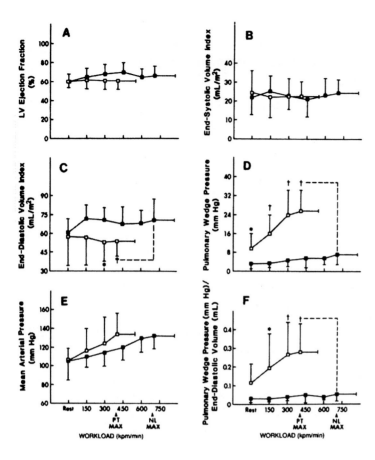

Figure 15.5 Response of left ventricular function to upright bicycle exercise in the patients with diastolic heart failure (□) and healthy controls (■) illustrated in Fig. 15.4. Pulmonary wedge pressure increases dramatically, but left ventricular end-diastolic volume fails to increase in the patients with heart failure, compared with healthy age- and gender-matched controls. LV ejection fraction remains normal. The intolerance to exercise is probably the result of increased pulmonary capillary wedge pressure and the resultant increased lung stiffness rather than decreased cardiac output or oxygen delivery to metabolizing tissues. PT MAX, patient maximum exercise; NL MAX, normal subject maximum exercise. (From Kitzman D, et al. Exercise tolerance in patients with heart failure and preserved left ventricular systolic function: failure of the Frank-Starling mechanism. *J Am Coll Cardiol* 1991;17:1065, with permission.)

are not limited by the ability to deliver oxygen to working skeletal muscle but by the rise in pulmonary capillary wedge pressure associated with exercise (Table 15.1). As illustrated in these examples, the relative contributions of

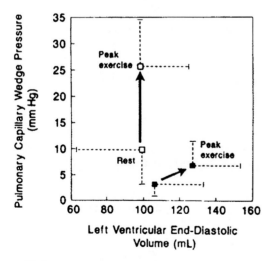

Figure 15.6 Plot of the relationship between changes in pulmonary capillary wedge pressure and left ventricular end-diastolic volume in the patients illustrated in Figs. 15.4 and 15.5. In patients with diastolic heart failure, the stiff left ventricle cannot dilate normally (□) in response to the increased venous return of exercise, leading to a marked rise in left ventricular filling pressure, compared with normal controls (■). (From Kitzman D, et al. Exercise tolerance in patients with heart failure and preserved left ventricular systolic function: failure of the Frank-Starling mechanism. *J Am Coll Cardiol* 1991;17:1065, with permission.)

the inability of the heart to augment cardiac output versus an exercise-induced rise in pulmonary capillary wedge pressure that could impair gas exchange are controversial. Exercise tolerance in patients with congestive heart failure is highly variable and correlates poorly with ejection fraction. Studies of the hemodynamic and ventilatory response to exercise have shown that as the clinical severity of congestive heart failure worsens, there is a progressive decrease in maximal O_2 consumption, premature onset of the anaerobic threshold, and declines in both maximal cardiac output and the cardiac output achieved at levels of submaximal O_2 consumption (18,19). Studies of brief exercise performed by patients with chronic congestive heart failure have shown that arterial oxygen saturation usually increases (presumably as a result of increased ventilation) despite elevation of the pulmonary capillary wedge pressure; maximal oxygen extraction is normal, and ventilatory mechanisms do not limit maximum O_2 consumption, so that both symptomatic limitation and the inability to normally increase oxygen delivery are caused by the failure to increase cardiac output adequately. Conversely, in patients with depressed LV ejection fraction who can achieve normal levels of exercise, factors that contribute to normal exercise capacity include normal augmentation of heart rate, the ability to increase cardiac output through further increases in LV end-diastolic volume and stroke volume, and tolerance of a high pulmonary venous pressure, possibly because of enhanced lymphatic drainage.

TABLE 15.1

RESPONSE TO SUPINE BICYCLE EXERCISE IN A 36-YEAR-OLD WOMAN WITH DILATED CARDIOMYOPATHY

Hemodynamic Parameter	Resting	Exercise (6 min)
Oxygen consumption index (mL/min per m^2)	117	504
Atrioventricular oxygen difference (mL/L)	34	75
Cardiac index (L/min per m^2)	3.4	6.7
Heart rate (beats per min)	80	140
Systemic arterial pressure (mm Hg), systolic/diastolic (mean)	130/70 (95)	142/83 (110)
Right atrial mean pressure (mm Hg)	6	7
Pulmonary capillary wedge mean pressure (mm Hg)	11	27
Left ventricular pressure (mm Hg)	130/17	142/28
Exercise index	—	1.1
Exercise factor	—	8.5

Therefore, in patients with severe depression of LV ejection fraction, the failure to increase cardiac output normally appears to be related both to the inability to increase stroke volume and to the inability to increase heart rate, compared with age-matched subjects (20). This *impaired chronotropic response* appears to be caused by an impaired postsynaptic response to β-adrenergic stimulation that may be related to several defects, including a reduced cardiac β-receptor density, "uncoupling" of the β-receptor and adenylate cyclase activity, and deficient production of cyclic adenosine monophosphate (21).

Evaluation of Valvular Heart Disease

Valvular Stenosis

Exercise may also be used in the cardiac catheterization laboratory to evaluate valvular heart disease. Gradients across the atrioventricular and semilunar valves may become apparent during exercise and may reach levels that account for the clinical symptoms of the patient. Exercise hemodynamics are especially useful when the resting transvalvular gradient or estimated valve area has borderline significance.

An example of the hemodynamic changes during supine dynamic exercise in a patient with moderate mitral stenosis is shown in Fig. 15.7 and Table 15.3. As the result of increased mitral valve flow and a decreased diastolic filling period, the pressure gradient increased significantly, producing left atrial pressures of sufficient magnitude to cause symptoms. Cardiac output increased normally, yielding an exercise index of 1.2 and an exercise factor of 5.8:

$$\frac{\Delta \text{ cardiac output}}{\Delta \text{ O}_2 \text{ consumption}} = \frac{2,800}{481} = 5.8 \qquad (15.5)$$

These data are compatible with mild mitral stenosis and illustrate the changes in a diastolic pressure gradient across the mitral valve required to produce an increase in cardiac output appropriate to the increased oxygen requirements of strenuous exercise.

TABLE 15.2

RESPONSE TO SUPINE BICYCLE EXERCISE IN A 60-YEAR-OLD MAN WITH DILATED CARDIOMYOPATHY

Hemodynamic Parameter	Resting	Exercise (6 min)
Oxygen consumption index (mL/min per m^2)	128	469
AV O$_2$ difference (mL/L)	40	96
Cardiac index (L/min per m^2)	3.2	4.9
Heart rate (beats per min)	90	141
Systemic arterial pressure (mm Hg), systolic/diastolic (mean)	91/62 (73)	107/67 (88)
Right atrial mean pressure (mm Hg)	5	20
Pulmonary capillary wedge mean pressure (mm Hg)	12	34
Left ventricular pressure (mm Hg)	91/16	107/34
Exercise index	—	0.85
Exercise factor	—	4.9

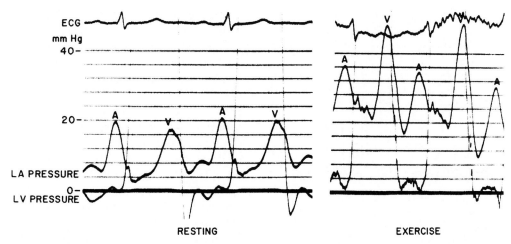

Figure 15.7 Simultaneous pressure recordings from left atrium and left ventricle at rest and at 5 minutes of bicycle ergometer exercise in a patient with mitral stenosis. The hemodynamic data for this patient are presented in Table 15.3.

In evaluating hemodynamic changes across stenotic valves during exercise, it is often found that the calculated valve area during exercise varies somewhat from that calculated on the basis of resting data (it is usually slightly larger). This variance is usually small and may be related to actual changes in the degree of valvular obstruction (i.e., a higher gradient and greater flow may force the stenotic leaflets to open farther), deficient data, or computational errors inherent in the assumptions applied to the equation for calculating valve orifice size.

Valvular Insufficiency

The hemodynamic consequences of valvular insufficiency with ventricular volume overload may be subtle at rest.

TABLE 15.3

HEMODYNAMIC CHANGES DURING SUPINE DYNAMIC EXERCISE IN A PATIENT WITH MITRAL STENOSIS[a]

Parameter	Resting	Exercise (5 min)
Left atrial pressure (mm Hg)		
A	20	34
V	18	46
Mean diastolic	10	26
Left ventricular mean diastolic pressure (mm Hg)	1	4
Oxygen consumption (mL/min)	207	688
Atrioventricular oxygen difference (mL/L)	31	74
Cardiac output (L/min)	6.5	9.3
Heart rate (beats per min)	72	108
Mitral value area (cm^2)	1.6	1.8
Exercise index	—	1.2
Exercise factor	—	5.8

[a]Same patient as in Fig. 15.7.

Dynamic exercise, by calling on the heart to substantially augment its forward cardiac output, may elicit changes in LVEDP and volume (preload) and in systemic vascular resistance (afterload) that are useful in assessing the cardiovascular limitations imposed by the valve lesion. Of particular importance here is the inability of many patients with valvular insufficiency to increase forward cardiac output in an appropriate manner, resulting in a low exercise index and an abnormal exercise factor. Dynamic exercise testing is especially valuable in such patients because the qualitative assessment of valvular insufficiency from angiograms may be unreliable and does not correlate well with the extent of functional impairment.

Figure 15.8 shows the hemodynamic response to dynamic bicycle exercise for a 55-year-old man with rheumatic heart disease and mitral regurgitation. The patient was able to increase cardiac output normally, but mean pulmonary capillary wedge pressure increased from 18 to 30 mm Hg, with V waves to 60 mm Hg, during 6 minutes of supine bicycle exercise. This patient had successful mitral valve replacement with relief of symptoms.

Performing a Dynamic Exercise Test

Dynamic exercise during cardiac catheterization is easily performed with a bicycle ergometer while the patient is supine. A protocol detailing the exercise test should be prepared beforehand to ensure that all essential data are obtained. Pressures should be obtained so that the appropriate valve gradients can be evaluated, and LV pressure should be monitored if LV performance is in question.

Supine bicycle exercise tests are performed most easily when catheterization is done by the arm (e.g., brachial, radial) and/or neck (e.g., jugular vein) approach. However, supine bicycle exercise tests can also be done with safety when catheterization is by the femoral approach if care is taken to place the right and left heart manifolds and

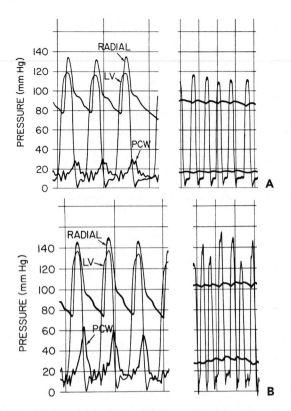

Figure 15.8 Hemodynamic findings during exercise in a 55-year-old man with mitral regurgitation. Left ventricular (LV), pulmonary capillary wedge (PCW), and radial artery pressure tracings are shown before **(A)** and during **(B)** the sixth minute of supine bicycle exercise. PCW mean pressure and V wave increased substantially with exercise.

transducers in a stable and accessible position on the chest, away from leg motion artifact, and if the femoral venous and arterial sheaths are visualized and secured in place by the hand of one operator during exercise to ensure that catheters and sheaths are not displaced by leg movement.

We usually carry out a supine bicycle exercise test immediately after baseline hemodynamic values and cardiac output have been measured, before contrast angiography. The patient's feet are secured in the bicycle stirrups, and the right heart, left heart, and systemic arterial catheters and attached manifolds are positioned so that they are not kinked or under tension and will not be disturbed during the exercise. Next, the system for measuring O_2 consumption is put in place (see Chapter 8). Alternatively, cardiac output can be assessed with the use of an indicator dilution technique (e.g., thermodilution), and O_2 consumption can be estimated as the quotient of cardiac output and AV O_2 difference.

Before beginning exercise, the patient is instructed that he or she will be coached to achieve a certain level of submaximal exercise over the first 1 minute that can be sustained for an additional 4 to 6 minutes. This detailed patient instruction is useful because some patients may be accustomed to the different format of progressively graded exercise aimed at achieving a transient level of maximal,

exhaustion-limited exercise used in upright treadmill tests. A sufficient number of syringes for measuring systemic arterial and mixed venous (pulmonary artery) blood oxygen saturation content should be at hand.

With the patient resting quietly and feet positioned on the bicycle, all manometers are zeroed, phasic and mean pressures are recorded at 25 or 50 mm/second paper speed (or electronic equivalent) and at the gain to be used during exercise, and cardiac output measurements are repeated to obtain an accurate pre-exercise baseline with legs elevated in the stirrups. Manometers are zeroed once again, all pressures are then redisplayed, and paper speed is slowed (to 5 to 10 mm/second). Exercise is then begun with all pressures displayed continuously on the monitor and recorded at slow speed. We generally record LV phasic pressure, systemic arterial (e.g., radial or femoral artery) mean pressure, and pulmonary capillary mean pressure simultaneously. It is desirable to choose a gain setting on the recorder such that all pressures may be visualized simultaneously (as shown in Fig. 15.8). At each 1-minute interval, a brief recording of all three pressures on phasic at 25 to 50 mm/second paper speed is accomplished, after which the pulmonary capillary and systemic arterial pressures are returned to mean and the paper speed is slowed to 5 to 10 mm/second. The continuous observation and recording of pressures is important because it permits the accurate monitoring of any rise in filling pressure or fall in arterial pressure during exercise and ensures that catheters remain in correct position for measurements at peak exercise.

After the patient has achieved a steady state level of exercise for 4 minutes, simultaneous LV-systemic arterial, LV-PCW, and PCW-to-pulmonary artery pullback pressures are recorded during minutes 4 to 6, after increasing the recorder speed to 50 mm/second without attempting to rezero the transducers. The right heart catheter is pulled back to the pulmonary artery, and exercise cardiac output is measured by the Fick or thermodilution technique, at which time systemic arterial and pulmonary artery blood samples are drawn for measurement of oxygen saturation.

Precautions should be taken during exercise to ensure patient safety. The duration and intensity of the exercise must be tailored to fit the needs of the individual patient. The electrocardiogram (ECG) should be monitored constantly to avoid serious arrhythmias, and exercise should be terminated if significant symptoms or greatly abnormal hemodynamic alterations occur. Little additional diagnostic information can be obtained by continuing the exercise to the point of producing pulmonary edema.

ISOMETRIC EXERCISE

Sustained isometric contraction of the forearm flexor muscles produces a cardiovascular reflex consisting of increases in heart rate, arterial blood pressure, and cardiac output.

The precise nature of this reflex is not completely understood, but it appears to require afferent neural impulses from the exercising extremity and may be related to inhibition of vagal activity. Although the cardiac output response may be blunted, the anticipated responses in heart rate and blood pressure are not blocked by administration of propranolol, indicating that more is involved than a simple increase in β-adrenergic stimulation.

Hemodynamic Response

The hemodynamic response to isometric handgrip exercise has been studied in a series of normal subjects and patients with heart disease (22). In normal adult subjects, heart rate, systemic arterial pressure, and cardiac output increase, whereas systemic vascular resistance shows no change, indicating that the increase in systemic arterial pressure is caused by the increased cardiac output rather than by a vasoconstrictor response. No significant or consistent change in LVEDP or stroke volume occurs, whereas stroke work, a function of both arterial pressure and stroke volume, usually increases. The augmentation of LV performance during isometric exercise may be caused by both increased LV myocardial contractility (22) and the Frank-Starling mechanism.

Patients with heart disease and decreased LV function or inotropic reserve commonly show an abnormal hemodynamic and contractile response to isometric exercise (22). Although the maximum rate of rise of LV pressure, peak dP/dt, may increase in diseased hearts, the change is of less magnitude than in normal subjects. LV stroke work may increase, remain unchanged, or decrease in response to isometric exercise in pathologic states. This may itself be evidence of compromised LV function but is more apparent when the change in stroke work is compared with the change in LVEDP. Significant increases in LVEDP are seen commonly in the abnormal response to isometric exercise (22) and indicate decreased inotropic reserve, dependence on the Frank-Starling mechanism to augment LV performance, and probably some component of diastolic dysfunction.

Performing an Isometric Exercise Test

Isometric exercise is most commonly performed as sustained handgrip. The subject is first tested to evaluate maximal voluntary contraction strength. A partially inflated sphygmomanometer cuff or a specially designed handgrip dynamometer may be used. This testing may be done before cardiac catheterization and should be done well before the actual handgrip test. The patient must be coached and encouraged to grip as hard as possible when maximal voluntary contraction strength is determined. Baseline resting hemodynamic data should include heart rate, systemic arterial pressure (phasic and mean), LV pressure, and cardiac output. Cardiac output is most easily determined for this form of exercise by the indicator dilution method (e.g.,

thermodilution) or by the Fick method with the continuous O_2 consumption measurement technique.

Once baseline data are collected, the subject is asked to grip the dynamometer at a level 30% to 50% of the previously determined maximal voluntary contraction. Some coaching is usually required to ensure that the patient sustains the grip. It is important that the patient not do a Valsalva maneuver during handgrip exercise, and the respiratory pattern should be closely observed. Valsalva maneuver may be avoided simply by engaging the patient in conversation during the test. We have used 50% maximal voluntary contraction for 3 minutes, with repeat measurements of pressures and cardiac output beginning at 2.5 minutes, so that measurements are completed by 3 minutes and the test may be terminated. The ECG should be monitored continuously to exclude the appearance of arrhythmias.

PACING TACHYCARDIA

Graded tachycardia induced by atrial pacing was first introduced in 1967 by Sowton et al. (23) as a stress test that could be used in the cardiac catheterization laboratory to evaluate patients with ischemic heart disease. They noted that artificially increasing the heart rate by pacing the right atrium usually could induce angina in patients with symptomatic coronary artery disease. Moreover, they found that the degree of pacing stress needed to produce ischemia, defined in terms of pacing rate and duration, was more or less reproducible in any given patient. Since this original report, numerous investigators have described characteristic pacing-induced ECG changes (24–30), alterations in adenosine production (31,32) and myocardial lactate metabolism (25,26), hemodynamic abnormalities (33–39), regional wall motion abnormalities (40,41), and defects in thallium scintigraphy (42,43). Although agreement on the overall usefulness of atrial pacing has not been universal, it is clear that the technique can safely and reliably induce ischemia in most patients with coronary artery disease and that information obtained during the pacing-induced ischemic state is often helpful in the diagnosis and treatment of the patient's underlying disease.

Hemodynamic Effects of Pacing Tachycardia

The principal form of stress that accompanies pacing tachycardia is an increase in myocardial O_2 consumption secondary to the increased heart rate and an increase in myocardial contractility because of the treppe effect (44). Associated with this increase in myocardial O_2 consumption is a reflex coronary vasodilation with an increase in myocardial blood flow. Apart from these changes in oxygen demand and supply, pacing tachycardia appears to be associated with no major hemodynamic stress, at least in patients with normal coronary arteries. Artificially increasing the heart rate by pacing the right atrium is accompanied by a concomitant decrease in ventricular stroke volume with little or no overall change in cardiac output. Moreover, there appears to be no significant change in ventricular afterload, venous return, or circulating catecholamines during pacing tachycardia.

Differences Between Pacing Tachycardia and Exercise Stress

The physiology of pacing is distinctly different from that of dynamic or isometric exercise, in which there are not only increases in heart rate and myocardial contractility but also major changes in ventricular loading conditions and cardiac output in response to increased metabolic demands from the periphery. Because of the differences in physiology between atrial pacing and exercise, each technique has relative advantages and disadvantages as a form of stress testing in the catheterization laboratory. Unlike pacing, exercise is associated with an increase in both heart rate and systolic blood pressure. As a result, exercise is usually capable of achieving a higher rate-pressure product (i.e., heart rate $\times$ peak systolic pressure) and represents a more severe form of stress with greater increases in myocardial O_2 consumption. On the other hand, pacing is not associated with exercise-induced changes in cardiac output or ventricular loading conditions, and, as a result, the characterization of ventricular function is easier. In addition, atrial pacing is superior to exercise for evaluating myocardial metabolic function, because the rapid rise in arterial blood lactate and adenosine levels that accompanies exercise may obscure alterations of myocardial lactate metabolism and adenosine production. Finally, unlike exercise, with the termination of pacing and the rapid diminution of myocardial oxygen requirement, myocardial ischemia almost always resolves rapidly (i.e., within 1 to 2 minutes). As a result, the physician has more control over the amount of stress that the patient experiences, with very little prolonged ischemia occurring in the poststress period.

Pacing tachycardia has been used as a form of stress testing in patients with heart disease for more than 30 years. The technique has been most useful in the assessment of patients with coronary artery disease.

Method for a Pacing Stress Test

Atrial pacing protocols usually can be conducted in the cardiac catheterization laboratory without undue prolongation of the routine catheterization procedure or significant added risks to the patient. In our experience, pacing is best conducted after the routine diagnostic aspects of catheterization and usually extends the procedure by no more than 15 to 30 minutes, depending on the details of the protocol. It is important that detailed planning of the protocol be made before the catheterization is begun to help incorporate the atrial pacing into the routine catheteriza-

tion as much as possible without unnecessary repetition of maneuvers and excessive prolongation of arterial time.

The type of catheter used for the pacing protocol can vary depending on the type of information that is to be evaluated during the pacing procedure. In general, the pacing catheter can be either unipolar or bipolar. If pacing is to be conducted with simultaneous myocardial metabolic assessment, a Gorlin or Baim-Turi pacing catheter that allows simultaneous pacing and coronary sinus lactate sampling is ideal. Sampling of both coronary sinus lactate and adenosine has been accomplished (32,45) with the use of a specially designed catheter placed in the coronary sinus. If assessment of myocardial O_2 consumption is to be made, a coronary sinus pacing catheter with the capability of measuring coronary blood flow, such as the Baim catheter (Elecath, Rahway, NJ), may be used. If pacing is to be conducted with simultaneous measurement of left heart filling pressures and cardiac output, then both a pacing catheter and a second right heart catheter (typically a thermodilution flow-directed catheter) may be inserted into the right side of the heart.

The pacing catheter may be inserted by either venous cutdown or percutaneous technique from the groin, the antecubital fossa, or the neck. Use of a coronary sinus pacing catheter usually requires a neck or arm approach for easier access into the coronary sinus.

Perhaps the most critical part of the atrial pacing technique is proper placement of the pacing lead because accidental displacement of the pacing tip during pacing can disrupt the protocol. The pacing lead can be placed at the junction of the superior vena cava and right atrium, at the lateral right atrial wall, or in the coronary sinus. Placement of the pacing lead is most stable at either the first or last of these positions because displacement of the lead commonly occurs from the lateral atrial wall during respiration. Stimulation of the phrenic nerve with subsequent diaphragmatic stimulation also occurs commonly with placement of the catheter against the lateral atrial wall. To avoid problems with displacement of the pacing tip, we have used a bipolar flared pacing catheter (Atri-Pace I, Mansfield Scientific, Mansfield, MA).

Once the pacing catheter is positioned in the right atrium, it is connected to the pulse generator unit. This unit should be equipped with a fixed-rate mode, pacing at least to 170 beats per minute (bpm), and a variable output from 0.5 to 10 mA. Bipolar pacing catheters may be connected directly to the pacemaker unit or attached through extension wires with alligator clamps. Unipolar catheters should have their negative pole grounded to the skin via either a needle electrode or standard ECG plates. Once the pacing catheter has been positioned properly and connected to the pulse generator, the ability of the pacemaker to stimulate the atrium and to control ventricular rate should be assessed. Initially, the output of the generator is set at 2 to 3 mA, and the pacing rate is adjusted to 10 bpm faster than the sinus rate. Pacing is then begun, and if there is atrial and ventricular capture, the pacing rate is increased by 10 bpm every 5 seconds until a rate of 150 to 160 bpm is reached. Inadequate pacing may occur secondary to an inadequate output of the pulse generator, improper lead positioning, or the development of atrioventricular block. The output of the pulse generator may be increased, but, in general, stimulating energies in excess of 7 to 8 mA frequently result in painful phrenic nerve stimulation. If excessively high energies are required for capture, the electrode lead should be repositioned. If atrioventricular block develops at high stimulatory rates, 1 mg atropine may be administered intravenously: This usually ensures adequate atrioventricular conduction up to rates of 140 bpm or more.

After the lead has been properly positioned and an adequate trial of pacing to assess capture has been performed, the actual pacing protocol may be done. A pacing stress test usually begins with pacing at approximately 20 bpm above the baseline rate, with increases of 20 bpm every 2 minutes, until angina pectoris or characteristic hemodynamic alterations occur, or until 85% of maximum age-predicted heart rate is achieved. Placement of a thermodilution balloon-tip flow-directed catheter, a left heart catheter, and a radial arterial cannula (or femoral arterial sheath side arm) before pacing allows simultaneous assessment of right- and left-sided heart pressures, cardiac output measurement by thermodilution and/or Fick method, and determination of systemic and pulmonary vascular resistances. Assessment of LV volumes also may be accomplished with standard angiographic, echocardiographic, or radionuclide techniques.

Following the induction of chest pain during pacing tachycardia, pacing may be continued at the same heart rate safely for up to 3 to 5 minutes, during which hemodynamic, metabolic, and ECG data may be obtained. After cessation of pacing, chest pain usually resolves quickly, but it may occasionally persist for up to 1 to 2 minutes after the return to sinus rhythm.

Pacing-Induced Angina

Initial reports on the use of atrial pacing tachycardia suggested that pacing-induced angina was a sensitive marker for the presence of ischemic heart disease and could serve as a suitable ischemic end point of pacing protocols (23). Specifically, the induction of angina was thought to mark a highly reproducible anginal threshold defined in terms of pacing rate and duration. Subsequent investigators have found, however, that chest pain is neither a sensitive nor a specific indicator of the presence of coronary artery disease. For example, Robson et al. (28) demonstrated that chest pain could be elicited in 80% of patients with normal coronary arteries if they were paced at extremely high rates (in excess of 180 bpm). Moreover, Chandraratna et al. (46) demonstrated the absence of angina in some patients with coronary artery disease who were stressed with pacing

tachycardia at a high rate. Similarly, in terms of defining anginal threshold according to the pacing rate and duration, as many as 20% of individuals have been shown to have considerable variation in these parameters (47). In view of these results, it is clear that chest pain alone should not be used as a reliable marker for the presence of pacing-induced ischemia. However, improved sensitivity and specificity of pacing-induced chest pain are noted when additional evidence of ischemia, such as pacing-induced ECG changes or myocardial metabolic abnormalities, is present.

Electrocardiographic Changes in Response to a Pacing Stress Test

Like pacing-induced angina, the presence of ischemic ST-segment depression during pacing tachycardia has not been regarded previously as a sensitive or specific marker for the presence of coronary artery disease. For example, in terms of sensitivity, Rios and Hurwitz (27) compared pacing tachycardia and exercise in 50 patients and found diagnostic ECG changes with pacing in only 20% with pacing tachycardia, compared with 83% with exercise. Similarly, in terms of specificity, Robson et al. (28) reported ST-segment depression of 1.5 mm or more during pacing tachycardia in as many as 80% of patients with normal coronary arteries. In addition to poor overall sensitivity and specificity, pacing tachycardia is associated with certain distortions of the ECG that sometimes make interpretation of ischemic ST-segment changes difficult or impossible. Pacing is associated with prolongation of the PR interval in most patients, and extreme prolongation of this interval can cause the pacemaker spike to fall within the ST segment of the preceding paced complex, thereby obscuring potential ST-segment changes.

Despite the previously reported poor utility of pacing-induced ECG changes, work from our laboratory (29) has suggested an improved sensitivity and specificity of ischemic ST-segment depression during pacing tachycardia if certain technical guidelines of the pacing protocol are followed. Several earlier pacing trials that reported a low sensitivity of pacing ECG changes used only limited three-lead recording, and it is clear, at least with standard exercise testing, that sensitivity can be improved substantially with full 12-lead monitoring.

To maximize the utility of pacing-induced ECG changes, pacing trials should be conducted with the use of the following guidelines. First, a 12-lead ECG is used for monitoring, and the ECG is regarded as positive for myocardial ischemia if ≥1 mm of horizontal or downsloping ST-segment depression is produced. Second, pacing tachycardia is terminated when 85% of maximal age-predicted heart rate is achieved or when typical ischemic chest pain is accompanied by diagnostic ECG changes. Finally, if marked prolongation of the PR interval distorts the preceding ST-segment changes, the ECG is considered positive for ischemia *only if there is ST-segment depression in the first five beats after the discontinuation of the pacing stimulus.*

Using these guidelines, actual pacing protocols conducted in our experience had an overall sensitivity and specificity of 94% and 83%, respectively, with regard to pacing-induced ECG changes. In addition, distortion of the ST segment by the pacing stimulus because of marked prolongation of the PR interval appeared to occur infrequently when the peak pacing rate was no higher than 85% of the maximum age-predicted heart rate. Moreover, in at least one subgroup of patients who were tested with both atrial pacing and standard treadmill exercise (29), the

concordance between pacing-induced and exercise-induced ECG changes was 90%. Examples of pacing-induced and exercise-induced ECG changes are shown for a patient with normal coronary arteries in Fig. 15.9A and for a patient with coronary artery disease in Fig. 15.9B.

The sensitivity of pacing-induced ECG changes may be further improved with the use of endocardial electrograms obtained during the pacing stress test. Nabel et al. (30) reported on the use of local unipolar electrograms recorded from the tip of a 0.064-cm-diameter guidewire positioned against the endocardial surface of potentially ischemic regions. Endocardial electrograms, LVEDP, and multiple

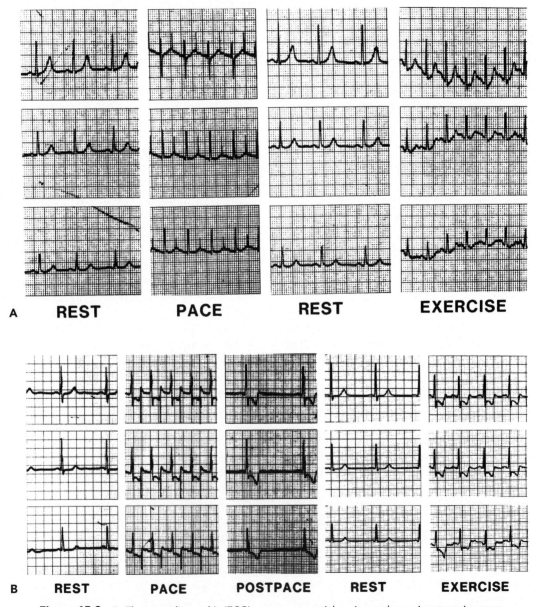

Figure 15.9 A. Electrocardiographic (ECG) response to atrial pacing and exercise stress in a man with normal coronary arteries. From top to bottom, leads V4, V5, and V6 are monitored. **B.** Comparison of ECG response to atrial pacing and exercise stress in a man with severe three-vessel coronary artery disease. Leads V4, V5, and V6 are monitored (top to bottom) as in **A.** ST depression occurs to the same degree with both types of stress. (From Heller GV, et al. The pacing stress test: a reexamination of the relation between coronary artery disease and pacing-induced electrocardiographic changes. *Am J Cardiol* 1984;54:50, with permission.)

surface ECG leads were recorded before, during, and after rapid atrial pacing in 21 patients with coronary artery disease. Before pacing, endocardial electrograms in all 21 patients were free of ST-segment elevation. After rapid atrial pacing, marked ST-segment elevation was apparent in 17 of the 21 patients. This ST-segment elevation could be abolished in all patients with the use of nitroglycerin. Moreover, in several patients, endocardial ST-segment elevation after pacing was abolished by successful percutaneous coronary angioplasty of the critically stenosed artery supplying the ischemic region of myocardium. The authors concluded that endocardial electrographic changes are a reliable marker of pacing-induced myocardial ischemia and may be more sensitive than angina, pacing-induced hemodynamic changes, or ST-segment depression on the surface ECG.

Myocardial Metabolic Changes Induced by a Pacing Stress Test

Abnormal myocardial metabolism has been documented during pacing-induced ischemia by means of coronary sinus sampling and the subsequent measurement of coronary arterial and venous blood lactate. Because lactate production is a byproduct of anaerobic glycolysis, its production by the heart and appearance within the coronary sinus is a sign of myocardial ischemia. Previous investigators have noted rapid increases in coronary sinus lactate levels during pacing tachycardia in patients with coronary artery disease, often before the appearance of angina (25,26). With cessation of pacing, the elevated coronary sinus lactate concentrations fall rapidly, representing a washout of the accumulated myocardial lactate and diminished lactate production as normal oxygenation is restored. Monitoring of arterial lactate levels while coronary sinus lactate levels are rising usually shows little or no elevation, in marked contrast to arterial lactate levels during exercise. As a result, atrial pacing tachycardia is superior to exercise for evaluating abnormal myocardial metabolic function because rapidly rising arterial lactate levels during exercise may obscure abnormal patterns of myocardial lactate metabolism.

Monitoring of coronary sinus lactate during pacing protocols is most easily accomplished with a Gorlin pacing catheter. Placement of the Gorlin catheter in the coronary

sinus usually can be confirmed by injection of a small amount of contrast medium. Care must be taken not to perforate either the coronary sinus or the great cardiac vein, and not to place the pacing tip of the catheter too distally because placement of the distal catheter into the great cardiac vein may result in ventricular rather than atrial pacing.

Arterial and coronary venous blood lactate concentrations in response to a pacing stress test are illustrated in Fig. 15.10. In the control state, the concentration of coronary sinus blood lactate is lower than lactate concentration in arterial blood, reflecting the fact that the heart normally consumes lactate as a fuel. During pacing tachycardia, coronary sinus blood lactate concentration rises progressively and exceeds arterial blood lactate concentration, reflecting a shift to anaerobic metabolism of the ischemic myocardium. The lactate falls rapidly after discontinuation of pacing because the heart rate returns to control immediately.

There has been renewed interest in using coronary sinus adenosine as a marker of myocardial ischemia. Adenosine, a metabolite released by ischemic myocardium, elicits an increase in coronary artery blood flow in response to a decrease in the ratio of myocardial oxygen supply to demand. As a result, adenosine should be a more sensitive marker of myocardial ischemia than lactate, which requires anaerobic glycolysis. An early report demonstrated that adenosine is increased in the coronary sinus blood of patients with ischemic heart disease during pacing tachycardia (31), and later Feldman et al. (32) made several methodologic improvements regarding adenosine measurements. A double-lumen "metabolic" catheter was used that allowed the addition and mixing of a solution to stop adenosine metabolism at the tip of the catheter. Adenosine has a half-life of less than 1.5 seconds in human blood. Furthermore, there are numerous sources of artifactual adenosine production in human blood. It is therefore essential that a solution that inhibits both the breakdown and the production of adenosine be mixed with human blood at the site of collection. Using this technique, adenosine was demonstrated to be a more sensitive marker of myocardial ischemia than lactate (32). Each patient with coronary artery disease ($N = 9$) atrially paced to ischemia demonstrated at least a 1.5-fold increase in coronary sinus adenosine. In contrast, only three of these nine patients had lactate production. In a subsequent

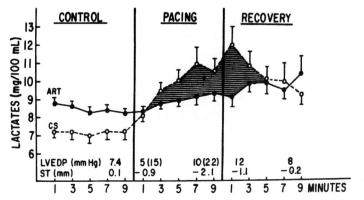

Figure 15.10 Mean values for arterial (ART) and coronary sinus (CS) blood lactate concentrate before (control), during (pacing), and after (recovery) tachycardia in 17 patients with coronary artery disease. Left ventricular end-diastolic pressure (LVEDP) changed little during pacing tachycardia but was elevated during brief periods of interruption of pacing (values in parentheses). ST-segment depression developed progressively during pacing tachycardia and resolved in recovery. Lactate extraction shifted to lactate production during ischemia, and this persisted into recovery for a brief period. (From Parker JO, Chiong MA, West RO, et al. Sequential alterations in myocardial lactate metabolism, S-T segments, and left ventricular function during angina induced by atrial pacing. *Circulation* 1969;40: 113, with permission.)

study with improved methodology (48), patients with coronary artery disease ($N = 17$) were found to have higher coronary sinus adenosine concentrations than a control group of patients ($N = 6$) at rest. This finding provides evidence that release of endogenous adenosine may be an intrinsic homeostatic mechanism to maintain resting flow distal to a stenotic coronary artery.

Hemodynamic Changes During a Pacing Stress Test

Patients without ischemic heart disease who are stressed by atrial-paced tachycardia generally demonstrate no significant change in cardiac output, mean arterial pressure, AV O_2 difference, or systemic vascular resistance. LVEDP and pulmonary capillary wedge pressure usually fall during pacing tachycardia and then return to prepacing baseline levels in the immediate postpacing period. LV end-diastolic and end-systolic volumes fall during pacing tachycardia, with a decrease in stroke volume and no significant change in ejection fraction.

Patients with coronary artery disease who are paced to ischemia likewise manifest no significant change in cardiac output, mean arterial pressure, AV O_2 difference, or systemic vascular resistance. Some investigators have documented slight decreases in cardiac output with slight increases in mean arterial pressure, AV O_2 difference, and systemic resistance. However, these differences are probably related to the intensity of pacing-induced ischemia, its duration before the measurement of hemodynamic variables, and the amount of myocardium that has become ischemic, with more extensive hemodynamic abnormalities occurring in the setting of more extensive myocardial ischemia. The most dramatic differences in pacing hemodynamics between patients with

normal coronary arteries and those with coronary artery disease are seen in terms of LV pressure-volume relationships during pacing tachycardia and in the immediate postpacing period. Of note, LV filling pressures do not show the progressive decrease seen in nonischemic patients, and elevations in pulmonary capillary wedge, mean pulmonary artery, and occasionally LV end-diastolic pressures occur at maximum pacing. Most important, there is an abrupt rise in LVEDP in the immediate postpacing period. Similarly, LV end-diastolic and end-systolic volumes decrease less during pacing-induced tachycardia in patients with ischemic heart disease compared with normal subjects, and there is often a significant decrease in LV ejection fraction.

A study looking at pressure-volume relationships during pacing tachycardia conducted by us (49) illustrates well the differences between nonischemic and ischemic hemodynamic responses to pacing. In this study, 22 patients, including 11 patients with normal coronary arteries and 11 with significant coronary artery disease, underwent sequential atrial pacing with simultaneous monitoring of LV pressure and ventricular volume measured by gated radionuclide ventriculography. Using synchronized LV pressure tracings and radionuclide time-activity volume curves, three sequential pressure-volume diagrams were constructed for each patient, corresponding to baseline, intermediate, and maximum pacing levels. All 11 patients with coronary artery disease demonstrated angina and significant ST-segment depression at maximum pacing, but none of the 11 patients with normal coronary arteries showed any evidence of pacing-induced ischemia.

Figure 15.11 shows typical LV pressure-volume curves for a patient with normal coronary arteries stressed with pacing tachycardia. Notably, there is a progressive leftward shift for the loop, with an increased heart rate and a pro-

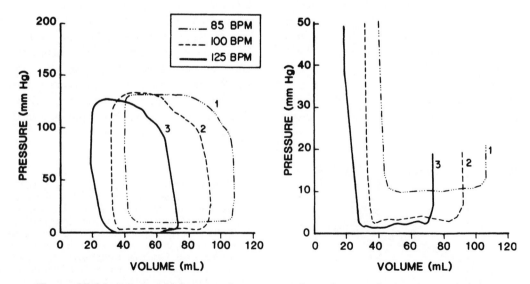

Figure 15.11 Sequential left ventricular pressure-volume diagrams for a patient with normal coronary arteries in response to atrial pacing tachycardia at three increasing heart rates (see text for discussion). (From Aroesty JM, et al. Simultaneous assessment of left ventricular systolic and diastolic dysfunction during pacing-induced ischemia. *Circulation* 1985;71:889, with permission.)

gressive downward shift in the LV diastolic pressure-volume limb of each pressure-volume curve. It is clear that changes in both systolic and diastolic function have occurred in these patients during pacing tachycardia. In terms of systolic function, the progressive leftward shift of the end-systolic portion of the loop presumably represents increased contractility secondary to a treppe effect. Other investigators (44) have likewise demonstrated a positive inotropic stimulus in response to increased heart rate, with increases in isovolumetric contraction indices (e.g., dP/dt) and ejection-phase indices (e.g., circumferential fiber shortening) during pacing tachycardia. With respect to diastolic function, the progressive downward shift of the diastolic limbs seen in Fig. 15.11 suggests that LV distensibility has increased slightly during pacing tachycardia. Whether this downward shift is related to an increase in myocardial relaxation, an alteration in viscoelastic properties, or a change in factors extrinsic to the myocardium (e.g., right ventricle, pericardium) is not known. It is notable that some investigators have documented small increases in markers of diastolic relaxation during pacing-induced tachycardia, such as peak negative dP/dt (50) and the time constant tau (51) in normal animals and the peak rate of posterior wall thinning (52) and LV internal dimension changes in humans.

Figure 15.12 shows sequential LV pressure-volume diagrams for a patient with coronary artery disease whose heart rate was increased progressively by atrial pacing. All patients in our study who developed chest pain and ischemic ECG changes demonstrated a similar pressure-volume pattern with an initial shift of the pressure-volume loop to the left at an intermediate heart rate, followed by a

rightward shift at peak pacing when ischemia developed. In terms of systolic function, it is clear that pacing resulted in an initial treppe effect with a leftward shift of the end-systolic portion of the diagram at intermediate pacing, followed by systolic failure at peak pacing with an increase in ventricular volumes and a rightward shift in the end-systolic portion of the curve. Similarly, in terms of diastolic function, it is evident that the patient did not show a progressive downward shift of the diastolic limb of the LV pressure-volume curve, but actually experienced an upward shift at intermediate and peak pacing. In part, the increase in LVEDP at peak pacing is related to systolic failure with an increase in ventricular volume. Because the patient did not experience evidence of systolic failure at the intermediate pacing level, however, it is also clear that this patient has experienced a primary decrease in LV diastolic distensibility so that pressure is higher at any given chamber volume throughout diastole.

Speculation has continued over the last three decades as to whether the increase in diastolic pressures during pacing-induced ischemia is related to a primary decrease in distensibility or is secondary to systolic failure with increases in ventricular volume. At present, it seems clear that both mechanisms play some role in creating the elevated diastolic pressures. The evidence, however, suggests that changes in diastolic distensibility actually precede altered systolic function (49).

The cause of the altered diastolic distensibility during pacing-induced ischemia has been debated, and a number of different mechanisms (35–38,53,54) have been proposed, including incomplete myocardial relaxation, altered diastolic tone, partial ischemic contracture of some

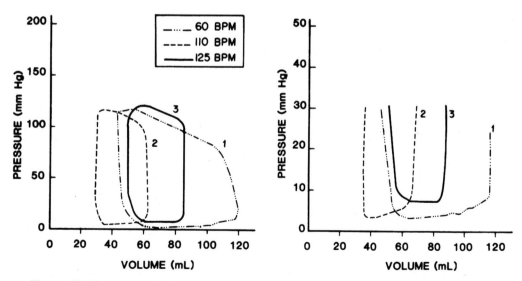

Figure 15.12 Sequential left ventricular pressure-volume diagrams in a patient with three-vessel coronary artery disease who was paced at three increasing heart rates. The patient developed angina and ischemic ST depression at peak pacing. (See text for discussion.) (From Aroesty JM, et al. Simultaneous assessment of left ventricular systolic and diastolic dysfunction during pacing-induced ischemia. *Circulation* 1985;71:889, with permission.)

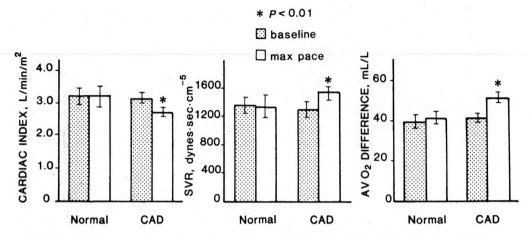

Figure 15.13 Changes in cardiac index, systemic vascular resistance (SVR), and arteriovenous oxygen (AV O₂) difference in 5 patients with normal coronary arteries and 20 patients with coronary artery disease (CAD) during pacing tachycardia. Patients with CAD showed a significant decrease in cardiac index and increases in SVR and AV O₂ difference during maximum pacing tachycardia. (From McKay RG, et al. The pacing stress test reexamined: correlation of pacing-induced hemodynamic changes with the amount of myocardium at risk. *J Am Coll Cardiol* 1984;3:1469, with permission.)

myofibrils within the distribution of the stenotic or occluded coronary artery, altered right ventricular loading, and influence of the pericardium. At present, it seems likely that relaxation of myocardial cells within the reversibly ischemic region is slowed and does not proceed to completion by end-diastole (53,54). This may be related to impaired diastolic calcium sequestration by sarcoplasmic reticulum, but data are insufficient to permit a firm conclusion.

The postpacing rise in LVEDP is perhaps the most concrete evidence of pacing-induced ischemia during atrial pacing protocols. In our protocols, this postpacing rise has been calculated on beats 5 through 15 after discontinua-

tion of pacing, with >5 mm Hg increase in LVEDP in comparison with the prepacing baseline being considered abnormal. Figures 15.13 and 15.14 summarize hemodynamic changes in patients with normal coronary arteries and in those with ischemic heart disease in response to a pacing stress test.

Quantification of the hemodynamic alterations induced by pacing tachycardia may also be useful in assessing myocardial performance in patients with other forms of cardiac disease. Feldman et al. (55) used atrial pacing tachycardia to evaluate the systolic and diastolic myocardial reserve of patients with dilated cardiomyopathy. Pacing-induced changes in LV pressure and volume in

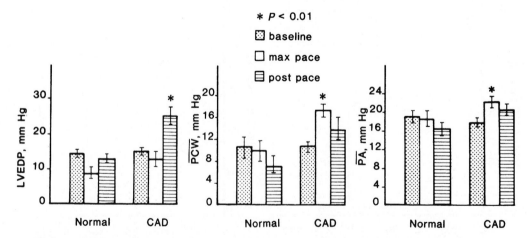

Figure 15.14 Changes in left ventricular end-diastolic pressure (LVEDP), mean pulmonary capillary wedge pressure (PCW), and mean pulmonary artery pressure (PA) in 5 patients with normal coronary arteries and 20 patients with coronary artery disease (CAD) during maximum pacing tachycardia and immediately after pacing. Patients with CAD showed significant elevations of PA and PCW at maximum pacing and of LVEDP immediately after pacing. (From McKay RG, et al. The pacing stress test reexamined: correlation of pacing-induced hemodynamic changes with the amount of myocardium at risk. *J Am Coll Cardiol* 1984;3:1469, with permission.)

seven patients with dilated cardiomyopathy (mean LV ejection fraction, 19%) were compared with findings in six patients with normal coronary arteries and normal LV function (mean LV ejection fraction, 69%). The patients with normal LV function demonstrated significant increases in LV peak positive dP/dt, LV end-systolic pressure-volume ratio, and LV peak filling rate during graded increases in heart rate with atrial pacing. They also exhibited a progressive leftward and downward shift of their pressure-volume diagrams, compatible with increased contractility and enhanced diastolic distensibility in response to pacing tachycardia. In contrast, patients with dilated cardiomyopathy demonstrated no increase in either LV peak positive dP/dt or the end-systolic pressure-volume ratio and absence of a progressive leftward shift of their pressure-volume diagrams. Moreover, patients with dilated cardiomyopathy demonstrated no increase in LV peak filling rate and a blunted downward shift of the diastolic limb of their pressure-volume diagrams. These data suggest that patients with dilated cardiomyopathy demonstrate little or no enhancement of systolic and diastolic function during atrial pacing tachycardia, indicating a depression of both inotropic and lusitropic reserve.

Regional Wall Motion Abnormalities During a Pacing Stress Test

Regional wall motion abnormalities during pacing-induced ischemia have been noted with contrast ventriculography, gated radionuclide ventriculography, and transesophageal echocardiography. Using contrast ventriculography, Dwyer (40) studied eight patients with coronary artery disease who were paced to angina and found that three developed regional hypokinesis in one area, while the remaining five developed at least two separate areas of hypokinesis or akinesis. In all cases, an associated coronary artery lesion could be identified in the vessel that supplied the area of the new regional wall motion abnormality. Similarly, Tzivoni et al. (41), using radionuclide ventriculography, found that 9 of 11 patients developed new regional wall motion abnormalities in response to pacing-induced ischemia.

The overall specificity and sensitivity of pacing-induced regional wall motion abnormalities have been defined with the development of simultaneous transesophageal two-dimensional echocardiography and atrial pacing. Lambertz et al. (56) first developed an ultrasound system in which an atrial pacing facility was incorporated. Fifty patients were evaluated prospectively by cardiac catheterization and pacing echocardiography; 44 had correlative exercise testing. Nine patients were found to have normal epicardial coronary arteries and normal pacing results (100% specificity). Thirty-eight of the 41 patients with significant coronary artery disease developed regional wall motion abnormalities with pacing (93% sensitivity). In contrast, the specificity and sensitivity for exercise testing were 50% and 53%, respectively.

Thallium Scintigraphy and the Pacing Stress Test

The incorporation of thallium scintigraphy into pacing protocols has improved the overall utility of atrial pacing as a stress test. In patients with normal coronary arteries, pacing tachycardia is associated with a homogeneous increase in myocardial O_2 consumption and a secondary increase in coronary blood flow. In patients with coronary artery disease, however, regional increases in myocardial blood flow may be limited by critical coronary stenoses. Because initial myocardial uptake of thallium 201 has been shown to reflect myocardial perfusion and viability, myocardial ischemia induced by pacing tachycardia theoretically should be detectable by thallium scintigraphy. Although early reports on the simultaneous use of atrial pacing and thallium scintigraphy suggested serious limitations (41), studies with improved methodology indicate that this approach is successful in detecting both reversible ischemia and infarcted myocardium (42,43).

To assess the utility of combined atrial pacing and thallium scintigraphy, our laboratory researchers (42) examined the correlation between pacing-induced and exercise-induced thallium defects in patients referred for evaluation of chest pain. The overall sensitivity and specificity of thallium imaging after atrial pacing were excellent. Moreover, segment-by-segment comparison of the thallium scans after either pacing or exercise stress testing revealed a correlation of 83%.

Simultaneous use of thallium scintigraphy and atrial pacing tachycardia can be accomplished by injection of 1.5 to 2.0 mCi of thallium 201 intravenously at peak pacing, followed by continued pacing for at least an additional 5 minutes. In routine thallium exercise testing, exercise is maintained for only 30 to 60 seconds after injection of the radionuclide to allow the thallium to reach the myocardium. However, because of the rapid decrease in heart rate after discontinuation of pacing and the subsequent rapid diminution of myocardial oxygen requirements, pacing is extended to 5 minutes. After discontinuation of the pacing stimulus, while the patient is in the supine position, standard anterior, 40°, and 70° left anterior oblique views are obtained immediately in the catheterization laboratory with a mobile scintillation camera. Repeat standard views are obtained 4 hours after termination of the pacing protocol.

Clinical Uses of Atrial Pacing

The complete evaluation of a patient's cardiac function in the catheterization laboratory often requires an examination of the patient's performance under stressed conditions, when ECG, metabolic, and hemodynamic abnormalities may manifest themselves fully. The role of stress testing is particularly important in the evaluation of patients with ischemic heart disease, in whom, for example, it may be useful to determine the anginal threshold, the magnitude of hemodynamic impairment during ischemia, and the efficacy of antianginal therapy and to establish a need for coronary revascularization. Although standard dynamic and isometric exercise may serve as a form of stress for many patients, not all patients are able to exercise because of physical disabilities, old age, pulmonary disease, peripheral vascular disease, and possibly beta-blockade. In each of these situations, atrial pacing may be used as a suitable form of stress.

REFERENCES

1. Weiner DA. Normal hemodynamic, ventilatory, and metabolic response to exercise. *Arch Intern Med* 1983;143:2173.
2. Dexter L, et al. Effects of exercise on circulatory dynamics of normal individuals. *J Appl Physiol* 1951;3:439.
3. Donald KW, Bishop JM, Cumming G, et al. The effect of exercise on the cardiac output and circulatory dynamics of normal subjects. *Clin Sci* 1955;14:37.
4. Higginbotham MB, et al. Regulation of stroke volume during submaximal and maximal upright exercise in normal man. *Circ Res* 1986;58:281.
5. Plotnick GD, et al. Use of the Frank-Starling mechanism during submaximal versus maximal upright exercise. *Am J Physiol* 1986;251:H1101.
6. Braunwald E, Sonnenblick EH, Ross J Jr, et al. An analysis of the cardiac response to exercise. *Circ Res* 1967;20(suppl I):44.
7. Ross J Jr, Linhart JW, Braunwald E. Effects of changing heart rate in man by electrical stimulation of the right atrium: studies at rest, during exercise, and with isoproterenol. *Circulation* 1965;32:549.
8. Thadani U, Parker JO. Hemodynamics at rest and during supine and sitting bicycle exercise in normal subjects. *Am J Cardiol* 1978;41:52.
9. Rodeheffer RJ, et al. Exercise cardiac output is maintained with advancing age in healthy human subjects: cardiac dilatation and increased stroke volume compensated for a diminished heart rate. *Circulation* 1984;69:203.
10. Port S, Cobb FR, Coleman RE, et al. Effect of age on the response of the left ventricular ejection fraction to exercise. *N Engl J Med* 1980;303:133.
11. McAllister BD, et al. Left ventricular performance during mild supine leg exercise in coronary artery disease. *Circulation* 1968;37:922.
12. Gerstenblith D, Renlund DG, Lakatta EG. Cardiovascular response to exercise in younger and older men. *Fed Proc* 1987;46:1834.
13. Higginbotham MB, et al. Sex-related differences in the normal cardiac response to upright exercise. *Circulation* 1984;70:357.
14. Murgo JP, Craig WE, Pasipoularides A. Evaluation of time course of left ventricular isovolumic relaxation in man. In: Grossman W, Lorell BH, eds. *Diastolic Relaxation of the Heart.* Boston: Martinus Nijhoff, 1986:217.
15. Aroesty JM, McKay RG, Heller GV, et al. Simultaneous assessment of left ventricular systolic and diastolic dysfunction during pacing-induced ischemia. *Circulation* 1985;71:89.
16. Carroll JD, Hess OM, Krayenbuehl HP. Diastolic function during exercise-induced ischemia in man. In: Grossman W, Lorell BH, eds. *Diastolic Relaxation of the Heart.* Boston: Martinus Nijhoff, 1986:217.
17. Kitzman D, Sullivan MJ. Exercise intolerance in patients with heart failure: role of diastolic dysfunction. In: Lorell BH, Grossman W, eds. *Diastolic Relaxation of the Heart,* 2nd ed. Boston: Kluwer, 1994:295.
18. Higginbotham MB, et al. Determinants of variable exercise performance among patients with severe left ventricular dysfunction. *Am J Cardiol* 1983;51:52.
19. Weber KT, Kinasewitz GT, Janicki JS, et al. Oxygen utilization and ventilation during exercise in patients with chronic cardiac failure. *Circulation* 1982;65:1213.
20. Colucci WS, et al. Impaired chronotropic response to exercise in patients with congestive heart failure. *Circulation* 1989;80:314.
21. Bristow MR, et al. Decreased catecholamine sensitivity and β-adrenergic receptor density in failing human hearts. *N Engl J Med* 1982;307:205.
22. Grossman W, et al. Changes in the inotropic state of the left ventricle during isometric exercise. *Br Heart J* 1973;35:697.
23. Sowton GE, Balcon R, Cross D, et al. Measurement of the angina threshold using atrial pacing. *Cardiovasc Res* 1967;1:301.
24. Lau SH, et al. Controlled heart rate by atrial pacing in angina pectoris: a determinant of electrocardiographic S-T depressions. *Circulation* 1968;38:711.
25. Parker JO, Chiong MA, West RO, et al. Sequential alterations in myocardial lactate metabolism, S-T segments, and left ventricular function during angina induced by atrial pacing. *Circulation* 1969;40:113.
26. Helfant RH, et al. Differential hemodynamic, metabolic, and electrocardiographic effects in subjects with and without angina pectoris during atrial pacing. *Circulation* 1970;42:601.
27. Rios JC, Hurwitz LE. Electrocardiographic responses to atrial pacing and multistage treadmill exercise testing: correlation with coronary anatomy. *Am J Cardiol* 1976;34:986.
28. Robson RH, Pridie R, Fluck DC. Evaluation of rapid atrial pacing in diagnosis of coronary artery disease: evaluation of atrial pacing test. *Br Heart J* 1976;38:986.
29. Heller GV, et al. The pacing stress test: a reexamination of the relation between coronary artery disease and pacing induced electrocardiographic changes. *Am J Cardiol* 1984;54:50.
30. Nabel EG, et al. Detection of pacing-induced myocardial ischemia by endocardial electrograms recorded during cardiac catheterization. *J Am Coll Cardiol* 1988;11:983.
31. Fox AC, Reed GE, Glassman E, et al. Release of adenosine from human hearts during angina induced by rapid atrial pacing. *J Clin Invest* 1974;53:1447.
32. Feldman MD, Ayers CR, Lehman MR, et al. Improved detection of ischemia-induced increases in coronary sinus adenosine in patients with coronary artery disease. *Clin Chem* 1992;38:256.
33. Parker JO, Ledwich JR, West RO, et al. Reversible cardiac failure during angina pectoris. *Circulation* 1969;34:745.
34. McCans JL, Parker JO. Left ventricular pressure-volume relationships during myocardial ischemia in man. *Circulation* 1973;48:775.
35. McLaurin LP, Rolett EL, Grossman W. Impaired left ventricular relaxation during pacing induced ischemia. *Am J Cardiol* 1973;32:751.
36. Mann T, Brodie BR, Grossman W, et al. Effect of angina on the left ventricular diastolic pressure-volume relationship. *Circulation* 1977;55:761.
37. Barry WH, Brooker JZ, Alderman EL, et al. Changes in diastolic stiffness and tone of the left ventricle during angina pectoris. *Circulation* 1974;49:225.
38. Mann T, Goldberg S, Mudge GH, et al. Factors contributing to altered left ventricular diastolic properties during angina pectoris. *Circulation* 1979;59:14.
39. Thadani U, et al. Clinical hemodynamic and metabolic responses during pacing in the supine and sitting postures in patients with angina pectoris. *Am J Cardiol* 1979;44:249.
40. Dwyer EM. Left ventricular pressure-volume alterations and regional disorders of contraction during myocardial ischemia induced by atrial pacing. *Circulation* 1970;42:1111.
41. Tzivoni D, et al. Diagnosis of coronary artery disease by multigated radionuclide angiography during right atrial pacing. *Chest* 1981;80:562.
42. Heller GV, et al. The pacing stress test: thallium 201 myocardial imaging after atrial pacing. *J Am Coll Cardiol* 1984;3:1197.
43. McKay RG, et al. The pacing stress test reexamined: correlation of pacing-induced hemodynamic changes with the amount of myocardium at risk. *J Am Coll Cardiol* 1984;3:1469.
44. Ricci D, Orlick A, Alderman E. Role of tachycardia as an inotropic stimulus in man. *J Clin Invest* 1979;63:695.
45. Shryock JC, Boykin MT, Hill JA, et al. A new method of sampling blood for measurement of plasma adenosine. *Am J Physiol* 1990;258:H1232.
46. Chandraratna PAN, et al. Spectrum of hemodynamic responses to atrial pacing in coronary artery disease. *Br Heart J* 1973;35:1033.

47. Thadani U, et al. Are the clinical and hemodynamic events during pacing in patients with angina reproducible? *Circulation* 1979;60: 1036.

48. McLaughlin DP, Beller GA, Linden J, et al. Hemodynamic and metabolic correlates of dipyridamole-induced myocardial thallium 201 perfusion abnormalities in multivessel coronary artery disease. *Am J Cardiol* 1994;74:1159.

49. Aroesty JM, et al. Simultaneous assessment of left ventricular systolic and diastolic dysfunction during pacing-induced ischemia. *Circulation* 1985;71:889.

50. Karliner JS, et al. Pharmacological and hemodynamic influences on the rate of isovolumetric left ventricular relaxation in the conscious dog. *J Clin Invest* 1977;60:511.

51. Weiss JL, Fredericksen JW, Weisfeldt ML. Hemodynamic determinants of the time-course of fall in canine left ventricular pressure. *J Clin Invest* 1976;58:751.

52. Fifer MA, Borow KM, Colan S, et al. Early diastolic left ventricular function in children and adults with aortic stenosis. *J Am Coll Cardiol* 1985;5:1147.

53. Grossman W. Diastolic dysfunction in congestive heart failure. *N Engl J Med* 1991;325:1557.

54. Paulus WJ. Upward shift and outward bulge: divergent myocardial effects of pacing angina and brief coronary occlusion. *Circulation* 1990;81:1436.

55. Feldman MD, Alderman JD, Aroesty JM, et al. Depression of systolic and diastolic myocardial reserve during atrial pacing tachycardia in patients with dilated cardiomyopathy. *J Clin Invest* 1988;82:1661.

56. Lambertz H, Kreis A, Trumper H, et al. Simultaneous transesophageal atrial pacing and transesophageal two-dimensional echocardiography: a new method of stress echocardiography. *J Am Coll Cardiol* 1990;16:1143.

Measurement of Ventricular Volumes, Ejection Fraction, Mass, Wall Stress, and Regional Wall Motion

16

Michael A. Fifer   *William Grossman*

Cardiac angiography was introduced initially to provide qualitative information regarding anatomic abnormalities of the cardiovascular system. Subsequently, it became apparent that quantitative information derived from cineangiography could provide insight into *functional* abnormalities of the heart as well. Direct measurements of ventricular dimension, area, and wall thickness allow calculation of volume, ejection fraction, mass, and wall stress. Assessment of pressure-volume relationships provides additional information regarding systolic and diastolic function of the ventricular chambers. Finally, techniques developed to assess *regional* left ventricular wall motion have proved useful in the evaluation of patients with coronary artery disease. Therefore, the ventricular angiograms obtained by the techniques described in Chapter 12 can be used to derive quantitative descriptors of geometry and function.

VOLUMES

Technical Considerations

As discussed in detail in Chapter 12, ventriculograms are generally recorded on cine film or in digital format at 15 to 60 frames per second (fps), and radiographic contrast material is usually injected into the left ventricle at rates of 7 to 15 mL/second for a total volume of 30 to 50 mL. Alternatively, the left ventricle may be visualized from contrast injections into the pulmonary artery, the left atrium (by the trans-septal technique), or, in cases of severe aortic insufficiency, the aortic root. Attention to catheter position and injection rate minimizes the occurrence of ventricular ectopy during contrast studies; this is important because analysis of extrasystoles and postextrasystolic beats cannot be used for proper assessment of basal ventricular function.

With the widespread availability of computer systems, the technique of determining ventricular volumes has evolved from a handheld planimeter with pencil and paper (or a calculator) to semiautomated software packages. The principles important in accurate volume determination, however, apply equally to manual and computer-based techniques. For example, the need for magnification correction applies to both manual and automated techniques of volume determination.

In the first step in assessing left ventricular chamber volume, the left ventricular outline or silhouette is traced. The ventricular silhouette should be traced at the *outermost margin of visible radiographic contrast* so as to include trabeculations and papillary muscles within the perimeter

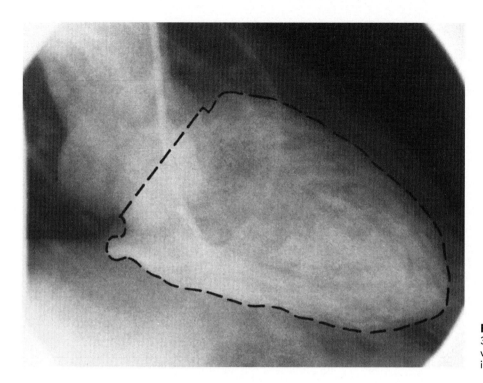

Figure 16.1 Left ventriculogram in the 30° right anterior oblique projection. The ventricular outline has been traced, as indicated by the *broken line*.

(Fig. 16.1). The aortic valve border is defined as a line connecting the inferior aspects of the sinuses of Valsalva. Some computer-based systems require that the entire ventricular silhouette be traced manually; others incorporate a semi-automated edge-detection algorithm, wherein some points on the ventricular silhouette are entered manually and others are supplied by the computer software.

To facilitate the calculation of left ventricular volume, the ventricle is usually approximated by an ellipsoid (1,2). Alternatively, techniques based on Simpson's rule, which is independent of assumptions regarding ventricular shape, may be used (3). Because the x-rays emanate from a point source, they are nonparallel; correction must therefore be made for magnification of the ventricular image onto the image intensifier. A further complicating factor is so-called pincushion distortion, which causes greater magnification at the periphery than in the center of the image, as a result of spherical aberration of the electromagnetic lens system (4). Finally, ventricular volumes calculated by most mathematical techniques overestimate true ventricular chamber volume, so that regression equations must be used to correct for the overestimation.

Biplane Formula

Biplane left ventriculography may be performed in the anteroposterior (AP) and lateral projections (2), the 30° right anterior oblique (RAO) and 60° left anterior oblique (LAO) projections (5), or angulated projections (e.g., 45° RAO and 60° LAO-25° cranial; 6). Although it is a complex geometric shape, the left ventricle can be approximated

with considerable accuracy by an ellipsoid (2; Fig. 16.2). The volume of an ellipsoid is given by the equation

$$V = \frac{4}{3} \pi \frac{L}{2} \frac{M}{2} \frac{N}{2} = \frac{\pi}{6} LMN \qquad (16.1)$$

where V is volume, L is the long axis, and M and N are the short axes of the ellipsoid. The long axis, L, is taken practically to be L_{max}, the longest chord that can be drawn within the ventricular silhouette in either projection. To determine M and N, each of the biplane projections of the left ventricle is approximated by an ellipse. M and N are taken to be the minor axes of these ellipses. They are calculated

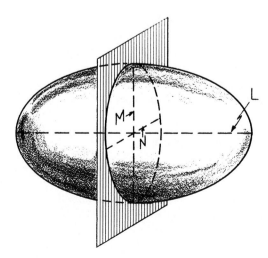

Figure 16.2 Ellipsoid used as a reference figure for the left ventricle. The long axis, *L*, and the short axes, *M* and *N*, are shown.

by the *area-length method*, as introduced by Dodge et al. (2) from the silhouette areas and long-axis lengths in each projection, using the standard geometric formula for the area of an ellipse as a function of its major and minor axes. For biplane oblique (RAO/LAO) left ventriculography, for example, the areas of the two ventricular silhouettes are given as

$$A_{RAO} = \pi \frac{L_{RAO}}{2} \frac{M}{2} \text{ and} \qquad (16.2)$$
$$A_{LAO} = \pi \frac{L_{LAO}}{2} \frac{N}{2}$$

L_{RAO} and L_{LAO} are the longest chords that can be drawn in the RAO and LAO silhouettes, respectively. The area of each traced silhouette (Fig. 16.1) is obtained by planimetry, and M and N are calculated by rearrangement as follows:

$$M = \frac{4A_{RAO}}{\pi L_{RAO}} \text{ and } N = \frac{4A_{LAO}}{\pi L_{LAO}} \qquad (16.3)$$

Combining Equations (16.1), (16.2), and (16.3),

$$V = \frac{\pi}{6} L_{max} \left(\frac{4A_{RAO}}{\pi L_{RAO}} \right) \left(\frac{4A_{LAO}}{\pi L_{LAO}} \right) \qquad (16.4)$$
$$= \frac{8}{3\pi} \frac{A_{RAO} A_{LAO}}{L_{min}}$$

where L_{min} is the shorter of L_{RAO} and L_{LAO}. Because L_{RAO} is almost always greater than L_{LAO}, L_{LAO} is usually substituted for L_{min}.

Equation (16.4) is derived for projections at right angles, or *orthogonal* projections, and is applicable to biplane oblique ventriculography in the 30° RAO and 60° LAO views, as just described, or for the older AP and lateral format. Although it is not valid theoretically for nonorthogonal projections (e.g., RAO and angulated LAO), it has been demonstrated empirically to be useful in those situations as well (6).

Right ventricular volumes have been calculated from biplane AP and lateral films using a modification of the Dodge area-length technique (7,8) or Simpson's rule (8–10). Because right ventricular volumes are rarely calculated from cineangiographic studies today, the reader is referred elsewhere for methodologic details (7–10).

Single-Plane Formula

The area-length ellipsoid method for estimating left ventricular chamber volume has been modified for use when only single-plane measurements obtained in the AP or RAO projection are available (4,11–13). Inherent in single-plane methods is the assumption that the left ventricular shape may be approximated by a prolate spheroid—that is, an ellipsoid in which the two minor axes are equal (12). It is assumed that the minor axis of the ventricle in the

projection used is equal to the minor axis in the orthogonal plane, which was not filmed. Recalling Eq. (16.1) for the general case of an ellipsoid:

$$V = \frac{\pi}{6} LMN \qquad (16.5)$$

If only single-plane (e.g., RAO) ventriculography is done, we assume that $M = N$ and that L in the plane presented is the true long axis of the ellipsoid. M is calculated from the single-plane silhouette area (A) and L by the area-length method as $M = 4A/\pi L$. Therefore, the single-plane volume calculation becomes

$$V = \frac{\pi}{6} LM^2 = \frac{\pi}{6} L \left(\frac{4A}{\pi L} \right)^2 = \frac{8A^2}{3\pi L} \qquad (16.6)$$

Magnification Correction: Single Plane

Correction accomplished by filming a calibrated grid at the estimated level of the ventricle (11) and submitting the grid to the same magnification process as the ventricle accounts for both linear magnification and pincushion distortion. Use of x-ray systems in which the center of the ventricle can be positioned at a fixed point (isocenter), around which the x-ray tubes and image intensifiers rotate, allows for magnification correction without the use of grids but does not correct for pincushion distortion.

The use of grids and other means of calculating magnification correction factors has been reassessed by Sheehan and Mitten-Lewis (14). They found that the error introduced by considering a large central square area of the grid rather than the portion encompassing a particular ventricular silhouette was negligibly small. Replacement of the grid by a circular disk did not significantly alter the calculated correction factor. Alternatively, the use of catheters with radiopaque markers separated by 1 cm also yielded accurate correction factors.

An approximation of the magnification correction may be obtained by considering the diameter of the catheter used for left ventriculography. However, there is a large potential percentage error in measurement of this small dimension, and the percentage error in volumes derived from it is roughly triple that in the linear correction factor. Furthermore, there is no correction for pincushion distortion. On the other hand, the error introduced into calculation of ejection fraction by this technique is much smaller than that in the calculation of ventricular volume; if it were not for the need for regression formulas (see later discussion), ejection fraction could be determined without regard to magnification.

In the single-plane formula, the cube of the linear correction factor adjusts the volume for magnification:

$$V = \frac{8}{3\pi} (CF)^3 \frac{A^2}{L} \qquad (16.7)$$

Magnification Correction: Biplane

In biplane studies, a correction factor (CF) must be calculated separately for each projection, yielding, in the case of biplane oblique cineangiography, CF_{RAO} and CF_{LAO}. The linear correction factor is multiplied by the measured lengths, and the square of this correction factor is multiplied by planimetered areas to convert to true lengths and areas. Accordingly, the corrected volume of the ventricle is

$$V = \frac{8}{3\pi} \frac{(CF_{RAO})^2 (CF_{LAO})^2}{CF_{LAO}} \frac{A_{RAO} A_{LAO}}{L_{LAO}}$$

$$= \frac{8 CF_{RAO}{}^2 CF_{LAO}}{3\pi} \frac{A_{RAO} A_{LAO}}{L_{LAO}} \qquad (16.8)$$

Regression Equations

Postmortem studies of hearts injected with contrast material have demonstrated that angiographic volumes calculated by Eq. (16.8) overestimate true left ventricular cavity volumes (2,4,5). This overestimation results in large part from the papillary muscles and trabeculae carneae, which do not contribute to blood volume but are nevertheless included within the traced left ventricular silhouette. Regression equations derived from these studies are used to adjust the calculated volumes. A list of the most commonly used regression equations is given in Table 16.1. For biplane studies in AP and lateral projections using large-film techniques, the regression equation of Dodge and Sandler (15) is used. For children (in whom this regression equation may yield a negative volume), another formula has been suggested (16). For cine studies in the 60° RAO/30° LAO projections, Wynne et al. (5) used postmortem casts, as shown in Fig. 16.3, to derive the regression equation shown in Table 16.1.

Single-plane techniques tend to overestimate volume significantly, compared with biplane methods, and this is reflected in the single-plane regression equations (Table 16.1). Regression equations are incorporated into commercial catheterization laboratory packages.

EJECTION FRACTION AND REGURGITANT FRACTION

Visual inspection of the cine film allows selection of frames depicting maximum (end-diastolic) and minimum (end-systolic) ventricular volumes. The ejection fraction (*EF*) is then calculated as follows (17,18):

$$EF = (EDV - ESV)/EDV = SV/EDV \qquad (16.9)$$

where *EDV* is end-diastolic ventricular volume, *ESV* is end-systolic ventricular volume, and *SV* is the angiographic stroke volume.

In patients with aortic and/or mitral regurgitation, comparison of the angiographically determined stroke volume with the forward stroke volume determined by the Fick technique or (in the absence of concomitant tricuspid regurgitation) the thermodilution technique yields the regurgitant stroke volume, that portion of the ejected volume that is regurgitated and therefore does not contribute to the net cardiac output (15). The regurgitant fraction (*RF*) is defined as follows (17–19):

$$RF = \frac{SV_{angiograhic} - SV_{forward}}{SV_{angiographic}} \qquad (16.10)$$

An assumption of this calculation is constancy of heart rate between the determination of forward cardiac output and the performance of left ventriculography. If the heart rate (*HR*) is substantially different at these two times, a modified method for calculating *RF* must be used, wherein the angiographic minute output ($SV_{angiographic} \times HR$) is substituted for angiographic stroke volume and the forward minute output or cardiac output is substituted for the forward stroke volume. This calculation is based on the assumption that cardiac output is independent of heart rate to a first approximation.

Because the derivation of *RF* involves the difference between the two stroke volume measurements, both of which contain some degree of error, the error in *RF* itself may be significant; interpretation of this number should be influenced by qualitative assessment of the degree of

TABLE 16.1

REGRESSION EQUATIONS TO CORRECT FOR OVERESTIMATION IN CALCULATION OF LEFT VENTRICULAR VOLUMES

Investigator	Angiographic Method	Age Group	Regression Equation
Wynne et al. (5)	Biplane cine RAO and LAO	Adults	$V_A = 0.989V_C - 8.1$
	Single-plane cine RAO	Adults	$V_A = 0.938V_C - 5.7$
Kennedy et al. (13)	Single-plane cine RAO	Adults	$V_A = 0.81V_C + 1.9$
Dodge et al. (2,15)	Biplane serial AP and lateral	Adults	$V_A = 0.928V_C - 3.8$
Graham et al. (16)	Biplane cine AP and lateral	Children	$V_A = 0.733V_C$
Sandler and Dodge (12)	Single-plane serial AP	Adults	$V_A = 0.951V_C - 3.0$

AP, anteroposterior; LAO, left anterior oblique; RAO, right anterior oblique; V_A, actual volume; V_C, calculated volume.

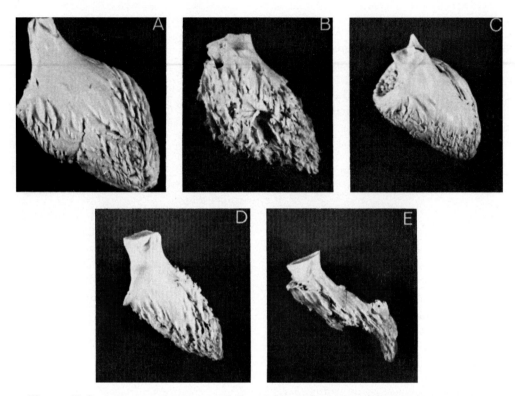

Figure 16.3 Left ventricular casts made from fresh postmortem specimens of human hearts, using an encapsulant mixed with barium sulfate powder. The shape of the left ventricle only roughly approximates an ellipsoid of revolution; nevertheless, amazingly good correlation was obtained between true volume of these casts (measured by water displacement of the actual cast) and calculated volume. (From Wynne J, Green LH, Grossman W, et al. Estimation of left ventricular volumes in man from biplane cineangiograms filmed in oblique projections. *Am J Cardiol* 1978;41:726, with permission.)

regurgitation seen on the angiogram. In cases of combined aortic and mitral regurgitation, estimation of the relative contribution of the two lesions must be made from the cineangiograms.

OTHER TECHNIQUES FOR MEASURING VENTRICULAR VOLUME AND EJECTION FRACTION

Image enhancement by computerized digital subtraction techniques can be used to obtain left ventriculograms after peripheral intravenous administration of contrast material (20,21). Peripheral injection of the contrast agent eliminates the problem of ventricular extrasystoles sometimes associated with direct injection of contrast material into the ventricular chamber. Alternatively, the image enhancement provided by the digital subtraction process permits direct left ventricular injections with small volumes of contrast agents (20), possibly allowing multiple ventriculograms under varying conditions during a single catheterization procedure. Ventricular volume and ejection fraction may be calculated from digital subtraction ventriculograms using the area-length method (20), as described for standard ventriculograms. Alternatively, ejection fraction may be determined by computer analysis of the attenuation of x-rays by the contrast agent within the ventricle (21,22). This technique is independent of geometric assumptions regarding the shape of the ventricle.

A multielectrode catheter capable of measuring intracavitary electrical impedance has been introduced (23–25) and has proved useful for the measurement of ventricular volume and ejection fraction without the use of contrast agents. An early version of the catheter, consisting of 12 platinum ring electrodes mounted at 1-cm intervals along the distal end of an 8F or 9F end-hole catheter, is shown in Fig. 16.4. A 4-mA current flows through the blood of the ventricular chamber between selected ring electrodes, and the voltage needed to drive this current reflects the instantaneous electrical impedance of the blood, which has been shown to be a direct function of the blood volume. Newer catheters, only 6F in diameter, combine impedance, volume, and micromanometer pressure measurements. Validation studies (23,24) indicate that both left and right ventricular volumes can be measured by this technique. An illustration of the potential usefulness of this catheter in assessing left ventricular pressure-volume relationships is shown in Fig. 16.5.

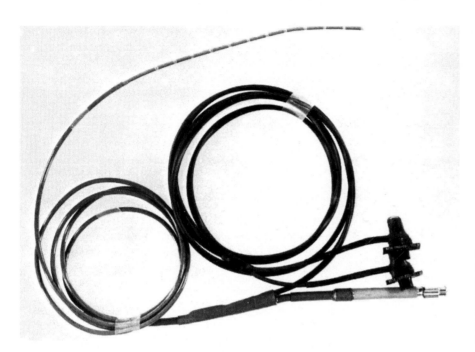

Figure 16.4 Multielectrode impedance catheter for measurement of instantaneous chamber blood volume (see text for description). (From McKay RG, et al. Instantaneous measurement of left and right ventricular stroke volume and pressure-volume relationships with an impedance catheter. *Circulation* 1984;69:703.)

LEFT VENTRICULAR MASS

Measurement of left ventricular wall thickness, in addition to the parameters measured for volume determination, allows calculation of left ventricular wall volume and estimation of left ventricular mass (LVM). For these calculations, it is assumed that wall thickness is uniform throughout the ventricle. Wall thickness (h) is measured at end-diastole at the left ventricular free wall roughly two

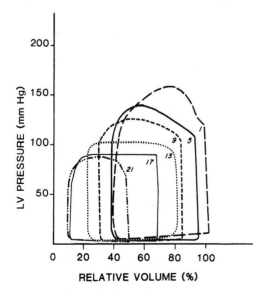

Figure 16.5 Use of multielectrode impedance catheter, shown in Fig. 16.4, to obtain left ventricular pressure-volume loops every fourth beat during inhalation of amyl nitrate. (From McKay RG, et al. Instantaneous measurement of left and right ventricular stroke volume and pressure-volume relationships with an impedance catheter. *Circulation* 1984;69:703, with permission.)

thirds of the distance from the aortic valve to the apex in the AP (26) or RAO (13) projection. Appropriate magnification correction is applied. For biplane methods, the total volume of left ventricular chamber and wall, V_{c+w}, is approximated by that of the corresponding ellipsoid:

$$V_{c+w} = \frac{4}{3}\,\pi\left(\frac{L+2h}{2}\right)\left(\frac{M+2h}{2}\right)\left(\frac{N+2h}{2}\right)$$

$$= \frac{\pi}{6}\,(L+2h)\left(\frac{4A_{\text{RAO}}}{\pi L_{\text{RAO}}}+2h\right) \quad (16.11)$$

$$\cdot\left(\frac{4A_{\text{LAO}}}{\pi L_{\text{LAO}}}+2h\right)$$

As with h, appropriate correction for magnification must be applied to A and L so that V_{c+w} represents the total volume of the left ventricular chamber and wall corrected for magnification. For single-plane methods, it is assumed that $M = N$, yielding the single-plane formula:

$$V_{c+w} = \frac{\pi}{6}\,(L+2h)\left(\frac{4A}{\pi L}+2h\right)^2 \quad (16.12)$$

The volume of the chamber is calculated by the biplane or single-plane technique. To exclude the volume of the papillary muscles and trabeculae from the chamber volume (and thus include their mass in *LVM*), the appropriate regression equation is applied, so that V_c is the regressed value for chamber volume. *LVM*, then, is calculated as follows:

$$\begin{aligned}LVM &= 1.050\,V_w\\ &= 1.050(V_{c+w}-V_c)\end{aligned} \quad (16.13)$$

where V_w is wall volume, and 1.050 is the specific gravity of heart muscle. This method has been validated by postmortem examination of hearts (26,27); however, it may not be accurate in the presence of marked right ventricular hypertrophy or pericardial effusion or thickening, where accurate measurement of wall thickness from the RAO silhouette may be impossible. The left ventricular wall thickness may sometimes be seen well in the LAO projection in the region of the posterior wall, or it may be measured accurately by echocardiography, computed tomography, or magnetic resonance imaging. Values obtained by any of these methods may be used for calculation of *LVM*.

NORMAL VALUES

A number of investigators have reported normal values in adults and children for left ventricular volume, ejection fraction, wall thickness, and mass (5,16,28–30). These are summarized in Table 16.2.

WALL STRESS

Whereas consideration of ventricular pressure and volume is useful for assessment of *ventricular* performance, direct evaluation of *myocardial* function requires attention to forces acting at the level of the individual myocardial fiber. In particular, correction must be made for differences in ventricular wall thickness and chamber radius (R), which modify the extent to which intraventricular pressure (P) is borne by the individual fiber; this is especially important in disease states characterized by ventricular hypertrophy or dilation or both. Such a correction may be achieved by consideration of wall stress (σ) (29,31–33). Several formulas are commonly used to calculate stress, all related to the basic Laplace relation:

$$\sigma = \frac{PR}{2h} \qquad (16.14)$$

Assumptions of the shape of the ventricular chamber and the properties of the ventricular wall have led to a number of such formulas for wall stress components in the circumferential, meridional, and radial directions (Fig. 16.6). Consideration of circumferential and meridional stress has been particularly useful for clinical applications. A representative formula for calculation of circumferential stress, σ_c is

$$\sigma_c = \frac{Pb}{h}\left(1 - \frac{h}{2b}\right)\left(1 - \frac{hb}{2a^2}\right) \qquad (16.15)$$

where a and b are the major and minor semiaxes, respectively, at the midwall. Meridional stress, σ_m, may be calculated as follows (32):

$$\sigma_m = \frac{PR}{2h(1 + h/2R)} \qquad (16.16)$$

where R is the internal chamber radius as bounded by the endocardial surface. For more detailed consideration of

TABLE 16.2

NORMAL AVERAGE VALUES FOR LEFT VENTRICULAR PARAMETERS BY ANGIOCARDIOGRAPHY (MEAN ± SD)

Investigator	Angiographic Method	Number of Patients	Age Group	End-Diastolic Volume (mL/m²)	End-Systolic Volume (mL/m²)	Ejection Fraction	Wall Thickness (mm)	Mass (g)
Wynne et al. (5)	Biplane cine RAO-LAO	17	Adults	72 ± 15	20 ± 8	0.72 ± 0.08	—	—
Kennedy et al. (27)	Biplane serial AP and Lat	16	Adults	70 ± 20	24 ± 10	0.67 ± 0.08	10.9 ± 2.0	167 ± 42
Hood (29)	Biplane serial AP and Lat	6	Adults	79 ± 11	28 ± 6	0.67 ± 0.07	8.5 ± 1.3	164 ± 35
Hermann and Bartle (30)	Biplane serial AP and Lat	6	Adults	71 ± 20	30 ± 10	0.58 ± 0.05	—	—
Graham et al. (16)	Biplane cine AP and Lat	19	Children younger than 2 yr	42 ± 10	—	0.68 ± 0.05	—	96 ± 11[a]
Graham et al. (16)	Biplane cine AP and Lat	37	Children older than 2 yr	73 ± 11	—	0.63 ± 0.05	—	86 ± 11[a]

[a]g/m².
AP, anteroposterior; LAO, left anterior oblique; RAO, right anterior oblique.

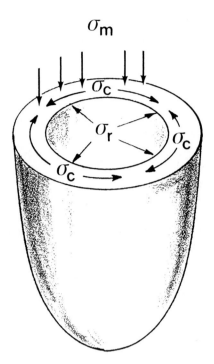

Figure 16.6 Circumferential (σ_c), meridional (σ_m), and radial (σ_r) components of left ventricular wall stress for an ellipsoid model. The three components of wall stress are mutually perpendicular.

wall stress formulas, the reader is referred to reviews of the subject (33).

Calculation of wall stress in disease states has provided information not apparent from consideration of pressure and volume data alone. For example, it has been demonstrated that peak stress does not necessarily occur at the same time in the cardiac cycle as does peak pressure and that, in compensated pressure overload, the increase in ventricular pressure is offset by a proportional increase in wall thickness, so that wall stress remains normal (Fig. 16.7; 32).

PRESSURE-VOLUME CURVES

Simultaneous measurement of ventricular pressure and volume allows construction of the pressure-volume diagram (Fig. 16.8; 34–37). The position and slope of the diastolic portion of the pressure-volume curve provide information regarding diastolic properties of the ventricle (35,38). Construction of the systolic portion of the curve is useful for analysis of the end-systolic pressure-volume relation, a measure of ventricular contractile function (see Chapter 17).

REGIONAL LEFT VENTRICULAR WALL MOTION

The recognition that left ventricular regional dys-synergy is a more sensitive marker of coronary artery disease than is depression of global function has led to attempts to quantify abnormalities of regional wall motion. Left ventriculography is performed in the RAO or RAO and LAO projections. The ventricle is divided into regions by one of two methods: (a) construction of lines perpendicular to the major axis that divide the major axis into equal segments (39,40) or (b) construction of lines drawn from the midpoint of the major axis to the ventricular outline at intervals of a fixed number of

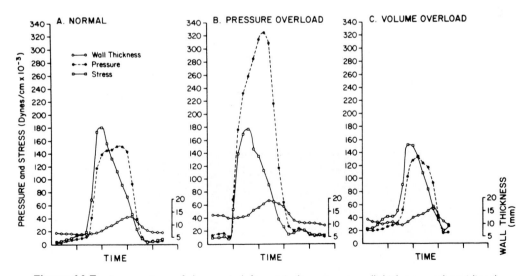

Figure 16.7 A comparison of changes in left ventricular pressure, wall thickness, and meridional stress throughout the cardiac cycle for representative normal **(A)**, pressure-overloaded **(B)**, and volume-overloaded **(C)** ventricles. These parameters are plotted at 40-msec intervals. In all three types of ventricles, peak stress occurs earlier than peak pressure. In the pressure-overloaded ventricle, peak pressure is markedly elevated, but peak systolic stress and end-diastolic stress are normal. In the volume-overloaded ventricle, peak systolic stress is normal, but end-diastolic stress is elevated. (From Grossman W, Jones D, McLaurin LP. Wall stress and patterns of hypertrophy in the human left ventricle. *J Clin Invest* 1975;56:56, with permission.)

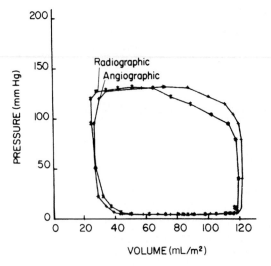

Figure 16.8 Pressure-volume diagram for the left ventricle. In this example, the diagram derived from single-plane cineangiography is compared with that constructed from radionuclide volume data. (From McKay RG, et al. Left ventricular pressure-volume diagrams and end-systolic pressure-volume relations in human beings. *J Am Coll Cardiol* 1984;3:301, with permission.)

degrees (39). Extent of inward (or outward) movement of individual segments can then be measured, usually with the aid of computer techniques, providing quantitative measures of hypokinesis, akinesis, and dyskinesis.

An automated method of processing the left ventricular cineangiogram was reported by Sasayama et al. (41–43). End-diastolic and end-systolic ventricular silhouettes are superimposed (Fig. 16.9), and 128 radial grids are drawn from the center of gravity of the end-diastolic silhouette to the endocardial margins. Measurement of the length of each radial grid between end-diastolic and end-systolic silhouettes measures segmental systolic and diastolic function. Figure 16.9 illustrates this technique in a patient with coronary disease before and after induction of angina pectoris by rapid atrial pacing. Simultaneous measurements of left ventricular pressure permit construction of segmental left ventricular pressure-length loops for both normally perfused myocardial regions (Fig. 16.9, c and d), and regions perfused by stenotic coronary arteries (Fig. 16.9, a and b). Depressed wall motion develops during angina in the latter, and compensatory hyperkinesis develops in the former.

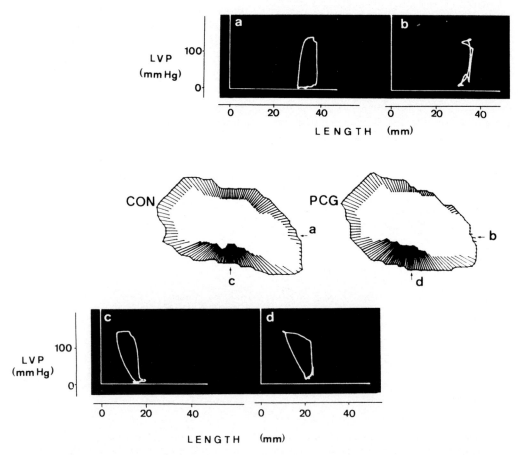

Figure 16.9 Assessment of regional wall motion in the control state (CON) and after induction of angina pectoris by atrial pacing tachycardia (PCG). Left ventricular pressure (LVP)–length loops are plotted for a myocardial region distal to a stenotic coronary artery **(a and b)** and for a normally perfused region **(c and d)**. (From Sasayama S, et al. Changes in diastolic properties of the regional myocardium during pacing-induced ischemia in man. *J Am Coll Cardiol* 1985;5:599, with permission.)

Another approach has been used by Sheehan et al. (44,45). Wall motion is measured along 100 chords constructed as perpendiculars to a line drawn midway between the end-diastolic and end-systolic left ventricular contours (Fig. 16.10). The motion of each chord is compared with a normal range established from analysis of ventriculograms from patients without heart disease. Deviations from the normal range indicate hypokinesis or hyperkinesis. In studies of wall motion after thrombolysis, availability of the LAO in addition to the RAO projection proved particularly useful in patients with left circumflex coronary artery thrombosis (45).

Software for regional wall motion analysis is now available in commercial catheterization laboratory computer systems.

REFERENCES

1. Arvidsson H. Angiocardiographic observations in mitral disease with special reference to volume variations in the left atrium. *Acta Radiol* 1958;49(suppl 158):1–124.
2. Dodge HT, Sandler H, Ballew DW, et al. The use of biplane angiocardiography for the measurement of left ventricular volume in man. *Am Heart J* 1960;60:762.
3. Chapman CB, Baker O, Reynolds J, et al. Use of biplane cinefluorography for measurement of ventricular volume. *Circulation* 1958;18:1105.
4. Greene DG, Carlisle R, Grant C, et al. Estimation of left ventricular volume by one-plane cineangiography. *Circulation* 1967;35:61.
5. Wynne J, Green LH, Grossman W, et al. Estimation of left ventricular volumes in man from biplane cineangiograms filmed in oblique projections. *Am J Cardiol* 1978;41:726.
6. Rogers WJ, et al. Quantitative axial oblique contrast left ventriculography: validation of the method by demonstrating improved visualization of regional wall motion and mitral valve function with accurate volume determinations. *Am Heart J* 1982;103:185.
7. Arcilla RA, Tsai P, Thilenius O, et al. Angiographic method for volume estimation of right and left ventricles. *Chest* 1971;60:446.
8. Graham TP Jr, Jarmakani JM, Atwood GF, et al. Right ventricular volume determinations in children: normal values and observations with volume or pressure overload. *Circulation* 1973;47:144.
9. Goerke RJ, Carlsson E. Calculation of right and left cardiac ventricular volumes: method using standard computer equipment and biplane angiocardiograms. *Invest Radiol* 1967;2:360.
10. Gentzler RD, Briselli MF, Gault JH. Angiographic estimation of right ventricular volume in man. *Circulation* 1974;50:324.
11. Kasser IS, Kennedy JW. Measurement of left ventricular volumes in man by single-plane cineangiocardiography. *Invest Radiol* 1969;4:83.
12. Sandler H, Dodge HT. The use of single plane angiocardiograms for the calculation of left ventricular volume in man. *Am Heart J* 1968;75:325.
13. Kennedy JW, Trenholme SE, Kasser IS. Left ventricular volume and mass from single-plane cineangiocardiogram: a comparison of anteroposterior and right anterior oblique methods. *Am Heart J* 1970;80:343.
14. Sheehan FH, Mitten-Lewis S. Factors influencing accuracy in left ventricular volume determination. *Am J Cardiol* 1989;64:661.
15. Sandler H, Dodge HT, Hay RE, et al. Quantitation of valvular insufficiency in man by angiocardiography. *Am Heart J* 1963;65:501.
16. Graham TP Jr, Jarmakani JM, Canent RV Jr, et al. Left heart volume estimation in infancy and childhood: reevaluation of methodology and normal values. *Circulation* 1971;43:895.
17. Arvidsson H, Karnell J. Quantitative assessment of mitral and aortic insufficiency by angiocardiography. *Acta Radiol* 1964;2:105.
18. Miller GAH, Brown R, Swan HJC. Isolated congenital mitral insufficiency with particular reference to left heart volumes. *Circulation* 1964;29:356.
19. Jones JW, et al. Left ventricular volumes in valvular heart disease. *Circulation* 1964;29:887.
20. Sasayama S, et al. Automated method for left ventricular volume measurement by cineventriculography with minimal doses of contrast medium. *Am J Cardiol* 1981;48:746.
21. Nissen SE, Elion JL, Grayburn P, et al. Determination of left ventricular ejection fraction by computer densitometric analysis of digital subtraction angiography: experimental validation and correlation with area-length methods. *Am J Cardiol* 1987;59:675.
22. Tobis J, et al. Measurement of left ventricular ejection fraction by videodensitometric analysis of digital subtraction angiograms. *Am J Cardiol* 1983;52:871.

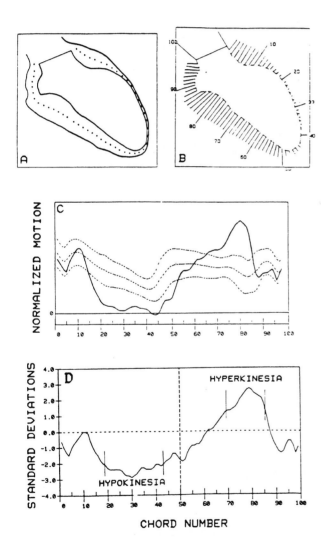

Figure 16.10 Wall motion as assessed by the center line method. The center line (**A,** *dotted line*) is constructed midway between the end-systolic and end-diastolic silhouettes. **B.** Chords are drawn at right angles to the center line. **C.** The percentage of systolic shortening along each chord is plotted and compared with normal mean and standard deviation values (*dashed and dotted lines*). **D.** Deviation from normal is replotted. (From Sheehan FH, Bolson EL, Dodge HT, et al. Advantages and applications of the center line method for characterizing regional ventricular function. *Circulation* 1986;74:293, with permission.)

23. McKay RG, Spears JR, Aroesty JM, et al. Instantaneous measurement of left and right ventricular stroke volume and pressure-volume relationships with an impedance catheter. *Circulation* 1984;69:703.

24. Kass DA, Midei M, Graves W, et al. Use of a conductance (volume) catheter and transient inferior vena caval occlusion for rapid determination of pressure-volume relationships in man. *Cathet Cardiovasc Diagn* 1988;15:192.

25. Odake M, Takeuchi M, Takaoka H, et al. Determination of left ventricular volume using a conductance catheter in the diseased human heart. *Eur Heart J* 1992;13(suppl E):57.

26. Rackley CE, Dodge HT, Coble YD Jr, et al. A method for determining left ventricular mass in man. *Circulation* 1964;29:666.

27. Kennedy JW, Reichenbach DD, Baxley WA, et al. Left ventricular mass: a comparison of angiocardiographic measurements with autopsy weight. *Am J Cardiol* 1967;19:221.

28. Kennedy JW, et al. Quantitative angiocardiography, I: the normal left ventricle in man. *Circulation* 1966;34:272.

29. Hood WP Jr. Wall stress in the normal and hypertrophied human left ventricle. *Am J Cardiol* 1968;22:550.

30. Hermann HJ, Bartle SH. Left ventricular volumes by angiocardiography: comparison of methods and simplification of techniques. *Cardiovasc Res* 1968;4:404.

31. Sandler H, Dodge HT. Left ventricular tension and stress in man. *Circ Res* 1963;13:91.

32. Grossman W, Jones D, McLaurin LP. Wall stress and patterns of hypertrophy in the human left ventricle. *J Clin Invest* 1974;56:56.

33. Yin FCP. Ventricular wall stress. *Circ Res* 1981;49:829.

34. Arvidsson H. Angiocardiographic determination of left ventricular volume. *Acta Radiol* 1961;56:321.

35. Dodge HT, Hay RE, Sandler H. Pressure-volume characteristics of diastolic left ventricle of man with heart disease. *Am Heart J* 1962;64:503.

36. Bunnell IL, Grant C, Greene DG. Left ventricular function derived from the pressure-volume diagram. *Am J Med* 1965;39:881.

37. McKay RG, Aroesty JM, Heller GV, et al. Left ventricular pressure-volume diagrams and end-systolic pressure-volume relations in human beings. *J Am Coll Cardiol* 1984;3:301.

38. Grossman W. Relaxation and diastolic distensibility of the regionally ischemic left ventricle. In: Grossman W, Lorell BH, eds. *Diastolic Relaxation of the Heart.* Boston: Martinus Nijhoff, 1988:193.

39. Herman MV, Heinle RA, Klein MD, et al. Localized disorders in myocardial contraction: asynergy and its role in congestive heart failure. *N Engl J Med* 1967;277:222.

40. Sniderman AD, Marpole D, Fallen EL. Regional contraction patterns in the normal and ischemic left ventricle in man. *Am J Cardiol* 1973;31:484.

41. Sasayama, S, Nonogi H, Kawm C. Assessment of left ventricular function using an angiographic method. *Jpn Circ J* 1982;46:1177.

42. Fujita M, et al. Automatic processing of cine ventriculograms for analysis of regional myocardial function. *Circulation* 1981;63:1065.

43. Sasayama S, et al. Changes in diastolic properties of the regional myocardium during pacing-induced ischemia in human subjects. *J Am Coll Cardiol* 1985;5:599.

44. Sheehan FH, Bolson EL, Dodge HT, et al. Advantages and applications of the centerline method for characterizing regional ventricular function. *Circulation* 1986;74:293.

45. Sheehan FH, Schofer J, Mathey DG, et al. Measurement of regional wall motion from biplane contrast ventriculograms: a comparison of the 30 degree right anterior oblique and 60 degree left anterior oblique projections in patients with acute myocardial infarction. *Circulation* 1986;74:796.

Evaluation of Systolic and Diastolic Function of the Ventricles and Myocardium

17

William Grossman

A critical aspect of most cardiac catheterization procedures is the evaluation of myocardial function. At its simplest, this consists of a visual assessment of the left ventricular (LV) contractile pattern from the left ventriculogram, together with measurements of LV end-diastolic pressure. In laboratories where most patients have right-sided heart catheterization and cardiac output measurement as part of a standard cardiac catheterization procedure, additional information about LV function may be gleaned from the cardiac output, stroke volume, and pulmonary capillary wedge pressure, whereas right ventricular (RV) function is reflected in the values for right ventricular end-diastolic pressure (RVEDP) and right atrial pressure. Measurements of pressures and cardiac output give important information about overall cardiac function, but may shed little light on whether dysfunction is caused by abnormal systolic or diastolic myocardial performance. This chapter describes some of the specific methods that can be used in the cardiac catheterization laboratory to examine myocardial performance in systole and diastole.

SYSTOLIC FUNCTION

Preload, Afterload, and Contractility

Systolic function of the myocardium is a reflection of the interaction of myocardial preload, afterload, and contractility. *Preload* is the load that stretches myofibrils during diastole and determines the end-diastolic sarcomere length.

For the left ventricle, this load is often quantified as the LV end-diastolic pressure (LVEDP). This pressure, taken together with LV wall thickness (h) and radius (R), determines LV end-diastolic *wall stress* ($\sigma \approx PR/h$), which is an estimate of the force stretching the myocardial fibers at end-diastole. The end-diastolic stress or stretching force is resisted by the intrinsic stiffness or elasticity of the myocardium, and the interaction of end-diastolic stretching force and myocardial stiffness determines the extent of end-diastolic sarcomere stretch. If the myocardium is diffusely fibrotic or infiltrated with amyloid, a very high end-diastolic stretching force may be required to produce even a normal end-diastolic sarcomere length. In such a case, LVEDP may be very high (e.g., >25 mm Hg), and attempts to lower it by diuretic or venodilator therapy may lead to reduction in end-diastolic sarcomere stretch to subnormal values and a concomitant fall in cardiac output.

Changes in preload influence both the extent and velocity of myocardial shortening in experiments using isolated cardiac muscle preparations. Increased preload augments the extent and velocity of myocardial shortening at any given afterload. In the intact heart, the relationship is more complex because increases in preload generally produce increases in LV chamber size and LV systolic pressure. Therefore, *afterload* (the force resisting systolic shortening of the myofibrils) is also increased, and this increase tends to blunt the increases in extent and velocity of myocardial shortening caused by increased diastolic fiber stretch. This point is discussed in more detail later in this chapter, under the section on ejection phase indices of systolic function.

Afterload varies throughout systole as the ventricular systolic pressure rises and blood is ejected from the ventricular chamber. LV systolic stress approximates the force resisting myocardial fiber shortening within the wall of the ventricle. The theory and methods for calculation of wall stress are described in Chapter 16. End-systolic wall stress is considered by many to be the final afterload that determines the extent of myocardial fiber shortening when preload and contractility are constant. An increase in end-systolic wall stress results in a decrease in myocardial fiber shortening. For the intact ventricle, an increase in afterload (end-systolic wall stress) therefore results in a fall in stroke volume and ejection fraction.

Contractility refers to the property of heart muscle that accounts for alterations in performance induced by biochemical and hormonal changes; it has classically been regarded as independent of preload and afterload. Contractility is generally used as a synonym for *inotropy*: both terms refer to the level of activation of cross-bridge cycling during systole. Contractility changes are assessed in the experimental laboratory by measuring myocardial function (extent or speed of shortening, maximum force generation) while preload and afterload are held constant. In contrast to skeletal muscle, the strength of contraction of heart muscle can be increased readily by a variety of biochemical and hormonal stimuli, some of which are listed in Table 17.1.

Increased myocardial contractility may be present in patients with hyperadrenergic states, thyrotoxicosis, or hypertrophic cardiomyopathy or in response to various drugs. It is manifested by an increase in the speed and extent of myocardial contraction at constant afterload and preload.

Experiments with isolated myocardial tissue have demonstrated that contractility is not truly independent of preload. Increased end-diastolic sarcomere stretch leads to an immediate increase in the strength of contraction owing to the Frank-Starling mechanism, followed by a gradual further increase in contractile strength over 5 to 10 minutes (1–3). Evidence supports a role for both increased intracellular calcium (Ca^{++}) release and increased myofilament sensitivity to any given level of cytosolic Ca^{++} as underlying factors in the length-dependent activation seen with increased preload (2).

Assessment of systolic function requires consideration of the simultaneous influence of afterload, preload, and contractility. Systolic function should *not* be regarded as synonymous with contractility. Major depression of systolic function can occur with normal contractility, as in conditions with so-called afterload excess (see later discussion).

Isovolumic Indices

One of the oldest and most widely used measures of myocardial contractility is the maximum rate of rise of LV systolic pressure, dP/dt. Wiggers noted more than 70 years ago that in animal experiments, the failing ventricle showed a reduced steepness of the upslope of the ventricular pressure pulse (4). In 1962, Gleason and Braunwald first reported measurement of dP/dt in humans (5). They studied 40 patients with micromanometer catheters. Maximum dP/dt in those patients without hemodynamic abnormalities

TABLE 17.1

HORMONES AND DRUGS THAT INFLUENCE MYOCARDIAL CONTRACTILITY

Agent	Presumed Mechanism	Influence on Contractility
Catecholamines with β-agonist activity	β-receptor stimulation → ↑ adenylate cyclase activity → ↑ cyclic AMP → ↑ Ca^{++} influx through sarcolemma → ↑ cytosolic Ca^{++}	+
Digitalis glycosides	Inhibition of Na^+-K^+ ATPase → ↑ intracellular Na^+ → ↑ Na^+/Ca^{++} exchange → ↑ cytosolic Ca^{++}	+
Calcium salts	↑ Extracellular Ca^{++} → ↑ Ca^{++} influx via slow channels and Na^+/Ca^{++} exchange → ↑ cytosolic Ca^{++}	+
Caffeine	Multiple actions: Local release of catecholamines Inhibition of sarcoplasmic reticular Ca^{++} uptake Inhibition of phosphodiesterase → ↑ cyclic AMP ↑ Sensitivity of contractile proteins of Ca^{++}	+
Milrinone, amrinone, other bipyridines	Phosphodiesterase inhibition → ↑ cyclic AMP → ↑ cytosolic Ca^{++}	+
Thyroid hormone	Increases myosin ATPase activity by altering production of certain myosin isozymes	+
Calcium-blocking agents (verapamil, nifedipine, D600, diltiazem)	Block Ca^{++} entry via slow channels	−
Barbiturates, ethanol	Depress contractility by unknown mechanism	−

AMP, adenosine monophosphate; ATPase, adenosine triphosphatase.

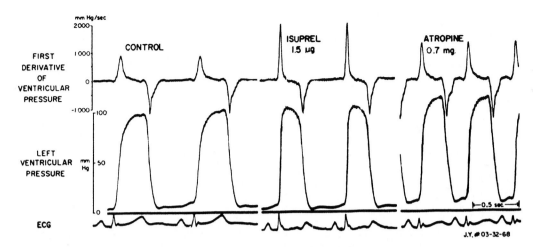

Figure 17.1 Micromanometer recordings of left ventricular pressure and its first derivative, d*P*/d*t*, in a patient with normal left ventricular function. Isoproterenol markedly increases contractility with large increments in positive d*P*/d*t*. Atropine produces tachycardia, which results in a treppe effect and a rise in +d*P*/d*t* above control. (From Gleason WL, Braunwald E. Studies on the first derivative of the ventricular pressure pulse in man. *J Clin Invest* 1962;41:80, with permission.)

ranged from 841 to 1,696 mm Hg/second in the left ventricle and 223 to 296 mm Hg/second in the right ventricle. Interventions known to increase myocardial contractility, such as exercise and infusion of norepinephrine or isoproterenol, caused major increases in d*P*/d*t*. Increased heart rate produced by intravenous atropine also caused a rise in maximum d*P*/d*t*, and the authors attributed this to the *treppe phenomenon* described by Bowditch. Acute increases in arterial pressure and afterload produced by infusion of the α-adrenergic vasoconstricting agent methoxamine produced little change in d*P*/d*t*. These points are illustrated in Figs. 17.1 and 17.2.

In normal subjects and in patients with no significant cardiac abnormality, maximum d*P*/d*t* increases significantly in response to isometric exercise (6), dynamic exercise (5), tachycardia by atrial pacing (7,8) or atropine (5), β-agonists (5), and digitalis glycosides (9). Relatively few studies have been done in humans to assess the changes in d*P*/d*t* induced by alterations in afterload and preload, but some studies do indicate that maximum positive d*P*/d*t* tends to increase slightly (6 to 8%) with moderate increases in LV preload (10) and shows little change with methoxamine-induced increases (5) or nitroprusside-induced decreases (11) in mean arterial pressure of 25 to 30 mm Hg. Extensive studies in animals have examined the influence of changes in afterload, preload, and contractility on maximum d*P*/d*t* (10,12–15). These studies generally show that maximum d*P*/d*t* rises with increases in afterload and preload,

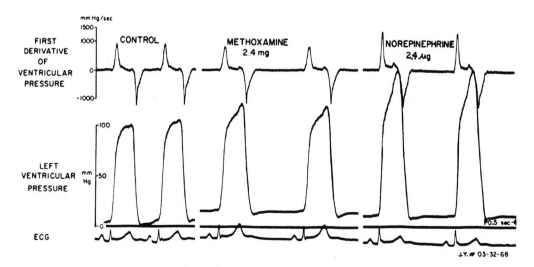

Figure 17.2 Micromanometer recordings of left ventricular (LV) pressure and d*P*/d*t*, as in Fig. 17.1. Methoxamine raises arterial and LV systolic pressure but does not increase +d*P*/d*t*. In contrast, the combined α- and β-adrenergic effects of norepinephrine increase LV systolic pressure and +d*P*/d*t*. (From Gleason WL, Braunwald E. Studies on the first derivative of the ventricular pressure pulse in man. *J Clin Invest* 1962;41:80, with permission.)

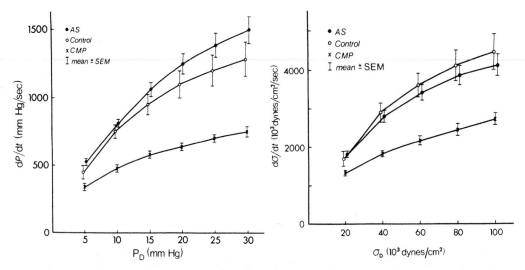

Figure 17.3 Left ventricular (LV) isovolumic indices of contractility. **A.** Rate of pressure development (dP/dt) as a function of LV-developed pressure (P_D). Mean values in control subjects (*open circles*), patients with aortic stenosis (AS, *closed circles*), and patients with dilated cardiomyopathy (CMP, *crosses*) are shown. Brackets represent standard errors of the mean (SEM). **B.** Rate of wall stress development ($d\sigma/dt$) as a function of LV-developed stress (σ_D) for the same groups. There are no significant differences for patients with AS compared with controls, although patients with CMP clearly show depressed values for dP/dt and $d\sigma/dt$ at all levels of P_D and σ_D. (From Fifer MA, Gunther S, Grossman W, et al. Myocardial contractile function in aortic stenosis as determined from the rate of stress development during isovolumic systole. *Am J Cardiol* 1979;44:1318, with permission.)

but the changes were quite small (<10%) in the physiologic range.

As discussed in Chapter 7, accurate measurement of dP/dt requires a pressure measurement system with excellent frequency-response characteristics. Micromanometer catheters are usually required to achieve this frequency-response range (16). Differentiation of the ventricular pressure signal can be achieved by (a) analog techniques online (Figs. 17.1 and 17.2), using a resistance capacitor (RC) differentiating circuit (5,10); (b) computer digitization of the analog LV pressure tracing and subsequent differentiation of a polynomial best fit to the averaged LV isovolumic pressure (17); or (c) computer digitization of the analog LV pressure tracing with subsequent Fourier analysis and differentiation (18).

In addition to dP/dt, several other isovolumic indices have been introduced in an attempt to obtain a "pure" contractility index, completely independent of alterations in preload and afterload (10,19,20). These indices include the maximum value of $(dP/dt)/P$, where P is LV pressure (the maximum value of $[dP/dt]/P$ is sometimes called V_{PM}); (peak dP/dt)/IIT, where IIT is the integrated isovolumic tension; $(dP/dt)/CPIP$, where $CPIP$ is the common developed isovolumic pressure; V_{max}, the extrapolated value of $(dP/dt)/P$ versus P, when $P = 0$; $(dP/dt)/P_D$ when the developed LV pressure, P_D, equals 5, 10, or 40 mm Hg; and the fractional rate of change of power, which involves the second derivative of LV pressure.

Although changes in dP/dt reflect acute changes in inotropy in a given individual, the usefulness of dP/dt is

reduced in comparisons between individuals, especially when there has been chronic LV pressure or volume overload. Peak dP/dt is generally increased in patients with chronic aortic stenosis, even though contractility is normal or decreased in most of these patients. To account for chronic changes in LV geometry and mass that occur with chronic LV overload, some investigators have examined the rate of rise of systolic wall stress (17). The peak value of $d\sigma/dt$ may be used as a contractility index, as may the spectrum plot that relates $d\sigma/dt$ to instantaneous σ (Fig. 17.3).

Pressure-Volume Analysis

Since the time of Frank and Starling, pressure-volume (PV) diagrams have been used to analyze ventricular function. The normally contracting left ventricle ejects blood under pressure, and the relationship of its pressure generation and ejection can be expressed in a plot of LV pressure against volume. As can be seen in Fig. 17.4, end-diastole is represented by point A, isovolumic contraction by line AB, aortic valve opening by point B, ejection by line BC, end-ejection and aortic valve closure by point C, isovolumic relaxation by line CD, mitral valve opening by point D, and LV diastolic filling by line DA.

Stroke Work

The area ABCD enclosed within the PV diagram in Fig. 17.4 is the external LV stroke work (SW), represented mathematically as $\int P dV$. Although the calculation of LVSW is most

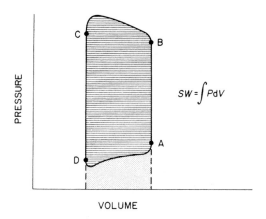

Figure 17.4 Diagram of ventricular pressure (*P*) plotted against simultaneous ventricular volume (*V*) for a single cardiac contraction. For the left ventricle, point A represents end-diastole, segment AB is isovolumic contraction, point B is aortic valve opening, segment BC is LV ejection, point C is aortic valve closure and represents end ejection, segment CD is isovolumic relaxation, point D is mitral valve opening, and segment DA is LV filling. LV stroke work (SW) is the cross-hatched area, and the stippled area is diastolic work done on the left ventricle by the right ventricle and left atrium. (See text for details.)

accurate when it is derived by integrating the area within complete PV diagrams, a practical approximation can be obtained as follows:

$$LVSW = (\overline{LVSP} - \overline{LVDP})SV(0.0136) \qquad (17.1)$$

where $\overline{LVSP}$ and $\overline{LVDP}$ are, respectively, the mean LV systolic and diastolic pressures (in mm Hg), *SV* is the LV total stroke volume (in mL), and 0.0136 is a constant for converting mm Hg-mL into g-m. $\overline{LVSP}$ and $\overline{LVDP}$ may be obtained from planimetry of direct pressure tracings, as shown in Fig. 17.5. When the total LV stroke volume is the same as the forward stroke volume, *SV* may be calculated as cardiac output divided by heart rate. In cases where LV total stroke volume differs from forward stroke volume (e.g., mitral or aortic regurgitation, ventricular septal defect), the P-V diagram may differ substantially in configuration from that shown in Fig. 17.4, and *LVSW* cannot be calculated from Eq. (17.1). Instead, planimetric integration of the entire P-V plot is required.

If LV pressure tracings are not available, in the absence of major regurgitation, *SW* can be approximated from the aortic and pulmonary capillary wedge pressures as follows:

$$LVSW = (\overline{AoSP} - \overline{PCW})SV(0.0136) \qquad (17.2)$$

where $\overline{AoSP}$ is the aortic systolic mean pressure (planimetered from the aortic pressure tracing, Fig. 17.5) and $\overline{PCW}$ is the mean pulmonary capillary wedge pressure. A further approximation may be made by substituting mean systemic arterial pressure for $\overline{AoSP}$, which it closely approximates.

LVSW is a reasonably good measure of LV systolic function in the absence of volume or pressure overload conditions, both of which may substantially increase calculated *LVSW*. The normal *LVSW* in adults is approximately 90 ± 30 g-m (mean ± SD); in adult patients with dilated cardiomyopathy or heart failure from extensive prior myocardial infarction, *LVSW* is often <40 g-m. Values ,<25 g-m indicate severe LV systolic failure, and when *LVSW* is <20 g-m, the prognosis is grave.

LVSW is a measure of total LV chamber function and can be considered to reflect myocardial contractility only when the ventricle is reasonably homogeneous in its composition, as in most patients with dilated cardiomyopathy. For patients with coronary artery disease and extensive myocardial infarction, *LVSW* may be depressed even though well-perfused areas of the myocardium with normal contractility remain.

Because power is the rate at which work is done, LV power in the normal heart is the integral of the product of LV pressure during ejection and aortic flow. LV power may be regarded as a measure of overall LV contractile function; with refinement (such as the measurement of preload-adjusted maximal power), it can be used as a measure of the inotropic state (21).

Ejection Phase Indices

LV systolic function can be assessed using only the volume data from the P-V diagram. One of the most widely used

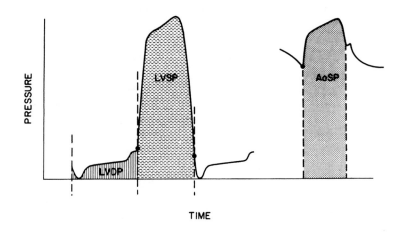

Figure 17.5 Left ventricular (LV) and aortic pressure tracings illustrate areas planimetered to measure LV mean systolic pressure (*LVSP*), LV mean diastolic pressure (*LVDP*), and aortic mean systolic pressure (*AoSP*). *LVSP* is the area contained under the LV pressure curve, bounded by perpendicular lines defining end-diastole and mitral valve opening; *LVDP* is the diastolic area, similarly defined. *AoSP* is the area contained under the aortic pressure curve, bounded by perpendicular lines defining aortic valve opening and closure.

TABLE 17.2

EVALUATION OF LEFT VENTRICULAR SYSTOLIC PERFORMANCE: NORMAL VALUES FOR SOME ISOVOLUMIC AND EJECTION PHASE INDICES

Contractility Indices	Normal Values (mean ± SD)	References
Isovolumic indices		
Maximum dP/dt	1610 ± 290 mm Hg/sec	7
	1670 ± 320 mm Hg/sec	23
	1661 ± 323 mm Hg/sec	19
Maximum (dP/dt)P	44 ± 8.4 sec^{-1}	19
V_{PM} or peak $\left[\dfrac{dP/dt}{28P}\right]$	1.47 ± 0.19 ML/sec	23
dP/dt/P_D at P_D = 40 mm Hg	37.6 ± 12.2 sec^{-1}	19
Ejection phase indices		
LVSW	81 ± 23 g-m	6
LVSWI	53 ± 22 g-m/m^2	24,25
	41 ± 12 g-m/m^2	26
EF (Angiographic)	0.72 ± 0.08	27
MNSER		
Angiographic	3.32 ± 0.84 EDV/sec	19
Echographic	2.29 ± 0.30 EDV/sec	28
Mean V_{CF}		
Angiographic	1.83 ± 0.56 ED circ/sec	19
	1.50 ± 0.27 ED circ/sec	22
Echographic	1.09 ± 0.12 ED circ/sec	28

dP/dt, rate of rise of left ventricular (LV) pressure; P_D, developed LV pressure; ML, muscle lengths; MNSER, mean normalized systolic ejection rate; ED, end-diastolic; V, volume; circ, circumference; EF, ejection fraction.

indices of LV systolic performance is the ejection fraction (EF), which is defined as follows:

$$EF = (LVEDV - LVESV)/LVEDV \qquad (17.3)$$

where *LVEDV* and *LVESV* are the LV end-diastolic and end-systolic volumes, respectively. In the cardiac catheterization laboratory, left ventricular *EF* (*LVEF*) is most often derived from the LV angiogram, as discussed in Chapter 16. If the *EF* is divided by the ejection time (*ET*), measured from the aortic pressure tracing, the quotient is called *mean normalized systolic ejection rate* (*MNSER*).

$$MNSER = \frac{(LVEDV - LVESV)}{(LVEDV)(ET)} \qquad (17.4)$$

Finally, another ejection phase index of LV systolic function is the velocity of circumferential fiber shortening, V_{CF} (22). This is calculated as the rate of shortening of a theoretic LV myocardial fiber in a circumferential plane at the midpoint of the long axis of the ventricle. For convenience, mean V_{CF} is used most often, rather than instantaneous or peak V_{CF}. Mean V_{CF} is obtained by subtracting the end-systolic endocardial circumferential fiber length (πD_{ES}) from the end-diastolic endocardial circumferential fiber length (πD_{ED}), then dividing by *ET* and normalizing for end-diastolic circumferential fiber length:

$$\begin{aligned} V_{CF} &= (\pi D_{ED} - \pi D_{ES})/\pi D_{ED}(ET) \\ &= (D_{ED} - D_{ES})/D_{ED}(ET) \end{aligned} \qquad (17.5)$$

D_{ED} and D_{ES} are end-diastolic and end-systolic minor axis dimensions. Although V_{CF} can be calculated from angiographic data using the area-length method ($D = 4\,A/\pi L$), it is most commonly calculated from values for D measured by M-mode echocardiography. Normal values for isovolumic and ejection phase indices are given in Table 17.2.

Ejection phase indices are obtained easily from LV angiography and can also be derived reliably from a variety of noninvasive techniques such as radionuclide ventriculography and echocardiography. The most widely used ejection phase index, the *EF*, is generally depressed when myocardial contractility is diminished. However, the ejection indices depend heavily on preload and afterload and cannot be regarded as reliable indices of contractility in conditions associated with altered loading conditions. For example, increases in preload cause the *EF* (and other ejection indices) to rise; consequently, *LVEF* may be increased in patients with mitral or aortic regurgitation, severe anemia, or other causes of increased diastolic LV inflow and may mask underlying deterioration of myocardial contractility. Conversely, increases in afterload cause the *EF* to fall; consequently, *LVEF* may be low in patients with severe aortic stenosis or other causes of increased resistance to systolic ejection and may falsely suggest underlying depression of myocardial contractility.

In practice, acute elevation of LV preload causes some increase in LV chamber size and aortic pressure, and these increases in afterload (systolic σ resisting shortening) tend

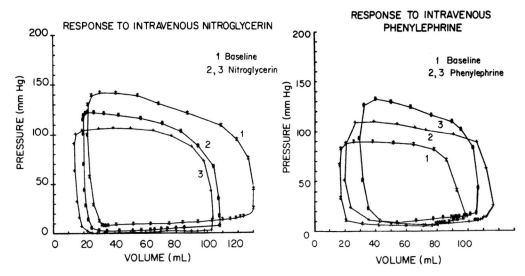

Figure 17.6 Left ventricular (LV) pressure-volume (P-V) plots constructed using radionuclide ventriculography to measure LV volume simultaneously with measurement of LV pressure during cardiac catheterization. **A.** Three sequential plots measured during baseline and at two sequential doses of intravenous nitroglycerin to lower LV pressure. **B.** Similar plots in a patient whose baseline LV systolic pressure was low: In this case, phenylephrine was used in increasing doses to produce three levels of systolic loading. The upper left (end-systolic) corners of the three P-V plots in each view define a straight line, the LV end-systolic P-V line. (See text for discussion.) (From McKay RG, Aroesty JM, Heller GV, et al. Left ventricular pressure-volume diagrams and end-systolic pressure relations in human beings. *J Am Coll Cardiol* 1984;3:301, with permission.)

to decrease the *EF* and other ejection indices, offsetting the rise in *EF* that a pure rise in preload would produce. Rankin and coworkers (28) produced changes in venous return by total body tilt in normal subjects; despite substantial changes in LV end-diastolic dimension and volume, there were no significant changes in *EF, MNSER,* or V_{CF}. Similarly, acute elevation of afterload caused by raising aortic pressure causes an increase in *LVEDP,* and the resultant rise in preload (end-diastolic fiber stretch) tends to increase the *EF* and other ejection indices, offsetting the fall in *EF* produced by a pure rise in afterload (25). These physiologic adjustments explain why the ejection indices are much more useful clinically than might be expected on the basis of studies in the isolated heart or muscle preparation.

An *LVEF* of <0.40 indicates depressed LV systolic pump function, and if there is no abnormal loading to account for it, an *LVEF* of ≤0.40 can be taken to signify depressed myocardial contractility. An *LVEF* <0.20 corresponds to severe depression of LV systolic performance and is usually associated with a poor prognosis. Interpretation of *EF* and other ejection indices is improved by consideration of the ventricular preload and afterload, and the latter values are defined most precisely by end-diastolic and end-systolic wall stresses, respectively.

End-Systolic Pressure-Volume and σ-Length Relations

Over the past 20 years, several groups have shown that the LV end-systolic P-V, pressure-diameter, and σ-length relationships accurately reflect myocardial contractility, independent

of changes in ventricular loading. This has been established in a series of studies in animals (29–35) and humans (36–42). The fundamental principle of end-systolic PV analysis is that at end-systole there is a single line relating LV chamber pressure to volume, unique for the level of contractility and independent of loading conditions. The LV end-systolic PV line can be generated by producing a series of P-V loops (such as the one in Fig. 17.4) over a range of loading conditions (Figs. 17.6 and 17.7). The line connecting the upper left corners of the individual P-V diagrams is the end-systolic P-V line, characterized by a slope and by an x-axis intercept, called V_0 (the extrapolated end-systolic volume when end-systolic pressure is zero). Current evidence indicates that an increase in contractility shifts the end-systolic P-V line to the left with a steeper slope, and a depression in contractility is associated with a displacement of the line downward and to the right, with a reduced slope. Although there is some uncertainty as to the meaning of V_0, it is generally agreed that an increase in slope of the end-systolic P-V line is a sensitive indicator of an increase in contractility. However, the technique of end-systolic analysis may not be as useful in comparisons among subjects as it is in comparisons of values in a single subject measured before and after an intervention. The end-systolic P-V lines for groups of patients with normal, intermediate, and depressed LV contractility are shown in Fig. 17.8.

To measure the end-systolic PV line, one can use aortic dicrotic notch pressure as end-systolic LV pressure and minimum LV chamber volume as end-systolic volume. LV volume can be measured by angiography, using either direct LV injection or right-sided injection with image enhancement

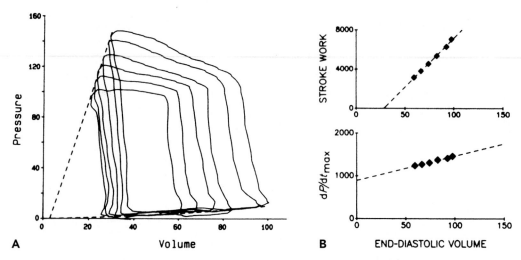

Figure 17.7 A. Left ventricular (LV) pressure-volume loops obtained during rapid LV unloading achieved by inferior vena cava (IVC) balloon occlusion in a patient undergoing cardiac catheterization. Volume was obtained by a conductance catheter technique. **B.** Relationships between stroke work, maximum rate of rise of LV systolic pressure, dP/dt, and LV end-diastolic volume. (From Kass DA, Maughan WL. From E_{Max} to pressure-volume relations: a broader view. *Circulation* 1988;77: 1203, with permission.)

by digital subtraction angiography. Alternatively, LV volume can be measured by radionuclide techniques, ultrasonic techniques, or a specially designed impedance (conductance) catheter (42,43).

Relationship Between Peak dP/dt and End-Diastolic Volume

Little and coworkers (44) have examined the relationship between LV dP/dt_{max} and end-diastolic volume and have

proposed the slope of this relationship as an index of contractile state. They have shown that, on theoretic grounds, this relationship can be derived from the LV end-systolic P-V relationship; both provide estimates of maximal myocardial elastance. This relationship is simpler to derive because both LV end-diastolic volume and dP/dt_{max} are more readily defined than either end-systolic pressure or volume. One does not need to be concerned about a lack of coincidence between end-systole and maximal elastance, as with the end-systolic P-V relationship.

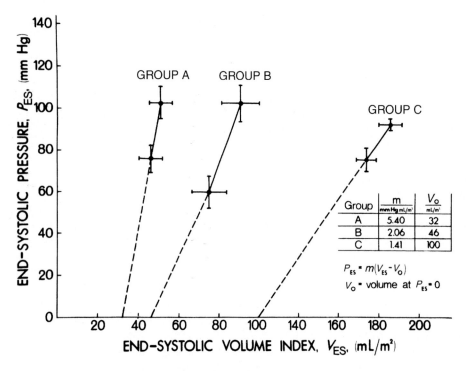

Figure 17.8 Left ventricular (LV) end-systolic pressure (P_{ES}) plotted against end-systolic volume index (V_{ES}) at two levels of loading for each of three patient groups: Group A, patients with normal LV contractile function; Group B, patients with moderate depression of LV contractile performance; Group C, patients with marked depression of LV contractility. Depressed contractility shifts the P_{ES}-V_{ES} relation to the right, with a reduced slope (m) and increased intercept (V_0). (From Grossman W, Braunwald E, Mann JT, et al. Contractile state of the left ventricle in man as evaluated from end-systolic pressure relations. *Circulation* 1977;45:845, with permission.)

Group	m (mm Hg mL/m')	V_0 (mL/m')
A	5.40	32
B	2.06	46
C	1.41	100

$$P_{ES} = m(V_{ES} - V_0)$$
$$V_0 = \text{volume at } P_{ES} = 0$$

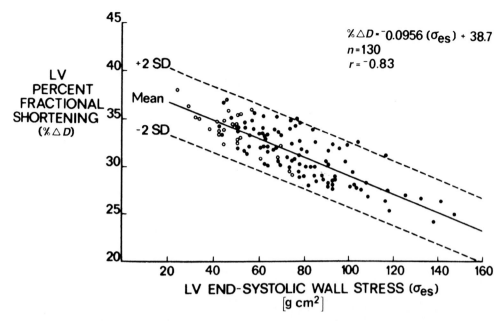

Figure 17.9 Relationship between left ventricular (LV) end-systolic wall stress (σ_{ES}) and % fractional shortening (%ΔD) measured by echocardiography for 130 control points, at rest *(open circles)* or during methoxamine infusion *(solid circles)*. The inverse relationship defines normal LV myocardial contractility. (From Borow KM, Green LH, Grossman W, et al. Left ventricular end-systolic stress-shortening and stress-length relations in humans. *Am J Cardiol* 1982;50:1301, with permission.)

The dP/dt_{max}–end-diastolic volume relationship, however, has yet to be evaluated extensively in the clinical setting. Also, the end-systolic P-V relationship can be estimated clinically by entirely noninvasive methods (45). Nevertheless, the relationship between dP/dt_{max} and end-diastolic volume represents an intriguing concept and may prove a valuable index of contractile state.

Stress-Shortening Relationships

Another approach to the assessment of LV systolic performance and myocardial contractility involves measuring the extent of cardiac muscle shortening and relating this shortening to the systolic wall stress (σ) resisting shortening.

If a ventricle is presented with progressively increasing resistance to ejection, σ rises while the extent of myocardial shortening declines. Therefore, a plot of systolic σ on the horizontal axis against myocardial shortening expressed as EF, V_{CF}, or percent fractional shortening (%ΔD) on the vertical axis yields a tight inverse relationship (Fig. 17.9). Data from studies of individual patients may then be compared with these normal values. In Fig. 17.9, if the point relating end-systolic σ (σ_{ES}) and %ΔD for a given patient lies within the confidence lines of the normal population, myocardial contractility is likely to be normal; however, if the σ_{ES}-%ΔD point lies below the normal range, contractility is depressed even if %ΔD is normal. Figure 17.10 shows that the σ_{ES}-%ΔD relationship is shifted upward by an increase in contractility resulting from a dobutamine infusion. One caution concerning the σ_{ES}-%ΔD relationship is

that it is preload sensitive. That is, increases in preload will increase %ΔD for any level of σ_{ES}. There is some evidence that when V_{CF} is substituted for %ΔD, the preload dependence of the stress-shortening relationship is attenuated or abolished.

Plots of systolic wall stress against *LVEF* have been analyzed for patients with a variety of conditions, including LV

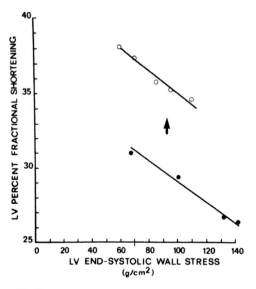

Figure 17.10 Upward shift in the left ventricular (LV) end-systolic stress-shortening relation resulting from dobutamine infusion (see text). (From Borow KM, et al. Left ventricular end-systolic stress-shortening and stress-length relations in humans. *Am J Cardiol* 1982;50:1301, with permission.)

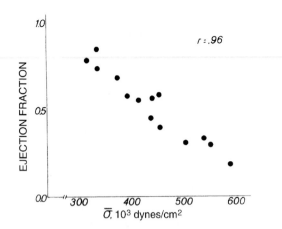

Figure 17.11 Left ventricular (LV) ejection fraction plotted against mean systolic circumferential wall stress, σ, for 14 patients with pure aortic stenosis (normal coronary arteries, no other valve disease) and varying degrees of LV decompensation. The inverse relationship is consistent with afterload excess as a principal cause of the decreased ejection fraction. (From Gunther S, Grossman W. Determinants of ventricular function in pressure-overload hypertrophy in man. *Circulation* 1979;59:679, with permission.)

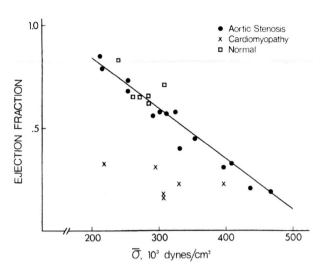

Figure 17.12 Plot of left ventricular (LV) ejection fraction against systolic σ, similar to Fig. 17.11 but including patients with aortic stenosis (*solid circles*), dilated cardiomyopathy (*crosses*), and normal ventricular function (*open squares*). The regression line was constructed from the patients with normal LV function and those with aortic stenosis (see text for discussion). (From Gunther S, Grossman W. Determination of ventricular function in pressure overload hypertrophy in man. *Circulation* 1979;5:679, with permission.)

pressure overload (Fig. 17.11). In these plots, comprised of multiple individual data points (each point relating LV wall σ and *EF* for an individual patient) an inverse systolic σ-*EF* relationship is apparent for patients with chronic LV pressure overload. This suggests that the depressed *LVEF* in some of these individuals is caused by excessive systolic σ; that is, the load resisting systolic shortening is abnormally high and is responsible for a reduced extent of shortening. This combination of high σ and low *EF* is sometimes referred to as *afterload mismatch* (46–48), and it implies that hypertrophy has been inadequate to return systolic wall stress to its relatively low normal level. Patients in whom *LVEF* is diminished out of proportion to any increase in systolic wall stress can be assumed to have depressed myocardial contractility (Fig. 17.12).

A refinement of this approach involves measuring the relation between end-systolic LV wall stress and the heart rate–corrected velocity of fiber shortening. This approach was found to be sensitive and preload independent in an assessment of LV response to nitroprusside and dopamine infusions in patients with dilated cardiomyopathy (49). In that study, this approach was more sensitive to detecting increased contractility than was LV dP/dt.

The advantage of σ-shortening analysis over P-V diagram analysis is that wall σ takes into consideration changes in LV geometry and muscle mass that occur in response to chronic alterations in loading. For example, a systolic pressure of 250 to 300 mm Hg imposed acutely on a normal left ventricle would result in considerable reduction in *LVEF*, perhaps down to the 20 to 30% range. This change occurs because, in the absence of any increase in LV wall thickness or decrease in chamber radius, systolic σ would more than double in response to such an acute pressure overload, and this would lead to a major reduction in

LVEF. However, if the increase in systolic pressure to 250 to 300 mm Hg occurs gradually and is matched by the development of sufficient hypertrophy in the appropriate pattern, systolic wall σ remains normal and fiber shortening and *LVEF* do not decrease. Therefore, in the presence of significant hypertrophy and/or altered LV geometry, σ-shortening analysis may have considerable value.

DIASTOLIC FUNCTION

Left Ventricular Diastolic Distensibility: Pressure-Volume Relationship

As pointed out by Henderson in 1923, "In the heart, diastolic relaxation is a vital factor and not merely the passive stretching of a rubber bag. Being vital, it is variable" (50). Analysis of diastolic function today requires appreciation that diastolic compliance is variable and may change substantially in a given patient from one minute to the next. Diastolic function is summated physiologically in the relation between LV pressure and volume during diastole (Fig. 17.4, segment DA). Traditionally, an upward shift in this diastolic PV relation is regarded as indicating increased LV diastolic chamber stiffness, and a downward shift indicates decreased stiffness or increased LV diastolic chamber compliance. In the terminology of physics and engineering, stiffness, and its opposite, compliance, relate a change in pressure (ΔP) to a change in volume (ΔV); therefore, some investigators have restricted these terms to refer to the slope of the diastolic P-V relation. In this regard, as

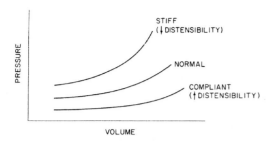

Figure 17.13 Diagrammatic representation of ventricular diastolic pressure-volume relations for normal, stiff, and compliant ventricles (see text for discussion).

seen in segment DA of Fig. 17.4, LV diastolic stiffness ($\Delta P/\Delta V$) is low early in diastole and rises steadily throughout diastolic filling.

Figure 17.13 shows theoretic LV diastolic PV plots for patients with normal, stiff, and compliant ventricular chambers. Several problems arise when stiffness and compliance are defined strictly in terms of the slope of the diastolic P-V diagram, and these problems are illustrated in Fig. 17.14. First, in some clinical conditions (e.g., angina pectoris), the LV diastolic P-V plot shifts upward in a parallel fashion, without a noticeable change in slope. These patients have increased LV filling pressure, often with normal chamber volumes, and from a hydrodynamic point of view the LV chamber must be regarded as presenting increased resistance to diastolic filling. To say that LV diastolic stiffness and compliance are normal in such patients because the upward shift has been a parallel one (without slope change) seems inappropriate. In other cases (e.g.,

after nitroprusside infusion in patients with heart failure), there is a downward shift in the LV diastolic PV plot, with an increase in the steepness of the plot; again, to say that such patients exhibit increased LV diastolic stiffness seems inappropriate, because they require a lower filling pressure to achieve the same diastolic chamber dimension and fiber stretch. Therefore, the LV diastolic P-V plot can show changes of two types: displacement (movement of the entire relationship upward, downward, or laterally) and configuration change (including change in curvature). In our studies, we have referred to upward or downward displacement changes as being associated with a change in ventricular distensibility (51). Therefore, if the LV diastolic PV plot shifts upward, we say that the LV chamber has become less distensible; a higher diastolic pressure is required to fill or distend the chamber to its earlier volume (Fig. 17.14). Similarly, a downward shift in the diastolic PV plot is said to indicate an increase in LV diastolic distensibility. The changes in curvature and/or configuration that may accompany these displacement changes are difficult to quantify and to interpret.

Various formulas have been developed for analyzing the curvature of the LV diastolic P-V plot (52–55). These generally assume that the curvature is exponential, an assumption that is often but not always reasonable. Diastolic P-V and P-segment length (SL) plots constructed from a series of end-diastolic points have been used in animal experiments to assess LV diastolic compliance (56), and this technique has been applied to clinical studies. When a series of end-diastolic P-V or P-SL points are plotted, the relation is more strictly exponential, and application of

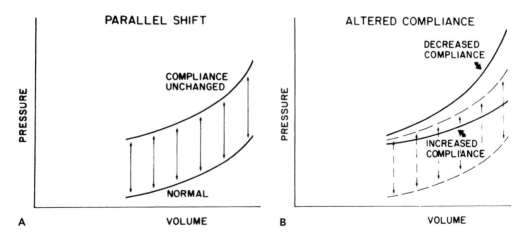

Figure 17.14 Schematic illustration of the difference between diastolic distensibility and compliance. **A.** The left ventricular diastolic pressure-volume (P-V) relation has undergone a parallel upward shift. Distensibility is decreased (higher diastolic pressure required to fill the ventricle to the same chamber volume), but compliance, defined as the slope of the P-V relation, is unchanged. On the right, superimposed on the parallel upward shift, are curves whose slopes are steeper (decreased compliance) or less steep (increased compliance) than either of the two parallel P-V curves. This illustrates the importance of distinguishing distensibility from compliance, because the curve labeled "increased compliance" nevertheless exhibits decreased diastolic distensibility, compared with the normal PV relation. (From Grossman W. Relaxation and diastolic distensibility of the regionally ischemic left ventricle. In: Grossman W, Lorell BH, eds. *Diastolic Relaxation of the Heart.* Boston: Martinus Nijhoff, 1988:193.)

TABLE 17.3

FACTORS THAT INFLUENCE LEFT VENTRICULAR (LV) DIASTOLIC CHAMBER DISTENSIBILITY

I. Factors extrinsic to the LV chamber
  A. Pericardial restraint
  B. Right ventricular loading
  C. Coronary vascular turgor (erectile effect)
  D. Extrinsic compression (e.g., tumor, pleural pressure)
II. Factors intrinsic to LV chamber
  A. Passive elasticity of LV wall (stiffness or compliance when myocytes are completely relaxed)
    1. Thickness of LV wall
    2. Composition of LV wall (muscle, fibrosis, edema, amyloid, hemosiderin) including both endocardium and myocardium
    3. Temperature, osmolality
  B. Active elasticity of LV wall owing to residual cross-bridge activation (cycling and/or latch state) through part or all of diastole
    1. Slow relaxation affecting early diastole only
    2. Incomplete relaxation affecting early-, middle-, and end-diastolic distensibility
    3. Diastolic tone, contracture, or rigor
  C. Elastic recoil (diastolic suction)
  D. Viscoelasticity (stress relaxation, creep)

mathematical models and analysis is more easily justified by the good agreement of measured data and mathematical predictions.

Clinical Conditions Influencing Diastolic Distensibility

Factors that influence the position of the LV diastolic PV plot (that is, factors that influence LV diastolic *distensibility*) are listed in Table 17.3. *Constrictive pericarditis* and *pericardial tamponade* are associated with a striking upward shift in the diastolic PV relation. This upward shift is a parallel shift without substantial change in curvature. Pericardial restraint is also important in the mechanism whereby altered RV loading can alter the LV diastolic PV relation. When distended, the right ventricle can decrease LV diastolic distensibility by exerting an extrinsic pressure on the LV chamber in diastole through the shared interventricular septum, which may actually bulge into the LV chamber. *Acute RV infarction* causes dilatation of the RV chamber that, in the presence of an intact, previously unstressed pericardium, may lead to extrinsic compression of the LV in diastole with a hemodynamic pattern resembling cardiac tamponade (57). The effect of increased RV loading on LV diastolic distensibility is an example of ventricular interaction, which is more prominent in the presence of an intact and relatively snug pericardium. In animal experiments, it is difficult to demonstrate diastolic ventricular interaction once the pericardium has been opened wide (55).

Coronary vascular turgor can influence LV diastolic chamber stiffness (58). The LV wall has a rich blood supply, and engorgement of the capillaries and venules with blood makes the wall relatively stiff: For obvious reasons, this has been referred to as the erectile effect. Although the erectile effect is probably not of much importance when coronary blood flow and pressure (the two components determining the degree of turgor) are in the physiologic range, a marked fall in coronary flow and pressure (as occurs distal to a coronary occlusion when collateral flow is poor or absent) is associated with a decrease in stiffness of the affected myocardium and an increase in LV diastolic distensibility.

Experimental evidence (59) supports an important role for *increased coronary venous pressure* as a major determinant of coronary vascular turgor. Increases in right atrial pressure from 0 to 15 and 30 mm Hg led to substantial upward shifts in the LV end-diastolic PV relation that could not be attributed to right ventricular distention and a shift in the interventricular septum. Extrinsic *compression of the heart by tumor* may cause decreased LV diastolic distensibility and may mimic cardiac tamponade.

When an upward shift in the diastolic PV relation is present and the extrinsic factors listed in Table 17.3 cannot clearly explain the altered distensibility, a change in one of the intrinsic determinants of LV distensibility is likely to be present. Altered passive elasticity caused by *amyloidosis*, edema, or diffuse fibrosis may cause a restrictive cardiomyopathic pattern, with high LV diastolic pressure relative to volume in the presence of reasonably well-preserved systolic function. Clinically, heart failure may be present. Endomyocardial biopsy of the right or left ventricle may be needed to establish the diagnosis (see Chapter 20).

Myocardial Ischemia

Abnormal diastolic relaxation can cause the diastolic P-V relation to shift upward strikingly. During *angina pectoris*, a 10 to 15 mm Hg rise in average LV diastolic pressure may occur with little or no change in diastolic volume; if this persists for a sufficient duration (>10 to 20 minutes), pulmonary edema may occur. Such episodes of *flash pulmonary edema* in patients with essentially normal LV systolic function and normal LV chamber size generally indicate a large mass of ischemic myocardium (60) and suggest three-vessel or left main coronary artery obstruction. The decreased LV distensibility during ischemia may be prevented in many patients by a Ca^{++} channel blocking agent (61). The mechanism of impaired myocardial relaxation during the ischemia of angina pectoris is not understood completely, but may be associated with diastolic Ca^{++} overload of the ischemic myocytes, in part related to ischemic dysfunction of the sarcoplasmic reticulum (62). During the ischemia of acute coronary occlusion, an upward shift of the diastolic P-V relation may occur if sufficient collateral blood flow is present to permit continued systolic contraction of the ischemic segment. If ischemia is sufficiently severe to cause complete akinesis of the affected myocardium, however, altered distensibility does not occur: *incomplete relaxation* can occur only in myocytes when there has been systolic cross-bridge activation. Also, the marked decrease in coronary vascular turgor distal to a coronary occlusion with poor or absent collaterals, together with local accumulation of hydrogen ion (H^+), contributes to an increase in regional distensibility, so that the net effect on the ventricular diastolic PV relation may be one of no change.

Cardiac Hypertrophy

Impaired relaxation with decreased LV diastolic distensibility is also seen in patients with *hypertrophic cardiomyopathy* and during angina pectoris in patients with *aortic stenosis* and normal coronary arteries.

Indices of Left Ventricular Diastolic Relaxation Rate

Much attention has been given to measures of LV diastolic relaxation during the isovolumic relaxation period and during early, middle, and late diastolic filling. These indices may be considered as either pressure-derived or volume flow-derived and may assess either global or regional diastolic relaxation (63–83). A listing of some of these indices and their normal values is given in Table 17.4.

Isovolumic Pressure Decay

The time course of LV pressure decline after aortic valve closure is altered in conditions known to be associated with abnormalities of myocardial relaxation. One of the simplest ways of quantifying the time course of LV pressure decline is to measure the maximum rate of pressure fall, peak negative dP/dt. Although peak negative dP/dt is altered by conditions that change myocardial relaxation, it is also altered by changes in loading conditions. For example, LV peak negative dP/dt increases (i.e., rises in absolute value) when aortic pressure rises. For example, an increase in LV peak negative dP/dt from $-1,500$ to $-1,800$ mm Hg/second could be caused by an increase in the rate of myocardial relaxation, a rise in aortic pressure, or both. An increase in peak negative dP/dt when aortic pressure is unchanged or declining, however, signifies an improvement of LV relaxation. LV peak negative dP/dt is decreased during the myocardial ischemia of either angina pectoris or infarction and is increased in response to β-adrenergic stimulation and the phosphodiesterase inhibitor milrinone (63). It is not increased by digitalis glycosides.

Time Constant of Relaxation

Because of the load dependency of peak negative dP/dt and the fact that it uses information from only one point on the LV pressure-time plot, other indices have been introduced that analyze the time course of LV isovolumic pressure fall more completely. In 1976, Weiss and coworkers introduced the time constant T (or tau) of LV isovolumic pressure decline (64). First, LV isovolumic pressure decline is fit to the equation

$$P = e^{At+B} \tag{17.6}$$

where P is LV isovolumic pressure, e is a mathematical constant (natural logarithm base), t is time after peak

---

TABLE 17.4

EVALUATION OF LEFT VENTRICULAR DIASTOLIC PERFORMANCE: NORMAL VALUES FOR SOME INDICES OF RELAXATION AND FILLING

Parameter	Normal Values	Reference
Peak $- dP/dt$	$2,660 \pm 700$ mm Hg/sec	7
	$2,922 \pm 750$ mm Hg/sec	80
	$1,864 \pm 390$ mm Hg/sec	81
	$1,825 \pm 261$ mm Hg/sec	82
T [logarithmic method, Eq. (17.7)]	38 ± 7 msec	80
	33 ± 8 msec	81
	31 ± 3 msec	82
T [derivative method, Eqs. (17.8) and (17.9)]	55 ± 12 msec	82
	47 ± 10	83
P_B [derivative method, Eqs. (17.8) and (17.9)]	-25 ± 9 mm Hg	82
PFR	3.3 ± 0.6 EDV/sec	73
Time-to-PFR	136 ± 23 msec	73
Peak $- dh/dt$ (posterior wall)	8.4 ± 3.0 cm/sec	77
	8.2 ± 3.7 cm/sec	78

LV, left ventricular; peak $- dP/dt$ = maximum rate of LV isovolumic pressure decline; T = time constant of LV isovolumic relaxation, calculated assuming both zero pressure intercept [Eq. (17.7)] and variable pressure (*PB*) intercept [Eqs. (17.8) and (17.9)]; PFR = LV peak filling rate, from radionuclide ventriculography, normalized to end-diastolic volumes (EDV)/sec; peak $- dh/dt$ = maximum rate of posterior wall thinning, measured by echocardiography.

negative dP/dt, and A and B are constants. This can also be expressed as

$$\ln P = At + B \qquad (17.7)$$

Then the natural logarithm of LV pressure versus time is plotted to allow calculation of the slope A, a negative number whose units are seconds^{-1}. The time constant T of isovolumic pressure fall is then defined as $-1/A$ (expressed in milliseconds) representing the time that it takes P to decline to $1/e$ of its value.

Studies by the Johns Hopkins group have suggested that myocardial relaxation is normally complete by approximately 3.5T after the onset of isovolumic relaxation. The normal value for T as calculated using a plot of $\ln P$ versus t is 25 to 40 milliseconds in humans. Therefore, by 140 milliseconds after the dicrotic notch, LV diastolic P-V relations should be determined primarily by passive elastic properties of the myocardium. Because the normal LV diastolic filling period is >400 milliseconds, it is unlikely, according to this concept, that late- and end-diastolic PV relations are still influenced by the relaxation process. However, there is now considerable evidence that even in the normal myocardium, cross-bridge cycling persists to some extent throughout diastole. This resting myocardial activity or tone makes it difficult to know what significance to apply to the concept that relaxation is complete at 3.5T. Nevertheless, it is important to emphasize that the relaxation process does progress with time through diastole, so that slowing of the process (prolongation of T) or shortening of the diastolic filling period (e.g., tachycardia) results in a greater resistance to early and even late diastolic filling.

Another approach to the measurement of T uses a more general equation to describe LV isovolumic pressure decline (65):

$$P = P_o e^{-t/T} + P_B \qquad (17.8)$$

In this formulation, if diastole were infinite in duration ($t = \infty$), P would decay to a residual pressure, P_B. In the initial formulation by Weiss and coworkers (64), P always declines toward zero in long diastoles. The more general formula allows for two variables: T (which equals $-1/A$) and P_B. Work by Carroll and coworkers (66), as well as other groups (63), has shown that both P_B and T can vary with physiologic maneuvers (e.g., exercise, ischemia). The biologic meaning of P_B is uncertain, although there has been speculation that it may reflect the level of diastolic myocardial tone. A problem with both P_B and T is that there is experimental evidence that the speed of the relaxation process itself is altered by myofiber stretch that occurs after mitral valve opening.

When T is to be derived from the formulas that assume a variable pressure intercept (P_B), the calculation is often accomplished by taking the first derivative (65):

$$P = P_o e^{-t/T} + P_B$$
$$dP/dt = -\frac{1}{T}(P - P_B) \qquad (17.9)$$

Here, a plot of dP/dt versus ($P - P_B$) has the slope $-1/T$.

Normal values in humans for T calculated by either the logarithmic method (asymptote = 0) or the derivative method (variable asymptote) are listed in Table 17.4.

Interesting experimental data comparing the two methods of calculating T with a gold standard were published by Paulus and coworkers (67). They measured LV pressure decay with a micromanometer catheter during isovolumic beats generated using an Inoue balloon to occlude the mitral valve orifice in patients with mitral stenosis who were undergoing balloon valvuloplasty. LV pressure declined to an asymptote of 2 ± 3 mm Hg, and T was calculated from a monoexponential curve fit using the measured asymptote pressure. This T was considerably shorter than the T calculated by the derivative (variable asymptote) method and was much closer to the value obtained by the original Weiss logarithmic method (64), which assumes a zero asymptote.

Not only slow myocardial relaxation but also asynchrony of the relaxation process within the ventricular chamber results in a prolongation of T. In addition, T is probably not completely independent of loading conditions, although the influence of altered loading is relatively small. Measurement of T should be attempted only from LV pressure tracings obtained with high-fidelity, micromanometer-tipped catheters, or from fluid-filled systems with demonstrated optimal damping and high (>25 Hz) natural frequencies (see Chapter 7). Of interest, investigators have reported the *noninvasive assessment* of LV relaxation by continuous-wave Doppler echocardiography in patients with some degree of mitral regurgitation (68,69). The Doppler mitral regurgitant velocity profile is recorded, digitized, and converted to ventriculoatrial pressure gradient curves with the use of the simplified Bernoulli equation and differentiated into instantaneous dP/dt. The relaxation time constant is then calculated assuming a zero-pressure asymptote (Fig. 17.15). In general, close correlations are seen between measurements of T made by this technique and those made from simultaneous LV micromanometer pressure measurements (68,69). However, accurate prediction of actual T was improved substantially when a measure of left atrial pressure was incorporated in the analysis.

Volume-Derived Indices of Relaxation

Peak Filling Rate

After mitral valve opening, ventricular filling usually proceeds briskly with an initial rapid filling phase, a middle slow filling phase, and a terminal increase in filling rate associated with atrial systole. The rapid filling phase may be characterized by a maximum or peak filling rate (PFR) and time-to-PFR. PFR is usually determined by plotting LV volume against time, fitting the initial portion of this plot after mitral valve opening to a third- (or higher-) order polynomial, and solving for the first derivative of this polynomial. LV volume for this calculation may be

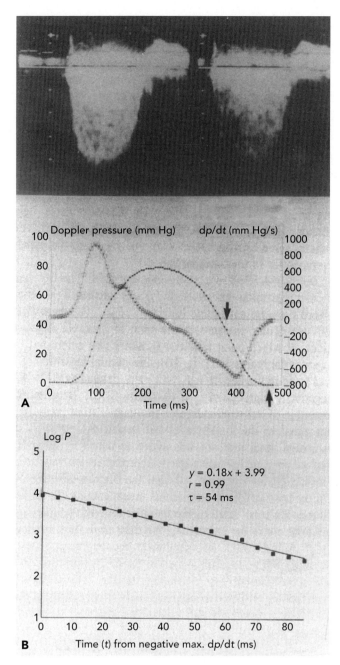

Figure 17.15 Doppler technique for measuring left ventricular (LV) rate of pressure fall, dP/dt, and the time constant of LV relaxation (*T*), using Doppler mitral regurgitant velocity spectrum (**A,** *top*), LV-left atrial pressure gradient and its first derivative (**A,** *bottom*), and linear plot of log LV-estimated pressure (*P*) versus time (**B**), with *T* = 1/slope. (From C Chen, et al. Doppler derived dP/dt and T in mitral regurgitation. *J Am Coll Cardiol* 1994;23:970, with permission.)

obtained from the LV cineangiogram or from radionuclide techniques.

As one might expect, PFR is preload dependent: interventions that raise left atrial pressure increase PFR, and interventions that reduce pulmonary venous return and left atrial pressure cause PFR to decrease (70). However, an increase in PFR that occurs when LV filling pressure (pul-

monary capillary wedge pressure, left atrial pressure, or LV diastolic pressure) is unchanged or falling can reasonably be taken as an indication that LV relaxation has improved. For example, PFR has been shown to decrease during angina pectoris (71) when LV filling pressure is increasing. Because the rise in LV filling pressure by itself would cause an increase in PFR, the fall in PFR that is actually observed most likely indicates slowed relaxation of the myocardium, consistent with the other findings in this condition (fall in peak negative dP/dt, prolongation of *T*) that suggest impaired relaxation of the ischemic myocardium. PFR is reduced in patients with coronary stenoses, even in the absence of overt ischemia, and improves after coronary angioplasty (72). PFR is also reduced in patients with hypertrophic cardiomyopathy and improves after administration of a calcium-blocking agent (73). PFR is usually normalized for end-diastolic volume (EDV) and expressed as EDV/second. Cardiac dilatation by itself tends to depress PFR, exaggerating its preload dependence.

Regional Diastolic Dysfunction

Diastolic dysfunction of specific regions of the left ventricle may be difficult to assess solely by examination of a global parameter of LV diastolic function such as the time constant of relaxation or the PFR. As pointed out by Pouleur and Rousseau (74), the time course of LV isovolumic pressure decline underestimates the severity of regional impairment in the rate of relaxation. Marked slowing of regional relaxation in an area of myocardial ischemia is partially masked by normal or enhanced rates of relaxation in adjacent normal regions of myocardium. Regional wall stress measurements have been proposed as an ideal way to assess regional rates of relaxation, but these can be made only by having knowledge of simultaneous LV pressure wall thickness and geometry (74).

A more practical way of assessing regional LV myocardial relaxation involves measurement of changes in regional LV chamber volume during isovolumic relaxation (Fig. 17.16) as well as regional PFR (75–77). Regional LV area may not be constant for each segmental area during "isovolumic" relaxation in the dysfunctional ventricle. Instead, some regions may increase while others decrease in area, owing to either asynchrony or regional slowing of the relaxation process, with resultant differences in active wall tension in different parts of the left ventricle. An example of the application of this approach to measurement of regional myocardial relaxation is seen in a hemodynamic study by Friedrich and coworkers (75) of 20 adult patients with LV hypertrophy resulting from aortic stenosis (mean aortic valve area, 0.7 ± 0.2 cm^2). LV global diastolic function was abnormal, with a *T* of 58 ± 4 milliseconds and a time-to-PFR of 378 ± 63 milliseconds. Enalaprilat, an angiotensin-converting enzyme inhibitor, was infused into the left coronary artery, and regional LV

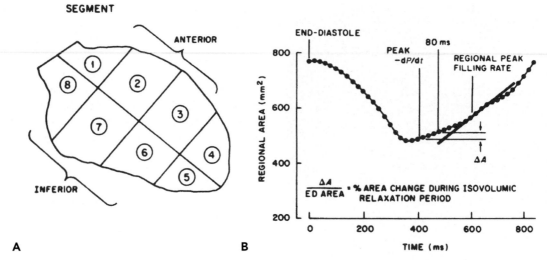

Figure 17.16 Analysis of diastolic left ventricular (LV) regional wall motion. **A.** The LV silhouette is divided into eight segments. **B.** The regional area is plotted throughout the cardiac cycle, and the change in area (ΔA) during isovolumic relaxation (defined as the first 80 milliseconds after peak rate of LV pressure fall) and regional peak filling rate are calculated. $-dP/dt$, maximum rate of LV pressure fall; ED, end-diastolic. (From Friedrich S, Lorell BH, Rousseau M, et al. Intracardiac angiotensin-converting enzyme inhibition improves diastolic function in patients with LV hypertrophy due to aortic stenosis. *Circulation* 1994;90:2761, with permission.)

diastolic function was assessed in both the anterior wall (perfused by enalaprilat) and the inferior wall. LV area change during isovolumic relaxation increased in anterior segments and decreased in inferior segments (Fig. 17.17), suggesting improved diastolic relaxation of the hypertro-

phied myocardium in response to angiotensin-converting enzyme inhibition (75), something seen previously only in animal experiments (76).

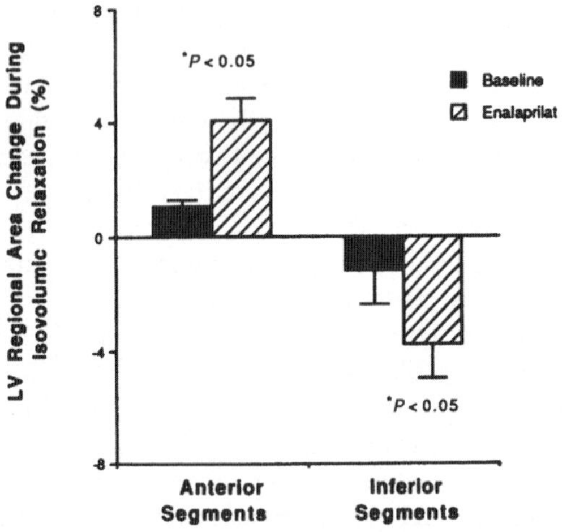

Rate of Wall Thinning

Another index of diastolic function, similar in some ways to PFR, is the peak rate of diastolic LV wall thinning. This can be measured echocardiographically by plotting posterior or septal wall thickness against time, fitting the data to a polynomial, and taking the first derivative (77–79). The posterior wall thickness, h, and its first derivative, dh/dt, reflect regional diastolic function of the posterior wall myocardium. An advantage of peak negative dh/dt over PFR is that it assesses regional myocardial function, whereas PFR describes behavior for the whole ventricle and is insensitive when equal and opposite changes in diastolic function are occurring in different parts of the LV chamber. Peak negative dh/dt decreases during angina, even though LV filling pressure rises (79).

Various other indices of diastolic myocardial relaxation have been proposed. Most are imperfect, as are the ones discussed here. However, important information about diastolic relaxation and distensibility usually can be gleaned from examination of the parameters discussed in this chapter, taken in the context of the clinical setting and other hemodynamic findings in an individual patient.

Figure 17.17 Left ventricular (LV) regional area change during isovolumic relaxation before and after selective left intracoronary angiotensin-converting enzyme (ACE) inhibition with enalaprilat in patients with marked LV hypertrophy and normal coronary arteries. Because total LV volume is constant during isovolumic relaxation, the increase in anterior segment area (presumably caused by improved myocardial relaxation owing to regional ACE inhibition) is exactly counterbalanced by a decrease in inferior segment area. (From Friedrich S, et al. Intracardiac angiotensin-converting-enzyme inhibition improves diastolic function in patients with LV hypertrophy due to aortic stenosis. *Circulation* 1994;90:2761, with permission.)

REFERENCES

1. Parmley WW, Chuck L. Length-dependent changes in myocardial contractile state. *Am J Physiol* 1973;224:1194.

2. Lakatta EG. Starling's Law of the Heart is explained by an intimate interaction of muscle length and myofilament calcium activation. *J Am Coll Cardiol* 1987;10:1157.

3. Lew WYW. Time-dependent increase in left ventricular contractility following acute volume loading in the dog. *Circ Res* 1988; 63:635.

4. Wiggers CJ. Studies on the cardiodynamic actions of drugs. I: the application of the optical methods of pressure registration in the study of cardiac stimulants and depressants. *J Pharmacol Exp Ther* 1927;30:217.

5. Gleason WL, Braunwald E. Studies on the first derivative of the ventricular pressure pulse in man. *J Clin Invest* 1962;41:80.

6. Grossman W, McLaurin LP, Saltz S, et al. Changes in inotropic state of the left ventricle during isometric exercise. *Br Heart J* 1973;35:697.

7. McLaurin LP, Rolett EL, Grossman W. Impaired left ventricular relaxation during pacing induced ischemia. *Am J Cardiol* 1973; 32:751.

8. Feldman MD, Alderman J, Aroesty JM, et al. Depression of systolic and diastolic myocardial reserve during atrial pacing tachycardia in patients with dilated cardiomyopathy. *J Clin Invest* 1988;82: 1661.

9. Mason DT, Braunwald E. Studies on digitalis, IX: effects of ouabain on the nonfailing human heart. *J Clin Invest* 1963;42:1105.

10. Grossman W, Haynes F, Paraskos J, et al. Alterations in preload and myocardial mechanics. *Circ Res* 1972;31;83.

11. Brodie BR, Grossman W, Mann T, et al. Effects of sodium nitroprusside on left ventricular diastolic pressure-volume relations. *J Clin Invest* 1977;59:59.

12. Wallace AG, Skinner NS, Mitchell JH. Hemodynamic determinants of the maximal rate of rise of left ventricular pressure. *Am J Physiol* 1963;205:30.

13. Zimpfer M, Vatner SF. Effects of acute increases in left ventricular preload on indices of myocardial function in conscious, unrestrained and intact, tranquilized baboons. *J Clin Invest* 1981;67:430.

14. Broughton A, Korner PI. Steady-state effects of preload and afterload on isovolumic indices of contractility in autonomically blocked dogs. *Cardiovasc Res* 1980;14:245.

15. Barnes GE, Horwitz LD, Bishop VS. Reliability of the maximum derivatives of left ventricular pressure and internal diameter as indices of the inotropic state of the depressed myocardium. *Cardiovasc Res* 1979;13:652.

16. Gersh BJ, Hahn CEW, Prys-Roberts C. Physical criteria for measurement of left ventricular pressure and its first derivative. *Cardiovasc Res* 1971;5:32.

17. Fifer MA, Gunther S, Grossman W, et al. Myocardial contractile function in aortic stenosis as determined from the rate of stress development during isovolumic systole. *Am J Cardiol* 1979;44:1318.

18. Arentzen CE, et al. Force-frequency characteristics of the left ventricle in the conscious dog. *Circ Res* 1978;42:64.

19. Peterson KL, et al. Comparison of isovolumic and ejection phase indices of myocardial performance in man. *Circulation* 1974;49: 1088.

20. Grossman W, Brooks HL, Meister SG, et al. New technique for determining instantaneous myocardial force-velocity relations in the intact heart. *Circ Res* 1971;28:290.

21. Sharir T, Feldman MD, Haber H, et al. Ventricular systolic assessment in patients with dilated cardiomyopathy by preload-adjusted maximal power. *Circulation* 1994;89:2045.

22. Paraskos JA, et al. A non-invasive technique for the determination of velocity of circumferential fiber shortening in man. *Circ Res* 1971;29:610.

23. Krayenbuehl HP, et al. High-fidelity left ventricular pressure measurements for the assessment of cardiac contractility in man. *Am J Cardiol* 1973;31:415.

24. Ross J Jr, et al. Left ventricular performance during muscular exercise in patients with and without cardiac dysfunction. *Circulation* 1966;34:597.

25. Ross J Jr, Braunwald E. The study of left ventricular function in man by increasing resistance to ventricular ejection with angiotensin. *Circulation* 1964;29:739.

26. McLaurin LP, Grossman W, Stefadouros M, et al. A new technique for the study of left ventricular pressure-volume relations in man. *Circulation* 1973;48:56.

27. Wynne J, Green LH, Grossman W, et al. Estimation of left ventricular volumes in man from biplane cineangiograms filmed in oblique projections. *Am J Cardiol* 1978;41:726.

28. Rankin LS, Moos S, Grossman W. Alterations in preload and ejection phase indices of left ventricular performance. *Circulation* 1975;51:910.

29. Suga H, Sagawa K, Shoukas AA. Load independence of the instantaneous pressure-volume ratio of the canine left ventricle and effects of epinephrine and heart rate on the ratio. *Circ Res* 1973;32:314.

30. Weber KT, Janicki JS, Reeves RC, et al. Factors influencing left ventricular shortening in isolated canine heart. *Am J Physiol* 1976; 230:419.

31. Maughan WL, Sunagawa K, Burkhoff D, et al. Effect of heart rate on the canine end-systolic pressure-volume relationship. *Circulation* 1985;72:654.

32. Kass DA, Yamazaki T, Burkhoff D, et al. Determination of left ventricular end-systolic pressure-volume relationships by the conductance (volume) catheter technique. *Circulation* 1986;73:586.

33. Burkhoff D, Sugiura S, Yue DT, Sagawa K. Contractility-dependent curvilinearity of end-systolic pressure-volume relations. *Am J Physiol* 1987;252:H1218.

34. McKay RG, Miller MJ, Ferguson JJ, et al. Assessment of left ventricular end-systolic pressure-volume relations with an impedance catheter and transient inferior vena cava occlusion: use of this system in the evaluation of the cardiotonic effects of dobutamine, milrinone, Posicor and epinephrine. *J Am Coll Cardiol* 1986;8:1152.

35. Sagawa K, Suga H, Shoukas AA, et al. End-systolic pressure/volume ratio: a new index of ventricular contractility. *Circulation* 1981;63:1223.

36. Grossman W, Braunwald E, Mann JT, et al. Contractile state of the left ventricle in man as evaluated from end-systolic pressure-volume relations. *Circulation* 1977;45:845.

37. McKay RG, Aroesty JM, Heller GV, et al. Assessment of the end-systolic pressure-volume relationship in human beings with the use of a time-varying elastance model. *Circulation* 1986;74:97.

38. Aroney CN, Herrmann HC, Semigran M, et al. Linearity of the left ventricular end-systolic pressure-volume relation in patients with severe heart failure. *J Am Coll Cardiol* 1989;14:127.

39. Starling MR, Walsh RA, Dell'Italia LJ, et al. The relationship of various measures of end-systole to left ventricular maximum time-varying elastance in man. *Circulation* 1987;76:32.

40. Borow KM, Neumann A, Wynne J. Sensitivity of end-systolic pressure-dimension and pressure-volume relations to the inotropic state in humans. *Circulation* 1982;65:988.

41. Konstam MA, Cohen SR, Salem DN, et al. Comparison of left and right ventricular end-systolic pressure-volume relations in congestive heart failure. *J Am Coll Cardiol* 1985;5:1326.

42. Kass DA, Midei M, Graves W, et al. Use of a conductance (volume) catheter and transient inferior vena caval occlusion for rapid determination of pressure-volume relationships in man. *Cathet Cardiovasc Diagn* 1988;15:192.

43. McKay RG, Spears JT, Aroesty JM, et al. Instantaneous measurement of left and right ventricular stroke volume and pressure-volume relationships with an impedance catheter. *Circulation* 1984;69:703.

44. Little WC. The left ventricular dP/dt$_{MAX}$–end-diastolic volume relation in closed-chest dogs. *Circ Res* 1985;56:808.

45. Marsh JD, Green LH, Wynne J, et al. Left ventricular end-systolic pressure-dimension and stress-length relations in normal human subjects. *Am J Cardiol* 1979;44:1311.

46. Ross J Jr. Afterload mismatch and preload reserve: a conceptual framework for the analysis of ventricular function. *Prog Cardiovasc Dis* 1976;18:255.

47. Gunther S, Grossman W. Determinants of ventricular function in pressure-overload hypertrophy in man. *Circulation* 1979;59:679.

48. Grossman W. Cardiac hypertrophy: useful adaptation or pathologic process? *Am J Med* 1980;69:576.

49. Borow KM, Neumann A, Marcus RH, et al. Effect of simultaneous alterations in preload and afterload on measurements of left ventricular contractility in patients with dilated cardiomyopathy: comparisons of ejection phase, isovolumetric and end-systolic force-velocity indexes. *J Am Coll Cardiol* 1992;20:787.

50. Henderson Y. Volume changes of the heart. *Physiol Rev* 1923; 3:165.
51. Grossman W. Relaxation and diastolic distensibility of the regionally ischemic left ventricle. In: Grossman W, Lorell BH, eds. *Diastolic Relaxation of the Heart: Basic Research and Current Applications for Clinical Cardiology.* Boston: Martinus Nijhoff, 1988:193.
52. Glantz SA. Computing indices of diastolic stiffness has been counterproductive. *Fed Proc* 1980;39:162.
53. Zile MR. Diastolic dysfunction: detection, consequences, and treatment. Part 1. Definition and determinants of diastolic function. *Mod Concepts Cardiovasc Dis* 1989;58:67.
54. Gaasch WH, et al. Left ventricular stress and compliance in man: with special reference to normalized ventricular function curves. *Circulation* 1972;45:746.
55. Glantz SA, et al. The pericardium substantially affects the left ventricular diastolic pressure-volume relationship in the dog. *Circ Res* 1978;42:433.
56. Momomura SI, Bradley AB, Grossman W. Left ventricular diastolic pressure-segment length relations and end-diastolic distensibility in dogs with coronary stenoses: an angina physiology model. *Circ Res* 1984;55:203.
57. Lorell BH, et al. Right ventricular infarction: clinical diagnosis and differentiation from cardiac tamponade and constriction. *Am J Cardiol* 1979;43:465.
58. Vogel WM, et al. Acute alterations in left ventricular diastolic chamber stiffness: role of the "erectile" effect of coronary arterial pressure and flow in normal and damaged hearts. *Circ Res* 1982; 51:465.
59. Watanabe J, Levine MJ, Bellotto F, et al. Effects of coronary venous pressure on left ventricular diastolic chamber distensibility. *Circ Res* 1990;67:923.
60. McKay RG, Aroesty JM, Heller GV, et al. The pacing thallium test reexamined: correlation of pacing-induced hemodynamic changes with the amount of myocardium at risk. *J Am Coll Cardiol* 1984; 3:1469.
61. Lorell BH, Turi Z, Grossman W. Modification of left ventricular response to pacing tachycardia by nifedipine in patients with coronary artery disease. *Am J Med* 1981;71:667.
62. Paulus WJ, Serizawa T, Grossman W. Altered left ventricular diastolic properties during pacing-induced ischemia in dogs with coronary stenosis: potentiation by caffeine. *Circ Res* 1982;50:218.
63. Monrad ES, McKay RG, Baim DS, et al. Improvements in indices of diastolic performance in patients with congestive heart failure treated with milrinone. *Circulation* 1984;70:1030.
64. Weiss JL, Frederiksen JW, Weisfeldt ML. Hemodynamic determinants of the time-course of fall in canine left ventricular pressure. *J Clin Invest* 1976;58:751.
65. Raff GL, Glantz SA. Volume loading slows left ventricular isovolumic relaxation rate. *Circ Res* 1981;48:813.
66. Carroll JD, Hess OM, Hirzel HO, et al. Exercise-induced ischemia: the influence of altered relaxation on early diastolic pressure. *Circulation* 1983;67:521.
67. Paulus WJ, Vantrimpont PJ, Rousseau MF. Diastolic function of the nonfilling human left ventricle. *J Am Coll Cardiol* 1992;20:1524.
68. Chen C, et al. Continuous wave Doppler echocardiography for noninvasive assessment of left ventricular dP/dt and relaxation time constant from mitral regurgitant spectra in patients. *J Am Coll Cardiol* 1994;23:970.
69. Nishimura RA, Schwartz RS, Tajik AJ, et al. Noninvasive measurement of rate of left ventricular relaxation by Doppler echocardiography: validation with simultaneous cardiac catheterization. *Circulation* 1993;88:146.
70. Chong CY, Herrmann HC, Weyman AE, et al. Preload dependence of Doppler-derived indexes of left ventricular diastolic function in humans. *J Am Coll Cardiol* 1987;10:800.
71. Aroesty JM, McKay RG, Heller GV, et al. Simultaneous assessment of left ventricular systolic and diastolic dysfunction during pacing-induced ischemia. *Circulation* 1985;71:889.
72. Bonow RO, et al. Improved left ventricular diastolic filling in patients with coronary artery disease after percutaneous transluminal coronary angioplasty. *Circulation* 1982;66:1159.
73. Bonow RO, et al. Effects of verapamil on left ventricular systolic function and diastolic filling in patients with hypertrophic cardiomyopathy. *Circulation* 1981;64:787.
74. Pouleur H, Rousseau M. Regional diastolic dysfunction in coronary artery disease: clinical and therapeutic implications. In: Grossman W, Lorell BH, eds. *Diastolic Relaxation of the Heart: Basic Research and Current Applications for Clinical Cardiology.* Boston: Martinus Nijhoff, 1988:245.
75. Friedrich SP, Lorell, BH, Rousseau MF, et al. Intracardiac angiotensin-converting enzyme inhibition improves diastolic function in patients with left ventricular hypertrophy due to aortic stenosis. *Circulation* 1994;90:2761.
76. Hayashida W, Kumada T, Kohno F, et al. Left ventricular regional relaxation and its nonuniformity in hypertrophic nonobstructive cardiomyopathy. *Circulation* 1991;84:1496.
77. Mason SJ, et al. Exercise echocardiography: detection of wall motion abnormalities during ischemia. *Circulation* 1979;59:50.
78. St. John Sutton MG, Tajik AJ, Smith HC, et al. Angina in idiopathic hypertrophic subaortic stenosis. *Circulation* 1980;61:561.
79. Bourdillon PD, Lorell BH, Mirsky I, et al. Increased regional myocardial stiffness of the left ventricle during pacing-induced angina in man. *Circulation* 1983;76:316.
80. Pouleur H, et al. Force-velocity-length relations in hypertrophic cardiomyopathy: evidence of normal or depressed myocardial contractility. *Am J Cardiol* 1983;52:813.
81. Hirota Y. A clinical study of left ventricular relaxation. *Circulation* 1980;62:756.
82. Thompson DS, et al. Analysis of left ventricular pressure during isovolumic relaxation in coronary artery disease. *Circulation* 1982;65:690.
83. Nonogi H, Hess OM, Bortone AS, et al. Left ventricular pressure-length relation during exercise-induced ischemia. *J Am Coll Cardiol* 1989;13:1062.

Special Catheter Techniques

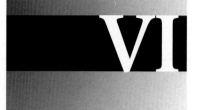

Evaluation of Myocardial Blood Flow and Metabolism

18

Morton J. Kern, MD   *Michael J. Lim, MD*

Fundamental concepts of coronary physiology and myocardial blood flow, once the subject of research studies, are now used in daily clinical practice. Despite the excellent imaging provided by coronary angiography and intravascular ultrasound, the weak correlation between luminal anatomy and coronary blood flow reserve makes such direct measurements of coronary flow physiology in the catheterization laboratory very valuable in evaluating angiographically borderline lesions and other phenomena such as no reflow. This chapter thus reviews the physiology of coronary flow regulation and the techniques most widely used to evaluate myocardial blood flow and metabolism, emphasizing catheter-based methods such as the intracoronary pressure and Doppler flow velocity guidewires.

CONTROL OF MYOCARDIAL BLOOD FLOW: THE MYOCARDIAL OXYGEN SUPPLY AND DEMAND RELATIONSHIP

The control of myocardial blood flow is based on balancing the myocardial oxygen supply and demand relationship, which states that the heart requires a sufficient quantity (supply) of oxygen for any given oxygen need (demand), to prevent ischemia or infarction. The heart is an aerobic organ that relies almost exclusively on the real-time oxidation of substrates for energy generation, with little ability to accumulate an oxygen debt as is seen with skeletal muscle. In a steady state, cardiac metabolic activity is thus accurately measured by myocardial oxygen demand

(MVO_2). The total metabolism of an arrested, quiescent heart is approximately 1.5 mL/minute per 100 gm, as required to support those physiologic processes not directly associated with contraction. In contrast, a beating canine heart has MVO_2 ranging from 8 to 15 mL/minute per 100 gm (1–3).

The heart is a relative omnivore, metabolizing substrates such as glucose, free fatty acids, lactate, amino acids, and ketones. These substrates are critical for the generation of high-energy phosphates (ATP and creatine phosphate; 3,4) that supply the energy requirements of the myocardium. At rest, the rate of force development and the frequency of force generation per unit time accounts for approximately 60% of myocardial energy use; myocardial relaxation accounts for approximately 15% of energy use; electrical activity accounts for 3 to 5%; and basal cellular metabolism accounts for the remaining 20% of energy use (5) (Fig. 18-1, Table 18-1). As workload increases, myocardial contractile function consumes an even greater fraction of high-energy phosphate availability. Any compromise in substrate availability causes the myocardium to minimize energy expenditure on mechanical work and divert the remaining high-energy substrates for the continued maintenance of cellular integrity, thus setting the stage for myocardial "hibernation" (6,7).

Under normal aerobic conditions, several substrates contribute simultaneously to meeting myocardial energy needs: free fatty acid (65%), glucose (15%), lactate and pyruvate (12%), and amino acids (5%; 3,4). Under aerobic conditions, glycolysis plays only a minor role. In fact,

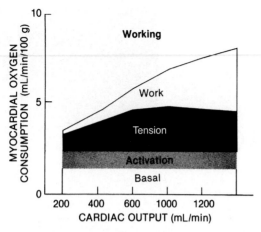

Figure 18.1 Basal metabolism, activation energy, tension-related energy, and energy for external work as components of myocardial oxygen consumption at various levels of cardiac output. (With permission from Ando H, Nakano E, Ueno Y, Tokunaga K. New techniques for analysis of cardiac energetics using a modified Fenn equation. *J Thorac Cardiovasc Surg* 1989;97:565.)

lactate is actually extracted by the myocardium, converted into pyruvate, and oxidized by way of the Krebs cycle. In the fasting state, when serum fatty acids are high, myocardial glucose uptake tends to be suppressed in favor of fatty acid utilization. But after an oral glucose load, or when a fall in myocardial blood flow or oxygen supply leads to a reduction or loss in mechanical function, glucose uptake is enhanced and fatty acid oxidation declines. Whereas glucose metabolism is preferentially aerobic, decreasing oxygen availability decreases high-energy phosphate and leads to the accumulation of ATP breakdown products (ADP, AMP, and other nucleosides). The myocardium then turns toward enhancing glycogenolysis and glycolysis to augment ATP production. In doing so, the pyruvate–lactate equilibrium is shifted toward lactate formation, causing net transmyocardial lactate production rather than extraction. Under extreme conditions, increasing cytosolic lactate and

TABLE 18.1

MYOCARDIAL OXYGEN CONSUMPTION COMPONENTS TOTAL: 6–8 ML/MIN PER 100 GM

Distribution			
Basal	20%	Volume work	15%
Electrical	1%	Pressure work	64%
Effects on $\dot{M}VO_2$ of 50% increases in			
Wall stress	25%	Heart rate	50%
Contractility	45%	Volume work	4%
Pressure work	50%		

The table demonstrates the dominant contribution to myocardial oxygen consumption ($\dot{M}VO_2$) made by pressure work and prominent effects of increasing pressure work and heart rate on $\dot{M}VO_2$. (Reproduced with permission from Gould KL. Coronary Artery Stenosis. New York: Elsevier, 1991:8.)

TABLE 18.2

DETERMINANTS OF MVO_2

Heart Rate
Contractile state
Tension development
Activation
Depolarization
Direct metabolic effect of catecholamines
Family history of coronary artery disease
Fatty acid uptake
Maintenance of active state
Maintenance of cell viability in basal state
Shortening against a load (Fenn effect)

hydrogen ion concentrations leads to inhibition of residual glycolysis, deprives the cell of even anaerobic ATP production, and begins a sequence of biochemical events that may lead to complete cessation of energy production with irreversible cellular injury.

The three major physiologic determinants of MVO_2 are heart rate, myocardial contractility, and myocardial wall tension or stress (2). Additional factors are shown in Table 18.2.

1. Heart rate is the most important determinant of MVO_2. When heart rate doubles, myocardial oxygen uptake approximately doubles. Heart rate is a dominant factor in the supply and demand ratio for two reasons: Increases in heart rate also increase oxygen consumption, and increases in heart rate reduce subendocardial coronary flow owing to shortening of the diastolic filling period. Subendocardial ischemia thus may occur during tachycardia because of simultaneously increasing demand (tachycardia) and compromised flow for the subepicardium (3).

2. Myocardial contractility is related to myocardial oxygen consumption by the degree of pressure work per heart beat. The net effect of positive inotropic stimuli (e.g., Ca^{++} and catecholamines) on MVO_2 is the result of wall tension (which declines with a reduction in heart size), and myocardial contractility (which is increased by inotropic stimuli). The decrease in MVO_2 that might be expected to result from falling ventricular wall tension is opposed by the increase in contractility, which tends to augment MVO_2. In the absence of heart failure, drugs that stimulate myocardial contractility elevate MVO_2 because heart size and therefore wall tension is not reduced substantially and does not offset the effect of enhanced contractility.

3. Myocardial wall tension is proportionate to the aortic pressure, myocardial fibril length, and ventricular volume. Myocardial oxygen consumption doubles as mean aortic pressure increases from 75 to 175 mm Hg, at constant heart rate and stroke volume. Comparing the relative effects of ventricular pressure, stroke volume,

and heart rate on MVO_2, researchers found that ventricular pressure development is a key determinant of MVO_2. MVO_2 per beat correlated well with the area under the LV pressure curve (time × pressure), termed the *tension-time index*, a more accurate determinant of MVO_2 than is the developed pressure alone (3,5). Tachycardia elevates MVO_2 by increasing the frequency of tension development per unit time, as well as by increasing contractility.

MVO_2 is also influenced by the degree of myocardial shortening during stroke volume ejection, although less so than by tension development. The systolic pressure-rate product (also known as the double product) can be used as an estimate of MVO_2 in a clinical setting, such as exercise or pacing tachycardia, recognizing the limited accuracy. MVO_2 closely correlates with the LV systolic pressure-volume loop area, the external mechanical work, the end-systolic elastic potential energy in the ventricular wall, the area enclosed by the systolic pressure-volume trajectory, and the E_{max} line.

Determinants of Myocardial Oxygen Supply

Myocardial oxygen supply is provided by blood transiting the coronary and capillary circuit at an adequate perfusion pressure (mean arterial pressure) and with a satisfactory hemoglobin function and concentration to carry and deliver oxygen to the myocardial cells. A breakdown in any linkage of the supply side factors can result in an inadequate myocardial oxygen supply and myocardial ischemia.

Regulation of Coronary Blood Flow and Resistance

Coronary arterial resistance (R, pressure/flow) is the summed resistances of the epicardial coronary conductance (R1), precapillary-arteriolar (R2), and intramyocardial capillary (R3) resistance circuits (8; Fig. 18.2). Normal epicardial coronary arteries in humans are typically 0.3 to 5 mm in caliber and do not offer appreciable resistance to blood flow. Even at the highest level of blood flow, there is no detectable resistance as would be manifest as a pressure drop along the length of human epicardial arteries (9), making large epicardial vessel resistance (R1) trivial until atherosclerotic obstructions develop. Most of the epicardial vessel wall consists of a muscular media that responds to changes in aortic pressure and modulates coronary tone in response to flow-mediated endothelium dependent vasodilators, circulating vasoactive substances, and neurohumoral stimuli. Large conduit arteries are unaffected by myocardial metabolites because of their extramural location, but can produce episodic increases in resistance during severe focal or diffuse contraction (vasospasm) in the absence of atherosclerosis. One exception is myocardial bridging, in which intramyocardial vessel segments may

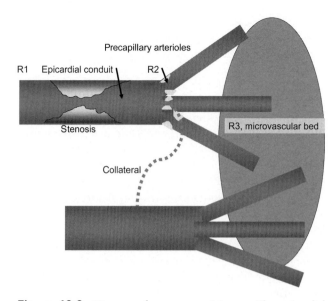

Figure 18.2 Diagram of coronary resistances. The epicardial arteries (R1) normally have negligible resistance until an atherosclerotic narrowing occurs (top artery). The precapillary arterioles (R2) regulate most of the coronary flow to the microvascular bed (R3). Diseased epicardial vessels are often connected to normal blood flow regions by collateral channels. (Modified from Dr. Bernard DeBruyne with permission.)

offer increased resistance during systole owing to mechanical compression of the bridged segment during ventricular contraction.

Changes in epicardial and arteriolar coronary resistances during physiologic or pharmacologic stimuli can be considered either primary or secondary vasomotor events (Fig. 18-3). Primary vasodilation signifies an alteration in myocardial vessel tone and perfusion with no preceding

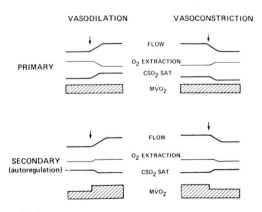

Figure 18.3 Primary and secondary coronary vasomotion as determined by the simultaneous measurement of coronary blood flow (FLOW) and coronary venous oxygen saturation (CSO$_2$ SAT). Primary vasodilation causes a rise in flow at constant myocardial oxygen consumption (MVO$_2$), resulting in lower transmyocardial oxygen extraction. In contrast, in secondary coronary vasodilation, an increase in myocardial oxygen consumption obliges a secondary rise in coronary blood flow with either constant or reduced coronary sinus oxygen saturation. (With permission from Baim DS, Rothman MT, Harrison DC. Simultaneous measurement of coronary venous blood flow and oxygen saturation during transient alterations in myocardial oxygen supply and demand. *Am J Cardiol* 1982;49:743.)

change in myocardial oxygen demand. Secondary vasodilation refers to changes in vessel tone and blood flow that occur in response to alterations in myocardial oxygen consumption (10).

Precapillary arterioles (R2) are resistive vessels connecting epicardial arteries to myocardial capillaries and are the principal controllers of coronary blood flow (8). Precapillary arterioles (100 to 500 microns in size) contribute approximately 25 to 35% of total coronary resistance. The prearteriolar resistance function autoregulates the driving pressure at the origin of the precapillary arterioles within a finite pressure range. This regulatory function is also influenced by myogenic and flow-dependent vasodilatation related to shear stress.

The microcirculatory resistance (R3) consists of a dense network of about 4,000 capillaries per square millimeter, which ensures that each myocyte is adjacent to a capillary. Capillaries are not uniformly patent because precapillary sphincters regulate flow according to oxygen demand. Several conditions, such as LV hypertrophy, myocardial ischemia, or diabetes, can impair the microcirculatory resistance (R3) and blunt the normal maximal increases in coronary flow. Increased R3 resistance may also be associated with elevated resting blood flow above that expected for the existing myocardial oxygen demand, resulting in reduced coronary flow reserve (i.e., the hyperemic/basal flow ratio).

As in any vascular bed, blood flow to the myocardium depends on the coronary artery driving pressure and the resistance produced by the serial vascular components. Coronary vascular resistance, in turn, is regulated by several inter-related control mechanisms that include myocardial metabolism (metabolic control), endothelial (and other humoral) control, autoregulation, myogenic control, extravascular compressive forces, and neural control. These control mechanisms may be impaired in diseased states, thereby contributing to the development of myocardial ischemia (Tables 18.3, 18.4).

Coronary vasodilator reserve is the ability of the coronary vascular bed to increase flow above the basal level in response to a mechanical or pharmacologic stimuli, to a maximal (or near maximal) hyperemic level. Such stimuli include the reactive hyperemia that follows transient coronary occlusion, exercise, or the administration of various pharmacologic agents. Coronary flow reserve is expressed as the ratio of maximal hyperemic flow to resting coronary flow—a ratio that averages from 4 to 7 in experimental animals and from 2 to 5 in man (11,12). In experimental animal studies, increasing conduit stenosis (R1) produces a predictable decline in coronary flow reserve, beginning at about a 60% artery diameter narrowing. At diameter stenoses >80 to 90%, all available coronary reserve has been exhausted and resting flow begins to decline (13–15; Fig. 18.4). This relationship between increasing stenosis severity and reduced available flow reserve has been used in assessing the effective physiologic severity of any given coronary lesion and forms the basis of many noninvasive test modalities for ischemia. In clinical practice for an individual patient, however, this relationship is unpredictable given complex three-dimensional anatomy, imprecise correlation between angiographic estimate of diameter stenosis reduction, and true lumen cross-sectional area.

TABLE 18.3
REGULATION OF CORONARY CIRCULATION

Mechanism	Effector
Autoregulation	Intrinsic vasoconstrictor tone
Perfusion pressure	Aortic or poststenotic pressure
Metabolic activity	Exercise, ischemia
Myocardial compression and myogenic mechanisms	Systolic-diastolic interaction
Neural control	Sympathetic, parasympathetic, pain
Endothelium	EDRF, EDCF
Pharmacologic	Dipyridamole, adenosine, acetylcholine, α-, β-agonists and antagonists, and so on

EDRF, endothelial derived relaxing factor; EDCF, endothelial derived constricting factor. Modified from Gould L. *Coronary Artery Stenosis and Reversing Atherosclerosis*, 2nd ed. New York: Arnold and Oxford University Press, 1998.

TABLE 18.4
MEDIATORS OF CORONARY VASODILATION[a]

Stimulus / Arterioles, increased flow	Epicardial arteries
Acetylcholine	
Endothelial*	Nitric oxide*
Flow shear	
Nitric oxide*	Endothelial*
Exercise	
Metabolic,* nitric oxide, neural	Nitric oxide,* neural
Pacing	
Nitric oxide,* metabolic	Nitric oxide*
Ischemia or hypoxia	
Metabolic,* nitric oxide	Metabolic,* nitric oxide
Perfusion pressure	
Myogenic*	Myogenic*
Reactive hyperemia	Myogenic, flow shear
Myogenic,* flow shear, metabolic, nitric oxide, prostacyclin	
Dipyridamole, adenosine	
Direct dilator,* nitric oxide	No direct effect
Nitroglycerine	
No direct effect	Direct dilator
Collaterals	
Nitric oxide,* prostaglandin	—

[a] Primary mechanism* followed by secondary or contributing mechanisms; endothelial, unknown mediator, not oxide; metabolic, unknown mediators or mechanisms or mechanisms but in part mediated by adenosine.
From Gould L. *Coronary Artery Stenosis and Reversing Atherosclerosis*, 2nd Ed. New York: Arnold and Oxford University Press, 1998.

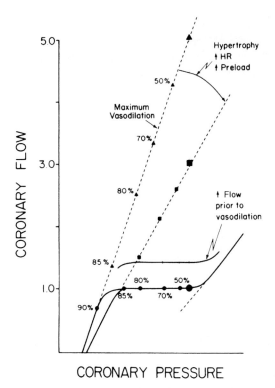

Figure 18.4 Resting and maximally vasodilated coronary pressure-flow relationships. Coronary flow reserve, the ratio of maximally vasodilated flow to resting flow, is a complex function of the actual position of the maximally vasodilated and resting flow curves. The slope of maximal vasodilation can be shifted by hypertrophy and changes in hemodynamics as can the basal flow be altered by similar events, thus explaining different CFR (maximal vasodilation/basal flow ratio) under different conditions and in different patients. (With permission from Klocke FJ. Measurements of coronary flow reserve: defining pathophysiology versus making decisions about patient care. *Circulation* 1987;76:1183.)

Furthermore, the influence of a stenosis on coronary blood flow is related principally to the morphologic features of the stenosis with resistance to flow changing exponentially with lumen cross-sectional area (the most commonly used measure of severity) and linearly with lesion length (Fig. 18.5). Additional factors contributing to stenosis resistance include the shape of the entrance and exit orifices, vessel stiffness, distensibility of the diseased segment (permitting active or passive vasomotion), and the variable lumen obstruction that may be superimposed by platelet aggregation and thrombosis compromising lumen area, a process active in acute coronary syndromes (16).

As blood traverses a diseased arterial segment, turbulence, friction, and separation of laminar flow causes energy loss resulting in a pressure gradient (ΔP) across the stenosis. Using a simplified Bernoulli formula for fluid dynamics, pressure loss across a stenosis can be estimated from blood flow as follows:

$$\Delta P = fQ + sQ^2 \tag{18.1}$$

$$\Delta P = \frac{1.8Q}{d_{sten}^4} + \frac{6.1Q^2}{d_{sten}^4} \tag{18.2}$$

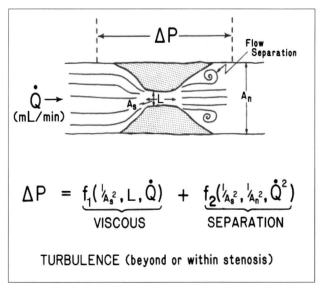

Figure 18.5 Diagrammatic illustration of the Bernoulli equation. ΔP, pressure gradient; A_s, area of the stenosis; A_n, area of the normal segment; L, stenosis length; $\dot{Q}$, flow; f_1, viscous friction factor (f); f_2, separation coefficient (s). See text for details.

where ΔP is the pressure drop across a stenosis in millimeters of mercury (mm Hg), Q is the flow across the stenosis in milliliters per second, and d_{sten} is the minimal diameter of the stenosis lumen in millimeters. In equation (18.1), the first term (f) accounts for energy losses owing to viscous friction between laminar layers of fluid and the second term (s) reflects energy loss when normal arterial flow is transformed first to high-velocity flow in the stenosis and then to the turbulent nonlaminar distal flow eddies at the exit from the stenosis (inertia and expansion).

$$f = \frac{8\pi\mu L}{A_s^2} \quad \text{and} \quad s = \frac{P}{2}\left(\frac{1}{A_n^2} - \frac{1^2}{A_s^2}\right)$$

Where A_s = stenotic segment cross-sectional area, p = blood density, μ = blood viscosity, L = stenosis length, A_n = normal artery cross-sectional area.

It is important to note that the separation energy loss term (s) increases with the square of the flow while viscous energy loss (f) becomes negligible. Thus, increases in coronary blood flow increase the associated pressure gradient in an exponential manner. Despite augmentation of coronary blood flow, the increasing pressure loss across the stenotic segment reduces myocardial perfusion pressure and lowers the threshold for myocardial ischemia relative to demand (17).

From equation (18.2), the trans-stenotic pressure drop is inversely proportional to the fourth power of the lumen radius. As a consequence, in a severe stenosis, relatively small change in luminal diameter (such as caused by active or passive vasomotion or transient obstruction by thrombus) can produce marked hemodynamic effects. For example, when the diameter stenosis is increased from 80 to 90%, the resistance of a stenosis rises nearly threefold. For most stenoses, the length of the narrowing has only a modest effect on its physiologic significance. However, in very long narrowed segments, significant turbulence occurs along the walls of the stenotic segment and energy is dissipated as heat when eddies form and impact on the vessel wall. In addition, a preserved arc of vascular smooth muscle in some diseased arteries may be compliant and subject to dynamic changes that can alter luminal caliber and stenosis resistance. Dynamic changes in stenosis severity and resistance can also occur passively in response to changes in intraluminal distending pressure or selective dilation of distal resistance vessels. Thus for a given stenosis, there is a family of pressure-flow relationships reflecting altered stenosis diameter and variable distending pressure.

Despite mild or moderate epicardial stenoses, coronary blood flow is maintained by compensatory vasodilatory regulation of the microcirculation (autoregulation). Resting coronary blood flow remains constant until epicardial luminal narrowing exceeds 85 to 90% diameter. However, unlike resting flow, maximal hyperemic coronary blood flow is attenuated when diameter stenosis approaches 45 to 60% (Fig. 18.6). The capacity to increase coronary blood flow in response to a hyperemic stimulus, called *coronary reserve* (CVR), is abolished when diameter stenosis >90%. Factors responsible for reduced CVR in absence of epicardial stenosis are shown in Table 18.5.

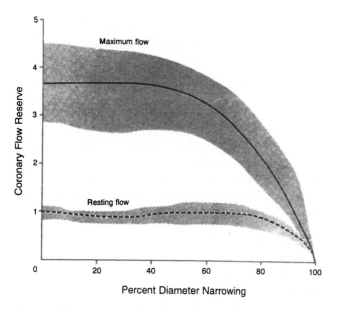

Figure 18.6 Coronary flow reserve expressed as ratio of maximum to resting flow plotted as a function of percent diameter narrowing. With progressive narrowing, resting flow does not change (*dashed line*, where as maximum potential increase in flow and coronary flow reserve begins to be impaired at approximately 50% diameter narrowing). The *shaded area* represents the limits of variability of data about the mean. (From Gould KL, Lipscomb K, Hamilton GW. Physiologic basis for assessing critical coronary stenosis: instantaneous flow response and regional distribution during coronary hyperemia as measures of coronary flow reserve. *Am J Cardiol* 1974;33:87–94.)

TABLE 18.5
FACTORS RESPONSIBLE FOR MICROVASCULAR DISEASE AND REDUCTION OF CORONARY FLOW RESERVE

Abnormal vascular reactivity
Abnormal myocardial metabolism
Abnormal sensitivity toward vasoactive substances
Coronary vasospasm
Myocardial infarction
Hypertrophy
Vasculitis syndromes
Hypertension
Diabetes
Recurrent ischemia

From Baumgart D, et al. Current concepts of coronary flow reserve for clinical decision making during cardiac catheterization. *Am Heart J* 1998; 136:136–149.

MEASUREMENT OF MYOCARDIAL METABOLISM

Measurement of myocardial metabolism may be performed noninvasively (i.e., positron emission tomography scanning) or invasively by transmyocardial sampling techniques that involve acquisition of simultaneous arterial and coronary venous (i.e., coronary sinus) blood. Specialized blood products commonly used in the determination of changes in myocardial metabolism include serum pyruvate, lactate, oxygen, and other metabolic or hematologic blood components. The transmyocardial extraction of pharmaceutical agents after systemic or intracoronary delivery can also be determined by the transmyocardial sampling for measurement of the arterial-venous concentration difference, along with measurement of blood flow per unit time.

In studies involving ischemic myocardial metabolism, the most commonly measured products are lactate and oxygen. Specialized chilled collection tubes containing an agent (perchloric acid) to stop red cell metabolism and prevent clotting are prepared. Samples should be obtained in pairs and serial containers labeled in advance of the procedure. Chemical assays need to be able to measure small differences in normal lactate levels across the myocardium. Clinical laboratory tests calibrated to high lactate levels for lactate acidosis are unsuitable for the small differences of transmyocardial measurements. Myocardial catecholamines (norepinephrine, epinephrine) and other vasoactive mediator products, such as prostaglandins, can be measured if sample tubes are placed immediately in ice to prevent platelet activation after blood withdrawal through a long narrow catheter lumen. Large-bore (≥6F) heparin-coated catheters may be required to assess platelet products.

In the setup of any measurement system for myocardial metabolism, advanced preparation of the sampling tubes and collection method should be made. Additional equipment, such as an iced bath, a centrifuge (in the laboratory), or a series of dilutional tubes may be needed. Although the techniques are not complicated, advanced preparation will facilitate studies without error or unnecessary prolongation of the study.

MEASURING MYOCARDIAL BLOOD FLOW IN THE CARDIAC CATH LAB

Historically, noninvasive techniques for measuring myocardial blood flow in patients included radionuclide tracer clearance and positron emission tomography, but recently magnetic resonance imaging has become increasingly important in the determination of myocardial blood flow and function. Catheter-based methods used in the evaluation of coronary flow include angiography, intracoronary pressure and Doppler sensor-guidewires, and coronary venous (sinus) efflux measurements.

ANGIOGRAPHIC BLOOD FLOW ESTIMATION

Since its introduction by the Thrombolysis in Myocardial Infarction (TIMI) investigators in 1985 (18), a simple, qualitative grading of angiographic coronary flow rates (Table 18.6) to assess the efficiency of reperfusion therapy has been widely used to gauge the restoration of perfusion in clinical trials. Improved TIMI flow grades are associated with improved outcomes (19–21).

A quantitative method of TIMI flow counts the number of cine frames from the introduction of dye in the coronary artery to a predetermined distal landmark. Cineangiography is performed with 6-French catheters and filming at 30 frames per second. The TIMI frame count for each major vessel is thus standardized according to specific distal landmarks. The first frame used for TIMI frame counting is that

in which the dye fully opacifies the artery origin and in which the dye extends across the width of the artery, touching both borders with antegrade motion of the dye. The last frame counted is when dye enters the first distal landmark branch. Full opacification of the distal branch segment is not required. Distal landmarks used commonly in analysis are the following: (1) for the left anterior descending (LAD), the distal bifurcation of the left anterior descending artery; (2) for the circumflex (CFX) system, the distal bifurcation of the branch segments with the longest total distance; (3) for the right coronary artery (RCA), the first branch of the posterolateral artery (22; Fig. 18.7).

The TIMI frame count (TFC) can further be corrected (corrected TIMI frame count, or CTFC) by normalizing for the length of the left anterior descending coronary artery for comparison with the two other major arteries; CTFC thus accounts for the distance the dye has to travel in the LAD relative to the other arteries (22). The average LAD coronary artery is 14.7 cm long, the right 9.8 cm, and the circumflex 9.3 cm. CTFC divides the absolute frame count in the LAD by 1.7 to standardize the distance of dye travel in all three arteries. Normal TFC and CTFC for LAD is 36 ± 3; for the CFX TFC, 22 ± 4; for the RCA TFC, 20 ± 3, but each has a CTFC of 21 ± 2. Table 18.7 provides reference values for CTFC. High CTFC may be associated with microvascular dysfunction despite an open artery, whereas CTFCs of <20 frames are associated with normal microvascular function and a low risk for adverse events in patients following myocardial infarction (Table 18.7).

The TIMI frame count method has several limitations. Gibson et al. (23) and Kern et al. (24) suggested that visual estimates of TIMI flow in the usual clinical setting bear little relationship to the quantitative TIMI frame count or measured Doppler flow velocity and that even noninfarct-related coronary arteries may show prolonged frame counts compared with normal values. Most likely, these prolonged TIMI frame counts are associated with microvascular dysfunction, even in the presence of an open artery (25). CTFCs >20 but <40 frames per second (the cutoff value for TIMI grade 3 flow) showed a higher risk for adverse outcome (26). Prolonged CTFCs 4 weeks after myocardial infarction appear to be associated with impaired infarct-artery-related flow at 1 year (26).

Injection technique can also impact on the CTFC. Using 7F diagnostic catheters, a mean increase of 1.0 mL/second of standard hand injections (10th to 90th percentile of left coronary injections: 1.5 to 2.5 mL/second; right coronary injections: 1.1 to 2.1 mL/second) induced a decrease of two frames in the CTFC (27).

To measure absolute angiographic coronary flow velocity, a guidewire can be used to determine the intravascular distance between ostium and TIMI landmark (23). The guidewire tip is positioned distally and marked with one Kelly clamp. The wire is withdrawn to the coronary ostium and marked with a second clamp, and the distance between clamps is measured. Velocity is then calculated

TABLE 18.6
TIMI FLOW GRADES

Normal distal runoff (TIMI 3) Contrast material flows briskly into and clears rapidly from the distal segment

Good distal runoff (TIMI 2) Contrast material opacifies the distal segment, but flow is perceptibly slower than in more proximal segments and/or contrast material clears from the distal segment slower than from a comparable segment in another vessel

Poor distal runoff (TIMI 1) A portion of contrast material flows through the stenosed arterial segment, but the distal segment is not fully opacified

Absence of distal runoff (TIMI 0) No contrast material flows through the stenosis

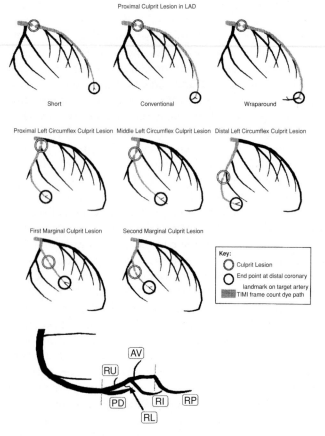

Figure 18.7 **Top.** Anatomic landmarks used for TIMI frame counting in the left anterior descending coronary artery. **Second row.** Anatomic landmarks used for TIMI frame counting in the left circumflex coronary artery. The artery used for TIMI frame counting is the artery with the longest total distance along which dye travels in the left circumflex coronary artery system and yet passes through the culprit lesion. When the culprit lesion is proximal to two arteries with equal total dye-path distances, the artery that arises more distally from the left circumflex coronary artery is used. The anatomic end point is the distalmost branch in the target artery. Usually, this end point branch can be found at approximately the midpoint of the distal third of the artery (five sixths of the distance down the vessel from its origin), but occasionally is located just before the termination of the artery. **Third row.** Anatomic landmarks used for TIMI frame counting in the RCA. (Adapted with permission from Gibson CM, Cannon CP, Daley WL, et al. TIMI frame count: a quantitative method of assessing coronary artery flow. *Circulation* 1996;93:879–888.)

using the following formula:

Velocity (cm/second)
= Distance (cm)/(frame count/frames per second)

The angioplasty guidewire velocity takes into account specific artery length in a particular patient, but its usefulness in clinical practice remains to be evaluated.

In general, TIMI frame counting is a simple, reproducible method for the assessment of angiographic coronary flow that is widely applicable and provides additional information related to treatment success and clinical outcome.

TIMI Blush Score

Angiographic successful reperfusion in acute myocardial infarction has been defined as TIMI 3 flow. However, TIMI 3 flow does not always result in effective myocardial

TABLE 18.7
REFERENCE VALUES FOR TIMI FRAME COUNTS

	Average	RCA	LCx	CTFC (LAD)	LAD
Normal	21.0 ± 3.1 (16–31)	20.4 ± 3.0 (16–26)	22.2 ± 4.1 (16–31)	21.1 ± 1.5 (18.8–24.1)	36.2 ± 2.6 (32–41)
Nonculprit at 90 minutes	25.5 ± 9.8 (10–57)	24.6 ± 7.1 (13–36)	22.5 ± 8.3 (10–52)	30.6 ± 11.5 (16.5–57.1)	52.0 ± 19.6 (28–97)
Culprit at 90 minutes	39.2 ± 20.0 (13–164.7)	37.2 ± 19.3 (13–112)	33.7 ± 9.0 (19–51)	43.8 ± 22.6 (17.1–164.7)	74.5 ± 38.4 (29–280)

TIMI Frame Counts and Corrected TIMI Frame Counts (CTFC) in coronary arteries without epicardial stenoses (normal) and in non-culprit and culprit arteries 90 minutes after myocardial infarction. Where RCA is right coronary artery, LCx is left circumflex coronary artery, and LAD is left anterior descending coronary artery. Values are expressed as frames ± standard deviation and 95% confidence intervals. (Adapted with permission from Gibson CM, Cannon CP, Daley WL, et al: TIMI frame count: a quantitative method of assessing coronary artery flow. Circulation 1996;93:879–888.)

reperfusion. Myocardial blush grade (MBG) is an angiographic measure of myocardial perfusion at the capillary level (28). MBG is defined as follows: 0 indicates no myocardial blush or contrast density; 1 indicates minimal myocardial blush or contrast density; 2 indicates moderate myocardial blush or contrast density, but less than that obtained during angiography of a contralateral or ipsilateral non–infarct-related coronary artery; and 3 indicates normal myocardial blush or contrast density, comparable with that obtained during angiography of a contralateral or ipsilateral non–infarct-related coronary artery (29). When myocardial blush is persistent (staining), this suggests leakage of contrast medium into the extravascular space and is also graded 0. To determine blush grading, the length of the angiographic run is needed to visualize the venous phase of the contrast passage. When the left coronary artery is involved, use the left lateral view. When the right coronary artery is involved, use the right oblique view. MBG after primary angioplasty for acute myocardial infarction appears to be an important prognostic feature and should be added to the commonly used TIMI flow grading to define successful angiographic reperfusion with primary angioplasty for acute myocardial infarction (29).

Coronary Venous Efflux

The measurement of coronary venous flow can be performed using coronary sinus thermodilution technique with only right heart cardiac catheterization. Coronary sinus blood flow (CSBF) is an approximation of blood flow to the left ventricle. Approximately two thirds of left anterior descending coronary artery flow drains into the great cardiac vein, the continuation of the anterior intraventricular vein as it reaches the atrioventricular groove. The great cardiac vein then becomes the coronary sinus at the point marked by the valve of Vieussens and the oblique vein of Marshall (a left atrial venous remnant of the embryonic left-sided superior vena cava). The remaining portion of left anterior descending venous drainage enters the coronary sinus along with blood from the circumflex territory by way of the left marginal vein and circumflex venous branches. Great cardiac vein flow thus represents primarily left anterior descending venous outflow, whereas coronary sinus flow represents a mixture of both left anterior descending and left circumflex coronary artery outflow, accounting for 80 to 85% of total left coronary outflow drained by this route (30).

Measurement of coronary venous flow is based on the principle of thermodilution, which states that the heat loss by the blood equals the heat gained by a cold indicator solution (Fig. 18.8). Room temperature fluid (5% dextrose or normal saline) is continuously infused by a control pump upstream in the coronary sinus. Coronary venous flow is then computed by the temperature reduction of blood indicator mixture flowing over the proximal catheter thermistor. A full discussion of CSBF is available elsewhere (31–33).

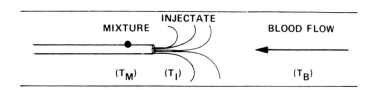

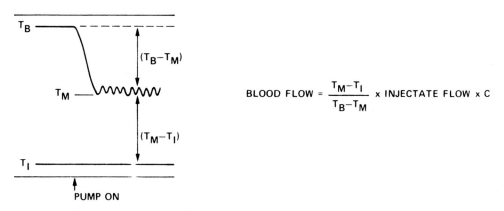

$$\text{BLOOD FLOW} = \frac{T_M - T_I}{T_B - T_M} \times \text{INJECTATE FLOW} \times C$$

Figure 18.8 Schematic diagram of the thermodilution technique. The thermal indicator (injectate) at temperature T_I is infused at a fixed rate, typically 50 mL/minute. The ensuing turbulence causes mixing of the injectate with coronary venous blood at temperature T_B, resulting in a mixture at temperature T_M. The temperatures monitored by the catheter tip (T_B and T_M) and injectate thermistors (T_I) are recorded continuously on a uniform temperature scale. Because the heat lost by blood is gained by the injectate, coronary venous flow can be calculated using the respective measured temperatures, the rate of indicator injection, and a constant derived from the specific heats of blood and injectate. (With permission from Bradley BA, Baim DS. Measurement of coronary blood flow in man: methods and implication for clinical practice. *Cardiovasc Clin* 1984;14:67.)

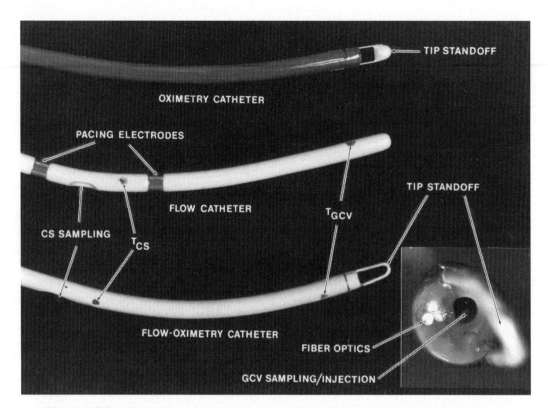

Figure 18.9 Coronary venous oximetry, thermodilution flow, and combined flow-oximetry catheters **(top to bottom).** The flow and flow-oximetry catheters have the following features in common: two lumina for indicator injection or sampling at the great cardiac vein (see inset) and coronary sinus sites and two great cardiac vein (T_{GCV}) and coronary sinus (T_{CS}) thermistors for regional flow determinations. The flow catheter additionally has two pacing electrodes. The oximetry and flow-oximetry catheters have fiberoptic bundles for the continuous measurement of great cardiac vein oxygen saturation. (With permission from Baim DS, Rothman MT, Harrison DC. Simultaneous measurement of coronary venous flow and oxygen saturation during transient alterations in myocardial oxygen supply and demand. *Am J Cardiol* 1982;49:743.)

Coronary sinus catheters are available only on special request for investigational studies (Cordis Webster, Baldwin Park, CA; Baim Electro-catheter, Rahway, NJ; Fig. 18.9). Special features of these catheters include pacing electrodes to facilitate the measurements at a constant heart rate by coronary sinus pacing, or reflectance oximetry sensors allowing the continuous measurement of great cardiac vein oxygen saturation and permitting online determination of regional myocardial oxygen consumption (MVO_2) computed as follows (10):

$$MVO_2 = Q \times (AO_2 - CSO_2)$$

where Q equals coronary venous flow, AO_2 is arterial oxygen content, and CSO_2 is coronary sinus oxygen content.

Coronary Sinus Cannulation Technique

The coronary sinus is located posteriorly and slightly caudal to the tricuspid annulus. The CS catheter with a single curve easily enters the ostium of the coronary sinus from a superior approach. The left brachial vein access is thus often preferred. Although a right brachial or femoral venous approach is feasible using a reverse loop technique, the easiest approach to the coronary sinus is still through the right internal jugular vein. After entering the right atrium, the catheter is rotated counterclockwise and advanced slightly until it just enters the right ventricle (detected by pressure waves or premature ventricular contractions). After slight additional counterclockwise rotation, the catheter is then withdrawn slowly until an atrial pressure tracing is restored. Gentle readvancement of the catheter from this position leads to cannulation of the coronary sinus. Should the right ventricle be re-entered, the same maneuver is repeated with accentuation of counterclockwise rotation.

Successful coronary sinus entry is confirmed by the maintenance of a right atrial pressure waveform as the catheter is smoothly advanced across the plane of the tricuspid valve. During catheter advancement, catheter resistance suggests impingement on venous branches or the valve of Vieussens. If slight catheter repositioning fails to correct the situation, the anatomic obstacle can usually be crossed with a 0.014-inch soft-tipped angioplasty guidewire, allowing advancement of the catheter over this wire to reach the desired sampling site in the great cardiac vein. The coronary sinus is a thin-walled venous structure

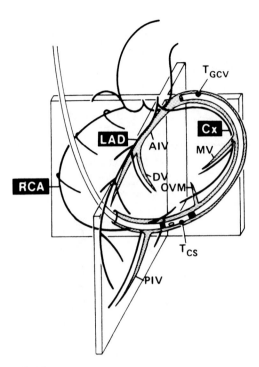

Figure 18.10 Schematic diagram of the cannulated coronary venous system in relation to the coronary artery anatomy: diagonal vein (DV), anterior interventricular vein (AIV), marginal vein (MV), oblique vein of Marshall (OVM), posterior interventricular vein (PIV), and the right, left anterior descending, and circumflex coronary arteries (RCA, LAD, Cx, respectively). (With permission from Baim DS, Rothman MT, Harrison DC. Simultaneous measurement of coronary venous flow and oxygen saturation during transient alterations in myocardial oxygen supply and demand. *Am J Cardiol* 1982;49:743.)

that can be easily perforated with the application of force. Correct intravascular position should be confirmed before catheter manipulation.

Reproducible coronary sinus or venous flow measurements require a stable catheter position, avoiding variable inclusion of blood entering from venous tributaries adjacent to the temperature thermistor. The most stable position for the catheter tip is near the point where the anterior interventricular vein meets the great cardiac vein, providing a selective measurement of left anterior descending coronary artery territory outflow (Fig. 18.10). The principal use of coronary venous measurements is determination of transmyocardial metabolism of blood products or drugs using the arterial-coronary sinus differences per unit flow.

MEASUREMENTS OF INTRACORONARY PRESSURE AND FLOW VELOCITY USING SENSOR-TIPPED GUIDEWIRES

Measurements of intracoronary blood flow velocity or translesional pressure can be used to determine the functional significance of a coronary stenosis. Directly measured physiologic data provide critical information, complementary

to the anatomic information and often useful for clinical decision-making (34).

Technique of Angioplasty Sensor-Guidewire Use

After diagnostic angiography or during angioplasty, the sensor angioplasty guidewire is passed through a standard Y connector attached to either the diagnostic or guiding catheter (5 or 6F catheters are suitable). Intravenous (IV) heparin 40 to 60 units/kg is given before introducing the guidewire. Intracoronary (IC) nitroglycerin (100 to 200 μg) is also given several minutes before the guidewire is advanced to minimize coronary vasomotion.

For flow velocity, the Doppler sensor, located at the very distal guidewire tip (Fig. 18.11A–C) is advanced at least 5 to 10 artery-diameter lengths (>2 cm) beyond the stenosis to measure laminar flow (otherwise the turbulent flow close to the stenosis may underestimate true velocity). Resting flow velocity is recorded, and then coronary hyperemia is induced by IC or IV adenosine with continuous recording of the flow velocity. Coronary vasodilatory reserve (CVR) is computed as the ratio of maximal hyperemic to basal average peak velocity (APV; Fig. 18.12). Because of the highly position-dependent signal, poor signal acquisition may occur in 10 to 15% of patients even within normal arteries. As with transthoracic echo Doppler studies, the operator must adjust the guidewire position (sample volume) to optimize the velocity signal.

To measure translesional pressure gradients for the calculation of the pressure-derived fractional flow reserve (FFR; 34), the pressure sensor, located 3 cm *proximal* to the wire tip, is advanced in the guide catheter to the coronary ostium. The sensor pressure is matched to the guide catheter pressure. The guidewire is then advanced into the artery with the sensor beyond the stenosis. The distance beyond the stenosis is not critical. Baseline pressure is recorded, followed immediately by induction of coronary hyperemia with IC or IV adenosine, continuously recording both guide catheter and sensor-wire pressures. FFR is computed as the ratio distal coronary to aortic pressure at maximal hyperemia occurring at the lowest distal coronary pressure (Fig. 18.13). For small guide catheters, flushing with saline will reduce pressure wave damping. Signal drift can be detected by observation of the pressure waveform (35). The safety of intracoronary sensor-wire measurements is excellent, with benign problems related mostly to adenosine. Severe transient bradycardia after IC adenosine occurs in <2.0% of patients, coronary spasm during passage of the Doppler guide wire in 1%, and ventricular fibrillation during the procedure in 0.2% of patients (36).

Coronary Hyperemia

Stenosis severity should always be assessed using measurements obtained during maximal hyperemia. At maximal

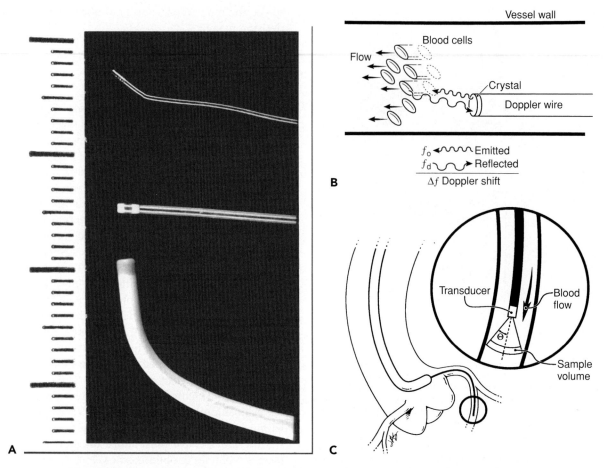

Figure 18.11 **A.** Top to bottom: sensor angioplasty guidewire, 1F tracking catheter, 6F diagnostic angiographic catheter. Ruler is in 1-mm divisions. **B.** Diagram of the Doppler concept. High-frequency ultrasound (f_o) is admitted from the Doppler crystal and is reflected off the moving red cell at frequency f_d. The difference between these two frequencies is termed the *Doppler shift* and is directly related to the velocity of red cells moving. (With permission from Kern MJ, Aguirre FV, Bach RG, Caracciolo EA, Donohue TJ, Labovitz AJ. Fundamentals of translesional pressure-flow velocity measurements. *Cathet Cardiovasc Diagn* 1994;31:137–143.) **C.** Diagram of coronary Doppler FloWire placed in the proximal segment of a coronary artery through a diagnostic catheter. The 12-MHz transducer has a sample volume located approximately 5.2 mm from the tip with a beam spread of 27°. The angle of incidence (theta) is <17°. Magnitude and direction of flow are easily determined by the spectral flow velocity. (With permission from Ofili EO, Kern MJ, Labovitz AJ, et al. Analysis of coronary blood flow velocity dynamics in angiographically normal and stenosed arteries before and after endolumen enlargement by angioplasty. *J Am Coll Cardiol* 1993;21:308–316.)

hyperemia, autoregulation is abolished and coronary blood flow is directly related to the driving pressure. Therefore, maximal hyperemic coronary blood flow is closely dependent on the coronary arterial pressure at the time of the measurement, a fact that is used in the derivation of pressure-derived fractional coronary flow reserve of the myocardium.

The most basic form of coronary hyperemia is reactive hyperemia. When a coronary artery is transiently occluded, release of the occlusion (reperfusion) is followed by a marked increase in coronary flow, a response termed *reactive hyperemia*. Reactive hyperemia follows an occlusion as short as 200 milliseconds. Maximal reactive hyperemia occurs after coronary occlusion of 20 seconds. Longer occlusion periods increase the duration but not the amplitude of hyperemia.

The most widely used pharmacologic agents to induce coronary hyperemia in the cath lab are papaverine and adenosine. The hyperosmolar ionic and low-osmolar, nonionic contrast media do not produce maximal vasodilatation. Nitrates increase volumetric flow, but since these agents also dilate epicardial conductance vessels, the increase in coronary flow velocity is less than with adenosine or papaverine. Intracoronary papaverine (8 to 12 mg) increases coronary blood flow velocity four to six times over resting values in patients with normal coronary arteries (37) and produces a response equal to that of an IV infusion of dipyridamole in a dose of 0.56 to 0.84 mg/kg

Coronary Flow Velocity and Reserve

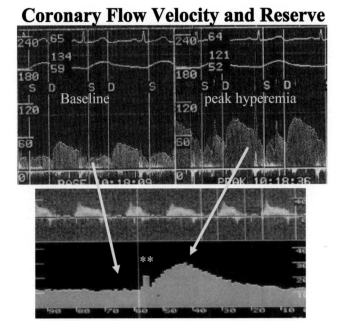

Figure 18.12 Coronary Doppler flow velocity signals used for the measurement of coronary flow velocity reserve in the cardiac cath lab. **Top.** Baseline signals *(left)* and peak hyperemic velocity signals *(right)*. Phasic flow velocity tracing is demarcated by systolic (S) and diastolic (D) markers, corresponding to the electrocardiogram and aortic pressure at top. Diastolic flow predominates over systolic flow. (The flow velocity scale is from 0 to 240 cm per second. **Bottom.** Continuous trend plot of average peak velocity showing the baseline and time course of peak hyperemia. The intracoronary bolus adenosine injection can be seen by the square wave signal preceding the rapid increase in average peak velocity. The phasic peak hyperemic velocity signal was captured and displayed in the upper right panel. In the bottom view, the trend plot scale is from 0 to 60 cm per second with a time base of 0 to 90 seconds. In this example, baseline flow is 13 cm per second and peak hyperemic flow is 30 cm per second for a coronary flow reserve of 2.3.

of body weight, but can cause QT prolongation occasionally and ventricular tachycardia or fibrillation (38).

Adenosine is a potent short-acting hyperemic stimulus with the total duration of hyperemia only 25% that of papaverine or dipyridamole (39). Adenosine is benign in the appropriate dosages (20 to 30 μg in the right coronary artery and 30 to 60 μg in the left coronary artery or infused intravenously at 140 μg/kg per minute). Because of a sustained hyperemia, some investigators prefer IV to IC adenosine. Jeremias et al. (40) compared IC (15 to 20 μg in the right and 18 to 24 μg in the left coronary artery) with IV adenosine (140 μg/kg per minute) and found a strong linear relationship between the two methods (r = 0.978 and P < 0.001). The mean measurement difference for FFR was −0.004 +/− 0.03. In 8% of cases, IC adenosine FFR was >0.05 units different from IV FFR. Thus, in a small percentage of cases, maximal coronary hyperemia requires increased IC adenosine doses. Table 18.8 lists the characteristics of adenosine and papaverine for use in coronary flow studies.

Other agents that produce maximal coronary hyperemia include ATP and dobutamine. Coronary flow reserve

was equivalent with ATP and papaverine (41) with IC ATP doses >15 μg. IV dobutamine (10 to 40 μg/kg per minute) has also been used to assess lesion severity with FFR (42). Compared with IV adenosine, peak dobutamine infusion produced similar distal coronary pressure and pressure ratios (P_d/P_a 60 ± 18 versus 59 ± 18 mm Hg; FFR 0.68 ± 0.18 and 0.68 ± 0.17, respectively; all P = NS). Moreover, high-dose IV dobutamine did not modify the angiographic area of the epicardial stenosis, and much like adenosine, fully exhausted myocardial resistance regardless of inducible left ventricular dysfunction.

MEASUREMENT OF CORONARY FLOW RESERVE

Coronary flow reserve (CFR), also known as coronary vasodilatory reserve (CVR) or coronary flow velocity reserve (CFVR), is defined as the ratio of maximal to basal coronary flow and is a measure of the ability of both the epicardial artery and the microvascular resistances to achieve maximal blood flow. There are two methods available for measuring coronary blood flow reserve in the catheterization laboratory: intracoronary Doppler flow velocity and coronary thermodilution.

Coronary Doppler Flow Velocity

Coronary Doppler measures the velocity of red blood cells moving past the ultrasound emitter/receiver on the end of a Doppler-tipped angioplasty guidewire (Fig. 18.11A). Coronary flow velocity is calculated from the difference between the transmitted and returning frequency (called the *Doppler frequency shift*), using the following equation:

$$V = \frac{(F_1 - F_0)C}{2F_0 (\cos \phi)}$$

where V is the velocity of blood flow, F_0 is the transmitting (transducer) frequency, F_1 is the returning frequency, C is a constant (speed of sound in blood), and ϕ is the angle of incidence.

When the transducer beam is nearly parallel to blood flow (cosine ϕ = 1), velocity can be accurately measured. Changes in blood flow velocity are reflected by changes in the Doppler frequency shift. The Doppler technique measures red blood cell velocity directly so that, unlike thermodilution, indicator-dilution markers are not required. Because the Doppler guidewire has a cross-sectional area of 0.164 mm^2, it is generally considered to be nonobstructive within any but the tightest coronary lesions. Easily recognized phasic coronary flow-velocity measurements are useful for assessing physiologic responses to mechanical and pharmacologic interventions in any small vessel (<5 to 6 mm diameter) without complex technical maneuvers (Fig 18.14). Volumetric flow can be estimated as the product of vessel area (cm^2) and flow velocity

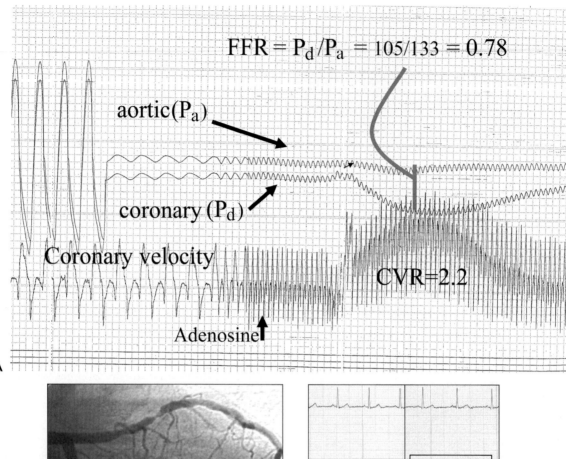

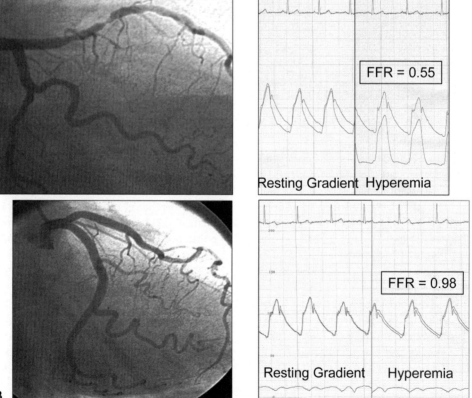

Figure 18.13 **A.** Pressure-derived fractional flow reserve (FFR) is the ratio of distal coronary pressure (P_d) divided by aortic pressure (P_a) at maximal hyperemia. In this example, a coronary flow velocity tracing is also provided demonstrating the maximal decline P_d occurs at peak velocity after intracoronary adenosine. FFR = 0.78 while coronary vasodilating reserve (CVR) = 2.2, both values above the ischemic threshold. (Courtesy of Dr. B. DeBruyne.) **B.** *Top left*: Angiogram of LAD with midvessel stenosis. *Top right*: Resting and Hyperemia gradient with FFR calculated at 0.55 (55/100 mm Hg). *Bottom left*: Angiogram after LAD stent. *Bottom right*: Resting and hyperemia gradients with FFR now normal (0.98). (Courtesy of Dr. B. DeBruyne.)

TABLE 18.8

CHARACTERISTICS OF PAPAVERINE AND ADENOSINE FOR CORONARY FLOW STUDIES

Drug	Dose	Plateau	T1/2	Side Effect	Pitfall
Papaverine IC	15 mg LCA 10 mg RCA	30–60 sec	2 min	Transient QT prolongation and T-wave abnormalities; very rarely. Ventricular tachycardia/torsade des pointes	Do not use guiding catheter with side holes.
Adenosine IC	30–50 mg LCA 20–30 mg RCA	5–10 sec	30–60 sec	No side effects: sometimes AV block during a few seconds after Injection in RCA	Submaximum stimulus in some patients interruption of aortic pressure Peak hyperemia may already have passed before arterial pressure has adjusted. Maximum gradient underestimated when calculated from mean signal, unless it is taken on beat-to-beat basis. No pullback curve possible. Guiding catheters with side holes confound calculation and may underestimate maximum gradient.
Adenosine IV	140 mg/kg per min	≤1–2 min	1–2 min	Decrease of blood pressure by 10–15%. Burning or angina-like chest pain during Infusion. (harmless, not ischemia) Not to be used in patients with severe Obstruction lung Disease. (bronchospasm)	If peripheral vein is used, avoid kinking of arm/elbow and avoid Valsalva maneuvers Withdraw guiding catheter slightly out of ostium if any sign of obstruction of the ostium is observed, or if guiding catheter with side holes is used.

Modified from Pijls NHJ, Kern MJ, Yock PG, De Bruyne B. Practice and potential pitfalls of coronary pressure measurement. *Cathet Cardiovasc Intervent* 2000;49:1–16.

(cm/second), yielding a value in cm^3/sec. Absolute Doppler flow velocities represent changes in volumetric coronary flow when the vessel cross-sectional area remains constant over the measurement period. Compared with volumetric measurements, velocity may underestimate the volumetric flow reserve in some vessels that demonstrate intact endothelial mediated vasodilation.

Guidewire Thermodilution Blood Flow Technique

The coronary thermodilution technique uses thermistors on a pressure-sensor angioplasty guidewire and measures the arrival time of room temperature saline bolus indicator injections through the guiding catheter into the coronary artery (43,44). The shaft of the angioplasty pressure-monitoring guidewire (PressureWire 3, Radi Medical Systems) has a temperature-dependent electrical resistance and acts as a proximal thermistor, which allows for the detection of the start of the indicator (saline) injection (Fig. 18.15A). A microsensor mounted 3 cm from the tip also enables simultaneous high-fidelity pressure measurements. Pressure and temperature are sampled at a frequency of 500 Hz. The wire is connected to a dedicated interface (RADI Analyzer, Radi Medical Systems) with modified software for online analysis of the thermodilution curves (Fig. 18.15B).

Thermodilution CFR (CFR$_{thermo}$) is defined as the ratio of hyperemic flow divided by resting coronary flow (F).

$$CFR = \frac{F \text{ at hyperemia}}{F \text{ at rest}} \qquad (18.3)$$

Flow is the ratio of the volume (V) divided by transit time (T$_{mn}$). Thus, CFR can be expressed as follows.

$$CFR = \frac{\left(\dfrac{V}{T_{mn}}\right) \text{ at hyperemia}}{\left(\dfrac{V}{T_{mn}}\right) \text{ at rest}} \qquad (18.4)$$

Assuming the epicardial volume (V) remains unchanged, CFR can be calculated as follows.

$$CFR = \frac{T_{mn} \text{ at rest}}{T_{mn} \text{ at hyperemia}} \qquad (18.5)$$

In animal experiments, a significant linear relation was found between flow velocity and $1/T_{mn}$. A significant correlation was found between CFR$_{Doppler}$, which was calculated from the ratio of hyperemic to resting flow velocities, and CFR$_{thermo}$, which was calculated from the ratio of resting to hyperemic T$_{mn}$ ($r = 0.76$; SEE (standard error of the estimate) $= 0.24$; $P < 0.001$; 44). Simultaneous measurements of CFR and FFR are thus obtained for research

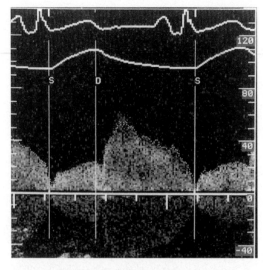

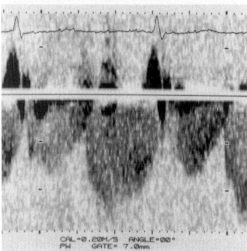

Figure 18.14 Comparison of coronary spectral flow velocity by two Doppler techniques. **Top.** Flow velocity spectra in a normal coronary artery using the intracoronary Doppler guidewire. **Bottom.** Flow velocity in the left anterior descending artery obtained with transesophageal echocardiography. Note the similarities of phasic pattern, although the direction of flow is inverted for the transesophageal Doppler signal. Scale for top view is 0 to 160 cm/second; scale for bottom view is 20 cm/division. Peak flow velocity for both signals is approximately 50 cm/second.

studies on coronary resistance. When combined with post-stenotic pressure measurements, coronary flow reserve measurements can provide a complete description of the pressure-flow relationship and the response of the microcirculation.

Normal Coronary Flow Velocity

Because the microvascular circulation is subject to biological variations between individuals, the range of normal coronary flow velocities at baseline and during hyperemia is large. In one study, simultaneous flow-velocity measurements were performed in the proximal and distal segments of 55 angiographically normal coronary arteries (45). The normal proximal left anterior descending and

circumflex time-averaged peak velocity was approximately 25 to 30 cm/second with peak diastolic velocity ranging from 40 to 50 cm/second and peak systolic velocity ranging from 10 to 20 cm/second. In the right coronary artery and in some distal left coronary locations, flow velocity values may be reduced by 15 to 20%. There was no difference in the phasic patterns of flow in the proximal and distal velocities in normal arteries at baseline or during hyperemia, with a diastolic predominant pattern (diastolic/systolic flow velocity ratio >1.5) in all arterial segments.

Normal CFR in young patients with normal arteries commonly exceeds 3.0 (Fig. 18.16; 46). In adult patients with chest pain undergoing cardiac catheterization with angiographically normal vessels, the CFR averages 2.7 ± 0.64 and is related, in part, to comorbid conditions such as hyperlipidemia, hypertension, or diabetes mellitus (47). CFR values <2.0 have been associated with inducible myocardial ischemia on stress testing (48). Changes in heart rate, blood pressure, and contractility alter CFR by changing resting basal flow or maximal hyperemic flow or both. Tachycardia increases basal flow, reducing CFR. Increasing mean arterial pressure reduces maximal vasodilatation, reducing hyperemic flow more than basal flow. CFR may be reduced in patients with essential hypertension and normal coronary arteries and in patients with aortic stenosis and normal coronary arteries. Diabetes mellitus increases basal flow and independently reduces coronary flow reserve, especially in patients with diabetic retinopathy owing to reduced volumetric coronary blood flow (velocity times vessel cross-sectional area) during hyperemia and higher baseline flow in diabetic patients with and without retinopathy compared with controls (49).

Relative Coronary Flow Velocity Reserve

Because CVR is the summed response of the two major coronary flow resistances (epicardial and microvascular), an abnormal value cannot distinguish between increased epicardial resistance or microvascular flow impairment (Fig. 18.17). To identify the site of flow impairment, a relative CVR (rCVR) can be calculated as the ratio of maximal flow in the coronary with stenosis (Q_S) to flow in a normal coronary without stenosis (Q_N), assuming basal flows are the same. The rCVR is independent of the aortic pressure and heart rate pressure product and is well suited to assess the physiologic significance of coronary stenoses. Using coronary flow velocity in the catheterization laboratory, rCVR is defined as the ratio of CVR$_{target}$ to CVR in an angiographically normal reference vessel, (rCVR = $(Q_s/Q_{base})/(Q_N/Q_{base})$ = (CVR$_{target}$/CVR$_{reference}$)). Use of this ratio assumes that basal flow in the two vessels is similar and that the microcirculatory response is uniform in the regions measured (Fig. 18.18). A normal range for rCVR is 0.8 to 1.0 (50). rCVR cannot be used in patients with three-vessel coronary disease who have no suitable reference vessel. Because it relies on the assumption that the

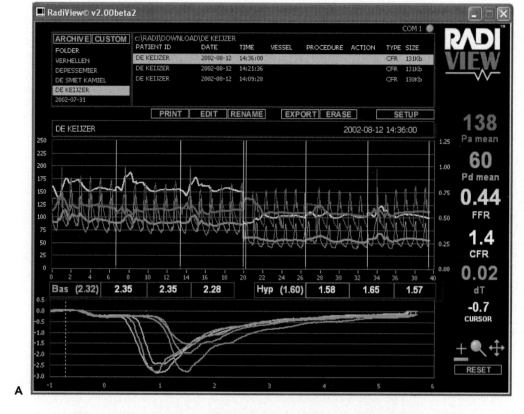

Simultaneous Pressure-Derived FFR and Thermodilution CFR

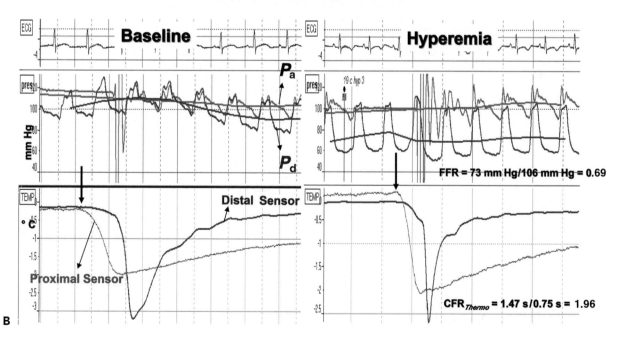

Figure 18.15 Simultaneous pressure **(A)** and temperature **(B)** signal for calculation of FFR and thermodilution coronary flow reserve (CFR). The top tracings represent central aortic pressure (Pa), distal coronary pressure (Pd), and FFR (Pd/Pa). The lower tracings are temperature tracings recorded by the proximal (shaft) and distal sensors. The half-time of injection was derived from the proximal thermodilution curve. CFR is calculated from the distal thermodilution. (Courtesy of Radi Medical, Uppsala, Sweden.)

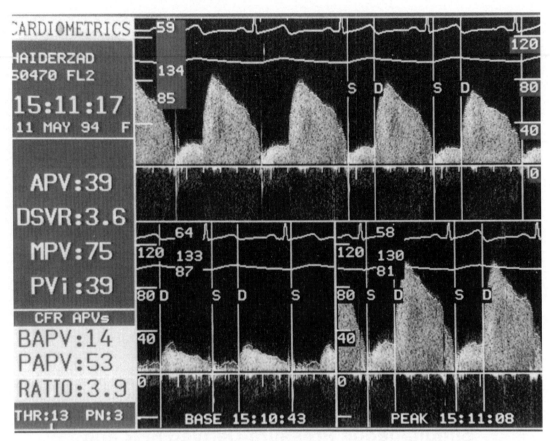

Figure 18.16 Measuring coronary vasodilatory reserve using flow velocity. Spectral flow-velocity signals are displayed in a continuous strip along the top view with heart rate and systolic and diastolic blood pressure displayed in the upper left corner box. The phasic signal demonstrates a normal hyperemic velocity with a small systolic component and a large diastolic component. Systolic and diastolic periods are demarcated by the S and D, respectively. The lower view is split into two sections: baseline *(left)* and hyperemic response *(right)*. Baseline average peak velocity (BAPV) is 14 cm/second. The peak hyperemic flow velocity obtained 25 seconds later after 18 µg of intracoronary adenosine is a peak average peak velocity (PAPV) of 53 cm/second, producing a coronary vasodilatory reserve (ratio) of 3.9. The diastolic/systolic velocity ratio (DSVR) is 3.6. The maximal peak velocity (MPV) is 75 cm/second, and the peak velocity integral (PVi) is 39 units.

microvascular circulation is uniformly distributed, rCVR is of no value in patients with myocardial infarction, LV regional dysfunction, or patients in whom the microcirculatory responses are heterogeneous. Continuous measurement of coronary flow velocity is useful for pharmacologic studies in patients during cardiac catheterization (Fig. 18.19). Because of the inherent difficulties and variability of both absolute and relative coronary flow velocity measurements, pressure-derived measurements are the preferred invasive method of physiologic stenosis assessment.

Measurement of Translesional Pressure-Derived Fractional Flow Reserve

Using coronary pressure distal to a stenosis measured at constant and minimal myocardial resistances (i.e., maximal hyperemia), Pijls et al. (51) derived an estimate of the percentage of normal coronary blood flow expected to go through a stenotic artery. This pressure-derived ratio is called the fractional flow reserve (FFR) and can be subdivided into three components describing the flow contributions by the coronary artery, the myocardium, and the collateral supply. FFR of the coronary artery (FFR_{cor}) is defined as the maximum coronary artery flow in the presence of a stenosis divided by the theoretic normal maximum flow of the same artery (i.e., the maximum flow in that artery if no stenosis were present). Similarly, FFR of the myocardium (FFR_{myo}) is defined as maximum myocardial (artery and bed) flow distal to an epicardial stenosis divided by its value if no epicardial stenosis were present. Stated another way, FFR represents that fraction of normal maximum flow that remains despite the presence of an epicardial lesion. The difference between FFR_{myo} and FFR_{cor} is FFR of the collateral flow.

The following equations are used to calculate the FFR of a coronary artery and its dependent myocardium:

$$FFR_{cor} = (P_d - P_w)/(P_a - P_w)$$

$$FFR_{myo} = (P_d - P_v)/(P_a - P_v)$$

$$FFR_{collateral} = FFR_{myo} - FFR_{cor}$$

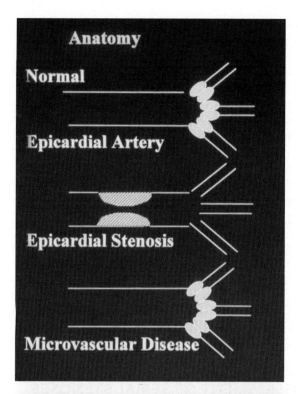

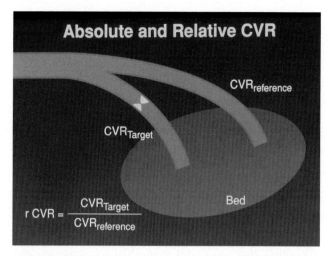

Figure 18.18 Relative coronary flow reserve (rCVR) is equal to $CVR_{target}/CVR_{reference}$. rCVR depends on the assumption that the microvascular bed is the same for both arteries and will therefore permit distinguishing the impact of a stenosis on the target vessel coronary reserve compared with CVR in an unobstructed reference vessel.

where P_a, P_d, P_v, and P_w are pressures of the aorta, distal artery, venous (or right atrial), and coronary wedge (during balloon occlusion) pressures, respectively; because FFR_{cor} uses P_w, it can be calculated only during coronary angioplasty. FFR_{myo} can be readily calculated during either diagnostic or interventional procedures (Fig. 18.13). FFR reflects both antegrade and collateral myocardial perfusion rather than merely trans-stenotic pressure loss (i.e., a stenosis pressure gradient). Because it is calculated only at peak hyperemia, FFR is differentiated from CVR by being largely independent of basal flow, driving pressure, heart rate, systemic blood pressure, or status of the microcirculation (52).

In contrast to the resting or hyperemic pressure gradient, FFR is strongly related to provocable myocardial ischemia demonstrated by comparisons with different clinical stress testing modalities in patients with stable angina. The nonischemic threshold value of FFR is >0.75. In patients with an abnormal microcirculation, it can be

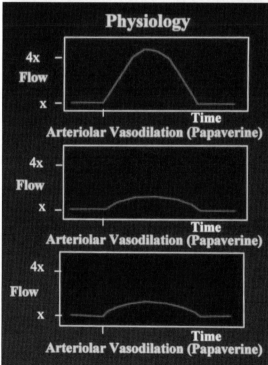

Figure 18.17 Interaction of the two major components of coronary flow reserve. **Top.** The two components, the epicardial artery and microcirculation, when both are normal produce a normal coronary flow velocity reserve greater than three times basal flow. **Center.** When there is an epicardial stenosis and normal microcirculation, coronary flow reserve is impaired. **Bottom.** When there is microvascular disease and a normal epicardial, coronary artery flow reserve is also impaired. Coronary flow reserve alone thus cannot differentiate between an epicardial stenosis and an impaired microvascular disease. (Modified from Wilson RF and Laxson DD. Caveat emptor–a clinician's guide to assessing the physiologic significance of arterial stenoses. Cathet Cardiovasc Diagn 1993, 29:93–98).

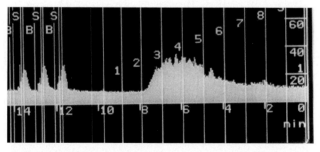

Figure 18.19 Continuous Trent plot of Doppler average peak velocity. Time base is in 2-minute intervals from 0 to 14 minutes. Vertical velocity axis is 0 to 60 cm/second. On the left side are three intracoronary adenosine hyperemic responses. B, baseline point; S, search point; and the following line is the peak velocity point. Numbered lines are event markers for minutes after intravenous bolus of adenosine A2a agonist drug.

argued that a normal FFR indicates the conduit resistance is not a major contributing factor to perfusion impairment, and that focal conduit enlargement (e.g., stenting) would not restore normal perfusion. FFR is thus specific for stenosis resistance and by design excludes the assessment and influence of the microcirculation.

Pijls et al. (35) reviewed potential pitfalls of coronary pressure measurements. Suitable guide catheters can be as small as 5F and commonly 6F guides, preferably without side holes. For best pressure fidelity, contrast should be flushed out of the catheter and replaced with normal saline. If catheter side holes are present, increasing intracoronary bolus doses of adenosine may be needed since excess drug can exit the side holes.

Verification and matching of pressures between the ascending aorta and sensor wire is important prior to crossing the lesions. Both pressure signals should be equal prior to crossing the lesion. Adjustment of fluid-filled transducer height to match the wire signal can be made before crossing the lesion. Matching of pressure transducer zero positions is also important. The guide catheter pressure zero is generally fixed to a reference height estimated to be approximately 5 cm below the sternum at the level of the right atrium. However, this estimation may be incorrect; the real aortic pressure may be different from the sensor wire when measured below the level of the atrium, depending on the course of the artery being studied. Decreasing the transducer level will increase the aortic pressure, thus assisting in the match when these two signals are not identical.

Validation of matched pressures after lesion assessment by pullback pressure recordings will identify signal drift. The withdrawal of the sensor proximal to the stenosis in question with the distal wire across the lesion will identify proximal signal equivalency to eliminate questions of drift. Often pressure waveforms (especially the dicrotic notch) across a critical stenosis will be changed and thus further identify the presence of signal drift.

Other pitfalls include pressure leakage through retained guidewire introducer or a loose Y connector. Damping of the pressure by the guiding catheter may occur with contrast media within the small guiding catheters (Fig. 18.20). With regard to guide catheter side holes, the pressure signal recorded to a side-hole guide catheter does not necessarily correspond to the proximal segment of the coronary artery since aortic pressure enters the guide through these holes. Because of the presence of the catheter, the actual proximal coronary pressure may be lower than that recorded by the catheter.

ASSESSMENT OF SERIAL STENOSES

An essential prerequisite for the calculation of FFR is the achievement of maximum transstenotic flow. In case of two consecutive stenoses, the blood flow interaction

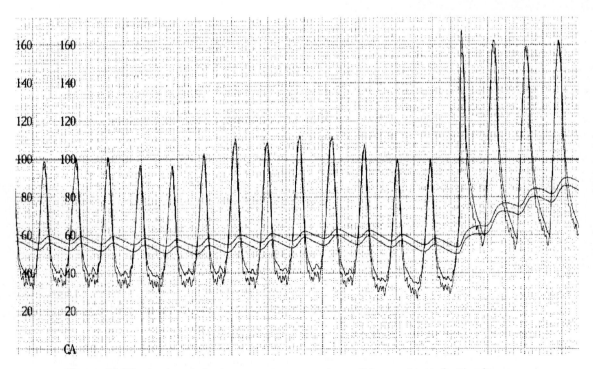

Figure 18.20 Aortic and distal coronary pressure across ostial narrowing. Left side of pressure tracings show features of guide catheter damping, which is also reflected in the distal pressure. On withdrawal of the guide catheter (toward right side of tracing), normal pressure waveforms can be seen.

between the stenoses limits the applicability of the simple FFR ratio (P_d/P_a) for a single stenosis. When a second stenosis is present in the same epicardial vessel, flow through one stenosis will be submaximal because of the second stenosis. The extent to which both stenoses influence each other is thus unpredictable. In this case, the simple FFR does not predict to what extent a proximal lesion will influence myocardial flow until complete relief of the second stenosis and restoration of maximal hyperemia. The simple FFR can assess the summed effect across any series of stenosis, but individual lesions in the series will be more difficult to appreciate without special calculations (53).

Individual FFR of each stenosis separately can be predicted by different equations using P_a, pressure between the two stenoses (P_m), P_d, and P_w, recorded during maximum hyperemia, thus reducing the error of FFR calculation in the presence of a second stenosis (Fig. 18.21A,B; 54). The serial FFR formula requires P_w obtained during coronary balloon occlusion and thus is not applicable for diagnostic studies alone.

In the examination of a single stenosis out of several in series, the worst stenosis, as indicated by the largest pressure drop during hyperemia, may not occur where it would have been expected from angiography. In that case, the equations for FFR_{pred} can be applied to each stenosis rather than the simple ratio P_d/P_a to determine the severity of each. In clinical practice, the measurements of P_a, P_m, and P_d can be obtained during a simple pullback of the pressure sensor from the distal to the proximal part of the vessel under maximum hyperemia (Fig. 18.21C).

SIMULTANEOUS PRESSURE-FLOW VELOCITY (P-V) RELATIONSHIPS

In a manner similar to that proposed by Gould et al., Marques et al. (55) showed that the pressure-velocity flow relationships (P-V) could effectively characterize mild, moderate, and severe human coronary stenoses. P-V data demonstrated that the variability of microvascular resistance contributed to discrepancies between fractional flow reserve and coronary blood flow velocity reserve in intermediate coronary lesions (56) with concordance between FFR and CFR occurring in 73% of patients (Fig. 18.22). Minimum microvascular resistance (the ratio of mean distal pressure to average peak blood flow velocity during hyperemia) was significantly higher in patients with FFR >0.75 and CFR <2.0. A hyperemic stenosis resistance index (defined as the ratio of hyperemic stenosis pressure gradient [mean aortic minus mean distal pressure] divided by hyperemic average peak velocity) had better agreement with single photon emission computed tomography (SPECT) scanning in lesions with discordant FFR and CFR (57). Thus, combined P-V measurements for research

describe the contribution of both the epicardial and microvascular resistance to myocardial perfusion.

CLINICAL APPLICATIONS OF CORONARY BLOOD FLOW MEASUREMENTS

The physiologic criteria for a hemodynamically significant coronary lesion include one or more of the following when using flow velocity: (a) poststenotic absolute coronary flow reserve (CVR) <2.0; (b) relative coronary flow reserve (rCVR) <0.8; (c) proximal-to-distal flow velocity ratio (P/D) <1.7; (d) diastolic-to-systolic velocity ratio (DSVR) <1.8; (e) when using pressure-sensor guidewires, the fractional flow reserve (FFR) threshold is <0.75.

Strong correlations exist between myocardial ischemic stress testing and FFR or CFR. An FFR of <0.75 identified physiologically significant stenoses associated with inducible myocardial ischemia with high (>90%) sensitivity, specificity, positive predictive value, and overall accuracy (58–60). An abnormal CFR (<2.0) corresponded to reversible myocardial perfusion imaging defects with high (>90%) sensitivity, specificity, predictive accuracy, and positive and negative predictive values (33). The AHA/ACC recommendations (61) for use of physiologic measurements during invasive procedures are provided in Table 18.9.

Deferral of Coronary Intervention

For intermediate stenoses, FFR or CFR values above the ischemic thresholds have been used to safely defer coronary interventions with adverse clinical event rates of <10% over a 2-year follow-up period (62–65). Despite excellent safety, some patients with deferred procedures may still have recurrent angina, but when physiologically normal, the functional and clinical impact of angiographically intermediate stenoses is associated with an excellent clinical outcome. As with other tests at a single point in time, in-laboratory translesional hemodynamics may not reflect the episodic ischemia-producing conditions of daily life related to changes in vasomotor changes, exercise, or emotional stress.

Fractional flow reserve can be used to determine the appropriateness of angioplasty. Bech et al. (65) studied 325 patients with intermediate coronary stenosis without documented myocardial ischemia. When FFR was >0.75, patients were randomly assigned to a percutaneous coronary intervention (PCI) deferral group ($n = 91$) or a performance group ($n = 90$). If FFR was <0.75, PTCA was performed as planned and these patients ($n = 144$) were followed as the reference group. At clinical follow-up, the event-free survival was similar between the deferral and performance groups (92% versus 89% at 12 months; 89% versus 83% at 24 months), but significantly lower in the

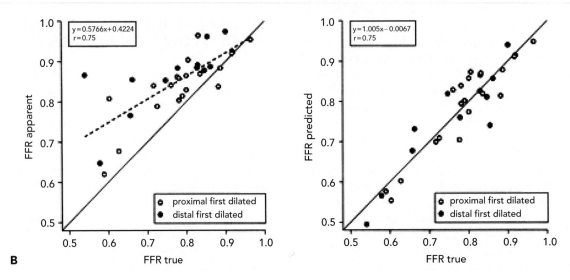

A

$$FFR(A)_{pred} = \frac{P_d - [(P_m/P_a) \times P_w]}{(P_a - P_m) + (P_d - P_w)}$$

B

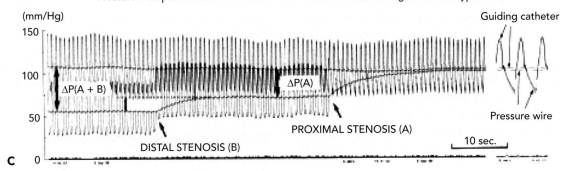

C

Pressure wire pulled back from distal LAD in ostium of I.CA during sustained hypercmia

Figure 18.21 A. Formulas for predicted FFR for lesions A and B in series, P_a, aortic pressure; P_m, pressure between A and B; P_d, distal artery pressure; P_w, coronary occlusion pressure. **B.** Influence of the presence of one stenosis within a coronary artery on the hemodynamic effect of the other. *Filled circles* indicate patients in whom the proximal stenosis was treated first; *open circles* indicate patients in whom the distal stenosis was treated first. *Left:* With increasing severity of one stenosis, the underestimation of the hemodynamic severity of the other stenosis becomes more pronounced. The solid line is the line of identity, and the dashed line is the regression line for measured data. *Right:* the regression line almost coincides with the line of identity and therefore is not visible. (From Pijls NHJ, de Bruyne B, Bech GJ, et al. Pressure measurement to assess the hemodynamic significance of serial stenoses within one coronary artery validation in humans. *Circulation* 2000;102:2371, with permission.) **C.** Example of coronary pressure measurement in patient with two stenoses within same artery. During sustained maximum coronary hyperemia, the pressure wire is pulled back slowly from the distal coronary artery to the tip of the guiding catheter. Phasic and mean aortic pressures are measured by the guiding catheter, and phasic and mean coronary pressures by the pressure wire. When the pressure sensor crosses either of the stenoses, a pressure gradient is registered *(arrows)*. Both the location and severity of each stenosis can be determined precisely by such a hyperemic pullback pressure recording. LAD, left anterior descending artery; LCA, left coronary artery; P, change in pressure. (From Pijls NHJ, de Bruyne B, Bech GJ, et al. Pressure measurement to assess the hemodynamic significance of serial stenoses within one coronary artery validation in humans. *Circulation* 2000;102:2371, with permission.)

reference group (80% at 12 months and 78% at 24 months). The percentage of patients free from angina was similar between the deferral and the performance group at 24 months, but there was a significantly higher incidence of angina in the reference (PCI) group (67% versus 50% at 12 months and 80% versus 50% at 24 months). In patients with coronary stenosis, FFR identifies those patients who will benefit from PCI and also indicates that performance of PCI in physiologic nonischemic lesions provides no additional benefit.

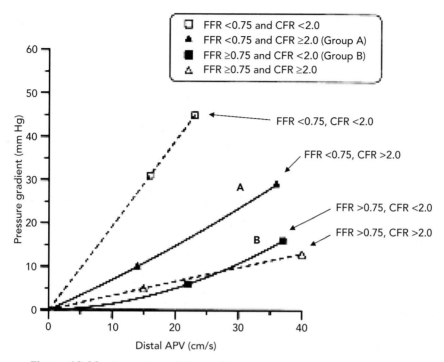

Figure 18.22 Comparison of FFR and CFR in 150 patients. Data are categorized on the basis of threshold values. Group A, FFR <0.75 and CFR >2.0. Group B, FFR >0.75 and CFR l<2. (From Meuwissen M, Chamuleau S, Siebes M, et al. Role of variability in microvascular resistance on fractional flow reserve and coronary blood flow velocity reserve in intermediate coronary lesions. *Circulation* 2001;103:184–187.)

TABLE 18.9

RECOMMENDATIONS FOR INTRACORONARY PHYSIOLOGIC MEASUREMENTS (DOPPLER ULTRASOUND, FFR)

Class IIa	Level of Evidence
1. Assessment of the physiologic effects of intermediate coronary stenosis (30–70% luminal narrowing) in patients with anginal symptoms. Coronary pressure of Doppler velocimetry may also be useful as an alternative to performing noninvasive functional testing (e.g., when the functional study is absent or ambiguous) to determine whether an intervention is warranted.	B

Class IIb	
1. Evaluation of the success of percutaneous coronary revascularization in restoring flow reserve and to predict the risk of restenosis	C
2. Evaluation of patients with anginal symptoms without an apparent angiographic culprit lesion	C

Class III	
1. Routine assessment of the severity of angiographic disease in patients with a positive, unequivocal noninvasive function study.	C

Smith SC Jr, et al. ACC/AHA Guidelines for Percutaneous Coronary Intervention. (Revision of the 1993 PTCA guidelines)—executive summary. *J Am Coll Cardiol* 2001;37:2215–2238.

FFR after stenting also predicts adverse cardiac events at follow-up. Pijls et al. (66) examined 750 patients from a multicenter study. Postprocedural FFR >0.90 was associated with the lowest 2-year event rate (<10%). In 36% of patients, FFR normalized after stenting (>0.95) with an event rate of 5%. In 32% of patients with post-FFR between 0.90 and 0.95, the event rate was 6%. In the remaining 32% with FFR <0.90, event rates were 20%. In 6% of patients with FFR <0.80, the event rate was 30% (Fig. 18.23). The lower FFRs may be owing to either edge stent subnormalization and/or diffuse disease and were associated with worse long-term outcome.

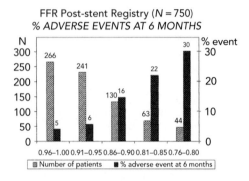

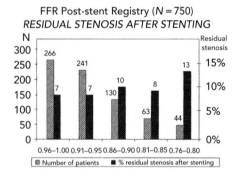

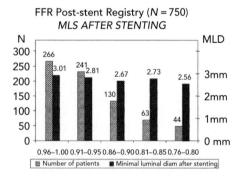

Figure 18.23 Clinical outcome of stenting and relationship to FFR. **Top.** Distribution of the study population over the five FFR categories. A strong inverse correlation was present between FFR after stenting and event rate at 6-month follow-up. **Center.** Distribution of percentage residual stenosis in the five FFR categories. **Bottom.** Minimal luminal diameter (MLD) in the five FFR categories. (Reproduced with permission from Pijls NHJ, Klauss V, Siebert U, et al. Coronary pressure measurement after stenting predicts adverse events at follow-up. A multicenter registry. *Circulation* 2002;105:2950–2954.)

Normalization of CFR occurs in only 50% of patients after PTCA alone owing to angiographically inapparent residual lumen obstruction. After stenting, CFR may normalize in 80% of patients corresponding to improved lumen area as the mechanism responsible for improved coronary blood flow (67). The remaining 20% of patients with widely patent stents had impaired CFR (<2.0) attributed to microvascular disease and/or transient emboli from PCI. A low post procedural CFR has been associated with a worse periprocedural outcome (68).

Assessment of Diffuse Atherosclerosis

A diffusely diseased atherosclerotic coronary artery can be viewed as a series of branching resistance units diverting and gradually distributing flow and reducing perfusion pressure along the length of the conduit. Diffuse atherosclerosis, in contrast to a focal narrowing, is characterized by a continuous and gradual pressure recovery as the sensor moves from the distal to proximal arterial region without a localized abrupt increase in pressure related to an isolated stenosis. De Bruyne et al. (10) examined FFR in normal and diffusely atherosclerotic nonstenotic arteries (Fig. 18.24A,B). FFR in the normal group was 0.97 ± 0.02 and was significantly lower, 0.89 ± 0.08, in the diffuse disease group. In 8% of arteries in the diffusely diseased group without a focal narrowing, FFR was <0.75, a value below the ischemic threshold (Fig. 18.24C). For diffuse atherosclerosis, mechanical therapy to treat impaired flow would be futile.

Acute Myocardial Infarction

Measurements of coronary blood flow or pressure during or immediately after treatment of acute myocardial infarction may not represent true lesion physiology because of the dynamic nature of both the stenosis and recovery response of the microcirculation. In patients with acute myocardial infarction studied no earlier than 6 days, De Bruyne et al. (69) found that a normal FFR was indicative of reversal of myocardial perfusion defects. Excluding false-positive and negative studies, the corresponding sensitivity, specificity, and predictive accuracy of acute MI FFR values were 87%, 100%, and 94%, respectively. A FFR >0.75 distinguished patients after myocardial infarction with negative perfusion scintigraphic imaging.

Postinfarction myocardial viability is associated with preservation of the microcirculation as reflected by characteristic phasic flow velocity patterns (Fig. 18.25; 70–72). After acute MI, recanalization phasic patterns of coronary flow differentiated the patients with TIMI 2 versus TIMI 3 angiographic flow. Patients with reduced average peak velocity (APV) and prolonged diastolic deceleration time and small diastolic-to-systolic velocity ratio had better LV recovery than those with systolic flow reversal, a rapid deceleration time, and negative diastolic-to-systolic flow

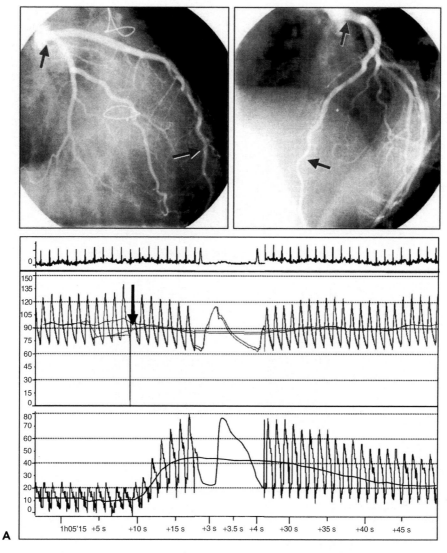

Figure 18.24 **A.** Angiograms, FFR, and coronary flow-velocity data in normal artery. Coronary pressure and aortic pressure remain identically matched during maximal hyperemia in arteries without evidence of atherosclerosis. **B.** Example of a 44-year-old man with stable angina pectoris. A tight stenosis in the mid-RCA was treated by angioplasty. The coronary angiogram of the LAD *(top)* did not show any focal stenosis, but luminal irregularities suggested diffuse atherosclerosis. Aortic (red) and distal coronary pressure (blue) recordings *(bottom)* during adenosine-induced maximal hyperemia show a pressure gradient of 23 mm Hg (corresponding to a FFR of 0.76) when the pressure sensor is located in the distal LAD. This pressure gradient indicates that the diffusely atherosclerotic artery is responsible for approximately one fourth of the total resistance to blood flow. When the sensor is slowly pulled back, a graded, continuous increase in distal coronary pressure is observed, which indicates diffuse atherosclerosis, not focal stenosis. The exact locations of aortic and distal coronary pressure measurements are indicated by the *arrows*. **C.** Graphs of individual values of FFR in normal arteries and in atherosclerotic coronary arteries without focal stenosis on arteriogram. The upper dotted line indicates the lowest value of FFR in normal coronary arteries. The lower dotted line indicates the 0.75 threshold level. (Reproduced with permission from De Bruyne B, Hersbach F, Pijls NHJ, et al. Abnormal epicardial coronary resistance in patients with diffuse atherosclerosis but "normal" coronary angiography. *Circulation* 2001;104:2401–2406.

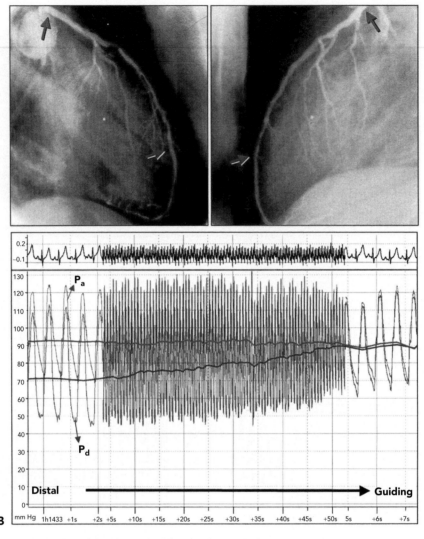

B

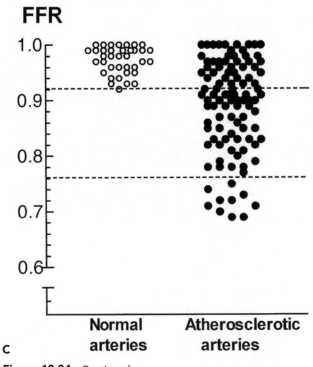

FFR

C   **Normal arteries**   **Atherosclerotic arteries**

Figure 18.24 Continued.

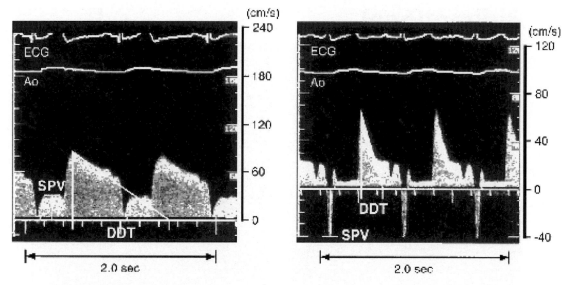

Figure 18.25 Phasic flow-velocity signals in patients with acute myocardial infarction demonstrating diastolic deceleration time (DDT) and systolic flow reversal (SPV). A rapid DDT and the presence of SPV is associated with poor myocardial functional recovery after infarction. (From Kawamoto T, et al. Can coronary blood flow velocity pattern after primary percutaneous transluminal coronary angioplasty predict recovery of regional left ventricular function in patients with acute myocardial infarction? *Circulation* 1999;100:339, with permission.)

velocity ratio. Similarly, after acute myocardial infarction, patients in whom APV increased after only a transient decline had better LV systolic functional recovery (ejection fraction increased 17 ± 9%) than those in whom the APV progressively decreased throughout the next day (ejection fraction increased only 4 ± 9%; $P = 0.007$; 70). These findings suggest that maneuvers that might maintain or augment coronary blood flow (e.g., an intra-aortic balloon pumping or adenosine) could be monitored to determine the impact on myocardial salvage.

QUANTITATIVE ASSESSMENT OF COLLATERALS IN THE CATH LAB

The four methods for assessing collaterals in the living patient are angiography, sensor-tipped flow and pressure angioplasty guidewire measurements, and noninvasive perfusion imaging techniques. Angiography and noninvasive perfusion techniques are discussed elsewhere (73–75).

Intracoronary Doppler Flow Velocity

Intracoronary doppler flow velocity measurements provide a quantitative estimate of epicardial detectable coronary flow. The physiologic response of the coronary collateral circulation to various drugs, maneuvers, and interventions can thus be determined by flow changes in patients during coronary balloon angioplasty.

Collateral flow velocity can be measured in either the ipsilateral or contralateral artery during coronary balloon occlusion. During angioplasty, the sensor guidewire is advanced into either the target (ipsilateral) artery beyond the stenosis (at least 5 to 10 arterial diameters, approximately 2 cm) or into an unobstructed contralateral reference vessel. For ipsilateral flow, an angioplasty balloon is then advanced and inflated, occluding any antegrade flow (Fig. 18.26A). Ipsilateral flow-velocity changes during balloon occlusion demonstrate different types of collateral flow (76). The most commonly observed types of flow are divided into combinations of monophasic or biphasic and antegrade or retrograde (Fig. 18.26B). The largest angiographic collaterals generally have the greatest ipsilateral flow velocity. However, acutely recruited epicardial collateral flow (i.e., not previously visualized by angiography) is also easily detected with this method (77).

Alternatively, collateral flow can be quantified by measuring velocity change in a nondisease contralateral artery during brief balloon occlusion of the diseased vessel. This approach also permits calculation of collateral vascular bed resistance. Piek et al. (78) examined contralateral artery velocity in 38 patients undergoing single vessel coronary angioplasty. Mean aortic pressure and coronary occlusion (wedge, P_w) pressure were used for the calculation of collateral vascular resistance ($R = P_w/P_a$). A significant transient increase in flow velocity during brief occlusion was noted in 15 patients with collateral vessels compared with 8 patients without (5 ± 1% versus 23 ± 17%, $P < 0.001$). The relative resistance of the collateral vascular bed was significantly reduced when collateral vessels were present during coronary occlusion (4 ± 4 versus 17 ± 5 units, $P < 0.001$). Electrocardiographic signs of ischemia

Bidirectional

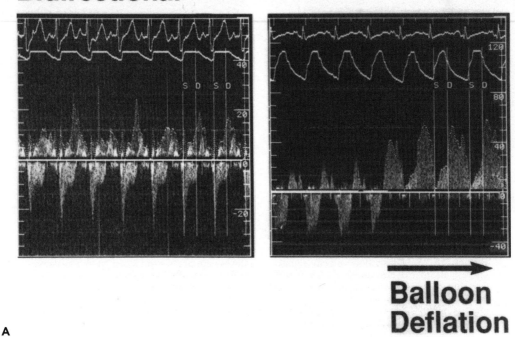

**Balloon
Deflation**

A

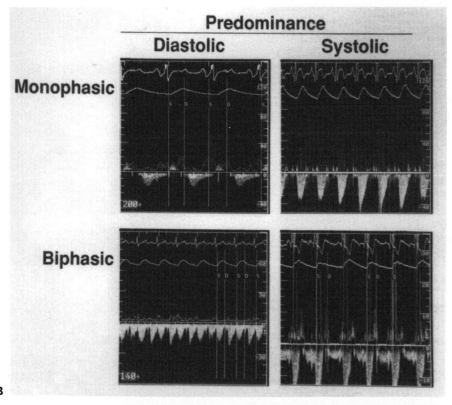

B

Figure 18.26 **A.** Changes in coronary flow velocity before, during and after balloon occlusion in a patient undergoing coronary angioplasty of the right coronary artery. *Left:* Bidirectional collateral flow during occlusion. *Right:* Large retrograde flow velocity that quickly changes to antegrade flow on balloon deflation. **B.** The four types of phasic epicardial collateral flow velocity seen during balloon occlusion. *Top:* Monophasic signals with systolic and diastolic predominance. *Bottom:* Biphasic flow demonstrates systolic and diastolic predominance. The direction of flow depends on the location of the wire relative to the input source of collateral flow. If a septal connection to an epicardial vessel is proximal to the wire, flow will be antegrade. If distal to the flow velocity tip of the guidewire, the flow may well be retrograde.

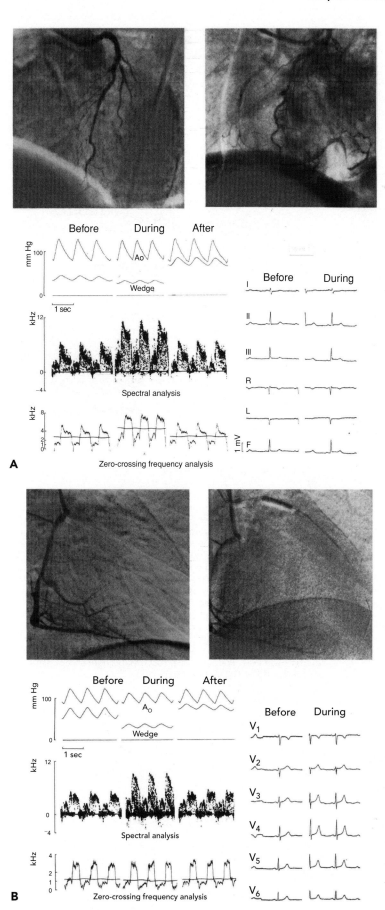

Figure 18.27 **A.** *Top:* Contrast injection of the left anterior descending coronary artery, LAO projection, before *(left)* and during *(right)* occlusion of the right coronary artery. Distal opacification of collateral vessels is evident. *Bottom left:* Aortic pressure, AO, distal coronary lesion pressure before, during (wedge), and after balloon inflation as well as simultaneously obtained Doppler tracings. *Bottom right:* Electrocardiogram before inflation and at 1 minute of coronary occlusion of the right coronary artery. The presence of collateral vessels during balloon occlusion coincide with 50% change in flow velocity of left anterior descending coronary artery from baseline values during coronary occlusion. (Piek JJ, van Liebergen RAM, Koch KT, et al. *Circulation* 1997;96:106–115.) **B.** *Top:* Contrast injection in the right coronary artery before *(left)* and during *(right)* occlusion of the LAD. *Bottom left:* The distal vessel is opacified by collaterals. Aortic and distal coronary artery pressure and Doppler flow velocity tracings during coronary occlusion. *Bottom right:* ECG before balloon inflation at 1 minute coronary occlusion of the LAD demonstrates collateral vessels during balloon inflation produces 65% change in flow velocity in the right coronary artery from baseline values. There are no ECG changes at 1 minute of coronary occlusion in this patient. (Piek JJ, van Liebergen RAM, Koch KT, et al. *Circulation* 1997;96:106–115.)

were less present in 15 patients with collateral vessels (Fig. 18.27A,B); that is, they demonstrated contralateral collateral flow during balloon occlusion.

Another calculation to quantify the presence and degree of collaterals is a Doppler-derived *collateral flow index* (CFI; 79–81), defined as the amount of flow via collaterals to a vascular region (velocity during occlusion, V_{occl}), divided by the amount of flow to the same region via the normally patent vessel (velocity, V_o). The velocity is the integral of both systolic and diastolic flow velocities during balloon occlusion. Bidirectional flow velocity signals, (the antegrade and retrograde velocity integrals) are added together. V_{occl}/V_o after successful PCI is the formula for CFI. A Doppler CFI >0.30 accurately predicts a collateral circulation sufficient to prevent myocardial ischemia during PCI (Fig. 18.28). The Doppler CFI is also a more sensitive determinant of collateral flow compared with angiographically visible collateral circulation.

Additional calculations of collateral flow can be derived from velocity and pressure and include the velocity integral (Vi) during balloon occlusion, the ratio of coronary wedge pressure to aortic pressure (Pw/Pa) during balloon occlusion, and the collateral resistance index (R_{coll}) calculated as aortic pressure minus wedge pressure divided by the flow-velocity integral. In patients with acutely recruitable collateral flow, in contrast to spontaneously visible collaterals, pharmacologic challenge with adenosine and nitroglycerin did not induce spontaneous change in diastolic velocity integral or the Pw/Pa ratio (82,83). The predominant mechanism of the improved collateral function is a decrease in the resistance in collateral vascular resistance and increase in vascular resistance of the recipient coronary artery.

Quantitatively determined collateral flow, specifically the CFI, also relates to future ischemic events. In 450 patients with stable coronary artery disease over a 2-year follow-up period (84), patients with CFI >0.25 had substantially reduced events compared with those with CFI <0.25 (2.2% of patients with good CFI had major cardiac events versus 9% among patients with poorly developed collaterals).

Intracoronary Pressure

Coronary back pressure during coronary occlusion reflects the degree of collateral filling. Collateral flow contribution to overall myocardial blood flow has been described by Pijls et al. (85,86). The fractional flow reserve (FFR) calculations account for coronary, myocardial, and collateral blood flow. The calculation of collateral fraction flow reserve is determined as follows:

Compute myocardial fraction flow reserve (FFR_{myo}):

$$FFR_{myo} = 1 - \Delta P/P_a - P_v$$
$$= P_d - P_v/P_a - P_v$$
$$= P_d/P_a$$

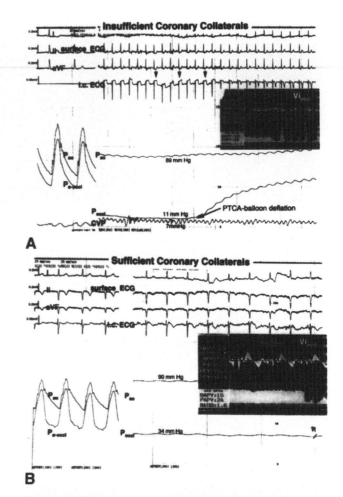

Figure 18.28 Schematic of occluded collateralized coronary artery on the left and of a pressure and Doppler flow velocity recording for the calculation of CFI and pressure CFI. Pressure and Doppler derived CFI, CFIp, and CFIv are determined by measuring intracoronary pressure during coronary occlusion, P_{occl} equals 46 mm Hg on right and blood flow velocity $V_{subocclusion}$ equals 11 cm/second in trend on lower right distal to balloon occluded artery. For CFIp aortic pressure of 93 mm Hg in tracing on right is simultaneously obtained via angioplasty guidewire. CVP is assumed to be 5 mm Hg. CFIv for nonocclusive intracoronary flow velocity after PTCA and after cessation of reactive hyperemia, V0 minus occlusion illustrates the ratio of CFIv obtained before occlusion 25 cm/second in this example and is determined by Doppler guidewire in the same position. (Fleisch M, Billinger M, Eberli F, et al. *Circulation* 1999;100:1945–1950.)

Compute coronary fractional flow reserve (FFR_{cor}):

$$FFR_{cor} = 1 - \Delta P/(P_a - P_w)$$

Calculate collateral fractional flow reserve (FFR_{coll}):

$$FFR_{coll} = FFR_{myo} - FFR_{cor}$$

where P_d is distal coronary pressure; ΔP, mean translesional pressure gradient; P_v, mean right atrial pressure; P_w, mean coronary wedge pressure of distal coronary pressure during balloon inflation; P_a. mean aortic pressure. All measurements except P_w are made during hyperemia.

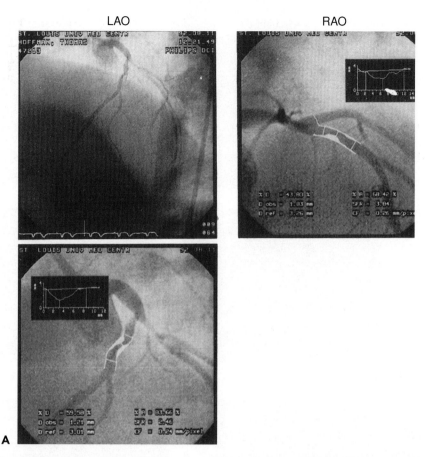

Figure 18.29 Case study 1 **A.** Angiogram of a left anterior descending (LAD) stenosis graded at 60% diameter reduction by quantitative coronary angiography. (LAO, left anterior oblique projection; RAO, right anterior oblique projection.) 6 days after an anterior myocardial infarction. In-laboratory assessment of the stenosis was performed before and after angioplasty. Basal and hyperemic flow velocity data were obtained 1 cm proximal and >10 artery diameters (or 2 cm) distal to the stenosis, using intracoronary adenosine (12 to 18 μg) administered through the guide catheter to evaluate flow reserve.
B. Coronary flow velocity assessment of the proximal (left) and distal LAD (right). The middle panels show coronary flow following hyperemia induced by intracoronary adenosine. The lower panels show the basal and hyperemic flow in the distal LAD following angioplasty.
C. Coronary pressure gradient in the LAD at rest and at hyperemia pre (left) and post (right) angioplasty. (With permission from Kern MJ, Flynn MS, Caracciolo EA, Bach RG, Donohue TJ, Aguirre FV. Use of translesional coronary flow velocity for interventional decisions in a patient with multiple intermediately severe coronary stenoses. *Cathet Cardiovasc Diagn* 1993;29:148–153.)

For FFR$_{collat}$, a coronary balloon is used to occlude the vessel and the mean coronary occlusion or wedge pressure (P$_w$, distal coronary pressure during balloon occlusion) is measured and divided by the mean aortic pressure (FFR$_{collat}$ = P$_w$/P$_a$). If the central venous pressure is abnormal, then it should be subtracted from both the wedge and aortic pressures. A FFR$_{collat}$ ≥0.25 suggests sufficient collaterals to prevent ischemia during PCI (81–82). FFR$_{collat}$ has also been studied in patients with acute myocardial infarction and shown to be the major determinant of left ventricular recovery after primary PCI. The study of collateral flow and function in patients is thus greatly facilitated by the use of sensor-wire measurements.

Case Studies in Coronary Blood Flow

Coronary angiography was performed and revealed a 60% diameter narrowing in the proximal left anterior descending coronary artery in this young man 6 days after an anterior myocardial infarction (panel A). In-laboratory assessment of the stenosis was performed before and after angioplasty (panel B). Basal and hyperemic flow velocity data were obtained 1 cm proximal to the stenosis. The Doppler guidewire was advanced across the stenosis. Distal (>10 artery diameters or 2 cm) basal and hyperemic flow responses were obtained. Intracoronary adenosine (12–18 μg) was administered through the guide catheter to evaluate

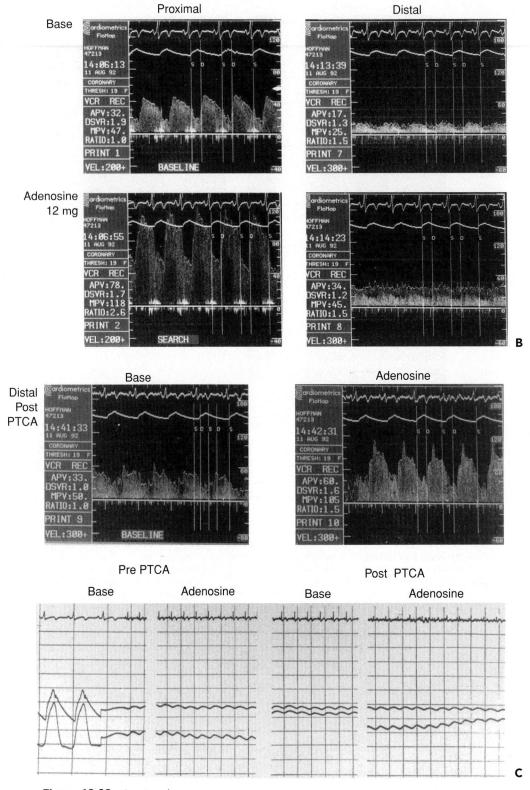

Figure 18.29 Continued.

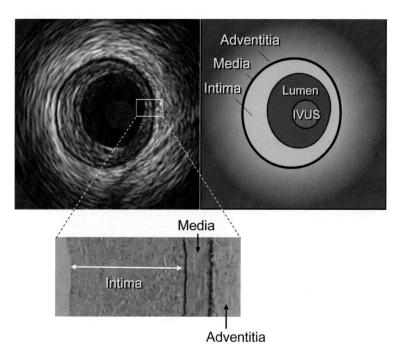

Figure 19.1 Cross-sectional format of a typical IVUS image. The bright-dark-bright, three-layered appearance is seen in the image with corresponding anatomy as defined. "IVUS" represents the imaging catheter in the blood vessel lumen. Histologic correlation with intima, media, and adventitia are shown. The media has lower ultrasound reflectance owing to less collagen and elastin compared with neighboring layers. Because the intimal layer reflects ultrasound more strongly than the media, there is a spillover in the image, which results in a slight overestimation of the thickness of the intima and a corresponding underestimation of the medial thickness.

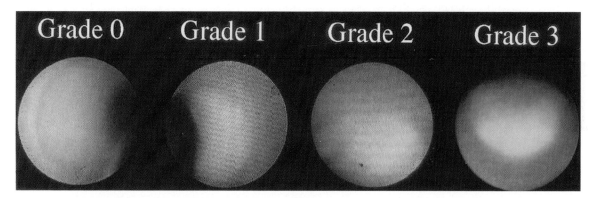

Figure 19.8 An example of yellow plaque grading by angioscopy. The surface color represents a lipid-rich core seen through a fibrous cap, and its intensity rises as the fibrous cap thins and becomes increasingly transparent. (From Ueda Y, et al. The healing process of infarct-related plaques. Insights from 18 months of serial angioscopic follow-up. *J Am Coll Cardiol* 2001;38:1916–1922.)

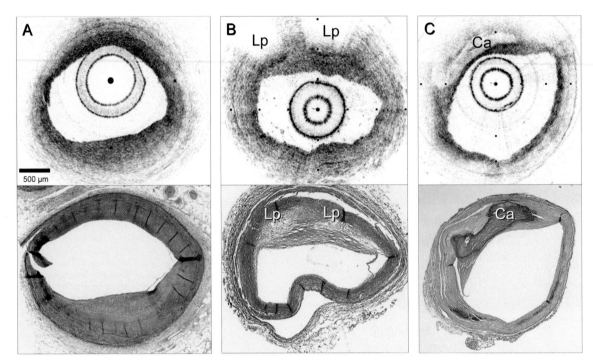

Figure 19.9 OCT images *(top)* and corresponding histology *(bottom)* for fibrous **(A)**, lipid-rich **(B)**, and calcific **(C)** plaques. In fibrous plaques, the OCT signal is observed to be strong and homogenous. In comparison, both lipid-rich (Lp) and calcific (Ca) regions appear as a signal-poor region within the vessel wall. Lipid-rich plaques have diffuse or poorly demarcated borders, whereas the borders of calcific nodules are sharply delineated. (Histologic stainings: Movat Pentachrome, Masson trichromed, and hematoxylin and eosin from left to right; original magnification 40×). (Courtesy of Bouma BE, Jang IK, and Tearney GJ.)

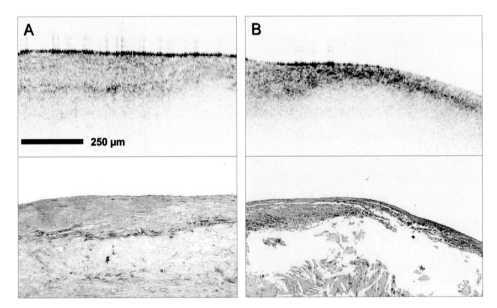

Figure 19.10 Raw OCT images *(top)* and corresponding histology (CD68 immunoperoxidase; original magnification 100×, *bottom)* of a fibroatheroma with a low macrophage density within the fibrous cap **(A)**; and a fibroatheroma with a high macrophage density within the fibrous cap **(B)**. (Tearney GJ, et al. *Circulation* 2003;107:113–119.)

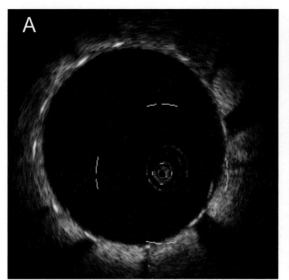 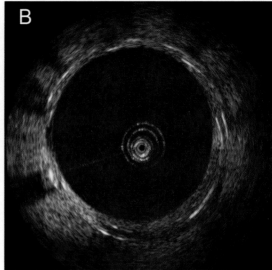

Figure 19.11 Follow-up OCT images of drug-eluting stents for de novo **(A)** and instent restenosis **(B)** lesions. The high resolution of OCT allows clear visualization of the stents, distinctly identifying each stent strut as well as a very thin neointimal layer covering the drug-eluting stent struts. (Courtesy of Grube E, and LightLab Imaging, Inc.)

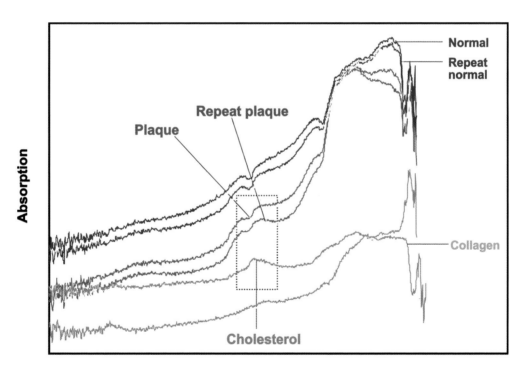

Figure 19.12 Diffuse reflectance NIR spectroscopy. Differences in individual chemical component spectra drive differences in the spectra of tissue samples, as shown on this diagram. The top 2 spectra are repeated measurements of a single normal sample, and middle 2 spectra are repeated measurements of a plaque. The cholesterol peak adds an additional feature to the plaque spectrum. Consequently, different tissue types can be recognized by examining these spectral patterns. (Courtesy of Muller JE, and InfraReDx, Inc.)

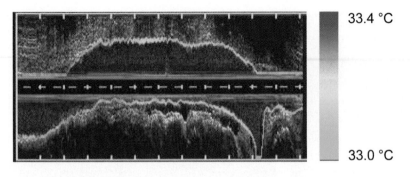

33.4 °C

33.0 °C

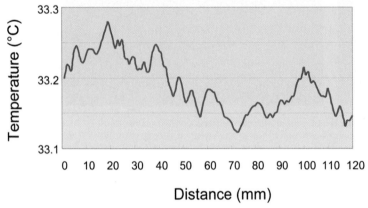

Figure 19.13 Intravascular thermography with an integrated thermography/IVUS catheter. The system displays a longitudinal color-coded thermal map of the studied vessel, superimposed on the lumen border of the IVUS image *(top)*. (Courtesy of Akasaka T, and Terumo Corp.)

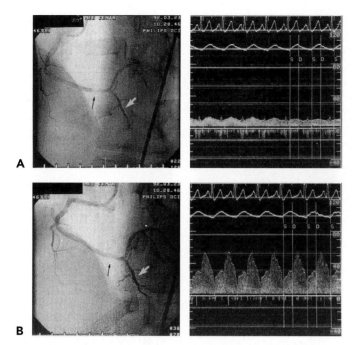

Figure 18.30 Case study 2. **Left.** Angiograms before and after angioplasty. **Right.** Poststenotic flow velocity in the posterior descending artery in the location of the *white arrow* demonstrating poor phasic flow and reduced mean velocity before angioplasty and increased mean velocity and normalized distal coronary flow after coronary angioplasty. Flow velocity measurements reflect the region in which velocity data is acquired. (With permission from Segal J, Kern MJ, Scott NA, et al. Alterations of phasic coronary artery flow velocity in man during percutaneous coronary angioplasty. *J Am Coll Cardiol* 1992;20:276–286.)

post-stenotic coronary reserve. Analysis of the flow velocity data revealed normal mean proximal velocity (32 cm/sec), with a normal phasic pattern and coronary flow reserve (2.5 × basal). Post-stenotic flow velocity, however, was abnormal (reduced mean velocity 17 cm/sec), with a proximal:distal velocity ratio of 32 : 17 = 1.9 (top right). In addition, the ratio of phasic diastolic/systolic velocity was abnormally low (1.3 in the distal vessel; a normal left coronary ratio >1.5), Distal coronary flow reserve was also impaired (1.42 × basal flow). These findings were associated with a basal translesional pressure gradient of 40 mmHg (increasing to 48 mmHg during maximal hyperemia). Coronary angioplasty was successfully performed. The stenosis was reduced (<30% diameter narrowing) with normalization of the distal phasic flow velocity pattern (diastolic/ systolic ratio = 1.6), augmentation of basal mean velocity (33 cm/sec), and an increase in distal flow reserve (−1.96) (panel C). The velocity data corresponded to a post-angioplasty translesional pressure gradient of 8 mmHg (20 mmHg during maximal hyperemia).

A 62 year old man presents to the catheterization laboratory and angiography shows an intermediate stenosis of the distal right coronary artery. A Doppler tipped flow wire was then placed past the stenosis (and into the mid portion of the posterior descending artery) in question and flow-velocity was assessed. The tracing obtained reveals poor phasic flow and a reduced mean velocity. Subsequent coronary flow reserve was assessed after adenosine hyperemia and found to be markedly abnormal. Angioplasty was performed on the distal right coronary artery, with resolution of the

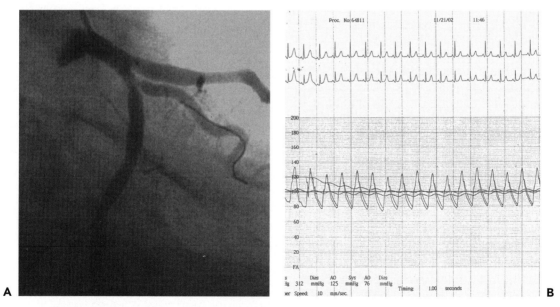

Figure 18.31 **A.** Case study 3. Ostial first obtuse marginal branch lesion is found in 54-year-old women with atypical angina and no stress testing. The operator must select best options for management. Although one could treat or defer for a stress test (returning to the lab if positive), an FFR was performed. **B.** FFR of OM stenosis was measured at 0.94. Medical therapy was recommended for hiatal hernia discomfort.

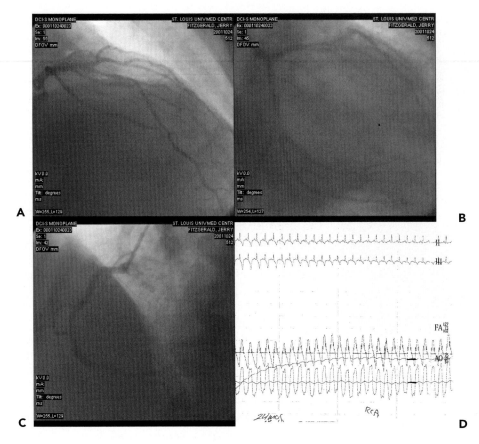

Figure 18.32 A. RAO cranial angiogram showing a diffusely diseased LAD with a moderate mid-vessel stenosis. **B.** RAO caudal angiogram showing a tightly stenosed circumflex coronary artery. **C.** RAO angiogram of the right coronary artery showing mild angiographic disease, **D.** FFR of the distal right coronary artery at maximal hyperemia revealing a physiologically significant gradient (FFR = 0.62).

stenosis. Subsequent assessment of coronary flow revealed restoration of the phasic flow, improvement in the mean flow velocity, and normalization of the coronary flow reserve.

Ostial first obtuse marginal branch lesion is found in 54 year old women with atypical angina and no antecedent stress test. The operator must select best options for management: Treat, refer for stress testing and return to lab if positive for ischemia, or measure FFR? In this case, FFR was performed utilizing a Doppler pressure wire and intra-coronary adenosine for hyperemia. The FFR of this lesion was found to be 0.94 with multiple doses of adenosine and the patient was discharged on medical therapy without angioplasty.

A 59 year old man presents for catheterization after being admitted for unstable angina. Angiography revealed a significant circumflex artery lesion, a diffusely diseased LAD with an intermediate stenosis of the mid-portion of the vessel and minimal angiographic disease in the right coronary artery. The operators were faced with percutaneous treatment of the circumflex artery or assessment of the other vessels with FFR. FFR assessment of the LAD was performed and was 0.78. Subequent FFR evaluation of the right coronary artery revealed an FFR of 0.62. By utilizing the intracoronary pressure-wire in this way, the patient was referred for coronary artery bypass grafting of all three vascular territories rather than undergoing incomplete percutaneous intervention of a single coronary lesion.

REFERENCES

1. Weber KT, Janicki JS. The metabolic demand and oxygen supply of the heart: physiologic and clinical considerations. *Am J Cardiol* 1979;44:722–729.
2. Rooke GA, Feigl EO. Work as a correlate of canine left ventricular oxygen consumption, and the problem of catecholamine oxygen wasting. *Circ Res* 1982;50:273–286.
3. Spaan, JAE. *Coronary Blood Flow; Mechanics, Distribution and Control.* Dordrecht, The Netherlands: Kluwer, 1991.
4. Braunwald E. Myocardial oxygen consumption: the quest for its determinants and some clinical fallout. *J Am Coll Cardiol* 1999;34:1365–1369.
5. Kal JE, Van Wezel HB, Vergroesen I. A critical appraisal of the rate pressure product as index of myocardial oxygen consumption for the study of metabolic coronary flow regulation. *Int J Cardiol* 1999;71:141–148.
6. Kloner RA, Bolli R, Marban E, et al. Medical and cellular implications of stunning, hibernation, and preconditioning: an NHLBI workshop. *Circulation* 1998;97:1848–1867.
7. Elsasser A, Schlepper M, Klovekorn WP, et al. Hibernating myocardium: an incomplete adaptation to ischemia. *Circulation* 1997;96:2920–2931.
8. Chilian WM. Coronary microcirculation in health and disease. Summary of an NHLBI workshop. *Circulation* 1997;95: 522–528.
9. De Bruyne B, Hersbach F, Pijls NHJ, et al. Abnormal epicardial coronary resistance in patients with diffuse atherosclerosis but "normal" coronary angiography. *Circulation* 2001;104: 2401–2406.
10. Baim DS, Rothman MT, Harrison DC. Simultaneous measurement of coronary venous blood flow and oxygen saturation during transient alterations in myocardial oxygen supply and demand. *Am J Cardiol* 1982;49:743–752.
11. Wilson RF, Marcus ML, White CW. Prediction of the physiologic significance of coronary arterial lesions by quantitative lesion

geometry in patients with limited coronary artery disease. *Circulation* 1987;75:723–732.

12. McGinn AL, Wilson RF, Olivari MT, Homans DC, White CW. Coronary vasodilator reserve after human orthotopic cardiac transplantation. *Circulation* 1988;78:1200–1209.
13. Gould KL, Lipscomb K, Hamilton GW. Physiologic basis for assessing critical coronary stenosis. Instantaneous flow response and regional distribution during coronary hyperemia as measures of coronary flow reserve. *Am J Cardiol* 1974;33:87–94.
14. Gould KL, Kelley KO. Physiological significance of coronary flow velocity and changing stenosis geometry during coronary vasodilation in awake dogs. *Circ Res* 1982;50:695–704.
15. Gould KL, Kirkeeide RL, Buchi M. Coronary flow reserve as a physiologic measure of stenosis severity. *J Am Coll Cardiol* 1990;15:459–474.
16. Siebes M, Campbell CS, D'Argenio DZ. Fluid dynamics of a partially collapsible stenosis in a flow model of the coronary circulation. *J Biomech Eng* 1996;118:489–497.
17. Pijls NHJ, De Bruyne B. Coronary Pressure. Dodrecht, The Netherlands: Kluwer, 1997:12–13.
18. The Thrombolysis in Myocardial Infarction (TIMI) trial. Phase I findings. TIMI Study Group. *New Engl J Med* 1985;312:932–936.
19. Cannon CP, Sharis PJ, Schweiger MJ, et al. Prospective validation of a composite end point in thrombolytic trials of acute myocardial infarction (TIMI 4 and 5). Thrombosis in Myocardial Infarction. *Am J Cardiol* 1997;80:696–699.
20. Barbagelata NA, Granger CB, Oqueli E, et al. TIMI grade 3 flow and reocclusion after intravenous thrombolytic therapy: a pooled analysis. *Am Heart J* 1997;133:273–282.
21. Simes RJ, Topol EJ, Holmes DR Jr, et al. Link between the angiographic substudy and mortality outcomes in a large randomized trial of myocardial reperfusion. Importance of early and complete infarct artery reperfusion. GUSTO-I Investigators. *Circulation* 1995;91:1923–1928.
22. Gibson CM, Cannon CP, Daley WL, et al. TIMI frame count: a quantitative method of assessing coronary artery flow. *Circulation* 1996;93:879–888.
23. Gibson CM, Dodge JT Jr, Goel M, et al. Angioplasty guidewire velocity: a new simple method to calculate absolute coronary blood velocity and flow. *Am J Cardiol* 1997;80:1536–1539.
24. Kern MJ, Moore JA, Aguirre FV, et al. Determination of angiographic (TIMI grade) blood flow by intracoronary Doppler flow velocity during acute myocardial infarction. *Circulation* 1996;94:1545–1552.
25. Uren NG, Crake T, Lefroy DC, de Silva R, Davies GJ, Maseri A. Reduced coronary vasodilator function in infarcted and normal myocardium after myocardial infarction. *New Engl J Med* 1994;331:222–227.
26. French JK, Ellis CJ, Webber BJ, et al. Abnormal coronary flow in infarct arteries 1 year after myocardial infarction is predicted at 4 weeks by corrected Thrombolysis in Myocardial Infarction (TIMI) frame count and stenosis severity. *Am J Cardiol* 1998;81: 665–671.
27. Dodge JT Jr, Rizzo M, Nykiel M, et al. Impact of injection rate on the Thrombolysis in Myocardial Infarction (TIMI) trial frame count. *Am J Cardiol* 1998;81:1268–1270.
28. van't Hof AWJ, Liem A, Suryapranata H, et al. Angiographic assessment of myocardial reperfusion in patients treated with primary angioplasty for acute myocardial infarction: myocardial blush grade: Zwolle Myocardial Infarction Study Group. *Circulation* 1998;97:2302–2306.
29. Henriques JPS, Zijlstra F, van't Hof AWJ, et al. Angiographic assessment of reperfusion in acute myocardial infarction by myocardial blush grade. *Circulation* 2003;107:2115.
30. Nakazawa HK, Roberts DL, Klocke FJ. Quantitation of anterior descending vs. circumflex venous drainage in the canine great cardiac vein and coronary sinus. *Am J Physiol* 1978;234:H163–166.
31. Ganz W, Tamura K, Marcus HS, Donoso R, Yoshida S, Swan HJ. Measurement of coronary sinus blood flow by continuous thermodilution in man. *Circulation* 1971;44:181–195.
32. Baim DS, Rothman MT, Harrison DC. Improved catheter for regional coronary sinus flow and metabolic studies. *Am J Cardiol* 1980;46:997–1000.
33. Pepine CJ, Mehta J, Webster WW Jr, Nichols WW. In vivo validation of a thermodilution method to determine regional left ventricular blood flow in patients with coronary disease. *Circulation* 1978;58:795–802.
34. Kern M. Curriculum in interventional cardiology: coronary pressure and flow measurements in the cardiac catheterization laboratory. *Cathet Cardiovasc Intervent* 2002;54:378–400.
35. Pijls NHJ, Kern MJ, Yock PG, De Bruyne B. Practice and potential pitfalls of coronary pressure measurement. *Cathet Cardiovasc Intervent* 2000;49:1–16.
36. Qian J, Ge J, Baumgart D, et al. Safety of intracoronary Doppler flow measurement. *Am Heart J* 2000;140:502–510.
37. Wilson RF, White CW. Intracoronary papaverine: an ideal coronary vasodilator for studies of the coronary circulation in conscious humans. *Circulation* 1986;73:444–451.
38. Wilson RF, White C. Serious ventricular dysrhythmias after intracoronary papaverine. *Am J Cardiol* 1988;62:1301–1302.
39. Wilson RF, Wyche K, Christensen BV, Zimmer S, Laxson DD. Effects of adenosine on human coronary arterial circulation. *Circulation* 1990;82:1595–1606.
40. Jeremias A, Whitbourn RJ, Filardo SD, et al. Adequacy of intracoronary versus intravenous adenosine-induced maximal coronary hyperemia for fractional flow reserve measurements. *Am Heart J* 2000;140:651–657.
41. Sonoda S, Takeuchi M, Nakashima Y, Kuroiwa A. Safety and optimal dose of intracoronary adenosine 5'-triphosphate for the measurement of coronary flow reserve. *Am Heart J* 1998;135: 621–627.
42. Bartunek J, Winjs W, Heyndrickx GR, de Bruyne B. Effects of dobutamine on coronary stenosis. Physiology and morphology comparison with intracoronary adenosine. *Circulation* 1999;100: 243–249.
43. Pijls NH, De Bruyne B, Smith L, et al. Coronary thermodilution to assess flow reserve: validation in humans. *Circulation* 2002;105: 2482–2486.
44. De Bruyne B, Pijls NHJ, Smith L, Wievegg M, Heyndrickx GR. Coronary thermodilution to assess flow reserve: experimental validation. *Circulation* 2001;104:2003.
45. Ofili EO, Kern MJ, Labovitz AJ, et al. Analysis of coronary blood flow velocity dynamics in angiographically normal and stenosed arteries before and after endolumen enlargement by angioplasty. *J Am Coll Cardiol* 1993;21:308–316.
46. Baumgart D, Haude M, Liu F, Ge J, Goerge G, Erbel R. Current concepts of coronary flow reserve for clinical decision making during cardiac catheterization. *Am Heart J* 1998;136:136–149.
47. Kern MJ, Bach RG, Mechem C, et al. Variations in normal coronary vasodilatory reserve stratified by artery, gender, heart transplantation and coronary artery disease. *J Am Coll Cardiol* 1996;28:1154–1160.
48. Kern MJ. Coronary physiology revisited: practical insights from the cardiac catheterization laboratory. *Circulation* 2000;101:1344–1351.
49. Akasaka T, Yoshida K, Hozumi T, et al. Retinopathy identifies marked restriction of coronary flow reserve in patients with diabetes mellitus. *J Am Coll Cardiol* 1997;30:935–941.
50. Baumgart D, Haude M, Goerge G, et al. Improved assessment of coronary stenosis severity using the relative flow velocity reserve. *Circulation* 1998;98:40–46.
51. Pijls NH, Van Gelder B, Van der Voort P, et al. Fractional flow reserve: a useful index to evaluate the influence of an epicardial coronary stenosis on myocardial blood flow. *Circulation* 1995;92: 3183–3193.
52. De Bruyne B, Bartunek J, Sys SU, et al. Simultaneous coronary pressure and flow velocity measurements in humans: feasibility, reproducibility, and hemodynamic dependence of coronary flow velocity reserve, hyperemic flow versus pressure slope index, and fractional flow reserve. *Circulation* 1996;94:1842–1849.
53. Pijls NHJ, de Bruyne B, G. Bech GJ, et al. Pressure measurement to assess the hemodynamic significance of serial stenoses within one coronary artery validation in humans. *Circulation* 2000; 102:2371.
54. De Bruyne B, Pijls NHJ, Heyndrickx GR, Hodeige D, Kirkeeide R, Gould KL. Pressure-derived fractional flow reserve to assess serial epicardial stenoses; theoretical basis and animal validation. *Circulation* 2000;101:1840.
55. Marques KMJ, Spruijt HJ, Boer C, Westerhof N, Visser CA, Visser FC. The diastolic flow-pressure gradient relation in coronary stenoses in humans. *J Am Coll Cardiol* 2002;39:1630–1636.

56. Meuwissen M, Chamuleau S, Siebes M, et al. Role of variability in microvascular resistance on fractional flow reserve and coronary blood flow velocity reserve in intermediate coronary lesions. *Circulation* 2001;103:184–187.

57. Meuwissen M, Siebes M, Chamuleau SAJ, et al. Hyperemic stenosis resistance index for evaluation of functional coronary lesion severity. *Circulation* 2002;106:441–446.

58. Pijls NH, De Bruyne B, Peels K, et al. Measurement of fractional flow reserve to assess the functional severity of coronary-artery stenoses. *N Engl J Med* 1996;334:1703–1708.

59. Chamuleau SAJ, Meuwissen M, van Eck-Smit BLF, et al. Fractional flow reserve, absolute and relative coronary blood flow velocity reserve in relation to the results of technetium-99m sestamibi single-photon emission computed tomography in patients with two-vessel coronary artery disease. *J Am Coll Cardiol* 2001;37:1316–1322.

60. Bartunek J, Marwick TH, Rodrigues AC, et al. Dobutamine-induced wall motion abnormalities: correlations with myocardial fractional flow reserve and quantitative coronary angiography. *J Am Coll Cardiol* 1996;27:1429–1436.

61. Smith SC Jr, et al. ACC/AHA Guidelines for Percutaneous Coronary Intervention (revision of the 1993 PTCA guidelines)—executive summary. *J Am Coll Cardiol* 2001;37:2215–2238.

62. Kern MJ, Donohue TJ, Aguirre FV, et al. Clinical outcome of deferring angioplasty in patients with normal translesional pressure-flow velocity measurements. *J Am Coll Cardiol* 1995;25:178–187.

63. Bech GJ, De Bruyne B, Bonnier HJRM, et al. Long-term follow-up after deferral of percutaneous transluminal coronary angioplasty of intermediate stenosis on the basis of coronary pressure measurement. *J Am Coll Cardiol* 1998;31:841–847.

64. Bech GJW, Pijls NHJ, De Bruyne B, et al. Usefulness of fractional flow reserve to predict clinical outcome after balloon angioplasty. *Circulation* 1999;99:883–888.

65. Bech GJW, De Bruyne B, Pijls NHJ, et al. Fractional flow reserve to determine the appropriateness of angioplasty in moderate coronary stenosis. A randomized trial. *Circulation* 2001;103:2928–2934.

66. Pijls NHJ, Klauss V, Siebert U, et al. Coronary pressure measurement after stenting predicts adverse events at follow-up. A multicenter registry. *Circulation* 2002;105:2950–2954.

67. Kern MJ, Dupouy P, Drury JH, et al. Role of coronary artery lumen enlargement in improving coronary blood flow after balloon angioplasty and stenting: a combined intravascular ultrasound Doppler flow and imaging study. *J Am Coll Cardiol* 1997;29:1520–1527.

68. Serruys PW, di Mario C, Piek J, et al. Prognostic value of intracoronary flow velocity and diameter stenosis in assessing the short- and long-term outcomes of coronary balloon angioplasty: the DEBATE Study (Doppler Endpoints Balloon Angioplasty Trial Europe). *Circulation* 1997;96:3369–3377.

69. De Bruyne B, Pijls NHJ, Bartunek J, et al. Fractional flow reserve in patients with prior myocardial infarction. *Circulation* 2001;104:157–162.

70. Akasaka T, Yoshida K, Kawamoto T, et al. Relation of phasic coronary flow velocity characteristics with TIMI perfusion grade and myocardial recovery after primary percutaneous transluminal coronary angioplasty and rescue stenting. *Circulation* 2000;101:2361–2367.

71. Yamamuro A, Akasaka T, Tamita K, et al. Coronary flow velocity pattern immediately after percutaneous coronary intervention as a predictor of complications and in-hospital survival after acute myocardial infarction. *Circulation* 2002;106:3051–3056.

72. Kawamoto T, Yoshida K, Akasaka T, et al. Can coronary blood flow velocity pattern after primary percutaneous transluminal coronary angiography predict recovery of regional left ventricular function in patients with acute myocardial infarction? *Circulation* 1999;100:339–345.

73. Cohen M, Rentrop KP. Limitation of myocardial ischemia by collateral circulation during sudden controlled coronary artery occlusion in human subjects: a prospective study. *Circulation* 1986;74:469–476.

74. Rentrop KP, Cohen M, Blanke H, Phillips RA. Changes in collateral channel filling immediately after controlled coronary artery occlusion by an angioplasty balloon in human subjects. *J Am Coll Cardiol* 1985;5:587–592

75. Rentrop KP, Thornton JC, Feit F, et al. Determinants and protective potential of coronary arterial collaterals as assessed by an angioplasty model. *Am J Cardiol* 1988;61:677–684.

76. Tron C, Donohue TJ, Bach RG, et al. Differential characterization of human coronary collateral blood flow velocity. *Am Heart J* 1999;132:508–515.

77. Yamada T, Okamoto M, Sueda T, et al. Relationship between collateral flow assessed by Doppler guide wire and angiographically collateral grades. *Am Heart J* 1995;130:32–37.

78. Piek JJ, Koolen JJ, et al. Spectral analysis of flow velocity in the contralateral artery during coronary angioplasty: a new method for assessing collateral flow. *J Am Coll Cardiol* 1993;21:1574–1582.

79. van Liebergen RAM, Piek JJ, Koch KT, et al. Quantification of collateral flow in humans: a comparison of angiographic, electrocardiographic and hemodynamic variables. *J Am Col Cardiol* 1999;33:670–677.

80. Seiler C, Fleisch M, Garachemani A, Meier B. Coronary collateral quantitation in patients with coronary artery disease using intravascular flow velocity or pressure measurements. *J Am Coll Cardiol* 1998;32:1272–1279.

81. Seiler C, Fleisch M, Billinger M, Meier B. Simultaneous intracoronary velocity- and pressure-derived assessment of adenosine-induced collateral hemodynamics in patient with one- to two-vessel coronary artery disease. *J Am Coll Cardiol* 1999;34:1985–1994.

82. Fleisch M, Billinger M, Eberli F, et al. Physiologically assessed coronary collateral flow and intracoronary growth factor concentrations in patients with 1- to 3-vessel coronary artery disease. *Circulation* 1999;100:1945–1950.

83. Piek JJ, van Liebergen RAM, Koch KT, et al. Pharmacological modulation of the human collateral vascular resistance in acute and chronic coronary occlusion assessed by intracoronary blood flow velocity analysis in an angioplasty model. *Circulation* 1997;96:106–115.

84. Pohl T, Seiler C, Billinger M, et al. Frequency distribution of collateral flow and factors influencing collateral channel development. Functional collateral channel measurement in 450 patients with coronary artery disease. *J Am Coll Cardiol* 2001;38:1872–1878.

85. Pijls NH, Bech GJ. el Gammal MI, et al. Quantification of recruitable coronary collateral blood flow in conscious humans and its potential to predict future ischemic events. *J Am Coll Cardiol* 1995;1522–1528.

86. Pijls NHJ, van Som AM, Kirkeeide RL, DeBruyne B, Gould KL. Experimental basis of determining maximum coronary, myocardial and collateral blood flow by pressure measurements for assessing functional stenosis severity before and after percutaneous transluminal coronary angioplasty. *Circulation* 1993;87:1354–1367.

Intravascular Imaging Techniques

19

Yasuhiro Honda   Peter J. Fitzgerald   Paul G. Yock[a]

Angiography remains the clinical standard for coronary and peripheral vascular imaging to identify significant arterial narrowing and to guide both catheter-based and surgical interventions (see Chapters 11 and 14). Although angiography provides a highly accurate picture of the vessel lumen, it provides very little information about the diseased arterial wall. The other catheter-based imaging tools described in this chapter—intravascular ultrasound, angioscopy, optical coherence tomography, spectroscopy, thermography, and intravascular MRI—provide supplemental and novel insights into vascular disease and the mechanisms of therapeutic intervention.

INTRAVASCULAR ULTRASOUND

Intravascular ultrasound (IVUS) catheters use reflected sound waves to visualize the arterial wall in a two-dimensional, tomographic format, analogous to a histologic cross section. They use significantly higher frequencies than noninvasive echocardiography (20 to 40 compared with 2 to 5 MHz). This provides high resolution (150 μm for the coronary catheters) at the expense of limited beam penetration (4 to 8 mm from the catheter tip). Since the initial clinical experience with IVUS in 1988 (1), this technique has gained acceptance as both a research method and as a clinical tool for situations in which the angiogram is unclear or unable to make precise measurements via visual estimate or computer-assisted techniques.

Imaging Systems

There are two approaches to IVUS imaging—solid state dynamic aperture and mechanical scanning. Both approaches generate a 360°, cross-sectional image plane perpendicular to the catheter tip. In the solid state approach, the individual elements of a circumferential array of transducer elements mounted near the tip of the catheter are activated with different time delays to create an ultrasound beam that sweeps the circumference of the vessel. As the number of elements has increased (now 64), there have been progressive improvements in lateral resolution. Complex miniaturized integrated circuits in the catheter tip control the timing and integration of the transducer activation and route the resulting echo information to a computer where cross-sectional images are reconstructed and displayed in real time. The length of the target vessel is scanned by a motorized or manual withdrawal of the entire catheter over a standard 0.014-inch angioplasty guidewire.

In the mechanical approach, a single transducer element is rotated inside the tip of a catheter via a flexible torque cable spun by an external motor drive unit attached to the proximal end of the catheter. Images from each angular position of the transducer are collected by a computerized image array processor, which synthesizes a cross-sectional ultrasound image of the vessel. The length of the target vessel is scanned by moving the rotating transducer back and forth manually or mechanically within the distal end of the catheter, rather than moving the catheter itself.

Both designs are commercially available in the United States. The solid state coronary catheter system (Volcano Therapeutics, Inc., Rancho Cordova, CA) has 64 transducer elements arranged around the catheter tip and uses a

[a] Tony M. Chou was a coauthor of this chapter in the previous edition. The assistance of Ali H.M. Hassan and Akiko Honda with the figures in this chapter is gratefully acknowledged.

center frequency of 20 MHz. The current coronary catheters in a rapid exchange configuration are 2.9F and thus compatible with a 5F guiding catheter. Larger peripheral imaging catheters are produced in both over-the-wire and rapid-exchange configurations. On the other hand, a 10F phased-array catheter for intracardiac echo (ICE) imaging (Siemens Medical Solutions USA, Inc., Malvern, PA) uses a different technology adapted from transesophageal echocardiography, providing a sector ultrasound image with color and spectral Doppler capabilities. The catheter is compatible with multiple-frequency imaging (5.0 to 10 MHz) so that the operator can determine the desired trade-off between resolution and penetration (up to 15 cm).

The mechanical IVUS system manufactured in the United States (Boston Scientific Corp., Natick, MA) uses 40-MHz coronary catheters that are 2.5F at the tip and 3.2F at the largest dimension, compatible with a 6F guiding catheter. Larger catheters with lower center frequencies are also available for peripheral and ICE imaging. The catheters are advanced over a guidewire using a short rail section at the catheter tip, just beyond the 15-cm-long segment within which the spinning transducer can be advanced or withdrawn. The fact that the guidewire runs outside the catheter parallel to the imaging segment results in a shadow artifact in the image (the so-called guidewire artifact). Mechanical catheters are slightly more difficult to prepare for use than the solid state catheters, since the imaging lumen must be carefully preflushed with saline to remove any air bubbles that might degrade the image and since the short rail design does not track as well as the longer rapid exchange systems. Nonuniform rotational distortion (NURD) can occur when bending of the drive cable interferes with uniform transducer rotation, causing a wedge-shaped, smeared image to appear in one or more segments of the image. This may be corrected by straightening the catheter and motor drive assembly and lessening tension on the guiding catheter.

In head-to-head comparisons, mechanical transducers have traditionally offered advantages in image quality compared with the solid state systems, although this gap has narrowed in recent years. Both systems continue to make image improvements, and good quality images can be achieved by either in most cases. The solid state system has a color flow display that shows blood flow in red, which can be useful particularly for novice IVUS interpreters. With both systems, serial cross-sectional images can be reconstructed into a longitudinal display mode (i.e., in a plane that runs along the axis of the vessel), and both still frames and video images can be digitally archived on local storage memory or a remote server using DICOM Standard 3.0.

Basic Procedures

The technique for delivering IVUS catheters is generally similar to that used for standard angioplasty/stent catheters (see Chapter 22). Prior to IVUS imaging, an intravenous injection of 5,000- to 10,000-unit heparin or equivalent anticoagulation (see Chapter 3) should be administered, as well as intracoronary nitroglycerine (100 to 300 µg) to reduce the potential for spasm. The image integrity should be checked before inserting the catheter, recognizing that the image in air will appear as a central catheter mask with concentric bright echo rings radiating outward from the center (caused by reverberations from the catheter–air interface). With the solid state catheter, the catheter tip is first positioned in the aorta or large proximal coronary vessel (i.e., not adjacent to any vessel wall) so that the ring-down artifact (a halo surrounding the catheter) can be electronically subtracted from the image before entering the coronary artery. The zoom, gain, gray scale (contrast), and noise elimination threshold (reject) can be adjusted if necessary.

Although it can be useful to watch the images as the catheter is advanced into the artery, it is generally best to advance the imaging element distal to the area of interest and perform a systematic examination during pullback. Automated pullback devices withdraw the imaging element at a steady rate of 0.5 or 1.0 mm/second, which allows accurate axial registration of each cross section and thus, precise longitudinal distance measurements.

Image Interpretation

Interpretation of the images begins with the identification of two key landmarks: the blood/intima (luminal) border and the media/adventitia interface (Fig. 19.1). The luminal border is the first bright interface beyond the catheter and is generally easy to locate on IVUS images. However, blood within the lumen exhibits a speckled low-intensity pattern that is more prominent at higher ultrasound frequencies and may make recognition of the intimal border more difficult. Signal-processing software can color code or subtract the blood signal so that it does not obscure the intimal interface. If the blood signal is still confusing, saline can be injected through the guiding catheter to reduce blood speckle and help to delineate the true lumen border.

The second key IVUS landmark is the media/adventitia border. In muscular arteries such as the coronary tree, the media may stand out as a thin dark band since it contains much less echo-reflective material (collagen and elastin) than the neighboring intima and adventitia. This provides a characteristic three-layered (bright-dark-bright) appearance on IVUS images (2). However, the stronger echo-reflectivity of the intimal layer often causes a spillover effect, known as *blooming*, resulting in a slight overestimation of the intimal thickness with a corresponding underestimation of the medial thickness. Also, this three-layered appearance may be undetectable in truly normal coronary arteries of which the intimal thickness is below the effective resolution of IVUS.

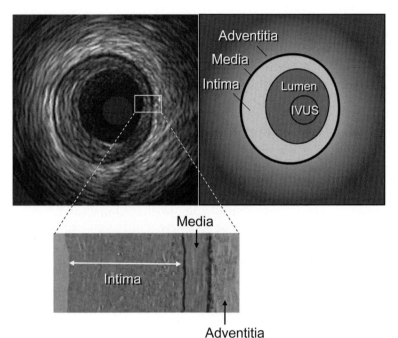

Figure 19.1 Cross-sectional format of a typical IVUS image. The bright-dark-bright, three-layered appearance is seen in the image with corresponding anatomy as defined. "IVUS" represents the imaging catheter in the blood vessel lumen. Histologic correlation with intima, media, and adventitia are shown. The media has lower ultrasound reflectance owing to less collagen and elastin compared with neighboring layers. Because the intimal layer reflects ultrasound more strongly than the media, there is a spillover in the image, which results in a slight overestimation of the thickness of the intima and a corresponding underestimation of the medial thickness. (See Color Plate)

In atherosclerotic disease where the media has been destroyed, the media may not appear as a distinct layer around the full circumference of the vessel. In the proximal vessel segments and at branch points, the media contains relatively high amounts of collagen and elastin, frequently causing it to blend with the surrounding layers. Even in these cases, however, the boundary between the outer media and adventitia (the outer perimeter of plaque-plus-media zone) is generally identifiable owing to a step-up in echo-reflectivity at this boundary without blooming. In most cases, the IVUS beam penetrates beyond the arterial wall, providing images of perivascular structures such as the cardiac veins, the myocardium, and pericardium (Fig. 19.2). These structures have characteristic appearances when viewed from different positions within the arterial tree and can provide useful landmarks regarding the position of the imaging plane (3).

Quantitative Assessment

Unlike coronary angiograms, IVUS images have an intrinsic distance calibration, which is usually displayed as a grid

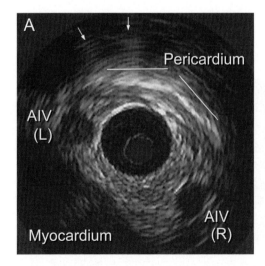
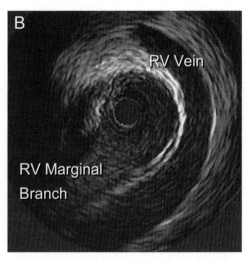

Figure 19.2 Perivascular landmarks. **A.** A distal cross section of the left anterior descending artery. The right and left branches of the anterior interventricular vein (AIV) are seen framing the coronary artery. The pericardium appears as a bright arc with spokes emitting from it *(arrows)*. **B.** A cross section of the mid right coronary artery. Bridging veins arch over the artery, typically at a position just adjacent to the right ventricular (RV) marginal branches.

on the image. Electronic caliper (diameter) and tracing (area) measurements can be performed at the tightest cross section (maximum stenosis), as well as at reference segments located proximal and distal to the lesion (4). In general, the reference segment is selected as the most normal-looking (largest lumen with smallest plaque burden) cross section within 10 mm from the lesion with no intervening major side branches.

Vessel and lumen diameter measurements are important in everyday clinical practice where accurate sizing of devices is needed. The maximum and minimum diameters (the major and minor axes of an elliptical cross section) are the most widely used. The ratio of maximum to minimum diameter defines a measure of symmetry. Area measurements are performed with computer planimetry; lumen area is determined by tracing the leading edge of the blood/intima border (Fig. 19.1), whereas total vessel (or external elastic membrane, EEM) area is defined as the area enclosed by the outermost interface between media and adventitia. Plaque area (or more accurately, the plaque plus media area) is calculated as the difference between vessel and lumen areas; the ratio of plaque to total vessel area is termed the percent plaque area, plaque burden, or percent cross-sectional narrowing.

Arterial Disease

The early changes of atherosclerotic disease, so-called fatty streaks, are too thin to be visualized with IVUS. As plaque continues to develop, it can be resolved on IVUS with different acoustic properties. A plaque with extensive lipid infiltration has low echo-reflectivity (less than the adventitia) on IVUS. Plaques with predominantly fibrous tissue are more echogenic than the fat-laden plaques and can cause signal attenuation to some degree. Calcified plaque is recognized by a bright interface that overlies a dark shadow extending radially outward (Fig. 19.3). This acoustic shadowing, often accompanied by reverberations or ghost

images of the calcium (regularly spaced arcs deep to the initial bright interface), obscures the true depth of the calcified plaque as well as any deeper tissue. Calcium is seen by IVUS in 60 to 80% of lesions undergoing intervention, only half of which are detected by fluoroscopy/angiography (5,6). A rough rule of thumb is that an arc of calcium must occupy two quadrants (180°) on IVUS to be visible on fluoroscopy. Calcium on IVUS is seen more frequently with increasing age and in patients with stable (as opposed to unstable) angina and correlates more with plaque burden than lesion severity (6).

One of the major limitations of IVUS in tissue identification is the difficulty in discriminating thrombus from soft plaque, because both have similar signals or "texture" and brightness. IVUS clues to the presence of thrombus include (a) a nodular appearance or clefts in the tissue, (b) small channels within the mass, (c) scintillating appearance (reminiscent of amyloidosis on transthoracic echocardiography). or (d) tissue that moves (wiggles) in response to motion of the vessel wall (4).

The application of IVUS in clinical practice has given us several unique insights into the nature of coronary disease. For example, IVUS generally reveals a much larger plaque burden than would be estimated by angiography. When a vessel appears to have a discrete stenosis by angiography, IVUS almost invariably shows that there is considerable atherosclerotic disease present throughout the entire length of the vessel. Even a reference that is normal or near normal angiographically has on average 35 to 51% of cross-sectional area plaque burden (Fig. 19.4; 7,8).

IVUS also gives a precise representation of the distribution of plaque within the vessel wall—specifically the eccentricity or concentricity of atherosclerotic plaque—and the relationship of plaque volume to vessel wall area. Plaques that appear to be concentric by angiography are often eccentric by IVUS and vice versa (5,9). Remodeling—localized expansion of the vessel wall in areas of high plaque burden as originally described by Glagov—occurs

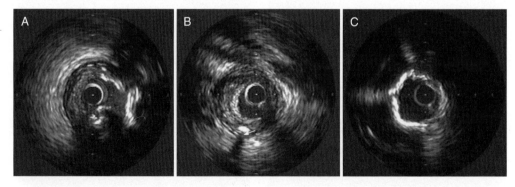

Figure 19.3 Examples of coronary calcification. **A.** A complex calcified plaque is seen between 12 and 6 o'clock. There is superficial and deep calcium with a disrupted appearance. **B.** Heterogeneous tissue density is shown with a rim of fibrofatty plaque and a deep deposit of calcium at 7 o'clock. **C.** Superficial circumferential calcification gives a napkin ring appearance. A faint reverberation is seen between 5 and 10 o'clock. The deeper vessel structure and external elastic membrane are obscured by the shadowing of the calcium layer.

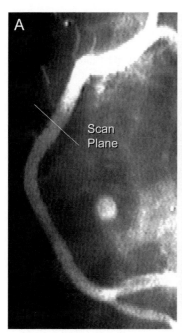

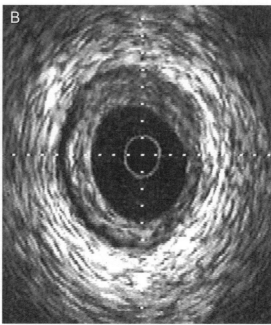

Figure 19.4 Angiographically silent disease. The angiogram of the right coronary artery suggests minimal disease **(A)**. IVUS images **(B)**, however, show significant circumferential plaque ranging from 0.5- to 1.5-mm thickness throughout its length. The lumen is large, round, and regular, accounting for the benign angiographic appearance.

as if the vessel were stretching to accommodate the accumulation of plaque so as to avoid narrowing its lumen. The remodeling response may be heterogeneous, with some segments showing the positive Glagov remodeling as others show negative remodeling (shrinkage or constriction that works in conjunction with plaque burden to accentuate luminal stenosis; 10,11). Consistent with postmortem studies, IVUS has demonstrated that proximal LAD lesions are localized on the opposite wall from the flow divider between the LAD and circumflex (12), supporting the theory that abnormally low shear forces contribute to plaque formation. Similarly, studies have shown that atherosclerotic plaque tends to form more on the inner curvature of the vessel arc (the wall opposite the pericardium when seen on IVUS; 13).

Diagnostic Applications

IVUS has been used to clarify situations in which angiography is equivocal or difficult to interpret (especially ostial lesions or tortuous segments where the angiogram may not lay out the vessel well for interpretation). For intermediate lesions, careful IVUS measurement is made of the minimum lumen area (MLA) compared with the proximal and distal reference lumen areas. A 60 to 70% area stenosis or an absolute lumen cross-sectional area <3 to 4 mm^2 indicates a hemodynamically significant stenosis (14–16). Alternatively, physiologic assessment with fractional flow reserve (FFR) provides a more direct measure of hemodynamic significance (see Chapter 18). The mere presence of plaque in coronary arteries by IVUS does not justify coronary interventions or bypass surgery, as plaque burden can be high in areas of minimal stenosis that do not warrant treatment.

One of most intriguing areas of current IVUS research is the attempt to identify the vulnerable plaque. Low echogenicity of plaque (an index correlated to its lipid content) has not been shown convincingly to predict clinical events, nor does IVUS imaging have sufficient resolution to identify the classic configuration of a thin fibrous cap overlying a lipid pool. Identification of lipid may be improved by the addition of tissue characterization methods (17,18), involving analysis of the raw radiofrequency signals in the reflected ultrasound beam (e.g. virtual histology, Volcano Therapeutics, Inc., Rancho Cordova, CA). Another application of the radiofrequency signal analysis is IVUS palpography that measures motion (strain) patterns of the arterial wall in response to the change between systolic and diastolic arterial pressure. In this technique, the local strain of the tissue is displayed color coded on the luminal boundaries of the IVUS image. A recent clinical study using three-dimensional IVUS palpography showed that the number of highly deformable plaques correlated with both unstable clinical presentation and levels of C-reactive protein (19). Plaque activity also appears to correlate with the extent of positive remodeling (20–23). It is plausible that there may be a pathophysiologic link between remodeling and plaque rupture, since increased activity of inflammatory cells and matrix metalloproteinases are linked both to both processes.

IVUS has also been used to assess the accelerated coronary artery disease seen after heart transplantation (24–26). The vasculopathy typically consists of concentric intimal proliferation that progresses to diffuse arterial obliteration within the first 2 years after transplantation. More complex plaques with calcification and little or no positive remodeling may develop subsequently, and contribute to hemodynamically significant stenosis.

Guidance for Interventions

IVUS imaging has proven useful in selecting appropriate catheter-based intervention as well as in optimizing the results of coronary procedures. With current IVUS catheters, most lesions intended for treatment can be imaged before intervention, providing information about the true size of the vessel, the distribution of plaque, and the nature of the involved tissue. Early observational studies suggested that this leads to a change in interventional strategy in 20 to 40% of cases (27,28), notably use of rotational atherectomy for calcified lesions or changes in balloon or sent sizing based on a larger EEM diameter than estimated from angiography.

Balloon Angioplasty

Tearing or dissection of plaque is a frequent and important feature of PTCA (see Chapter 22) and occurs in 45 to 70% of cases interrogated by IVUS imaging, compared with 20 to 45% by angiography (5,29–31). IVUS has shown that dissections are often located at the junction of calcified and noncalcified plaque (where shear forces from dilation are high) or at the junction between eccentric plaque and normal vessel wall (as the elastic, nondiseased wall separates away from the more rigid plaque). The depth of dissections relative to the media or adventitia can also be accurately evaluated (Fig. 19.5). IVUS has been used effectively to guide balloon sizing in PTCA, as in CLOUT (CLinical Outcomes with Ultrasound Trial) where IVUS guidance led oversizing of the balloon by 0.5 mm compared with angiography (32). This strategy leads to a low postprocedure residual stenosis without increased complication rates and 6-month restenosis rates in the 20% range (33,34). A serial IVUS study demonstrated that most late lumen loss following nonstent intervention was owing to negative arterial remodeling (a decrease in vessel cross-sectional area), with only about a quarter of the late loss owing to tissue proliferation (35–37).

Atherectomy

IVUS studies have demonstrated that plaque removal accounts for only 40 to 80% of lumen gain with directional coronary atherectomy (DCA), with the remainder owing to mechanical expansion by the device and balloon dilatation (see Chapter 23; 38,39). In addition, impressively high residual plaque burden has been demonstrated following even optimal DCA (an average of 60% residual plaque burden in vessels with angiographic residual stenosis <20%). IVUS imaging has also been used successfully as an adjuvant to DCA. The presence of superficial calcium substantially reduces tissue retrieval, and serial IVUS can be used as a directional aid to facilitate more accurate and complete plaque removal.

Studies in which IVUS was used in conjunction with DCA suggested that restenosis correlates with the residual plaque burden following atherectomy. In the Optimal Atherectomy Restenosis (OARS) trial, residual plaque burden was thus 57% with a restenosis rate of 29% (39), whereas an average postprocedure plaque burden of 46% in the Adjunctive Balloon Angioplasty following Coronary Atherectomy Study (ABACAS) resulted in a 6-month angiographic restenosis of 21% (40). As with PTCA, late lumen loss following DCA is owing predominantly to negative remodeling, with a smaller component of intimal proliferation (35–37,41).

Stents

Stent struts are easily visualized on IVUS examination as a collection of bright, distinct echoes, characteristic for each stent type. IVUS also reveals that part of the mechanism of lumen enlargement following stent placement is the axial extrusion of noncalcified plaque into the adjacent reference zones (42,43). Plaque volume is thus driven out of the stented region and gained in the distal and proximal reference sites, a phenomenon that possibly contributes to the angiographic step-up/step-down appearance poststenting.

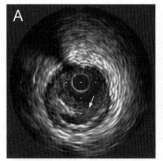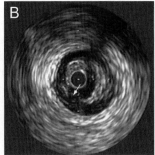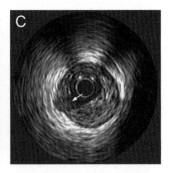

Figure 19.5 Examples of dissections. **A.** A superficial dissection starting at 6 o'clock and extending clockwise. The dissection flap does not extend far into the vessel lumen. **B.** A deeper dissection with dissection flap that extends into the lumen and may compromise flow or precede abrupt closure. Injection of contrast in this setting can demonstrate free fluid flow behind the flap to better define the extent of tear. **C.** Eccentric plaque with a deep dissection at 8 o'clock that penetrates the external elastic lamina and extends into the adventitia.

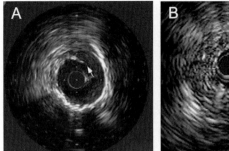
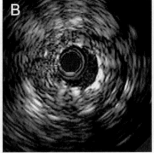
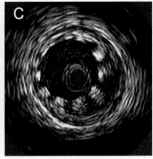

Figure 19.6 IVUS-detected problems with stent deployment. **A.** An edge tear, or a disruption of plaque, at the stent margin with little compromise of the lumen. **B.** Incomplete stent expansion relative to the vessel size. **C.** Incomplete stent apposition, where there is a gap between a portion of the stent and the vessel wall (between 12 and 7 o'clock on the IVUS image). The apparent thickness of the stent struts in this area is owing to reverberations. Injection of contrast/saline or blood speckling on a dynamic image can help define the lumen boundary behind the struts.

IVUS has identified several stent deployment issues, including incomplete expansion and incomplete apposition (Fig. 19.6). Incomplete expansion occurs when a portion of the stent is inadequately expanded compared with the distal and proximal reference dimensions, as may occur where dense fibrocalcific plaque is present. Incomplete apposition (seen in 3 to 10% of stent cases) occurs when part of the stent structure is not fully in contact with the vessel wall, possibly increasing local flow disturbances and the potential risk for subacute thrombosis. IVUS observation of incomplete expansion and apposition by Colombo and Tobis led to their development of the current high-pressure deployment techniques (see Chapter 24; 44,45).

Subsequent studies have shown that IVUS-guided stent placement improves the clinical outcome of bare metal stents. In the Multicenter Ultrasound guided Stent Implantation in Coronaries (MUSIC) trial, IVUS-guided stenting required (a) complete apposition over the entire stent length, (b) instent minimum stent area (MSA) ≥90% of the average of the reference areas or 100% of the smallest reference area, and (c) symmetric stent expansion with minimum/maximum lumen diameter ≥0.7 (46). Subacute thrombosis of <2% was felt to represent a reduction over nonguided deployment, although with current antiplatelet regimens, similar results can usually be achieved by high pressure postdilation without IVUS confirmation.

Nevertheless, a number of studies have suggested a link between suboptimal stent implantation and stent thrombosis, including the Predictors and Outcomes of Stent Thrombosis (POST) registry, which demonstrated that 90% of thrombosis patients had suboptimal IVUS results—incomplete apposition (47%), incomplete expansion (52%), and evidence of thrombus (24%)—even though only 25% of patients had abnormalities on angiography (47). These observations were replicated in a more recent study by Cheneau and colleagues, suggesting that mechanical factors continue to contribute to stent thrombosis even in this modern stent era with optimized antiplatelet regimens (48). Although the use of IVUS in all

patients for the sole purpose of reducing thrombosis is clearly not warranted from a cost standpoint, IVUS imaging should be considered in patients at particularly high risk for thrombosis (e.g., slow flow) or in whom the consequences of thrombosis would be severe (left main).

Over the past decade, a number of studies have shown that MSA as measured by IVUS is one of the strongest predictors for both angiographic and clinical restenosis. Kasaoka and colleagues (50) indicated that the predicted risk of restenosis decreases 19% for every 1-mm^2 increase in MSA and suggested that stents with MSA >9 mm^2 have a greatly reduced risk of restenosis (49). In the Can Routine Ultrasound Improve Stent Expansion (CRUISE) trial, IVUS guidance by operator preferences increased MSA from 6.25 to 7.14 mm^2, leading to a 44% relative reduction in target vessel revascularization at 9 months compared with angiographic guidance alone. In the Angiography Versus IVUS-Directed stent placement (AVID) trial, IVUS-guided stent implantation resulted in larger acute dimensions than angiography alone (7.54 versus 6.94 mm^2) without an increase in complications and lower 12-month TLR rates for vessels with angiographic reference diameter <3.25 mm, severe stenosis at preintervention (>70% angiographic diameter stenosis), and vein grafts (51). However, controversial results were also reported in some IVUS-guided stent trials (52,53), presumably owing to differing procedural end points for IVUS-guided stenting as well as various adjunctive treatment strategies that were used in these trials in response to suboptimal results.

Instent restenosis is owing to intimal proliferation (Fig. 19.7); there is no evidence for stent recoil or late compression (37,54). Growth of neointima is generally greatest in the areas with the largest present plaque burden (55,56), and the intimal growth process seems to be more aggressive in diabetic patients (57). In the treatment of instent restenosis, IVUS can be helpful in distinguishing pure intimal ingrowth from poor stent expansion, especially if ablative therapies are being considered. Using serial IVUS immediately before and after balloon angioplasty for

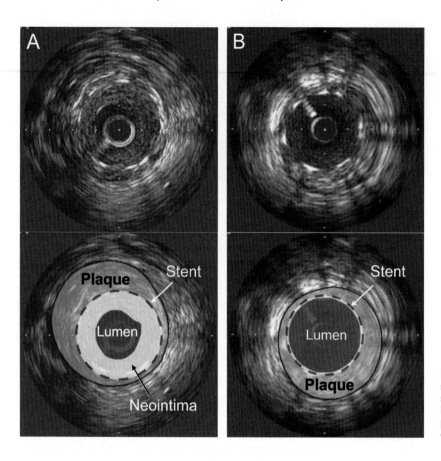

Figure 19.7 IVUS images 8 months after stent deployment. A conventional bare metal stent shows a considerable amount of neointima inside the stent **(A)**. In contrast, a significant suppression of instent neointimal proliferation is observed with a sirolimus-eluting stent **(B)**.

instent restenosis, Castagna and colleagues (58) have shown that in 1,090 consecutive instent restenosis lesions, 38% of lesions had a MSA <6.0 mm². Stent underexpansion can result in clinically significant lumen compromise even with minimal neointimal hyperplasia. For this type of instent restenosis, mechanical optimization will be appropriate in most cases. IVUS can also track the response to treatment, with evidence that angioplasty of instent restenosis is followed by reintrusion of tissue within 40 minutes after intervention (59). This finding may help explain why it appears that ablative therapies appear to have better outcomes than balloon angioplasty for instent restenosis (see Chapter 23).

Drug-Eluting Stents

In the drug-eluting stent (DES) era, the fact that the drugs dramatically reduce the variability of the biologic response (intimal proliferation) further strengthens the prognostic value of the MSA as a powerful predictor for instent restenosis. This is well illustrated in recent IVUS work by Sonoda and colleagues (60), in which sirolimus-eluting stents showed a stronger positive relation with a greater correlation coefficient between baseline MSA and 8-month MLA compared with control bare metal stents (0.8 versus 0.65 and 0.92 versus 0.59, respectively).

The discovery of edge effects associated with intracoronary radiation therapy raised the concern of lumen narrowing in adjacent reference segments as a potential limitation of

DES as well. Fortunately, clinical experience so far with sirolimus and paclitaxel-eluting stents has shown no accelerated edge restenosis overall when compared with conventional bare metal stents. Detailed serial IVUS analysis of the SCORE trial revealed that the favorable edge effect was primarily owing to the lack of vessel shrinkage despite similar amounts of plaque proliferation compared with the control group (61). A similar vessel response has also been reported in ASPECT and TAXUS-II (62,63). On the other hand, several DES trials demonstrated less effective suppression of late lumen loss at the proximal peristent segment compared with the distal edge, possibly providing an important clue for optimal deployment of DES. These findings suggest that less aggressive stent dilatation and complete coverage of reference disease may be beneficial, as long as significant underexpansion and incomplete strut apposition to the vessel wall are avoided.

Recurrent restenosis following DES implantation for instent restenosis was also recently investigated using IVUS (64). In a series of 48 instent restenosis lesions treated with sirolimus-eluting stents, 82% of recurrent lesions had a MSA <5.0 mm² compared with 26% of nonrecurrent lesions (P = 0.003). In addition, a gap between sirolimus-eluting stents was identified in 27% of recurrent lesions versus 5% of nonrecurrent lesions. These observations further emphasize the importance of procedural optimization at the DES implantation for both de novo and instent restenosis lesions.

Late acquired incomplete apposition of DES has also been reported in both experimental (paclitaxel) and clinical studies (sirolimus and paclitaxel). Importantly, several IVUS studies have indicated that the main mechanism is focal, positive vessel remodeling, as in the case of brachytherapy (65). Furthermore, there is a strong suggestion that incompletely apposed struts are seen primarily in eccentric plaques, with gaps developing mainly on the disease-free side of the vessel wall, suggesting that the combination of mechanical vessel injury combined with the reduced healing caused by pharmacologic agents in the setting of little underlying plaque may predispose the vessel wall to chronic, pathologic dilatation.

Safety

As with other interventional procedures, the possibility of spasm, dissection, and thrombosis exists when intravascular imaging catheters are used. In a retrospective study of 2,207 patients, Hausmann and colleagues (66) identified spasm in 2.9% of patients and other complications including dissection, thrombosis, and abrupt closure with "certain relation" to IVUS in 0.4%. This study was performed with first-generation catheters in the early 1990s, and it is likely (though not documented) that the incidence of spasm and other complications is substantially lower with the current-generation catheters.

Usage and Costs

In 2003–2004, it is estimated by the U.S. manufacturers that IVUS catheters are used in approximately 4 to 5% of coronary interventional cases in the United States. A significant—but unknown—proportion of current IVUS usage is for clinical studies, such as trials of drug-eluting stents. Over the past 5 years, the use of catheters has increased at approximately 5% per year. In Europe, IVUS usage is considerably lower (1%), whereas in Japan >30% of coronary interventions use IVUS guidance. These international differences in usage reflect not only practice patterns but also significant differences in reimbursement for IVUS imaging (highest in Japan).

In the United States, current retail sales prices for the stand-alone single-use imaging catheters range between $600 and $850. The retail price of the IVUS imaging console is between $150,000 and $250,000, though the actual prices paid by hospitals vary widely depending on bundling deals and other special arrangements. The Health Care Financing Administration approved reimbursement for the IVUS procedure and interpretation for Medicare patients in 1997, based on the number of vessels imaged. A number of other carriers have also approved reimbursement for IVUS, although payment is on a region-by-region basis. In most places, the total reimbursement is less than the cost of the catheters.

ANGIOSCOPY

Percutaneous coronary angioscopy is an endoscopic technology adapted from the gastrointestinal to the endovascular domain. It provides real-time, full-color images of the luminal surface of coronary arteries to visualize the surface color and superficial morphology of atherosclerotic plaque, thrombus, and intimal flaps. Since the initial clinical experience in percutaneous coronary angioscopy reported in 1985 (67), significant technical improvement has been achieved with image quality enhancement, catheter miniaturization, and development of subselective catheterization systems. Although the Food and Drug Administration has not yet approved any coronary angioscopy system for use in the United States, clinical investigators worldwide have been using this diagnostic modality to offer unique insights into the pathophysiology of coronary lesions, particularly in the field of acute coronary syndromes.

Imaging Systems and Procedures

In general, intracoronary angioscopy consists of an external optical engine incorporating a light source and a Charge Coupled Device (CCD) camera; a fiberoptic catheter for illumination and imaging; a subselective delivery catheter system; and a video monitor with an image recording system. The light source emits a high-intensity white light to illuminate the target object through the fiberoptic catheter. The imaging catheter contains a flexible fiberoptic bundle of several thousand pixels; the latest generation catheter, incorporating 6,000 fibers, is 0.75 mm in outer diameter with a microlens providing a 70° field of view and a focused depth ranging from 1 to 5 mm. The delivery catheter system for the imaging catheter serves two roles: subselective delivery of the angioscope to the target segment, and the creation of a blood-free field for optical imaging. Conventional delivery systems were equipped with a distal balloon or cuff for occluding blood flow; an alternative system uses a smaller catheter to continuously flush an optically clear liquid in front of the tip of the angioscope for blood displacement. This approach precludes possible complications related to the balloon occlusion (coronary rupture, dissection, or thrombosis) and minimizes ischemic time as blood flow is restored immediately as the flush pressure is reduced.

Prior to the procedure, "white balancing" by imaging a reference white surface is required to adjust the internal circuitry of the video camera for the correct white level. The occlusion cuff system requires an 8F guiding catheter whereas the nonocclusion/flush approach is compatible with a 6F guiding catheter; both delivery designs accept a standard 0.014-inch angioplasty guidewire. The angioscope with the cuff occlusion design (4.5F) is advanced to the region of interest using a double monorail technique (inner optical bundle and outer delivery catheter) under fluoroscopy. As warm Ringer lactate is infused (0.3 to 1.0 mL/second) through the distal guidewire lumen, the occlusion cuff is gently inflated with a saline/contrast mixture until a satisfactory blood-free imaging is obtained. The monorail optical bundle is then advanced or withdrawn along the guidewire as needed to bring the target lesion into the optimal view.

In contrast, the angioscope with the noncuff approach uses an over-the-wire technique to advance the delivery system (4.0F) to the target site. After removal of a 2.9F inner catheter together with the guidewire (a secondary guidewire thus may be required to protect the target lesion), the fiberoptic probe is advanced within the outer delivery catheter. To avoid vessel injury, the probe tip should be placed immediately proximal to the exit of the delivery catheter under real-time angioscopy. The segment of interest is then imaged by pullback of the entire system with continuous flush through the delivery catheter. Some operators experienced in this technique prefer warm low-molecular weight dextran for safe and effective irrigation.

Image Interpretation

Similar to gastrointestinal angioscopy, coronary angioscopic images are interpreted based on the surface color and endoluminal morphology of vessel walls or structures. The normal coronary artery surface appears as grayish white and smooth in contour without any protruding structure, whereas atherosclerotic plaques can show varying degrees of yellowish color (Fig. 19.8) with or without visible irregularities on the luminal surface. The yellow plaque surface signifies a lipid-rich core seen through a fibrous cap, and the yellow intensity rises as the fibrous cap thins and becomes increasingly transparent. Dissections are characterized as visible cracks or fissures on the luminal surface and/or sail-like white protruding structures that can be loose or immobile inside the lumen. Intimal flaps are visualized as thin, faint, highly mobile fronds of white tissue. Both structures are generally contiguous and of similar appearance to the adjacent vessel wall. Thrombi are recognized as masses that are red, white, or mixed in color, which adhere to the intima or protrude into the lumen. Red masses, not dislodged by flushing, are considered as fibrin/erythrocyte-rich thrombi, whereas white granular or cottonlike appearances are characteristics of platelet-rich thrombi. Subintimal hemorrhage may be detected as distinct, demarcated patches of red coloration that are clearly within the vessel wall.

A histopathologic basis for angioscopic image interpretation has been provided by several investigators. In an ex vivo study of 70 postmortem human arterial segments, Siegel and colleagues (68) classified angioscopic findings as normal artery, stable atheroma, disrupted atheroma, and thrombus. Compared with the histologic reference, angioscopy demonstrated a high sensitivity, specificity, and accuracy (each >90%) for all categories but disrupted atheroma. For this type of lesion, the sensitivity was only moderate (73%), whereas the specificity, accuracy, and predictive values were still high (>90%). Importantly, the sensitivity of angioscopy for thrombus was 100% and significantly superior to that of IVUS (57%). Other investigators validated in vivo angioscopic findings using corresponding tissue materials retrieved by DCA (69). This study concluded that yellow plaque color was closely related to degenerated plaque or atheroma and was associated with unstable coronary syndromes.

To alleviate subjectivity in reporting angioscopic interpretation, several investigators have proposed classification systems for angioscopic findings with reproducibility evaluation. The Ermenonville classification was established by a European coronary angioscopy working group, featuring several parameters, such as image quality, lumen diameter, surface color, atheroma, dissection, and thrombus, graded in 3 to 5 categories (70). However, κ values for chance-corrected intraobserver and interobserver agreements of the diagnostic items were low at 0.51 to 0.67 and 0.13 to 0.29, respectively. On the other hand, the important items, such as red thrombus and dissection, were

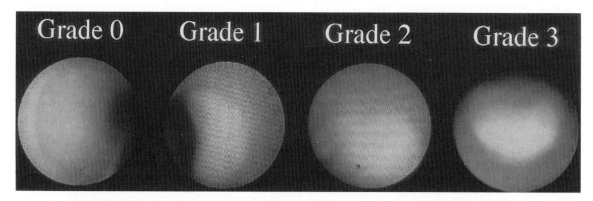

Figure 19.8 An example of yellow plaque grading by angioscopy. The surface color represents a lipid-rich core seen through a fibrous cap, and its intensity rises as the fibrous cap thins and becomes increasingly transparent. (From Ueda Y, et al. The healing process of infarct-related plaques. Insights from 18 months of serial angioscopic follow-up. *J Am Coll Cardiol* 2001;38:1916–1922.) (See Color Plate)

shown to have a good intraobserver and acceptable inter-observer agreements when recoded more simply as either present or absent. Similarly, relatively simple classifications by other investigators resulted in good reproducibility (71). Quantitative evaluation of lumen narrowing is also limited with current angioscopy, although a total occlusion and the presence or absence of lumen narrowing can be recognized.

Clinical Experience

Acute Coronary Syndromes

Driven by the high sensitivity of angioscopy to detect intraluminal thrombus in vivo, a number of clinical studies have investigated morphologic characteristics of culprit lesions responsible for acute coronary syndromes. By angioscopy, most culprit lesions show occlusive or mural thrombi frequently overlying disrupted yellow plaque (69,72,73). The thrombi are predominantly white, but can turn into red or mixed once they become occlusive. In some cases, the thrombi look yellow where they are mixed with exposed materials from a lipid core of disrupted plaque. One investigator group suggests that this type of culprit lesions may have a higher risk of distal embolization at PCI than purely thrombotic lesions with no visible plaque content protrusion (74). In a small percentage of acute myocardial infarction cases, neither yellow plaque nor adhering thrombus is detected after reperfusion; in these situations, secondary thrombosis after vasospasm or other mechanisms may be suspected.

The detailed healing process of infarct-related, disrupted plaques has also been evaluated in vivo by serial angioscopy. In a study by Ueda and colleagues (75), culprit lesions were examined immediately after PCI and/or thrombolysis and at 1, 6, and 18-month follow-up. Thrombus was detected in 93% at baseline and in 64% even 1 month after the onset of acute myocardial infarction, suggesting long persistent thrombogenicity at the culprit lesion. The prevalence of thrombus, however, markedly decreased at the following time points, accompanied by a significant reduction in visually graded yellow color intensity of the plaque. Interestingly, these stabilization processes were significantly impaired in patients with diabetes mellitus or hyperlipidemia.

Detection of Vulnerable Plaque

To date, a number of angioscopic studies have suggested that intensive yellow surface color of plaque is associated with unstable lesion morphology or clinical presentations. An early clinical study showed that yellow plaques were more common in patients with acute coronary disorders (50%) than in those with stable angina (15%) or old myocardial infarction (8%; 72). In a more recent study of 843 patients who underwent catheterization for suspected coronary disease, 1,253 yellow plaques were detected at nonstenotic (diameter stenosis <50%) segments and were graded as 1 to 3 (from light to intensive yellow) using prespecified color samples (Fig. 19.8; 76). This extensive series reported that intraluminal thrombus was detected more frequently on the plaque of higher yellow color grade (15%, 26%, and 52% on the plaque of color grade 1, 2, and 3, respectively, $P <$ 0.0001).

Pathophysiologic mechanisms for this association may be partly explained by structural and mechanical characteristics of yellow plaques. An experimental study using a bovine model of lipid-rich plaque showed an inverse correlation between angioscopic percent yellow saturation and histologic plaque cap thickness (77). A similar correlation was also reported in a clinical study by comparing angioscopic surface colors and plaque cap thickness measured by integrated backscatter analysis of IVUS signals (78). Furthermore, another clinical angioscopic study with conventional IVUS and simultaneous intracoronary pressure measurement demonstrated that yellow plaques had higher distensibility and greater remodeling ratio (more compensatory enlargement) than white plaques (23), both suggesting increased vulnerability of angioscopic yellow plaques.

On the other hand, yellow surface color of individual plaques alone may not have a sufficiently high predictive value for future clinical events, presumably owing to the presence of "silent" plaque rupture as well as the need of additional factors for triggering the events. Uchida and colleagues (79) reported the first prospective 12-month follow-up study and found that acute coronary syndromes occurred more frequently in patients with yellow plaques than in those with white plaques. Moreover, the syndromes occurred more frequently in patients with glistening yellow plaques than in those with nonglistening yellow plaques, but the positive predictive values of overall yellow and glistening yellow plaques were only 28% and 69%, respectively. More recently, Asakura and colleagues performed extensive angioscopic examination of all three major coronary arteries in patients undergoing follow-up catheterization 1 month after myocardial infarction (80). Both infarct-related and non–infarct related coronary arteries showed equally prevalent, multiple yellow plaques (3.7 ± 1.6 versus 3.4 ± 1.8 plaques per artery, respectively), indicating a pan-coronary process of vulnerable plaque development. Clinical follow-up (931 ± 107 days) of the enrolled patients showed a secondary event rate of only 20%. On this basis, the same investigator group proposed a plaque index (number of yellow plaques multiplied by maximum color grade) and found that patients who suffered another acute event during 5-year follow-up had a higher index at baseline than patients who did not (9.5 ± 6.8 versus 4.4 ± 4.0, $P = 0.02$; 74). Although whole coronary tree examination by angioscopy is not practical in clinical settings, angioscopic plaque characterization has the potential to offer unique complementary information in the field of vulnerable plaque/patient investigation.

Interventional Applications

Assessment of lesions before or after coronary intervention represents another commonly reported application of coronary angioscopy. One early study, for example, evaluated 122 patients undergoing conventional PTCA and revealed that angioscopic thrombus was strongly associated with in-hospital adverse outcomes (either a major complication or a recurrent ischemic event) after PTCA (relative risk, 3.11; 95% CI, 1.28 to 7.60; $P = 0.01$; 81). Another study also showed a similar correlation between the presence of red thrombus and early closure following laser-assisted coronary angioplasty (82).

Coronary angioscopy may significantly contribute to our understanding of new interventional devices or pharmacologic interventions. In coronary stenting, for example, several investigators have evaluated in vivo vessel response to bare metal stent implantation by serial angioscopy. Unlike animal models, these human studies suggested that, in some cases, several months may be required for visible completion of neointimal coverage over the metal struts. Instent neointima became thick and nontransparent until 6 months and, thereafter, became thinner and transparent by 3 years (83). Similarly, thrombus was observed up to 6 months but completely disappeared by 3 years, indicating that functional neointimal maturation may require up to several months following stent implantation. A more recent study investigated the effect of stenting on infarct-related lesions as well (84). At baseline, most lesions had complex morphology (96%) and yellow plaque color (96%), most of which were still observed even 1 month after stenting. At 6-month follow-up, however, the plaque shape and color mostly turned into smooth (97%) and white (93%), suggesting that stent implantation may lead to sealing of unstable plaque with neointimal proliferation. Similar changes in plaque color have also been reported with lipid-lowering interventions (85).

Safety and Limitations

The light source of angioscopy provides a high intensity but "cold" light (low infrared content) to avoid thermal damage to the illuminated vessel wall. On the other hand, mechanical designs of the angioscope and its delivery catheter can significantly affect the safety profile of this invasive imaging tool. To date, several complications have been reported, related to the occlusion cuff of the delivery catheter or transient ischemia owing to flow obstruction during imaging. Another complication is so-called wire-trapping caused by a loop formation of the guidewire between the two monorail wire channels of a certain angioscopy system. With the new over-the-wire system with no occlusion cuff, one experienced group reported a

complication rate of <1% during 1,200 procedures, but no comprehensive report of a large multicenter experience is yet available.

Despite recent technical advances, angioscopy is still limited in evaluating small vessel segments or imaging across tight stenoses. Also, at the presence of protruding structures, only the proximal aspect of the target may be visualized. Other technical limitations include its limited capability to assess inner tissue structures and the subjectivity of qualitative interpretation that potentially results in relatively large intraobserver and/or interobserver variability.

Future Directions

One technical solution to the subjective color interpretation is a quantitative colorimetric analysis of angioscopic images. In addition to the variability of human color perception, hardware-induced chromatic distortions can occur depending on angioscopic systems, individual catheters, illuminating light settings, and spatial location of the object within the view field. Quantitative colorimetric methods can overcome these limitations, and excellent measurement reproducibility with this technique has been reported in experimental studies (86).

Another interesting area in technical advancement may be integration of the angioscope into other catheter-based devices. The unique capability of angioscopy, particularly in the detection of thrombus and yellow plaques, can complement other imaging modalities and may enhance the efficacy of a certain type of treatment modality, such as thrombectomy catheters or devices for chronic total occlusion (CTO).

OPTICAL COHERENCE TOMOGRAPHY

Optical coherence tomography (OCT) generates real-time tomographic images from backscattered reflections of infrared light. This use of optical echoes thus can be regarded as an optical analog of IVUS. The greatest advantage of this light-based imaging technology is its significantly higher resolution (10 times or greater) than that of conventional pulse-echo, ultrasound-based approaches. The principal technology was developed and first described by researchers at the Massachusetts Institute of Technology in 1991 (87) and has been applied clinically in ophthalmology, dermatology, gastroenterology, and urology.

Imaging Systems and Procedures

The intravascular OCT imaging system consists of an optical engine emitting and receiving infrared light signals; a catheter interface unit including a motor drive; a fiberoptic imaging catheter; and a computer processor and display console for system control, image reconstruction, and digital recording. The optical engine includes a super-luminescent diode as a source of low coherent, infrared light, with a wavelength of approximately 1,300 nm to minimize light absorption by vessel wall and blood cell components (protein, water, hemoglobin, and lipids). The high propagation speed of light requires OCT to use interferometric techniques to determine the depth of the reflector. The emitted light is thus split into a sample beam (that travels through the imaging catheter to the scanning tissue and is reflected back to the interferometer) and a reference beam (reflected from a moving reference mirror whose distance within the system is accurately known). When these beams are recombined, positive interference occurs only when the two paths are matched—only the tissue plane that corresponds exactly to the reference arm length is recorded for image reconstruction. The motion of the reference beam mirror allows variable tissue depths to be interrogated, and rotation of the imaging lens allows circumferential data to be collected and passed to the processor for reconstruction of a cross-sectional image. Pullback of the imaging lens allows for a longitudinal scan. Current intravascular OCT systems have an axial resolution of 10 to 12 μm and lateral and out-of-plane resolution of 20 to 25 μm each at the focus. Inverse or pseudocolor OCT images are displayed in a real time format with video scanning rates of up to 30 frames per second.

The imaging procedure of intravascular OCT is similar to that of IVUS, except that (as in angioscopy) blood must be displaced by saline or a contrast medium while imaging. Technically, this is because the dominant mode of signal attenuation in OCT is multiple scattering, so that additional scattering by red blood cells results in very large signal loss.

At this point, only one company (LightLab Imaging Inc., Westford, MA) has commercialized the intravascular applications of OCT. This company produces dedicated imaging wires and occlusion balloon catheters for intravascular use. The 0.014-inch imaging wire with an atraumatic spring mounted on its tip is inserted distally to the occlusion balloon through the guidewire lumen. During the imaging, blood flow is interrupted by inflating the balloon with a modest amount of saline flush from its distal flush exit ports. The balloon inflation is performed at a low pressure to avoid unnecessary vessel stretching. Since the original guidewire is exchanged for the image wire, there is no guidewire artifact on the image plane. A second research group in the Wellman Labs at Massachusetts General Hospital uses custom-built OCT catheters modified from commercially available 3.2F mechanical IVUS catheters by substituting an optical imaging core for the IVUS core. With this approach, OCT images are acquired during intermittent 8- to 10-mL saline flushes through the guiding catheter. Since this design has a short guidewire lumen at the distal portion of the catheter tip, the guidewire is always seen by OCT as a point artifact with shadowing.

Experimental Data

Several experimental studies have demonstrated that intravascular OCT can reliably visualize the microstructure (i.e., 10 to 50 micron, versus 150 to 200 micron for IVUS) of normal and pathologic arteries. Typically, the media of the vessel appears as a lower signal intensity band than the intima and adventitia, giving a three-layered appearance similar to that seen by IVUS. The higher resolution of OCT, however, can often provide superior delineation of each structure with visualization of internal and external elastic membranes as separate thin high-intensity layers. Fibrous plaques exhibit homogeneous, signal-rich (highly backscattering) regions; lipid-rich plaques exhibit signal-poor regions (lipid pools) with poorly defined borders and overlying signal-rich bands (corresponding to fibrous caps); and calcified plaque exhibits signal-poor regions with sharply delineated upper and/or lower borders (Fig. 19.9; 88). Thus OCT has the advantage of being able to image through calcium without shadowing, as seen with IVUS. On the other hand, signal penetration through the diseased arterial wall is generally more limited (no more than 2 mm with current OCT devices), making it difficult to investigate deeper portions of the artery or to track the entire circumference of the media–adventitia interface (Fig. 19.9).

The diagnostic accuracy of OCT for the above plaque characterization criteria was confirmed by an ex vivo study of 307 human atherosclerotic specimens including aorta, carotid, and coronary arteries (88). Independent evaluation by two OCT analysts demonstrated a sensitivity and specificity of 71 to 79% and 97 to 98% for fibrous plaques; 90 to 94% and 90 to 92% for lipid-rich plaques; and 95 to 96% and 97% for fibrocalcific plaques, respectively (overall agreement versus histopathology, κ = 0.83 to 0.84). The interobserver and intraobserver reproducibility of OCT assessment was also high (κ values of 0.88 and 0.91, respectively). In addition, ex vivo measurement of fibrous cap thickness (<500 μm) showed a high degree of correlation between OCT and histomorphometry (r = 0.91, P < 0.0001).

One interesting approach by OCT to in-depth plaque characterization is macrophage quantification in the fibrous cap of atherosclerotic plaques. This signal-processing technique is based on the hypothesis that macrophage-infiltrated caps may have a higher heterogeneity of optical index of refraction, exhibiting stronger optical scattering with a higher signal variance than less infiltrated fibrous caps (Fig. 19.10). In an ex vivo study of 26 lipid-rich atherosclerotic arterial segments, Tearney and colleagues (89) compared the standard deviation of the OCT signal intensity with cap macrophage density quantified by immunohistochemistry. Prior to the computation, background and speckle noises were filtered out, and the standard deviation was normalized by the maximum and minimum OCT signals in the image. There was a high degree of

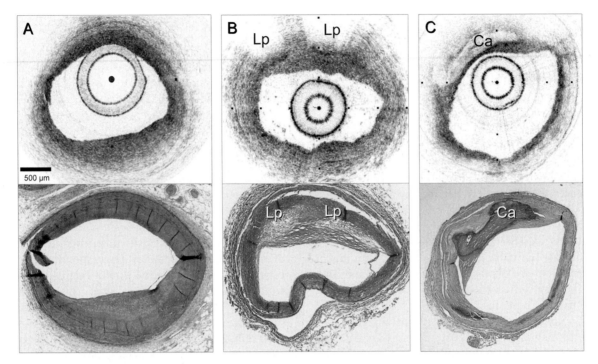

Figure 19.9 OCT images *(top)* and corresponding histology *(bottom)* for fibrous **(A)**, lipid-rich **(B)**, and calcific **(C)** plaques. In fibrous plaques, the OCT signal is observed to be strong and homogenous. In comparison, both lipid-rich (Lp) and calcific (Ca) regions appear as a signal-poor region within the vessel wall. Lipid-rich plaques have diffuse or poorly demarcated borders, whereas the borders of calcific nodules are sharply delineated. (Histologic stainings: Movat Pentachrome, Masson trichromed, and hematoxylin and eosin from left to right; original magnification 40×). (Courtesy of Bouma BE, Jang IK, and Tearney GJ.) (See Color Plate)

positive correlation between OCT and histologic measurements of fibrous cap macrophage density (r = 0.84, P < 0.0001). A range of OCT signal standard deviation thresholds (6.15% to 6.35%) yielded 100% sensitivity and specificity for identifying caps containing >10%

CD68 staining. Although direct visualization of individual mononuclear macrophages is limited with current intravascular OCT devices, advanced image-processing algorithms as shown in this study may be of great utility in the assessment of plaque instability.

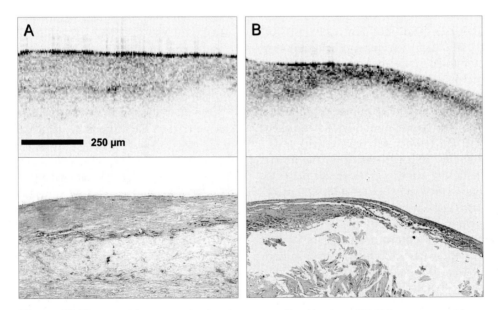

Figure 19.10 Raw OCT images *(top)* and corresponding histology (CD68 immunoperoxidase; original magnification 100×, *bottom)* of a fibroatheroma with a low macrophage density within the fibrous cap **(A);** and a fibroatheroma with a high macrophage density within the fibrous cap **(B).** (Tearney GJ, et al. *Circulation* 2003;107:113–119.) (See Color Plate)

Clinical Experience

Although in vivo experience in intravascular OCT is still limited, several single-center studies have demonstrated promising results of coronary imaging in clinical settings. In the first coronary OCT study in humans reported by Jang and colleagues (90), 17 coronary segments in 10 patients were imaged with 3.2F OCT catheters (modified IVUS catheters) during intermittent saline flushes through the guiding catheter. The duration of clear OCT imaging after each saline purge was approximately 2 seconds, and all patients tolerated the procedure well without complications. The maximum penetration depth of OCT imaging measured 1.25 mm versus 5 mm for IVUS. In vivo axial resolutions, determined by measuring the full-width half-maximum of the first derivative of a single axial reflectance scan at the surface of the tissue, were 13 ± 3 μm with OCT versus 98 ± 19 μm with IVUS. All fibrous plaques, macro-calcifications, and echolucent regions identified by IVUS were visualized in corresponding OCT images. However, intimal hyperplasia and echolucent regions, which may correspond to lipid pools, were identified more frequently by OCT than by IVUS.

In addition, recent clinical reports by the same investigator group showed that intravascular OCT had detected lipid-rich plaques and thrombus more frequently in acute myocardial infarction or unstable angina than in stable angina lesions (91). Similar feasibility results were also reported by other investigator groups using a different OCT system with dedicated catheters and image wires (a 3.7F monorail flush catheter with the image wire integrated into a saline flush lumen). In a pilot series of 16 patients scheduled for percutaneous coronary intervention, preinterventional OCT imaging with motorized pullback

was successfully performed and well tolerated in all patients (92). Two plaques showed inhomogeneous, low-reflecting areas (necrotic cores) covered by highly backscattering fibrous caps with a thickness of 45 and 50 μm.

Encouraging preliminary results were reported in the assessment of coronary interventions as well. Using 3.0 or 3.2F modified imaging catheters, Bouma and colleagues (93) successfully imaged 42 coronary lesions before and immediately after stenting. In this series, OCT detected dissections, instent tissue prolapse, and incomplete stent apposition more often than IVUS. With a dedicated OCT catheter, Grube and colleagues (94) also reported a follow-up OCT examination 6 months after drug-eluting stent implantation for the treatment of instent restenosis. The high resolution of OCT allowed clear visualization of the overlapped stents (stent-in-stent), distinctly identifying each stent strut as well as a very thin neointimal layer covering the drug-eluting stent struts (Fig. 19.11). Although exact clinical impact of intravascular OCT needs to be systematically evaluated, these preliminary reports confirmed that this new imaging technology has the potential to provide a new level of anatomic detail not only as a research technique but also as a clinical tool, particularly for evaluation of vulnerable plaque.

Safety and Limitations

Because the biologic safety of applied energies in OCT has been well established in other medical fields, potential issues predominantly derive from the mechanical designs of intravascular devices (imaging catheters and saline delivery system) and transient ischemia during coronary imaging. Although preliminary clinical experience suggests equivalent safety properties of intravascular OCT to early

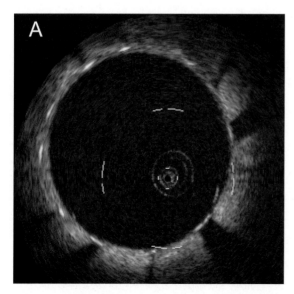 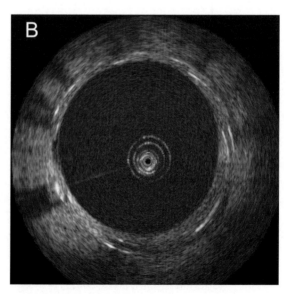

Figure 19.11 Follow-up OCT images of drug-eluting stents for de novo (**A**) and instent restenosis (**B**) lesions. The high resolution of OCT allows clear visualization of the stents, distinctly identifying each stent strut as well as a very thin neointimal layer covering the drug-eluting stent struts. (Courtesy of Grube E, and LightLab Imaging, Inc.) (See Color Plate)

IVUS or angioscopy systems, large multicenter registries are required to determine the exact incidence and severity of possible complications in various clinical settings.

At present, the major technical limitations of intravascular OCT are significant blood interference and shallow signal penetration through vessel walls. Thus, current in vivo imaging requires the displacement of blood from the imaging field and is restricted to the visualization of superficial vessel structures.

Future Directions

Several image improvement methods are being investigated, including index matching (to improve imaging through blood; 95) and frequency domain imaging (to increase the acquisition rate and radial scan range). Other technical enhancements currently being explored consist of various signal processing techniques to provide additional biochemical or functional information to the structural details of OCT. Spectroscopic analysis uses a spectrum of the infrared light reflected from the structures and color codes the information on the tomographic images, providing insights into the biochemical contents of the tissue. Polarization analysis, measuring the degree of birefringence in the tissue, may also be helpful in plaque component discrimination, since regions with highly oriented fibrous or smooth muscle cell components are more sensitive to the polarity of the imaging light than degenerated atheromatous regions with randomly oriented cells. OCT Doppler and elastography are analogous to those of ultrasound-based approaches but may offer improved sensitivity, owing to its higher resolution and contrast. In addition, viscoelasticity of the structure may be accurately assessed based on its intrinsic properties using laser speckle analysis.

SPECTROSCOPY

Spectroscopy determines the chemical composition of plaque substances, based on the analysis of spectra induced by interaction of electromagnetic radiation, or light, with the tissue materials. To date, several forms of photonic spectroscopy have been adapted for characterization of atherosclerotic plaques, including diffuse reflectance near-infrared (NIR), Raman, and fluorescence spectroscopy. When tissues are exposed to a light beam containing a broad mixture (spectrum) of wavelengths, wavelengths absorbed by the illuminated molecules will be missing from the spectrum of the original light after it has traversed the tissue. *Diffuse reflectance NIR spectroscopy* analyzes the amount of this absorbance as a function of wavelengths within the NIR window (700 to 2,500 nm; Fig. 19.12). On

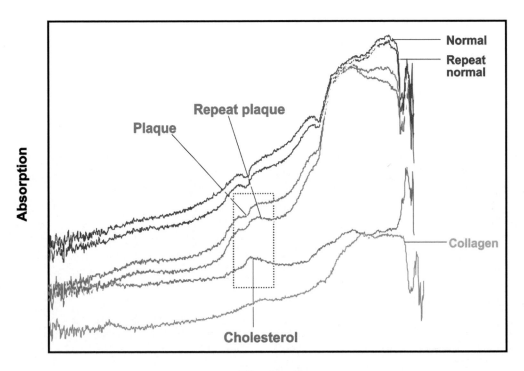

Figure 19.12 Diffuse reflectance NIR spectroscopy. Differences in individual chemical component spectra drive differences in the spectra of tissue samples, as shown on this diagram. The top 2 spectra are repeated measurements of a single normal sample, and middle 2 spectra are repeated measurements of a plaque. The cholesterol peak adds an additional feature to the plaque spectrum. Consequently, different tissue types can be recognized by examining these spectral patterns. (Courtesy of Muller JE, and InfraReDx, Inc.) (See Color Plate)

the other hand, *Raman spectroscopy* uses a light beam of a single wavelength and monitors shifts in wavelength as some of the incident photons interact with the molecules so as to gain or lose energy (i.e., shift in wavelength). Raman spectroscopy measures this inelastic scattering, or so-called Raman scattering, since it contains unique information on the substance with which the photons interacted. Under a certain condition, the photons can excite molecules to a higher energy level, the decay from which releases the energy difference in the form of light. *Fluorescence spectroscopy* uses photoluminescence or luminescent emission to identify the properties of the tissue being illuminated. Each technique has shown promising ex vivo results and is under active investigation for in vivo coronary applications.

Imaging Systems and Procedures

Like other light-based diagnostic techniques, the development of a catheter-based spectroscopy system for percutaneous coronary applications faces several technical challenges in terms of rapid signal acquisition with adequate signal-to-noise ratio and tissue penetration through blood. At present, one coronary catheter system has been successfully developed for in vivo diffuse reflectance NIR spectroscopy and is under clinical evaluation for commercial use (InfraReDx, Inc., Cambridge, MA). The 3.2F NIR catheter contains fiberoptic bundles for delivery and collection of light within a protective outer sheath. The latest generation catheter in a rapid-exchange design can be advanced to the coronary segment of interest using a standard interventional technique. The catheter directs the light to the vessel wall with a mirror located at the tip to acquire spectra within 20 milliseconds through flowing blood. This configuration allows not only a circumferential data collection but also a complete longitudinal scan of the target segment using controlled pullback of the probe. The collected light is analyzed by a spectrometer; using a diagnostic algorithm, the processed data are color coded and displayed in a grid pattern with the spatial (circumferential and longitudinal) information.

Although further improvement is still required prior to clinical testing, a miniaturized fiberoptic probe with a real-time analysis system has been developed for future intravascular application of Raman spectroscopy as well. The probe (Visionex, Atlanta, GA) consists of a central fiber (core diameter: 400 μm) for laser delivery and seven collection fibers (core diameter: 300 μm) around the central fiber. Both fibers have a dielectric filter to block the Raman signal generated by the fiber material. The system uses an 830-nm diode laser (Process Instruments Diode Laser, Salt Lake City, Utah) as a light source, and spectra acquisition times were reported to be 3 to 5 seconds for reliable detection of cholesterol and 1 second for calcium in an ex vivo setting. Although this prototype is a forward-viewing system, other investigators are also developing side-viewing catheter probes suitable for intravascular Raman scattering or fluorescence measurements.

Experimental Data

Over the past decade, a number of experimental studies have reported the ability of biospectroscopy (reflectance, Raman, and fluorescence) to identify the basic chemical components of atherosclerotic plaques in animal models or human arterial samples (Fig. 19.12). Particularly, intensive efforts are now focused on the characterization of the specific features of plaque vulnerability. Using diffuse reflectance NIR spectroscopy, Moreno and colleagues (96) recently examined 199 human aortic samples and compared the findings with corresponding histology. A diagnostic algorithm was constructed with 50% of the samples used as a reference set; blinded predictions of plaque composition were then performed on the remaining samples. The sensitivity and specificity of NIR spectroscopy for histologic plaque vulnerability were 90% and 93% for lipid pool, 77% and 93% for thin fibrous cap (<65 μm), and 84% and 89% for inflammatory cell infiltration, respectively. Similar promising results of NIR spectroscopy to identify lipid-rich plaques have been reported in human carotid endoatherectomy (97) and coronary autopsy specimens (98) as well. Whereas these ex vivo studies were performed in a blood-free laboratory setup, a recent in vivo study using a 1.5-mm fiber-bundle NIR catheter system also showed the feasibility of intravascular NIR spectroscopy through blood (99). In this rabbit aortic model, the catheter-based system identified lipid areas >0.75 mm^2 with 78% sensitivity and 75% specificity.

Although Raman spectroscopy has a theoretical advantage in direct quantification of individual plaque components, only a small percentage of photons are recruited into the Raman shift, resulting in a low signal-to-noise ratio and poor tissue penetration. However, recent exclusive use of the NIR wavelength laser (750 to 850 μm), coupled with enhanced CCD array cameras, could significantly improve the signal-to-noise ratio. In addition, mathematical tools have been developed to separate the contribution of background fluorescence in the Raman spectrum. In an ex vivo study of human coronary specimens, Romer and colleagues also demonstrated that a tissue layer of 300 μm attenuates the Raman cholesterol signals by 50% at 850 nm excitation (100), indicating that a lipid core up to 1 to 1.5 mm from the lumen could still be detected with this technique. Accordingly, the first in vivo application of catheter-based, intravascular Raman spectroscopy was demonstrated by Buschman and colleagues (101). This experimental study showed that the in vivo intravascular Raman signal obtained from an aorta was a simple summation of signal contributions of the vessel wall and blood.

On the other hand, the strong fluorescence of arterial tissue is a potential advantage of fluorescence spectroscopy over Raman analysis, permitting good signal-to-noise ratio with rapid spectra acquisition. Nevertheless, the encouraging ex vivo studies with fluorescence spectroscopy have not been translated into successful in vivo applications of this technique. This is in part owing to the significant spectra attenuation and distortion by the interplay of absorption and scattering at the presence of hemoglobin. Recently, a combined approach using fluorescence and diffuse reflectance spectroscopy has been proposed to minimize this technical limitation.

Safety and Limitations

At present, no published clinical experience is available in intravascular spectroscopy. In a swine coronary model, however, a prototype over-the-wire 3.2F NIR catheter system showed no evidence of vessel wall injury, including dissection, thrombus, and perforation, in any of the coronary vessels studied. The second-generation, rapid-exchange NIR catheter is currently under Phase I clinical evaluation.

Spectroscopic techniques provide no anatomical or depth information. Another important limitation is the relatively long acquisition time, resulting in substantial motion artifact in clinical settings. The second-generation NIR system, however, achieved a significantly shorter acquisition time (20 milliseconds) that is sufficient for intravascular use.

Future Directions

A catheter-based spectroscopy device combined with another structural imaging modality, such as IVUS or OCT, may allow comprehensive plaque evaluation by providing both chemical and anatomical information. The theoretical synergy of these two different modalities was demonstrated in an ex vivo human coronary study by Romer and colleagues (102). Although the spectroscopic and IVUS data were collected separately, Raman spectroscopy accurately identified and quantified cholesterol and small calcium deposits that were not detected by IVUS. Other investigators also reported a combined side-viewing Raman and IVUS experiment in a transluminal ex vivo setup (103). Current efforts are aimed at the simultaneous acquisition of IVUS images and Raman spectra through an integrated IVUS/Raman spectroscopic side-viewing catheter.

Another interesting attempt is to use diffuse reflectance NIR spectroscopy for in situ measurement of tissue pH or lactate concentration in atherosclerotic plaques. These metabolic parameters may indicate the activity of macrophages and other inflammatory cells, offering additional functional measures of plaque vulnerability. The feasibility of this technique has been demonstrated in an ex vivo study using human carotid endoatherectomy specimens (104), and further technical refinements are awaited for the clinical applications.

INTRAVASCULAR THERMOGRAPHY

The concept of plaque temperature measurement as a marker of local inflammation process was originally proposed by Casscells and colleagues (105), using human carotid endoatherectomy specimens. In this ex vivo study with a needle thermistor, intimal surface temperature correlated positively with cell density (mostly macrophages) and inversely with the distance of the cell clusters from the luminal surface. This is clinically important because a dense infiltration by active macrophages can destabilize plaque by secretion of cytokines, growth factors, or matrix metalloproteinases (MMP), ultimately leading to plaque rupture or erosion. Accordingly, several catheter-based devices have been developed for in vivo temperature measurement of human coronary arteries.

Imaging Systems and Procedures

The local temperature of the vessel wall can be assessed by two approaches: thermocouple-based and infrared-based measurements. The first approach incorporates a single or multiple thermal sensor(s) at the catheter tip and requires the contact of the thermal sensor(s) on the vessel wall. To date, several designs have been proposed to achieve this contact and have been tested in clinical studies. One system (Medispes SW A.G., Zug, Switzerland) has a single thermistor at the distal end of a 3F rapid-exchange polyurethane shaft (4F at the thermistor level). On the back of the thermistor, a specially designed hydrofoil is embedded so that the bloodstream drives the thermistor against the vessel wall. The same investigator group also developed a similar temperature probe but with a noncompliant semi-balloon, instead of the hydrofoil to minimize the cooling artifact by coronary blood flow. Two other systems have multiple sensors on a self-expanding nitinol five-wire basket (Volcano Therapeutics, Inc., Rancho Cordova, CA) or four self-expanding nitinol arms (Thermocore Medical Ltd., Guildford, UK) for the vessel wall contact, allowing simultaneous, circumferential temperature acquisitions. These over-the-wire systems have a protective outer sheath to expand/close the temperature sensing assembly. Using automated pullback, both systems can display a longitudinal color-coded thermal map of the studied vessel. Other investigators embedded a thermocouple in the most distal end of a 0.014-inch guidewire (Imetrx, Mountain View, CA). The wire tip is preshaped into a gentle angle, causing the thermosensitive tip of the wire to contact the vessel wall. A motor drive unit is designed for a combination of rotation and pullback motions so that the sensor tip travels a spiral path along the vessel wall.

A second approach uses an infrared fiberoptic catheter provides thermal imaging without direct vessel wall contact. The 4F prototype side-viewing catheter has 19 chalcogenide fibers with a wedge-shaped mirror at the tip. The heat reflected from the vessel wall is detected by a focal plane array cooled infrared camera connected to the proximal end of the imaging catheter, generating real-time color-coded thermographic images of the lumen. This system is still in an ex vivo testing phase but may have the potential for less invasive intravascular thermography.

Experimental Data

The feasibility of intravascular thermography for the in vivo assessment of local inflammatory foci has been validated in a rabbit aortic model. Using a thermography catheter with the self-expanding arm design, Verheye and colleagues (106) demonstrated that temperature heterogeneity was not present in the aortic segments of normal rabbits. In contrast, the aortic segments of hypercholesterolemic rabbits showed significant temperature heterogeneity (up to >1°C) that was associated with increased plaque thickness as assessed by IVUS. After 3 months of dietary cholesterol lowering, however, this temperature heterogeneity significantly decreased while the plaque thickness remained unchanged. Importantly, the reduced temperature heterogeneity paralleled the changes in plaque histology, which showed a marked loss of macrophages. Additional ex vivo experiments of the samples confirmed the positive relation between the local temperature and the local total macrophage mass.

Clinical Experience

The first clinical study with intravascular thermography was reported by Stefanadis and colleagues (107) in 1999, in which temperature difference between atherosclerotic plaques and the adjacent healthy vessel wall increased progressively from control subjects to patients with stable angina, unstable angina, and acute myocardial infarction (mean difference: 0.004 ± 0.009°C, 0.106 ± 0.110°C, 0.683 ± 0.347°C, and 1.472 ± 0.691°C, respectively). This study also showed significant intraplaque temperature heterogeneity, particularly in patients with unstable angina and acute myocardial infarction. In addition, there were significant positive correlations between the temperature difference and local morphologic (positive remodeling as assessed by IVUS) and systemic markers (C-reactive protein, serum amyloid A, and serum MMP-9 levels) of potential plaque vulnerability as well (108–110). A recent clinical study by Akasaka and colleagues (111) directly confirmed the initial preclinical observations by demonstrating a significant correlation of in vivo temperature data with corresponding histopathology (macrophage density) of the coronary specimens obtained by DCA.

Importantly, increased local temperature in atherosclerotic plaques may also have a strong impact on clinical outcomes of PCI. In a prospective series of 86 successful PCI patients (82 were treated with stenting), the temperature difference (ΔT) was shown as a strong predictor of adverse cardiac events (odds ratio 2.14, $P = 0.043$) during the follow-up period (18 ± 7 months; 112). The incidence of adverse cardiac events in patients with ΔT ≥ 0.5°C was 41%, as compared with 7% in patients with ΔT <0.5°C ($P < 0.001$). Another study showed that the administration of statins was associated with decreased ΔT in patients with coronary artery disease (113). In this series, the ΔT did not correlate with the cholesterol level at hospital admission, possibly suggesting a direct anti-inflammatory effect of statins. Although the clinical impact of this finding remains to be investigated, in vivo plaque temperature measurement may be useful not only for risk stratification but also as a surrogate end point of therapeutic interventions.

Safety and Limitations

The intravascular thermography devices are still under clinical evaluation, and at present, no acute or short-term adverse safety issues have been reported. One important concern is, however, possible vessel wall injury owing to the direct contact of the thermocouple-based devices. A recent animal study of pig coronary arteries evaluated endothelial damages by a thermography catheter with the self-expanding arm design, using Evans blue, scanning electron microscopy (SEM), and factor VIII antibody (114). Intracoronary pullback of the catheter was associated with acute and partial de-endothelialization, which normalized within 2 weeks and paralleled the findings observed with a standard IVUS catheter. It remains to be seen whether these favorable observations can be extrapolated to vulnerable plaques for which this technique was originally designed.

Another technical consideration is the potential influence of coronary flow on measured temperature. Using a bench-top model of a focal, eccentric, heat-generating lesion and a guidewire-based thermography system, Courtney and colleagues (115) demonstrated that the measured temperature increased linearly with source temperature and decreased with flow rates by an exponent of -0.33 ($P < 0.001$ for both). This "cooling effect" of blood flow has also been shown by several other investigators in both experimental and clinical settings, although the reported effects significantly differed in degree (114,116). It could explain the lack of heterogeneity in plaque temperature in recent studies using nonocclusive thermography catheters and will likely limit the diagnostic potential of thermography.

Future Directions

Similar to the spectroscopic techniques, intravascular thermography provides no anatomical information. Thus, combining thermography with other structural imaging techniques may offer an attractive synergy of metabolic and anatomic predictors of plaque vulnerability. Several investigators are currently developing integrated

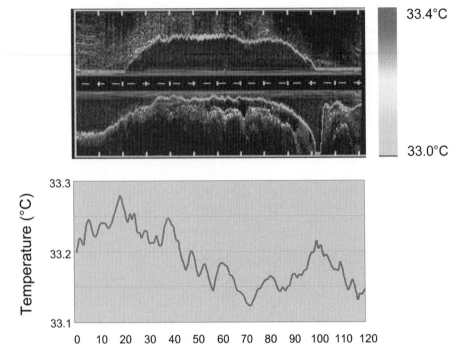

Figure 19.13   Intravascular thermography with an integrated thermography/IVUS catheter. The system displays a longitudinal color-coded thermal map of the studied vessel, superimposed on the lumen border of the IVUS image *(top)*. (Courtesy of Akasaka T, and Terumo Corp.) (See Color Plate)

thermography/IVUS catheters, providing a real-time color-coded thermal map on the IVUS image (Fig. 19.13). This approach may also allow additional functional information by incorporating new ultrasound-based signal analysis techniques, such as intravascular elastography.

INTRAVASCULAR MR IMAGING

Magnetic resonance imaging (MRI) is capable of providing both anatomical and compositional information on soft tissues, which makes it unique among all other imaging modalities. In the cardiovascular field, several investigators have shown that standard noninvasive MRI techniques can identify and characterize atherosclerotic lesions in humans and animal models. However, this plaque component characterization is currently limited to relatively large or superficial arteries, such as the aorta and carotid arteries, owing to the significant falloff of signal-to-noise ratio in deeper artery imaging by the external coil. One possible solution to this limitation is the placement of a MRI probe within the artery, allowing a high signal-to-noise ratio at the level of the artery wall. Accordingly, several intravascular MRI probes have been developed, each demonstrating improved resolution over external coils for in vivo imaging of atherosclerotic lesions.

Imaging Systems and Procedures

The most common approach to intravascular MRI is a combination of an intravascular receiver coil and an external MRI scanner. One company (Surgi-Vision, Inc., N. Chelmsford, MA) is commercializing a 0.030-inch intravascular MRI coil for peripheral imaging. This wire-based device is made from nitinol tubing with mechanical properties similar to standard stainless steel guidewires. The device is used in conjunction with an existing standard MRI scanner to image midsize vessels such as the renal arteries. For integration of the imaging wire with interventional procedures, a 0.014-inch intravascular MRI coil is also being developed.

Another company (Magna-Laboratory, Inc., Syosset, NY) is planning to release a 4.3F intravascular MRI probe with a single-loop receiver coil design. The device includes a lumen for a 0.014-inch guidewire and can be positioned using a standard interventional technique. In a preclinical rabbit study using a 1.5-tesla MRI system, the intravascular coil allowed aortic images to be obtained with 156×156 µm in-plane resolution (versus 352×352 µm with a standard external phased array coil; 117). No significant motion artifacts were noted, despite the continuation of arterial blood flow during image acquisition.

Experimental Data

Several experimental studies have confirmed the ability of intravascular MRI coils to accurately identify and quantify components of complex atherosclerotic plaques. In an early study using a 5F receiver coil with a 1.5-tesla scanner, Correia and colleagues (118) investigated 11 thoracic human aortas obtained at autopsy. In this study, the arterial wall composition analysis was performed using T2-weighted images, on which thickened intima, fibrous cap, and aortic adventitia showed low signal intensities, while the necrotic core and aortic media appeared bright. The intravascular MRI showed an agreement of 80% with histopathology in intimal thickness, 75% in fibrous cap grading, and 74% in necrotic core grading.

Zimmermann-Paul and colleagues used heritable hyperlipidemic rabbits to evaluate the feasibility of intravascular MRI in the study of atherosclerotic plaque progression (119). The MRI was performed using an intravascular coil consisting of a single-loop copper wire integrated in a 5F balloon catheter and a 1.5-tesla scanner, allowing an in-plane resolution of 117 × 156 μm. In this study, the progression of atherosclerotic changes over time was clearly visible. A good correlation was observed between the histologic AHA plaque characterization and MRI classifications, with an overall agreement of 88%.

More recently, in a study of human carotid endoatherectomy specimens, Rogers and colleagues (120) demonstrated a standard 0.5-tesla scanner could still achieve a reasonable degree of resolution (156 × 250 μm) with a 5F intravascular MRI coil. This study also suggested that various pulse sequences (magnetization transfer contrast, inversion recovery, and gradient echo sequences) taking advantage of differences in biochemical structure of individual plaque components may provide a more efficient method of MRI plaque characterization, compared with the conventional determination of absolute T1 and T2 values.

Safety and Limitations

Current intravascular MRI probes still require technical improvements for clinical coronary applications, and therefore, no comprehensive safety report is available at this point. Except for the guidewire-based design, most prototypes are 4 to 5F in diameter, which are not optimized for small-caliber arteries or lesions with significant stenosis. Another theoretical safety issue is possible heat generation during the imaging. Inserted metallic objects have the potential to couple with the transmitting radiofrequency coil and amplify the electric field in their vicinity, which results in radiofrequency heating of the surrounding tissue. However, a recent experimental study using a guidewire-based intravascular MRI in a rabbit model showed no abnormal changes of the coagulation factors, clinical manifestations of blood coagulation disorders, or histopathologic thermal damage in target vessels (121).

Other technical limitations include limited axial resolutions for thin fibrous cap detection, possible motion artifact owing to a long acquisition time, reduced image quality when the catheter coil moves off-axis from the external magnet field, and the requirement of an external scanner and MRI-compatible equipment in the catheterization laboratory.

Future Directions

Efforts are ongoing to develop more effective and user-friendly systems and to enhance the image-processing software. Rivas and colleagues (122) reported their real-time intravascular MRI system designed to overcome the artifact originating from the catheter and cardiac motion during the intravascular imaging. In a continuous flow phantom and in vivo in the rabbit aorta, the real-time intravascular imaging sequence achieved 120 to 440 μm resolutions at up to 16 frames per second. Other investigators (TopSpin Medical, Lod, Israel) have developed an intravascular MRI probe incorporating both magnets and coils within the catheter tip, permitting stand-alone catheter-based imaging with no external MRI scanner. The system is specifically designed for tissue characterization (lipid, fibrous tissue, and thrombi of varying ages), rather than simple anatomic imaging. The prototype providing a color-coded tissue component map is currently under phase 1 clinical evaluation. Finally, the combined use of targeting contrast agents, such as super paramagnetic iron oxide (SPIO), may further enhance the efficacy of intravascular MRI in the functional assessment of vulnerable plaques.

REFERENCES

1. Yock P, et al. Intravascular two-dimensional catheter ultrasound: initial clinical studies. *Circulation* 1988;78:II-21.
2. Fitzgerald PJ, et al. Intravascular ultrasound imaging of coronary arteries. Is three layers the norm? *Circulation* 1992;86:154–158.
3. Fitzgerald PJ, et al. Orientation of intracoronary ultrasonography: looking beyond the artery. *J Am Soc Echocardiogr* 1998;11:13–19.
4. Mintz GS, et al. American College of Cardiology Clinical Expert Consensus Document on Standards for Acquisition, Measurement and Reporting of Intravascular Ultrasound Studies (IVUS). A report of the American College of Cardiology Task Force on Clinical Expert Consensus Documents. *J Am Coll Cardiol* 2001;37:1478–1492.
5. Fitzgerald PJ, et al. Mechanisms and outcomes of angioplasty and atherectomy assessed by intravascular ultrasound imaging. *J Clin Ultrasound* 1993;21:579–588.
6. Mintz GS, et al. Determinants and correlates of target lesion calcium in coronary artery disease: a clinical, angiographic and intravascular ultrasound study. *J Am Coll Cardiol* 1997;29:268–274.
7. St Goar FG, et al. Intravascular ultrasound imaging of angiographically normal coronary arteries: an in vivo comparison with quantitative angiography. *J Am Coll Cardiol* 1991;18:952–958.
8. Mintz GS, et al. Atherosclerosis in angiographically "normal" coronary artery reference segments: an intravascular ultrasound study with clinical correlations. *J Am Coll Cardiol* 1995;25:1479–1485.
9. Mintz GS, et al. Limitations of angiography in the assessment of plaque distribution in coronary artery disease: a systematic study of target lesion eccentricity in 1446 lesions. *Circulation* 1996;93:924–931.
10. Nishioka T, et al. Contribution of inadequate compensatory enlargement to development of human coronary artery stenosis: an in vivo intravascular ultrasound study. *J Am Coll Cardiol* 1996;27:1571–1576.
11. Mintz GS, et al. Contribution of inadequate arterial remodeling to the development of focal coronary artery stenoses. An intravascular ultrasound study. *Circulation* 1997;95:1791–1798.

12. Kimura BJ, et al. Atheroma morphology and distribution in proximal left anterior descending coronary artery: in vivo observations. *J Am Coll Cardiol* 1996;27:825–831.

13. Jeremias A, et al. Spatial orientation of atherosclerotic plaque in non-branching coronary artery segments. *Atherosclerosis* 2000; 152:209–215.

14. Abizaid A, et al. Clinical, intravascular ultrasound, and quantitative angiographic determinants of the coronary flow reserve before and after percutaneous transluminal coronary angioplasty. *Am J Cardiol* 1998;82:423–428.

15. Takagi A, et al. Clinical potential of intravascular ultrasound for physiological assessment of coronary stenosis: relationship between quantitative ultrasound tomography and pressure-derived fractional flow reserve. *Circulation* 1999;100:250–255.

16. Briguori C, et al. Intravascular ultrasound criteria for the assessment of the functional significance of intermediate coronary artery stenoses and comparison with fractional flow reserve. *Am J Cardiol* 2001;87:136–141.

17. Komiyama N, et al. Tissue characterization of atherosclerotic plaques by intravascular ultrasound radiofrequency signal analysis: an in vitro study of human coronary arteries. *Am Heart J* 2000;140:565–574.

18. Nair A, et al. Coronary plaque classification with intravascular ultrasound radiofrequency data analysis. *Circulation* 2002;106: 2200–2206.

19. Schaar JA, et al. Incidence of high-strain patterns in human coronary arteries: assessment with three-dimensional intravascular palpography and correlation with clinical presentation. *Circulation* 2004;109(22):2716–2719.

20. Schoenhagen P, et al. Extent and direction of arterial remodeling in stable versus unstable coronary syndromes: an intravascular ultrasound study. *Circulation* 2000;101:598–603.

21. Gyongyosi M, et al. Arterial remodelling of native human coronary arteries in patients with unstable angina pectoris: a prospective intravascular ultrasound study. *Heart* 1999;82:68–74.

22. von Birgelen C, et al. Plaque distribution and vascular remodeling of ruptured and nonruptured coronary plaques in the same vessel: an intravascular ultrasound study in vivo. *J Am Coll Cardiol* 2001;37:1864–1870.

23. Takano M, et al. Mechanical and structural characteristics of vulnerable plaques: analysis by coronary angioscopy and intravascular ultrasound. *J Am Coll Cardiol* 2001;38:99–104.

24. Lim TT, et al. Role of compensatory enlargement and shrinkage in transplant coronary artery disease. Serial intravascular ultrasound study. *Circulation* 1997;95:855–859.

25. Pethig K, et al. Mechanism of luminal narrowing in cardiac allograft vasculopathy: inadequate vascular remodeling rather than intimal hyperplasia is the major predictor of coronary artery stenosis. Working Group on Cardiac Allograft Vasculopathy. *Am Heart J* 1998;135:628–633.

26. Yeung AC, et al. Incidence and progression of transplant coronary artery disease over 1 year: results of a multicenter trial with use of intravascular ultrasound. Multicenter Intravascular Ultrasound Transplant Study Group. *J Heart Lung Transplant* 1995;14(6 Pt 2):S215–220.

27. Mintz GS, et al. Impact of preintervention intravascular ultrasound imaging on transcatheter treatment strategies in coronary artery disease. *Am J Cardiol* 1994;73:423–430.

28. Gorge G, et al. Role of intravascular ultrasound in the evaluation of mechanisms of coronary interventions and restenosis. *Am J Cardiol* 1998;81:91G–95G.

29. Honye J, et al. Morphological effects of coronary balloon angioplasty in vivo assessed by intravascular ultrasound imaging. *Circulation* 1992;85:1012–1025.

30. Athanasiadis A, et al. Lesion morphology assessed by pre-interventional intravascular ultrasound does not predict the incidence of severe coronary artery dissections. *Eur Heart J* 1998;19:870–878.

31. Fitzgerald PJ, et al. Contribution of localized calcium deposits to dissection after angioplasty. An observational study using intravascular ultrasound. *Circulation* 1992;86:64–70.

32. Stone GW, et al. Improved procedural results of coronary angioplasty with intravascular ultrasound-guided balloon sizing: the CLOUT Pilot Trial. Clinical Outcomes With Ultrasound Trial (CLOUT) Investigators. *Circulation* 1997;95:2044–2052.

33. Colombo A, et al. Intravascular ultrasound-guided PTCA. *Eur Heart J* 1998;19:196–198.

34. Haase KK, et al. Acute and one year follow-up results after vessel size adapted PTCA using intracoronary ultrasound. *Eur Heart J* 1998;19:263–272.

35. Kimura T, et al. Remodeling of human coronary arteries undergoing coronary angioplasty or atherectomy. *Circulation* 1997; 96:475–483.

36. Mintz GS, et al. Arterial remodeling after coronary angioplasty: a serial intravascular ultrasound study. *Circulation* 1996;94:35–43.

37. Mintz GS, et al. Intravascular ultrasound to discern device-specific effects and mechanisms of restenosis. *Am J Cardiol* 1996; 78:18–22.

38. Braden GA, et al. Qualitative and quantitative contrasts in the mechanisms of lumen enlargement by coronary balloon angioplasty and directional coronary atherectomy. *J Am Coll Cardiol* 1994;23:40–48.

39. Simonton CA, et al. 'Optimal' directional coronary atherectomy: final results of the Optimal Atherectomy Restenosis Study (OARS). *Circulation* 1998;97:332–339.

40. Suzuki T, et al. Effects of adjunctive balloon angioplasty after intravascular ultrasound-guided optimal directional coronary atherectomy: the result of Adjunctive Balloon Angioplasty After Coronary Atherectomy Study (ABACAS). *J Am Coll Cardiol* 1999;34:1028–1035.

41. Lansky AJ, et al. Remodeling after directional coronary atherectomy (with and without adjunct percutaneous transluminal coronary angioplasty): a serial angiographic and intravascular ultrasound analysis from the Optimal Atherectomy Restenosis Study. *J Am Coll Cardiol* 1998;32:329–337.

42. Ahmed JM, et al. Mechanism of lumen enlargement during intracoronary stent implantation: an intravascular ultrasound study. *Circulation* 2000;102:7–10.

43. Maehara A, et al. Longitudinal plaque redistribution during stent expansion. *Am J Cardiol* 2000;86:1069–1072.

44. Colombo A, et al. Intracoronary stenting without anticoagulation accomplished with intravascular ultrasound guidance. *Circulation* 1995;91:1676–1688.

45. Nakamura S, et al. Intracoronary ultrasound observations during stent implantation. *Circulation* 1994;89:2026–2034.

46. de Jaegere P, et al. Intravascular ultrasound-guided optimized stent deployment. Immediate and 6 months clinical and angiographic results from the Multicenter Ultrasound Stenting in Coronaries Study (MUSIC Study) [see comments]. *Eur Heart J* 1998;19:1214–1223.

47. Uren NG, et al. Predictors and outcomes of stent thrombosis: an intravascular ultrasound registry. *Eur Heart J* 2002;23:124–132.

48. Cheneau E, et al. Predictors of subacute stent thrombosis: results of a systematic intravascular ultrasound study. *Circulation* 2003;108:43–47.

49. Kasaoka S, et al. Angiographic and intravascular ultrasound predictors of in-stent restenosis. *J Am Coll Cardiol* 1998;32: 1630–1635.

50. Fitzgerald PJ, et al. Final results of the Can Routine Ultrasound Influence Stent Expansion (CRUISE) study. *Circulation* 2000; 102:523–530.

51. Russo RJ, et al. Angiography Versus Intravascular Ultrasound-Directed stent placement: final results from AVID. *Circulation* 1999;100:I-234.

52. Mudra H, et al. Randomized comparison of coronary stent implantation under ultrasound or angiographic guidance to reduce stent restenosis (OPTICUS Study). *Circulation* 2001;104: 1343–1349.

53. Schiele F, et al. Impact of intravascular ultrasound guidance in stent deployment on 6-month restenosis rate: a multicenter, randomized study comparing two strategies—with and without intravascular ultrasound guidance. RESIST Study Group. REStenosis after Ivus guided STenting. *J Am Coll Cardiol* 1998; 32:320–328.

54. Hoffmann R, et al. Patterns and mechanisms of in-stent restenosis. A serial intravascular ultrasound study. *Circulation* 1996;94: 1247–1254.

55. Prati F, et al. In-stent neointimal proliferation correlates with the amount of residual plaque burden outside the stent: an intravascular ultrasound study. *Circulation* 1999;99:1011–1014.

56. Shiran A, et al. Effect of preintervention plaque burden on subsequent intimal hyperplasia in stented coronary artery lesions. *Am J Cardiol* 2000;86:1318–1321.

57. Kornowski R, et al. Increased restenosis in diabetes mellitus after coronary interventions is due to exaggerated intimal hyperplasia. A serial intravascular ultrasound study. *Circulation* 1997;95:1366–1369.

58. Castagna MT, et al. The contribution of "mechanical" problems to in-stent restenosis: an intravascular ultrasonographic analysis of 1090 consecutive in-stent restenosis lesions. *Am Heart J* 2001;142:970–974.

59. Shiran A, et al. Early lumen loss after treatment of in-stent restenosis: an intravascular ultrasound study. *Circulation* 1998;98:200–203.

60. Sonoda S, et al. Impact of final stent dimensions on long-term results following sirolimus-eluting stent implantation: serial intravascular ultrasound analysis from the SIRIUS trial. *J Am Coll Cardiol* 2004;43:1959–1963.

61. Kataoka T, et al. Three-dimensional IVUS assessment of edge effects following drug-eluting stent implantation. *J Am Coll Cardiol* 2002;39:70A.

62. Hong MK, et al. Paclitaxel coating reduces in-stent intimal hyperplasia in human coronary arteries: a serial volumetric intravascular ultrasound analysis from the ASian Paclitaxel-Eluting Stent Clinical Trial (ASPECT). *Circulation* 2003;107:517–520.

63. Serruys PW, et al. Vascular responses at proximal and distal edges of paclitaxel-eluting stents: serial intravascular ultrasound analysis from the TAXUS II trial. *Circulation* 2004;109:627–633.

64. Fujii K, et al. Contribution of stent underexpansion to recurrence after sirolimus-eluting stent implantation for in-stent restenosis. *Circulation* 2004;109:1085–1088.

65. Serruys PW, et al. Intravascular ultrasound findings in the multicenter, randomized, double-blind RAVEL (RAndomized study with the sirolimus-eluting VElocity balloon-expandable stent in the treatment of patients with de novo native coronary artery lesions) trial. *Circulation* 2002;106:798–803.

66. Hausmann D, et al. The safety of intracoronary ultrasound. A multicenter survey of 2207 examinations. *Circulation* 1995;91:623–630.

67. Spears JR, et al. Coronary angioscopy during cardiac catheterization. *J Am Coll Cardiol* 1985;6:93–97.

68. Siegel RJ, et al. Histopathologic validation of angioscopy and intravascular ultrasound. *Circulation* 1991;84:109–117.

69. Thieme T, et al. Angioscopic evaluation of atherosclerotic plaques: validation by histomorphologic analysis and association with stable and unstable coronary syndromes. *J Am Coll Cardiol* 1996;28:1–6.

70. den Heijer P, et al. The 'Ermenonville' classification of observations at coronary angioscopy—evaluation of intra- and interobserver agreement. European Working Group on Coronary Angioscopy. *Eur Heart J* 1994;15:815–822.

71. de Feyter PJ, et al. Ischemia-related lesion characteristics in patients with stable or unstable angina. A study with intracoronary angioscopy and ultrasound. *Circulation* 1995;92:1408–1413.

72. Mizuno K, et al. Angioscopic coronary macromorphology in patients with acute coronary disorders. *Lancet* 1991;337:809–812.

73. Ueda Y, et al. Intracoronary morphology of culprit lesions after reperfusion in acute myocardial infarction: serial angioscopic observations. *J Am Coll Cardiol* 1996;27:606–610.

74. Ueda Y, et al. Coronary atherosclerosis and acute coronary syndrome: new insights from angioscopic viewpoints. *Vasc Dis Prev* 2004;1:53–57.

75. Ueda Y, et al. The healing process of infarct-related plaques. Insights from 18 months of serial angioscopic follow-up. *J Am Coll Cardiol* 2001;38:1916–1922.

76. Ueda Y, et al. Assessment of plaque vulnerability by angioscopic classification of plaque color. *Am Heart J* 2004;148:333–335.

77. Miyamoto A, et al. Atheromatous plaque cap thickness can be determined by quantitative color analysis during angioscopy: implications for identifying the vulnerable plaque. *Clin Cardiol* 2004;27:9–15.

78. Kawasaki M, et al. In vivo quantitative tissue characterization of human coronary arterial plaques by use of integrated backscatter intravascular ultrasound and comparison with angioscopic findings. *Circulation* 2002;105:2487–2492.

79. Uchida Y, et al. Prediction of acute coronary syndromes by percutaneous coronary angioscopy in patients with stable angina. *Am Heart J* 1995;130:195–203.

80. Asakura M, et al. Extensive development of vulnerable plaques as a pan-coronary process in patients with myocardial infarction: an angioscopic study. *J Am Coll Cardiol* 2001;37:1284–1288.

81. White CJ, et al. Coronary thrombi increase PTCA risk. Angioscopy as a clinical tool. *Circulation* 1996;93:253–258.

82. Larrazet FS, et al. Angioscopy variables predictive of early angiographic outcome after excimer laser-assisted coronary angioplasty. *Am J Cardiol* 1997;79:1343–1349.

83. Asakura M, et al. Remodeling of in-stent neointima, which became thinner and transparent over 3 years: serial angiographic and angioscopic follow-up. *Circulation* 1998;97:2003–2006.

84. Sakai S, et al. Morphologic changes in infarct-related plaque after coronary stent placement: a serial angioscopy study. *J Am Coll Cardiol* 2003;42:1558–1565.

85. Takano M, et al. Changes in coronary plaque color and morphology by lipid-lowering therapy with atorvastatin: serial evaluation by coronary angioscopy. *J Am Coll Cardiol* 2003;42:680–686.

86. Lehmann KG, et al. Composition of human thrombus assessed by quantitative colorimetric angioscopic analysis. *Circulation* 1997;96:3030–3041.

87. Huang D, et al. Optical coherence tomography. *Science* 1991;254:1178–1181.

88. Yabushita H, et al. Characterization of human atherosclerosis by optical coherence tomography. *Circulation* 2002;106:1640–1645.

89. Tearney GJ, et al. Quantification of macrophage content in atherosclerotic plaques by optical coherence tomography. *Circulation* 2003;107:113–119.

90. Jang IK, et al. Visualization of coronary atherosclerotic plaques in patients using optical coherence tomography: comparison with intravascular ultrasound. *J Am Coll Cardiol* 2002;39:604–609.

91. Jang IK, et al. In-vivo coronary plaque characteristics in patients with various clinical presentations using optical coherence tomography: comparison with intravascular ultrasound. *Circulation* 2003;108:373.

92. Regar E, et al. Real-time, in vivo optical coherence tomography of human coronary arteries using a dedicated imaging wire. *Am J Cardiol* 2002;90:129H.

93. Bouma BE, et al. Evaluation of intracoronary stenting by intravascular optical coherence tomography. *Heart* 2003;89:317–320.

94. Grube E, et al. Images in cardiovascular medicine. Intracoronary imaging with optical coherence tomography: a new high-resolution technology providing striking visualization in the coronary artery. *Circulation* 2002;106:2409–2410.

95. Brezinski M, et al. Index matching to improve optical coherence tomography imaging through blood. *Circulation* 2001;103:1999–2003.

96. Moreno PR, et al. Detection of lipid pool, thin fibrous cap, and inflammatory cells in human aortic atherosclerotic plaques by near-infrared spectroscopy. *Circulation* 2002;105:923–927.

97. Wang J, et al. Near-infrared spectroscopic characterization of human advanced atherosclerotic plaques. *J Am Coll Cardiol* 2002;39:1305–1313.

98. Moreno PR, et al. Identification of lipid-rich plaques in human coronary artery autopsy specimens by near-infrared spectroscopy. *J Am Coll Cardiol* 2001;37:356A.

99. Moreno PR, et al. Identification of lipid-rich aortic atherosclerotic plaques in living rabbits with a near infrared spectroscopy catheter. *J Am Coll Cardiol* 2001;37:3A.

100. Romer TJ, et al. Raman spectroscopy for quantifying cholesterol in intact coronary artery wall. *Atherosclerosis* 1998;141:117–124.

101. Buschman HP, et al. In vivo determination of the molecular composition of artery wall by intravascular Raman spectroscopy. *Anal Chem* 2000;72:3771–3775.

102. Romer TJ, et al. Intravascular ultrasound combined with Raman spectroscopy to localize and quantify cholesterol and calcium salts in atherosclerotic coronary arteries. *Arterioscler Thromb Vasc Biol* 2000;20:478–483.

103. de Korte CL, et al. Vascular plaque characterization using intravascular ultrasound elastography and NIR Raman spectroscopy in vitro. *Proc SPIE* 2000;3982:180–186.

104. Naghavi M, et al. pH Heterogeneity of human and rabbit atherosclerotic plaques; a new insight into detection of vulnerable plaque. *Atherosclerosis* 2002;164:27–35.

105. Casscells W, et al. Thermal detection of cellular infiltrates in living atherosclerotic plaques: possible implications for plaque rupture and thrombosis. *Lancet* 1996;347:1447–1451.

106. Verheye S, et al. In vivo temperature heterogeneity of atherosclerotic plaques is determined by plaque composition. *Circulation* 2002;105:1596–1601.

107. Stefanadis C, et al. Thermal heterogeneity within human atherosclerotic coronary arteries detected in vivo: a new method of detection by application of a special thermography catheter. *Circulation* 1999;99:1965–1971.

108. Stefanadis C, et al. Heat production of atherosclerotic plaques and inflammation assessed by the acute phase proteins in acute coronary syndromes. *J Mol Cell Cardiol* 2000;32:43–52.

109. Toutouzas K, et al. The temperature of atherosclerotic plaques is correlated with matrix metalloproteinases concentration in patients with acute coronary syndromes. *J Am Coll Cardiol* 2001;37:356A.

110. Toutouzas K, et al. Positive arterial remodeling is associated with increased temperature of atherosclerotic plaques in patients with acute coronary syndromes. *J Am Coll Cardiol* 2001;37:4A.

111. Akasaka T, et al. Relation between plaque temperature and histology. *Eur Heart J* 2003;24:153.

112. Stefanadis C, et al. Increased local temperature in human coronary atherosclerotic plaques: an independent predictor of clinical outcome in patients undergoing a percutaneous coronary intervention. *J Am Coll Cardiol* 2001;37:1277–1283.

113. Stefanadis C, et al. Statin treatment is associated with reduced thermal heterogeneity in human atherosclerotic plaques. *Eur Heart J* 2002;23:1664–1669.

114. Verheye S, et al. Intravascular thermography: immediate functional and morphological vascular findings. *Eur Heart J* 2004; 25:158–165.

115. Courtney BK, et al. Validation of a thermographic guidewire for endoluminal mapping of atherosclerotic disease: an in vitro study. *Cathet Cardiovasc Interv* 2004;62:221–229.

116. Stefanadis C, et al. Thermal heterogeneity in stable human coronary atherosclerotic plaques is underestimated in vivo: the "cooling effect" of blood flow. *J Am Coll Cardiol* 2003;41:403–408.

117. Worthley SG, et al. A novel nonobstructive intravascular MRI coil: in vivo imaging of experimental atherosclerosis. *Arterioscler Thromb Vasc Biol* 2003;23:346–350.

118. Correia LC, et al. Intravascular magnetic resonance imaging of aortic atherosclerotic plaque composition. *Arterioscler Thromb Vasc Biol* 1997;17:3626–3632.

119. Zimmermann-Paul GG, et al. High-resolution intravascular magnetic resonance imaging: monitoring of plaque formation in heritable hyperlipidemic rabbits. *Circulation* 1999;99:1054–1061.

120. Rogers WJ, et al. Characterization of signal properties in atherosclerotic plaque components by intravascular MRI. *Arterioscler Thromb Vasc Biol* 2000;20:1824–1830.

121. Yang X, et al. Thermal effect of intravascular MR imaging using an MR imaging-guidewire: an in vivo laboratory and histopathological evaluation. *Med Sci Monit* 2002;8:MT113–117.

122. Rivas PA, et al. In vivo real-time intravascular MRI. *J Cardiovasc Magn Reson* 2002;4:223–232.

Endomyocardial Biopsy

20

Kenneth L. Baughman, MD   *Donald S. Baim, MD*

Heart muscle disorders remain one of the most poorly understood areas in cardiology. Although right heart catheterization can define the severity of congestion, depression of cardiac output, and response to therapy, and left heart catheterization and angiography can identify some specific causes of heart failure (e.g., coronary artery, valvular or pericardial disease), more than half of the patients presenting with new onset heart failure remain classified as idiopathic. It stands to reason that myocardial biopsy should allow more precise characterization of the underlying primary myocardial pathology in such patients, provide prognostic guidance, and monitor therapy. In reality, however, these benefits have been established for relatively few myocardial pathologies (such as transplant rejection and doxorubicin toxicity). But as more precise molecular and genetic analysis are now applied to myocardial biopsy specimens (beyond the standard histologic, immunohistochemical, and electron microscopic analysis currently available), the prognostic value of myocardial biopsy should improve. This chapter will thus review the history of endomyocardial biopsy, available devices, biopsy techniques and complications, guidance for post procedure care, and indications for endomyocardial biopsy in the current era, tools, and techniques for obtaining and analyzing myocardial biopsy specimens.

HISTORICAL APPROACHES

In 1958, Weinberg, Fell, and Lynfield (1) performed biopsies through an incision in the left intercostal space at the costochondral junction. The pericardium was identified after dissection of the cartilage and the pleura and partially resected to allow an incisional biopsy of the epicardium and myocardium. In reality, the pericardial biopsy was of as much or greater value than myocardial biopsy revealing inflammatory, tuberculosis, and traumatic causes of pericardial constriction, but two of the patients displayed myocardial pathology (lupus myocarditis and nonamyloid restrictive heart disease). Because of the need for an open incision and surgical extraction, however, this technique was not widely adopted.

In 1960, Sutton and Sutton (2) reported their experience with percutaneous heart biopsy performed at the left ventricular apex or peristernal region in the fifth intercostal space, using a modified flexible thin walled Terry needle. One hundred and fifty biopsies were performed in 54 patients with myocardial disease of unknown cause. With this technique, 13 of 54 patients had inadequate specimens for diagnosis, 13 of 54 had no abnormality, and 16 displayed nuclear enlargement and/or fibrosis compatible with idiopathic cardiomyopathy. But 12 of the 54 patients had specific etiologic findings including myocarditis, sarcoidosis, rheumatic heart disease, and fibroelastosis. One patient died 11 days after biopsy, and frequent ventricular premature contractions were reported.

Timmis and colleagues (3) used a percutaneous Vim-Silverman or Menghini needle in 20 dogs, using electrocardiographic monitoring via the needle to signal epicardial contact. Whereas diagnostic material was obtained in 60.5% of the attempts, these animals developed signs and symptoms suggestive of pneumothorax or hemopericardium, and most displayed an inflammatory pericarditis within 2 weeks of the puncture. Even so, in 1972 Shirey and colleagues (4) reported similar use of a Silverman needle to obtain specimens percutaneously from 198 patients with heart disease, of whom 36% had primary myocardial disease whereas the others had coronary or valvular heart disease. The needle was inserted at the left ventricular apex under fluoroscopy until premature beats and pulsation through the needle indicated contact with the left ventricular wall. With the cannula held in position, the obturator was replaced with a cutting stylet or cutting needle and the elongated specimen obtained was then sectioned for appropriate examination. Nearly all (192 of 198) of these patients had tissue recovered, with half showing nonspecific hypertrophy and interstitial fibrosis, 13% small vessel disease, and the rest showing nonspecific basophilic degeneration, amyloidosis, rheumatic heart disease, or myocarditis. The validity of the percutaneous biopsy was confirmed in 11 patients who later died, allowing full postmortem examination of the heart. Complications of this technique included pericardial tamponade in eight and postpericardioectomy syndrome in an additional four patients.

In 1965, Bulloch (5) introduced the concept of percutaneous insertion of a heart biopsy needle through the right external or internal jugular vein to allow sampling of the right interventricular septum. In this technique, cutting blades were inserted through a 16-gauge, 50-cm-long curved shaft positioned in the right ventricle through a large-bore radiopaque catheter. Although this techniques is no longer used, it established several principles that are still used today: (1) percutaneous access, (2) use of the right internal jugular vein, (3) definition of right heart boundaries by right heart catheterization before an endomyocardial attempt, (4) rotation of the curved biopsy sheath counterclockwise (anteriorly) to avoid the coronary sinus or tricuspid valve, and (5) advancing the tip of the biopsy forceps toward the interventricular septum (posterior medially). Although the 20 human specimens revealed no specific diagnosis, the authors reported no serious complications.

The Konno biopsy techniques were introduced by Sakakibara and Konno (6). Their original device consisted of a 100-cm shaft equipped at its tip with two sharpened cups (diameter either 2.5 or 3.5 mm). The cups were opened and closed under the control of a single wire, activated by a sliding assembly attached to the proximal end of the catheter. This flexible bioptome thus allowed endomyocardial sampling by pinching rather than advancement of a cutting needle. The authors demonstrated the relative ease of the obtaining samples in five patients, with establishment of a specific diagnosis in three. Because of the large size of the catheter head, however, it was usually introduced by a cutdown technique through a large vein or artery. The Konno bioptome is currently used infrequently because of its relatively large size, stiff shaft, and lack of durability with repeated usage (7,8).

In 1972, Caves modified the Konno biopsy for use through the right internal jugular vein (9,10). This modification allowed the bioptome to be inserted percutaneously, but the large diameter of the bioptome head required use of a large (nonvalved) sheath that placed the patient at risk for bleeding or air embolization at the time of bioptome insertion or removal. The technique did allow several advantages

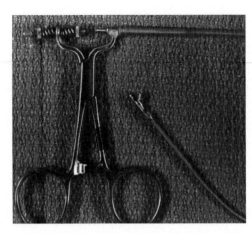

Figure 20.1   Stanford (Caves-Schulz) bioptome. The surgical clamp drives a control wire to which it is connected via two adjustable nuts, thereby controlling the position of the single mobile jaw at the distal end of the catheter.

including percutaneous insertion, use of local anesthetic allowing minimal discomfort to the patient, rapid performance, direct passage of the bioptome to the right ventricular apex, and repeated entry and exit through the same sheath.

Caves (11) subsequently introduced the Stanford modification to the previous Konno Bioptome (Fig. 20.1). The Stanford (or Caves-Shulz) bioptome served as the industry standard from approximately 1975 to 1995 (12). It was 50 cm long and had a moderately flexible coil shaft fabricated from stainless steel wire coated by a clear plastic tubing (Scholten Surgical Supply, Palo Alto, CA). Two hemispheric cutting jaws with a combined diameter of 3 mm (9 French) were mounted on the catheter tip. One of the jaws remained stationary while the other opened and closed under the control of a mosquitolike clamp at the proximal end of the catheter. The degree of curvature of the bioptome could be modified between 45 and 90° by preshaping the shaft and adjusting the degree of closure of the handle ratchet mechanism. Spring-loaded adjustable nuts allowed the operator to adjust the amount of force applied with opening and closing of the surgical-like clamp. Because this bioptome was reusable, it required careful cleaning after each use and ultimately the need for retooling and sharpening of the cutting edges of the jaws after 50 procedures.

Richardson (13) of Kings College Hospital in London introduced a smaller-diameter (1.8-mm) bioptome in 1974 that was more flexible and could be inserted percutaneously into jugular, femoral, or even subclavian veins. In 1977, Kawai and Kitaura designed a bioptome with a more flexible tip controlled by rotation of a knob on the operating handle (7,8; Fig. 20.2). A modification of this bioptome allowed intracardiac electrocardiographic monitoring (1980). Although the bioptome allowed easy maneuverability through the vasculature and across the tricuspid or aortic valve, the flexible tip required a stylet to be advanced into the bioptome shaft before an endomyocardial biopsy could be performed.

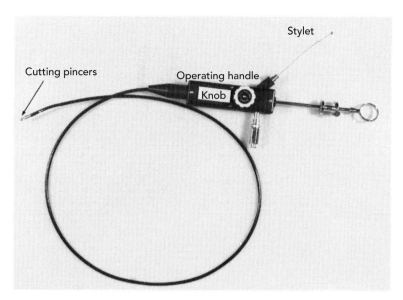

Figure 20.2 The Kawai flexible endomyocardial biopsy catheter. (From Kawai C, Matsumori A, Kawamura K. Myocardial biopsy. Ann Rev Med 31: 139, 1980, with permission)

MODERN BIOPTOMES

Currently, biopsy forceps draw heavily on the early instruments described above. They are, however, single-use and disposable devices that eliminate the risk of patient-to-patient disease transmission, pyrogen reaction, need for retooling and resharpening of the cutting edges, and mechanical malfunction sometimes seen in the earlier reusable devices. They follow either a preshaped or flexible (long-sheath) format (Fig. 20.3).

The unshaped flexible bioptomes are inserted through a preformed sheath that directs the head of the instrument toward the desired portion of the right ventricular septum or left ventricular wall. The preformed sheath is generally advanced over an angled pigtail or balloon flotation

catheter and remains in the ventricular cavity throughout the biopsy procedure. This increases the risk for ventricular arrhythmia or perforation and reduces the operator control of the site and direction of the bioptome's path.

In contrast, the preshaped bioptomes are introduced through a short venous sheath and maneuvered as independent catheters to access the right ventricle. They are stiffer and allow greater control by the operator of the course and direction of the instrument. The degree of curvature of the preshaped bioptome can be modified by the operator to suit the angulation required to traverse the tricuspid valve. For the rare patient in whom the relatively stiff preshaped bioptome fails to enter the right ventricle, biopsy can still be performed by advancing a preformed sheath into the ventricle over either a guidewire or a ballooned-tipped catheter. Disposable bioptomes and sheaths are available for use from the right or left jugular vein, subclavian vein, femoral vein, or femoral arteries and vary in length, shape, jaw size, and diameter.

BIOPSY TECHNIQUE

Right ventricular heart biopsy can be performed percutaneously from the right internal jugular vein, left internal jugular vein, right subclavian, and right or left femoral veins. Left ventricular biopsy is usually performed from the right or left femoral artery; however, it can be accomplished from the right or left brachial artery. The necessary equipment is listed in Table 20.1.

Internal Jugular Access

Right ventricular endomyocardial biopsy procedures are most commonly performed via the right internal jugular vein. Patients usually fast for 8 hours prior to the procedure,

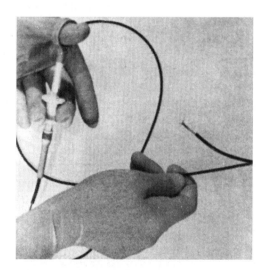

Figure 20.3 The Olympus bioptome positioned through a modified Stanford biopsy sheath. (From Anderson JL, Marshall HW. The femoral approach to endomyocardial biopsy: comparison with internal jugular and transarterial approaches. Am J Cardiol 53: 833, 1984, with permission).

TABLE 20.1
EQUIPMENT FOR ENDOMYOCARDIAL BIOPSY

Continuous electrocardiographic monitor
Automatic intermittent cutaneous or invasive blood pressure
   monitor
Continuous oxygen saturation monitor
Ether screen or drape support
Povidone-iodine, alcohol, or both
Plastic or cloth drape set
Two 20-mL syringes
One 10-mL syringe
One 25-, one 22-, and three or four 18-gauge needles
250 mL of flush solution (with heparin)
18-gauge Amplatz needle or 22-gauge micropuncture needle
7, 8, or 9F self-sealing introducer with 0.038-inch guidewire
Micropuncture wire, 0.021 inch
4 or 5F micropuncture sheath
No. 11 surgical blade and handle
Mosquito clamp or small-tipped instrument
   Tissue preservative
   Formalin
   Glutaraldehyde
   Dry ice
Lidocaine: 1 or 2%, 15 mL
Emergency equipment
   Defibrillator
   Pacemaker and wire
   Pericardiocentesis set
   Resuscitation drugs and equipment

From Baughman KL: *History and Current Techniques of Endomyocardial Biopsy.* W. B. Saunders, Philadelphia, 2002 Fig. 25.1, p. 269.

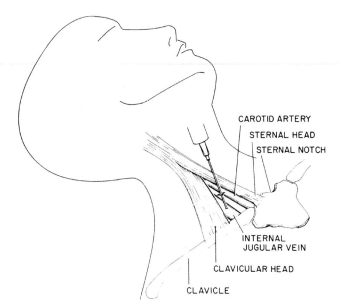

Figure 20.4 Regional anatomy for internal jugular puncture. With the patients head rotated to the left, the sternal notch, clavicle, as well as the sternal and clavicular heads of the sternocleidomastoid muscle are identified. A skin nick is made between the two heads of this muscle, and two fingerbreadths above the top of the clavicle (near the top of the anterior triangle). The needle is inserted at an angle of 30-40 degrees from vertical, at 20-30 degrees right of saggital, aiming the needle away from the more medially located carotid artery.

but sedative premedications are generally not required for this outpatient procedure. Monitoring during the procedure includes continuous electrocardiogram, pulse oximetry, and blood pressure. For patients who are in decompensated heart failure, continuous arterial pressure monitoring (using a small-bore catheter or a commercially available noninvasive instrument) is recommended.

The patient's head is turned 30 to 45° to the left to facilitate evaluation and preparation of the venous cannulation site. The internal jugular is located lateral to the carotid artery, within the *anterior triangle* formed by the sternal and clavicular head of the sternocleidomastoid muscle and top of the clavicle (Fig. 20.4). These anatomical features can be identified more easily by having the patient briefly lift his or her head just off the table. Internal jugular venous cannulation should be attempted in the middle third of the triangle outlined by the landmarks noted above. This allows compression of venous or arterial structures should bleeding persist after the procedure or if carotid artery puncture occurs during the procedure. Additionally, this higher location in the anterior triangle lessens the risk of pneumothorax. If the location of the internal jugular vein is not readily apparent, we routinely evaluate the neck vasculature echocardiographically, using a 7.5-MHz dedicated sector scanner (Site Rite, Dynamax Corporation, Pittsburgh,

PA) or a conventional echo transducer encased in a sterile sheath. The jugular vein can be distinguished from the more medial carotid artery by location, the pulsatility of the artery, and the compressibility of the vein (Fig. 20.5). Use of echo guidance has been demonstrated to increase the frequency of vein cannulation, decrease access time, and decrease complication rates (14,15).

After the patient's landmarks have been identified, the neck is prepared with a standard povidone-iodine and alcohol preparation. The field is isolated using sterile towels and/or plastic drapes. An ether screen or similarly fashioned device can be used to isolate this area and to protect the patient's face from the drapes. Successful puncture of the internal jugular is facilitated by distension of the vein—in patients with low venous pressure or a small internal jugular vein, this can be achieved by placing the patient in a head-down Trendelenburg position, elevating the legs on a wedge, or having the patient perform a Valsalva maneuver during needle advancement.

A 25-gauge needle is used to apply a small interdermal bleb of 2% Xylocaine at the site of planned sheath entry. A 22-gauge needle is then used to anesthetize the area from the superficial bleb toward the internal jugular vein. After the area is successfully anesthetized, a small (2 mm) incision is made at the superficial site of initial infiltration with a no. 11 surgical blade. The incision is then expanded with the tip of a mosquito clamp to ensure that the skin will accommodate the 7F venous sheath. In the classic approach, the 22-gauge anesthesia needle is directed toward the anticipated venous

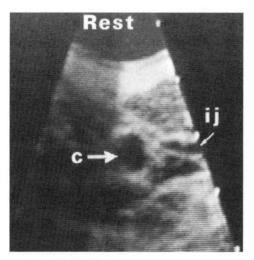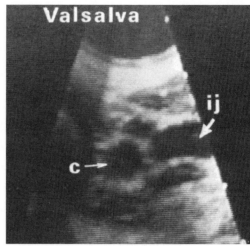

Figure 20.5 Two-dimensional echo of the carotid artery (c) and the internal jugular vein (ij) at rest (left) and during Valsalva maneuver (right), showing the maked enlargement in jugular venous caliber with increased distending pressure.

pathway at an angle of approximately 30 to 40° from vertical and 20° right of the sagittal plane and is advanced in small increments, aspirating before infiltration of small amounts of lidocaine to provide local anesthesia. Excess lidocaine infiltration should be avoided, since it may result in venous compression or infiltration of vocal cords or carotid sheath resulting in transient hoarseness or Horner syndrome.

Once venous blood is aspirated, indicating entry into the internal jugular vein, the operator notes the position and direction of the needle as a second 18-gauge single-wall puncture needle with syringe is advanced parallel to the "finder" needle. Continuous aspiration is applied as the needle is advanced in small increments, particularly in individuals with small internal jugular veins or low central venous pressures. Usually the "give" of the vein wall is palpable, even before blood return is evident. A J-tip guidewire is then introduced, followed by the necessary sheath.

If the initial attempts at venous entry are unsuccessful, the probing needle is retracted to just beneath the skin level and redirected more laterally. If venous return is still not achieved, the needle may be directed more medially (toward the plane of the carotid artery). Should arterial puncture occur, the probing needle and syringe will fill spontaneously with well-oxygenated blood, and the needle must be removed and compressed for 5 minutes or until hemostasis is obtained. As described above, this problem can be avoided by using echo guidance when the initial puncture attempt is unsuccessful.

An alternative approach that we now use routinely at the Brigham and Women's Hospital is to use a 22-gauge micropuncture needle (Fig. 20.6), as the deep anesthesia, probing, and definitive entry device for internal jugular vein cannulation. This needle is very atraumatic and accepts a special 0.021-inch mandril guidewire over

which a special coaxial double dilator is advanced. Once this has entered the jugular vein and superior vena cava, the inner cannula and 0.021-inch guidewire are removed and a conventional 0.038-inch guidewire is inserted through the outer cannula. The cannula is then removed, and a 7 or 8 French self-sealing sheath is inserted over the guidewire. This is facilitated by passing the wire from the superior vena cava, across the right atrium, and into the inferior vena cava, avoiding runs of ventricular ectopy seen when the wire tips enters the right ventricle. Once the sheath is in the appropriate position, the guidewire is removed, the

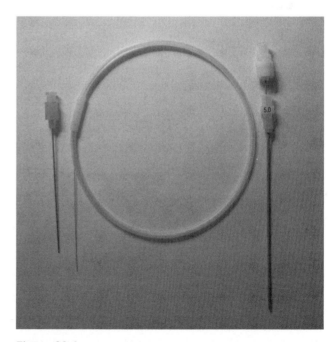

Figure 20.6 Micropuncture apparatus: 22-gauge micropuncture needle, 0.021-inch guidewire, 5F guided sheath, and obturator.

sheath is aspirated and flushed, and the heart biopsy procedure can proceed.

Right Subclavian Vein Access

Rarely, the right subclavian vein is used when patient anatomic factors make the internal jugular and femoral veins inappropriate for access (16). The entry site into the subclavian vein should be somewhat more lateral than is routinely the case for subclavian venous catheterization, as a superior vena cava/subclavian vein angle that is too acute will prevent the relatively stiff bioptome from negotiating this angle into the right heart. The standard site of entry for subsequent heart biopsy is in the infraclavicular region, lateral to the area of the bend of the clavicle. The preceding recommendations of anesthesia application and vein entry apply. The needle is directed medially in a plane virtually parallel to the surface of the x-ray table toward the region of the supraclavicular notch. If this is unsuccessful, approaches more inferiorly or at a steeper angle to the chest wall can be attempted. The standard single-wall or micropuncture technique is used, as noted above. All intravascular catheters should move without obstruction. In both the internal jugular and subclavian techniques, fluoroscopy should be used to ensure that the guidewire is directed downward toward the inferior vena cava or right atrium rather than upward toward the head.

Femoral Vein Approach

Although entry into the femoral vein is technically less challenging, biopsy from the femoral vein is more difficult. In a series of biopsy patients reported by Anderson and Marshall (17), the internal jugular vein could not be cannulated in 12% of patients, whereas all had successful femoral vein insertion. The femoral vein is located just medial to the femoral artery and the site of entry should be inferior to the inguinal ligament. The femoral artery can serve as a constant landmark for orientation. The Amplatz, Seldinger, or micropuncture techniques are all used for the femoral venous approach. Ultimately, a guiding sheath of variable length is inserted in the inferior vena cava from the femoral venous site.

The femoral artery is approached in a fashion very similar to the femoral vein. Left ventricular biopsies are occasionally indicated in patients with specific left ventricular masses or local pathology, isolated ventricular dysfunction, or an infiltrative process specific to the left ventricle (18). The risks of embolization and perforation are somewhat greater for patients submitted to left ventricular endomyocardial biopsy as evidenced by higher incidence of pain, low blood pressure, and pericardial effusions after left as opposed to right ventricular endomyocardial biopsy. After femoral sheath insertion, a constant infusion drip should be maintained through the sheath to avoid clot formation within the lengthy catheters.

Biopsy Methods

Fluoroscopy guidance has proven most beneficial in the performance of endomyocardial biopsies. Nonetheless, some investigators (19) have described the use of two-dimensional echocardiography, as opposed to fluoroscopy, which the authors believe reduces the risk of perforation. Visualization of the biopsy forceps is technically difficult and requires considerable operator and technician experience. We and others (19–21) have used echocardiography to biopsy intracardiac masses in the right or left heart, but standardly perform endomyocardial biopsy under fluoroscopy.

Right Internal Jugular Venous Approach—Preshaped Bioptome

The preshaped 50-cm bioptome is inserted through the venous sheath with the tip of the bioptome pointing toward the lateral wall of the right atrium. In the mid right atrium, the bioptome is advanced slowly as it is turned counterclockwise. This is facilitated by the fact that the direction of the bioptome head is concordant with that of the handle, but free motion and the desired orientation should always be confirmed fluoroscopically. The anterior rotation of the bioptome head allows the tip to cross the tricuspid valve while it avoids the coronary sinus and tricuspid apparatus. Continued advancement and counterclockwise rotation then allows the bioptome to advance farther into the right ventricle and orient toward the septum (Fig. 20.7). Extreme care must be applied during this maneuver to avoid perforation of the vena cava, right atrium, or right ventricular free wall by the relatively stiff bioptome. If resistance is encountered, the bioptome should be pulled back and a different angle of entry attempted— the biopsy forceps should *never* be forced or prolapsed into the ventricle. If entry of the right ventricle remains difficult, a Swan-Ganz catheter or other balloon flotation device may be used to define the pathway across the tricuspid valve into the right ventricle.

Once in the right ventricle, the bioptome should lie against the midportion of the interventricular septum. On fluoroscopy, the bioptome should lie across the patient's spine and is usually directed inferiorly below the plane of the tricuspid valve. If there is any question as to the bioptome's position, fluoroscopy in the 30° right anterior oblique (RAO) and 60° left anterior oblique (LAO) projections will confirm that the catheter is on the ventricular side of the atrioventricular groove and pointed toward the septum. The correct position is also marked by ventricular ectopy, so that absence of such ectopy and fluoroscopy showing the catheter to lie in the atrioventricular groove suggests that the bioptome has entered the coronary sinus

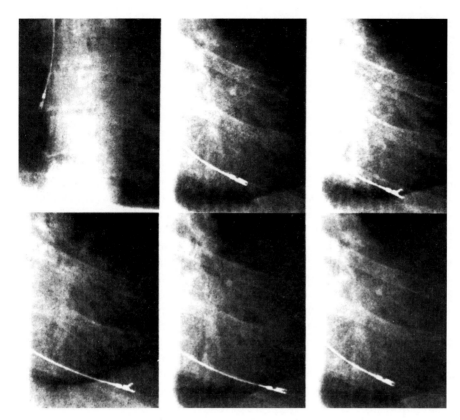

Figure 20.7 Cineangiographic frames obtained during right ventricular endomyocardial biopsy using the Stanford bioptome. From left to right, the top row shows the bioptome against the lateral right atrial wall, against the ventricular septum, and withdrawn slightly with jaws open. In the bottom row, the jaws are reapplied to the septum, closed, and withdrawn with the sample contained.

or the infradiaphragmatic venous system. It must be withdrawn and repositioned before the jaws are opened and an attempt is made to retrieve tissue!

Even within the right ventricle, it is important to avoid the relatively thin right ventricular free wall (Fig. 20.8) by directing the head of the biopsy forceps toward the interventricular septum. The interventricular septum lies in a plane approximately 45° diagonal to the plane of the patient's chest wall and corresponds to orientation of the instrument handle leftward and posteriorly. In patients with cardiomyopathy, especially those with elevated pulmonary pressure

or right ventricular enlargement, the orientation of the handle may be straight posterior.

Contact with the interventricular septum is confirmed by the appearance of premature ventricular contractions. The biopsy forceps are then withdrawn 1 to 2 cm, opened, and advanced slowly to engage the septum. The biopsy head is slowly closed to encapsulate the endomyocardial specimen. Because of the trabeculated nature of the endomyocardial surface, gentle forward pressure should be maintained while the jaws are being closed to ensure myocardial contact. Patients with restrictive heart disease

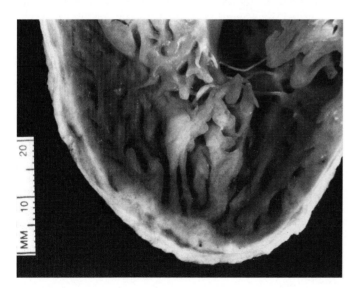

Figure 20.8 Postmortem specimen shows heavy trabeculation of the interior surface of the right ventricle, and the thinness of the right ventricular free wall.

or following transplant often demonstrate a pulsatile transmission of ventricular contractility through the course of the bioptome, whereas those with idiopathic dilated cardiomyopathy are often "soft" and engagement of the ventricular septum is confirmed only by ventricular premature contractions.

After the biopsy has been secured, the operator must maintain pressure on the forceps closure device to make sure the jaws remain closed while the specimen is withdrawn from the right ventricle, right atrium, and superior vena cava. There may be some slight "give" as the specimen is released from the myocardium. Specimens that require excessive force to remove suggest entrapment of the tricuspid apparatus, transmural biopsy, or biopsy of a scar focus. In these circumstances, the bioptome head is released by opening the jaws, the bioptome is withdrawn, and another biopsy site selected. Once removed, the specimen must be scooped from the forceps and placed in the appropriate preservative.

Patients not infrequently experience a pulling or tugging sensation as the specimen is withdrawn from the heart surface. Sharp chest pain during bioptome insertion or the performance of an endomyocardial biopsy implies cardiac perforation. Other clues to possible perforation include persistent ventricular premature contractions, excessive retraction of the ventricular wall during biopsy withdrawal, or a biopsy specimen that floats in formalin (suggesting epicardial fat content). Any of these markers should prompt blood pressure checks and fluoroscopy of the heart borders to detect signs of pericardial tamponade (see Chapter 32). This risk is lowest in patients with prior cardiac surgery or advanced cardiomyopathy and greatest in nonsurgical patients with relatively normal chamber size and systolic function.

Patients with heart transplantation who undergo repeated heart biopsies may require variation in the direction of the biopsy forceps to avoid scarred areas of prior biopsy. This may include some anterior or posterior angulation or alteration of the degree of curvature in the bioptome. The number of specimens taken per biopsy procedure is variable and dependent on the patient's clinical status. The operator must balance the pathologists desire to have adequate tissue and risks involved with performance of the procedure. We usually take three to five samples to yield adequate tissue for examination and to detect focal pathology that might not be evident in a single sample.

At the conclusion of the procedure, the heart border should be examined fluoroscopically to exclude tamponade before the venous sheath is removed and the puncture site is dressed. Patients who have had serial biopsies (e.g., transplant patients) can be discharged home within 1 hour of uncomplicated biopsy.

Right Internal Jugular—Preformed Sheath

The disposable preformed sheath technique can also be used from the internal jugular approach. It differs from the preformed bioptome technique as described above, since the sheath (rather than the bioptome itself) is advanced into the right ventricle. This directs the bioptome, which is very flexible and lacking in inherent shape. A 7 French 45-cm preformed sheath can be inserted into the superior vena cava and right atrium through a short 9 French self-sealing sheath. Insertion of a smaller sheath through a larger sheath allows greater torque control and decreases the risk of biopsy sheath kinking. The preformed sheath is guided into the right ventricle by use of a guidewire or a balloon-tipped flotation catheter. Once the sheath is in the right ventricle, the catheter or wire guide is removed while the sheath remains in position. If there is any question as to the right ventricular placement, the side arm of the guiding sheath can be attached to a pressure monitor and right ventricular pressure demonstrated, or a gentle contrast injection can be performed. The tip of the preformed sheath should be free floating rather than positioned against the ventricular myocardium or trabeculated portion of the right ventricle muscle. Once in a stable position, the sheath should be aspirated and flushed with heparinized solution. The sheath should be connected to a constant infusion port to maintain patency and avoid clot formation.

The flexible biopsy catheter is then inserted through the disposable sheath. The distal portion of the biopsy forceps can be manually curved before entry into the sheath to avoid straightening of the sheath during insertion of the bioptome and disturbing the appropriate angle for biopsy performance. The jaws of the bioptome should be opened immediately on exiting the sheath to increase cross-sectional area and thereby reduce the risk of perforating the myocardial wall. The bioptome is directed posteriorly and perpendicular to the plane of the septum. Gentle pressure is applied as the jaws are slowly closed. Once the bioptome has been removed from the sheath, the jaws are opened and the specimen removed. The bioptome jaws are flushed with saline, and repeated biopsies are taken as indicated clinically. Repeated biopsy attempts may require alteration in the direction of the sheath or angulation of the bioptome.

Femoral Vein Approach—Preformed Sheath

As with the right internal jugular venous approach, we prefer to insert a 9 French self-sealing sheet in the femoral vein through which the 7 French guiding sheath is inserted. All guiding sheaths have an angle of curvature, which varies from a 135° straight angle to a gentle 180° curvature or multiangulated curvature (Baim guiding sheath; 22,23). Each is inserted into the right ventricular cavity with the assistance of an internal dilator, wire guide, pigtail catheter, or flotation balloon–tipped catheter. Rarely, the femoral venous approach is used to biopsy the left ventricle in children via a trans-septal approach (24). The femoral approach allows the operator less control over the site and location of the endomyocardial biopsy, which may increase the risk for perforation.

The 130°-angle femoral sheath must be evaluated before insertion to ensure that the length of the sheath extension from the right atrium to right ventricular biopsy site does not exceed the anatomic distance from the right atrial border to the right ventricular apex. (This can be done by placing the sheath on the exterior portion of the patient's chest under fluoroscopy. If the postangled portion of the bioptome is too long, it should be shortened before insertion.)

As with the internal jugular approach using a preformed sheath, insertion of the bioptome may straighten the sheath, altering the ideal angle for performance of the biopsy. If this is the case, the distal portion of the otherwise unformed 104-cm bioptome can be preshaped manually before insertion into a curve similar to that of the sheath to decrease the chance of losing the ideal biopsy angle. Out-of-plane posterior angulation of the tip of the bioptome relative to the broad more proximal curve can help direct the tip toward the ventricular septum as it exits the sheath.

Once the preformed sheath is inserted, it should be continuously flushed to avoid clot formation or thromboembolic complications. If there is a question of biopsy sheath tip location, a hand flush of contrast dye may be helpful (Fig. 20.9). The 104-cm bioptome is inserted through the disposable sheath. The biopsy jaws should be opened just as the bioptome exits the preformed sheath, decreasing the potential for perforation by the bioptome. The biopsy forceps are advanced to the myocardial border with the jaws open. The jaws are slowly closed while gentle pressure is maintained against the septum. If the tip of the preformed sheath lies against the septum, the biopsy forceps can be unsheathed by retracting the sheath while maintaining the biopsy forceps in a stable position. This decreases the potential for perforation. After the specimen is obtained, as the biopsy forceps are withdrawn, the sheath is advanced slightly to restore its original position in the ventricle. Once the biopsy specimen has been removed from the preformed sheath, the forceps are opened and the specimen scooped from the jaws and placed in the appropriate preservative.

Left Ventricular Biopsy—Femoral Artery Preformed Sheath

As with the femoral venous approach, the femoral artery requires insertion of a larger preformed short sheath to maintain artery patency and allow biopsy sheath manipulation. The short and long (98-cm) femoral artery disposable sheath must be maintained under constant pressurized infusion with a heparinized solution to maintain patency and avoid embolic phenomenon. The preformed sheath is inserted into the left ventricular cavity using a guidewire and pigtail catheter. The wire, pigtail catheter, and preformed sheath are gently manipulated to cross the aortic valve and enter the left ventricular cavity. Once in the left ventricle, an area of acceptable irritability is established. The inferior posterior portions of the left ventricular cavity as well as areas of previous myocardial infarction should be avoided to reduce the risk of perforation because of the relatively thin muscle in these sites.

The sheath is cleared of debris by aspirating and flushing before the 104-cm bioptome is inserted through the sheath and into the left ventricular cavity. The biopsy forceps should be directed away from the mitral valve apparatus. The jaws are opened and directed to the left ventricular wall, the specimen is encapsulated, and the jaws are closed firmly with extraction of the sample. Because of the increased contraction of the left ventricle, less forward pressure is applied during performance of the biopsy. The sheath is maintained in the left ventricular cavity and its position adjusted to ensure sampling from several sites.

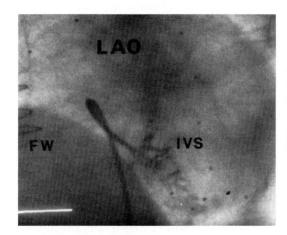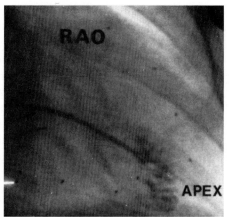

Figure 20.9 Right ventricular biopsy from the femoral vein using a double-angulated sheath. (Left) In the left anterior oblique projection, contrast injection demonstrates how the terminal sheath curve orients the tip towards the septum (IVS) and away from the free wall (FW). (Right) In the right anterior oblique position, contrast injection demonstrates a suitable position about mid-way from the atrial-ventricular groove to the apex.

BIOPSY COMPLICATIONS

Virtually all complications associated with endomyocardial biopsy occur during the procedure itself, that is, while the patient is still in the catheterization laboratory. Potential complications include ventricular perforation and pericardial tamponade, malignant ventricular arrhythmias, transient complete heart block, pneumothorax, carotid artery puncture, supraventricular arrhythmias, nerve paresis, and venous hematoma (25,26).

Perforation

The greatest risk to patients from the performance of endomyocardial biopsy is ventricular perforation (27; Fig. 20.8). This may result in pericardial tamponade and death. Patients with a prothrombin time >18 seconds or who have received heparin without reversal within the last 2 hours should probably not be submitted to endomyocardial biopsy. Perforation is usually a complication of injury to the right ventricular free wall, which is only 1 to 2 mm thick. Patients with pulmonary hypertension, a bleeding diathesis, or right ventricular enlargement may be at increased risk for right ventricular perforation. Any patient complaining of sharp pain during the performance of the endomyocardial biopsy should be considered to have experienced cardiac perforation. Patients with perforation immediately complain of a visceral pain and within 1 to 2 minutes may develop bradycardia and hypotension. This is in part owing to an exaggerated vagal response, but limited benefit is achieved by atropine administration. No further biopsy attempts should be performed until the importance of the patient's complaints has been fully investigated. This may include fluoroscopy of the heart border, measurement of the right atrial pressure waveform, or performance of a portable echocardiogram. Patients with suspected perforation should have their right atrial pressure and the pulsatility of the right and left heart borders continuously evaluated. Loss of pulsation of heart borders and increased right atrial pressure are strong indicators for pericardial tamponade. Echocardiography should be obtained immediately to determine the presence and severity of pericardial blood accumulation. Cardiovascular collapse or electrical mechanical disassociation in the setting of a biopsy should be considered to be presumptive evidence of pericardial tamponade, and the operator must be prepared to do an immediate pericardiocentesis, even before echocardiographic confirmation of tamponade.

Occasionally, acute bleeding into the pericardial space will clot and prevent adequate draining by pericardiocentesis. Persistent hemodynamic compromise and an inability to drain the pericardium percutaneously mandate that the patients be explored immediately, occasionally in the catheterization laboratory. Because of the risk of tamponade, a pericardiocentesis tray should be always available in the procedure room where biopsies are performed.

Malignant Ventricular Arrhythmias

Premature ventricular contractions are anticipated when the right or left ventricular cavities are entered, and in fact are indications of appropriate placement of the bioptome or sheath. Occasionally, ventricular couplets or triplets may be seen. Rarely, in patients with cardiomyopathy and pre-existent ventricular arrhythmias, sustained malignant ventricular arrhythmia may occur. This can usually be terminated by removing the biopsy sheath or forceps from the ventricular cavity. If this does not stop the ventricular ectopy, medical therapy with antiarrhythmic agents or cardioversion may be necessary.

Supraventricular Arrhythmias

During cannulation of the right atrium, the atrial wall may be stimulated, causing atrial arrhythmias, particularly in those who have had a history of these rhythm disturbances in the past. Atrial arrhythmias are more likely to occur in patients with elevations of right atrial pressure. In patients with high filling pressures or a history of arrhythmia, right atrial wall contact should be avoided if possible. Occasionally, atrial tachycardia can be mechanically interrupted by touching the right atrial wall with the bioptome, interrupting the circus rhythm. This may increase the risk of perforation, however.

Heart Block

Patients with pre-existent left bundle branch block may be at risk for complete heart block during manipulation of catheters or bioptomes in the right heart. Pressure against the septum near the tricuspid apparatus may stun the right bundle, delay conduction through the interventricular septum (a new right bundle branch block), or cause progression of prior left bundle branch block to complete heart block. Removal of the offending bioptome or catheter usually resolves the complete heart block. If this is not the case, a temporary pacing catheter can be inserted after removal of the biopsy forceps. Particularly in patients with pre-existing bundle branch block, a temporary pacemaker and pacemaker wire should be immediately available in the catheterization laboratory for emergent use if needed.

Pneumothorax

Laceration of the lung pleura during performance of right internal jugular or right subclavian venous entry may result in a pneumothorax. This risk can be minimized by performing the internal jugular approach in the midneck region and by continuously aspirating during every attempt at venous entry. Patients who complain of shortness of breath should be investigated immediately with fluoroscopy of the lung margins and urgent pneumothorax evacuation as needed.

Puncture of the Carotid Artery or Subclavian Artery

The internal jugular and subclavian veins lie adjacent to both the carotid and subclavian arteries. Even with sonographic guidance, occasional arterial puncture may occur. Puncture of an artery using the guiding needle, micropuncture needle, or even an 18-gauge needle can be addressed by immediate recognition of the complication, withdrawal of the needle, and compression until homeostasis is obtained. This does not preclude performance of a safe venous approach, but bleeding in and around the site of arterial puncture may tamponade the venous system in the carotid sheath and make this site unusable. Cannulation of an artery with a large (7 to 9 French) sheath is a more serious error that requires urgent surgical consultation.

Pulmonary Embolization

Patients with preformed sheaths may develop clot within the sheath during the performance of the endomyocardial biopsy if not continuously flushed (28). This may result in recurrent thromboembolic phenomena (pulmonary embolization or potentially paradoxical embolization into the systemic arterial circuit). Additionally, patients who develop a clot in the sheath not infrequently have that clot pushed forward and wedged against the endomyocardial surface of the heart by the bioptome resulting in a clot biopsy as opposed to endomyocardial tissue.

Nerve Paresis

Excessive or ill-directed infiltration of lidocaine in and around the jugular vein and carotid sheath may result in Horner syndrome, vocal cord paresis, and rarely, diaphragmatic weakness. These complications are short lived, lasting 1 to 2 hours, if owing to lidocaine infiltration rather than direct nerve trauma.

Venous Hematoma

A venous hematoma may form as a result of the excessive movement of the venous sheath during the procedure, inadequate compression of the venous entry site after the procedure, or late venous bleeding owing to a transient or sustained increase in right atrial pressure or coagulopathy. This may result in local bleeding, but rarely results in long-term complications that prevent subsequent use of this site for venous entry. Nonetheless, appropriate attention to the site of venous entry cannot be overemphasized, particularly in those patients who must return repeatedly for endomyocardial biopsies.

Arterial Venous Fistula

Occasionally, arterial fistulas develop between small branches of the coronary artery and the right ventricle in a heart transplant patient. These are caused by biopsy of septal coronary branch with subsequent arterial communication into the cavity from which the biopsy was performed. A multitude of long-term studies have demonstrated that these coronary AV fistula are of no hemodynamic or clinical consequence and can be followed conservatively (29–31).

POSTPROCEDURE CARE

After the biopsy sheath is removed, appropriate pressure should be applied to avoid local bleeding complications. Patients undergoing biopsy by jugular venous access can usually be discharged from the biopsy suite or recovery room immediately if no bleeding occurs within 5 to 10 minutes. Patients with femoral venous entry require 2 to 3 hours of supine bed rest before attempted ambulation. Patients with arterial entry require several hours of bed rest with or without arterial closure devices.

Patients should be monitored for bleeding and any change in hemodynamics. We do not routinely obtain postprocedure chest radiographs unless there is a suggestion of pneumothorax during the procedure. The Band-Aid applied to their entry site can be removed after 24 hours, and patients can have oral intake within minutes of the performance of their procedure if they can sit up.

TISSUE PROCESSING

The operator has the responsibility for obtaining adequate tissue for analysis and for performing the initial preparations that permit subsequent pathologic evaluation. It is generally recommended that at least five separate specimens be obtained to minimize sampling error. Most myocardial diseases affect both ventricles, so that either chamber may be sampled, depending on operator experience and preference. Selective left ventricular involvement may be present in certain diseases (endomyocardial fibrosis, scleroderma, left heart radiation, and cardiac fibroelastosis of infants and newborns). Left ventricular biopsy may be performed in these conditions, or in patients in whom right ventricular biopsy has been unsuccessful or nondiagnostic. In the remaining patients, we generally prefer right (rather than left) ventricular biopsy because of greater ease and speed and less likelihood of morbidity.

The safest and most eloquent techniques of endomyocardial biopsy and sample preparation are useless without expert pathologic interpretation. The availability of the cardiac pathologist who is fully trained in the evaluation of biopsy-obtained tissue and conversant with the latest classification schemes is mandatory in any biopsy program.

Artifacts such as crushing or contraction bands are frequently present in endomyocardial biopsy specimens and may be overinterpreted by an inexperienced pathologist or one used to evaluating only postmortem specimens. The operator may assist the pathologist by appropriate handling of the tissue in the catheterization laboratory. The specimen should be removed gently from the jaws of the bioptome with a fine needle and placed immediately in the appropriate fixative. Frozen specimens may be prepared in the catheterization laboratory by placing samples in a suitable fluid-embedding medium and immersing them in a liquid nitrogen and dry ice isopentane mixture to allow immediate interpretation. Additional special sample preparation or staining (iron, amyloid) may be indicated for evaluation for specific disease states.

It is the operator's responsibility to ensure that the heart biopsy specimens obtained are delivered to the appropriate laboratory for analysis. Preferably, the operator should review the slide material obtained and assist the pathologist with an appropriate history and ensure that special studies are obtained as needed.

Patients with idiopathic dilated cardiomyopathy display a specific pathologic pattern including myocyte hypertrophy and interstitial fibrosis. These findings may allow the clinician to rule out other entities, help define the severity, and judge the duration of the patient's cardiomyopathic condition. In a large series of patients submitted into myocardial biopsy (32–34), approximately 20% have a specific cause identified. Taking the biopsy and clinical information together, a diagnosis can be made on virtually all patients presenting with heart failure (Table 20.2). But the threshold for performing endomyocardial biopsy clearly depends on the operator's experience, the availability of pathology expertise, and the institutional view of how important the findings are for the diagnosis and management of individual patients. Increasingly, molecular techniques are available that will dramatically enhance the value of endomyocardial biopsy performance, above and beyond the simple histologic, immunohistochemical, and biochemical analysis that has been available to this point. Polymerase chain reaction techniques will allow pathologists to determine whether or not the patient's myopathic process is associated with a pre-existent or ongoing viral infection (35). Similarly, other immune markers, such as HLA upregulation and immune deposition, will help to identify those patients who suffer from some form of an autoimmune process that may be perpetuating ventricular dysfunction (36).

Given that the presence of severe heart muscle disease reduces life expectancy by as much as many malignancies, we believe it is important to attempt to obtain tissue in patients who present to the catheterization laboratory and are not found to have valvular, coronary, or pericardial disease to account for their ventricular dysfunction or heart failure. The utility and findings in specific disease states are summarized below.

TABLE 20.2
MYOCARDIAL BIOPSY INDICATIONS AND FINDINGS

Current Indications
  Cardiac allograft rejection monitoring
  Cardiomyopathy of unknown cause
  Severe ventricular arrhythmias of unknown cause
  Drug induced cardiomyopathy (anthracycline)
  Restrictive or constrictive heart disease
  Research interests
Cardiac Disorders with Specific Findings (see also Table 20.3)
  Immune or inflammatory disease states
  Myocarditis
  Cardiac allograft rejection
  Sarcoidosis
  Cytomegalovirus infection
  Toxoplasmosis
  Rheumatic carditis
  Chagas disease
  Kawasaki disease
Degenerative
  Idiopathic cardiomyopathy
  Anthracycline cardiomyopathy
  Radiation cardiomyopathy
  Infiltrative
  Amyloidosis
  Gaucher Disease
  Hemochromatosis
  Fabry Disease
  Glycogen storage disease
Ischemic
  Acute myocardial infarction
  Chronic ischemic cardiomyopathy
  Schönlein-Henoch purpura
Cancer
  Primary cardiac cancer
  Metastatic cardiac cancer

Transplant Rejection

Endomyocardial biopsy has been the cornerstone of monitoring of antirejection therapy in patients with heart or heart–lung transplants (37,38). Biopsy allows the detection of early rejection before the clinical findings of advanced cardiac damage (arrhythmias, third heart sound, congestive heart failure) become manifest and confirms the adequacy of pulsed immunosuppressive therapy to control each acute rejection episode. Surveillance biopsies are performed frequently during the first 6 months after transplantation because of the high incidence of rejection during this early period. No methodology thus far investigated has demonstrated a sensitivity or predictive accuracy high enough to replace endomyocardial biopsy in the detection of rejection in adults, although scintigraphy after the administration of indium 111-labeled antimyosin Fab fragments may correlate best with biopsy findings (39). Because immunologic transplant rejection is a diffuse process, sampling errors are rare. The light-microscopic histologic features of rejection include interstitial edema, inflammatory infiltration, and immunoglobulin deposition. More severe rejection is marked by myocytolysis and even interstitial hemorrhage.

The original Stanford grading system (1981) defined absent, mild, moderate, and severe grades of rejection, the later two showing both lymphocytic infiltrates and myocyte damage. The newer (1989) grading scale of the International Society of Heart and Lung Transplantation (27) distinguishes four grades of rejection. *Milder rejection*—grade 1 (focal perivascular [1A] or diffuse [1B] sparse infiltrate without necrosis) and grade 2 (single focus of aggressive infiltration and/or myocyte damage) do not warrant active treatment. In contrast, *more severe rejection*—grade 3 (multifocal aggressive infiltrates and/or myocyte damage [3A] or diffuse inflammation with necrosis [3B]) or grade 4 (diffuse polymorphous infiltrate with necrosis and a variable degree of edema, hemorrhage, or vasculitis) warrant aggressive immunosuppression even if the patient is asymptomatic.

Adriamycin Cardiotoxicity

Doxorubicin hydrochloride (Adriamycin) is a potent anthracycline antibiotic that is active against many tumors, but whose usefulness is limited by its tendency to cause progressive and irreversible dose-related cardiotoxicity (40). The incidence is 4% at doses <500 mg/m^2, 18% between 500 and 600 mg/m^2, and 36% >600/m^2. One approach to safe clinical use has thus been to limit the total cumulative dose to 500 mg/m^2, but this constitutes an unnecessary limitation in patients who can tolerate substantially higher doses without cardiotoxicity and who depend on the drug for tumor control. At the same time, this approach fails to protect patients with pre-existing heart disease, prior radiotherapy or cyclophosphamide administration, or who are older than age 70, who may develop cardiac toxicity at substantially lower doses. Because overt impairment of cardiac function is a relatively late finding in Adriamycin toxicity, noninvasive testing may fail to disclose whether additional doses of Adriamycin can be given safely.

Bristow and coworkers (41), however, have demonstrated that a progressive series of histologic changes (including electron microscopic evidence of myofibrillar loss and cytoplasmic vacuolization) takes place during the development of Adriamycin cardiotoxicity. The extent of these changes can predict whether a patient is likely to develop clinical cardiotoxicity during the subsequent chemotherapy cycle. The 5-step grading system relates grade to the percent of cells that show these histology changes (1 = <5%, 1.5 = 5 to 15%, 2 = 16 to 25%, 2.5 = 26 to 35%, and 3 = >35%). A biopsy score of 2.5 or higher indicates that doxorubicin therapy should be terminated, whereas lower scores allow administration of the next cycle of therapy followed by rebiopsy, thus permitting maximal yet safe dosing with Adriamycin while

substantially decreasing the incidence of morbidity and mortality from Adriamycin cardiotoxicity.

Dilated Cardiomyopathy

Dilated cardiomyopathy—primary myocardial failure in the absence of underlying coronary, valvular, or pericardial disease—has an age-adjusted prevalence of 36 per 100,000 population in the United States and causes approximately 10,000 deaths each year (42). The prevalence is 2.5 times higher in blacks and males. The clinical syndrome, which includes advanced congestive heart failure with dilation of both ventricles, chest pain, and arrhythmias, can be owing to a variety of toxins, metabolic abnormalities, inflammatory or infectious causes, neuromuscular diseases, or familial syndromes. The classification scheme was updated by the World Health Organization in 1995 (43).

By the time of clinical presentation, most patients with dilated cardiomyopathy already have well-established cardiac damage. Although the course is highly variable and may include transient periods of improvement, the 1-year mortality may be as high as 25 to 30% (42). Since dilated cardiomyopathy carries a substantial mortality, our approach to any young or middle-aged patient who presents with dilated cardiomyopathy consists of an invasive evaluation that includes both coronary angiography and endomyocardial biopsy. The former may be helpful, because clinical signs and symptoms (chest pain or a history of myocardial infarction) are neither sensitive nor specific for distinguishing idiopathic dilated from ischemic cardiomyopathy—both factors may be present in patients with classic dilated cardiomyopathy (with angiographically normal coronaries) or may be absent in up to half of patients with ischemic cardiomyopathy (despite a high incidence of triple vessel disease). Since some patients with a myopathic presentation of extensive coronary artery disease do well with revascularization, coronary angiography is an important part of the evaluation.

Unfortunately, endomyocardial biopsy in patients with dilated cardiomyopathy generally displays only the monotonous histologic findings of myocyte hypertrophy, interstitial and replacement fibrosis, and endocardial thickening (34,42). Occasional small clusters of lymphocytes (<5 per high-power [300 to 400×] field) may be present, without meeting criteria for diagnosing myocarditis. The amount of collagen—particularly rigid type I collagen—is increased, potentially accounting for an increase in diastolic stiffness (44). As such, the histologic findings in dilated cardiomyopathy generally do not aid in establishing cause, long-term prognosis, or appropriate specific therapy. However, there are clearly patients with otherwise garden-variety dilated cardiomyopathy, in whom *specific processes* can be diagnosed by endomyocardial biopsy (Table 20.3). The yield of endomyocardial biopsy findings that will significantly alter either therapy or long-term prognosis in dilated cardiomyopathy, however, is admittedly low (32,34,45).

TABLE 20.3

FINAL CLINICAL PLUS BIOPSY DIAGNOSIS FROM 1,278 PATIENTS WITH DILATED CARDIOMYOPATHY

Diagnosis	Frequency	%
Idiopathic dilated cardiomyopathy	654	51.2
Myocarditis (2/3 active, 1/3 borderline)	117	9.2
Coronary artery disease	98	7.7
Peripartum cardiomyopathy	58	4.5
Hypertension	54	4.2
Human immunodeficiency virus infection	46	3.6
Amyloidosis	41	3.2
Connective tissue disease (mostly scleroderma/lupus)	40	3.1
Drug-induced (mostly adriamycin)	30	2.3
Chronic alcohol abuse	30	2.3
Familial cardiomyopathy	25	2.0
Valvular heart disease	19	1.5
Sarcoid	16	0.9
Endocrine (mostly thyroid)	11	0.9
Hemochromatosis	9	0.7
Neoplastic	6	0.5

Modified from Felker GM, Hu W, Hare JM, Hruban RH, Baughman KL, Kasper EK. The spectrum of dilated cardiomyopathy. The Johns Hopkins experience with 1,278 patients. *Medicine* (Baltimore) 1999; 78:270.

Myocarditis

In contrast to the "burned-out" condition of the myocardium in dilated cardiomyopathy, myocarditis is an acute or subacute inflammatory illness in which there is variable lymphocytic infiltration in conjunction with myocardial cell damage (42,46,47). Epidemiologic studies suggest that approximately 5% of a Coxsackie B virus-infected population show some evidence of cardiac involvement (42), and replicating enteroviral RNA may be recovered in myocardial samples (35,48–50). Infection and inflammation may resolve spontaneously or may become chronic with perpetuation of an autoimmune process that causes ongoing myocardial damage (51,52). Similar processes can result from various viral, protozoal, metazoal, or bacterial infections. Patients with myocarditis typically present with symptoms of chest pain, arrhythmias, or heart failure, with a clinical course that may vary from days to months. Newer noninvasive tests such as scintigraphy after administration of indium 111-labeled antimyosin Fab (where a ratio of counts over the heart to counts over the lung in the anterior view >1.6 is positive) may help identify cases of myocarditis, but it has a low sensitivity (66%) compared with endomyocardial biopsy (47). In patients in whom myocarditis is strongly suspected but not confirmed by scintigraphy, biopsy should still be performed.

Much of the confusion in this field stemmed from use of various definitions for *myocarditis*, some of which (e.g., more than five lymphocytes per high-power field) were fairly liberal. In contrast, the Dallas criteria (53) adopted in 1986 require that infiltrating lymphocytes be adjacent to myocyte necrosis or degeneration to diagnose *active myocarditis*. If lymphocyte infiltration is present without adjacent myocyte damage, the diagnosis is *borderline myocarditis*. Roughly 9% of biopsies done for the evaluation of dilated cardiomyopathy will show myocarditis (about two thirds active and one third borderline; 33). Biopsy samples that were previously read as showing myocarditis may now be read as borderline or even frankly negative using the Dallas criteria. If the biopsy shows nondiagnostic abnormalities (particularly if borderline changes are present), the patient may still turn out to have active myocarditis on a repeat biopsy (54). If confirmation of active myocarditis is clinically relevant, repeat right ventricular biopsy is generally sufficient, since the incidence of right versus left ventricular discordance in myocarditis is apparently low (54,55).

Using both clinical and histopathologic criteria (33,56,57), the Hopkins group has classified myocarditis as *fulminant* (intense infiltration, acute onset with progression to death or recovery within 1 month, poor response to immunosuppressives); *subacute* (less distinct onset, active inflammation, potentially good response to immunosuppressives); *chronic active* (progressive decline in cardiac function, a biopsy that shows mixed inflammation and fibrosis, and only a brief response to immunosuppressives); or *chronic persistent* myocarditis (histologic evidence of myocarditis, near normal ventricular function, unaffected by immunosuppressives). Positive biopsies for myocarditis may thus be found in patients presenting with new- or recent-onset congestive heart failure, including patients with peripartum cardiomyopathy during the last month of pregnancy or within the 5 months after delivery (58) and in survivors of cardiac arrest who have no other evident organic heart disease (59). Several recent series of patients with AIDS have shown serious clinical cardiac abnormalities associated with myocarditis (60–62).

Given this high apparent prevalence of myocarditis among patients with both acute and chronic illness, uncontrolled use of immunosuppressive treatment (analogous to that used for transplant rejection) was reported in the 1980s (63,64). Patients with active inflammation appeared to show histologic and some clinical improvement. However, immunosuppressive therapy also caused significant complications, and it was not clear that the frequency of improvement exceeded that seen spontaneously in many patients with myocarditis.

This general confusion about the prevalence and optimal treatment for myocarditis led to the conduct of the Myocarditis Treatment Trial (65). Between October 1986 and October 1990, 2,233 patients who underwent nontransplant endomyocardial biopsy within 2 years of symptom onset at one of 30 participating centers were screened. Histopathologic evidence of myocarditis was found in 214 (10%), of whom 111 with a left ventricular ejection fraction <45 and no medical contraindication were randomized to either placebo or 24 weeks of cyclosporine/prednisone (after an initial azathioprine/prednisone arm was dropped). There was no significant benefit in the primary end point (improvement in left ventricular ejection fraction from baseline to 28 weeks) between the patients receiving immunosuppression and those receiving conventional stepped drug therapy for congestive heart failure. Despite initial screening by expert pathologists, only 66% of baseline biopsies met rigorous Dallas criteria for active myocarditis when over-read by the core laboratory, and the trial was seriously underpowered to detect even substantial clinical benefit. Some physicians thus still consider use of immunosuppressives in patients with biopsy-proven myocarditis and a deteriorating clinical picture, particularly in the clinical picture of active myocarditis. Of course, such patients should also be screened for cardiac transplantation, should their condition continue to deteriorate.

Recent studies by Martin, Wojinick, and Frustaci have raised questions as to the validity of the Dallas Criteria as the exclusive marker of myocarditis. Martin (49) demonstrated that children with a viral syndrome and positive endomyocardial biopsies by PCR for viral genetic sequences often fail to demonstrate myocarditis by the histologic Dallas criteria. Wojinick (36) demonstrated that HLA upregulation in patients with a clinical syndrome compatible with myocarditis was a marker for patients who respond to immunosuppressive therapy, whereas Dallas criteria myocarditis was found in only 16% of this population. Frustaci (48), in a series of patients with dilated cardiomyopathy and presumed myocarditis that failed to improve with standard medical therapy, showed that those who responded to immunosuppressives with an improvement in ejection fraction had anti-heart antibodies and no viral persistence by PCR. Therefore, the absence of persistent virus, the presence of immune upregulation by anti-heart antibodies, and HLA upregulation may better define a population with immune-related heart dysfunction responsive to immunosuppressive therapy.

Restrictive Versus Constrictive Disease

Heart failure caused by impaired diastolic functioning of a normal-sized or mildly dilated left ventricle is an uncommon but important clinical entity (see Chapters 31 and 32). In some cases, this may be owing to pericardial constriction, in which instance endomyocardial biopsy would offer no further information. A restrictive pattern (43,66,67) may be seen in some patients with hypertrophic myopathy, associated with a pattern of myocyte fiber disarray. More important, diastolic dysfunction may also be caused by one of a series of diseases that can be readily diagnosed with endomyocardial biopsy, thus sparing the patient from inappropriate medical or surgical therapy (i.e., pericardial stripping; 66). These disorders include primary amyloidosis, Loeffler endomyocardial fibrosis, carcinoid-related damage, Fabry disease, and the glycogen storage diseases (67a).

Of these, amyloid (AL) is one of the most common (1,000 to 3,000 new U.S. cases per year; 67–69). It also has one of the worst prognoses (typical survival for amyloid patients of 12 months is reduced to 5 months in patients with cardiac involvement). Recent trials suggest that treatment with melphalan and prednisone significantly prolongs survival (70), so definitive diagnosis is important. Although most patients with cardiac amyloidosis have evidence on biopsy of more accessible organs or urinary light chain excretion, about 10% do not. Cardiac biopsy should be performed in patients with thick walls and a small hypokinetic ventricle, particularly if the myocardium has the characteristic speckled appearance on echocardiography.

Sarcoid is also relatively common (>10,000 new U.S. cases per year; 71,72). Although serious cardiac dysfunction is detected in only 5 to 10% of patients, more than three fourths have cardiac involvement on autopsy. About half of the patients have electrocardiographic abnormalities of conduction, or repolarization, whereas some have papillary muscle dysfunction, infiltrative cardiomyopathy, or pericarditis (71,72).

Hemochromatosis may present with either a dilated or restrictive pattern. It is found in roughly 1% of endomyocardial biopsies (34,73), but is important to identify given the benefits of iron chelation therapy.

FUTURE DIRECTIONS

Endomyocardial biopsy remains the gold standard for the diagnosis of transplant rejection and anthracycline cardiotoxicity and a highly valuable tool for the diagnosis of myocarditis. The recent use of highly specific molecular probes to look for virus genetic material or autoimmune activity in endomyocardial biopsy material promises to further sharpen the diagnostic potential of this technique. Although the lack of positive findings in the Myocarditis Treatment Trial dampened enthusiasm for widespread performance of endomyocardial biopsy in patients presenting with congestive heart failure, the procedure remains safe and helpful. With newer techniques to define immune upregulation and viral persistence, there is no question that endomyocardial biopsies will again define myocarditis and its appropriate treatment. Furthermore, molecular and genetic analysis will identify patients in the current idiopathic cardiomyopathy category who have an infectious or inherited cause for their cardiac dysfunction. Once we understand the pathophysiology for patients' cardiac conditions, we will be in a much stronger position to appropriately identify therapy. Despite ongoing uncertainty of its correct place in the clinical workup (74), endomyocardial biopsy plays an important role in the evaluation of patients with recent onset or rapidly deteriorating cardiomyopathy or potential cardiac involvement of certain systemic diseases, as well as in furthering our understanding of the pathophysiology and treatment of diseases of the heart muscle.

REFERENCES

1. Weinberg M, Fell EG, Lynfield J. Diagnostic biopsy of the pericardium and myocardium. *Arch Surg* 1958;76:825.
2. Sutton DC, Sutton GC. Needle biopsy of the human ventricular myocardium: review of 54 consecutive cases. *Am Heart J* 1960; 60:364.
3. Timmis GC, Gordon S, Baron RH. Percutaneous myocardial biopsy of the left ventricle: experience in 198 patients. *Circulation* 1972;46:112.
4. Shirey EK, Hawk WH, Mukerji D. Percutaneous myocardial biopsy. *Am Heart J* 1965;70:449.
5. Bulloch RT, Murphey ML, Pearce MB. Intracardiac needle biopsy of the ventricular septum. *Am J Cardiol* 1965;16:227.
6. Sakakibara S, Konno S. Endomyocardial biopsy. *Jpn Heart J* 1962; 3:537–543.
7. Kawai C, Kitaura Y. New endomyocardial biopsy catheter for the left ventricle. *Am J Cardiol* 1977;40:63.
8. Kawai C, Matsumori A, Kawamura K. Myocardial biopsy. *Annu Rev Med* 1980;31:139.
9. Caves PK, Stinson EB, Graham AF. Percutaneous transvenous endomyocardial biopsy. *JAMA* 1973;225:288.
10. Caves PK, Stinson EB, Dong EJ. New instrument for transvenous cardiac biopsy. *Am J Cardiol* 1974;33:264.
11. Caves PK, Coltart J, Billingham M. Transvenous endomyocardial biopsy—application of a method for diagnosing heart disease. *Postgrad Med J* 1975;51:286.
12. Mason JW. Techniques for right and left ventricular endomyocardial biopsy. *Am J Cardiol* 1978;41:887.
13. Richardson PJ. King's endomyocardial bioptome. *Lancet* 1974;1:660.
14. Denys BG, Uretsky BF, Reddy PS, Ruffner RJ, Sandhu JS, Breishlatt WM. An ultrasound method for safe and rapid central venous access. *N Engl J Med* 1991;324:566.
15. Denys BG, Uretsky BF, Reddy PS. Ultrasound-assisted cannulation of the internal jugular vein. A prospective comparison to the external landmark-guided technique. *Circulation* 1993;87:1557–1562.
16. Corley DD, Strickman N. Alternative approaches to right ventricular endomyocardial biopsy. *Cathet Cardiovasc Diagn* 1994;31:236–239.
17. Anderson JL, Marshall HW. The femoral venous approach to endomyocardial biopsy: comparison with internal jugular and transarterial approaches. *Am J Cardiol* 1984;53:833–837.
18. Brooksby IAB. Left ventricular endomyocardial biopsy. *Lancet* 1974;2:1222.
19. Pierard L, El Allaf D, D'Orio V, Demoulin JC, Carlier J. Two-dimensional echocardiographic guiding of endomyocardial biopsy. *Chest* 1984;85:759–762.
20. Copeland JG, Valdes-Cruz L, Sahn DJ. Endomyocardial biopsy with fluoroscopic and two-dimensional echocardiographic guidance: case report of a patient suspected of having multiple cardiac tumors. *Clin Cardiol* 1984;7:449–452.
21. Miller LW, Labovitz AJ, McBride LA, Pennington DG, Kanter K. Echocardiography—guided endomyocardial biopsy. A 5-year experience. *Circulation* 1988;78:III99–102.
22. Anastasiou-Nana MI. Validation of a new femoral venous method of endomyocardial biopsy: comparison with internal jugular approach. *J Intervent Cardiol* 1988;53:833.
23. Canedo MI. Tampa Bay catheter: a new guiding catheter for endomyocardial biopsy via femoral approach. *Cathet Cardiovasc Diagn* 1992;25:71–75.
24. Rios B, Nihill MR, Mullins CE. Left ventricular endomyocardial biopsy in children with the transseptal long sheath technique. *Cathet Cardiovasc Diagn* 1984;10:417–423.
25. Sekiguchi M, Take M. *World Survey of Catheter Biopsy of the Heart. Cardiomyopathy: Clinical, Pathological, and Theoretical Aspects.* Baltimore: University Park Press 1980:217.
26. Deckers JW, Hare JM, Baughman KL. Complications of transvenous right ventricular endomyocardial biopsy in adult patients with cardiomyopathy: a seven-year survey of 546 consecutive diagnostic procedures in a tertiary referral center. *J Am Coll Cardiol* 1992;19:43–47.
27. Friedrich SP, Berman AD, Baim DS, Diver DJ. Myocardial perforation in the cardiac catheterization laboratory: incidence, presentation, diagnosis, and management. *Cathet Cardiovasc Diagn* 1994; 32:99–107.
28. Kreher SK, Ulstad VK, Dick CD, DeGroff R, Olivari MT, Homans DC. Frequent occurrence of occult pulmonary embolism from venous sheaths during endomyocardial biopsy. *J Am Coll Cardiol* 1992;19:581–585.
29. Henzlova MJ, Nath H, Bucy RP, Bourge RC, Kirklin JK, Rogers WJ. Coronary artery to right ventricle fistula in heart transplant recipients: a complication of endomyocardial biopsy. *J Am Coll Cardiol* 1989;14:258–261.
30. Fitchett DH, Forbes C, Guerraty AJ. Repeated endomyocardial biopsy causing coronary arterial-right ventricular fistula after cardiac transplantation. *Am J Cardiol* 1988;62:829–831.
31. Sandhu JS, Uretsky BF, Zerbe TR, et al. Coronary artery fistula in the heart transplant patient. A potential complication of endomyocardial biopsy. *Circulation* 1989;79:350–356.
32. Kasper EK, Agema WR, Hutchins GM, Deckers JW, Hare JM, Baughman KL. The causes of dilated cardiomyopathy: a clinicopathologic review of 673 consecutive patients. *J Am Coll Cardiol* 1994;23:586–590.
33. Felker GM, Thompson RE, Hare JM, et al. Underlying causes and long-term survival in patients with initially unexplained cardiomyopathy. *N Engl J Med* 2000;342:1077–1084.
34. Felker GM, Hu W, Hare JM, Hruban RH, Baughman KL, Kasper EK. The spectrum of dilated cardiomyopathy. The Johns Hopkins experience with 1,278 patients. *Medicine* (Baltimore) 1999;78: 270–283.
35. Pauschinger M, Doerner A, Kuehl U, et al. Enteroviral RNA replication in the myocardium of patients with left ventricular dysfunction and clinically suspected myocarditis. *Circulation* 1999; 99:889–895.
36. Wojnicz R, Nowalany-Kozielska E, Wojciechowska C, et al. Randomized, placebo-controlled study for immunosuppressive treatment of inflammatory dilated cardiomyopathy: two-year follow-up results. *Circulation* 2001;104:39–45.
37. Billingham ME, Cary NR, Hammond ME, et al. A working formulation for the standardization of nomenclature in the diagnosis of heart and lung rejection: Heart Rejection Study Group. The International Society for Heart Transplantation. *J Heart Transplant* 1990;9:587–593.
38. Miller LW, Schlant RC, Kobashigawa J, Kubo S, Renlund DG. 24th Bethesda conference: Cardiac transplantation. Task Force 5: Complications. *J Am Coll Cardiol* 1993;22:41–54.
39. Ballester M, Bordes R, Tazelaar HD, et al. Evaluation of biopsy classification for rejection: relation to detection of myocardial damage by monoclonal antimyosin antibody imaging. *J Am Coll Cardiol* 1998;31:1357–1361.
40. Singal PK, Iliskovic N. Doxorubicin-induced cardiomyopathy. *N Engl J Med* 1998;339:900–905.
41. Bristow MR, Mason JW, Billingham ME, Daniels JR. Doxorubicin cardiomyopathy: evaluation by phonocardiography, endomyocardial biopsy, and cardiac catheterization. *Ann Intern Med* 1978; 88:168–175.
42. Dec GW, Fuster V. Idiopathic dilated cardiomyopathy. *N Engl J Med* 1994;331:1564–1575.
43. Richardson P, McKenna W, Bristow M, et al. Report of the 1995 World Health Organization/International Society and Federation of Cardiology Task Force on the Definition and Classification of Cardiomyopathies. *Circulation* 1996;93:841–842.
44. Marijianowski MM, Teeling P, Mann J, Becker AE. Dilated cardiomyopathy is associated with an increase in the type I/type III collagen ratio: a quantitative assessment. *J Am Coll Cardiol* 1995; 25:1263–1272.
45. Mason JW. Endomyocardial biopsy and the causes of dilated cardiomyopathy. *J Am Coll Cardiol* 1994;23:591–592.
46. Herskowitz A, Campbell S, Deckers J, et al. Demographic features and prevalence of idiopathic myocarditis in patients undergoing endomyocardial biopsy. *Am J Cardiol* 1993;71:982–986.
47. Kuhl U, Lauer B, Souvatzoglu M, Vosberg H, Schultheiss HP. Antimyosin scintigraphy and immunohistologic analysis of endomyocardial biopsy in patients with clinically suspected

myocarditis—evidence of myocardial cell damage and inflammation in the absence of histologic signs of myocarditis. *J Am Coll Cardiol* 1998;32:1371–1376.

48. Frustaci A, Chimenti C, Calabrese F, Pieroni M, Thiene G, Maseri A. Immunosuppressive therapy for active lymphocytic myocarditis: virological and immunologic profile of responders versus nonresponders. *Circulation* 2003;107:857–863.

49. Martin AB, Webber S, Fricker FJ, et al. Acute myocarditis. Rapid diagnosis by PCR in children. *Circulation* 1994;90:330–339.

50. Pauschinger M, Bowles NE, Fuentes-Garcia FJ, et al. Detection of adenoviral genome in the myocardium of adult patients with idiopathic left ventricular dysfunction. *Circulation* 1999;99: 1348–1354.

51. Kawai C. From myocarditis to cardiomyopathy: mechanisms of inflammation and cell death: learning from the past for the future. *Circulation* 1999;99:1091–1100.

52. Why HJ, Meany BT, Richardson PJ, et al. Clinical and prognostic significance of detection of enteroviral RNA in the myocardium of patients with myocarditis or dilated cardiomyopathy. *Circulation* 1994;89:2582–2589.

53. Aretz HT, Billingham ME, Edwards WD, et al. Myocarditis. A histopathologic definition and classification. *Am J Cardiovasc Pathol* 1987;1:3–14.

54. Dec GW, Fallon JT, Southern JF, Palacios I. "Borderline" myocarditis: an indication for repeat endomyocardial biopsy. *J Am Coll Cardiol* 1990;15:283–289.

55. Hauck AJ, Kearney DL, Edwards WD. Evaluation of postmortem endomyocardial biopsy specimens from 38 patients with lymphocytic myocarditis: implications for role of sampling error. *Mayo Clin Proc* 1989;64:1235–1245.

56. Lieberman EB, Hutchins GM, Herskowitz A, Rose NR, Baughman KL. Clinicopathologic description of myocarditis. *J Am Coll Cardiol* 1991;18:1617–1626.

57. McCarthy RE 3rd, Boehmer JP, Hruban RH, et al. Long-term outcome of fulminant myocarditis as compared with acute (nonfulminant) myocarditis. *N Engl J Med* 2000;342:690–695.

58. Midei MG, DeMent SH, Feldman AM, Hutchins GM, Baughman KL. Peripartum myocarditis and cardiomyopathy. *Circulation* 1990;81:922–928.

59. Frustaci A, Bellocci F, Olsen EG. Results of biventricular endomyocardial biopsy in survivors of cardiac arrest with apparently normal hearts. *Am J Cardiol* 1994;74:890–895.

60. Reilly JM, Cunnion RE, Anderson DW, et al. Frequency of myocarditis, left ventricular dysfunction and ventricular tachycardia in the acquired immune deficiency syndrome. *Am J Cardiol* 1988;62:789–793.

61. Herskowitz A, Vlahov D, Willoughby S, et al. Prevalence and incidence of left ventricular dysfunction in patients with human immunodeficiency virus infection. *Am J Cardiol* 1993;71: 955–958.

62. Barbaro G, Di Lorenzo G, Grisorio B, Barbarini G. Incidence of dilated cardiomyopathy and detection of HIV in myocardial cells of HIV-positive patients. Gruppo Italiano per lo Studio Cardiologico dei Pazienti Affetti da AIDS. *N Engl J Med* 1998; 339:1093–1099.

63. Kereiakes DJ, Parmley WW. Myocarditis and cardiomyopathy. *Am Heart J* 1984;108:1318–1326.

64. Mason JW, Billingham ME, Ricci DR. Treatment of acute inflammatory myocarditis assisted by endomyocardial biopsy. *Am J Cardiol* 1980;45:1037–1044.

65. Mason JW, O'Connell JB, Herskowitz A, et al. A clinical trial of immunosuppressive therapy for myocarditis. The Myocarditis Treatment Trial Investigators. *N Engl J Med* 1995;333: 269–275.

66. Keren A, Popp RL. Assignment of patients into the classification of cardiomyopathies. *Circulation* 1992;86:1622–1633.

67. Schoenfeld MH, Supple EW, Dec GW, Jr., Fallon JT, Palacios IF. Restrictive cardiomyopathy versus constrictive pericarditis: role of endomyocardial biopsy in avoiding unnecessary thoracotomy. *Circulation* 1987;75:1012–1017.

67a. Arad M, et al. Glycogen storage diseases presenting as hypertrophic cardiomyopathy. *N Engl J Med* 2005; 352:362–72.

68. Kyle RA. Amyloidosis. *Circulation* 1995;91:1269–1271.

69. Falk RH, Comenzo RL, Skinner M. The systemic amyloidoses. *N Engl J Med* 1997;337:898–909.

70. Kyle RA, Gertz MA, Greipp PR, et al. A trial of three regimens for primary amyloidosis: colchicine alone, melphalan and prednisone, and melphalan, prednisone, and colchicine. *N Engl J Med* 1997;336:1202–1207.

71. Newman LS, Rose CS, Maier LA. Sarcoidosis. *N Engl J Med* 1997; 336:1224–1234.

72. Yazaki Y, Isobe M, Hiramitsu S, et al. Comparison of clinical features and prognosis of cardiac sarcoidosis and idiopathic dilated cardiomyopathy. *Am J Cardiol* 1998;82:537–540.

73. Olson LJ, Edwards WD, Holmes DR Jr, Miller FA Jr, Nordstrom LA, Baldus WP. Endomyocardial biopsy in hemochromatosis: clinicopathologic correlates in six cases. *J Am Coll Cardiol* 1989;13: 116–120.

74. Williams JF, Bristow MR, Fowler MC. Guidelines for the evaluation and management of heart failure (ACC/AHA Task Force). *Circulation* 1995;92:2764.

Intra-Aortic Balloon Counterpulsation and Other Circulatory Assist Devices

21

Daniel Burkhoff[a]

Significant hemodynamic embarrassment (owing to cardiogenic shock in the setting of acute myocardial infarction, decompensated chronic heart failure, and acute mitral valve regurgitation, or ventricular septal defect) clearly increases the risk of any diagnostic or interventional procedure. Right heart catheterization is valuable for excluding the possibility of occult hypovolemia or high-output failure (owing to sepsis or a vasodilator response to agents such as milrinone) and for measuring the extent of cardiogenic shock and its response to treatment. Pharmacologic therapy (arterial and venous vasodilators, vasoconstrictors, positive inotropes (see Chapter 2) may be helpful, but is often not sufficiently potent to normalize hemodynamics or has undesirable side effects (increased arrhythmias, worsened tissue perfusion). Accordingly, various devices have been developed to provide hemodynamic support to patients in various acute and chronic clinical settings. This includes treatment of patients with baseline hemodynamic compromise, as well as the prophylactic stabilization of patients with borderline ventricular function and large portions of the remaining viable myocardium at risk during percutaneous coronary interventions or cardiac surgical procedures. To the extent that some of these support devices favorably alter the relationship between myocardial oxygen supply and oxygen demand (see Chapter 18), these devices may be the treatment of choice

in medically refractory unstable angina when definitive revascularization procedure is delayed. This chapter will review the design, indications, and technique for use for these hemodynamic support devices.

INTRA-AORTIC BALLOON COUNTERPULSATION

The first device developed for use in all of these settings was the *intra-aortic balloon pump* (IABP) which uses counterpulsation to increase aortic pressure during diastole while decreasing aortic pressure during ejection. This enhances the pressure gradient for coronary artery blood flow (which occurs primarily during diastole) while decreasing the impedance for ejection of blood from the ventricle during systole. Despite the advent of increasingly sophisticated left ventricular assist devices (LVADs) and cardiopulmonary support (CPS) systems that are designed to provide more complete circulatory support, IABP remains the most practical and widely used form of circulatory support.

The intra-aortic balloon pump system consists of a balloon-tipped catheter that is connected to a console that controls the timing and volume of balloon inflation and deflation during the cardiac cycle. The concept of using timed inflation of a balloon to generate a positive pressure pulse during diastole (to improve coronary flow) and then rapidly deflating the balloon to withdraw that volume during systole (to reduce resistance to systolic ejection) was

---

[a] This chapter contains significant portions of the material contributed by Fayaz Shawl and Julian M. Aroesty to previous editions.

first conceived by Clauss in 1961 (1,2) and applied clinically by Kantrowitz in 1968 (3). At first, the practice was confined to patients with cardiogenic shock (1,2), but this was soon followed by successful use in patients with medically refractory unstable angina (4). Insertion of a balloon catheter was initially performed surgically (the first IAB catheters measured 12 to 14 French in diameter), but most insertions today are done percutaneously, thanks to smaller diameter (8 to 9 French) over-the-wire catheters (5,6). The popularity of IABP stems from its ease of use, safety, and the perception of clinical effectiveness.

IABP Catheter

The intra-aortic balloon (IAB) catheter consists of a long cylindrical polyurethane balloon (length roughly 10 cm, inflated volume 30 to 50 mL) that is mounted on a flexible shaft. The tip of the IAB is ideally positioned in the descending thoracic aorta, 1 to 2 cm beyond the origin of the left subclavian artery. This balloon is abruptly inflated with helium immediately after aortic valve closure, causing an increase in aortic diastolic pressure. Inflation is maintained until just before the beginning of systolic ejection (i.e., the opening of the aortic valve), when the helium is abruptly withdrawn to rapidly deflate the balloon and thereby produce a sharp fall in systolic aortic pressure with a resultant decrease in the impedance to left ventricular ejection. The inflation–deflation cycle is generally triggered (timed) relative to the R wave of the surface ECG. If use of the ECG is not possible or the ECG signal itself is inade-

quate, alternative triggering options are available (e.g., pacer, pressure, or a fixed internal trigger for patients in ventricular fibrillation or on cardiopulmonary bypass). The console allows for adjustment of the timing of balloon inflation and deflation to optimize the hemodynamic effect, as reflected in the arterial pressure waveform.

Most IABs are dual-lumen catheters. One lumen is used to shuttle gas to and from the balloon. The second (central) lumen allows delivery of the catheter over a guidewire and subsequent monitoring of central aortic pressure. A 40-mL balloon is used in most adults, and a 30- or 34-mL balloon is reserved for smaller patients (approximately 5 feet to 5 feet 4 inches). A 50-mL balloon is available for patients $\geq$6 feet. Pediatric balloons are also available in 2.5, 5.0, 12.0, and 20-mL sizes (Table 21.1). Early balloon consoles used CO_2 gas because of its excellent solubility in blood in the event that the balloon membrane developed a leak. As the shaft size of balloon catheters decreased, it became desirable to use gas with a lower molecular weight (i.e., helium) to maintain the fast gas shuttle speeds needed for crisp inflation and deflation.

Percutaneous Insertion

With rare exceptions, such as the presence of severe peripheral vascular disease, the IAB catheter is inserted percutaneously through the femoral artery. If femoral insertion is not possible, the clinician may opt for insertion using a subclavian or brachial artery approach. Percutaneous IAB insertion can be performed via femoral artery grafts if special

TABLE 21.1

SUMMARY OF AVAILABLE IABS BY MANUFACTURER AND SIZE

Manufacturer	Balloon Catheter Size (F)	Dual Lumen or Single Lumen	Balloon Volume (mL)	Sheathed/ Sheathless Insertion or Both	Sheath Provided (F)	Guidewire (in./cm)
Datascope Corp.						
Linear 7.5F IAB catheters	7.5	Dual lumen	25, 34, & 40	Both	7.5	0.25/0.064
Fidelity 8F IAB catheters	8	Dual lumen	25, 34, & 40	Both	8	0.25/0.064
True Sheathless 9.5F IAB catheters	9.5	Dual lumen	25, 34, & 40	Both	10	0.30/0.077
Percor Stat DL 10.5F IAB catheter	10.5	Dual lumen	50	?	11.5	0.30/0.077
Pediatric IAB catheter	4.5	Single lumen	2	Available for surgical insertion only		
Pediatric IAB catheter	5.5	Single lumen	5			
Pediatric IAB catheter	5.5	Single lumen	7			
Pediatric IAB catheter	7.0	Single lumen	12			
Pediatric IAB catheter	7.0	Single lumen	20			
Arrow International						
UltraFlex 7.5F IAB Catheters	7.5	Dual lumen	30 & 40	Both	8	0.25/0.064
Ultra 8F IAB Catheters	8	Dual lumen	30 & 40	Both	8	0.25/0.064m
NarrowFlex 8F IAB Catheters	8	Dual lumen	30 & 40	Both	9.5	0.30/0.077
Rediguard 9F IAB Catheters	9	Dual lumen	50	Both	10.5	0.30/0.077
8F 40 mL sheathless IAB catheter	8	Dual lumen	40	Both	9	0.25/0.064
7F 30 mL sheathless IAB catheter	7	Dual lumen	30	Both	8	0.25/0.064

attention is paid to puncture technique (7). Although the reduction in the diameter of IAB catheters in recent years (8F is the predominant size today) has reduced the incidence of serious vascular complications, a careful preprocedure clinical evaluation can minimize the risk of complications. Clotting parameters (prothrombin time, partial thromboplastin time, and platelet count) should be checked, and a clinical evaluation of the possible peripheral vascular disease should be performed prior to IAB insertion.

IABs are generally inserted percutaneously over a guidewire using either a small (8 to 9F) sheath or a sheathless (over-the-wire) technique. The technique for preparation and puncture of the common femoral artery is described in Chapter 4. If balloon placement is being performed as a stand-alone procedure, the artery is predilated using a 7 or 8F dilator after the wire has been advanced to the level of the diaphragm. Firm pressure is maintained over the puncture site to prevent hematoma as the dilator is removed and the wire wiped clean. Next, the appropriate-size sheath (or the balloon catheter itself if the sheathless insertion is chosen) is introduced over the wire. When balloon placement is being performed at the conclusion of a catheterization procedure, the new low-profile Datascope 8F IAB catheters can often be placed via an existing 8F sheath. (Note: current Arrow 8F catheter kits contain a 9 or 9.5F introducer sheath.) In this case, it is helpful to insert the special IAB catheter guidewire up to the level of the diaphragm before removing the final diagnostic or interventional guiding catheter to eliminate the need to renegotiate tortuous iliac vessels.

The IAB catheter should be dipped in saline prior to insertion. Air is then evacuated from the balloon, using a large (60-mL) syringe attached to the one-way valve supplied in the kit, to maintain the lowest possible IAB profile during introduction. The guidewire lumen should then be flushed with a heparin–saline solution and the balloon loaded onto the guidewire supplied with the IAB insertion kit. Maintaining the guidewire above the carina (bifurcation of the trachea into left and right mainstem bronchi, which is generally just distal to the left subclavian artery), the balloon should be advanced to that level with minimal resistance. Alternatively, fluoroscopy in the left anterior oblique projection usually allows direct visualization of the upper mediastinal density that corresponds to the left subclavian takeoff. When the radiopaque tip-marker reaches this level, the guidewire is removed, the central lumen of the balloon catheter is aspirated and flushed, and the guidewire lumen is attached to either the coronary manifold or a pressurized flushing device equipped with a pressure transducer (Intraflo) that delivers 3 mL/hour to maintain lumen patency. Special care must be taken to prevent inadvertent injection of air bubbles or thrombi through the guidewire lumen, since its tip is only a short distance below the aortic arch. The balloon shaft may be equipped with a protective plastic outer sleeve that can be advanced to mate with the hub of the introducer sheath to maintain sterility if subsequent adjustment is required. If a long (23-cm) sheath has been used to negotiate a tortuous iliac artery, the sheath must be partially withdrawn prior to initiation of counterpulsation so that the distal end of the sheath does not overlie and trap the distal end of the balloon.

Sheathless Insertion

Although insertion through a sheath is quite easy, most current balloons have a tapered nose to allow them to be inserted directly over a guidewire (i.e., without use of a sheath). Because the balloon shaft is roughly 1.5F (0.5 mm) smaller than the corresponding sheath's outer diameter, sheathless insertion results in less femoral arterial trauma and less obstruction to the limb circulation in patients with small or atherosclerotic arteries. Care must be taken to adequately predilate the soft-tissue track and to avoid kinking either the guidewire or balloon catheter during insertion. Additionally, the balloon catheter should *not* be rotated as it is passed through the soft tissues, as this will produce unnecessary tissue trauma. If undue resistance is encountered while advancing the catheter, consideration should be given to reverting to a sheathed insertion.

Initiation of Counterpulsation

Following connection to the console, the system is purged with helium inflation gas. The console can be set so that the balloon will be inflated to approximately half its rated volume with each inflation, and counterpulsation is begun at the 1:2 or 1:3 setting (every other or every third beat) so that preliminary timing adjustments can be made (see below). Fluoroscopy can be used to confirm appropriate placement of the balloon proximally, full exit from the sheath distally, and uniform expansion without twists or kinks. Balloon volume is then increased to its full rated value, and fluoroscopy is performed again to verify that the balloon position is appropriate and that the balloon has assumed a uniform symmetric cylindrical shape at full inflation. The balloon shaft and sheath (if used) are sewn to the skin, povidone-iodine (Betadine) solution is applied to the entrance site, a mark is placed across the balloon shaft and the skin to detect any subsequent balloon migration, and a sterile dressing is applied. If the patient is not already anticoagulated, heparin (5,000 units intravenously) should be given intravenously as soon as the balloon is inserted, followed by continuous intravenous heparin titrated to maintain an activated clotting time (ACT) of 1.5 to 2.0 times normal.

Adjusting Counterpulsation Timing

Maximal benefit depends on proper timing of balloon inflation and deflation. Timing should be done by inspection of the central aortic pressure tracing through the balloon central lumen, since the change in contour and the timing of the pulse wave as it moves from the central aorta to the periphery can make accurate timing of counterpulsation difficult. Optimal waveform interpretation is also facilitated by having the transducer as close as possible to the hub of the balloon, connected by a short relatively stiff tubing (see Chapter 7, Pressure Measurement). Timing is best done with the console set at 1:2 or 1:3 pumping (i.e., counterpulsation of every other or every third beat) so that arterial pressure tracings from consecutive beats with and without counterpulsation can be compared (Fig. 21.1). The newest IABP systems (the CS100 manufactured by Datascope Corp. and the AutoCat 2 Wave manufactured by Arrow International) use tip pressure measurements to set proper timing automatically and require little, if any, manipulation of the console controls by the operator to maintain correct timing.

When appropriately timed, the effect of IABP is to reduce ventricular afterload and increase cardiac output, as shown in the example of Fig. 21.1B, obtained from a patient with chronic heart failure. The aortic and ventricular pressure and ventricular volume measurements shown in this figure illustrate these points, particularly as shown by the corresponding pressure-volume loops shown in the bottom panel (note that ventricular volume was measured using the conductance catheter technique). Initiation of

IABP reduced peak aortic and ventricular pressure, decreased end-diastolic volume, and increased stroke volume, which are collectively indicative of both preload and afterload reduction.

Inflation

As stated above, the newest systems set proper inflation timing automatically. In older systems, however, it is necessary for the operator to look at a central aortic pressure tracing and slowly adjust the inflation timing later until the dicrotic notch becomes visible. Inflation should then be moved back to a slightly earlier time until the inflation upstroke fuses with the central aortic dicrotic notch to form a "U" (see Fig. 21.2). Earlier inflation should be avoided, because this will increase aortic pressure during left ventricular ejection, resulting in decreased stroke volume.

Deflation

As with inflation, the newest systems set deflation timing automatically. In older systems, deflation should be timed to take place just before the opening of the aortic valve. Starting with deflation that is clearly too early (before the R wave), the timing of deflation is delayed progressively until

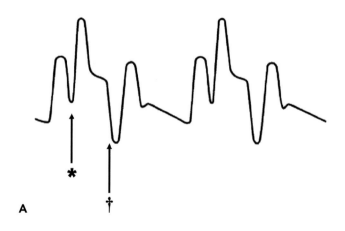

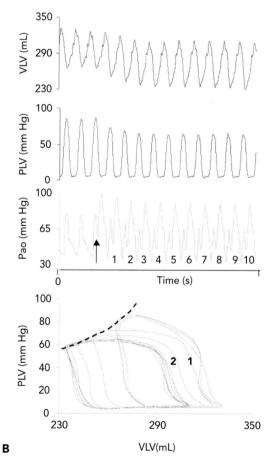

Figure 21.1 **A.** Central aortic waveform with properly timed intra-aortic balloon pump (IABP) operating in 1:2 mode (i.e., balloon pumping every other beat). Balloon inflation (*→) occurs at the dicrotic notch, and diastolic pressure is augmented compared with the normal beat. Balloon deflation (†→) occurs just prior to ejection, and there is a drop in aortic pressure, signifying reduction of the impedance to ejection. **B.** Aortic pressure (Pao), LV pressure (PLV), and LV volume (VLV) measured from a heart failure patient at the initiation of 1:1 IAB pumping (arrow). Characteristic changes in diastolic Pao are apparent. IABP induced diastolic unloading (decreased end-diastolic volume), afterload reduction (marked decreases in end-systolic volume and decreased systolic pressure) while increasing stroke volume. These hemodynamic changes are readily demonstrated in the pressure-volume loops in the lower part of the figure. (View B tracings courtesy of Dr. Jan Schreuder, Department of Cardiac Surgery, San Raffaele University Hospital, Milan.)

Balloon Timing

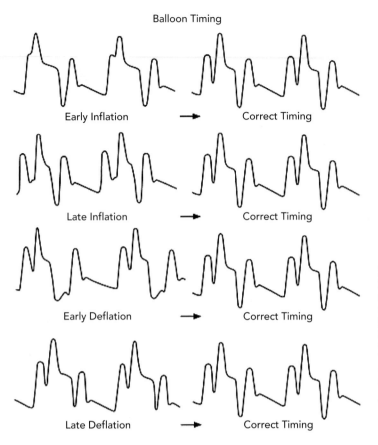

Early Inflation ➝ Correct Timing

Late Inflation ➝ Correct Timing

Early Deflation ➝ Correct Timing

Late Deflation ➝ Correct Timing

Figure 21.2 The timing of balloon inflation and deflation is adjusted in the 1:2 mode. The inflation point is moved rightward (later) until it occurs in late diastole, and the dicrotic notch is uncovered. The inflation timing is moved progressively earlier in the cardiac cycle until the dicrotic notch on the central aortic tracing just disappears. Examples of early, late, and correct inflation are shown in the top two tracings. Similarly, the deflation knob is moved leftward (earlier) and then slowly advanced toward the right (later in the cardiac cycle) until the end-diastolic pressure dips 10 to 15 mm Hg below the patient's unassisted diastolic pressure. This will produce a maximal lowering of the patient's unassisted systolic pressure. Examples of early, late, and correct deflation timing are shown in the bottom two traces.

the maximum reduction of aortic systolic pressure is observed in the subsequent beat. This is usually accompanied by a parallel 10 to 15 mm Hg decrease in the nadir of central aortic diastolic pressure (Fig. 21.2). Recent data suggest that later deflation approaching left ventricular ejection is not detrimental and may, in fact, enhance stroke volume (8); however, the clinical implications of variation of deflation timing have not been studied systematically in controlled clinical trials.

Timing in the Presence of Arrhythmias

In the presence of *atrial fibrillation* or marked *irregularity of the cardiac rhythm*, balloon timing is best adjusted so that deflation occurs on the peak of the R wave to avoid left ventricular ejection against an inflated balloon during the occasional short R-R intervals. *Atrial pacing* may also produce timing difficulties if the console misinterprets the atrial pacing spike as the peak of the R wave. This can be overcome either by timing the balloon off the arterial pressure contour, by choosing a monitor lead that magnifies the difference between the ECG R wave and the atrial pacing spike, or by setting the console to the mode that discriminates between the pacing spike and R wave by sensing both the height and duration of the signal. Manual adjustment of timing with today's state-of-the-art systems, however, is rarely required as

these systems adapt automatically to irregularly timed beats as encountered in atrial fibrillation and other rhythm abnormalities by continuously seeking the best available trigger source and making the appropriate timing adjustments.

Angiography During Counterpulsation

Whenever possible, it is desirable to perform angiography or percutaneous coronary intervention prior to balloon placement so that a single femoral access site can be used. In hemodynamically unstable patients, however, counterpulsation can be used *during* such procedures. In this case, the balloon catheter is placed first and cardiac angiography is then performed via the opposite femoral artery or the radial artery. If the contralateral femoral approach is used for angiography, a few precautions should be taken to avoid damaging the balloon membrane. The guidewire and catheters should be advanced beyond the level of the balloon with inflation suspended briefly and with the tip of the catheter pointed away from the balloon toward the wall of the aorta (9). Once the interventional catheter is in the ascending aorta, counterpulsation can be resumed. Inflation and deflation of the IAB does not interfere with manipulation of the interventional catheter. However, the operator should remember to suspend balloon operation temporarily during catheter exchanges.

Patient Management During Counterpulsation

Patients having an IAB are maintained in an intensive care unit and therefore receive a high level of medical care and observation. During counterpulsation, it is particularly important that patients undergo specific evaluations at least daily for evidence of sepsis, thrombocytopenia, blood loss, hemolysis, vascular obstruction (i.e., distal leg ischemia), thrombus, embolus, and vascular dissection. Mild to moderate thrombocytopenia may occur owing to platelet destruction, but the platelet count rarely falls below 50,000 to 100,000/mL unless there is some other problem such as heparin-induced thrombocytopenia or disseminated intravascular coagulation. Following balloon removal, the platelet count should rapidly return to normal (10).

The level of heparin anticoagulation should be monitored closely, with partial thromboplastin time (PTT) maintained at 50 to 70 seconds to prevent thrombotic or embolic complications. Evaluation of the circulation to the involved limb should be done as often as every 2 hours. Dorsalis pedis and posterior tibial pulses should be palpated at least every 6 to 8 hours. Use of Doppler probe to confirm presence of distal pulses is mandatory if these are not palpable. A chest radiograph should be reviewed daily during IABP support to ensure that the catheter tip is properly located at the level of the carina. If balloon position has migrated, presence of the protective sheath allows for repositioning to avoid potential complications of improper balloon position. If the IAB sits below the recommended position, renal arteries may be blocked during inflation. IAB positioning above the recommended position can block the subclavian artery or can cause damage to the aortic arch.

Weaning from Counterpulsation and Balloon Removal

Balloon counterpulsation is a temporary support measure. The balloon is usually removed once the patient's condition has stabilized after the acute insult (usually after 24 to 48 hours of pumping). Before removal of an intra-aortic balloon, patients are weaned progressively from support by decreasing the counterpulsation mode from 1:1 to 1:2 and then 1:3 counterpulsation. Sufficient time should elapse between stages to ensure the patient will tolerate a progressive decrease in the level of hemodynamic support without exhibiting clinical deterioration. Once the decision has been made to discontinue IABP support, pumping should be maintained at 1:3 until a clinician is available to remove the balloon. Once heparin has been stopped, continuous pumping in the 1:3 mode will reduce the chance of clot formation, until the clotting parameters have fallen an ACT <160 seconds or a PTT <50 seconds, allowing the device to be removed safely.

At the point when the IAB is to be removed, the pump should be shut off and a 50-mL syringe with stopcock attached to the balloon inflation port to create a vacuum. The balloon is then withdrawn. The site is then firmly compressed by hand or with a mechanical compression device for 30 to 60 minutes. The patient is kept at bed rest, avoiding hip flexion on the involved side, for the next 24 hours. If the balloon is placed only during an interventional procedure, the groin site can be managed by use of one of the groin closure devices or by "pre-close" of the puncture site with the Perclose suture device (see Chapter 5).

Complications

Data on 16,909 patients undergoing IABP therapy, collected by the Benchmark Counterpulsation Outcomes Registry (sponsored by Datascope Corp.) between 1996 and 2000 and published in the Journal of the American College of Cardiology in 2001, showed the incidence of major complications resulting from the use of an intra-aortic balloon pump to be 2.8%. The incidence of minor complications was 4.2%. Major complications were defined as limb ischemia resulting in a loss of pulse or sensation or abnormal limb temperature or pallor requiring surgical intervention, severe bleeding requiring transfusion or surgical intervention, and balloon leak and death directly attributable to IAB catheter insertion or failure. Minor complications included such things as limb ischemia (evidenced by a diminished pulse) that resolves after catheter removal and nonsevere bleeding involving either a minor hematoma or some degree of puncture site oozing (11; Table 21.2). Independent predictors of a major complication were female gender, age (75 years or older), and peripheral vascular disease. IABP-related mortality was 0.5% (11; Table 21.3).

Overall complication rates associated with the use of IABP therapy appear to have declined over the course of the last 25 years. The introduction of low-profile 8 French IAB catheters in the late 1990s, no doubt, accelerated this drop (12). A single-center study of 240 patients receiving IABP treatment between 1985 and 1990 (10 years prior to the first publication of the Benchmark Registry data) showed a 7.5% rate of major complications and an overall complication rate of 13% (13). Another single-center European study of patients receiving IABP treatment between 1989 and 1996 showed the rates to be 4.7% and 10.4%, respectively (14). Despite the significant decline in balloon-related complication rates, however, complications can be serious and therefore it is incumbent on operators to take all possible measures to avoid balloon-related complications.

Indications and Contraindications

The changing clinical applications for intra-aortic balloon counterpulsation have, in many ways, paralleled the

TABLE 21.2

SUMMARY OF COMPLICATIONS FROM BENCHMARK REGISTRY

	Total Population (*n* = 16,909)	Diagnostic Catheterization Only (*n* = 1,576)	Catheterization and PCI Only (*n* = 3,882)	Surgery CABG (*n* = 9,179)	Non-CABG (*n* = 1,086)	No Intervention or Revascularization Noted (*n* = 1,186)
In hospital mortality (%)	21.2	32.2	18.4	16.8	37.8	34.1
Mortality—balloon in place (%)	11.6	17.6	10.1	9.2	19.8	20.2
IABP-related mortality[a] (%)	0.05	0.1	0.1	0.0	0.0	0.1
Amputation[b]	0.1	0.0	0.1	0.1	0.1	0.0
Major limb ischemia[c] (%)	0.9	0.6	0.5	1.2	1.0	0.5
Any limb ischemia (%)	2.9	3.2	1.9	3.5	2.5	1.7
Severe access site bleeding (%)	0.8	0.8	1.2	0.7	0.7	0.3
Any access site bleeding (%)	2.4	2.7	4.4	1.7	1.3	1.4
Balloon leak (%)	1.0	0.9	0.8	1.1	0.5	1.6
Composite outcomes						
Major IABP complication[d] (%)	2.8	2.8	2.2	3.0	2.9	2.4
Any IABP complication[e] (%)	7.0	7.6	7.5	7.1	6.0	5.2
Any unsuccessful IABP[f](%)	2.3	2.5	1.7	2.5	2.4	2.7

[a] Death as direct consequence of IABP therapy. [b] All major limb ischemia. [c] Loss of pulse or sensation, abnormal limb temperature or pallor, requiring surgical intervention. [d] Balloon leak, severe bleeding, major limb ischemia, or death as a direct consequence of IABP therapy. [e] Any access site bleeding, any limb ischemia, balloon leak, poor inflation, poor augmentation, insertion difficulty, or death as direct result of IABP therapy. [f] Balloon leak, poor inflation, poor augmentation, or insertion difficulty.
CABG, coronary artery bypass graft; IABP, intra-aortic balloon pump; PCI, percutaneous coronary intervention.
From Ferguson JJ 3rd, Cohen M, Freedman RJ Jr, et al. The current practice of intra-aortic balloon counterpulsation: results from the Benchmark Registry. *J Am Coll Cardiol* 2001;38:1456–1462.

advances in cardiac surgery and interventional cardiology. Based on the initial experience by Kantrowitz and others, IABP was then used as a stand-alone treatment for patients who had suffered an acute myocardial infarction and had lapsed into cardiogenic shock. Long-term survival of these patients, however, was poor. It soon became clear, particularly after it was shown that cardiac catheterization and angiography could be performed safely during balloon pumping (15), that IABP plus revascularization might improve survival. This concept has been supported, but not proven, in several uncontrolled clinical studies (16–22). Over time, IABP was used in patients with poor left ventricular (LV) function undergoing coronary artery bypass grafting (CABG) or valvular surgery who experienced "stunned myocardium" and could not be weaned from cardiopulmonary bypass, as well high-risk CABG patients (e.g., those with critical left main stenoses). Today, intra-aortic balloon counterpulsation continues to be used prophylactically in high-risk surgical patients. Table 21.4 lists indications and Table 21.5 lists contraindications for IAPB.

TABLE 21.3

RISK FACTORS FOR COMPLICATIONS

Risk Factor	Estimated Odds Ratio (Presence/Absence)	95% Confidence Limits	P Value
PVD	1.968	1.557, 2.487	<0.001
Female	1.737	1.414, 2.134	<0.001
BSA <1.65 m²	1.453	1.095, 1.926	<0.05
Age ≥75 yr	1.289	1.048, 1.585	<0.05

The chi-square was highly significant ($P < 0.001$); however, the concordance index was only 61%. The following variables were rested, but were not significant: primary intervention, history of diabetes, previous myocardial infaction, previous coronary artery bypass graft, indications for use (cardiogenic shock, wean from cardiopulmonary bypass), primary/tertiary care institution, catheter size, and left vessel main involvement.
BSA, body surface area; IABP, intra-aortic balloon pump; PVD, peripheral vascular disease.
From Ferguson JJ 3rd, Cohen M, Freedman RJ Jr, et al. The current practice of intra-aortic balloon counterpulsation: results from the Benchmark Registry. *J Am Coll Cardiol* 2001;38(5):1456–1462.

TABLE 21.4
INDICATIONS

Hemodynamic compromise
Cardiogenic shock secondary to AMI with continuing ischemia, VSD, or MR
Cardiogenic shock due to transient ischemia, myocarditis, sepsis, drug toxicity, etc.
Inability to wean from bypass after cardiac surgery
Hemodynamic support while awaiting transplantation
Severe arrhythmia owing to refractory ischemia

Medically refractory ischemia
Medically refractory unstable angina
Failed PTCA with refractory ischemia

Prophylactic high-risk intervention
High-risk PTCA owing to LV dysfunction and/or large territory at risk
PTCA during acute myocardial infarction
Stabilization in patients with severe aortic stenosis
Severe multivessel or left main CAD requiring urgent cardiac or noncardiac surgery
Large myocardial infarction

AMI, acute myocardial infarction; CAD, coronary artery disease; LV, left ventricle; MR, mitral regurgitation; PTCA, percutaneous transluminal coronary angioplasty; VSD, ventricular septal defect.

Starting in the early 1980s, IABP was used in conjunction with angioplasty to stabilize patients prior to an interventional procedure or as a bailout measure following unsuccessful early or late closure of a vessel as a way of stabilizing patients for emergency bypass. As stents, platelet inhibitors, and other additions to the interventional cardiologist's armamentarium began to emerge in the 1990s, patients who only a few years earlier would have been deemed too high risk for angioplasty and referred to surgery were now treated in the catheterization laboratory. Here again, just as it had in the early days of surgical revascularization, the availability of balloon pumping played a role in allowing the clinician to treat many of these cardiac patients.

Today the most frequent indications for use of IABP are hemodynamic support during or after cardiac catheterization, particularly in the case of high-risk interventions, and

TABLE 21.5
CONTRAINDICATIONS FOR INTRA-AORTIC BALLOON PUMPING

Significant aortic regurgitation
Abdominal aortic aneurysm
Aortic dissection
Uncontrolled septicemia
Uncontrolled bleeding diathesis
Severe bilateral peripheral vascular disease uncorrectable by peripheral angioplasty or cross-femoral surgery
Bilateral femoral-popliteal bypass grafts for severe peripheral vascular disease

cardiogenic shock. The next most frequent indications are in patients failing to wean from cardiopulmonary bypass, preoperative management of high-risk surgical patients, and management of patients with refractory unstable angina (Table 21.6; 11).

The 1999 task force guideline of the American Heart Association and the American College of Cardiology listed Class I indications for use of intra-aortic balloon pump counterpulsation in the setting of acute myocardial infarction (MI) as follows: (1) cardiogenic shock as a stabilizing measure for angiography and prompt revascularization, (2) acute ventricular septal defect (VSD) or mitral regurgitation (MR) complicating acute MI as stabilizing therapy for angiography and repair/revascularization, (3) recurrent intractable ventricular arrhythmias with hemodynamic instability, and (4) refractory post-MI angina as a bridge to angiography and revascularization. These indications represent about half of the IAB usage noted in 5,495 acute MI patients in the Benchmark Registry reported by Stone et al. in 2003 (23). A detailed analysis of IABP usage in the largest series of patients receiving balloon pump support to date ($n = 16,909$) was published in 2001 (11).

Clinical Results

Many studies have been conducted to examine the hemodynamic effects of counterpulsation and its benefit in different clinical situations. The number of such studies is too large to review here, so only an overview of the salient findings shall be presented.

Support and Stabilization of Patients Undergoing Percutaneous Coronary Intervention

One of the main uses of IABP continues to be support and stabilization of patients undergoing percutaneous coronary interventions, particularly those considered at high risk for major adverse cardiac events (Table 21.6). In recent years, these risk criteria have included such things as poor LV function, multiple vessel and left main disease, age older than 70 years, and prior CABG surgery (24). As interventionalists have gained more experience in performing coronary interventions on increasingly complex lesions, multiple vessels, and in patients with heart failure, there is a perception among some that the overall need for prophylactic IABP support has declined. These advances notwithstanding, the benefit of IABP in preventing intraprocedural adverse events during high-risk percutaneous coronary interventions (PCIs) for patients with borderline hemodynamics, ongoing ischemia, or cardiogenic shock has been recognized by the ACC/AHA Guidelines for Percutaneous Coronary Interventional Procedures (25). These guidelines evolved from largely uncontrolled and/or retrospective analyses of single-center experiences in the use of IABP in this setting, as summarized below.

TABLE 21.6

USES OF IABP FROM THE REGISTRY

	Total Population (n = 16,909)	Diagnostic Catheterization Only (n = 1,576)	Catheterization and PCI Only (n = 3,882)	Surgery CABG (n = 9,179)	Surgery Non-CABG (n = 1,086)	No Intervention or Revascularization Noted (n = 1,186)
Suppurt and stabilization (%)	20.6	21.4	54.4	9.7	5.0	7.8
Cardiogenic shock (%)	18.8	33.1	23.7	12.3	23.8	29.4
Weaning from cardiopulmonary bypass (%)	16.1	0.4	0.1	24.9	31.4	7.1
Preop: high-risk CABG (%)	13.0	4.6	0.2	22.1	6.4	1.9
Refractory unstable angina (%)	12.3	15.3	8.3	15.8	2.2	3.0
Refractory ventricular failure (%)	6.5	9.1	2.5	5.9	15.7	12.7
Mechanical complication owing to AMI (%)	5.5	9.8	7.0	4.2	5.2	5.1
Ischemia related to intractable VA (%)	1.7	1.6	1.5	1.9	1.7	1.6
Cardiac support for high-risk general surgery patients (%)	0.9	2.1	0.2	0.5	4.3	1.1
Other (%)	0.8	0.7	0.2	0.8	2.5	2.0
IIntraoperative pulsatile flow (%)	0.4	0.1	0.1	0.7	0.5	0.2
Missing indication (%)	3.3	1.8	1.9	1.2	1.5	28.1

AMI, acute myocardial infarction; CABG, coronary artery bypass grafe; PCI, percutaneous coronary intervention; VA, ventricular arrhythmias.
From Ferguson JJ 3rd, Cohen M, Freedman RJ Jr, et al. The current practice of intra-aortic balloon counterpulsation: results from the Benchmark Registry. *J Am Coll Cardiol* 2001;38:5: 1456–1462.

In a study by Briguori et al. (26) of 133 consecutive elective PCI patients with left ventricle ejection fraction (LVEF) ≤30%, 61 received prophylactic IABP prior to the procedure. The remaining patients received elective IABP at the discretion of the operator. A jeopardy score based on coronary angiograms was calculated for each patient to quantify the amount of myocardium at risk. The overall incidence of intraprocedural major adverse cardiac events was significantly less in the group that received prophylactic IABP support (17% versus 0%). Among those patients in both groups with a jeopardy score of 6 or less, the rate of intraprocedural events was similar. Predictors of intraprocedural events were shown to be elective (versus prophylactic) IABP, female sex, and a jeopardy score of 6 or higher.

The National Registry of Supported Angioplasty reported the results in 801 patients with supported or standby supported angioplasty. Patients older than age 70 or with left main coronary artery (LMCA) stenosis are at higher risk, and those with LVEF <20% do better with prophylactic support. However, those with >50% of myocardium in jeopardy and low ejection fraction can undergo intervention with a 7.2% in-hospital mortality with either prophylactic or standby IABP support (27). With standby CPS support, the in-hospital mortality for a similar group of patients is 6.0% (28). A nonrandomized comparison of prophylactic intra-aortic balloon pumping with prophylactic cardiopulmonary support did not reveal any difference between the two support techniques in MI, stroke, emergency bypass surgery, or death, but did show a higher rate of peripheral vascular complication in the CPS group (29). This would seem to suggest that mortality is more a function of the baseline characteristics of the patient than of the particular support device used.

A retrospective analysis of 159 consecutive high-risk patients undergoing rotational atherectomy revealed that the 28 patients with elective preprocedure IABP placement had the same occurrence of slow flow (18% versus 17%), equal hospital stay, and similar vascular complication rate. However, among the patients developing slow flow, there were no non-Q wave MIs in the IABP group, as compared with 27% in the control group (30).

Cardiogenic Shock

Cardiogenic shock remains the leading cause of death in patients with acute MI who reach the hospital alive (31). In two large studies, the Worcester Heart Attack Study (n = 4,762) and the GUSTO-1 trial (n = 41,021), the incidence of cardiogenic shock in those acute MI patients who reached the hospital alive were 7.5% and 7.2%, respectively. In-hospital mortality among those with cardiogenic shock in the community-based Worcester Heart Attack Study was 77.7% compared with 13.5% for those without cardiogenic shock. In-hospital survival in this study did not improve during the time of the study (1975–1988). In-hospital mortality in the GUSTO-1 trial was 55% for those who arrived at the hospital in shock, 57% for those who developed shock after they were admitted, and 3% for those without shock (32,33). A subsequent analysis of the 89% of shock patients in GUSTO-1 who developed shock following their arrival at the hospital showed that age was the strongest predictor of shock after admittance. A 47% increased risk of developing shock was associated with each 10-year increase in age. A simple and reliable scoring algorithm for predicting the development of cardiogenic shock based on age and physical examination of the patient on arrival at the hospital resulted from the analysis (34).

Current treatment strategies for patients in cardiogenic shock in the setting of acute myocardial infarction usually include the use of (1) inotropes and pressor agents to counter LV dysfunction and hypotension and help stabilize the patient until hemodynamic support can be initiated; (2) IABP hemodynamic support, which increases coronary blood flow and collateral circulation; and finally, (3) definitive revascularization, either PCI or CABG. Use of IABP has been associated with improved survival in patients experiencing cardiogenic shock following acute MI (35). Other studies have shown a survival benefit in patients with cardiogenic shock who received thrombolytics and IABP versus thrombolytics alone (36).

Studies have shown a significant survival benefit in patients with acute infarction accompanied by cardiogenic shock who received IABP and thrombolytics compared with thrombolytics alone, 93% versus 37% (37), and 67% versus 49% (38). A subgroup analysis of 310 patients presenting with shock in the international multicenter GUSTO study revealed a wide disparity in the use of the IABP. This study revealed a trend toward a lower 30-day and 1-year mortality in patients receiving counterpulsation therapy, >80% of whom were from the centers in the United States. Despite the trend toward improved survival, however, IABP appears to be underused with only one third of cardiogenic shock patients presenting to U.S. centers undergoing IABP insertion (39). Aggressive diagnostic and therapeutic interventions in the United States compared with non-U.S. centers included IABP use (35% versus 7%), PTCA (26% versus 8%), and cardiac catheterization (58% versus 23%) and was accompanied by a lower 30-day mortality (50% versus 66%) and 1-year mortality (56% versus 70%; 40).

In the absence of early revascularization, mortality from cardiogenic shock remains high, approaching 85% in some reports. Even with early revascularization, mortality in those diagnosed with cardiogenic shock is approximately 50% (31). Patients with multiple infarctions or serious comorbidity, those requiring mitral valve replacement or repair for concomitant mitral regurgitation, and those with coronary anatomy that is unfavorable for bypass have the worst prognosis with surgery (41). Nonrandomized studies, in which the survival in patients with successful revascularization is compared with those patients in whom no attempt was made or the attempt failed, have all shown a much worse survival in the latter group.

Accordingly, the ACC/AHA Guidelines for the Management of Patients with Acute Myocardial Infarction rec-

ommend IABP when cardiogenic shock cannot be quickly reversed with pharmacologic therapy (42,43):

Class I
1. Cardiogenic shock not quickly reversed with pharmacologic therapy as a stabilizing measure for angiography and prompt revascularization
2. Acute mitral regurgitation or VSD complicating MI as a stabilizing therapy for angiography and repair/revascularization
3. Recurrent intractable ventricular arrhythmias with hemodynamic instability
4. Refractory post-MI angina as a bridge to angiography and revascularization

Class IIa
1. Signs of hemodynamic instability, poor LV function, or persistent ischemia in patients with large areas of myocardium at risk

Class IIb
1. In patients with successful PTCA after failed thrombolysis or those with three-vessel coronary disease to prevent reocclusion
2. In patients known to have large areas of myocardium at risk with or without active ischemia

Counterpulsation has also produced favorable responses in patients with shock owing to a nonischemic cause. In a reported series of noncoronary shock patients, most with acute myocarditis, IABP was inserted in ventilated patients failing pharmacologic support. Three to four days of counterpulsation was sufficient to allow adequate recovery of ventricular function in 25% of the patients. The remainder required a left ventricular assist device or biventricular support device for 3 to 79 days. At follow-up (7 to 54 months), all patients had recovered normal ventricular function and were asymptomatic, suggesting that patients with severe noncoronary shock may be supported for up to several weeks before transplantation is considered (44). However, it is emphasized that there are no prospective, randomized studies of IABP in this group of patients.

High-Risk CABG/Weaning from Cardiopulmonary Bypass

Almost from the outset and continuing to the present, balloon pumping has been used to support surgical patients who experience preoperative or postoperative hemodynamic instability and to improve clinical outcomes in high-risk patients undergoing coronary artery bypass grafting. Those CABG patients with poor LV function and left main disease have frequently been characterized as high risk. There continues to be some debate on benefits of preoperative versus perioperative or postoperative balloon pump support.

A study by Christenson et al. (45) defined high risk coronary surgical patients as those who present with two or more of the following preoperative criteria: left ventricular ejection fraction <0.30, left main stenosis >70%, unstable angina at the time of surgery despite optimal medical treatment, diffuse coronary disease requiring four or more distal anastomoses to achieve complete revascularization and reoperation. In this observational study, preoperative IABP was associated with lower in-hospital mortality compared with those receiving IABP postoperatively. Earlier studies by Christenson et al. demonstrated reduced ICU and hospital length of stay with preoperative IABP. More recently, preoperative IABP has also proved valuable in improving outcomes for high-risk patients undergoing off-pump coronary artery bypass grafting (OPCABG; 46,47).

Unstable Angina

Patients with medically refractory unstable angina continue to make up a large proportion of those treated by balloon pumping. During counterpulsation, they may exhibit only a modest decrease in peak systolic pressure and in left ventricular filling pressure with unchanged cardiac output, left ventricular volumes, ejection fraction, and regional contraction, as determined by angiographic chordal shortening (48). In patients with anterior wall ischemia, measurements of coronary sinus flow from the ischemic area may improve with counterpulsation, but this is not a uniform response (49).

There are two large multicenter randomized trials of counterpulsation to maintain patency of the infarct related artery. The first, reported in 1994, confirmed the benefit of this strategy (50). Patients with restored patency within 24 hours of their acute infarction were randomly assigned to standard therapy or to 48 hours of counterpulsation. Repeat angiography was performed on day 5. Reocclusion was present in 8% of the IABP patients, but in 21% of those receiving standard care who also were almost twice as likely to suffer death, stroke, or a recurrent ischemic event (50). These results were good news to cardiologists seeking methods to prevent abrupt vessel closure in the prestent era. Today, of course, the availability of stents and other new PCI-related treatment modalities have dramatically reduced the rate of abrupt vessel closure following PCI and hence the need for IABP as an adjunctive/protective measure to maintain patency of the treated vessel (51).

Emergent CABG for Failed PCI

The need for emergency CABG following PCI has decreased significantly over time (see Chapter 22). A review of 18,593 patients undergoing PCI between 1992 and 2000 showed the rate of emergency CABG falling from 1.5% in 1992 to 0.14% in 2000. A total of 113 (0.61%) patients required emergency CABG. Major indications were extensive dissection followed by perforation/tamponade and recurrent acute closure (52). An earlier analysis of 9,145 patients undergoing PTCA documented a decline in the incidence of emergency CABG from 3.8% to 2.3% between

1980 and 1990 and has decreased further (approximately 0.2% in the coronary stent era (see Chapters 22 and 23). Mortality associated with emergency bypass surgery here, however, rose from 4.6% to 7.6%. The major determinant of in-hospital mortality following emergent surgery for failed PTCA in this group was hemodynamic status at the time of surgery. Patients requiring cardiopulmonary resuscitation or those in shock had a mortality of 28% (13 of 46); whereas those with stable hemodynamics at the time of emergent CABG had a mortality of only 1.4% (3 of 207). Preoperative IABP use increased from 13% in the period 1980 to 1985 to 33% in the period 1985 to 1990. Late survival was excellent—92% at 2 years and 87% at 5 years (53).

Bridge to Cardiac Transplantation

The intra-aortic balloon has been successful in selected cases at maintaining severely decompensated patients awaiting suitable donor hearts. Although the support is less substantial than that delivered by the cardiopulmonary support system or ventricular assist device, IABP is more easily maintained over the intermediate term and may be enough to supply the required degree of hemodynamic support. IABP insertion techniques have been developed in recent years, including use of a vein cuff sewn to the axillary artery, that sidestep problems associated with long-term femoral IAB placement and preserve patient mobility during the waiting period for a donor heart (54–56).

Enhanced External Counterpulsation

Enhanced external counterpulsation (EECP; 57,58) is a noninvasive outpatient therapy used primarily today to treat patients with chronic stable angina. The therapy uses three pairs of large inflatable cuffs that are wrapped around a patient's calves, thighs, and buttocks and sequentially inflated at the onset of diastole in 50-millisecond intervals to produce a retrograde pressure wave back to the heart. The cuffs are then simultaneously and rapidly deflated just prior to the start of systole. Treatment is usually given 1 hour per day, 5 days a week for a period of 7 weeks for a total of 35 1-hour treatments. Inflation and deflation of the cuffs is triggered by the ECG and is based on the same timing principles as those used for intra-aortic balloon pumping. The hemodynamic effects of EECP have been shown to be similar to those of IABP, with EECP conferring the added benefit of increased venous return. A recent study documented the acute hemodynamic effects of EECP using invasive monitoring. This study showed that EECP increases diastolic and mean pressures and reduces systolic pressure in the central aorta and the coronary artery. The clinical effectiveness of EECP in chronic stable angina and other settings such as acute and chronic heart failure is currently under investigation. This technique may, in the future, find application in some settings where IABPs are now being used.

LEFT VENTRICULAR SUPPORT

Although intra-aortic balloon pumping is considered the standard of care for many conditions requiring hemodynamic support, there are no randomized studies in any setting to prove that this approach provides clinical benefit. This probably reflects the development and widespread adoption of IABP prior to the time when the U.S. Food and Drug Administration regulated the medical device industry. For the case of cardiogenic shock, however, it is widely appreciated that the amount of hemodynamic support provided by IABPs is not always sufficient to compensate for the impaired left and/or right ventricular pumping capacity. In addition, IABP is not generally suitable for long-term application in patients with chronic irreversible heart failure. This has motivated development of alternate approaches to providing short-term (several days) and long-term (weeks, months, or years) circulatory support.

Short-Term Circulatory Support

Over 50,000 patients with myocardial infarction surviving to hospital admission in the United States demonstrate significant hemodynamic compromise and are in need of hemodynamic support. Many of these patients are treated at tertiary care centers where advanced treatments are not available. In addition, increasing numbers of patients with chronic heart failure present with acute or subacute hemodynamic compromise in need of such support. Although, as detailed above, medical treatment with intravenous inotropes followed by use of the IABP is considered the first line of treatment, these strategies are frequently not effective. Because of the urgency of the situation, these patients are not readily eligible for treatment with advanced forms of ventricular assist (described below), nor are such treatments necessarily warranted. Therefore, several devices are in various phases of development to provide short-term ventricular assist. In addition to their possible use in patients with cardiogenic shock, such devices with increased flow capacity are also being studied to support the high-risk PCI procedures and to reduce infarct size in the setting of acute myocardial infarction.

Percutaneous Cardiopulmonary Support

Percutaneous cardiopulmonary support (CPS) is one form of mechanical circulatory assist that has been available for many years. It is analogous to the heart–lung machine used during open heart surgery in that a pump withdraws deoxygenated blood from a venous cannula and pumps it through a heat exchanger, a membrane oxygenator, and finally, through a femorally placed arterial cannula back to

the aorta. Both femoral and arterial cannulae can be inserted percutaneously. These devices can completely support the circulation for up to about 6 hours, after which platelet aggregation, hemolysis, bleeding, and increased capillary permeability with plasma loss may become problematic. Such devices have been used in the settings of cardiac arrest, cardiogenic shock, and high-risk PCI. In the latter application, it has been used both prophylactically (i.e., inserted electively prior to PCI) and in a standby mode in which CPS equipment and personnel are available in the cardiac catheterization laboratory should hemodynamic collapse develop. When inserted following development of hemodynamic collapse, the time delay prior to institution of hemodynamic support appears to be associated with a detrimental impact on survival (28,59–63). Accordingly, the application of CPS is most effective when used in the catheterization laboratory that is already prepared for insertion and technical support (63), and use in other settings is rare.

In addition, as interventional catheter techniques have advanced, the necessity for *prophylactic* support with a device that provides the magnitude of support provided by CPS has diminished. This reduction in use is substantiated by a retrospective comparison of outcomes in patients undergoing high-risk angioplasty who either received prophylactic CPS or were part of a control group for whom CPS was readily available (standby group). This study showed a need for use of CPS in <10% of patients in the standby group with comparable procedural success in both groups, but an increased rate of femoral access complications and the requirement for transfusion in the prophylactic group (28). *Thus, in the current interventional era, the full hemodynamic support provided by CPS is rarely necessary, and the continuous technical backup required for operation of the CPS device and availability of increasingly simpler devices are major impediments to widespread use.*

TandemHeart

Another device currently approved for short term (6 hours) support is the TandemHeart percutaneous ventricular assist device (Cardiac Assist, Pittsburgh PA, Fig. 21.3A). This device consists of an extracorporeal centrifugal (continuous flow) pump that withdraws blood from the left atrium (via a 21 French trans-septal cannula) introduced via the femoral vein (see Chapter 4). Blood is then pumped by the device (at ~3.5 L/minute), and delivered into one or both femoral arteries through 15 to 18F cannulae (64–66). The pump thus functions in parallel with the left ventricle in moving blood from the left atrium to the aorta.

Preliminary results showed that this device can improve hemodynamics in patients with cardiogenic shock caused by myocardial infarction and other causes. Studies also showed a reduction in serum lactate levels, an indication that there is improved tissue perfusion and oxygenation, and thus reversal of the cardiogenic shock state. In a more

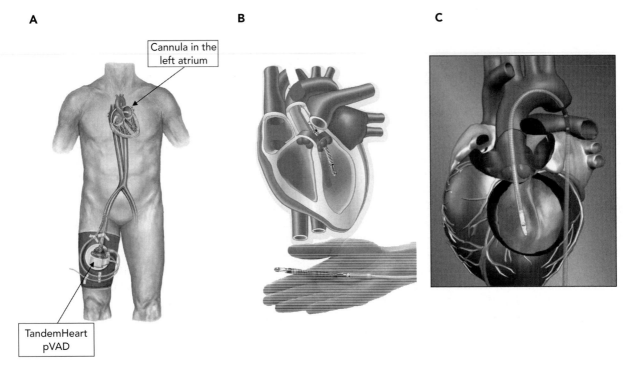

Figure 21.3 Three types of percutaneously deployable, catheter-based temporary ventricular assist devices that are in various stages of evaluation. **A.** The Cardiac Assist TandemHeart system uses a centrifugal pump connected to a trans-septal catheter to withdraw blood from the left atrium and pumps it back to the femoral artery. **B.** The Impella Recover system uses a miniature rotary motor that spins an impeller, all mounted on the tip of a catheter, to draw blood through a cannula with an inflow port in the LV and outflow port in the proximal aorta. **C.** The A-Med percutaneous ventricular assist device uses an externally powered motor to rotate a cable inside a catheter, which in turn rotates a propeller to draw blood through a distal cannula whose inflow port is positioned inside the LV and outflow port is positioned in the descending aorta.

recent study, 41 patients with cardiogenic shock owing to acute myocardial infarction failing medical treatment were randomized to treatment with either an IABP or the TandemHeart assist device (67). In both groups, patients were supported for an average of approximately 3.5 days. The IABP had almost no effect on hemodynamics, but the TandemHeart device significantly increased cardiac output and blood pressure while significantly decreasing pulmonary capillary wedge pressure and serum lactate. Despite these clear improvements in multiple clinically important parameters, however, short-term (i.e., death during support) and 30-day mortality rates were comparable: approximately 20% and approximately 43%, respectively, in both groups. Also, compared with IABP, use of the TandemHeart device was associated with a greater incidence of certain adverse effects (such as lower limb ischemia and bleeding); however, none of these adverse events appeared to contribute importantly to mortality.

Although that study was underpowered to detect what could be a clinically significant reduction in mortality (which could take as many as several hundred patients per group), it is also possible that lack of mortality benefit has potential important implications. Specifically, Hochman (68) has suggested that reversal of the *hemodynamic derange-*

ments of cardiogenic shock may not address all the critical underlying pathophysiologic abnormalities. Other abnormalities, such as elevated inflammatory cytokines and elevated inducible nitric oxide synthase (iNOS), with consequent increased levels of NO and peroxynitrite, could contribute importantly to morbidity and mortality in cardiogenic shock and do not appear to be reversed with restoration of a more normal hemodynamic state. This suggests that addition of other treatments in combination with effective hemodynamic support may yield better results.

Other Support Devices

Although the TandemHeart system is readily inserted by a skilled interventionalist trained in trans-septal puncture, other devices are being developed that do not require such puncture. One device, available in Europe and under study in the United States, is the Impella Recover System (Impella Cardio System AG, Aachen, Germany; Fig. 21.3B; 69–71). This system has an electromagnetic motor directly coupled to a helical impeller located near the tip of a catheter. When the "snorkel" at the tip of the catheter is placed across the aortic valve and into the left ventricular chamber, the motor rotates the impeller at $\sim$50,000 to 90,000 rpm, drawing left ventricular blood into the distal end of the catheter, passing it though a short cannula, and discharging it into the ascending aorta. Two systems are under development, a 20F device (capable of pumping 5.0 L/minute, via surgical insertion into the thoracic aorta) and a 12F device (capable of pumping 2.5 L/minute, via percutaneous insertion). Preliminary data suggest that this type of device provides better unloading of the left ventricle (more enhancement of forward flow and mean arterial pressure, and greater reduction in left ventricular systolic work/oxygen demand) than the IABP, and the clinical effects of this better unloading are currently under study.

Another percutaneously deployable device is the A-Med percutaneous ventricular assist device (A-Med System, West Sacramento, CA; Fig. 21.3C) that is based on an already available right heart support system (72). This device is fashioned after a prior system called the Hemopump (73–75) and consists of a percutaneously inserted cannula into which a driveline with distal propeller is inserted. The propeller sits approximately 10 cm from the distal tip. An electromagnetic motor that sits outside the body rotates the driveline, creating a pressure gradient between the left ventricle and aorta that pumps blood. The device is a 16F device that is designed to pump approximately 3.5L/minute.

Although we have thus far focused on the use of these percutaneously deployable devices to treat cardiogenic shock, these devices can also be used to provide hemodynamic support during high-risk percutaneous coronary interventions (66,74). The availability of drug-eluting stents has resulted in more widespread application of PCI, including in patients who would ordinarily be considered to be at high risk of adverse events during PCI, including left main lesions and multivessel disease in patients with impaired left ventricular function. As discussed above, IABPs have been used at the discretion of the operator for this application, and specific recommendations are available (25), although no randomized studies have yet been performed to indicate that this strategy improves patient outcomes. For more extreme cases, cardiopulmonary bypass has been used (28,76,77). However, availability of easily deployable, hemodynamically effective pumps could conceivably be used to support high-risk PCI cases.

Another potential application of percutaneous hemodynamic support is to unload the left ventricle during a myocardial infarction with the goal of reducing energy demands and thus reducing infarct size. Fig. 21.4A compares the effects of an IABP and a percutaneous ventricular assist device on ventricular and aortic pressures, ventricular volumes, and left ventricular pressure-volume loops. The IABP enhances blood pressure during diastole and reduces systolic ventricular pressure, but does not significantly influence ventricular volumes. In contrast, the percutaneous assist device markedly reduces ventricular volumes and preload, and reduces peak ventricular pressure while increasing aortic systolic and diastolic pressures. The marked difference in hemodynamic effects of these two types of devices is shown dramatically in the pressure-volume loops in Fig. 21.4B. Compared with the subtle effects of the IABP, the percutaneous assist device markedly unloads the heart (decreased preload and afterload volumes and pressures), reduces the work of the LV (area inside the loop), and therefore decreases myocardial oxygen consumption (78). Indeed, use of this device in an experimental model of acute coronary ligation has resulted in marked reduction in myocardial infarct size (71).

Thus, although IABP is commonly used in a number of clinical settings, efforts to develop devices that provide more potent hemodynamic support are under development. Such devices, possibly coupled with new medical approaches, may improve outcome in cardiogenic shock, a condition associated with mortality rates reported in the literature ranging between 40 and 80%. These devices have other potential applications and appear to more potently provide pressure and volume ventricular unloading. Whether the use of such devices will be associated with better clinical outcomes remains to be determined.

Long-Term Circulatory Support

A number of devices have been developed to provide full circulatory support for extended periods in patients with end-stage heart failure. These are electrically or pneumatically powered pumps that are implanted surgically. Several devices use extracorporeal systems (e.g., the Thoratec Ventricular Assist Device and the Abiomed BVS 5000, Abiomed, Danvers, MA) and are intended for intermediate-term applications (days to weeks). These devices can be used to provide left and/or right ventricular support as required by individual patient needs. Other devices use pumps that are implanted in the body (HeartMate II, Thoratec, Pleasanton, CA; Novacor Left Ventricular Assist System, Baxter Health Care Corp., Deerfield, IL; AbioCor, Abiomed, Danvers, MA; and others) and have been used for extended times (months to years). Although powered externally through lines that cross the skin, these pumps allow patients to ambulate with many patients able to enjoy an active lifestyle. Most left ventricular assist devices are connected to the left ventricle via an inflow conduit placed in the left ventricular apex, returning blood through an outflow conduit that is connected to the proximal aorta (Fig. 21.5).

Broadly speaking, there are three clinical applications of these devices: (1) bridge to transplant, (2) bridge to recovery, and (3) destination therapy. Two internally implanted devices are currently approved for the bridge to transplant indication (HeartMate and Novacor). When used in transplant-eligible patients at high risk of death, these devices are associated with improved survival to transplant (79). In the course of using devices in this manner, it was learned that hearts of patients supported could normalize size, structure, and function, on some occasions permitting

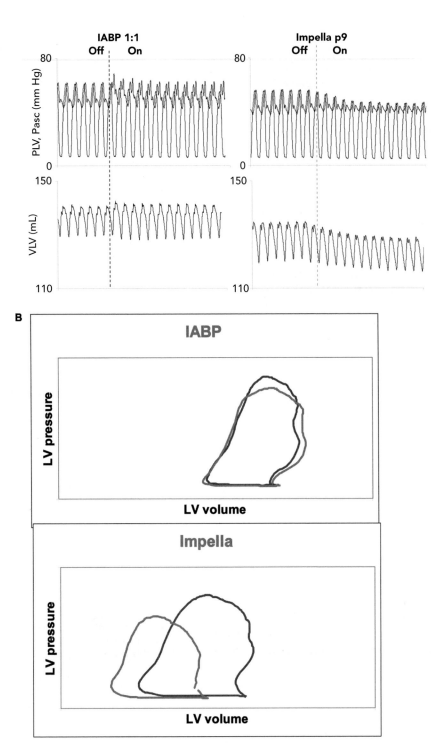

Figure 21.4   A. Aortic and left ventricle (LV) pressure *(top)*, LV volume *(center)*, and aortic flow *(bottom)* measured in an animal model prior to and during support with either an intra-aortic balloon pump or an Impella Recover system. IABP reduces systolic aortic and LV pressures but increases aortic pressure during diastole, thus improving coronary blood flow and oxygen supply. The continuous flow Impella system reduces systolic pressure with relatively little effect on diastolic pressure, but the LV volume is markedly reduced. **B.** Left ventricular pressure-volume loops corresponding to tracing of view A. The loops demonstrate the profound pressure and volume unloading provided by the continuous flow system, thus markedly reducing pressure-volume area (73) and thus reducing oxygen demands of the LV. This contrasts with the effects of the IABP, which, on the pressure-volume diagram, provides mainly a relatively small effect on peak systolic pressure and therefore relatively little influence on oxygen demand. (Tracing provided courtesy of Dr. FH van der Veen, PhD, Department of Cardiothoracic Surgery, Maastricht, The Netherlands.)

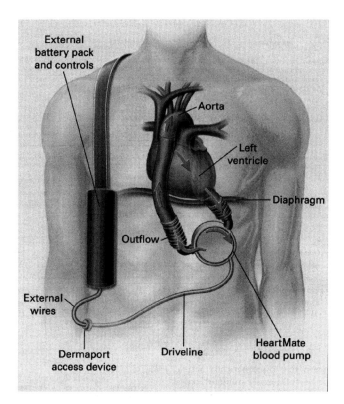

Figure 21.5 A schematic diagram showing the HeartMate left ventricular assist device and how it receives blood through a conduit connected to the LV apex and pumps through a second conduit connected to the proximal aorta.

device removal without the need for cardiac transplant (80–83). This remarkable phenomenon, referred to as *reverse remodeling*, has lead to the appreciation that even the end-stage failing heart has the capacity to recover function if the hemodynamic and neurohormonal stresses of chronic heart failure are relieved to a sufficient degree and for a sufficient time. This has lead to the concept that such devices can be used in a critically ill patient to allow recovery of heart function. Once the heart recovers, the device could be removed without the need for transplantation, the so-called bridge to recovery application. However, research has shown that the heart failure state recurs in many patients who have undergone device removal after showing recovery of ventricular function (84,85). There is no approved indication for the use of any ventricular assist device as a bridge to recovery, but this remains an area of active research. More recently, the HeartMate II ventricular assist device has been approved as a permanent treatment in critically ill patients not eligible for heart transplantation, the so-called destination therapy. It was shown that 2-year survival was improved from <10% to approximately 25% (86). However, this was at the cost of a relatively high rate of neurologic bleeding, strokes, peripheral embolic events, and infections, among other adverse effects. Therefore, use of this device as destination therapy is not currently widespread.

In an effort to improve outcomes in destination therapy, a number of new devices are currently under development

and in various stages of clinical testing. These include devices that are smaller (and therefore in principal involve less invasive implantation surgeries) and devices in which all components are implanted beneath the skin to eliminate the infections associated with lines crossing the skin. Finally, one device under development and testing (the AbioCor Implantable Replacement Heart) is a totally mechanical heart that replaces the entire heart (as with a transplant; 87). Early experience was associated with a high rate of adverse effects, and a second generation device is now being tested.

Development of permanent ventricular assist devices has been pursued for >30 years and in many ways can still be considered to be in its infancy. Remarkable progress has been made, and the lives of many patients have been influenced. Progress will continue to make these devices more reliable, less invasive, and therefore safer and more widely available to the increasing number of patients who could benefit from such technology.

REFERENCES

1. Clauss RH, Birtwell WC, Albertal G, et al. Assisted circulation, I: the arterial counterpulsator. *J Thorac Cardiovasc Surg* 1961;41:447–458.
2. Moulopoulos SD, Topaz S, Kolff WJ. Diastolic balloon pumping (with carbon dioxide) in the aorta—a mechanical assistance to the failing circulation. *Am Heart J* 1962;63:669–675.
3. Kantrowitz A, Tjonneland S, Freed PS, et al. Initial clinical experience with intraaortic balloon pumping in cardiogenic shock. *JAMA* 1968;203:113–118.
4. Weintraub RM, Aroesty JM, Paulin S, et al. Medically refractory unstable angina pectoris I: long-term follow-up of patients undergoing intraaortic balloon counterpulsation and operation. *Am J Cardiol* 1979;43:877–882.
5. Maccioli GA. *Intra-aortic Balloon Pump Therapy.* Baltimore: Williams & Wilkins, 1997:13.
6. Bregman D, Casarella WJ. Percutaneous intraaortic balloon pumping: initial clinical experience. *Ann Thorac Surg* 1980;29:153–155.
7. LaMuraglia GM, Vlahakes GJ, Moncure AC, et al. The safety of intraaortic balloon pump catheter insertion through suprainguinal prosthetic vascular bypass grafts. *J Vasc Surg* 1991;13:830–835.
8. Kern MJ, Aguirre FV, Caracciolo EA, et al. Hemodynamic effects of new intra-aortic balloon counterpulsation timing methods in patients: a multicenter evaluation. *Am Heart J* 1999;137:1129–1136.
9. Aroesty JM, Schlossman D, Weintraub RM, Paulin S. Transfemoral selective coronary artery catheterization during intra-aortic balloon by-pass pumping. *Radiology* 1974;111:307–309.
10. McCabe JC, Abel RM, Subramanian VA, Gay WA Jr. Complications of intra-aortic balloon insertion and counterpulsation. *Circulation* 1978;57:769–773.
11. Ferguson JJ 3rd, Cohen M, Freedman RJ Jr, et al. The current practice of intra-aortic balloon counterpulsation: results from the Benchmark Registry. *J Am Coll Cardiol* 2001;38:1456–1462.
12. Cohen M, Ferguson JJ 3rd, Freedman RJ Jr, et al. Comparison of outcomes after 8 vs. 9.5 French size intra-aortic balloon counterpulsation catheters based on 9,332 patients in the prospective Benchmark registry. *Cath Cardiovasc Interv* 2002;56:200–206.
13. Eltchaninoff H, Dimas AP, Whitlow PL. Complications associated with percutaneous placement and use of intraaortic balloon counterpulsation. *Am J Cardiol* 1993;71:328–332.
14. Arceo A. In-hospital complications of percutaneous intraaortic balloon counterpulsation. *Angiology* 2003;54:577–585.
15. Leinbach RC, Buckley MJ, Austen WG, et al. Effects of intra-aortic balloon pumping on coronary flow and metabolism in man. *Circulation* 1971;43(5 suppl):I77–81.

16. Willerson JT, Curry GC, Watson JT, et al. Intraaortic balloon counterpulsation in patients in cardiogenic shock, medically refractory left ventricular failure and/or recurrent ventricular tachycardia. *Am J Med* 1975;58:183–191.

17. Baron DW, O'Rourke MF. Long-term results of arterial counterpulsation in acute severe cardiac failure complicating myocardial infarction. *Br Heart J* 1976;38:285–288.

18. Hagemeijer F, Laird JD, Haalebos MMP, Hugenholtz PG. Effectiveness of intraaortic balloon pumping without cardiac surgery for patients with severe heart failure secondary to a recent myocardial infarction. *Am J Cardiol* 1977;40:951–956.

19. McEnany MT, Kay HR, Buckley MJ, et al. Clinical experience with intraaortic balloon pump support in 728 patients. *Circulation* 1978;58(3 pt 2):I124–132.

20. DeWood MA, Notshe RN, Hensley GR, et al. Intraaortic balloon counterpulsation with and without reperfusion for myocardial infarction shock. *Circulation* 1980;61:1105–1112.

21. Lorente P, Gourgon R, Beaufils P, et al. Multivariate statistical evaluation of intraaortic counterpulsation in pump failure complicating acute myocardial infarction. *Am J Cardiol* 1980;46:124–134.

22. Pierri MK, Zema M, Kligfield P, et al. Exercise tolerance in late survivors of balloon pumping and surgery for cardiogenic shock. *Circulation* 1980;62(2 pt 2):I138–141.

23. Stone GW, Ohman EM, Miller MF, et al. Contemporary utilization and outcomes of intra-aortic balloon counterpulsation in acute myocardial infarction. *J Am Coll Cardiol* 2003;41:1940–1945.

24. Hartzler GO, Rutherford BD, McConahay DR, Johnson WL, Giorgi LV. "High-risk" percutaneous transluminal coronary angioplasty. *Am J Cardiol* 1988;61:33G–37G.

25. ACC/AHA Guidelines for Percutaneous Coronary Intervention. *J Am Coll Cardiol* 2001;37:2215–2238.

26. Briguori C, Sarais C, Pagnotta P, et al. Elective versus provisional intra-aortic balloon pumping in high risk percutaneous transluminal coronary angioplasty. *Am Heart J* 2003;145:700–707.

27. Tommaso CL, Vogel RA. National Registry for Supported Angioplasty: results and follow-up of three years of supported and standby supported angioplasty in high-risk patients. *Cardiology* 1994;84:238–244.

28. Teirstein PS, Vogel RA, Dorros G, et al. Prophylactic versus standby cardiopulmonary support for high risk percutaneous transluminal coronary angioplasty. *J Am Coll Cardiol* 1993;21: 590–596.

29. Shreiber TL, Kodali UR, O'Neill WW, et al. Comparison of acute results of prophylactic intraaortic balloon pumping with cardiopulmonary support for percutaneous transluminal coronary angioplasty (PTCA). *Cathet Cardiovasc Diagn* 1998;45:115–119.

30. O'Murchu B, Foreman RD, Shaw RE, et al. Role of intraaortic balloon pump counterpulsation in high risk coronary rotational atherectomy. *J Am Coll Cardiol* 1995;26:1270–1275.

31. Hochman JS. Cardiogenic shock complicating acute myocardial infarction: expanding the paradigm. *Circulation* 2003;107:2998–3002.

32. Goldberg RJ, Gore JM, Alpert JS, et al. Cardiogenic shock after acute myocardial infarction. Incidence and mortality from a community-wide perspective, 1975 to 1988. *N Engl J Med* 1991; 325:1117–1122.

33. Holmes DR Jr, Bates ER, Kleiman NS, et al. Contemporary reperfusion therapy for cardiogenic shock: the GUSTO-I trial experience. The GUSTO-I Investigators. Global Utilization of Streptokinase and Tissue Plasminogen Activator for Occluded Coronary Arteries. *J Am Coll Cardiol* 1995;26:668–674.

34. Hasdai D, Califf RM, Thompson TD, et al. Predictors of cardiogenic shock after thrombolytic therapy for acute myocardial infarction. *J Am Coll Cardiol* 2000;35:136–143.

35. Data from Hudson RM, et al. presented at the American Heart Association 72nd Session 1999.

36. Sanborn TA, Sleeper LA, Bates ER, et al. Impact of thrombolysis, intra-aortic balloon pump counterpulsation, and their combination in cardiogenic shock complicating acute myocardial infarction: a report from the SHOCK Trial Registry. SHould we emergently revascularize Occluded Coronaries for cardiogenic shocK? *J Am Coll Cardiol* 2000;36(3 suppl A):1123–1129.

37. Kovack PJ, Rasak MA, Bates ER, et al. Thrombolysis plus aortic counterpulsation: improved survival in patients who present to community hospitals with cardiogenic shock. *J Am Coll Cardiol* 1997;29:1454–1458.

38. Barron HV. The Use of intra-aortic balloon counterpulsation in patients with cardiogenic shock complicating acute myocardial infarction: data from the National Registry of Myocardial Infarction 2. *Am Heart J* 2001;141:933–939.

39. Anderson RD, Ohman EM, Holmes DR Jr, et al. Use of intraaortic balloon counterpulsation in patients presenting with cardiogenic shock: observations from the GUSTO-I Study. Global Utilization of Streptokinase and TPA for Occluded Coronary Arteries. *J Am Coll Cardiol* 1997;30:708–715.

40. Holmes, DR Jr, Califf RM, van de Werf F, et al. Difference in countries' use of resources and clinical outcome for patients with cardiogenic shock after myocardial infarction: results from the GUSTO trial. *Lancet* 1997;349:75–78.

41. Dilley RB, Ross J Jr, Bernstein EF. Serial hemodynamics during intraaortic balloon counterpulsation for cardiogenic shock. *Circulation* 1973;48(1 suppl):III99–104.

42. Menon V, Fincke R. Cardiogenic shock: a summary of the randomized SHOCK trial. *Congest Heart Fail* 2003;9:35–39. Review.

43. 1999 ACC/AHA Guidelines for the Management of Acute Myocardial Infarction. *Circulation* 1999;100:1016–1030.

44. Dembitsky WP, Moore CH, Holman WL, et al. Successful mechanical circulatory support for noncoronary shock. *J Heart Lung Transplant* 1992;11:129–135.

45. Christenson JT, Cohen M, Ferguson JJ, et al. Trends in intraaortic balloon counterpulsation complications and outcomes in cardiac surgery. *Ann Thorac Surg* 2002;74:1086–1091.

46. Suzuki T, Okabe M, Handa M, Yasuda F, Miyake Y. Usefulness of preoperative intraaortic balloon pump therapy during off-pump coronary artery bypass grafting in high-risk patients. *Ann Thorac Surg* 2004;77:2056–2059; discussion 2059–2060.

47. Christenson JT, Licker M, Afksendiyos K. The role of intra-aortic counterpulsation in high-risk OPCAB surgery: a prospective randomized study. *J Card Surg* 2003;18:286–294.

48. Aroesty JM. Cardiogenic shock. *Curr Cardiovasc Top.* 1979;5:51–64.

49. Williams DO, Korr KS, Dewirtz H, Most AS. The effect of intraaortic balloon counterpulsation on regional myocardial blood flow and oxygen consumption in the presence of coronary artery stenosis in patients with unstable angina. *Circulation* 1982;66: 593–597.

50. Ohman EM, George BS, White CJ, et al. Use of aortic counterpulsation to improve sustained coronary artery potency during acute myocardial infarction. Results of a randomized trial: the Randomized IABP Study Group. *Circulation* 1994;90:792–799.

51. Srinivas VS, Brooks MM, Detre KM, et al. Contemporary percutaneous coronary intervention versus balloon angioplasty for multivessel coronary artery disease: a comparison of the National Heart, Lung and Blood Institute Dynamic Registry and the Bypass Angioplasty Revascularization Investigation (BARI) study. *Circulation* 2002;106:1627–1633.

52. Seshadri N. Emergency coronary bypass surgery in the contemporary percutaneous coronary intervention era. *Circulation.* 2002; 106:2346–2350.

53. Boylan MJ, Lytle BW, Taylor PC, et al. Have PTCA failures requiring emergent bypass operations changed? *Ann Thorac Surg* 1995;59:283–286.

54. Birovljev S, Radovancevic B, Burnett CM, et al. Heart transplantation after mechanical circulatory support: four years experience. *J Heart Lung Transplant* 1992;11:240–245.

55. H'Doubler PB Jr, A novel technique for intraaortic balloon pump placement via the left axillary artery in patients awaiting cardiac transplantation. *Cardiovasc Surg* 2000;8:463–465.

56. Cochran RP. Ambulatory intraaortic balloon pump use as a bridge to heart transplant. *Ann Thorac Surg* 2002;74:746–751.

57. Taguchi I, Ogawa K, Oida A, Abe S, Kaneko N, Sakio H. Comparison of hemodynamic effects of enhanced external counterpulsation and intra-aortic balloon pumping in patients with acute myocardial infarction. *Am J Cardiol* 2000;86:1139–1141, A9.

58. Michaels AD, Linnemeier G, Soran O, Kelsey SF, Kennard ED. Two-year outcomes after enhanced external counterpulsation for stable angina pectoris from the International Patient Registry [IEPR]. *Am J Cardiol* 2004;93:461–464.

59. Overlie PA, Walter PD, Hurd HP II, et al. Emergency cardiopulmonary support with circulatory support devices. *Cardiology* 1994;84:231–237.

60. Hill JG, Bruhn PS, Cohen SE, et al. Emergent applications of cardiopulmonary support: a multiinstitutional experience. *Ann Thorac Surg* 1992;54:699–704.

61. Dembitsky WP, Moreno-Cabral J, Adamson RM, Daily PO. Emergency resuscitation using portable extracorporeal membrane oxygenation. *Ann Thorac Surg* 1993;55:304–309.

62. Grambow DW, Deeb GM, Pavlides GS, et al. Emergent cardiopulmonary bypass in patients having cardiovascular collapse in the cardiac catheterization laboratory. *Am J Cardiol* 1994;73:872–875.

63. Overlie PA, Walter PD, Hurd HP, et al. Emergency cardiopulmonary support with circulatory support devices. *Cardiology* 1994;84:231–237.

64. Pitsis AA, Dardas P, Mezilis N, Nikoloudakis N, Filippatos G, Burkhoff D. Temporary assist device for postcardiotomy cardiac failure. *Ann Thorac Surg* 2004;77:1431–1433

65. Kar B, Butkevich A, Civitello AB, et al. Hemodynamic support with a percutaneous left ventricular assist device during stenting of an unprotected left main coronary artery. *Tex Heart Inst J* 2004;31:84–86.

66. Vranckx P, Foley DP, de Feijter PJ, Vos J, Smits P, Serruys PW. Clinical introduction of the TandemHeart, a percutaneous left ventricular assist device, for circulatory support during high-risk percutaneous coronary intervention. *Int J Cardiovasc Intervent* 2003;5:35–39.

67. Thiele H, Sick P, Boudriot E, et al. Randomized comparison of intra-aortic balloon support versus a percutaneous left ventricular assist device in patients with revascularized acute myocardial infarction complicated by cardiogenic shock. *J Am Coll Cardiol.* 2004; abstract.

68. Hochman JS. Cardiogenic shock complicating acute myocardial infarction: expanding the paradigm. *Circulation* 2003;107:2998–3002.

69. Jurmann MJ, Siniawski H, Erb M, Drews T, Hetzer R. Initial experience with miniature axial flow ventricular assist devices for postcardiotomy heart failure. *Ann Thorac Surg* 2004;77:1642–1647.

70. Siegenthaler MP, Brehm K, Strecker T, et al. The Impella Recover microaxial left ventricular assist device reduces mortality for postcardiotomy failure: a three-center experience. *J Thorac Cardiovasc Surg* 2004;127:812–822.

71. Meyns B, Stolinski J, Leunens V, Verbeken E, Flameng W. Left ventricular support by catheter-mounted axial flow pump reduces infarct size. *J Am Coll Cardiol* 2003;41:1087–1095.

72. Lima LE, Jatene F, Buffolo E, et al. A multicenter initial clinical experience with right heart support and beating heart coronary surgery. *Heart Surg Forum* 2001;4:60–64.

73. Sweeney MS. The Hemopump in 1997: a clinical, political, and marketing evolution. *Ann Thorac Surg* 1999;68:761–763.

74. Scholz KH, Dubois-Rande JL, Urban P, et al. Clinical experience with the percutaneous hemopump during high-risk coronary angioplasty. *Am J Cardiol* 1998;82:1107–1110, A6.

75. Scholz KH, Tebbe U, Chemnitius M, et al. Transfemoral placement of the left ventricular assist device "Hemopump" during mechanical resuscitation. *Thorac Cardiovasc Surg* 1990;38:69–72.

76. Schreiber TL, Kodali UR, O'Neill WW, Gangadharan V, Puchrowicz-Ochocki SB, Grines CL. Comparison of acute results of prophylactic intraaortic balloon pumping with cardiopulmonary support for percutaneous transluminal coronary angioplasty (PTCA). *Cathet Cardiovasc Diagn* 1998;45:115–119.

77. de Lezo J Sr, Pan M, Medina A, et al. Percutaneous cardiopulmonary support in critical patients needing coronary interventions with stents. *Cathet Cardiovasc Intervent* 2002;57:467–475.

78. Suga H. Ventricular energetics. *Phys Rev* 1990;70:247–277.

79. Frazier OH, Rose EA, McCarthy PM, et al. Improved mortality and rehabilitation of transplant candidates treated with a long-term implantable left ventricular assist device. *Ann Surg* 1995;222:327–326.

80. Levin HR, Oz MC, Chen JM, Packer MP, Rose EA, Burkhoff D. Reversal of chronic ventricular dilation in patients with end-stage cardiomyopathy by prolonged mechanical unloading. *Circulation* 1995;91:2717–2720.

81. Heerdt PM, D Burkhoff. Reverse molecular remodeling of the failing human heart following support with a left ventricular assist device. In: Dhalla NS. *Signal Transduction and Cardiac Hypertrophy.* Boston: Kluwer, 2002:19–35.

82. Barbone A, Holmes JW, Heerdt PM, et al. Comparison of right and left ventricular responses to left ventricular assist device support in patients with severe heart failure: a primary role of mechanical unloading underlying reverse remodeling. *Circulation* 2001;104:670–675.

83. Dipla K, Mattiello JA, Jeevanandam V, Houser SR, Margulies KB. Myocyte recovery after mechanical circulatory support in humans with end-stage heart failure. *Circulation* 1998;97:2316–2322.

84. Levin HR, Oz M, Catanese K, Rose EA, Burkhoff D. Transient normalization of systolic and diastolic function after LVAD support in a patient with dilated cardiomyopathy. *J Heart Lung Transplant* 1996;15:840–842.

85. Mancini DM, Beniaminovitz A, Levin H, et al. Low incidence of myocardial recovery after left ventricular assist device implantation in patients with chronic heart failure. *Circulation* 1998;98:2383–2389.

86. Rose EA, Gelijns AC, Moskowitz AJ, et al. Long-term mechanical left ventricular assistance for end-stage heart failure. *N Engl J Med* 2001;345:1435–1443.

87. Dowling RD, Gray LA Jr, Etoch SW, et al. Initial experience with the AbioCor implantable replacement heart system. *J Thorac Cardiovasc Surg* 2004;127:131–141.

Interventional
Techniques

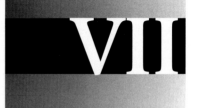

Percutaneous Balloon Angioplasty and General Coronary Intervention

22

Donald S. Baim

Dotter and Judkins (1) first proposed the concept of transluminal angioplasty—enlargement of the lumen of a stenotic vessel by a catheter technique in 1964. They advanced a spring-coil guidewire across an atherosclerotic arterial stenosis and left this wire in place to serve as a rail over which a series of progressively larger rigid dilators were advanced to enlarge the vessel lumen. This Dotter technique proved effective in peripheral arteries, but the need to insert large-caliber rigid dilators through the arterial puncture (and the high shear forces applied by the dilators as they crossed the atherosclerotic lesion) ultimately restricted clinical application. In 1974, Gruentzig (2) replaced the series of rigid dilators with an inflatable nonelastomeric balloon mounted on a comparatively smaller catheter shaft. As such, the tip of the balloon catheter could be introduced percutaneously, advanced across a vascular stenosis in its smaller (collapsed) state, and then inflated with sufficient force to enlarge the stenotic lumen. Although others had speculated about the possibility, Gruentzig was the first to refine balloon angioplasty into a usable clinical tool, through a series of experiments in animals, cadavers, peripheral arteries, and the coronary arteries of patients undergoing bypass surgery. This culminated in the first percutaneous transluminal coronary angioplasty (PTCA) of a stenotic coronary artery in a conscious human (September 16, 1977; 3).

PTCA remained the only catheter-based revascularization technique in widespread use until the mid-1990s, when a series of other modalities including atherectomy and stenting (see Chapters 23 and 24) were introduced. To recognize the inclusion of these additional modalities, the technique is now more commonly referred to as percutaneous coronary intervention (PCI) and now stands as the dominant form of coronary revascularization. Its widespread adoption has transformed the field of *invasive* cardiology (i.e., diagnostic cardiac catheterization as discussed in the initial chapters of this text), into the new field of *interventional* cardiology (use of cardiac catheters to deliver therapy). This chapter will review the basic equipment, techniques, and results of coronary angioplasty, as well as the utility of PTCA and PCI in specific clinical and anatomic situations, as a historical and conceptual foundation for the entire field of catheter-based percutaneous coronary intervention.

HISTORY

After Gruentzig's pioneering cases in 1977, most cardiologists viewed the new technique of balloon angioplasty with a great deal of skepticism. But a small group of cardiologists around the world recognized the great potential it might hold (4). In 1979, they met to form a registry of all coronary angioplasty cases worldwide under the sponsorship of the National Heart, Lung, and Blood Institute (NHLBI). That registry grew to 3,000 cases by 1981, although no more than 1,000 angioplasties were performed in any given year during that period. From these humble beginnings, progressive improvements in equipment and technique have produced dramatic growth in percutaneous

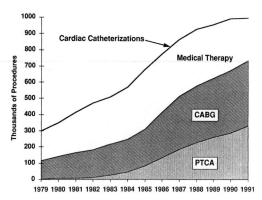

Figure 22.1 Early growth in the number of coronary angioplasty procedures (PTCA) is shown by the bottom *(stippled)* band, increasing from less than 1,000 per year in 1979–1981 to more than 300,000 per year by 1991. This was then similar to the annual number of bypass operations (CABG, *cross-hatched band*) and the number of patients remaining on medical therapy after roughly 1,000,000 diagnostic catheterizations. By 2004, the number of annual catheterizations in the United States had grown to approximately 2 million, with roughly 50% (1 million) of the patients who underwent diagnostic cardiac catheterization being referred for percutaneous coronary intervention and roughly 20% (400,000) being referred for bypass surgery. (From American College of Cardiology; also American Heart Association. *2004 Heart and Stroke Statistical Update.* Dallas, TX; American Heart Association, 2003.)

transluminal coronary angioplasty (PTCA) and transformed it into the dominant form of coronary revascularization (Fig. 22.1). By 1990, the annual number of coronary angioplasty procedures in the United States rose to 300,000, equaling the annual number of bypass surgeries. By 2000, catheter-based coronary revascularization was performed in more than 800,000 patients with ischemic syndromes owing to anatomically suitable coronary artery lesions, compared with some 350,000 who underwent bypass surgery. Currently, some 1,000,000 PCI procedures are performed annually in the United States (5), with a similar number of coronary interventions performed outside of the United States, making it one of the most common procedures worldwide.

Over the past decade, however, the central role of balloon dilation has become much less prominent as a stand-alone treatment. It now serves mostly as an *adjunctive* means of preparing for (i.e., predilating) or perfecting (i.e., postdilating) a coronary lesion during a stent placement or atherectomy procedure. Despite progressive broadening in its clinical and anatomic indications, the use of these newer interventional devices and adjunctive antithrombotic pharmacology (see Chapter 3) have improved the success rate of PCI to 98%, the procedural mortality to roughly 1%, the emergency bypass rate to <0.5%, and a 1-year recurrence rate to <10%.

EQUIPMENT

A coronary angioplasty system consists of three basic components (Fig. 22.2): (a) a guiding catheter, which provides

stable access to the coronary ostium, a route for contrast administration, and a conduit for the advancement of the dilatation equipment; (b) a leading guidewire that can be passed through the guiding catheter, across the target lesion, and well into the distal coronary vasculature to provide a rail over which a series of therapeutic devices can be advanced; and (c) a nonelastomeric balloon dilatation catheter filled with liquid contrast medium. Technologic advances generate improvements in specific equipment each year, so any detailed description of current products would be outdated too soon to be of value here, but some general principles remain.

Guiding Catheters

Guiding catheters remain a crucial component in PTCA. The original guiding catheters were thick-walled 10 and 11F tubes that had small lumens, minimal torque control, and sharp edges. In contrast, current guiding catheter designs more closely emulate the performance of diagnostic coronary angiographic catheters. To allow passage of therapeutic instruments, however, guiding catheters must have a lumen diameter at least twice that of a typical diagnostic

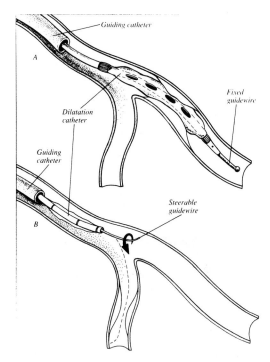

Figure 22.2 Components of the coronary angioplasty system. The original Gruentzig fixed guidewire balloon **(A)** compared with the steerable guide wire system **(B)**. Although both are advanced through a guiding catheter positioned in the coronary ostium, neither the wire shape nor its orientation could be changed once the original Gruentzig catheter was introduced, whereas the steerable design allows the guidewire to be advanced, withdrawn and reshaped, and steered independently of the balloon catheter to select the desired vessel. Once in place in the distal vessel beyond the target lesion, the guidewire serves as a rail over which the angioplasty balloon or other device can be advanced. (From Willerson JT, ed. *Treatment of Heart Diseases.* New York: Gower Medical, 1992.)

catheter (e.g., 0.076-inch [2 mm] versus 0.038-inch [1 mm]). To achieve this lumen in a catheter whose outer diameter is as small as 6F (2 mm, or 0.080 inch), the catheter walls must be very thin (<0.12 mm, or 0.005-inch). Yet the catheter must still incorporate a Teflon liner to reduce friction, metal or plastic braid to transmit torque and provide sufficient stiffness to offer backup support during device advancement, and a smooth outer coating to resist thrombus formation. The complexity of this design goal requires use of special materials whose properties are typically varied along the length of the catheter to optimize the balance between support and flexibility at each point. Most guiding catheters now also include a very soft material in the most distal 2 mm of the catheter to reduce the chance of vessel trauma during engagement of the nontapered tip.

Guiding catheters are now available in virtually all of the conventional Judkins and Amplatz curves, as well as a wide range of custom shapes (extra backup (XB), hockey stick, multipurpose, Voda, etc.) designed to ease engagement or provide better support during balloon advancement. As thin-wall technology has improved and balloon shaft diameters have decreased, the predominant size of guiding catheters has fallen progressively: 9F guiding catheters predominated in the early 1980s, with 8F (2.7-mm) catheters taking over in the late 1990s, and 6F guiding catheters in common use today. Although larger guiding catheters are sometimes still needed for bigger devices or treatment of bifurcation lesions, most procedures can be completed through a 6F guiding catheter introduced through the same sheath used to perform diagnostic coronary angiography. Some 5F guiding catheters are even available for use for radial artery access (see Chapter 4).

To function adequately, the guiding catheter must be able to selectively engage the ostium. This requires the selection of an appropriate catheter shape and the ability to manipulate the catheter under fluoroscopic guidance (see Chapter 11). Engagement of the desired vessel, however, should not interfere with arterial inflow. This is routinely possible in the left coronary artery, but damping of the guiding catheter pressure when the right coronary artery ostium is engaged was once a common and vexing problem. This has been overcome by the smaller diameter (i.e., 6F) guiding catheters and by the introduction of guiding catheters equipped with side holes that allow ongoing perfusion despite wedged engagement. Because the guiding catheter is also used to deliver small boluses of contrast medium into the involved vessel (as needed to visualize vascular side branches and the target lesion for angioplasty), however, contrast flow out of such side holes may increase the total contrast load used during a procedure.

A second important function of the guiding catheter is to provide adequate support for advancement of interventional devices across the target stenosis. This support derives from the intrinsic stiffness of the guiding catheter material, a catheter shape that buttresses it against the opposite aortic wall, and/or deep engagement of the guiding catheter into the coronary ostium (Fig. 22.3). While deep engagement of the guiding catheter is sometimes needed, it is also well-recognized as a potential cause of complications (i.e., ostial dissection). This complication has become far less frequent with incorporation of an atraumatic bumper on the tip of most guiding catheters and the performance of deep engagement only by coaxial advancement over the balloon catheter. After a deeply engaged guiding catheter

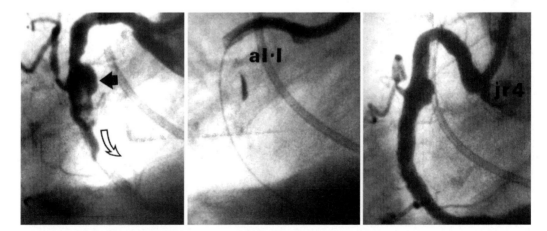

Figure 22.3 Use of deep guiding catheter engagement to facilitate coronary intervention. **Left.** Complex lesion in the right coronary artery including aneurysm *(dark arrow)* and diffuse distal disease *(open curved arrow)*. **Center.** Left Amplatz guiding catheter (AL-1) is deeply engaged to provide optimal support for stent placement. **Right.** After stent placement, the vessel is widely patent, but replacement of the Amplatz catheter with a conventional right Judkins catheter (JR4) shows how effective the Amplatz has been in straightening out a severe upward bend (shepherd's hook) in the proximal right coronary artery. Although progressive improvement in device profile and trackability has made such deep engagement less necessary, the technique is still of great value in selected cases. Deep seating of the guiding catheter needs to be done with great care and coaxial advancement of the guiding catheter over a balloon catheter to avoid injuring the proximal coronary artery.

has been used to push a dilatation balloon or other device across the lesion, the operator cannot forget to then withdraw the guiding catheter back to a more neutral position (just outside the vessel ostium) to avoid its migration into an even deeper position as the device is withdrawn. In this sense, the ability to use the guiding catheter actively constitutes one of the important skills required for effective management of the overall angioplasty equipment system.

Guidewires

The original dilatation catheter designed by Gruentzig had a short segment of guidewire (spring coil) attached to its tip to lead the balloon in the vessel lumen and help avoid subintimal passage as the catheter was passed across the stenosis (see Fig. 22.2). Because the shape or orientation of this leading wire could not be modified once the catheter had been introduced, it provided the operator no control over whether the catheter followed the desired path or was diverted into one or more side branches proximal to the lesion. In the early 1980s, Simpson designed a movable guidewire system in which a 0.018-inch Teflon-coated wire extended and moved freely through a central lumen within a coaxial dilatation catheter (6). If this guidewire selected the desired vessel, it was advanced until it crossed the target lesion. If the guidewire instead selected a more proximal side branch, the balloon catheter was advanced to a point just before the side branch as the wire was withdrawn and reshaped in an effort to choose the desired path beyond. By a series of such iterative advancements of wire and dilatation catheter, many lesions could be crossed with the guidewire and then with the dilatation catheter. In 1983, this concept advanced further with the introduction of the first steerable guidewires, whose rotational orientation could be controlled precisely using a "torquer" (pin vise) attached to the proximal end of the wire.

In contrast to crude early guidewires, modern guidewires are designed to combine tip softness, trackability around curves, radiographic visibility, and precise torque control, which together allow the guidewire to be steered past vascular side branches and through tortuous or stenotic segments. With these refinements, crossing a subtotal lesion with the guidewire has become a task that takes seconds rather than minutes to hours, opening up all portions of the epicardial coronary circulation to a variety of interventional devices. The basic guidewire consists of a solid core (stainless steel or superelastic nitinol) that is ground to a progressive taper in its distal portion. This taper helps retain torque control when the wire is steered around the series of bends located in the guiding catheter and proximal coronary anatomy and allows the stiffer proximal portions of the wire to follow the soft tip into side branches. This core is generally covered by a spring coil, which is usually Teflon-coated stainless steel on the body of the wire, and more radiopaque platinum on the distal 3 to 25 cm. A family of hydrophilic plastic-covered

guidewires (i.e., Choice PT, Boston Scientific, Natick, MA) are also available to aid in crossing vessels with extreme tortuosity or total occlusion, but the spring-coil design is still dominant.

There is substantial choice of tip stiffness, driven by the way the tapered core wire is attached to the outer coil at the wire tip. In soft wires, the tapered core is welded to the coil via a flattened intermediary shaping ribbon that allows the operator to kink or bend the tip of the wire into a shape that is appropriate for navigating the vessel features it must pass while maintaining the required level of atraumatic softness. Experienced interventional operators use their thumbnail or the shaft of the guidewire introducer to shape the guidewire tip to meet the challenges of anatomic navigation—larger-diameter bends are used for selecting left anterior descending (LAD) versus circumflex artery, whereas smaller kinks or bends are used for selecting branches (e.g., diagonal versus LAD).

When greater *probing force* is required (e.g., for probing a chronic total occlusion), stiffer tip designs are available. These core-to-tip guidewires are often graded by the force that the straight guidewire tip can apply to a strain gauge from a distance of 1 cm——wires are available with force increments from 3 gm, 4.5 gm, 6 gm, and ultrastiff 9 gm. Use of these stiff-tip guidewires requires a high degree of skill and feel to avoid unintentional vessel injury (dissection or perforation), and in general operators are well advised to start with soft conventional guidewires and work up to the specialty stiff wires progressively and only as needed.

Independent of the tip stiffness, advancing certain devices around bends may take more *shaft support* from the guidewire. This is provided by extra-support wires, which have a thicker and stiffer inner core. Alternatively, some operators prefer to place a second guidewire across the lesion in parallel (a "buddy" wire) to straighten vessel bends and facilitate device passage. The wire has a series of corrugations near its distal end (the Wiggle Wire Guidant, Santa Clara, CA) that can also be used to help deflect the leading edge of a device away from a calcified plaque or the leading edge of a previously placed stent when advancement over a conventional wire is difficult. With this variety of choices in 0.014-inch guidewires, it is currently rare to use larger-diameter guidewires in coronary work, although wires of 0.016 and 0.018 were previously used for this purpose (requiring, of course, the use of matching devices with larger internal lumen diameters). Smaller-diameter guidewires offer little advantage except with certain devices such as the 0.009-inch Rotablator wire (see Chapter 23), but some specialty total occlusion guidewires have a reduced diameter tip (reduced from 0.014 inch to 0.009–0.012 inch) to help them negotiate small residual lumens.

Standard coronary guidewires are 175 cm long, i.e., some 40 cm longer than the average balloon catheter. This allows the wire to be advanced across the lesion while the balloon catheter remains in the guiding catheter, but does not generally offer sufficient length for exchange of one device for another. Most guidewires are therefore also available in a double- (i.e., 300-cm) exchange length, or are extendable to that length by attachment of a proximal additional segment. Such wires can be passed independently through the guiding catheter and across the target lesion, to remain in place as a series of devices (balloons, rotational atherectomy burrs, stents) is employed, without the risk of subintimal passage of the second guidewire as it crosses the partially dilated segment (7). A similar strategy can be followed with shorter (175-cm) guidewires, provided that rapid-exchange or monorail balloon catheters and stent delivery systems are used (see below). Although the movable guidewire concept (implemented in the current spectrum of highly sophisticated steerable guidewires) has simplified, shortened, and improved the success rate of coronary angioplasty, it is still important to heed the advice of Dotter and Judkins (1) that *the guidewire is passed across the atheromatous block more by the application of judgment than of force.*

Dilatation Catheters

The dilatation catheters for coronary angioplasty have undergone radical evolution since 1977. As described above, the original Gruentzig catheters were designed with a short segment of guidewire permanently affixed to the catheter tip to decrease the risk of subintimal passage during advancement down the coronary tree. The shaft of this catheter had two lumens—one for inflation and deflation of the balloon and one for distal pressure measurement and/or contrast injection. This reflected the initial reliance on monitoring trans-stenotic (i.e., aortic root to distal coronary) pressure gradient as a way of assessing lesion severity, since it was very difficult to perform adequate contrast injections through small-lumen guiding catheters around the large (4.3F, 1.3-mm) shafts of early balloon catheters. In contrast, virtually all dilatation catheters now have an independently movable and/or steerable guidewire extending the entire length of the dilatation catheter, as described by Simpson and coworkers (see Fig. 22.2). The central lumen of such dilatation catheters must have a sufficient caliber to allow free movement of the guidewire, but is no longer generally used for either pressure measurement or contrast injection around the wire. The concept of using trans-stenotic pressure gradients to evaluate the significance and completeness of correction of coronary stenoses, however, has undergone renewed interest with the advent of solid state pressure measurement guidewires (see "Fractional Flow Reserve," Chapter 18). Occasionally, however, the distal balloon lumen is still used (after removal of the guidewire) for distal contrast or drug injection (i.e., for the treatment of no-reflow, see Chapter 3).

An important feature of the dilatation catheter is the diameter of the smallest opening through which the deflated balloon can be passed (its *profile*). The original

Gruentzig catheters had a 0.060-inch (1.5-mm) profile, but current over-the-wire dilatation catheters have profiles as small as 0.025 inch (0.6 mm). To preserve the best balloon profile, a "negative" or "aspiration" preparation should be performed in which a contrast-filled 20-mL syringe is attached to the balloon inflation hub, the plunger is pulled back to apply a vacuum, and gently released to allow the balloon to draw in a small volume of dilute (1:2 dilution with saline) contrast. A "positive" prep, in which the balloon is first aspirated and then actively inflated with contrast material, should generally be avoided to avoid compromising the best possible crossing profile. The magnitude of this issue is seen when one attempts to reuse a previously inflated balloon to cross a second lesion and finds that the secondary (or rewrap) profile is far less satisfactory than the primary (prior to inflation) profile.

The field of angioplasty balloon catheters is now bifurcated into *over-the-wire* (OTW) catheters in which the guidewire runs concentrically within the balloon shaft throughout its entire length and *monorail* (rapid-exchange, or Rx) catheters in which the wire is contained within the balloon shaft over only its distal 25 cm and then runs outside the balloon shaft more proximally. Such catheters can be exchanged quickly by a single operator over a standard length (175-cm) guidewire and generally have smaller shaft profiles to allow better contrast injection or simultaneous placement of two balloons for the treatment of bifurcation lesions. Specially designed *fixed-wire* devices, which consist of a balloon mounted directly on a steerable wire core, were developed and used widely in the late 1980s to provide deflated profiles as small as 0.020 inch (0.5 mm), but their use has become less common as refinements in balloon technology have allowed competitive performance from over-the-wire systems. Fixed-wire devices may still be of unique value in special situations (e.g., dilating side branches through the struts of a stent placed in the parent vessel).

Although profile is important, the ability of the balloon to bend so as to advance easily through tortuous vascular segments *(trackability)* and the presence of sufficient shaft stiffness *(pushability)* to force it through the stenosis are also important. Delivery of the balloon is also aided by the incorporation of a friction-resistant coating (silicone or a hydrophilic coating such as polyethylene oxide) to improve surface lubricity. Other specialized balloon catheters include perfusion balloon catheters, which have a series of side holes in the shaft proximal and distal to the balloon segment or a spiral channel within the balloon to allow ongoing antegrade blood flow and thereby mitigate myocardial ischemia during prolonged balloon inflations (Fig. 22.4). In an era where stents provide definitive control of elastic recoil and dissection, however, the use of perfusion balloons has become rare except for controlling hemorrhage from a coronary perforation without producing severe distal myocardial ischemia (see Chapter 3).

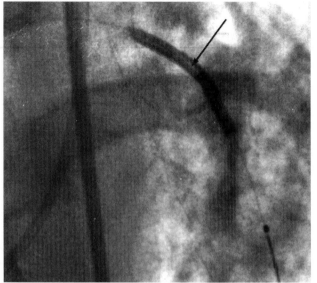

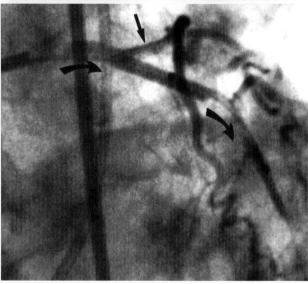

Figure 22.4 Use of a perfusion balloon catheter. **Top.** The inflated perfusion balloon *(arrow)* is shown in the left anterior descending artery and can be recognized by the presence of the non-contrast-filled *(white)* perfusion lumen running through the center of the balloon. **Bottom.** Injection through the guiding catheter *(left curved arrow)* shows direct opacification of the circumflex *(straight arrow)* as well as contrast flow into the distal left anterior descending: This flow enters through proximal side holes, passes through the perfusion lumen within the balloon, and flows out into the distal vessel *(right curved arrow)*. The 40- to 60-mL/minute flow to the distal vessel through the perfusion lumen helps mitigate myocardial ischemia during prolonged balloon inflations, but use of the high-profile devices has become less common with the advent of broad stent use.

Some special balloons exploit the concept of *focused force angioplasty,* in which a second guidewire or microblades on the balloon surface (cutting balloon, Boston Scientific, Natick, MA; Fx mini-rail Guidant, Santa Clara, CA) concentrate the delivery of dilating force from the balloon to the lesion to lower stenosis resolution pressure and reduce balloon slippage forward or backward during inflation (so-called watermelon seeding effect). These techniques have

not, however, improved the long-term patency compared with conventional PTCA (8,9), and the cutting balloon carries a small but real risk of perforation when oversized.

Other than these factors, the most important characteristic of the dilatation catheter is its ability to inflate to a precisely defined diameter despite application of pressures that average 10 to 16 atm. This was not possible with early balloons manufactured from polyvinyl chloride (PVC), whose compliance led to balloon oversizing and rupture at pressures as low as 6 atm. More suitable performance can be readily achieved today using balloons manufactured from high-density polyethylene, polyethylene terephthalate (PET), or nylon, despite balloon wall thickness as low as 0.0003 to 0.0005 inch (3 to 5 ten-thousandths of an inch). Based on material and wall thickness, each balloon has an individual compliance characteristic reflecting the pressure at which the balloon reaches its specified (nominal) diameter and how much that diameter increases as the balloon is inflated to even higher pressures. More compliant balloon materials tend to reach their rated (nominal) diameter at 6 atm and then grow by ≤20% above their nominal size (i.e., a 3.0-mm balloon growing to 3.5 mm) at 10 atm. Semicompliant balloon materials such as high-density polyethylene or nylon grow by <10% over this pressure range, whereas truly noncompliant balloon materials such as PET can retain their defined diameter up to 20 atm to allow dilatation of calcific stenoses or full expansion of coronary stents (Fig. 22.5).

Balloon compliance characteristics must be kept in mind especially when inflating a compliant or semicompliant balloon to pressures above nominal (usually roughly 8–10 atm) to avoid overdistending the adjacent normal vessel. Because the noncompliant balloon materials preclude growth in normal segments upstream and downstream of a rigid lesion, they may be desirable whenever high pressures are needed and may also help to treat resistant lesions by concentrating dilating force on the stenosis itself (rather than in balloon growth and dilatation of the adjacent vessel).

Regardless of which balloon type is used, it is important to stay within the prescribed range of inflation pressure is also important to prevent balloon rupture. This pressure range is specified in terms of the *rated burst pressure* (i.e., an inflation pressure at which the probability of balloon rupture is <0.1%). Taking any balloon catheter above its rated burst pressure (usually 16 to 20 atm) increases the risk of balloon rupture, with the potential for air embolization (if the balloon was incompletely purged), vessel rupture, local dissection, or difficulty in removing the balloon from an incompletely dilated lesion (10). This risk grows the further above rated burst pressure that the balloon is inflated, until it reaches 50% risk of rupture when the average burst pressure is reached. Instead of relying solely on high balloon inflation pressures, there are many other alternatives for dealing with the resistant lesion. It is usually better to use focused force angioplasty, rotational atherectomy, or

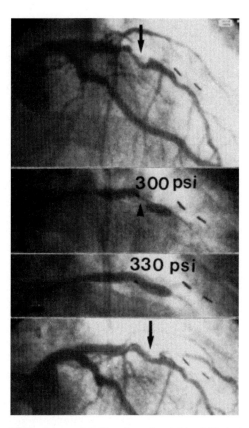

Figure 22.5 Successful dilatation of a rigid calcific lesion. This rigid lesion **(top)** in the midleft anterior descending coronary artery of a postbypass patient (note surgical clips) resisted dilatation at 300 lb/in² (20 atm), but yielded to an inflation pressure of 330 lb/in² (22 atm; **middle two views**) with an excellent angiographic result **(bottom)**. Such pressures are obtainable only with special high-pressure balloon construction because standard angioplasty balloons have rated rupture pressures of only 14 to 16 atm. In current practice, such lesions would more likely be treated by rotational atherectomy (see Chapter 23).

laser atherectomy, Chap. 24, rather than to inflate any balloon catheter to pressures more than 2 to 3 atm above its rated burst pressure. A rare exception to this rule is stent postdilatation in a calcified or fibrotic lesion that has not been adequately predilated or pretreated with rotational atherectomy before stent placement, and where there is no alternative for achieving full stent expansion.

Various manufacturers currently provide dilatation catheters that meet these design specifications with inflated diameters of 1.5, 2.0, 2.5, 3.0, 3.5, and 4.0 mm to match the size of the coronary artery in which the stenosis is located. Larger balloons (i.e., 4.5, 5.0, and 6.0 mm) are occasionally needed for treatment of large right coronary arteries or saphenous vein grafts. Quarter-sized balloons (e.g., 2.25, 2.75, and 3.25 mm) are also available, but that degree of precision probably exceeds the operator's ability to gauge vessel size, and stocking quarter-sizes tends unfavorably to increase the size of a laboratory's balloon inventory. The usual length of the inflatable balloon segment is either 15 or 20 mm, but balloons are also available in shorter (10 mm for dilating or postdilating focal lesions) or longer (30 or 40 mm for dilation of a diffusely diseased segment) inflated segment lengths (11). Although most lesions can be dilated effectively with balloon catheters from any of the several manufacturers, subtle differences in performance characteristics can make the difference between success and failure; therefore, each interventional laboratory still needs to stock a variety of balloon types. Although balloon prices were once nearly $700, competition has brought current prices down to $200 to $250, giving little incentive for resterilization and reuse, with the risk of infection, prolonged procedure time, and device failures with resterilized products (12,13).

PROCEDURE

A coronary angioplasty procedure bears a superficial resemblance to diagnostic cardiac catheterization in that catheters are introduced percutaneously under local anesthesia, However, since angioplasty involves superselective cannulation of diseased coronary arteries with guidewires and balloon catheters, temporary occlusion of antegrade coronary arterial flow, as well as manipulation of the offending atherosclerotic lesion by balloon inflation, the procedure is significantly more complicated and entails roughly 10 times the risk (i.e., 1% versus 0.1%) compared with a purely diagnostic catheterization (14). The risks of coronary angioplasty vary greatly with the baseline clinical condition of the patient, the characteristics of the lesion to be treated, and the techniques that are used (see "Complications" below and Chapter 3). When obtaining informed consent, the individual estimated risks should be discussed in detail with the patient and family prior to the procedure. To mitigate the very real risks of major complications, angioplasty should be attempted only by experienced personnel and generally only in a setting where full cardiac surgical and anesthetic support is available (15,16). One exception is the performance of emergency coronary angioplasty for the treatment of acute ST-elevation myocardial infarction (STEMI), where the need for rapid revascularization has led to the allowance of such procedures in approved catheterization laboratories staffed by experienced interventional operators, even when on-site cardiac surgery is not available (16,17). The practice of elective angioplasty without on-site surgery, however, remains outside the PCI Guidelines at this time (16a).

Patients were once admitted the night before elective angioplasty, but current cost-driven protocols call for admission on the morning of the procedure. Details of the patient evaluation, informed consent, and preprocedure laboratory work will thus generally have been completed in a separate outpatient visit or be compressed into a very brief encounter immediately prior to the procedure. This is particularly true for patients who come to catheter-based intervention at the conclusion of what began as a diagnostic catheterization that progressed to coronary intervention (so-called ad hoc angioplasty or cath with PCI stand-by; 18). If angioplasty is not available at the diagnostic catheterization facility, if the combined procedure is likely to exceed safe contrast loading limits, or if high anticipated procedural risk makes surgical consultation or additional discussions with the patient and family desirable before proceeding with a nonemergent intervention, the procedure may still be concluded after only the diagnostic portion with the PCI as a separate procedure. Similar considerations apply to the decision to stage a complex multivessel procedure into two or more sessions (i.e., patient tolerance, clinical stability, total contrast load, stability of the initial treatment results), but current techniques generally make staging (between diagnostic and interventional procedures, or between treatment of some lesions and others) an uncommon clinical necessity, the reason for which should be documented in the patient chart.

Oral intake should be restricted after midnight on the evening prior to the procedure, and the patient should be pretreated with *aspirin* 325 mg/day to diminish platelet deposition on the disrupted endothelium (19). In the aspirin-allergic patient, a graded aspirin desensitization protocol (20) may be used before PCI or immediately after PCI in which other antiplatelet therapy has been provided (see below). An *oral platelet ADP-receptor antagonist* (such as clopidogrel) may be administered prior to the procedure (21), often supplemented by intravenous platelet glycoprotein IIb/IIIa receptor blockers (22), to reduce the incidence of periprocedural myocardial infarction or repeat emergency revascularization for vessel closure or stent-thrombosis. Since aspirin reduces late cardiac mortality in patients with coronary disease, it is generally continued indefinitely after the procedure. Similar data now exist for longer-term clopidogrel treatment (23).

Angioplasty is generally done from the femoral approach, although brachial and radial approaches can be used based on considerations about vascular access, as well as operator and patient preference. Most catheter-based interventions can be performed safely without right heart catheterization, but a right heart catheter may provide potentially valuable measurements of both baseline filling pressures and intraprocedural hemodynamic deterioration in patients with abnormal baseline left ventricular function or treatment of major vascular territories. The venous sheath also allows rapid initiation of ventricular pacing, although placement of a prophylactic pacemaker is seldom needed except in cases where rotational atherectomy or rheolytic thrombectomy of vessels supplying the right or dominant circumflex coronary artery is planned (see Chapter 23).

After placement of the arterial sheath, intravenous antithrombin therapy is initiated (see Chapter 3). The most common agent is still *unfractionated heparin* (70 units/kg, or 7,000 to 10,000 units), which may be reduced to 50U/kg when administration of a platelet glycoprotein IIb/IIIa receptor blocker is planned. Alternatives include

low-molecular weight heparin (e.g., enoxaparin) in patients who have been on such agents preprocedure (24), or one of the *direct thrombin antagonists* (e.g., bivalirudin [Angiomax, the Medicines Company, Parsippany, NJ]; 25, 25a). If unfractionated heparin is used, it should be noted that there is wide patient-to-patient variability in heparin binding and activity, so that an ACT (activated clotting time) should be measured and additional heparin should be administered as needed to prolong the ACT to 275 to 300 seconds (reduced to 250 seconds if a platelet glycoprotein IIb/IIIa receptor blocker is to be given) *before any angioplasty devices are introduced*. Additional doses or an infusion of the antithrombotic agent may be required to maintain the ACT at this level throughout the case—ACTs <250 seconds are associated with a marked increase in the incidence of occlusive complications unless an adjunctive IIb/IIIa receptor blocker is used, whereas ACTs >300 to 350 seconds tend to increase the risk of bleeding (26). ACTs may also be used to monitor the effect of direct thrombin inhibitors such as bivalirudin, which have found increasing use during PCI based on more predictable dose-response characteristics than heparin, greater efficacy against clot-bound thrombin, reduced platelet activation, less bleeding, and lack of cross-reactivity in patients with the heparin-induced thrombocytopenia or thrombosis syndrome (HITTS, Chapter 3). Since low-molecular weight heparin has relatively more activity against factor Xa than against thrombin, it causes less prolongation of the ACT so that specialized anti-Xa assays are required to monitor low–molecular weight heparin effects.

Baseline angiograms are then obtained of one or both coronary arteries using either a standard diagnostic catheter or the angioplasty guiding catheter. Baseline angiography serves to (a) evaluate any potential changes in angiographic appearance (interval development of total occlusion, thrombus formation) since the prior diagnostic catheterization, (b) permit the selection of the angiographic views that allow optimal visualization of the stenoses, and (c) aid in planning of the detailed interventional strategy. Coronary injections should be repeated after the administration of 200 mg of intracoronary nitroglycerin to demonstrate that spasm is not a significant component of the target stenosis and to minimize the occurrence of coronary spasm during the subsequent angioplasty—we have seen cases where the intended target of a catheter-based intervention resolved with intracoronary nitroglycerin, and an unnecessary intervention was avoided! The best working views that show the target lesions and adjacent side branches most clearly and with the least foreshortening are recorded and transferred to the road-map monitor for reference during the procedure. The approximate reference diameter and length of each target lesion is estimated by comparing it to the 6F (2 mm) diagnostic catheter or selected guiding catheter. Decisions are then made regarding the sequence of lesions to be approached (integrating lesion severity, myocardial territory involved, and noninvasive test data) and the specific interventional approach that will be used. For example, a bifurcation lesion that may require kissing balloon inflations and a simultaneous kissing stents implantation (see Chapter 24) may suggest use of a guiding catheter larger than 6F.

The appropriate guiding catheter is connected to the pressure manifold (see Chapter 11) by way of an extension tube and a rotating hemostatic valve (Tuohy-Borst valve) and positioned in the appropriate coronary ostium. The hemostatic valve contains an adjustable O-ring that allows introduction and free movement of the angioplasty balloon while maintaining a sufficient seal around the balloon shaft to permit pressure measurement and contrast injection. The angioplasty guidewire is then introduced into the guiding catheter, either loaded into the initial angioplasty balloon or inserted through a needlelike guidewire introducer (*bare-wire* technique), and steered across the target lesion. The guidewire is advanced across the lesion with the aid of puffs of contrast material through the guiding catheter as the vessel is imaged fluoroscopically in a projection that shows the desired path free of foreshortening or overlapping side branches. Once the position of the wire tip in the distal vasculature has been confirmed by contrast angiography, the desired angioplasty balloon or other device is selected.

Experience has shown that the best and safest stand-alone angioplasty results were obtained using a balloon whose diameter closely approximates that of the presumably nondiseased reference segment adjacent to the site being treated (balloon/artery ratio 0.9:1.1; 27,28). Slightly larger balloons (approximately 1.1 to 1.2 times the size of the reference lumen) were sometimes used if intravascular ultrasound (see Chapter 19) showed that the outer vessel diameter in the reference segment (external elastic membrane [EEM]) diameter was significantly larger than the reference lumen. On the other hand, slightly smaller initial balloons were used when it was difficult to estimate the correct reference size of a diffusely diseased or rapidly tapering vessel, or when great difficulty was anticipated in crossing the lesion. In the era where stenting (especially drug-eluting stenting) has become the definitive treatment, however, it is routine to predilate the target lesion with a balloon that is slightly undersized relative to the reference vessel and roughly the same length as the target lesion (see Chapter 24). Modern low-profile stents can often be delivered without predilation of the target lesion (so-called *direct stenting*), but predilation makes delivery and accurate placement of the stent within the lesion easier, facilitates the selection of the correct stent diameter and length (by comparison with the diameter and length of the inflated predilating balloon), and ensures that lesion compliance is sufficient to allow full expansion of the stent without pretreatment by rotational atherectomy (see Chapter 23).

The selected balloon is prepared by flushing the central (guidewire) lumen with heparinized saline and filling the balloon inflation lumen with a dilute (1:2) radiographic contrast material. When balloon burst pressures were lower and rupture was more frequent, contrast filling was accomplished by a "positive prep" in which the balloon was aspirated, inflated with contrast, and then aspirated again to remove any air. With more robust balloon materials, however, it is now more common to perform only a "negative prep" in which a contrast-filled syringe is used to pull air from the balloon lumen and then let the balloon aspirate a small amount of contrast material when vacuum on the syringe is released. This method of preparing the balloon catheter avoids inflation before it is across the target lesion and thus helps maintain the lowest possible deflated profile for crossing a severe stenosis. Some operators prefer to prepare the balloon before introduction and attach a three-way stopcock to its inflation hub to maintain a vacuum, whereas others prefer to prep the balloon in the body just before crossing the lesion. The balloon catheter is then loaded onto the free end of the guidewire, advanced through the loosened O-ring, down the proximal vessel, and across the lesion.

Once the dilatation catheter has been positioned within the target stenosis, the balloon is inflated progressively using a screw-powered handheld inflation device equipped with a pressure dial. At low pressure (i.e., 2 to 4 atm), the balloon typically exhibits an hourglass appearance owing to central restriction by the coronary stenosis being treated. In soft lesions, this restriction (or "waist") may expand gradually as the inflation pressure is increased, allowing the balloon to assume its full cylindrical shape. In more rigid lesions, the restriction may remain prominent until the balloon expands abruptly at a *stenosis resolution pressure* that may be anywhere between 4 and 20 atm (29). Some operators prefer to increase pressure rapidly until all balloon deformity resolves, but this increases the risk of dissection when a fibrotic or calcified plaque yields suddenly or when the ends of a somewhat compliant balloon grow to excessive diameter on either side of the resistant lesion. If a calcified plaque resists expansion at 10 to 14 atm, one may thus prefer to consider use of the Rotablator (see Chapter 23) rather than pushing to the very high balloon inflation pressures ($\geq$20 atm, Fig. 22.5) that may be required for full dilation.

At the other extreme, elastic (usually eccentric) stenoses may allow full balloon expansion at low pressures but then tend to recoil promptly once the balloon is deflated. This type of lesion was once treated by repeated inflations, cautious use of oversized balloons, or directional atherectomy, but stent implantation is now the routine treatment. Focused force dilation (with a cutting balloon or external guidewire balloon may also be helpful in dilating the fibrotic or elastic lesion effectively (see below). There is little objective evidence that slower speed of inflation or prolonged (1 minute or more) inflations offer more benefit than the 30-second inflations (30). Exploration of even longer (15-minute) inflations using a perfusion balloon showed slightly better acute results with no difference in long-term patency (31).

Whatever inflation strategy is selected, the response of each lesion to balloon dilation must then be assessed individually so that the dilation protocol can be tailored to achieve the best possible result. The most common way to assess lesion response to balloon dilation is repeat angiography performed through the guiding catheter. By leaving the exchange-length guidewire in place during such angiography or using a rapid-exchange balloon catheter, the balloon can be removed from the guiding catheter without losing access to the distal vessel or the ability to perform additional intervention (repeat balloon inflation, stent placement, etc.). Complete normalization of the vessel lumen would be the ideal end result of coronary angioplasty, but a typical result of even a successful angioplasty is a 30% residual diameter stenosis (i.e., a 1.9-mm lumen in a 3-mm vessel) with some degree of intimal disruption (reflected as localized haziness, filling defect, or dissection). Although this once created a dilemma about whether to persist with additional balloon inflations (weighed against the risk of creating a vessel dissection), the need to obtain a perfect result with balloon angioplasty is now moot in the stent era—*any lesion that can be stented is stented.* In the current view, the best position for stand-alone balloon angioplasty is thus in lesions that are poorly suited to stenting owing to vessel size below 2 mm or branch ostial disease where bifurcation stenting is not contemplated.

Given the importance of achieving the best acute angiographic result, and the uncertainty inherent in angiographic assessment of the irregular lumen postangioplasty, a number of other techniques have been used to grade the quality of an angioplasty result. Initially, PTCA operators relied heavily on the trans-stenotic gradient as an index of dilatation adequacy, seeking a postdilation pressure difference of <15 mm Hg between the aortic pressure (measured through the guiding catheter) and the distal coronary artery pressure (measured through the tip of the dilatation catheter). In practice, such measurements were complicated by the presence of the dilatation catheter within the stenosis and the small size of the dilatation catheter lumen, which led to abandonment of the gradient measurement by 1988 (32). There has been some recent reawakened interest based on the availability of using newer solid state *pressure-measuring* guidewires that can be used to assess the trans-stenotic gradient at baseline flow and during maximal hyperemia (33; see Chapter 18). The goal is to achieve a fractional flow reserve (FFR)—defined as the ratio of distal coronary pressure to aortic pressure during adenosine-induced hyperemia—>0.95 in a successful PCI. The same type of physiologic assessment can be done using Doppler *flow-measuring* guidewires to assess diastolic/systolic flow ratios or coronary flow reserve (CFR) as an index of baseline lesion significance and a confirmation of adequate dilation. Alternatively, *intravascular ultrasound* (IVUS; see Chap. 19) can more accurately measure

lumen diameter and cross-sectional area after dilation, and can detect vessel dissection or hematoma more accurately. Although IVUS has provided important mechanistic insights into balloon angioplasty, it is not used in more than 5 to 10% of routine clinical cases because of the added procedural time and expense. In most laboratories, the postdilation angiogram thus remains the gold standard of whether or not an adequate result has been obtained.

Once adequate dilatation is deemed to have been achieved, it is common to withdraw the balloon catheter completely from the guiding catheter, leaving the guidewire across the dilated segment for several minutes to allow observation of the treated vessel for signs of angiographic deterioration. With more predictable interventions such as stenting, however, a single set of postprocedure angiograms in orthogonal views with the guidewire removed is usually sufficient to document a suitable result in the treated lesion and the absence of dissections, branch occlusions, or guidewire perforations in the adjacent portions of the vessel. At that point, other significant lesions may be dilated similarly, or the procedure may be concluded and the patient transferred to the recovery area.

POSTPROCEDURE MANAGEMENT

Postprocedure management after PCI has been progressively streamlined (14). It was once common to leave the arterial sheath in place overnight with continued heparin infusion, while perfusing the sheath lumen and monitoring for distal limb ischemia. This practice allowed prompt vascular reaccess should delayed abrupt closure occur (34). With the advent of stenting and IIb/IIIa receptor blocker, such delayed abrupt closures occur so infrequently that the practice shifted to removal of the sheaths later the same day as soon as the heparin effect wore off (ACT <160 seconds), with no postprocedure heparin infusion (35,36). In fact, now with the wide adoption of femoral puncture site closure devices, it is common to remove the arterial sheath in the cath lab at the end of the interventional procedure, despite a fully anticoagulated state (see Chapter 4).

After sheath removal, the patient typically remains at bed rest for 18 to 24 hours and then ambulates before discharge. The time to ambulation is reduced significantly, however, if a femoral closure device has been used. If a IIb/IIIa receptor blocker was used intraprocedurally, it is commonly infused for approximately 18 hours postprocedure. Aspirin (325 mg/day) is continued indefinitely, and patients who have received a stent are given clopidogrel (Plavix) as a 300–600 mg loading dose at the end of the procedure and 75 mg per day for 2 to 4 weeks (bare-metal stent) or 3 to 6 months (drug-eluting stent or brachytherapy). Beginning clopidogrel 3 to 6 hours before the intervention obviates the need for a postprocedure loading dose and may attenuate the additional benefit provided by a IIb/IIIa receptor blocker. Longer-term clopidogrel may also reduce the rates of death, myocardial infarction, or stroke out to 12 months following PCI (21,23).

With a good angiographic result in the treated lesions, marked relief of ischemic symptoms should be expected unless other significant disease has been left untreated. In the patient with multivessel disease (see below), it may thus be particularly helpful to evaluate the postangioplasty physiologic state by a maximal exercise test in the first few weeks after discharge. Earlier (i.e., predischarge) exercise testing was once performed on a routine basis, but has now been abandoned largely owing to the potential of groin rebleeding, delay of discharge, or the small risk of precipitating thrombotic closure of the dilatation site. Patients may return to full activity within 72 hours, by which time the groin puncture site should have healed sufficiently to allow even brisk physical activity.

Patients should expect to have no anginal symptoms early after discharge—ongoing anginal symptoms after discharge suggests persistent untreated disease or a poor result at the treatment site. A good initial result, with recurrent symptoms within the first weeks or 1 to 2 months may suggest *subacute stent thrombosis*, which usually presents as an acute STEMI requiring emergent recatheterization. On the other hand, initial symptomatic relief followed by recurrence of symptoms at between 2 and 6 months suggests restenosis of the dilated segment (this has been reduced markedly from 30% with PTCA to 15% with bare-metal stenting to <5% with drug-eluting stenting) (see Chapter 24). When symptoms recur 1 or more years after successful angioplasty, this suggests progression of disease at another site (37). This may become evident by symptoms or on a follow-up exercise test, which may be performed annually or as needed to evaluate recurrent symptoms after PCI. Along with education regarding these possibilities and their proposed management (including additional catheter intervention or bypass surgery, as needed), the acute angioplasty admission should also be viewed as an opportunity to educate the patient and family about changes in lifestyle (smoking, exercise) or drug therapy (to control hypertension or lipid abnormalities) to reduce the risk for the progression of atherosclerotic disease (38). Current lipid guidelines call for achieving a LDL level <70 mg/dL in patients with proven coronary artery disease, as would be the case for the post-PCI patient (39).

MECHANISM OF PTCA

According to the original explanation proposed by Dotter and Judkins (1) and by Gruentzig et al. (3), the enlargement of the vessel lumen following angioplasty was ascribed to *compression of the atheromatous plaque*—akin to footprints in the snow. In fact, true plaque compression accounts for the minority of the observed improvement (40). Extrusion of liquid components from the plaque does permit some compression of soft plaques but contributes

minimally to improvement in more fibrotic lesions, even when balloon inflation is prolonged to 1 minute. Absent significant reduction in plaque volume, most luminal improvement following PTCA seems to result from *plaque redistribution*—more like footprints in wet sand. Some of this takes place by longitudinal displacement of plaque upstream and downstream from the lesion, but most improvement in the lumen following balloon angioplasty or stenting results from controlled overstretching of the entire vessel segment by the PTCA balloon. This stretching leads to fracture of the intimal plaque, partial disruption of the media and adventitia, with consequent enlargement of both the lumen and the overall outer diameter of the vessel (40; Fig. 22.6).

Although use of a full-sized balloon (balloon/artery ratio of 1:1) should theoretically eliminate all narrowing at the treatment site, the overstretched vessel wall invariably exhibits elastic recoil (41,42) following balloon deflation, as well as some degree of local vasospasm (43). These processes typically leave the stretched vessel with a 30% residual stenosis (i.e., a 2-mm lumen in a 3-mm vessel that has been dilated with a 3-mm balloon). A typical balloon angioplasty result also shows evidence of localized trauma to more superficial plaque components as an almost universal haziness of the lumen (44). Greater degrees of disruption are reflected by intimal filling defects (Fig. 22.7), contrast caps outside the vessel lumen, or spiral dissections that may interfere with antegrade blood flow (Fig. 22.8). This local disruption has been seen on IVUS, angioscopy, and the histologic examination of postmortem angioplasty specimens, and its extent correlates with the risk of an occlusive complication (45). In contrast, stenting or directional atherectomy reduce or even eliminate this elastic recoil, dissection, and vascular tone, and thereby provide lower (0 to 10% rather than 30%) postprocedural residual stenosis, and a smooth and uniform lumen by angiography or IVUS, with less chance of acute or delayed closure.

Given the amount of "angio*blasty*" that takes place during balloon dilation, it is remarkable that dislodgment and distal embolization of plaque fragments seem to be infrequent in both experimental studies (46) and most clinical angioplasty procedures. There is increasing evidence, however, of distal atheroembolization during balloon angioplasty and stent placement. This is most clearly established in patients undergoing dilatation of a saphenous vein bypass graft or patients with large thrombi adherent to the lesion. Distal embolization of large (>1 mm) plaque elements is usually manifest as an abrupt cutoff of flow in the embolized distal vessel (47). In contrast, *micro*embolization of plaque debris or adherent thrombus may contribute to postprocedure chest pain, enzyme elevation, or the no-reflow phenomenon in which there is dramatic reduction in antegrade flow with manifestations of severe ischemia (chest pain and ST-segment elevation), in the absence of epicardial vessel stenosis, dissection, or macroembolic cutoff (48). No-reflow can usually be improved by

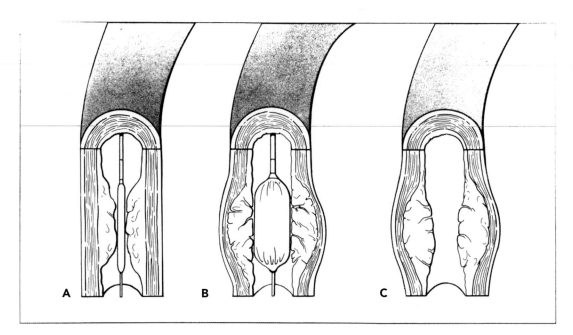

Figure 22.6 Proposed mechanism of angioplasty. **A.** Deflated balloon positioned across stenosis. **B.** Inflation of the balloon catheter within the stenotic segment causes cracking of the intimal plaque, stretching of the media and adventitia, and expansion of the outer diameter of the vessel. **C.** Following balloon deflation, there is partial elastic recoil of the vessel wall, leaving a residual stenosis of 30% and local plaque disruption that would be evident as haziness of the lumen contours on angiography. (From Willerson JT, ed. *Treatment of Heart Diseases*. New York: Gower Medical, 1992.)

distal intracoronary injection of an arterial vasodilator (nitroprusside 100 μg; verapamil 100 μg; diltiazem 250 μg; nicardipine 200 μg; adenosine 100 μg—but not nitroglycerin, which is more of an epicardial than arteriolar vasodilator). But such treatment does not prevent periprocedural myocardial infarction. In contrast, the use of a distal occlusion/aspiration embolic protection system (see Chapter 23) recovered atheroembolic debris and reduced the incidence of these complications by nearly half. The

SAFER trial of vein graft stenting thus showed that such enzyme elevations occurred in 17% of lesions, with evidence of no-reflow in 8% of lesions, which were reduced to 9.7 and 3.3%, respectively, through the use of distal embolic protection (49). Similar benefits have now been seen with the distal embolic filter devices (50), and in other vascular beds (carotid, renal, native coronary), suggesting that the use of embolic protection may become more widespread.

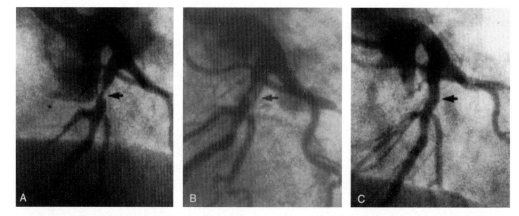

Figure 22.7 Normal healing of PTCA-related coronary dissection. Compared with the baseline angiogram **(A)**, the immediate post-PTCA angiogram **(B)** shows enlargement of the left anterior descending (LAD) lumen with two small filling defects typical of an uncomplicated coronary dissection. Follow-up angiogram 3 months later **(C)** shows preservation of luminal caliber with complete healing of the localized dissection. (From Baim DS. Percutaneous transluminal coronary angioplasty. In Braunwald E, ed. *Harrison's Principles of Internal Medicine: Update VI*. New York: McGraw-Hill, 1985.)

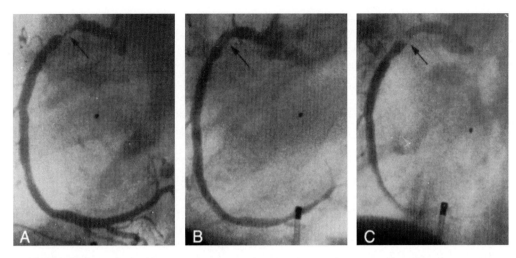

Figure 22.8 Coronary dissection leading to abrupt reclosure. The appearance of a right coronary stenosis prior to **(A)** and immediately following **(B)** coronary angioplasty, with an evident localized dissection. Within 15 minutes following removal of the dilatation catheter, the patient experienced chest pain associated with inferior ST-segment elevation and angiographic evidence of progressive dissection with impeded antegrade flow **(C)**. Standard management in 1980 (when this case was done) consisted of emergency bypass surgery, which was accomplished without complication. Current practice would be to attempt to recross the lesion and "tack down" the dissection by repeat balloon inflation, or more likely place one or more stents. (From Baim DS. Percutaneous transluminal angioplasty—analysis of unsuccessful procedures as a guide toward improved results. *Cardiovasc Intervent Radiol* 1982;5:186.)

Although it is a theoretical possibility with sufficient local stretching trauma, frank vessel rupture has turned out to be a fortunately rare consequence during conventional balloon angioplasty, barring the use of significantly oversized balloons (51). Vessel perforation is actually more common (approximately 1% incidence) when atherectomy devices such as directional atherectomy, rotational atherectomy, or laser angioplasty are used (52; see Chapter 23), when stents are post-dilated at high pressure (>18 atm) with oversized (>1.1:1) balloons, or when stiff hydrophilic wires are advanced into small distal branches. *Local vessel perforation or distal guidewire perforation in a patient on IIb/IIIa blocker agents usually constitutes a medical emergency* requiring prompt blockage of the perforation site with a balloon, drainage of hemopericardium, and definitive sealing of the perforation site with prolonged balloon inflation, a membrane-covered stent, an embolic coil, or emergency surgery (52,53; see Chapters 3 and 32).

ACUTE RESULTS OF ANGIOPLASTY

Early published data on coronary angioplasty success derive mostly from the 3,000-patient NHLBI Angioplasty Registry, which collected all procedures performed between 1977 and September of 1981 (54). Although case selection in the registry focused on "ideal" PTCA candidates—those with proximal, discrete, concentric, subtotal, noncalcified stenoses of a single vessel—the primary success rate of 61% would be considered disappointing by current standards. The main explanations for the low primary success rate in

the registry were failure to cross the lesion with the dilatation system (29% of cases) and failure to dilate the lesion adequately once having crossed (12% of cases). These failures were a result of two factors:) the relative lack of experience of operators contributing cases to the registry (the learning curve), and the use of original Gruentzig fixed-wire dilatation catheters with limited maneuverability, a comparatively high deflated balloon profile, and a low peak inflation pressure. Also sobering was the nearly 9% incidence of major complications, including a 6% incidence of emergency bypass surgery to treat abrupt vessel closure owing to local dissection, a 4.9% incidence of Q-wave myocardial infarction, and a 1.5% mortality rate.

Despite the inclusion of patients with more difficult coronary anatomy, progressive improvement in equipment (including the widespread availability of steerable guidewires since 1983), the second PTCA registry (1985–1986; 55,56), had a success rate of 78%, with reduction in the incidence of major complications to 7%, including emergency bypass surgery 3.5%, Q-wave myocardial infarction 4.3%, and the mortality for patients with single-vessel disease (from 0.85 to 0.2%). Overall procedural mortality, however, remained close to 1% because of the inclusion of greater numbers of patients with multivessel disease in the 1985–1986 registry.

In the new device era (late 1990s and early 2000s), the availability of stents, atherectomy devices, and better anticoagulant and antiplatelet regimens have boosted acute procedural success >95% and reduced major adverse cardiac events falling to roughly 3% (death 1%, emergency surgery 0.3%, and Q-wave or large non–Q-wave MI 1.5%; 57). But it is important to remember that significant complications continue to occur, and the burden remains on the operator to select patients carefully, choose the best approach, execute it well, and respond quickly to evolving complications to minimize their ultimate scope and clinical impact.

COMPLICATIONS

As a specialized form of cardiac catheterization, coronary angioplasty is attended by the usual risks related to invasive cardiac procedures (see also Chapter 3). In contrast with diagnostic procedures, the larger-caliber guiding catheter used for angioplasty is more likely to result in damage to the proximal coronary artery and cause local bleeding complications at the catheter introduction site. Selective advancement of guidewires and dilatation catheters into diseased coronary arteries may lead to vessel injury if they are manipulated too aggressively.

Several systems have been devised to predict risk, which may be useful in preprocedural discussions with the patient and family or in monitoring how actual procedural outcomes over time compare with what is predicted (risk adjustment, looking at the observed versus expected complication rate ratio). The risk of procedural or in-hospital mortality is driven mostly by clinical factors such as age, cardiogenic shock, congestive heart failure, renal failure, and urgent or emergent PCI; 58–61; Table 22.1; Fig. 22.9). Procedure success and overall complications, however, tend to be driven by lesion-related features. The original AHA/ACC Type A, B, and C lesion categorization (62; Table 22.2) was modified by Ellis (63) to discriminate between B1 and B2 lesions (i.e., those with one or more than one B characteristic), but the continued validity of this classification scheme has come into question in the stent era. The Society for Cardiac Angiography and Intervention has thus proposed a simplification into four risk categories (based on whether or not the lesion has a type C feature and whether it is patent or occluded; 64). This offers a somewhat better predictive value of both procedural success and major complications (death, myocardial infarction [CK elevation], emergency surgery, or emergency repeat angioplasty) and shows the potent effect of stenting in reducing those complications across the board (Fig. 22.10).

The potent effect of stenting (and potentially platelet glycoprotein IIb/IIIa blockers) on reducing the need for emergency surgery is shown clearly in the prospective Cleveland Clinic review of 18,593 PCIs performed from 1992 through 2000 (65). Emergency surgery was required in 113 (0.61%) cases, owing to extensive dissection ($n = 61$), perforation/tamponade ($n = 23$), and recurrent acute closure ($n = 23$), but its prevalence decreased from 1.5% of PCIs in 1992 to 0.14% in 2000 ($P < 0.001$), in parallel with increased stent use (Fig. 22.11). The consequences of emergency surgery for a PCI complication, however, are still daunting: of the 113 patients who underwent emergency CABG, there were 17 (15%) in-hospital deaths, 14 (12%) perioperative Q-wave myocardial infarctions, and 6 (5%) cerebrovascular accidents.

TABLE 22.1
MULTIVARIABLE PREDICTORS OF MORTALITY IN VARIOUS PUBLISHED INTERVENTIONAL MODELS

First author	Hannan	Kimmel	Ellis	O'Connor	Moscucci	Shaw	Qureshi
Database source	New York	SCAI	5 U.S. hospitals	NNE	8 Michigan hospitals	ACC-NCDR	Beaumont
Years of treatment	1991–1994	1992	1993–1994	1994–1996	1997–1999	1998–2000	1996–1998
Number of patients	62,670	10,622	12,985,	15,331	10,729	100,253	9,954
Age	×	×	×	×	×	×	×
MI <24 h	×	×	×	×	×	×	× (14 days)
Shock	×	×	×	×	×	×	
LV function	×			×	×	×	
Female	×		×			×	
Lesion complexity		×	×	×		×	
Diabetes	×					×	
Renal failure	×			×	×	×	×
Left main disease						×	
Proximal LAD						×	
Urgent procedure				×		×	
Preprocedure IABP				×		×	
PVD	×			×	×		
Multivessel disease		×			×		×

For each model, the multivariable correlates of mortality found are indicated by an X.
ACC-NCDR, American College of Cardiology–National Cardiovascular Device Registry; IABP, intraaortic balloon pump; LAD, left anterior descending; LV, left ventricular; MI, myocardial infarction; NNE, Northern New England; PVD, peripheral vascular disease; SCAI, Society for Cardiac Angiography and Intervention.
From Cutlip DE, Ho KKL, Kuntz RE, Baim DS. Risk assessment for percutaneous coronary intervention—our version of the weather report? *J Am Coll Cardiol* 2003;42:1986–1989.

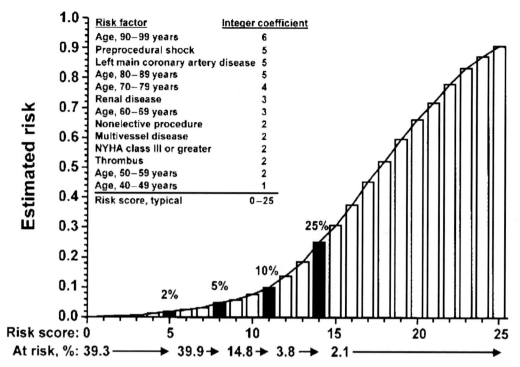

Risk factor	Integer coefficient
Age, 90–99 years	6
Preprocedural shock	5
Left main coronary artery disease	5
Age, 80–89 years	5
Age, 70–79 years	4
Renal disease	3
Age, 60–69 years	3
Nonelective procedure	2
Multivessel disease	2
NYHA class III or greater	2
Thrombus	2
Age, 50–59 years	2
Age, 40–49 years	1
Risk score, typical	0–25

Figure 22.9 Mayo Clinic risk score for mortality assigns integer coefficients for each named clinical variable so that one can read the estimated mortality risk that corresponds to the total of the integer coefficients from the curve and the value on the Y axis. The 2% of patients with a total score over 14 thus have an expected procedural mortality of 25%! (From Singh M, Lennon RJ, Holmes DR Jr, Bell MR, Rihal CS. Correlates of procedural complications and a simple integer risk score for percutaneous coronary intervention. *J Am Coll Cardiol* 2002;40:387–393, with permission.)

Coronary Artery Dissection

The most common complications of coronary angioplasty relate directly to local injury at the dilatation site caused as part of the angioplasty process, as described in the section concerning mechanisms. Although plaque disruption and dissection may be caused by the guiding catheter or overly vigorous attempts to pass the guidewire through a tortuous stenotic lumen, most dissections are actually the by-product of the "controlled injury" that is induced intentionally by inflation of the dilatation catheter (40). In fact, localized dissections can be found routinely in animal or cadaveric models of angioplasty and are evident angiographically in at least one half of patients immediately after balloon angioplasty (44). When these dissections are small and nonprogressive and do not interfere with antegrade flow in the distal vessel, they have no clinical consequence other than transient mild pleuritic chest discomfort. Follow-up angiography as soon as 6 weeks after the angioplasty procedure usually demonstrates complete healing of the dissected segment (see Fig. 22.7), although occasional localized formation of aneurysms has been described at the site of dissection (66,67).

Abrupt Closure

Prior to the era of widespread stent use, large progressive dissections not uncommonly interfered with antegrade

flow and led to total occlusion of the dilated segment (a phenomenon known as abrupt closure; see Fig. 22.8). With balloon angioplasty alone (before the advent of new devices), abrupt closure occurred in roughly 5% of patients as the result of compression of the true lumen by the dissection flap (45), with superimposed thrombus formation, platelet adhesion, or vessel spasm. In one study (68), postangioplasty dissections were evident angiographically in 40% of dilated lesions, with spiral (type D) dissections in 3.5% of patients. The presence of a type D dissection increased the risk of frank or "threatened" abrupt closure (residual stenosis >50%, with reduced antegrade flow) from a baseline of 6.1% to 28%. This finding supports the earlier findings of Ellis et al. (69) showing a fivefold increase in abrupt closure with postprocedure dissection and stressing the relative importance of the postprocedure result (as opposed to preprocedure clinical or angiographic variables) on the risk of abrupt closure Most abrupt closures after stand-alone balloon angioplasty developed within minutes of the final balloon inflation, so that it was the routine practice to observe the lesion for 10 minutes after the last balloon inflation, before leaving the catheterization laboratory. But abrupt closure also occurred up to several hours later (in 0.5 to 1% of cases) as the heparin anticoagulation wore off (particularly prior to the use of IIb/IIIa receptor blocker infusions in patients with marginal angiographic results of stand-alone balloon angioplasty).

TABLE 22.2

LESION MORPHOLOGIC PREDICTORS OF PROCEDURE SUCCESS AND COMPLICATION BASED ON THE AHA/ACC LESION CLASSIFICATION SYSTEM

Characteristics of type A, B1, B2, and C lesions
  Type A lesions (high success, >85%; low risk)
    Discrete (<10 mm length)
    Concentric
    Readily accessible
    Nonangulated segment <45°
    Smooth contour
    Little or no calcification
    Less than totally occlusive
    Not ostiol in location
    No major branch involvement
    Absence of thrombus
  Type B1 lesions (moderate success, 60 to 85%; moderate risk)
    Tubular (10–20 mm length)
    Eccentric
    Moderate tortuosity of proximal segment
    Moderately angulated segment, 45–90°
    Irregular contour
    Moderate to heavy calcification
    Ostial in location
    Bifurcation lesions requiring double guidewires
    Some thrombus present
    Total occlusion <3 months old
  Type B2 lesions (Ellis modification of AHA/AOC system)
    Two or more type B characteristics
  Type C lesions (low success, <60%; high risk)
    Diffuse (>2 cm length)
    Excessive tortuosity of proximal segment
    Extremely angulated segment >90°
    Inability to protect major side branches
    Degenerated vein grafts with friable lesions
    Total occlusion >3 months old

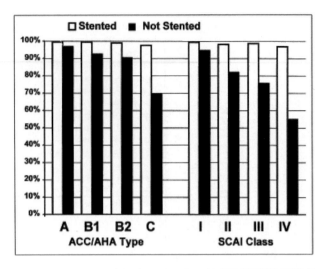

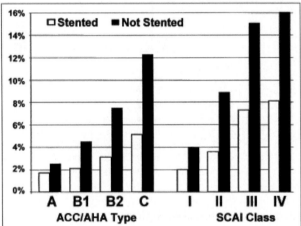

Figure 22.10   Lesion risk scores. **Top.** The probability of success by AHA type lesion *(left)* and the new SCAI class *(right)*, treated with (open bars) and without (closed bars) coronary stenting. **Bottom.** The probability of a major complication based on AHA lesion type *(left)* and the new SCAI class *(right)*, treated with (open bars) and without (closed bars) coronary stenting. The SCAI score, based simply on whether the vessel has one or more type C characteristics and is open or occluded, has a stronger predictive value of success and complications than the traditional AHA/ACC score. The beneficial effect of stenting on complications is evident. (See also Table 22.2; From Krone RJ, Shaw RE, Klein LW, Block PC, et al. Evaluation of the American College of Cardiology/American Heart Association and the Society for Coronary Angiography and Interventions lesion classification system in the current "stent era" of coronary interventions. (From the ACC-National Cardiovascular Data Registry). *Am J Cardiol* 2003; 92:389–394, with permission.)

Before 1985, most patients who experienced abrupt closure of a major epicardial coronary artery went directly to emergency surgery, in an effort to minimize the amount of consequent myocardial damage. The rate of emergency surgery was thus 5 to 6%, but even with emergency surgery within 90 minutes of the onset of vessel occlusion, up to 50% of patients sustained a Q-wave myocardial infarction (70). The development of perfusion catheters—infusion catheters or angioplasty balloons with multiple side holes along their distal shaft to allow 40 to 60 mL/minute of blood to enter proximal to the site of occlusion, flow through the central lumen, and re-exit into the lumen distal to the point of occlusion—allowed patients to go to the operating room in a nonischemic state (Fig. 22.4), and was shown to reduce the incidence of transmural infarction during emergency surgery to approximately 10% (71). Once it was realized that many abrupt closures can be reversed by simply readvancing the balloon dilatation catheter across the lesion to "tack up" the dissection via repeated

balloon inflation, the emergency surgery rate fell in half to roughly 3%. Prolonged balloon inflations (up to 20 minutes, using an autoperfusion balloon to limit ongoing ischemia) further improved the ability to reverse abrupt closure (72).

Since 1993, however, the availability of coronary stents has made the certainty of reversing abrupt closure >90% (73). This success has made it routine to stent any patient with a large postprocedure dissection as a pre-emptive

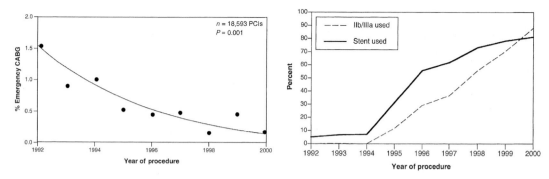

Figure 22.11 The Cleveland Clinic experience with 18,593 PCIs from 1992 through 2000 shows the progressive reduction in the risk of requiring emergency bypass as the result of PCI **(left)** as the institutional use of stents and glycoprotein IIb/IIIa receptor blockers increased over that period **(right).** (From Seshadri N, et al. Emergency coronary artery bypass surgery in the contemporary percutaneous coronary intervention era. *Circulation* 2002;106:2346–2350, with permission.)

treatment for threatened abrupt closure even when flow compromise is not apparent. Of course, with elective stenting of >90% of interventional procedures, this problem has been largely eliminated, with emergency surgery rates having fallen to <0.5%, as evidenced in the Cleveland Clinic series discussed above (65).

Beyond the mechanical issues of residual stenosis and local dissection, it is now clear that platelet-rich clots contribute significantly to the abrupt closure process. The presence of thrombus, reflected as a globular filling defect, increases the risk of abrupt closure from 7.2 to 27.8% (68). The role of thrombus in abrupt closure is further supported by an increased risk of abrupt closure in patients with a subtherapeutic ACT and the reduction of ischemic end points seen in patients treated with a bolus plus infusion of various platelet glycoprotein IIb/IIIa blockers (see Chapter 3; 22). Although platelets may adhere to damaged vessel wall through other receptors, activation of the 50,000 to 80,000 glycoprotein IIb/IIIa receptors on each platelet's surface allows them to bind avidly to fibrin to cause platelet aggregation and thrombosis (see Chapter 3). Vessels with moderate local dissection but preserved antegrade flow are thus more likely to stay patent in the presence of agents that reduce the affinity of the activated IIb/IIIa receptor for fibrinogen, thereby reducing the incidence of emergency surgery or unplanned (bailout) stent placement. These agents also significantly reduce the incidence of periprocedural myocardial infarction, particularly the incidence of CK elevations (non-Q-wave myocardial infarctions) that are seen in 10 to 30% of patients undergoing coronary intervention. Given their moderate expense and increased bleeding risk, there is still heterogeneity (see below) in whether these agents should be used in all coronary interventions or restricted to the 30 to 40% of patients who have high-risk lesion morphologies or a suboptimal mechanical result after mechanical intervention.

Other Complications

A number of other complications have been described as the result of coronary angioplasty. Q-wave myocardial infarction occurs in approximately 1% of patients (54), often as a result of abrupt closure or "snowplow" loss of a major side branch originating within or in close proximity to the lesion being treated. If creatinine phosphokinase (CPK) MB isoenzyme levels are measured routinely, however, 10 to 30% of patients will show some elevation following apparently uncomplicated procedures (74), generally as the result of distal microembolization or loss of smaller side branches. The importance of these "infarctlets" has been the subject of considerable debate. There is no dispute that larger non-Q-wave infarctions—those with total CK levels greater than twice normal or absolute CK-MB levels greater than five times the upper limit of normal, particularly if associated with new ST-T wave abnormalities—carry the same import as a periprocedural Q-wave infarction. The debate concerns whether smaller elevations of CK-MB (between one and five times normal, which do not significantly impair ventricular function) also increase late mortality. Several large studies have demonstrated that patients with even one and five times normal CK-MB elevation have an increased incidence of adverse events (in different studies, sometimes death, sometimes repeat MI, sometimes repeat revascularization) during the subsequent 3 to 5 years.

But is this a cause-and-effect relationship (the small MIs cause the late adverse outcomes) or the result of a confounder (both the CK elevations and the variety of late events are each related to a common factor such as the diffuseness of atherosclerotic disease)? Pooled analysis of more than 20,000 interventional patients enrolled in randomized trials of IIb/IIIa receptor blockers versus placebo (75) do show a modest 6 to 12 month mortality benefit, but one should note that most of the patients in those trials underwent balloon angioplasty (with a higher risk of

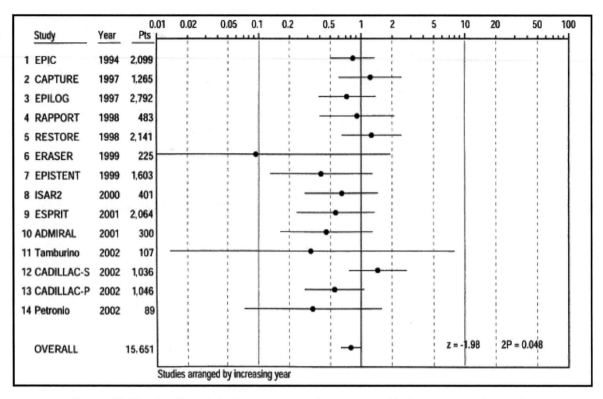

Figure 22.12 The effect of platelet glycoprotein IIb/IIIa receptor blockade on 6-month mortality in a pooled analysis of 15,651 patients treated with balloon angioplasty in various 14 randomized trials comparing the IIb/IIIa blockers with conventional heparin anticoagulation alone. (From Kelly D, Arora D. Prognostic significance of myocardial enzyme release after coronary interventions. *Cathet Cardiovasc Intervent* 1999;46:292, with permission.)

vessel closure against which the IIb/IIa receptor blockers would be protective) rather than stenting (where the protective effect is less certain), that patients with clear intraprocedural failures or complications were included in the study cohort along with patients who had a small incidental CK-MB elevation after an otherwise successful procedure in many of the studies, and that the mortality benefit is variable (Fig. 22.12).

Occlusion of branch vessels originating from within the stenotic segment occurs in 14% of vessels at risk during angioplasty of the main vessel, according to what has been called the *snowplow effect* (76). If the branch vessel is small, this event usually has no significant clinical sequelae and should not discourage attempted angioplasty. On the other hand, if a large branch vessel originates from within the stenotic segment, simultaneous dilatation of the main vessel and the involved branch with two separate dilatation systems (the kissing balloon technique) may be required for preservation of both vessels (77). This originally utilized two guidewires that could be inserted through a single guiding catheter (one guidewire placed into the main vessel and one into the involved side branch) to allow alternating advancement of a balloon catheter into one and then the other vessel (78). Current large-lumen guiding catheters and low-profile dilatation systems, however, now allow kissing balloon inflations through a single 7F or even 6F guiding

catheter. The effective side-by-side balloon diameter in the proximal vessel can be estimated as the square root of the sum of the squares of the individual balloon diameters (two 3.0 balloons have an effective combined diameter of 4.25 mm [square root of 18=9+9]). The results can be improved, however, by the use of various bifurcation stent strategies (see Chapter 24), or atherectomy of both the parent and branch vessel (79; see Chapter 23).

Perforation of the coronary artery with a stiff guidewire occurs rarely and does not necessarily have dire consequences, unless a device is passed over the wire or the wire perforation takes place in a patient receiving a platelet IIb/IIIa receptor blocker. Frank rupture of the coronary artery owing to use of too large a dilatation balloon or the use of an atherectomy device (see Chapter 23) can also cause vessel perforation that leads to rapid tamponade and hemodynamic collapse (52,53). Perforations may be classified based on angiographic appearance as type I—extraluminal crater without extravasation; type II—pericardial and myocardial blush without contrast jet extravasation; and type III—extravasation through a frank (1-mm) perforation. In the absence of extravasation (type III), most perforations may be effectively managed without urgent surgical intervention. Even type III perforations can be managed nonoperatively with the combination of: pericardiocentesis, reversal of anticoagulation, and either prolonged perfusion balloon inflation at the site of perforation or deployment of a covered stent. If these approaches are not successful, perforations usually require surgical repair.

Tamponade also may result from perforation of the right atrium or right ventricle during placement of temporary pacemaker electrode catheters, particularly in angioplasty patients who are receiving antiplatelet therapy in addition to full anticoagulation. This potential complication and the infrequency (<1%) of severe bradycardiac complications support the recommendation against prophylactic pacing during coronary angioplasty (15,16), although such pacing is required for certain atherectomy and thrombectomy procedures (see Chapter 23). Ventricular fibrillation occurs in approximately 1% of angioplasty procedures (54), usually as the result of prolonged ischemia during balloon advancement or inflation. In addition to causing electrical instability, ischemia during balloon inflation may cause marked electrocardiographic changes (80), abnormalities in regional left ventricular systolic and diastolic function, as well as regional myocardial lactate production (81,82).

Although angioplasty guidewires and catheters are extremely reliable, *device failures* can occur when any device is subjected to severe operating stresses (i.e., when a guidewire is rotated repeatedly in a single direction while its tip is held fixed in a total occlusion or when a balloon catheter is inflated past its operating pressure range in an attempt to dilate a resistant stenosis). In a small percentage of cases, this may lead to detachment of a part of the wire or dilatation catheter, with a fragment remaining in the coronary artery (83). In the stent era, this also includes dislodgment of a bare-mounted stent from its delivery balloon or failure of the stent delivery balloon to inflate or deflate properly. To avoid the need for surgical removal, the angioplasty operator should be familiar with various techniques (baskets, bioptomes, intertwined guidewires) for catheter retrieval (84). Although hard to remember in the heat of battle, any failed products should be saved, sealed in a bag, and returned to the manufacturer for structural analysis that may disclose a root cause manufacturing flaw. Device failures should also be reported to the Food and Drug Administration (FDA) *MAUDE* (Manufacturer user facility and distributor experience database) online at www.accessdata.fda.gov/scripts/medwatch to facilitate the recognition and tracking of patterns that may otherwise appear as just a random device failure event to a single operator.

THE HEALING RESPONSE TO CORONARY ANGIOPLASTY—RESTENOSIS

Following successful balloon angioplasty, the body attempts to repair the damage caused by the procedure-related mechanical injury (85). Within minutes, a carpet of platelets and fibrin is deposited. Within hour to days, inflammatory

cells begin to infiltrate the site, cytokines are released, and vascular smooth muscle cells begin to migrate from the media toward the lumen. These smooth muscle cells and fibroblasts convert from their normal phenotype to a synthetic phenotype and remain in this form as they undergo hypertrophy, proliferate, and begin to secrete extensive extracellular matrix (Fig. 22.13). The luminal surface is simultaneously colonized by endothelial cells that slowly regain their normal barrier function and secretory functions in making tissue plasminogen activator (t-PA) and endothelium-derived relaxation factor (EDRF). Along with this proliferative neointimal response, there may also be further elastic recoil and fibrotic contraction of the vessel wall (i.e., negative vessel remodeling) during this period. Different arteries and different interventions appear to undergo different degrees of proliferation and

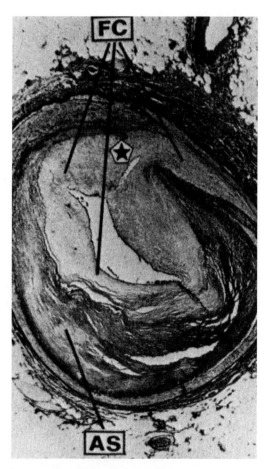

Figure 22.13 Mechanisms of restenosis: Cross section of a restenotic lesion in the left anterior descending artery 5 months after initial coronary angioplasty shows the original atherosclerotic plaque (AS), the crack in the medial layer induced by the original procedure *(star)*, and the proliferation of fibrocellular tissues (FC) that constitutes the restenotic lesion. In stent restenosis, the mechanism is purely such proliferation, whereas in nonstent interventions such as balloon angioplasty there is frequently also a component owing to shrinkage of the overall vessel diameter (unfavorable remodeling) at the treatment site. (From Serruys PW, et al. Assessment of percutaneous transluminal coronary angioplasty by quantitative coronary angiography: diameter versus videodensitometric area measurements. *Am J Cardiol* 1984;54:482.)

vessel contraction—for example, stents renarrow exclusively by neointimal hyperplasia, whereas nonstent devices also undergo a significant amount of late narrowing owing to contraction of the entire vessel wall (86). There are also significant patient-to-patient variations in the late healing response after coronary intervention, reflected in variable amounts of late loss in lumen diameter between the completion of the intervention and the time when the repair process stabilizes (roughly 6 months). Follow-up angiography shows continued maintenance of lumen diameter at the treated site beyond 6 to 9 months (87).

If the healing response is excessive, however, most or all of the gain in lumen diameter produced by the initial intervention may be lost to the healing process. This causes the return of a severe stenosis and ischemic symptoms—a phenomenon known as restenosis of the dilated segment (Fig. 22.14). Throughout the 1980s, restenosis was considered a dichotomous outcome (like death) that either did or did not develop. Although a great deal was learned about restenosis from the study of conventional angioplasty patients (e.g., its time course, histology, and various clinical factors that correlated with an increased incidence of restenosis; 88), data derived from stent and atherectomy procedures led to new paradigms for evaluating restenosis

(89). In this paradigm, it was more useful to consider restenosis as a continuous variable (like height), and to use cumulative distribution curves to show the ranked population distribution of the late result (expressed as either late lumen diameter or late percent diameter stenosis) for the whole treated population (Fig. 22.15). On the diameter stenosis curve, the percentage of the population that has a late diameter stenosis of >50% serves as a useful benchmark for comparing the angiographic restenosis rates between different populations or treatment groups.

Every treated lesion undergoes some degree of late loss, but fortunately late loss usually negates only part (roughly half) of the acute gain, so that a long-term net gain in lumen diameter results with alleviation of myocardial ischemia. In fact, there tends to be a roughly linear relationship between the acute gain in lumen diameter caused by the intervention, and late loss in lumen diameter (caused by the proliferative and fibrotic reaction of the artery during the healing phase), whose slope (the *loss index*) is roughly 0.5 for most interventions. This means that larger lumen diameters immediately after intervention translate into larger lumen diameters at 6-month angiographic restudy (the "bigger is better" dictum). Prior to drug-eluting stents (see below), all new mechanical devices

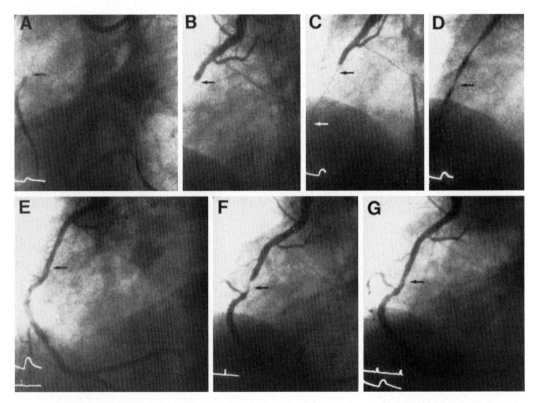

Figure 22.14   Clinical restenosis. **A–D.** A totally occluded right coronary artery with filling of the distal vessel by way of left to right collaterals. **E.** The essentially normal appearance of the right coronary artery following successful angioplasty. **F.** The appearance 6 weeks later when angina had recurred. **G.** The appearance following successful re-PTCA. Restenosis developed again 6 weeks following the second PTCA, but the patient was then asymptomatic for more than 6 years after a third PTCA procedure. (From Dervan JP, Baim DS, Cherniles J, Grossman W. Transluminal angioplasty of occluded coronary arteries: use of a moveable guide wire system. *Circulation* 1983;68:776.)

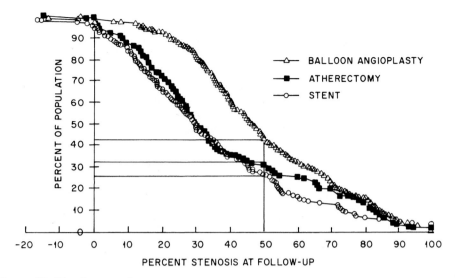

Figure 22.15 The view of restenosis as a continuous process that takes place to some degree in every treated segment favors displaying the late result (here, percent stenosis at follow-up) for the whole treated population. For patients treated by balloon angioplasty, directional atherectomy, or stenting, the Y axis shows the percent of patients who have a stenosis greater than the stenosis value on the X axis. The ability of stenting and atherectomy to lower restenosis is shown by a shift of their cumulative distribution function curves to the left. If a dichotomous definition of restenosis is applied, the intersection of each curve with a late diameter stenosis of 50% (vertical line) corresponds to a dichotomous restenosis rate of 43% for angioplasty, 31% for atherectomy, and 26% for stenting. (From Kuntz RE, et al. Novel approach to the analysis of restenosis. *J Am Coll Cardiol* 1992;19:1493.)

that have been able to deliver a lower restenosis rate than balloon angioplasty have done so by providing a larger acute lumen diameter (more acute gain), rather than by reducing the loss index (Fig. 22.16).

The central importance of the acute postprocedure geometry to the late result, however, does not reduce the importance of factors that modulate the loss index. Biologic variables such as diabetes have a major effect on increasing loss index and restenosis for any given postprocedure result, and there has been a relentless search for drugs or procedural variations that could decrease the loss index "tax" rate. Although manipulating procedure-related

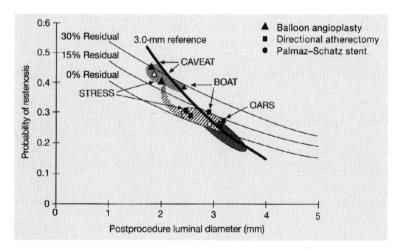

Figure 22.16 Except for anti-proliferative therapies (i.e., drug-eluting stents and brachytherapy), the strongest determinants of the probability of restenosis (late diameter stenosis of >50%) are a large postprocedure lumen diameter and a low residual percent stenosis. Once these variables are taken into account, it no longer matters which device had been used—it is the result and not the device that matters. Balloon angioplasty *(triangles)* thus has a 2- to 2.3-mm lumen with a 40% restenosis rate, whereas stenting has a 2.9- to 3.2-mm lumen with a 20% restenosis rate (slightly worse results with stenting in the STRESS study are shown, as well). Directional atherectomy *(squares)* has an angioplastylike result in CAVEAT but a more stentlike result in BOAT and OARS (see Chapters 23 and 24). (Modified from Kuntz RE, et al. A generalized model of restenosis following conventional balloon angioplasty, stenting, and directional atherectomy. *J Am Coll Cardiol* 1993;21:15.)

variables (such as duration of conventional balloon inflation) have been unrewarding, and while trials of numerous systemic drug regimens (aspirin, nifedipine, ticlopidine, steroids, prolonged heparin administration, fish oil, mevinolin, ketanserin, etc.) have shown little or no beneficial effect against restenosis, two modalities have now shown important benefits against late loss and consequently, restenosis.

Brachytherapy

The delivery of 2,000 cGy (see Chapter 2) of either beta (90) or gamma (91) radiation to the tissues of the coronary arterial wall greatly retards intimal proliferation and the recurrent restenosis rate within bare-metal coronary stents. While some benefit was seen in some studies of atherectomy debulking of in-stent restenosis, the combination of mechanical dilation plus catheter-delivered brachytherapy is an effective treatment for in-stent restenosis, although much of the benefit tends to be lost by 5-year follow-up. Trials of primary radiation at the time of stenting were less impressive, and the inhibition of stent endothelialization by radiation treatment clearly increases risk of delayed stent thrombosis, which may then occur up to 6 to 9 months after treatment. Since the release of drug-eluting stents in 2003, however, the clinical use of coronary brachytherapy has diminished markedly.

Drug-Eluting Stents

Contrary to the frustrations involved with finding an effective systemic drug to inhibit restenosis after angioplasty or stenting, it is now clear that the local release of rapamycin (sirolimus; 92,93) and its derivatives or of paclitaxel (94,95) from a polymer matrix over the 30 days after stent implantation can substantially reduce inflammation and smooth muscle cell proliferation within a stent (see Chapter 24). In this context, an effective drug reduces in-stent late loss from the usual 1 mm (500 microns on each side of the stent) to as little as 0.2 mm (100 micron on each side of the stent) (95a). This dramatically reduces the restenosis rate after initial stent implantation or after secondary implantation of a drug-eluting stent within an in-stent restenosis. To provide maximal benefit, the length of such drug-eluting stents should generally be somewhat (approximately 10 mm) longer than that of the lesion being treated to prevent injured but nontreated diseased areas at each end of a shorter stent. Because drug-eluting stents also have somewhat delayed endothelialization compared with bare-metal stents, anti-platelet therapy (aspirin and clopidogrel) must be extended (3 to 6 months versus 2 to 4 weeks).

LONG-TERM RESULTS OF ANGIOPLASTY

Although the preceding discussion of restenosis emphasizes mechanistic and quantitative angiographic analyses

of late outcome (with an emphasis on the status of the treated site), *the long-term clinical benefit of coronary angioplasty as a strategy for treating patients with coronary artery disease derives from its ability to prevent subsequent ischemic events.* The traditional measure of this ability has been the freedom of angioplasty patients from *any* subsequent events, including death, myocardial infarction, or a repeat revascularization procedure (either repeat PTCA or late bypass surgery). As trials of new devices have unfolded, however, it has become increasingly important to distinguish whether a late cardiac event consists of repeat target lesion or target vessel revascularization (i.e., TLR or TVR) owing to restenosis of the dilated segment, or whether the late event is a result of a non-TVR caused by he unchecked natural history of coronary artery disease (i.e., the persistence or progression of disease elsewhere in the coronary tree; 89). In general, the events that develop during the restenosis window—the first 8 to 12 months after successful angioplasty—reflect predominantly restenosis of the treated segment. Given the quiescence of the dilated lesion thereafter, most of the events that develop after 12 months reflect the progression of disease at other sites (Fig. 22.17; 37).

One-year data from 838 patients with single-vessel disease in the 1985–1986 registry (96) shows mortality in 1.6%, MI in 1.9%, repeat angioplasty in 18.1%, and bypass surgery in 6.2% after balloon angioplasty. In subsequent studies of bare-metal stenting, the incidence of repeat revascularization within the first year in patients with single vessel intervention fell to 12 to 15% (97). With current drug-eluting stents, the 1- and 2-year TLR rates are as low as

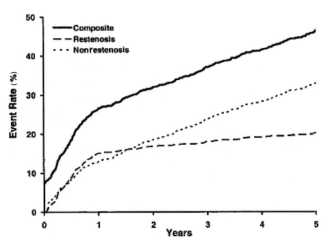

Figure 22.17   Five-year clinical follow-up after bare-metal stenting. This graph shows that the incidence of adverse clinical events owing to restenosis reaches its peak by 1 year and is then relatively flat to 5 years. Cumulative adverse events (solid line), however, continue to increase during years 2 through 5 and actually outnumber restenosis events by year 5. This illustrates the importance of aggressive risk factor modification on long-term clinical well-being, even if the incidence of restenotic events in the treated segments were to fall to zero. (From Cutlip DE, Chhabra A, Baim DS, et al. Beyond restenosis—five year clinical outcomes from second-generation coronary stent trials. *Circulation* 2004;110:1226–1230, with permission.)

4 and 6%, respectively, whereas bare-metal stents rates remain 16 and 20% at 1 and 2 years, respectively (92–95). No matter how low the in-stent restenosis rate falls, it is important to realize that this cannot address late failures of the nontarget lesion sites owing to progression of disease (37), and thus underscores the importance of aggressive attention to risk-factor reduction in the post-PCI patient.

The repeat revascularization rates for patients with diabetes or multivessel disease are clearly higher than those in nondiabetic patients with single-vessel disease (see below). In the 1985–1986 registry (96), patients with multivessel disease had a higher in-hospital mortality (1.7 versus 0.2%), more common adverse events within the first year after hospital discharge (mortality in 2.8%, MI in 3.4%), but a significantly higher need for repeat revascularization. This pattern has been borne out in the randomized trials comparing angioplasty with bypass surgery in patients with multivessel coronary artery disease, where up to 35% of angioplasty patients (but only 5% of surgery patients) require a repeat revascularization within the first year after treatment (98,99) Even with bare-metal stenting in the ARTS study (100), PCI patients with multivessel disease still showed a roughly 20% greater need for repeat revascularization than surgery patients (Fig. 22.18). By comparison, 4 to 6% TVR rates for drug-eluting stents should allow PCI to offer similarly low late repeat revascularization rates as surgery, although trials of drug-eluting stents in patients with multivessel disease are still in progress at this time.

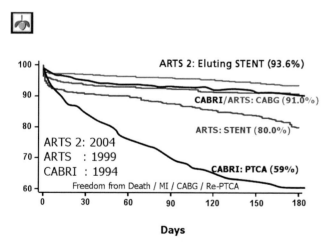

Figure 22.18 Improving results of PCI compared with bypass surgery (CABG). In a series of trials spanning a decade from 1994–2004, the 180-day event-free survival of bypass surgery has remained 91%. This was markedly superior to PTCA in CABRI (32% absolute difference) owing to the effect of restenosis. In ARTS, this deficit improved to 11% with the use of bare-metal stenting. In the ARTS 2 trial, the event-free survival of drug-eluting stents was actually superior to that of bypass by 2.6% at 180 deep, with major adverse clinical events of 10.4 and 11.6 respectively at 1 year follow-up. (Courtesy of Prof. Patrick Serruys and Legrand VM, Serruys PW, Unger F, et al. Three-year outcome after coronary stenting versus bypass surgery for the treatment of multivessel disease (ARTS). *Circulation* 2004;109:1114, with permission).

Special attention will need to be paid to patients with diabetes mellitus, since they have significantly higher TVR rates in both the drug-eluting and bare-metal stent arms (10 and 28.8%, respectively; 101).

CURRENT INDICATIONS

With the improvements in equipment and technique described above, coronary angioplasty has become the dominant form of coronary revascularization (1,000,000 PCI versus 350,000 CABG procedures; 5). This growth in PCI beyond the concomitant reduction in bypass surgery volume suggests that the use of angioplasty has moved beyond the narrow group of patients who would have undergone bypass surgery (as had been suggested in the original NHLBI registry guidelines), to the point where it is now also seen as an alternative to medical therapy in selected patients. Data from Emory between 1981 and 1988 (102) thus showed that the percent of diagnostic catheterization patients who went on to coronary angioplasty increased from 4.3 to 30.3%, whereas the percent undergoing bypass surgery decreased only from 44.0 to 28.5%. Nearly as much angioplasty growth over that period was thus explained by contraction of the fraction of patients treated medically (from 51.7 to 41.2%) as by the shift from surgery to angioplasty. Similar patterns are shown in a survey from 1989 to 1997 at the 17 U.S. sites that participated in the Bypass Angioplasty Revascularization Investigation (BARI), where the percent of all revascularizations that were catheter based (versus surgical) increased from 52.2% to 62% by 1997 (103).

Because the person who is responsible for case selection is often the person who will perform the angioplasty, it is critically important that operators have a full understanding of the indications and outcomes so that only suitable patients are treated. The issues that need to be addressed include the following: (a) How compelling is the clinical justification for revascularization, (b) do the "culprit" lesions have anatomic features that would give a reasonable level of safety and probability of successful PCI, (c) does PCI compare favorably (or at least equally) with the other therapeutic options such as bypass surgery or continued medical therapy in this patient, and (d) what combination of interventional devices would offer the best short- and long-term outcomes. This evaluation process thus involves integration of complex clinical, angiographic, pathophysiologic, and technical knowledge to decide that a particular patient is or is not an angioplasty candidate, and therefore constitutes an important component of angioplasty operator training (see Chapter 1).

With the rapid growth of coronary angioplasty, there have been a series of position papers outlining the "correct" use of this procedure (15–17,103a). The ACC/AHA first published Angioplasty Guidelines in 1988, revising them in 1993, 2001, and 2004. These statements are useful compilations that outline some well-accepted indications and contraindications for coronary angioplasty and are available online at http://www.acc.org/clinical/topic/topic.htm. It is beyond the scope of this chapter to review these guidelines in detail, and the reader is referred to this excellent source material and summaries (103a). The discussion below includes some general commentary on specific situations.

Mild Stable Angina or Asymptomatic Patients with Ischemia

Patients with stable angina or asymptomatic myocardial ischemia are considered as candidates for coronary intervention if they have objective evidence of ischemia, hemodynamically significant lesions in one or two coronary arteries that subtend a moderate or large area of viable myocardium, and a high likelihood of success and a low risk of morbidity and mortality for PCI (16). It is clear that most of these patients in this category could be treated medically, and it is important to note that randomized trials of medical therapy versus PCI such as RITA-2 have failed to show benefit in freedom from death and MI, although they have shown less angina and better exercise tolerance in the PCI group (104,105). The Asymptomatic Cardiac Ischemia Pilot (ACIP) study (106) randomized 558 patients suitable for revascularization by PTCA or CABG to three treatment strategies: angina-guided drug therapy, angina plus ischemia-guided drug therapy, and revascularization by PTCA or CABG (102 PTCA and 90 CABG). At 2 years of follow-up, the revascularization patients had less death or MI (4.7% versus 8.8% for the ischemia-guided group and 12.1% for the angina-guided group, $P < 0.01$). This suggests that outcomes of revascularization with PTCA are very favorable compared with medical therapy in patients with asymptomatic ischemia on treadmill testing or ambulatory monitoring and severe anatomic coronary disease favorable for PCI.

Of note (in contradistinction to the earlier version), the 2005 Guidelines no longer make the distinction between single-vessel and multivessel disease for nondiabetic patients. The issue of PCI versus CABG in multivessel disease has been addressed by several large randomized trials that demonstrate (in appropriately selected patients with multivessel coronary disease) that an initial strategy of standard PTCA yields similar overall outcomes (e.g., death, MI) compared with initial revascularization with coronary artery bypass (98,99). For example, in BARI the 5-year survival for those assigned to PTCA (note: performed with neither stents nor IIb/IIIa receptor blockers) was 86.3% versus 89.3% for those assigned to CABG ($P = 0.19$), with similar freedom from Q-wave MI of 78.7% and 80.4%, respectively. By 5 years of follow-up, however, nearly 54% of those assigned to PTCA had undergone additional revascularization procedures, compared with only 8% of the patients assigned to CABG. It is important to note that patients with diabetes mellitus were an important exception

to the survival neutrality of PCI versus CABG in BARI, having a significantly lower 5-year survival (65.5% versus 80.6% for CABG, $P = 0.003$) if they received at least one internal mammary artery graft (107). Interestingly, most of the mortality in the diabetic patients followed myocardial infarction, and one important difference between CABG and PCI is that only the former protects the distal myocardium against subsequent plaque rupture in untreated portions of the vulnerable proximal epicardial segments (108,109). Furthermore, the benefit of surgery is not absolute, since diabetic patients enrolled in the BARI registry failed to show a similar advantage for CABG over PCI (110), suggesting that physician judgment in the selection of diabetic patients for PCI may be an important factor. This important question regarding the management of diabetic patients with multivessel coronary artery disease will be addressed using drug-eluting stents in the upcoming FREEDOM trial.

Moderate Stable and Unstable Angina

It is recommended the PCI be done in patients with moderate or severe symptoms (angina Class II to IV, unstable angina or non–ST-elevation MI) with one or more significant lesions that subtend a moderate or large area of viable myocardium and are suitable for PCI with a high likelihood of success and low risk of morbidity or mortality. Although some studies of unstable angina such as TIMI-IIIB (111) and VANQWISH (112) have shown little benefit of routine PCI over aggressive medical therapy, more recent studies such as FRISC II (113), which used IIb./IIIa receptor blockers and stenting, have shown a 22% reduction (from 12.1 to 8.4%) in death or MI at 6 months and a 50% reduction in hospital readmission, compared with a conservative strategy in which PCI was reserved for strongly positive exercise test results. Similar benefit was seen in the TACTICS-TIMI 18 study (114), with a reduction in death, MI, and rehospitalization (from 19.4 to 15.9%, $P = 0.0025$), as well as death or MI (from 9.5 to 7.3%, $P < 0.05$) at 6 months.

ST-Elevation Myocardial Infarction

The treatment of acute MI has undergone a major revolution over the past 15 years, with the recognition that intracoronary thrombosis is the final mechanism of vessel occlusion and the understanding that prompt re-establishment of vessel patency offers significant clinical benefit (17,115). Although current thrombolytic regimens can open nearly 75% of infarct vessels within 90 minutes of intravenous administration, approximately 15% of vessels fail to open in response to thrombolytic therapy, only half the open vessels have normal (TIMI grade 3) flow, and at least 10% of vessels opened by thrombolysis either reocclude or cause recurrent angina during hospitalization owing to the persistence of an underlying high-grade atherosclerotic stenosis. On the other hand, trials comparing thrombolysis to primary angioplasty have consistently shown lower mortality (5.0 versus 7.0%, $P = 0.0002$), less nonfatal reinfarction (3.0% versus 7.0%, $P = 0.0003$), and less hemorrhagic stroke (0.05% versus 1%, $P = 0.0001$) with primary angioplasty (both PTCA and stenting) (Fig. 22.19; 116).

The current PCI guidelines thus recommend that primary PCI should be performed in patients with STEMI who present within 12 hours of symptom onset, if performed in a timely fashion (medical contact-to-balloon or door-to-balloon time ≤90 minutes) by persons skilled in the procedure, working in an appropriate laboratory environment (16). This includes patients with severe congestive heart failure and/or pulmonary edema (Killip Class 3) presenting within 12 hours of the onset of infarction, particularly if they are younger than 75 years old (116,117). It may be reasonable to perform primary PCI in older patients with good prior functional status, or patients with onset of symptoms within the prior 12 to 24 hours who present with severe congestive heart failure, hemodynamic or electrical instability, or persistent ischemic symptoms. Patients with an acute ST-elevation myocardial infarction may undergo primary PCI safely at community hospitals that do not offer elective angioplasty, as long as a trained team and trained operators are present (17,118). Studies such as DANAMI-2 (119) suggest alternatively that interhospital transfer for primary PCI at an angioplasty center is still preferred over thrombolysis, even if the treatment delay would be up to 45 minutes (frequently possible if the receiving hospital team uses the transfer time to come in and set up the cath lab). Patients with anterior wall STEMI who have failed to reperfuse after thrombolytic therapy have also been shown to benefit from salvage PCI performed within the first 8 hours after symptom onset, with a reduction in rates of in-hospital death and combined death and congestive heart failure up to 1 year in the Randomized Evaluation of Rescue PCI with Combined Utilization Endpoints (RESCUE) trial (120).

Although primary PCI can restore epicardial flow promptly, many patients fail to have complete restoration of myocardial perfusion (reflected by impaired or persistent myocardial blush and delayed resolution of ST-segment elevation). In fact, this is the original situation in which no-reflow was described. Although this may simply reflect myocardial, endothelial swelling, or white cell aggregation, it may also reflect distal embolization of thrombus or atherosclerotic debris released during treatment of the infarct lesion. Platelet glycoprotein IIb/IIIa receptor blockers have shown only modest benefit in this regard (121,122), and studies of routine thrombectomy or distal embolic protection with a distal occlusion/aspiration device have so far failed to show significant improvement in ST-segment resolution or radionuclide-measured myocardial infarct size as a percent of the left ventricle (see Chapter 23). This does not reduce the benefit of thrombectomy in vessels with a large thrombus burden or use of embolic protection in selected patients in patients. Other modalities such as

moderate systemic hypothermia (32 to 34°C), local infusion of hyperbaric oxygen, and metabolic support for the reperfused myocardium are still under study for their potential to reduce infarct size and enhance myocardial recovery after primary PCI for acute myocardial infarction (115).

Prior Coronary Bypass Surgery

Bypass surgery provides excellent early symptomatic benefit, but 40% of saphenous vein conduits will be occluded and many more will develop severe narrowing within 10 years of surgery (118). Although only 2% of such patients require angioplasty or repeat bypass surgery within the first 5 years, 31% will require a repeat revascularization by year 12 (including 20% reoperation and 15% PTCA; 123). Internal mammary conduits have a better long-term track record (124), but some of these grafts develop significant early stenosis at their distal anastomotic site. Finally, patients with previous bypass surgery frequently develop new or progressive disease beyond a graft insertion site or in a nongrafted vessel over time. By these various mechanisms, it is common for the patient who has undergone a previous bypass operation to develop recurrent angina.

Although recurrent angina can be managed by repeat bypass surgery, repeat surgery is a higher-risk procedure in a patient population that is older and sicker than those undergoing initial bypass. With the progressive growth of coronary angioplasty, many such patients can be managed by catheter-based intervention on the diseased graft or a stenotic native vessel, so angioplasty of postoperative patients accounts for approximately 20% of current volume. Although angioplasty has lower in-hospital mortality than reoperation (1.2 versus 6.8%), late mortality is similar, and angioplasty carries a higher incidence of repeat interventions including a 24% 5-year risk of requiring reoperation (125,126). The approach varies according to the timing and location of the culprit lesion.

Vein-graft stenoses that present within the first year after surgery are caused most commonly by intimal hyperplasia and respond quite well to balloon dilatation. Late vein-graft stenoses (average 8 years postsurgery) are caused more commonly by diffuse atherosclerosis that has a distinct tendency to fragment and/or embolize into the distal coronary bed during dilatation (127; Fig. 22.20). The SAFER trial using the PercuSurge distal occlusion aspiration embolic protection system showed that atheroembolic material was recovered routinely during SVG stenting and that embolic protection offered a 42% reduction in major adverse clinical events at 30 days compared with stenting over a conventional guidewire (49). The FIRE trial showed that similar benefit is provided by a distal filter device (50; see also Chapter 24). Stenting was shown to provide better freedom from saphenous vein graft (SVG) restenosis than PTCA in the small SAphenous VEin graft Disease (SAVED) trial (128), making stenting the preferred therapy for the

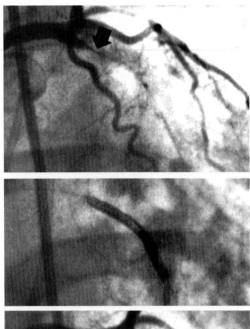

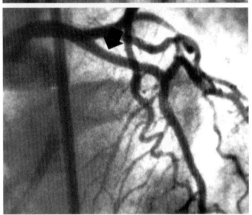

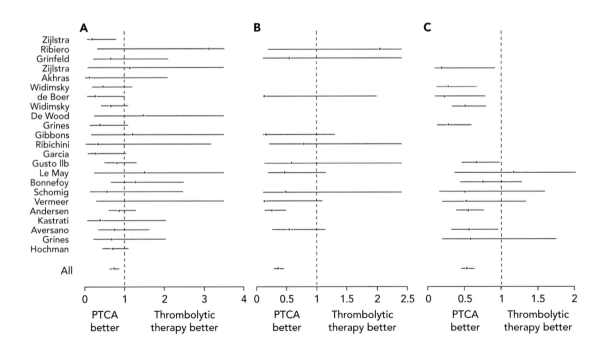

Figure 22.19 Primary angioplasty for acute myocardial infarction (MI). **Top frame.** A primary angioplasty procedure showing baseline total occlusion of the proximal left anterior descending (arrow). Two hours into acute anterior MI with cardiogenic shock. **Center frame.** Primary angioplasty is shown with placement of a perfusion balloon across the area of occlusion. **Bottom frame.** Postangioplasty, there is no residual stenosis (arrow) and brisk antegrade flow. Despite a peak CPK approaching 2,000, this patient's hemodynamic status recovered promptly, with normal wall motion on gated nuclear ventriculography 6 weeks later. **Bottom graphic.** Meta-analysis of 7,739 patients with acute STEMI randomized to thrombolysis or primary PCI in 23 trials, showing significant reduction in mortality (A, from roughly 7 to 5%), nonfatal reinfarction (B, from roughly 7 to 3%), and stroke (C, from 2 to 1%) for a reduction of combined adverse end points from 14 to 8% by primary angioplasty. (From Keeley EC, Boura JA, Grines CL. Primary angioplasty versus intravenous thrombolytic therapy for acute myocardial infarction: a quantitative review of 23 randomised trials. *Lancet* 2003;361:13–20, with permission.)

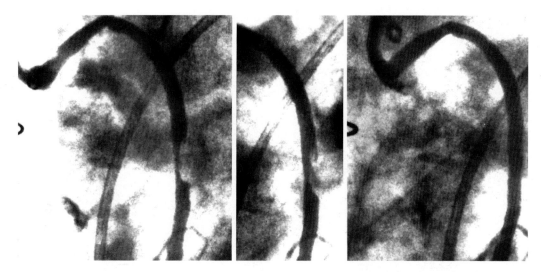

Figure 22.20 Saphenous vein graft intervention. **Left.** Eccentric stenosis in the midportion of an 8-year-old saphenous vein graft to the left anterior descending. **Center.** Following conventional balloon angioplasty, there is marked disruption of the plaque and elastic recoil, leaving a 70% residual stenosis. **Right.** Following placement of a single balloon-expandable stent, there is a smooth lumen with no residual stenosis. These excellent acute results, plus the favorable late restenosis rate, make stenting the treatment of choice for the focally diseased saphenous vein graft, although today stent placement would be performed in conjunction with distal embolic protection (see Chapter 23) and might make use of a drug-eluting stent (see Chapter 24).

treatment of the diseased vein grafts, and preliminary data with the drug-eluting stents in SVG are encouraging (93). But it is important to note that about half of the symptomatic recurrences in SVG stenting are owing to progression of disease at other nonstented portions of the SVG (129,130), begging the question as to whether the availability of low-restenotic-rate drug-eluting stents and distal embolic protection make it beneficial to "reline" much of the length of a graft with a focal stenosis and signs of more diffuse degeneration.

In addition to plaque friability, older grafts frequently contain thrombus, which may embolize during attempted angioplasty. Grafts with large thrombotic filling defects were once pretreated by intracoronary infusion of a thrombolytic agent (e.g., urokinase 50,000 to 100,000 IU/hour or recombinant tissue plasminogen activator [rt-PA] 20 mg over 20 minutes) to dissolve the clot and allow the underlying stenosis to be dilated (Fig. 22.21), but are now generally treated with rheolytic thrombectomy (Possis AngioJet) to remove thrombi before definitive mechanical intervention (131; see also Chapter 23). Of course, the other option in a patient with a failing high-risk vein graft lesion is to open the corresponding native vessel, which is more reasonable now with the availability of new technologies for crossing chronic total occlusions, but patients with multiple failed and/or totally occluded SVGs should generally be considered for reoperation.

Unlike saphenous veins, internal mammary artery grafts are generally resistant to disease, with a 10-year patency rate of greater than 90% (124). Still, some patients develop recurrent angina early (within 6 months) after bypass surgery owing to stenosis of the internal mammary/native artery anastomosis. These lesions can be dilated effectively using low-profile, trackable dilatation catheters (132) with a moderate (approximately 20%) restenosis rate (Fig. 22.21). Current bare metal and drug-eluting stents can track through internal mammary grafts to treat these distal anastomotic lesions as well. When evaluating patients with recurrent ischemia in the distribution of an internal mammary graft, it is also important to investigate the possibility of subclavian or brachiocephalic stenosis proximal to the internal mammary origin, which can now be treated by angioplasty or stent placement. Limited data regarding angioplasty of gastroepiploic artery grafts suggest similar results of angioplasty in these arterial conduits (133). Although technically also a graft, the response of the diffuse lesions characteristic of cardiac homografts (accelerated allograft vasculopathy) to coronary angioplasty have not been well characterized (134).

Total Coronary Occlusion

Although total occlusion was initially a contraindication to attempting angioplasty, it has been clear since the early to mid-1980s that many chronic total occlusions can be dilated successfully. The main reason to attempt such a procedure is to relieve angina caused by an inadequate collateral supply to viable distal myocardium (Fig. 22.22), but there is growing evidence that opening chronic total occlusions can also improve regional wall motion and perhaps even improve survival (perhaps by establishing another collateral source to protect against progression of

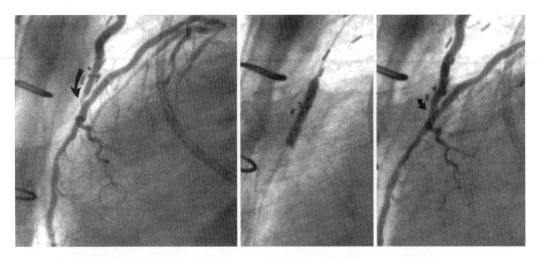

Figure 22.21   LIMA angioplasty. This 58-year-old man developed recurrent angina 5 months after bypass surgery that had involved grafting of the left internal mammary artery (LIMA) to the left anterior descending (LAD) coronary artery (whose proximal segments had exhibited early restenosis after two rotational atherectomy procedures). **Left.** In the left lateral projection, severe stenosis (*curved arrow*) is seen at the distal anastomosis where the IMA meets the LAD. **Center.** Inflation of a 3.0-mm over-the-wire angioplasty balloon at 70 psi. **Right.** Posttreatment angiography shows 20% residual stenosis. This site and timing (as well as the favorable response to conventional balloon angioplasty) are typical for postoperative problems with the internal mammary graft, although it would be more common now to use a drug-eluting stent to treat this type of lesion.

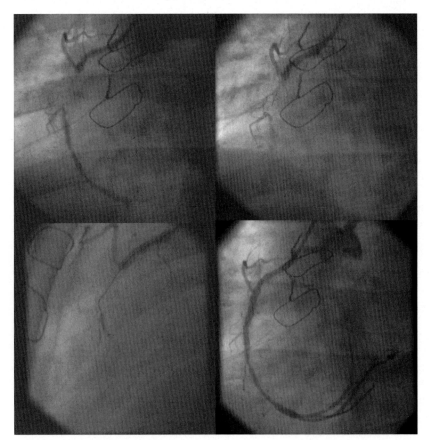

Figure 22.22   Chronic total occlusion of the right coronary in a patient with prior bypass surgery and an occluded graft. **Top left.** Some antegrade filling was evident owing to bridging collaterals, so that placement of a second catheter for contralateral injection of additional collateral-supplying vessels was not necessary. **Top right.** The IntraLuminal Therapeutics Safe-Cross guidewire was advanced, using optical guidance and radiofrequency (RF) ablation. **Bottom left.** A stiff (4.5 gm) conventional guidewire was substituted to make the sharp angulation into the distal vessel. **Bottom right**–Final result. (From Baim DS, et al. Utility of the Safe-Cross-guided radiofrequency total occlusion crossing system in chronic coronary total occlusions (results of the GREAT Registry Study). *Am J Cardiol* 2004;94: 853–858, with permission.)

contralateral disease; 135). The main challenge in angioplasty of a total occlusion is the need to pass a guidewire through the area of occlusion and into the vessel lumen beyond. This is best done by crossing through the path of least resistance, i.e., the "latent" true lumen, without causing vascular dissection or perforation in the attempt to do so. The traditional approach is to use a series of guidewires (progressing from soft- to stiff-tipped) to gently probe the stump of the occlusion. The wire is then rotated and advanced millimeter by millimeter through the total occlusion until it emerges into the distal coronary artery beyond. At each point, the direction of the wire tip is guided by feel as well as careful fluoroscopy (in multiple projections), and with simultaneous injection of the occluded vessel and the contralateral vessel, which supplies distal collaterals.

Even in experienced hands, this approach has a primary success rate in chronic total occlusion of only 60 to 70% (135,136), owing mostly to inability to advance the guidewire across the occlusion. The presence of one or more chronic total occlusions is thus one of the most common reasons for sending a patient to bypass surgery rather than attempting angioplasty (137). The success of crossing such lesions has improved with the introduction of stiffer and lubricious coated guidewires as described above. A variety of other approaches have been evaluated, including the low-speed rotational angioplasty, ultrasound vibrational angioplasty, and the excimer laser guidewire (138), but none has significantly increased the ability to cross the chronic total occlusion without increasing the incidence of vessel perforation or extensive local dissection. Still newer techniques have been introduced recently, including the LuMend Frontrunner (blunt microdissection with a 0.039-inch double-jaw catheter; 139) and the IntraLuminal Therapeutics Safe-Cross wire (optical computerized reflectometry to detect proximity to the vessel wall, plus the ability to deliver radiofrequency energy to the catheter tip to facilitate advancement of forward-looking imaging; 140). Each device has shown a roughly 70% secondary success rate after the failure of good-faith attempts using conventional guidewires, with low (1 to 2%) incidence of perforation.

Once the guidewire has been passed into the distal vessel, treatment of the total occlusion proceeds as does any other catheter-based intervention. Rarely, it may not be possible to pass even a 1.5-mm low-profile balloon through the occluded segment over the guidewire, and rotational atherectomy or a small (0.9-mm diameter) excimer laser catheter may be needed (see Chapter 23), followed by angioplasty and stenting. Randomized trials have shown that bare metal stents have a restenosis rate of 32% in chronic total occlusions, compared with 74% with balloon angioplasty alone (141,142) Preliminary data with drug eluting stents are encouraging, so that maintaining long-term patency should not be a challenge if primary wire crossing can be achieved.

Left Main Intervention

Significant left main (LM) disease has traditionally been an unequivocal indication for bypass surgery. One exception was "protected" left main lesions, in which the presence of a patent bypass graft to either the LAD or circumflex made the lesion functionally the proximal part of the other left coronary branch. While these lesions have been stented for a number of years, the "unprotected" left main has remained categorized as a high-risk procedure (143). Early work with PTCA showed that acute procedural success was favorable, particularly in patients with good LV function treated electively (144). But patients with poor LV function had acute in-hospital complications >20%. More concerning was the tendency for restenosis to present as sudden death, which has led to routine angiographic restudy at 2 to 3 months, followed by elective surgery for restenotic lesions (144–147). With the advent of DES, the concept of PCI of unprotected LM has gained further interest and is being explored in several small registries (148). Although placement of a drug-eluting stent in the ostial or midshaft portions of the left main is generally straightforward, treatment of distal bifurcation left main lesions requires special techniques (see Chapters 23 and 24) and often hemodynamic support (see Chapter 19). At the present time, however, such treatment should probably not be offered broadly to patients who have good surgical options.

FINANCIAL AND REGULATORY CONSIDERATIONS

Because coronary angioplasty is performed in a cardiac catheterization laboratory under local anesthesia, it is attended by substantially lower in-hospital costs than coronary bypass surgery. On the other hand, this cost benefit has been partially eroded by the greater need for repeat procedures to treat restenosis within the first year. Although drug-eluting stents decrease this need, they substantially increase the acute procedural costs. So the net cost savings thus depend on the balance among these variables. In general, however, current interventional practices have proven either cost-saving or cost-effective relative to surgery, and they offer less patient morbidity, faster return to work, equivalent mortality benefit and symptom relief (barring the restenosis). PCI is thus usually preferred when anatomically possible. Since the decision is being made by the same operator (the cardiologist who performs the diagnostic catheterization frequently makes the decision about treatment and then performs the coronary angioplasty), the large expense associated with catheter revascularization has increasingly made angioplasty a target for scrutiny in the managed-care environment.

In addition to issues about the appropriateness of angioplasty procedures and markedly different usage rates across the country, there is also a major question about whether every hospital should offer bypass surgery or angioplasty. In fact, only about 1,500 of the nation's 7,000 hospitals do so, but there is continued pressure on those that do not to open such programs. Data from a nationwide study of 217,836 Medicare beneficiaries who underwent coronary angioplasty (149) clearly show excess mortality and emergency surgery rates in hospitals that perform <200 angioplasty procedures per year.

These issues also apply to the training and continued caseload for angioplasty operators (150,151). Early in the development of coronary angioplasty, physicians active in diagnostic catheterization learned to perform angioplasty by attending live demonstration courses and watching or assisting on a small number of procedures (i.e., 10 to 20) under the guidance of a knowledgeable operator. Given the ever-increasing complexity of the procedure, however, virtually all new angioplasty operators since the mid-1980s have received formal training consisting of a third (or third and fourth) year of interventional fellowship beyond completion of their training in diagnostic coronary angiography. Those fellowships are now approved by the Accreditation Council for Graduate Medical Education (ACGME; see Chapter 1) and require the interventional trainee to perform a minimum of 250 procedures (152). After fellowship, operators who maintain an interventional load of >75 cases per year generally have a lower rate of risk-adjusted complications than lower-volume operators, including in the stent era (153). Although some data suggest that operators slightly below this number can maintain good outcomes by working in supportive very-high-volume centers (154), this may not extend to the many operators who perform less than half of the recommended annual caseload and work in less-supportive low-volume centers. Since the American Board of Internal Medicine began offering a Certificate of Additional Qualification in Interventional Cardiology to graduates of approved fellowships in 1999, fewer than 4,500 of an estimated 8,000 cardiologists who perform percutaneous coronary intervention have met the eligibility criteria, taken, and passed the certification exam. As catheter-based interventions continue to evolve toward progressively more challenging clinical and anatomic situations, and as the development of new technologies for coronary intervention continues, this gap between committed interventional cardiologists and casual practitioners is thus likely to continue to grow.

THE ROLE OF BALLOON ANGIOPLASTY IN THE NEW DEVICE ERA

Between its introduction in 1977 and 1990, conventional balloon angioplasty (POBA, or plain old balloon angioplasty) was the *only* mechanical intervention available for percutaneous coronary revascularization. The choice of devices was very much like the situation described by Mark Twain: "To the man with a hammer, everything looks like a nail." In contrast, the period from 1988 through 1994 saw unparalleled investigation of a wave of new stent and atherectomy devices. The first of the new devices (directional coronary atherectomy) was approved by the FDA in 1990, with approval of two other atherectomy devices (rotational and extraction atherectomy), excimer lasers, and two balloon-expandable stents by 1994. Newer classes of devices (thrombectomy, distal protection, brachytherapy, total occlusion crossing, etc.) have continued to be introduced, progressively reducing the role of conventional balloon angioplasty as a stand-alone tool for coronary intervention (Fig. 22.23).

Operators must master these new technologies if they provide advantages in terms of (a) the predictability of the

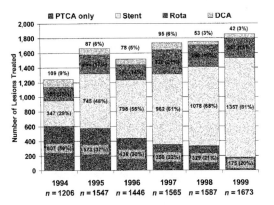

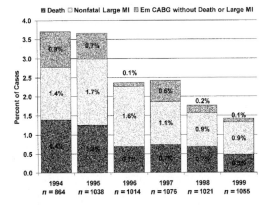

Figure 22.23 Rapid replacement of balloon angioplasty by stenting and atherectomy modalities in the early new device era (1994–1999). **Top.** During this 5-year period, there was a dramatic increase in the use of stenting (from 29 to 68% of interventions) as well as ongoing use of atherectomy (directional plus rotational atherectomy from approximately 22% of interventions), but a corresponding decrease in the use of stand-alone balloon angioplasty (from 50% to 21% of interventions). Stenting is now used in >98% of interventions, with atherectomy and stand-alone balloon angioplasty <5% each. **Bottom.** The clinical benefits of the new device trend were reflected in the ability to treat a broader range of lesion types, an increase in primary success rate (from 92 to 98%), and a halving in the incidence of major complications (death, large MI [Q-MI or CK greater than five times normal] or emergency surgery from 3.7 to 1.8%). The use of intravenous platelet glycoprotein IIb/IIIa receptor blockers in the approximately 20% of patients in whom a perfect mechanical result could not be achieved by catheter-based techniques may have also contributed to this improvement in adverse outcomes.

acute result, (b) the quality of the acute result (less residual stenosis), (c) the ability to treat a lesion that would have been refractory to conventional angioplasty, or (d) the ability to reduce the incidence of subsequent restenosis. The best example is the *balloon-expandable stent*, which triggered a paradigm shift, moving from a bailout device, to a provisional way to treat suboptimal PTCA results, to the default coronary treatment (now replaced by drug-eluting stents, as described above). Although this has reduced balloon angioplasty to more of an adjunctive treatment (for predilation to aid in device passage, or postdilation to improve the new device-created result) rather than a stand-alone treatment, I still believe that the skills, knowledge, and judgment derived from balloon angioplasty over the last 25 years will continue to form the foundation on which broader interventional skills are built during the years to come.

REFERENCES

1. Dotter CT, Judkins MP. Transluminal treatment of arteriosclerotic obstruction: description of a new technique and a preliminary report of its application. *Circulation* 1964;30:654.
2. Gruentzig A, Kumpe DA. Technique of percutaneous transluminal angioplasty with the Gruentzig balloon catheter. *AJR Am J Roentgenol* 1979;132:547.
3. Gruentzig AR, Senning A, Siegenthaler WE. Non-operative dilatation of coronary artery stenosis—percutaneous transluminal coronary angioplasty. *N Engl J Med* 1979;301:61.
4. King SB. Angioplasty from bench to bedside. *Circulation* 1996; 93:1621.
5. American Heart Association. *2004 Heart and Stroke Statistical Update.* Dallas, TX; American Heart Association, 2003.
6. Simpson JB, Baim DS, Robert EW, Harrison DC. A new catheter system for coronary angioplasty. *Am J Cardiol* 1982;49:1216.
7. Dervan JP, McKay RG, Baim DS. The use of an exchange wire in coronary angioplasty. *Cathet Cardiovasc Diagn* 1985;11:207.
8. Mauri L, Bonan R, Weiner BH, et al. Cutting balloon angioplasty for the prevention of restenosis: results of the Cutting Balloon Global Randomized Trial. *Am J Cardiol* 2002;90:1079–1083.
9. Albiero R, Silber S, Di Mario C, et al.; RESCUT Investigators. Cutting balloon versus conventional balloon angioplasty for the treatment of in-stent restenosis: results of the restenosis cutting balloon evaluation trial (RESCUT). *J Am Coll Cardiol* 2004;43: 943–949.
10. Carell ES, Schroth G, Ali A. Circumferential balloon rupture and catheter fracture due to entrapment in a calcified coronary stenosis. *Cathet Cardiovasc Diagn* 1994;32:346.
11. Tenaglia AN, Zidar JP, Jackman JD Jr, et al. Treatment of long coronary artery narrowings with long angioplasty balloon catheters. *Am J Cardiol* 1993;71:1274.
12. Plante S, Strauss BH, Goulet G, et al. Reuse of balloon catheters for coronary angioplasty: a potential cost-saving strategy? *J Am Coll Cardiol* 1994;24:1475.
13. Smith JJ, Henderson JA, Baim DS. The Food and Drug Administration and reprocessing of single-use medical devices: a revised policy and new questions. *J Vasc Intervent Radiol* 2002; 13:1179–1182.
14. Levine GN, Kern MJ, Berger PB, et al.; American Heart Association Diagnostic and Interventional Catheterization Committee and Council on Clinical Cardiology .Management of patients undergoing percutaneous coronary revascularization. *Ann Intern Med* 2003;139:123–136.
15. Guidelines for percutaneous transluminal coronary angioplasty. A report of the American College of Cardiology/ American Heart Association Task Force (Committee on Percutaneous Transluminal Coronary Angioplasty). *J Am Coll Cardiol* 1993;22:2033–2054.
16. Guidelines for percutaneous transluminal coronary angioplasty (update). A report of the American College of Cardiology/ American Heart Association Task Force (Subcommittee on Percutaneous Transluminal Coronary Angioplasty). 2005, in press.
16a. Wennberg DE, Lucas FL, Siewers AE, et al. Outcomes of percutaneous coronary interventions performed at centers without and with onsite coronary bypass graft surgery. *JAMA* 2004;292: 1961–8.
17. Antman EM, et al. ACC/AHA Guidelines for the Management of Patients With ST-Elevation Myocardial Infarction. A Report of the American College of Cardiology/American Heart Association Task Force on Practice Guidelines. Online @ Acc.org.
18. Blankenship JC, et al. Ad hoc coronary intervention. *Cathet Cardiovasc Intervent* 2000;49:130–134.
19. Fuster V, Dyken ML, Vokonas PS, Hennekens C. Aspirin as a therapeutic agent in cardiovascular disease: AHA medical scientific statement. *Circulation* 1993;87:659.
20. Solensky R. Drug allergy: desensitization and treatment of reactions to antibiotics and aspirin. *Clin Allergy Immunol* 2004;18: 585–606.
21. Early and sustained dual oral antiplatelet therapy following percutaneous coronary intervention: a randomized controlled trial. *JAMA* 2002;288:2411–2420.
22. Kong DF, Califf RA, Miller DP, et al. Outcomes of therapeutic agents that block the platelet glycoprotein IIb/IIIa integrin in ischemic heart disease. *Circulation* 1998;98:2829.
23. Effects of pretreatment with clopidogrel and aspirin followed by long-term therapy in patients undergoing percutaneous coronary intervention: the PCI-CURE study. *Lancet* 2001;358: 527–533.
24. Wong GC, Giugliano RP, Antman EM. Use of low-molecular-weight heparins in the management of acute coronary artery syndromes and percutaneous coronary intervention. *JAMA* 2003;289:331–342.
25. Lincoff AM, Kleiman NS, Kereiakes DJ, et al. Long-term efficacy of bivalirudin and provisional glycoprotein IIb/IIIa blockade vs heparin and planned glycoprotein IIb/IIIa blockade during percutaneous coronary revascularization: REPLACE-2 randomized trial. *JAMA* 2004;292:696–703.
25a. Gurm HS, et al. Effectiveness and safety of Bivalirudin during percutaneous coronary intervention in a single medical center. *Am J Cardiol* 2005;95:716–721.
26. Ferguson JJ, Dougherty KG, Gaos CM, et al. Relation between procedural activated coagulation time and the outcome after percutaneous transluminal coronary angioplasty. *J Am Coll Cardiol* 1994;23:1061.
27. Roubin GS, Douglas JS Jr, King SB 3rd, et al. Influence of balloon size on initial success, acute complications, and restenosis after percutaneous transluminal coronary angioplasty. *Circulation* 1988;78:557.
28. Nichols AB, Smith R, Berke AD. et al. Importance of balloon size in coronary angioplasty. *J Am Coll Cardiol* 1989;13:1094.
29. Chenu P, Zakhia R, Marchandise B, et al. Resistance of the atherosclerotic plaque during coronary angioplasty: a multivariable analysis of clinical and angiographic variables. *Cathet Cardiovasc Diagn* 1993;29:203.
30. Blankenship JC, Kruckoff MJ, Werns SW, et al. Comparison of slow oscillating versus fast balloon inflation strategies for coronary angioplasty. *Am J Cardiol* 1999;83:675.
31. Ohman EM, Marquis JF, Ricci DR, et al. A randomized comparison of the effects of gradual prolonged versus standard primary balloon inflation on early and late outcome: results of a multicenter clinical trial. *Circulation* 1994;89:1118.
32. Anderson HV, Roubin GS, Leimgruber PP, et al. Measurement of transstenotic pressure gradient during percutaneous transluminal coronary angioplasty. *Circulation* 1986;73:1223.
33. Bech GJW, Pijls NHJ, DeBruyne B, et al. Usefulness of fractional flow reserve to predict clinical outcome after balloon angioplasty. *Circulation* 1999;99:883.

34. Simpendorfer C, Belardi J, Bellamy G, et al. Frequency, management and follow-up of patients with acute coronary occlusions after percutaneous transluminal coronary angioplasty. *Am J Cardiol* 1987;59:267.

35. Rabah M, et al. Heparin after percutaneous intervention (HAPI): a prospective multicenter randomized trial of three heparin regimens after successful coronary intervention. *J Am Coll Cardiol* 1999;34:461–467.

36. Friedman HZ, Cragg DR, Glazier SM, et al. Randomized prospective evaluation of prolonged versus abbreviated intravenous heparin therapy after coronary angioplasty. *J Am Coll Cardiol* 1994;24:1214.

37. Cutlip DE, Chhabra A, Baim DS, et al. Beyond restenosis—five year clinical outcomes from second-generation coronary stent trials. *Circulation* 2004;110:1226–1230.

38. Herrmann HC. Prevention of cardiovascular events after percutaneous coronary intervention. *N Engl J Med* 2004;350: 2708–2710.

39. Grundy, SM, et al. Implications of recent clinical trials for the National Cholesterol Educational Program Adult Treatment Panel III Guidelines. *Circulation* 2004;110:227–239.

40. Sanborn TA, et al. The mechanism of transluminal angioplasty: evidence for formation of aneurysms in experimental atherosclerosis. *Circulation* 1983;68:1136.

41. Rensig BJ, et al. Quantitative angiographic assessment of elastic recoil after percutaneous transluminal coronary angioplasty. *Am J Cardiol* 1990;66:1039.

42. Rozenman Y, et al. Clinical and angiographic predictors of immediate recoil after successful coronary angioplasty and relation to late restenosis. *Am J Cardiol* 1993;72:1020.

43. Fischell TA, Derby G, Tse TM, Stadius ML. Coronary artery vasoconstriction after percutaneous transluminal coronary angioplasty: a quantitative arteriographic analysis. *Circulation* 1988; 78:1323.

44. Holmes DR Jr, Vlietstra RE, Mock MB, et al. Angiographic changes produced by percutaneous transluminal coronary angioplasty. *Am J Cardiol* 1983;51:676.

45. Black AJR, Namay DL, Niederman AL, et al. Tear or dissection after coronary angioplasty—morphologic correlates of an ischemic complication. *Circulation* 1989;79:1035.

46. Sanborn TA, Faxon DP, Waugh D, et al. Transluminal angioplasty in experimental atherosclerosis: analysis for embolization using an in vitro perfusion system. *Circulation* 1982;66: 917.

47. Saber RS, Edwards WD, Bailey KR, et al. Coronary embolization after balloon angioplasty or thrombolytic therapy—an autopsy study of 32 cases. *J Am Coll Cardiol* 1994;22:1283.

48. Piana R, Paik GY, Moscucci M, et al. Incidence and treatment of "no reflow" after percutaneous coronary intervention. *Circulation* 1994;89:2514.

49. Baim DS, Wahr D, George B, et al.; Saphenous vein graft Angioplasty Free of Emboli Randomized (SAFER) Trial Investigators. Randomized trial of a distal embolic protection device during percutaneous intervention of saphenous vein aorto-coronary bypass grafts. *Circulation* 2002;105:1285–1290.

50. Stone GW, et al. Randomized comparison of distal protection with a filter-based catheter and a balloon occlusion and aspiration system during percutaneous intervention of diseased saphenous vein aortocoronary bypass grafts. *Circulation* 2003;108: 548–553.

51. Saffitz JE, Rose TE, Oaks JB, Roberts WC. Coronary artery rupture during coronary angioplasty. *Am J Cardiol* 1983;51:902.

52. Ellis SG, Ajluni S, Arnold AZ, et al. Increased coronary perforation in the new device era: incidence, classification, management, and outcome. *Circulation* 1994;90:2725.

53. Fejka M, Simon R, Dixon SR, et al. Diagnosis, management, and clinical outcome of cardiac tamponade complicating percutaneous coronary intervention. *Am J Cardiol* 2002;90: 1183–1186.

54. Kent KM, Mullin SM, Passamani ER. Proceedings of the National Heart, Lung, and Blood Institute Workshop on the Outcome of Percutaneous Transluminal Angioplasty, June 7–8, 1983, *Am J Cardiol* 1984;53:1C.

55. Detre K, Holubkov R, Kelsey S, et al. Percutaneous transluminal coronary angioplasty in 1985–1986 and 1977–1981: the NHLBI Registry. *N Engl J Med* 1988;318:265.

56. Holmes DR Jr, Holubkov R, Vlietstra RE, et al. Comparison of complications during percutaneous transluminal coronary angioplasty from 1977 to 1981 and from 1985 to 1986: the NHLBI PTCA Registry. *J Am Coll Cardiol* 1988;12:1149.

57. Anderson HV, et al. A contemporary overview of percutaneous coronary interventions; The American College of Cardiology-National Cardiovascular Data Registry (ACC-NCDR). *J Am Coll Cardiol* 2002;39:1096–1103.

58. Cutlip DE, Ho KKL, Kuntz RE, Baim DS. Risk assessment for percutaneous coronary intervention—our version of the weather report? *J Am Coll Cardiol* 2003;42:1986–1989.

59. Shaw RE, Anderson HV, Brindis RG, et al. Development of a risk adjustment mortality model using the American College of Cardiology-National Cardiovascular Data Registry (ACC-NCDR) experience: 1998–2000. *J Am Coll Cardiol* 2002;39: 1104–1112.

60. Singh M, Lennon RJ, Holmes DR Jr, Bell MR, Rihal CS. Correlates of procedural complications and a simple integer risk score for percutaneous coronary intervention. *J Am Coll Cardiol* 2002;40: 387–393.

61. Queshi MA, et al. Simplified scoring system for predicting mortality after percutaneous coronary intervention. *J Am Coll Cardiol* 2003;42:1890–1895.

62. Ryan T, et al. Guidelines for percutaneous transluminal coronary angioplasty. A report of the American College of Cardiology/American Heart Association Task Force (Subcommittee on Percutaneous Transluminal Coronary Angioplasty). *J Am Coll Cardiol* 1988;12:529–545.

63. Ellis SG, Vandormael MG, Cowley MJ, and the POSCH Group. Coronary morphologic and clinical determinates of procedural outcome with angioplasty for multivessel coronary disease: implications for patient selection. *Circulation* 1990;82:1193–1202.

64. Krone RJ, Shaw RE, Klein LW, Block PC, et al. Evaluation of the American College of Cardiology/American Heart Association and the Society for Coronary Angiography and Interventions lesion classification system in the current "stent era" of coronary interventions (from the ACC-National Cardiovascular Data Registry). *Am J Cardiol* 2003;92:389–394.

65. Seshadri N, et al. Emergency coronary artery bypass surgery in the contemporary percutaneous coronary intervention era. *Circulation* 2002;106:2346–2350.

66. Hill JA, Margolis JR, Feldman RL, et al. Coronary arterial aneurysm formation after balloon angioplasty. *Am J Cardiol* 1983;52:261.

67. Vassanelli C, Turri M, Morando G, et al. Coronary artery aneurysm formation after PTCA—a not uncommon finding at follow-up angiography. *Int J Cardiol* 1989;22:151.

68. Ferguson JJ, et al. The relation of clinical outcome to dissection and thrombus formation during coronary angioplasty. *J Invasive Cardiol* 1995;7:2.

69. Ellis SG, Roubin GS, King SB 3rd, et al. Angiographic and clinical predictors of acute closure after native vessel coronary angioplasty. *Circulation* 1988;77:372.

70. Talley JD, Jones EL, Weintraub WS, et al. Coronary artery bypass surgery after failed elective percutaneous transluminal coronary angioplasty—a status report. *Circulation* 1989;79:I126.

71. Paik GY, Kuntz RE, Baim DS. Perfusion therapy to resolve myocardial ischemia en route to emergency bypass grafting for failed percutaneous transluminal angioplasty. *J Intervent Cardiol* 1995;8:319.

72. de Muinck ED, den Heijer P, van Dijk RB, et al. Autoperfusion balloon versus stent for acute or threatened closure during percutaneous transluminal coronary angioplasty. *Am J Cardiol* 1994;74:1002.

73. George BS, Voorhees WD 3rd, Roubin GS, et al. Multicenter investigation of coronary stenting to treat acute or threatened closure after percutaneous transluminal coronary angioplasty: clinical and angiographic outcomes. *J Am Coll Cardiol* 1993;22: 135.

74. Kelly D, Arora D. Prognostic significance of myocardial enzyme release after coronary interventions. *Cathet Cardiovasc Intervent* 1999;46:292.

75. Karvouni E, et al. Intravenous glycoprotein IIb/IIIa receptor antagonists reduce mortality after percutaneous coronary interventions. *J Am Coll Cardiol* 2003;41:26–32.

76. Meier B, Gruentzig AR, King SB 3rd, et al. Risk of side branch occlusion during coronary angioplasty. *Am J Cardiol* 1984;53:10.

77. Meier B. Kissing balloon coronary angioplasty. *Am J Cardiol* 1984;54:918.

78. Osterle SN, McAuley BJ, Buchbinder M, Simpson JB. Angioplasty at coronary bifurcations: single-guide, two-wire technique. *Cathet Cardiovasc Diagn* 1986;12:57.

79. Dauerman HL, Higgins PJ, Sparano AM, et al. Mechanical debulking versus balloon angioplasty for the treatment of true bifurcation lesions. *J Am Coll Cardiol* 1998;32:1845.

80. Wohlgelernter D, Cleman M, Highman HA, et al. Regional myocardial dysfunction during coronary angioplasty: evaluation by two-dimensional echocardiography and 12 lead electrocardiography. *J Am Coll Cardiol* 1986;7:1245.

81. Bertrand ME, Leblanche JM, Fourrier JL, et al. Left ventricular systolic and diastolic dysfunction during acute coronary artery balloon occlusion in humans. *J Am Coll Cardiol* 1988;12:341.

82. Serruys PW, Wijns W, van den Brand M, et al. Left ventricular performance, regional blood flow, wall motion, and lactate metabolism during transluminal angioplasty. *Circulation* 1984;70:25.

83. Hartzler GO, Rutherford BD, McConahay DR. Retained percutaneous transluminal coronary angioplasty equipment components and their management. *Am J Cardiol* 1987;60:1260.

84. Serota H, Deligonul U, Lew B, et al. Improved method for transcatheter retrieval of intracoronary detached angioplasty guidewire segments. *Cathet Cardiovasc Diagn* 1989;17:248.

85. McBride W, Lange RA, Hillis LD. Restenosis after successful coronary angioplasty. *N Engl J Med* 1988;318:1734.

86. Mintz GS, Popma JJ, Pichard AD, et al. Arterial remodeling after coronary angioplasty—a serial intravascular ultrasound study. *Circulation* 1996;94:35.

87. Serruys PW, Luijten HE, Beatt KJ, et al. Incidence of restenosis after successful coronary angioplasty: a time related phenomenon—a quantitative angiographic follow-up study of 342 patients. *Circulation* 1988;77:361.

88. Hirshfeld JW Jr, Schwartz JS, Jugo R, et al. Restenosis after coronary angioplasty: a multivariable statistical model to relate lesion and procedure variables to restenosis. *J Am Coll Cardiol* 1991;18:647.

89. Kuntz RE, Baim DS. Defining coronary restenosis: newer clinical and angiographic paradigms. *Circulation* 1993;88:1310.

90. Popma JJ, Suntharalingam M, Lansky AJ, et al.; Stents And Radiation Therapy (START) Investigators. Randomized trial of 90Sr/90Y beta-radiation versus placebo control for treatment of in-stent restenosis. *Circulation* 2002;106:1090–1096.

91. Leon MB, et al. Localized intracoronary gamma-radiation therapy to inhibit the recurrence of restenosis after stenting. *N Engl J Med* 2001;344:250–256.

92. Moses JW, et al. Sirolimus-eluting stents versus standard stents in patients with stenosis in a native coronary artery. *N Engl J Med* 2003;349:1315–1323.

93. Lemos PA, et al. Unrestricted utilization of sirolimus-eluting stents compared with conventional bare stent implantation in the "real world": the Rapamycin-Eluting Stent Evaluated At Rotterdam Cardiology Hospital (RESEARCH) registry. *Circulation* 2004;109:190–195.

94. Stone GW, Ellis SG, Cox DA, et al. A polymer-based paclitaxel-eluting stent in patients with coronary artery disease. *N Engl J Med* 2003;350:221–231.

95. Stone, GW, Ellis, SG, Cox, DA, et al. One-year clinical results with the slow release, polymer-based, paclitaxel-eluting TAXUS stent: the TAXUS-IV trial. *Circulation* 2004;109:1942.

95a. Lemos PA, et al. Comparison of late luminal loss response pattern after sirolimus-eluting stent implantation or conventional stenting. *Circulation* 2004;110:3199–3205.

96. Detre K, Holubkov R, Kelsey S, et al. One-year follow-up results of the 1985–1986 National Heart, Lung, and Blood Institute's percutaneous transluminal coronary angioplasty registry. *Circulation* 1989;80:421.

97. Cutlip DE, Chauhan MS, Baim DS, et al. Clinical restenosis after coronary stenting: perspectives from multicenter clinical trials. *J Am Coll Cardiol* 2002;40:2082–2089.

98. Pocock SJ, Henderson RA, Rickards AF, et al. Meta-analysis of randomised trials comparing coronary angioplasty with bypass surgery. *Lancet* 1995;346:1184.

99. Popma J, Kuntz RE, Baim DS. A decade of improvement in the clinical outcomes of percutaneous coronary intervention for multivessel coronary artery disease. *Circulation* 2002;106:1592–1594.

100. Legrand VM, Serruys PW, Unger F, et al. Three-year outcome after coronary stenting versus bypass surgery for the treatment of multivessel disease (ARTS). *Circulation* 2004;109:1114.

101. Moussa I, et al. Impact of sirolimus-eluting stents on outcome in diabetic patients: a SIRIUS substudy. *Circulation* 2004;109:2273–2278.

102. Weintraub WS, et al. Changing use of coronary angioplasty and coronary bypass surgery in the treatment of chronic coronary artery disease. *Am J Cardiol* 2990;65:183.

103. Holubkov R, et al. Trends in coronary revascularization 1989–1997—the Bypass Angioplasty Revascularization Investigation (BARI) survey of procedures. *Am J Cardiol* 1999;84:157.

103a. Silber S, et al. Guidelines for percutaneous coronary interventions: the Task Force for percutaneous coronary interventions of the European Society of Cardiology. *European Heart J* 2005;26:804–847.

104. Coronary angioplasty versus medical therapy for angina: the second Randomised Intervention Treatment of Angina (RITA-2) trial. RITA-2 trial participants. *Lancet* 1997;350:461–468.

105. Seven-year outcome in the RITA-2 trial: coronary angioplasty versus medical therapy. *J Am Coll Cardiol* 2003;42:1161–1170.

106. Davies RF, et al. Asymptomatic Cardiac Ischemia Pilot (ACIP) study two-year follow-up: outcomes of patients randomized to initial strategies of medical therapy versus revascularization. *Circulation* 1997;95:2037–2043.

107. Seven-year outcome in the Bypass Angioplasty Revascularization Investigation (BARI) by treatment and diabetic status. *J Am Coll Cardiol* 2000;35:1122–1129.

108. Kuntz RE. Importance of considering atherosclerosis progression when choosing a coronary revascularization strategy—the diabetes-percutaneous transluminal coronary angioplasty dilemma. *Circulation* 1999;99:847.

109. Wang JC, Normand SL, Mauri L, et al. Coronary artery spatial distribution of acute myocardial infarction occlusions. *Circulation* 2004;110:278–284.

110. Feit F, Brooks MM, Sopko G, et al. Long-term clinical outcome in the Bypass Angioplasty Revascularization Investigation Registry: comparison with the randomized trial. BARI Investigators. *Circulation* 2000;101:2795–2802.

111. Anderson HV, Cannon CP, Stone PH, e al. One-year results of the Thrombolysis in Myocardial Infarction (TIMI) IIIB clinical trial—a randomized comparison of tissue-type plasminogen activator versus placebo and early invasive versus early conservative strategies in unstable angina and non-Q-wave myocardial infarction. *J Am Coll Cardiol* 1995;26:1643.

112. Boden WE, O'Rourke RA, Crawford MH, et al. Outcomes in patients with acute non-Q-wave myocardial infarction randomly assigned to an invasive as compared with a conservative management strategy (VANQWISH). *N Engl J Med* 1998;328:1785.

113. Long-term low-molecular-mass heparin in unstable coronary-artery disease: FRISC II prospective randomised multicentre study. FRagmin and Fast Revascularisation during InStability in Coronary artery disease. Investigators. *Lancet* 354:701–709.

114. Cannon CP, Weintraub WS, Demopoulos LA, et al.; TACTICS (Treat Angina with Aggrastat and Determine Cost of Therapy with an Invasive or Conservative Strategy—TIMI 18 Investigators. Comparison of early invasive versus and conservative strategies in patients with unstable angina and non-ST elevation myocardial infarction treated with early glycoprotein IIb/IIIa inhibition. *N Engl J Med* 2001;344:1879–1887.

115. Van de Werf F, Baim DS. Reperfusion for ST-segment elevation myocardial infarction: an overview of current treatment options. *Circulation* 2002;105:2813.

116. Keeley EC, Boura JA, Grines CL. Primary angioplasty versus intravenous thrombolytic therapy for acute myocardial infarction: a quantitative review of 23 randomised trials. *Lancet* 2003;361:13–20.

117. Hochman JS. Cardiogenic shock complicating acute myocardial infarction: expanding the paradigm. *Circulation* 2003;107: 2998–3002.

118. Wharton TP, Grines LL, Turco MA, et al. Primary angioplasty in acute myocardial infarction at hospitals with no surgery on-site (the PAMI-No SOS study) versus transfer to surgical centers for primary angioplasty. *J Am Coll Cardiol* 2004;43:1943–1950.

119. Andersen HR, Nielsen TT, Rasmussen K, et al. A comparison of coronary angioplasty with fibrinolytic therapy in acute myocardial infarction (DANAMI-2). *N Engl J Med* 2003;349: 733–742.

120. Ellis SG, Da Silva ER, Spaulding CM, Nobuyoshi M, Weiner B, Talley JD. Review of immediate angioplasty after fibrinolytic therapy for acute myocardial infarction: insights from the RESCUE I, RESCUE II, and other contemporary clinical experiences. *Am Heart J* 2000;139:1046–1053.

121. Topol EJ, Neumann FJ, Montalescot G. A preferred reperfusion strategy for acute myocardial infarction. *J Am Coll Cardiol* 2003; 42:1886.

122. Stone GW, Grines CL, Cox DA, et al. Comparison of angioplasty with stenting, with or without abciximab, in acute myocardial infarction. *N Engl J Med* 2002;346:957.

123. Lau GT, Lowe HC, Kritharides L. Cardiac saphenous vein bypass graft disease. *Seminars in vascular medicine* 2004;4: 153–159.

124. Loop FD, Lytle BW, Cosgrove DM, et al. Influence of internal-mammary-artery graft on 10-year survival and other cardiac events. *N Engl J Med* 1986;314:1.

125. Weintraub WS, Jones EL, Morris DC, King SB, Guyton RA, Craver JM. Outcome of reoperative coronary bypass surgery versus coronary angioplasty after previous bypass surgery. *Circulation* 1997; 95:868.

126. Morrison DA, Sethi G, Sacks J, et al. Percutaneous coronary intervention versus repeat bypass surgery for patients with medically refractory myocardial ischemia: AWESOME randomized trial and registry experience with post-CABG patients. *J Am Coll Cardiol* 2002;40:1951–1954.

127. Waller BF, Rothbaum DA, Gorfinkel HJ, et al. Morphologic observations after percutaneous transluminal angioplasty of early and late aortocoronary saphenous vein bypass grafts. *J Am Coll Cardiol* 1984;4:784.

128. Savage MP, Douglas JS, Fishman DL, et al. Stent placement compared with balloon angioplasty for obstructed coronary bypass grafts. *N Engl J Med* 1997;337:740.

129. Ellis SG, Brener SJ, DeLuca S, et al. Late myocardial ischemic events after saphenous vein graft intervention—importance of initially "non-significant" vein graft lesions. *Am J Cardiol* 1997; 79:1460.

130. Baim DS. Percutaneous treatment of saphenous vein graft disease—the ongoing challenge. *J Am Coll Cardiol* 2003;42: 1370–1372.

131. Kuntz RE, Baim DS, Cohen DJ, et al. A trial comparing rheolytic thrombectomy with intracoronary urokinase for coronary and vein graft thrombus (the Vein Graft AngioJet Study [VeGAS 2]). *Am J Cardiol* 2002;89:326–330.

132. Hearne SE, et al. Internal mammary artery graft angioplasty—acute and long-term outcome. *Cathet Cariovasc Diagn* 1998;44:153.

133. Isshiki T, et al. Percutaneous angioplasty of stenosed gastroepiploic artery grafts. *J Am Coll Cardiol* 1993;22:727.

134. Topaz O, et al. Percutaneous revascularization modalities in heart transplant recipients. *Cathet Cardiovasc Intervent* 1999;46: 227.

135. Suero JA, et al. Procedural outcomes and long-term survival among patients undergoing percutaneous coronary intervention of a chronic total occlusion in native coronary arteries—a 20-year experience. *J Am Coll Cardiol* 2001;38:409–414.

136. Olivari Z, Rubartelli P, Piscione F, et al. Immediate results and one-year clinical outcome after percutaneous coronary interventions in chronic total occlusions: data from a multicenter, prospective, observational study (TOAST-GISE) *J Am Coll Cardiol* 2003;41:1672–1678.

137. Bourassa MG, et al. Bypass Angioplasty Revascularization Investigation: patient screening, selection and recruitment. *Am J Cardiol* 1995;75:3C–8C.

138. Serruys PW, Hamburger JN, Koolen JJ. Total occlusion trial with angioplasty by using laser guidewire—the TOTAL trial. *Eur Heart J* 2000;21:1797–1805.

139. Whitborn RJ, Cincotta M, Mossop P, Selmon M. Intraluminal blunt microdissection for angioplasty of chronic total occlusion. *Cathet Cardiovasc Intervent* 2003;58:194–198.

140. Baim DS, et al. Utility of the Safe-Cross-guided radiofrequency total occlusion crossing system in chronic coronary total occlusions (results of the GREAT Registry Study). *Am J Cardiol* 2004; 94:853–858.

141. Sirnes PA, Golf S, Myreng Y, et al. Sustained benefit of stenting chronic coronary occlusion: long-term clinical follow-up of the Stenting in Chronic Coronary Occlusion (SICCO) study. *J Am Coll Cardiol* 1998;32:305–310.

142. Rubartelli P, Verna E, Niccoli L, et al. Coronary stent implantation is superior to balloon angioplasty for chronic total occlusions—a six-year clinical follow-up of the GISSOC trial. *J Am Coll Cardiol* 2003;41:1498–1492.

143. Baim DS. Is it time to offer elective percutaneous treatment of the unprotected left main coronary artery? *J Am Coll Cardiol* 2000;35:1551–1553.

144. Ellis SG, Tamai H, Nobuyoshi, et al. Contemporary percutaneous treatment of unprotected left main coronary stenoses. *Circulation* 1997;96:3867.

145. Takagi T, Stankovic G, Finci L, et al. Results and long-term predictors of adverse clinical events after elective percutaneous interventions on unprotected left main coronary artery. *Circulation* 2002; 106:698–702.

146. Silvestri M, Barragan P, Sainsous J, et al. Unprotected left main coronary artery stenting: immediate and medium-term outcomes of 140 elective procedures. *J Am Coll Cardiol* 2000;35:1543–1550.

147. Park SJ, Lee CW, Kim YH, et al. Technical feasibility, safety, and clinical outcome of stenting of unprotected left main coronary artery bifurcation narrowing. *Am J Cardiol* 2002;90:374–378.

148. Chieffo A, et al. Early and mid-term results of drug-eluting stent implantation in unprotected left main. *Circulation* 2005;111: 791–795.

149. Jolis JG, Peterson ED, DeLong ER et al. The relation between the volume of coronary angioplasty procedures at hospitals treating Medicare beneficiaries and short-term mortality. *N Engl J Med* 1994;331:1625.

150. Hirshfeld JW, Ellis SG, Faxon DP. Recommendations for the assessment and maintenance of proficiency in coronary interventional procedures: statement of the American College of Cardiology. *J Am Coll Cardiol* 1998;31:722–743.

151. Ellis SG, Weintraub W, Holmes D, Shaw R, Block PC, King SB. Relation of operator volume and experience to procedural outcome of percutaneous coronary revascularization at hospitals with high interventional volumes. *Circulation* 1997;96: 2479.

152. Hirshfeld JW, Banas JS, Brundage BH, et al. American College of Cardiology training statement on recommendations for the structure of an optimal adult interventional cardiology training program: a report of the American College of Cardiology task force on clinical expert consensus documents. *J Am Coll Cardiol* 1999;34:2141–2147.

153. Ryan TJ. Stents—expanding the case for volume minimums in interventional cardiology. *J Am Coll Cardiol* 1998;32:977.

154. Harjai KJ, et al. Impact on interventionalist volume, experience, and board certification on coronary angioplasty outcomes in the era of stenting. *Am J Cardiol* 2004;94:421–426.

Coronary Atherectomy, Thrombectomy, and Embolic Protection

23

Campbell Rogers   *Donald S. Baim*[a]

Although balloon angioplasty (Chapter 22) and coronary stenting (Chapter 24) are the mainstays of coronary intervention, various adjunctive technologies have been used to augment their results. These include devices that remove plaque from lesions (atherectomy), devices that remove clots from vessels (thrombectomy), and devices that capture and remove embolic debris (embolic protection), which are the subject of this chapter.

Atherectomy devices widen the coronary lumen by removing rather than merely displacing atherosclerotic plaque. They include cut-and-retrieve devices (directional atherectomy; 1–3) as well as atheroablation without recovery of the resulting debris (rotational [4,5] and laser atherectomy [6]). These devices were originally developed as primary treatments to limit restenosis, but in current practice they are more commonly used to enhance the procedural outcome of balloon angioplasty or stent placement in certain complex lesion subsets (uncrossable or undilatable lesions, or bulky origin plaques). As such, the proportion of interventions that involve atherectomy has diminished (from a high of 30% in the early 1990s to 5 to 10% since the emergence of drug-eluting stents). Although stents generally provide equivalent or better short- and long-term results in addition to less complexity, time, and cost, the unique capabilities of the atherectomy devices make it important for the skilled interventionalist to understand the available techniques and be able to match available

devices with patient and lesion characteristics to optimize acute angiographic results and procedural safety.

This chapter will also review thrombectomy devices (including the Possis AngioJet Rheolytic thrombectomy catheter) and the rapidly proliferating class of embolic protection devices (which trap and recover atheroembolic particulate debris liberated from the lesion in the course of coronary intervention). The use of embolic protection has become routine during stenting of degenerated saphenous vein bypass grafts and is evolving rapidly in other coronary and peripheral interventional settings (see Chapters 22, 24, and 26).

ATHERECTOMY

Directional Coronary Atherectomy (DCA)

Device Description

The directional coronary atherectomy catheter (Simpson AtheroCath, Guidant, Santa Clara, CA) was first used in human peripheral vessels in 1985 (1) and in coronary arteries in 1986 (7). The coronary device was approved in 1990, following a large multicenter registry experience (8). Despite several minor improvements, the basic concept remains intact—a windowed steel housing is pressed up against the lesion by a low-pressure positioning balloon, allowing any plaque that protrudes into the window to be shaved from the lesion by a spinning cup-shaped cutter and trapped in the device nose cone. The coronary device

---

[a] Dr. Richard Kuntz was a coauthor of this chapter in previous editions.

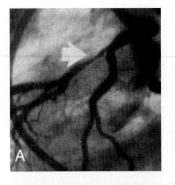
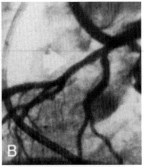
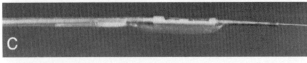
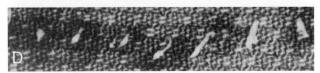

Figure 23.1 Directional coronary atherectomy. Left coronary angiography (lateral view) reveals a long eccentric stenosis in the mid–left anterior descending (LAD) artery **(A)**. After atherectomy, the lumen is smooth and there is no significant residual stenosis or dissection **(B)**. A 7F AtheroCath was used **(C)**, and several pieces of atheroma were retrieved **(D)**.

tracks over a 0.014-inch guidewire (Fig. 23.1), and wire braid in the shaft of the catheter allows the device to be rotated to facilitate its advancement across the lesion and to provide precise rotational orientation of the cutting window in the lesion. During cuts, a battery-powered motor drive unit spins the cup-shaped cutter at approximately 2,500 rpm as the cutter is manually advanced across the window using a small lever on the motor drive unit. The current design (Flexi-Cut) uses a single 6F housing with a wider window opening than on previous devices (160 versus 120°) and different-sized positioning balloons (2.5 to 2.9 mm, 3.0 to 3.5 mm, and 3.5 to 3.9 mm) to achieve different effective working diameters.

Procedure

The size of the atherectomy device is determined relative to the size of the normal vessel adjacent to the stenosis (the reference segment). Predilation with a small (e.g., 2.0-mm) conventional balloon may be used to facilitate passage of the AtheroCath, but larger predilating balloons should not be used to avoid causing dissections or expanding the outer vessel diameter, making recovery of tissue more difficult during subsequent cuts. The Flexi-Cut catheter can be delivered through an 8F guiding catheter. After flushing the central lumen and filling the balloon lumen with dilute contrast material, the device is passed into the guiding catheter over an exchange-length guidewire that has been positioned well across the target lesion. To cross

the target lesion, the device is advanced with gentle forward pressure during continuous rotation of the atherectomy catheter. If the device does not pass easily, attempts to force it into the lesion or around curves in the vessel should be avoided, since forceful advancement of the rigid housing through a stiff, calcified, tortuous vessel could traumatize the vessel wall (9).

Once the device is in position at the target lesion, the device is rotated until the cutting window is seen to point toward the greatest plaque burden in a fluoroscopic projection that maximizes visualization of the target lesion and its eccentricity. The positioning balloon is inflated to 5 psi, the motor is activated, and the cutter is withdrawn to the proximal end of the window. The positioning balloon is then inflated further to 10 to 20 psi before the cutter is advanced slowly (>5 seconds) across the window. After each cut, the balloon is deflated and the device is rotated by 60 to 90° to address another segment of remaining plaque burden. Balloon pressure during cutting may be escalated in 10-psi increments to a maximum of 40 to 50 psi to increase effective device size and plaque retrieval. Cuts oriented toward nondiseased walls, particularly toward the carina of bifurcations, should be avoided to minimize the risk of vessel perforation. After four to six cuts, or if incomplete cutter advancement indicates that the nose cone collecting chamber is becoming full, the device should be removed and emptied before additional cuts are made. Intravascular ultrasound (Chapter 19) may be helpful in assessing the lumen diameter, as well as the amount and location of residual plaque burden.

Although directional atherectomy was designed to enlarge the vessel lumen purely by excising atherosclerotic plaque (2), the acute result derives from a combination of plaque removal and dilation. Early data showed that the amount of plaque removed (averaging 18.5 mg) accounts for less than half the observed gain in volume seen at the lesion site (8,10), with the rest resulting from facilitated angioplasty. Owing to adaptive Glagov remodeling of the vessel wall, a substantial amount of plaque (40 to 50%, as a percent of the outer vessel [external elastic lamina, or EEL] cross-sectional area) remains even after a successful atherectomy that has normalized the angiographic vessel lumen relative to that of the adjacent reference segments (11). Since atherectomy improves the radial compliance of the diseased and stiff coronary segment, and since the mechanism of lumen enlargement is due in part to dilation, it stands to reason that postatherectomy balloon angioplasty and stenting should impart additional volume expansion, and optimal atherectomy practice thus makes routine use of postdilation and stenting to further enlarge the treated lumen (12–15).

Results

Published experience with directional atherectomy includes single-center reports (16,17), as well as results from multicenter registries (8,12,18) and multicenter randomized trials

(13,15,19–21). These trials show that atherectomy provides acute success and complication rates comparable with balloon angioplasty but with less residual stenosis. Procedural safety is also comparable, although there is a higher incidence of clinically silent elevations in creatine kinase myocardial band (CK-MB) following directional atherectomy. In the Balloon vs Optimal Atherectomy Trial (BOAT; 13), this was not associated with increased mortality at 1 or 3 years, with a trend toward more late deaths by 1 year in the balloon angioplasty compared with the DCA arm (eight deaths versus three deaths, $P = 0.14$).

There are significant differences among the stand-alone directional atherectomy trials in terms of angiographic restenosis. For the two early (1990–1991) randomized trials, high (>25%) residual stenoses (29% for CAVEAT I and 26% for CCAT; 19,20) reflected cautious tissue removal and the discouragement of adjunctive balloon postdilatation. In contrast, subsequent experiences performed more aggressive tissue removal and used routine balloon postdilation to obtain much lower residual stenoses (<15%). The benefit of this approach compared with stand-alone balloon angioplasty was confirmed in the OARS (15), BOAT (8), and ABACAS (21) studies, with angiographic restenosis rates of 21 to 31%, compared with the 46 to 50% restenosis rates in CAVEAT and CCAT. With the advent of coronary stenting in 1994, however, it became possible to achieve these excellent acute and long-term results with less procedural difficulty.

Some studies have suggested a benefit of DCA prior to adjunctive stenting in certain lesion types. In the SOLD (Stenting after Optimal Lesion Debulking) study (12), 71 patients underwent directional atherectomy of coronary lesions before stenting, achieving an angiographic restenosis rate of 11%. Interestingly, this was owing both to a slightly larger acute result as well as to a reduced late loss index (33% versus the more typical 50%) compared with stenting alone. A similar experience has been reported by Kiesz and coworkers (the ADAPTS study; 22), in which 89 lesions in 60 patients were treated with a combination of DCA debulking followed by stenting. These initial registry reports suggested that restenosis with this approach might be low, leading to the randomized AMIGO trial (23). While the AMIGO trial overall showed no net benefit in late lumen diameter for directional atherectomy before bare-metal stent placement, the subset of >100 patients treated by Colombo and the parallel 500-patient DESIRE trial (24) performed in Japan (both using more aggressive tissue removal) did show a significantly (approximately 20%) larger acute post-treatment and late follow lumen diameter for the debulk and stent approach. With the advent of drug-eluting stents (see Chapter 24), however, this small benefit is probably not sufficient to drive widespread lesion debulking before stent placement. There are to date no in-depth studies combining directional atherectomy with drug-eluting stents.

Tissue Analysis and Consequences of Deep Wall Resection

Atherectomy provides a unique opportunity for studying the pathophysiology of atherosclerosis and coronary restenosis in human coronary arteries (25). Standard light microscopy demonstrates that atherosclerotic plaque (97%), media (66%), adventitia (30%), and thrombus (43%) are commonly recovered. Histologic analysis of DCA specimens shows intimal hyperplasia in 93% of restenotic lesions, with proliferating-phenotype smooth-muscle cells interspersed with ground substance. Surprisingly, however, 44% of primary (de novo) lesions have intimal hyperplasia that is histologically indistinguishable from intimal hyperplasia seen in lesions with prior restenosis (26). Remarkably, retrieval of deep wall components seems to be well tolerated acutely. Although 6-month angiographic follow-up (27,28) showed no relationship between deep wall resection and restenosis, the risk of late aneurysm formation after stand-alone directional atherectomy may be increased (29,30). Some have speculated that this risk may be even higher with drug-eluting stents through impairment of vessel healing, although there is no evidence of this to date.

Use in Specific Lesion Types

Bifurcation Lesions

Plaque obstruction in large epicardial coronary arteries that involves the origin of a large branch—such as the left anterior descending/diagonal branch bifurcation or the distal portion of the left main coronary trunk—presents a special problem for the interventionalist. The treatment of true bifurcation lesions using conventional balloon angioplasty and stenting techniques is limited by the tendency for plaque to shift between the parent vessel and the ostium of the branch vessel (see Chapter 22). Directional atherectomy may enhance acute results in treatment of bifurcation lesions by excising the tissue that might otherwise be shifted into the branch ostium (31–33). The preferred technique involves sequential atherectomy of the main vessel and its branch, if the branch vessel is large enough (>2.5 mm) to accommodate the device (Fig. 23.2). The acute and long-term results of DCA for the treatment of true bifurcation lesions have not been compared with stenting, but were compared with balloon angioplasty by Dauerman (34). The atherectomy group had lower acute residual diameter stenosis and lower target vessel revascularization rate (28% for atherectomy versus 53% for balloon angioplasty, $P = 0.01$). We first position the 0.014-inch guidewire into the distal parent vessel and perform initial cuts directed toward the ostium of the branch vessel in an effort to minimize "snowplow" branch compromise. Next, the guidewire is withdrawn and redirected into the branch vessel, where additional cuts are performed. Finally, kissing balloon inflation in the parent and branch vessel is performed, followed by stent placement.

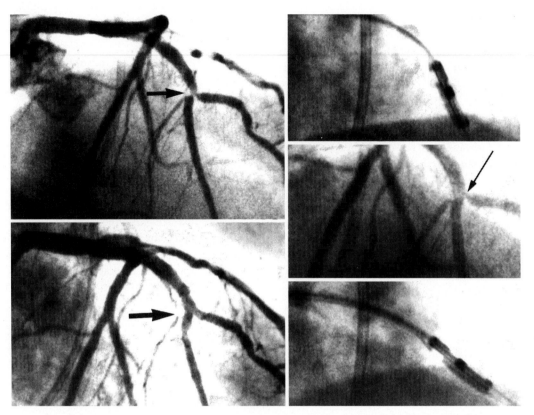

Figure 23.2 Bifurcation atherectomy. **Top left.** "Mercedes Benz" lesion involving the bifurcation of the left anterior descending (LAD) and diagonal branch *(arrow).* **Top right.** Directional atherectomy of LAD, leaving tight stenosis of the diagonal origin **(right center,** *arrow).* **Bottom right.** Atherectomy of the diagonal origin leaves excellent result **(bottom left).** (From Dauerman H, Baim D, Cutlip DE, et al. Mechanical debulking versus balloon angioplasty for the treatment of diffuse in-stent restenosis. *Am J Cardiol* 1998;82:277.)

In-Stent Restenosis

In the setting of in-stent restenosis with large neointimal tissue volume, DCA offers the most potent debulking capacity among the atherectomy and atheroablative devices and has been shown to be safe and effective in achieving <20% residual in-stent diameter stenosis with low subsequent clinical restenosis rates (20 to 30%; Fig. 23.3). In some atherectomy procedures for in-stent restenosis, the tissue sample may include a small section of stent struts although without apparent clinical consequence. Furthermore, analysis of DCA-recovered tissue from restenosis within drug-eluting stents may shed light on mechanisms of failure for these devices.

New Approaches to Directional Atherectomy

One new approach to coronary debulking is the Simpson Fox Hollow device. Compared with the AtheroCath, this device uses controlled deformation of the catheter tip (rather than inflation of a positioning balloon) to force atheroma into the cutting window. The entire device is moved forward with the cutter exposed to perform tissue resection (rather than just the cutter being moved forward

within a fixed-length window), although in both cases the resulting resected plaque is captured in a hollow nose cone. Initial reports indicate large amounts of tissue retrieved, and the ongoing COMBAT trial is examining the potential benefit of this device as a prelude to stenting in bifurcation settings, and in the periphery, where stenting is not always desirable.

High-Speed Mechanical Rotational Atherectomy (Rotablator)

Device Description

The high-speed mechanical rotational atherectomy device (Rotablator (Boston Scientific, Boston, MA; 4,5) consists of an olive-shaped stainless steel or brass burr whose surface is embedded with diamond chips each measuring 30 to 120 microns in diameter (Fig. 23.4). The burr is attached to a hollow flexible drive shaft that permits it to be advanced over a steerable 0.009-inch guidewire with a 0.014-inch platinum coil tip. The drive shaft is encased within a Teflon sheath through which flush solution (heparinized Ringer lactate, nitroglycerin, and Rotaglide

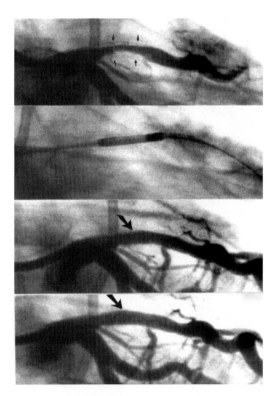

Figure 23.3 Directional atherectomy of in-stent restenosis. **Top.** Restenosis within stent in the mid–left anterior descending (*arrows* denote stent struts). **Upper center.** Directional atherectomy catheter positioned within stent. **Lower center.** Enlarged lumen following atherectomy *(arrow).* **Bottom.** Final result after balloon dilatation.

[a special low-friction emulsion]) is pumped to lubricate and cool the drive shaft and burr. Our preferred mixture is 4 mg of verapamil, 4 mg of nitroglycerin, 5,000 U of heparin, and 20 mL of Rotaglide mixed in a 1-liter bag of normal saline (NS).

The drive shaft is rotated at 140,000 to 200,000 rpm by a compressed air turbine during advancement across the lesion (Fig. 23.5). Burrs for coronary use are available in 1.25-, 1.5-, 1.75-, 2.0-, 2.15-, 2.25-, and 2.5-mm diameters. The selection of burr sizes is largely empirical, but should not exceed a final burr-to-artery ratio of 0.7 (i.e., 2.15-mm burr in a 3.0-mm vessel). In treating long segments of disease, heavily calcified lesions, and subtotal de novo lesions, it is generally advisable to start with a smaller (1.5- or 1.75-mm) burr, and step up to the final burr size in 0.5-mm increments. The Roto-Link system allows interchange of burrs without the need to replace the entire drive unit, offering some benefit in procedure speed and cost.

Procedure

Conventional angioplasty guiding catheters as small as 6F may be used for Rotablator atherectomy as long as their lumen is at least 0.020 inch larger than the largest burr to be used (see Table 23.1). Two guidewires are available, a floppy guidewire and an extra-support guidewire. The floppy wire has the advantage of minimizing guidewire bias—a phenomenon seen when a stiff guidewire straightens a curved vessel segment and causes deeper cuts or dissection as the burr is forced against the tautly stretched lesser curvature of the vessel. On the other hand, the floppy guidewire may fail to control adequately the travel of the burr around tight bends, leading to uncontrolled cutting on the greater curvature of the vessel. If difficulty is anticipated crossing the target lesion with the Rotablator guidewire using a bare-wire technique, the lesion may be crossed with a conventional 0.014-inch angioplasty wire and exchanged for the Rotablator guidewire using a suitable transport or low-profile balloon catheter. The

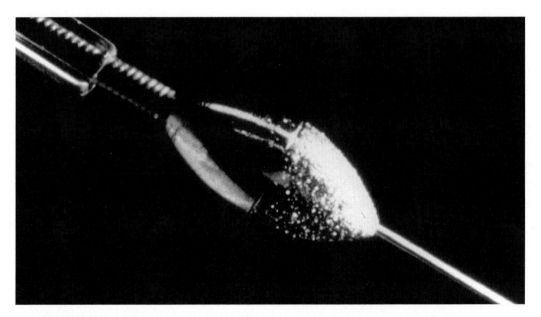

Figure 23.4 Close-up view of the Rotablator burr embedded with diamond chips and special 0.009-inch guidewire. (Reproduced with permission from Heart Technology, Inc., and Physician's Press.)

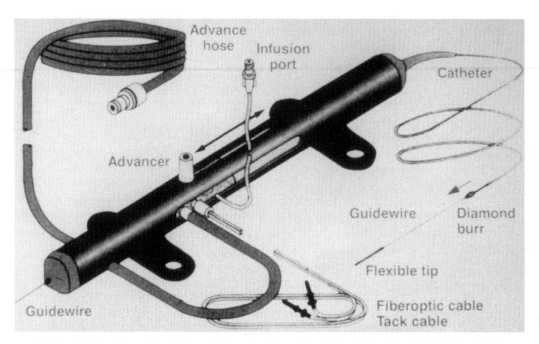

Figure 23.5 Schematic overview of the original Rotablator assembly. (Reproduced with permission from Heart Technology, Inc., and Physician's Press.) In the current Rota-link design, the drive unit is separate and can be used with a series of burr cables.

Rotablator guidewire has a dedicated torque clip that must be attached to the wire whenever the Rotablator is activated to prevent the wire from spinning and causing possible vessel trauma.

Once the guidewire is across the lesion, the burr should be advanced to within a few centimeters of the rotating hemostatic valve, with the lines for compressed air supply and tachometer readout attached to the drive console and the advancer lever locked in its midway position. While the operator holds the catheter carefully so that the burr tip is not in contact with the sterile drapes, the system should be tested by depressing the foot pedal and having an assistant adjust the turbine pressure to maintain burr speeds of 140,000 to 160,000 rpm. During the test, the operator should also confirm adequate flow of the pressurized

heparinized flush through the Teflon sheath, free motion of the advancer lever, and a firm grip of the wire brake during burr rotation. Once this test has been completed, the static burr can be advanced into and through the guiding catheter. Any resistance encountered as the burr is passed around the primary curve of the guiding catheter can be overcome by firm traction on the guidewire or gentle traction on the guiding catheter itself to lessen the curve slightly. Note, however, that the guiding catheter must remain well seated in the vessel ostium to prevent kinking or looping of the guidewire in the aortic root while the burr is advanced—such unrecognized loops in the radiolucent wire can lead to its transaction when the burr is activated at the ostium!

Once the burr has been advanced to 1 to 2 cm proximal to the target lesion, the advancer lever should be unlocked and pulled gently back to near to its proximal limit as the entire catheter is withdrawn gently by 1 or 2 mm. This relieves any compression in the drive shaft that might otherwise cause the burr to lurch forward into the lesion on activation. Under fluoroscopy, the burr is then activated by the foot pedal and adjusted to the desired "platform" speed (160,000 rpm for smaller burrs, 140,000 rpm for burrs >2.0 mm) before engaging the lesion. Advancement of the lever then brings the spinning burr slowly into contact with the lesion. It is important to be aware of the sound of the turbine, the rotational speed display, and tactile feedback during "rotablation." When the burr face encounters excessive resistance to rotation, the speed will fall, but it is essential to avoid speed drops of >5,000 rpm during advancement. Greater speed drops caused by excessive

TABLE 23.1

INNER DIAMETER OF GUIDING CATHETERS TO ACCOMMODATE ROTABLATOR BURRS

Rotablator Burr Size (mm)	Guiding Catheter ID
1.25	0.059
1.50	0.069
1.75	0.078
2.0	0.088
2.15	0.092
2.25	0.097
2.5	0.107

ID, inner diameter (inch).

pressure on the burr against the lesion may result in the liberation of larger particles, frictional heating of the plaque, or torsional dissection. We prefer advancing with a "pecking" motion in which brief (1- to 3-second) periods of plaque contact are alternated with longer (3- to 5-second) periods of reperfusion provided by pulling the burr back from the plaque face. This reduces speed drops and aids in the clearance of particulate debris through the distal circulation.

After 30 seconds of operation, the device should be withdrawn into the proximal vessel and rotation suspended for a similar time before reactivating and advancing the burr again. During each pause, a small test injection should be performed to ensure antegrade flow and absence of vascular trauma or perforation. This sequence should be repeated until the device can be advanced through the full length of the lesion without any fluoroscopic or tactile resistance to burr advancement and with no audible change in the pitch of the turbine or reduction in burr speed. The foot pedal is then used to activate the lower speed "dynaglide" mode, and the burr is removed while depressing the brake-release button. It is important to note that in dynaglide mode, the burr is not subject to pressure control (spinning at 90,000 rpm in all circumstances) and should never be advanced in this mode.

Unless contraindicated, a platelet glycoprotein (GP) Ib/IIIa receptor antagonist should be used in conjunction with rotational atherectomy, to limit the speed-dependent platelet activation and aggregation (35,36). Intravenous vasodilators, e.g. nitroglycerin, should be avoided prior to and during rotational atherectomy to minimize the risk of hypotension. For patients with target lesions in the distribution of the right coronary artery, prophylactic temporary pacemaker insertion, or at least femoral venous access, is recommended.

Mechanisms of Rotablator

Although directional atherectomy relies on tissue cutting and retrieval, high-speed mechanical rotational atherectomy relies on plaque abrasion and pulverization. The Rotablator selectively abrades inelastic tissue (i.e., plaque) by the principle of differential cutting while more tissue (i.e., normal vessel wall) tends to be deflected away from the burr (37). The abraded plaque is pulverized into particles 20 to 50 µm in diameter that can pass through the coronary microcirculation (4,38,39). Although these particles have long been felt not to interfere with the coronary microcirculation (40), the reported benefit of glycoprotein IIb/IIIa receptor blockers against transient hypoperfusion suggests a role for platelet-mediated microvascular flow reduction during rotational atherectomy (35). Reisman (36) has confirmed ex vivo platelet activation with greater activation and greater vessel heating at higher burr speeds. These findings have encouraged the use of lower (<160,000 rpm) speed during rotational atherectomy, although this necessitates longer cumulative burr time.

There is a significant incidence of non–Q-wave myocardial infarction and no reflow after rotational atherectomy (41), particularly in longer lesions. These problems may be secondary to particle embolization, spasm, or microcavitation caused when the burr surface velocity exceeds the speed of sound in water (42). Microcavitations or hemolysis of red blood cells with resultant local adenosine release may also contribute to transient bradycardia and atrioventricular (AV) block. Reassuringly, two studies have demonstrated no immediate or long-term impact of rotational atherectomy on left ventricular ejection fraction (43,44).

Results

Following Rotablator, the average residual diameter stenoses is 37 to 54% (41,44–49). However, Reisman and others demonstrated that the lesion site diameter was significantly larger 24 hours after rotational atherectomy than it was immediately postprocedure (50,51), implying that the high acute residual diameter stenosis may reflect an increase in vessel tone. Intravascular ultrasound may be useful for identifying which lesions are best suited for Rotablator and for guiding the use of larger burrs, balloon angioplasty, directional atherectomy, or stenting (51). In general, superficial calcium deposits that will come in contact with the burr surface are most amenable to Rotablator, whereas deep calcium deposits are not. However, most calcified lesions are not crossable by an intravascular ultrasound (IVUS) catheter before treatment.

Use of adjunctive low-pressure balloon angioplasty or stenting is standard after Rotablator (47). Rotablator pretreatment improves vessel compliance and therefore stent expansion so-called "plaque" modification (52), and quantitative angiographic studies using matching lesion subsets suggest that pretreating many types of lesions with Rotablator can facilitate the results of adjunctive angioplasty (53; Figs. 23.6–23.8). However, early studies also indicated significant angiographic complications in nearly 40% of lesions after Rotablator—including angiographic dissection in 29%, side-branch occlusion in 1.8%, distal embolization in 0.9%, no reflow in 6.1%, abrupt closure in 11.2%, severe spasm in 13.8%, and perforation in 1 to 2% of lesions. With modifications to technique as described above, current Rotablator complication rates are now comparable with other interventional modalities. As with directional atherectomy, however, there is a higher incidence of non–Q-wave myocardial infarction after Rotablator (19% in one study of long lesions; 41), although this tends to be reduced by adjunctive use of platelet GP IIb/IIIa receptor antagonists.

In the present era, the ERBAC (Excimer, Rotablator, Balloon Angioplasty for Complex Lesions) study randomized patients to rotational atherectomy, excimer laser angioplasty, or balloon angioplasty (see below in laser section), showing that the final-diameter stenosis after Rotablator and adjunctive angioplasty was significantly

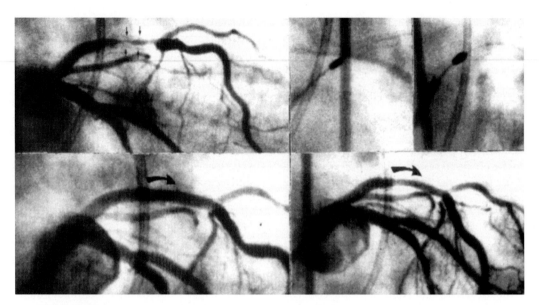

Figure 23.6 **Top left.** Rotablator for in-stent restenosis. Severe restenosis is present in the proximal left anterior descending (note stent struts, *small arrows*). **Top center and top right.** Rotational atherectomy with 1.75- and 2.15-mm burrs. **Bottom right.** Appearance post-Rotablator. **Bottom left.** Appearance after final balloon dilatation.

lower than after excimer laser or balloon angioplasty alone, yet 6-month angiographic restenosis was similar (45 to 50%; 54). Other observational studies suggest a clinical restenosis rate of 38% and an angiographic restenosis rate between 31 and 59%. The 500-patient randomized STRATAS trial compared aggressive rotational atherectomy, defined as burr-to-artery ratio >0.75, to standard burr sizing (<0.7) to evaluate the impact of

greater debulking (55). There was no difference in acute outcome, except for a trend towards more non–Q-wave myocardial infarction and a higher 6-month restenosis (58%, for the aggressive arm versus 52% for the conventional arm; $P = NS$). These findings thus favor single-burr plaque modification over a multi-burr debulking strategy. Finally, in small calcified coronaries, the randomized DART trial found no difference in angiographic or clinical

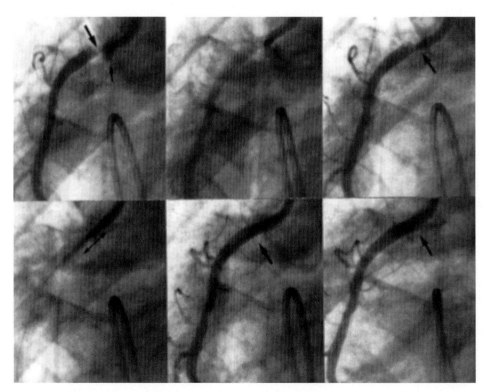

Figure 23.7 Ostial RCA rotastent. **Top left.** Severe ostial right coronary stenosis *(long arrow)* with heavy calcification *(short arrow)*. **Top center.** A 1.75-mm Rotablator burr positioned just outside the lesion. **Top right.** Modest lumen enlargement after rotational atherectomy. **Bottom left.** The resulting lumen, however, allowed advancement of a stent. **Bottom center.** Stent deployment. **Bottom right.** Final result post-dilatation.

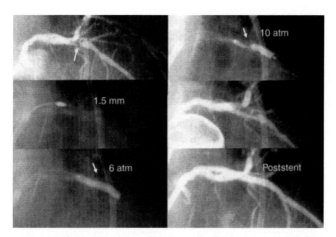

Figure 23.8 Resistant calcified lesion becomes responsive after Rotablator. **Top left.** Severe stenosis in the proximal left anterior descending *(arrow).* **Top right.** Persistent waist despite inflation of angioplasty balloon to 10 atm. **Center left.** Advancement of a 1.5-mm Rotablator burr (note the heavy calcium shadows). **Center right.** Modest lumen enlargement following Rotablator. **Bottom left.** Following Rotablator, however, the same balloon now expands completely at 6 atm. **Bottom right.** Final result after stent placement.

restenosis with or without use of Rotablator before balloon dilation (56).

In the stent era, Hoffman and coworkers (57) demonstrated that treatment of calcified lesions with rotational atherectomy before stenting resulted in larger post-treatment lumen diameters and higher 9-month event-free survival compared with historical controls undergoing stenting alone. The prospective SPORT trial (58) randomized 735 patients to Rotablator plus stenting or to stenting alone. Acute procedural success was improved for patients undergoing Rotablator and stenting (93.6% versus 88%, $P = 0.01$), but there was no difference found in subsequent restenosis (target lesion repeat [TLR] rates: 30.4 versus 27.6%, $P = $ NS). This "rota-stent" approach, however, remains our standard technique for calcified ostial and left main lesions (59,60). Data on Rotablator prior to drug-eluting stent implantation are lacking, although this may help in stent delivery and more uniform stent expansion resulting in more homogenous drug delivery.

Contraindications to Rotablator include the presence of visible thrombus or extremely eccentric lesions in a severe bend in which the normal vessel wall lies on the outer curve of the bend. Although Rotablator is technically feasible in long lesions, it may be associated with a significant incidence of no-reflow or non–Q-wave myocardial infarction, and there are no data to suggest superiority to conventional angioplasty using long balloons. Rotablator also has a clear operator learning curve to permit safe use and is further limited by the maximum 2.5-mm burr diameter, the frequent need for adjunctive balloon angioplasty or stenting, the high cost of procedures, and the lack of a confirmed impact on restenosis. Although the complications of distal embolization—no reflow, severe coronary vasospasm, brady-

cardia, and perforation—are uncommon with refinement in Rotablator technique as described above, they can clearly occur, making Rotablator use uncommon among low-volume interventional operators.

Use in Specific Lesion Types

Rotational atherectomy is particularly indicated for specific lesion subsets where stent delivery is difficult or known to be associated with suboptimal acute angiographic results. Among those are calcified, ostial nondilatable lesions or chronic total occlusions (Figs. 23.6–23.8). Although detailed randomized trial data are limited, we recommend the use of Rotablator for those lesions that are least likely to be treated optimally by conventional angioplasty and stenting, such as long, ostial and heavily calcified lesions including left main arteries, calcified bifurcation lesions (61), and the rare (1 to 2%) lesions that cannot be dilated successfully at inflation pressures of 10 to 12 atm. Also, lesions that cannot be crossed with a balloon or stent catheter owing to lesion rigidity or excessive calcification of the proximal vessel may be amenable to Rotablator (62) or excimer laser (see below).

Bifurcation Lesions

As with directional atherectomy, debulking of bifurcation lesions prior to stenting may lessen the risk of plaque shift and side-branch narrowing or occlusion. When the side branch or main branch is ≤2.5 mm in diameter and the angulation of the side branch origin is fairly obtuse (>120°), rotablation should be carried out in the main branch first. If the result is smooth and without dissection, the wire can then be repositioned into the side branch and rotablation performed. If a larger burr is then required, this same alternating process can be repeated.

Jailed Side Branches

A subset of bifurcation lesions is those where a stent has been previously placed across the origin of a side branch, which has subsequently become narrowed. Rotational atherectomy has been used in this setting to pass through a cell in the stent into the jailed side branch. This approach has been accomplished safely without burr entrapment, provided the stent cell overlying the side-branch ostium has been previously balloon dilated and a small initial burr size (1.25 or 1.5 mm) is chosen.

Calcified Lesions

Rotational atherectomy has become the standard approach for heavily calcified lesions or for lesions whose approach requires traversing heavily calcified, although not necessarily stenotic, segments. In these settings, small burr sizes (e.g., 1.5 mm) often provide adequate vessel preparation without the need for use of serial burrs.

Undilatable Lesions

Occasionally, severely stenotic lesions will not respond to initial balloon dilations at 10 to 12 atm. In this circumstance, rotational atherectomy, again often with a single small burr, will modify the vessel wall and allow dilation and stenting. Caution must be used to ensure that no dissection is present after the initial (unsuccessful) attempt at balloon dilation, and Rotablator should be avoided after attempted angioplasty if there is any evidence of local dissection.

Ostial Lesions

Aorto-ostial lesions of the RCA or left main, or lesions of the origin of the left anterior descending (LAD) or left circumflex (LCX) pose challenges for acute success as well as late restenosis that may be improved with rotational atherectomy. As sites of heavy elastin content and substantial plaque, bulk ostial lesions are frequently difficult to dilate. Furthermore, precise stent positioning is essential to ensure adequate coverage of the ostium. Rotational atherectomy can help by modifying plaque to allow initial dilation and debulking to allow smoother stent positioning and better contrast opacification around the stent as it is positioned.

In-Stent Restenosis

Rotational atherectomy was widely used in the treatment of bare-metal stent restenosis. Conflicting data existed regarding the merits of this approach, particularly in conjunction with vascular brachytherapy (34,63–66). In the prebrachytherapy era, the ROSTER trial, which used IVUS to exclude from randomization patients who had poorly dilated stents, showed a benefit to debulking with rotational atherectomy. The randomized ARTIST trial, however, which used only a single small burr and only low-pressure postdilation, failed to show benefit compared with high-pressure balloon dilation of in-stent restenosis (66). In the setting of vascular brachytherapy, no clear advantage to adjunctive rotational atherectomy has been demonstrated, and use of this approach has declined precipitously.

ABLATIVE LASER TECHNIQUES

It was hoped that laser angioplasty would permit precise plaque removal with fewer acute complications and lower incidence of clinical restenosis (67). Despite the evolution of catheter system designs over the years, restenosis rates following laser angioplasty have not been lower than with balloon angioplasty alone (6,54). Given the lack of clinical benefit over other mechanical therapies, and the significant capital cost ($100,000 to $250,000) for acquiring a laser system, hopes for laser coronary angioplasty have shifted from a mainstream stand-alone therapy to an infrequently used adjunctive treatment to debulk plaque before stenting in lesions with large atherosclerotic plaque burdens, or to debulk in-stent restenosis. Because laser systems are still in use in some laboratories, and newer applications may still be found, the body of theoretical and clinical data will be reviewed.

Laser Generation

Light amplification by stimulated emission of radiation (laser) is the process of creating an in-phase (coherent) beam of monochromatic light with high energy. The lasing medium is "pumped" by an external energy source to force most of the atoms or molecules from their lower-energy ground state to a higher-energy excited state. After a brief time—measured in nanoseconds—the atoms begin to relax to their ground state by giving off a photon whose wavelength is determined by the energy difference between the excited and ground states, by the equation $E = hv$, where h = Planck's constant and $v = c/l$ (c, speed of light; l, wavelength). One spontaneously released photon of precisely matched energy (hv) can induce other excited atoms in the lasing medium to relax to the ground state and emit photons that are identical in direction, wavelength, and phase to the stimulating photon (stimulated emission). As this wave passes through the laser cavity, light coalesces into a single wavefront whose intensity increases exponentially as it travels along the optical axis of the laser cavity and is reflected back and forth between the mirrors positioned at either end of the chamber. This standing wave of intense, monochromatic, coherent light then permeates the optical coupler, from which it travels down the optical fibers within the multifiber laser catheter whose other end is positioned within the coronary artery lumen to illuminate the obstructing plaque with a burst of laser light.

Laser–Tissue Interactions

The interaction between laser light and biologic tissue depends on the wavelength, the mode of laser operation (continuous wave or pulsed), the energy density of the laser light (fluence), as well as any interposed fluid medium (saline or blood) and the tissue's intrinsic absorption characteristics. For coronary laser angioplasty, lasers can be divided into ultraviolet lasers (e.g., XeCl excimer lasers, 300-nm wavelength) in which ablative energy is absorbed directly by atherosclerotic plaque absorption and near-infrared/infrared lasers (e.g., holmium or neodynium YAG [yttrium-aluminum-garnet], 2,000-nm wavelength) in which thermal energy produced by water absorption leads to secondary photocoagulation. It is also important to distinguish continuous-wave laser systems, in which laser light is emitted in an uninterrupted manner, from newer pulsed systems that deliver peak laser over a very short pulse followed by a long interpulse interval to reduce heating of surrounding tissue. Despite these theoretical advantages, all pulsed laser systems still produce some thermal effects that are detectable with histologic examination after holmium and excimer laser radiation (68,69).

Although water is almost completely transparent to ultraviolet light at wavelengths greater than 193 nm, it absorbs infrared light strongly owing to excitement of the

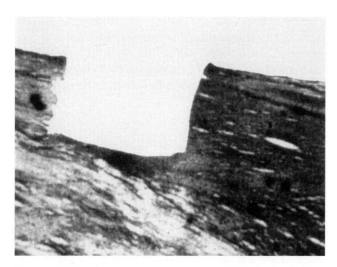

Figure 23.9 Ablation of postmortem human aortic tissue with pulsed excimer laser radiation at 193 nm under air.

translational, vibrational, and rotational frequencies of the H:O bond. On the other hand, blood, x-ray contrast agents, and tissue DNA absorb ultraviolet (UV) light avidly. When laser light encounters biologic tissue, tissue vaporization occurs if the light contains wavelengths that are absorbed by the tissue, and if the absorbed energy exceeds the threshold for triggering a phase transformation. Tissue ablation then takes place through one of three mechanisms: vaporization of tissue (photothermal effects), ejection of debris (photoacoustic effect), or direct breakdown of molecules (photochemical dissociation; 70). Because early experimental studies involving free-laser

beams in air (67) showed tidy ablation of biologic tissue with clean margins and no histologic evidence of thermal injury (Fig. 23.9), it was thought that photodissociation was the predominant mechanism of excimer laser ablation of atherosclerotic plaque in vivo. Studies under saline or blood, however, disclosed less efficient plaque ablation and significant dissection of adjacent tissue owing to formation and implosion of vapor bubbles at the impact site. The use of intracoronary saline infusion to displace blood and radiographic contrast in the excimer laser field may thus reduce the risk of vessel dissection during excimer laser angioplasty (Figs. 23.9, 23.10).

Catheter Delivery Systems

All current clinical laser systems share common elements: a laser generator, an energy coupler, and a catheter delivery system. Laser catheters have evolved from the initial single bare optical fibers to today's trackable, flexible, over-the-wire or monorail catheter systems that contain several hundred optical fibers. Each optical fiber is composed of a transmitting material (such as purified silica for excimer laser angioplasty) surrounded by a cladding. Since the cladding and silica fibers have different refractive indices, this creates an interface that promotes internal reflection and transmission of light down the length of fiber with negligible energy loss. The brittle fiber and cladding materials are surrounded by a flexible protective coating to allow bending without fissuring. Efficient coupling of energy between the laser generator and the optical fibers requires critical tolerances for alignment and precise polishing of the fiber ends.

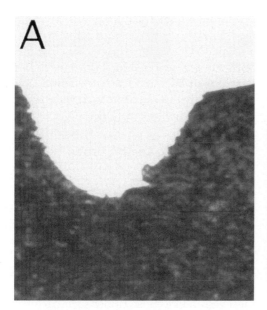
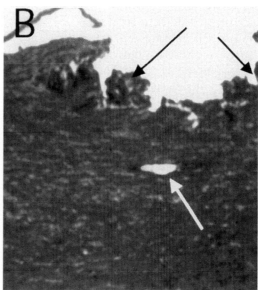

Figure 23.10 Ablation of porcine aortic tissue after pulsed excimer laser angioplasty at 308 nm with multifiber laser catheters under saline **(A)** or blood **(B)**. (Photomicrographs courtesy of L. Wells, Spectranetics, Colorado Springs, CO.)

Procedure

Conventional guiding catheters can be used for excimer laser angioplasty. Because laser catheters are stiffer than balloon catheters and have difficulty negotiating acute angles into the target vessel, coaxial alignment is imperative. Otherwise, firm guide support theoretically is not needed to advance the activated laser catheter through the target lesion, and excessive pushing of the catheter across the lesion may increase the risk of vessel dissection. To maximize the likelihood of a safe outcome and reduce the risk of vessel perforation with excimer laser angioplasty, it is important to select a laser catheter with a diameter at least 1.0 mm smaller than the reference diameter of the target vessel, e.g., a 2-mm catheter for a 3-mm vessel. For diffuse disease or total and subtotal occlusions, a smaller laser catheter (1.3 or 1.4 mm) should be used for initial crossing. In practice, we commonly use only the smallest (0.9-mm) laser catheter to cross lesions that cannot be crossed with a balloon catheter. In this context, it has the benefit of being advanced over a standard 0.014-inch guidewire, rather than requiring recrossing with the special Rotablator wire (see above).

After the target lesion is crossed with the guidewire, the laser catheter is advanced to lie at the proximal end of the lesion. Before activating the laser and beginning ablation of the lesion, every effort must be made to first remove all contrast medium from the target vessel by flushing the guide catheter with at least 30 mL of saline. This is important, because the interaction between excimer laser radiation and any retained contrast medium may increase the generation of shock waves with disruption of adjacent tissue planes (71).

During pulsed excimer laser angioplasty, laser energy is delivered at a fluence of 40 to 70 mJ/mm^2 at a frequency of 20 to 25 Hz for a duration of 1 to 5 seconds as the tip of the catheter is advanced through the lesion. For soft lesions such as saphenous vein graft lesions and restenosis lesions, laser ablation may commence at a fluence of 40 mJ/mm^2, but for calcified lesions and de novo lesions in the native coronary arteries, the initial fluence should be 50 mJ/mm^2. As the laser is activated, the catheter is advanced slowly under fluoroscopic guidance through the lesion at an average rate of 0.5 to 1.0 mm/second. After each 1- to 5-second train of laser pulses, the laser catheter should "rest" for 10 seconds to avoid potential attenuation of energy transmission through the optical fibers. If the laser catheter meets resistance and cannot pass through the lesion at the initial fluence, the energy output should be increased by increments of 10 mJ/mm^2 to a maximum of 60 or 70 mJ/mm^2. If the laser catheter still cannot be advanced at higher fluence levels, the repetition rate also can be increased by increments of 5 Hz to a maximum of 40 Hz. With the 0.9-mm laser catheter, fluence up to 80 mJ/mm^2 at a repetition rate of up to 80 Hz can be used. If the laser catheter still fails to make progress through a stenotic segment after 15 seconds of laser time, the temptation for forceful advancement of the catheter should be avoided, since this will only increase the risk of vessel perforation. Once the laser catheter has been advanced completely through the stenotic segment, adjunctive balloon dilation and stenting can be performed.

Results

Clinical success with the excimer laser, defined as less than 50% residual stenosis (after all treatments) and absence of major in-hospital complications, has been reported in 84 to 94% of patients with saphenous vein graft lesions, aorto-ostial stenoses, total occlusions, long lesions, and undilatable lesions (54,72–74). Early clinical experience with holmium laser coronary angioplasty in 331 patients demonstrated a procedural success rate of 94% and a perforation rate of 1.9% (73–75). Because of the similarities for both excimer laser and holmium laser interaction with tissue, the clinical results for the two systems are quite similar.

Despite increased clinical success with catheter improvements, the rates of vessel dissection and perforation have remained constant, with an incidence of propagating dissection as high as 22% (Fig. 23.11; 72,74). Although coronary artery dissection is not unique to laser angioplasty, extension of the dissection beyond the treated site is probably more common following laser angioplasty than after use of balloon angioplasty or other devices. Vessel perforation occurs during laser angioplasty in 1 to 2% of patients treated (76) and commonly leads to a major complication (death, MI, cardiac tamponade, or bypass surgery). Risk factors for perforation include the use of oversized laser catheters, bifurcation lesions, and diabetes mellitus (77). The use of a saline flush during lasing has been shown to reduce the incidence of dissection and perforation both experimentally (78) and clinically.

Although laser angioplasty was developed initially to reduce restenosis by ablating atheromatous plaque without injuring the normal components of the arterial wall, restenosis was reported in approximately 50% of patients treated with laser and balloon dilation Extensive data of outcomes after laser and stenting with bare-metal or drug-eluting stents are lacking (79).

Use in Specific Lesion Types

Undilatable Lesions

In a similar fashion to rotational atherectomy, excimer laser angioplasty is associated with successful treatment in 89% of 36 patients with lesions that could be crossed with a guidewire but could not be dilated with balloon angioplasty (80). Laser angioplasty should not be attempted, however, in cases where prior dilation attempts resulted in local vessel dissection. Under such circumstances, use of excimer laser angioplasty is invariably associated with worsened dissection or perforation.

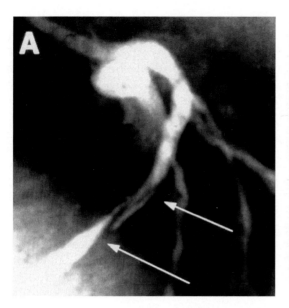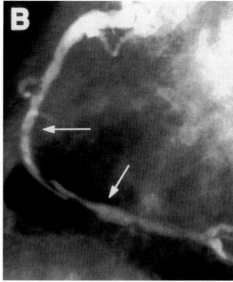

Figure 23.11   Coronary artery dissections after excimer laser angioplasty. Treatment of a long lesion in the left anterior descending artery (**A,** *proximal arrow*) was associated with propagating dissection (*distal arrow*). Treatment of a total occlusion in the midportion of the right coronary artery (**B,** *proximal arrow*) was associated with propagating dissection to the distal right coronary artery (*distal arrow*).

Total Occlusions

Total occlusions crossable with a guidewire are associated with procedural success rates of 84 to 90% with excimer laser angioplasty (81,82). Many dissections that occur with excimer laser angioplasty, especially in the treatment of total occlusions, arise because the guidewire has traveled along an extraluminal course. It is thus important to ensure that the guidewire is in the true lumen of the vessel by using IVUS or frequent contrast injections to confirm that the distal wire tip remains mobile before advancing the laser catheter. In the prestent era, long-term success after excimer laser treatment of total occlusions was limited by the development of restenosis in approximately 50% of patients. In the randomized AMRO trial (73), there was no restenosis benefit seen for excimer laser compared with balloon angioplasty in a subset of 103 patients who presented with total occlusions. With bare-metal or drug-eluting stents, there are no complete data.

For total occlusions not crossable with a conventional guidewire, a new approach with an excimer laser-based guidewire recently underwent clinical investigation. The Prima laser guidewire system (Spectranetics Corp., Colorado Springs, CO) consists of an 0.018-inch fiberoptic bundle coupled to a pulsed excimer laser operating at a tip fluence of 60 mJ/mm^2 at 25 to 40 Hz. The system uses a centering balloon to position the initial ablation trajectory through the obstruction. It was evaluated more formally in two prospective trials in which the laser guidewire was used only after conventional guidewire techniques were performed and documented to fail. The U.S. TOTAL trial evaluated the learning phase of the lasing strategy in a 179-patient registry

(83). Using the Prima catheter alone or in combination with a conventional guidewire, 61% of the refractory total occlusions were successfully crossed. Major complications were low, with a 1.1% death rate and 1.7% rate of perforation leading to tamponade. A similar European feasibility trial demonstrated a 59% successful recanalization rate in 39 patients who could not be treated with conventional guidewire techniques (84). The European TOTAL Surveillance Study was a multicenter trial done to evaluate the safety and performance of the excimer laser system in 345 patients with a median occlusion age of 29 weeks (85). The recanalization rate was 59%, with no deaths, emergency surgery, or Q-wave myocardial infarctions. Although coronary perforations (laser "exits") were seen in 21% of cases, only 1% had tamponade. The independent covariates associated with success were occlusion age <40 weeks and lesion length <30 mm.

Calcified Lesions

Calcified lesions initially were thought to be an indication for excimer laser angioplasty (86), but results of several studies tempered the enthusiasm for this indication. In the Excimer Laser Rotational Atherectomy Balloon Angioplasty Comparison involving 620 patients (ERBAC trial; 54), excimer laser angioplasty was compared with conventional balloon angioplasty and percutaneous transluminal rotational atherectomy for types B and C lesions and a high proportion of calcified lesions. The procedural success rate was 84% for balloon angioplasty, 88% for excimer laser angioplasty, and 93% for rotational atherectomy. The incidence of major complications (death, MI, or bypass surgery) was greater after excimer laser angioplasty than after rotational atherectomy or balloon angioplasty (6.2 versus 2.3% and 4.8%, respectively). At 6-month follow-up, the incidence of clinical events (death, MI, bypass surgery, or repeat intervention) was greater after treatment with rotational atherectomy than balloon angioplasty (53 versus 45%, $P < 0.05$), whereas treatment with excimer laser angioplasty was associated with an intermediate rate of clinical events (49%). These data do not support the use of laser in calcified lesions.

In-Stent Restenosis

Laser angioplasty may be used successfully as a debulking treatment for in-stent restenosis. Excimer laser angioplasty with adjunctive balloon dilatation was evaluated in 527 in-stent lesions in 440 patients previously treated with bare-metal stents (87). There was a 92% laser angioplasty success, with serious adverse events including death (1.6%), Q-MI (0.5%), perforation (0.9%), and dissections after laser (4.8%) or postdilatation (9.3%). Mehran and coworkers (88) compared the results of balloon angioplasty alone with excimer laser followed by balloon angioplasty in 98 cases of in-stent restenosis treated without vascular brachytherapy. By quantitative angiography and intravascular ultrasound, excimer laser was found to safely provide greater acute gain, plaque reduction, larger cross-sectional lumen area, and a trend for lower clinical restenosis than seen with balloon angioplasty.

MECHANICAL THROMBECTOMY

The pathogenesis of acute myocardial ischemic syndromes in native coronary arteries and saphenous aortocoronary vein grafts clearly involves thrombus formation (89–91). Often the amount of thrombus formation at the surface of a ruptured plaque required to interrupt coronary flow is so small as not to be evident on coronary angiography. Occasionally, however, larger thrombi propagate beyond the culprit plaque or into a proximal area of stagnant flow. Such large thrombi may be evident on angiography, and attempted intervention in such lesions tends to produce significant clinical problems (distal embolization, no reflow, abrupt closure). Historically, such cases with substantial intraluminal thrombus have been recognized by certain angiographic and clinical clues (recent onset of symptoms, a mobile, rat-tail filling defect) and treated by infusions of thrombolytic drugs. More recently, these large thrombi have been considered suitable targets for mechanical thrombectomy devices.

Pharmacologic Strategies Devised to Remove Thrombus

Before the development of mechanical thrombectomy, standard therapy involved direct intracoronary or intragraft infusion of urokinase (92–94). The safety and efficacy of this approach was evaluated in the ROBUST trial (95), in which 107 patients with occluded saphenous vein bypass grafts were treated with direct urokinase infusion through a 0.035-inch infusion wire. After 25.4 hours of urokinase infusion to a mean dosage of 3.7 million units, a 69% recanalization success rate was observed with major complications including a 3% stroke rate and a 6.5% death rate. Broader use of adjunctive urokinase infusion, however, during intervention in patients with unstable angina, was studied in the randomized TAUSA trial (96) and was associated with a worsening of clinical outcomes. In an attempt to avoid systemic lytic complications, urokinase has also been delivered directly to the thrombus surface using various specialized delivery catheters or hydrogel-coated balloons. Initial experience showed complete dissolution of thrombus in patients with angiographically evident thrombus in native coronary and vein graft obstructions (97–99).

Mechanical Thrombectomy

Limitations in speed, efficacy, and bleeding complications have fostered the development of catheter-based techniques for direct thrombus removal. Several catheter-based systems have been designed either to disintegrate thrombus or to aspirate and remove thrombus from the body.

Cut-and-Aspirate Devices

The mechanical cutting and aspirating transluminal extraction catheter (TEC) device was once advocated as a potential strategy for the treatment of thrombus-containing native coronaries and vein grafts (100–104), but its use has been associated with problems with distal embolization and vessel injury. More recently, the X-sizer device has used a rotating helical auger at its tip, combined with luminal suction, to remove clots. In the X-tract trial, there was no net benefit in the X-TRACT trial (105) except for a reduction in large myocardial infarction (CK-MB greater than eight times normal) in a subgroup with large baseline thrombi. The Pathways Medical device uses external vanes on a spinning catheter, combined with luminal suction, to remove clots and atherosclerotic debris from saphenous vein grafts, but remains investigational at this time.

Venturi/Bernoulli Suction

Another approach is to use a high-speed water jet to create suction via the Bernoulli/Venturi effect. The Cordis Hydrolyser used this approach, but had only limited European exposure in humans in peripheral vessels (106), hemodialysis shunts (107), and coronary arteries and vein grafts (108,109). By far, the dominant application of this principle, however, is the Possis AngioJet. This catheter has a stainless steel tip connected to a high-pressure hypotube

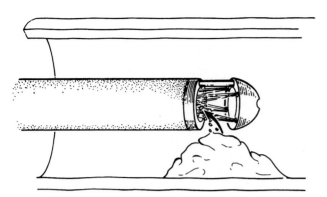

Figure 23.12 Principle of Rheolytic thrombectomy with the Possis AngioJet. High-speed saline jets exit orifices near the catheter tip and spray back into the mouth of the catheter. This creates intense local suction by the Venturi effect, which pulls thrombus into the jets, where the thrombus is macerated and propelled down the catheter lumen for external collection.

(Fig. 23.12). Saline is injected through the catheter via the hypotube into the tip, where it exits as a set of high-speed jets directed back through a small opening before re-entering the main catheter lumen and then being evacuated. By the Venturi/Bernoulli principle, this creates a low-pressure region at the tip within the small opening. Combined with a normal pressure in the arterial lumen of >100 mm Hg, a driving pressure of 860 mm Hg thus pulls surrounding fluid (blood, thrombus, and saline) into the tip opening. There, the jets break the thrombus into subcellular-sized particles and propel them proximally through the catheter lumen and out of the body. A hemostasis valve allows for the evacuation lumen to be sealed around a 0.014-inch-diameter guidewire, over which the catheter is advanced down the coronary vessel.

In the original AngioJet, the jet passed across a 1-m gap near the tip of the catheter, but in contemporary catheters the jet is encased in an outer catheter shaft that has two low-pressure orifices close to the jet and two higher-pressure orifices slightly more proximal. This design creates a circular vortex around the tip of the catheter that is more efficient in clot removal. This has allowed downsizing to the 4F XMI device, which is available in over-the-wire and rapid-exchange formats, each compatible with 6F guiding catheters and 0.014-inch guidewires. They are intended for use in vessels >2.0 mm in diameter, with a larger 5F XVG catheter requiring an 8F guiding catheter and best suited to large (>5.0 mm) saphenous vein bypass grafts or large peripheral arteries. Previous in vivo histologic studies have shown that the catheter produces minimal or no vessel wall damage (110).

Procedure

Once the culprit thrombotic lesion is crossed with a conventional guidewire, the AngioJet is advanced over that wire and distal to the thrombotic lesion. When the foot pedal is depressed, the high-pressure saline jets are activated.

During continued activation, the catheter is withdrawn slowly across the lesion at 0.5 to 1.0 mm/second. By activating the saline jets distal to the lesion, the risk of dislodgement and embolization of thrombotic debris may be reduced, although some operators still prefer to activate the AngioJet proximal to the occlusion as they approach and cross the lesion. Angiography is performed after the first AngioJet pass, and repeated passes are performed until there is no further evidence of improvement in the lumen diameter or thrombus burden between sequential passes.

Transient bradycardia almost always accompanies activation of the AngioJet catheter in the right coronary artery or dominant circumflex, most likely owing to local adenosine release by hemolysis. For this reason, placement of a temporary transvenous pacemaker is essential prior to AngioJet use.

Results

The AngioJet has been used successfully to remove thrombus in semielective situations such as thrombotic vein grafts (Fig. 23.13) as well as in acute coronary ischemic scenarios including acute myocardial infarction (Fig. 23.14; 111–113). It is most effective in removing thrombus <48 hours old. Cross-linking of fibrin and cellular organization make older thrombi less susceptible to fragmentation and removal by the AngioJet.

The Vein Graft AngioJet Study (VeGAS 1), a multicenter registry of 90 patients with acute ischemic syndromes, demonstrated that the AngioJet Rheolytic thrombectomy catheter reduced the angiographically measured thrombus burden within native coronary arteries or saphenous vein bypass grafts by an average of 86% (114). The Vein Graft AngioJet Study Randomized Trial (VeGAS 2) randomized 500 patient with angiographically evident thrombus to the AngioJet Rheolytic Thrombectomy System or selective overnight intracoronary urokinase infusion, do assess the safety and effectiveness of thrombus removal before stenting during the treatment of saphenous vein grafts or native coronaries (115). Because the 30-day event-free survival for major adverse cardiac events (defined as freedom from death, myocardial infarction, emergent bypass surgery, target lesion revascularization, or stroke) was significantly better for the AngioJet group after enrollment of 300 patients, the data safety committee recommended early termination at a final enrollment of 349 patients (180 in the AngioJet arm and 169 in the urokinase arm). The results of VeGAS 1 and VeGAS 2 were the basis of the Food and Drug Administration (FDA) approval of the device in June 1998.

More recently, the *AngioJet Rheolytic Thrombectomy In Patients Undergoing Primary Angioplasty for Acute Myocardial Infarction* (AIMI) trial tested the hypothesis that routine removal of coronary thrombus prior to definitive angioplasty and stenting in the setting of acute myocardial infarction would improve perfusion and myocardial salvage (115a) . In total, 480 patients with acute ST-segment

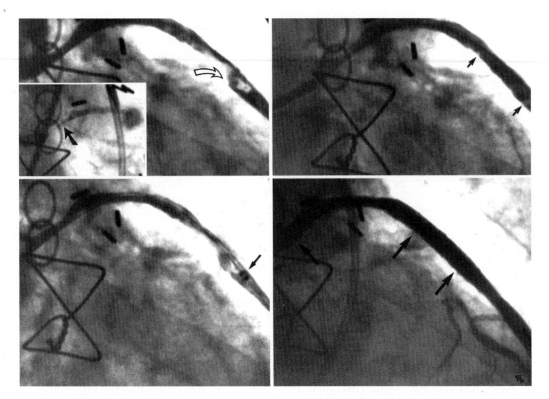

Figure 23.13   Top left insert. Rheolytic thrombectomy with the Possis AngioJet in a patient with an occluded saphenous vein graft. **Top left.** Following balloon angioplasty of the graft ostium, a large filling defect *(open arrow)* is apparent in the body of the graft. **Bottom left.** The AngioJet *(arrow)* is advanced beyond the presumptive thrombus, activated, and pulled back slowly. **Top right.** Following AngioJet treatment, only small defects remain. **Bottom right.** Placement of stents in the ostium and body of the graft provides near-normal appearance and antegrade flow.

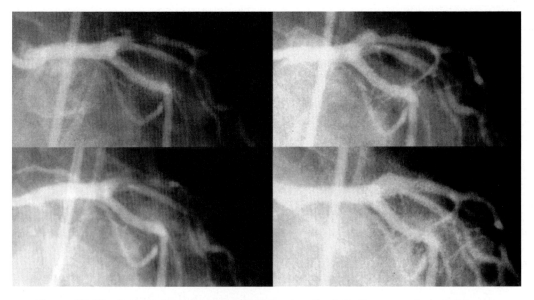

Figure 23.14 AngioJet for acute myocardial infarction. **Top left.** Primary angioplasty for acute anterior wall myocardial infarction shows thrombotic occlusion of the proximal left anterior descending. **Bottom left.** Passage of the AngioJet distal to thrombus. **Top right.** Following aspiration with the AngioJet, the thrombotic filling defect is gone. **Bottom right.** Following stent placement, a large smooth lumen and brisk antegrade flow are present.

elevation myocardial infarction within 12 hours of symptom onset were randomized to either conventional stenting or to AngioJet followed by stenting. The primary end point was infarct size measured 14 to 28 days after presentation by Tc-99m sestamibi single photon emission computed tomography (SPECT) imaging. Ninety-five percent of patients received adjunctive pharmacologic treatment with platelet GP IIb/IIIa receptor antagonists, and the AngioJet was delivered successfully to 95% of patients assigned to that therapy. Despite the fact that 53 to 55% of patients had occluded infarct-related arteries on initial angiography, and an additional 20 to 22% of patients had patent arteries with moderate or large thrombi, the primary end point showed that final infarct size was actually larger (12.5 versus 9.8% of the left ventricle, $P < 0.02$) and TIMI 3 flow was less often achieved (92 versus 97%, $P < 0.02$) in patients randomly assigned to thrombectomy. Finally, the 30-day end point of composite major adverse clinical events (MACEs; death, new Q-wave MI, stroke, TLR) was higher in the thrombectomy group (6.7 versus 1.7%, $P < 0.01$).

Although this suggests that AngioJet thrombectomy should not be performed routinely in patients undergoing primary angioplasty for acute myocardial infarction, there are several important limitations of the AIMI trial that merit mention. Since randomization took place after initial angiography, many patients with large thrombi were likely treated with open-label thrombectomy. Furthermore, delay in reperfusion to allow for setup of the AngioJet console and pacemaker insertion contributed to a total procedure time that was 16 minutes longer in the thrombectomy group than in the control group ($P < 0.0001$). Recognizing these limitations, our clinical practice continues to make use of this device in the setting of acute MI when a large thrombus is present.

Suction Thrombectomy

Several catheters are available for simple suction thrombectomy and may be of value in the management of thrombotic lesions. Although not subjected to controlled studies, these low-profile devices act through simple aspiration. Examples include the Export catheter (Medtronic, Inc.), originally designed as part of the PercuSurge embolic protection Guardwire device, the Rescue catheter (Boston Scientific), and the Pronto catheter (Vascular Solutions). The Rinspirator (Kerberos) has the added attribute of performing simultaneous saline infusion and aspiration to create turbulence that may improve the efficiency of thrombus removal compared with the laminar flow achieved with the simple tubular aspiration catheters.

Ultrasonic Thrombectomy

Ultrasonic vibration can induce cavitation that can fragment thrombus into small particulates. The Acolysis System

used therapeutic coronary ultrasound (at 41.9 kHz) delivered to the tip of a 5F catheter to produce this effect (116–119). In the initial experience, 20 patients were treated with the coronary ultrasound thrombolysis for saphenous vein graft (SVG) disease (75% had total occlusions); there was a 70% device success, with only one patient (5%) having evident distal embolization. However, in the ATLAS trial, 118,181 patients undergoing SVG stenting were randomized to receive Acolysis or abciximab. Angiographic procedural success was achieved in 63% of Acolysis patients and 82% of abciximab patients ($P = 0.008$), and the incidence of major adverse cardiac events at 30 days was 25% with Acolysis and 12% with abciximab ($P = 0.036$), owing primarily to a more frequent non–Q-wave MI with Aacolysis (19.6% versus 7.9%, $P = 0.03$). An ultrasonic guidewire (OmniSonics), which produces a similar effect to Acolysis in vitro, is still in clinical testing.

EMBOLIZATION PROTECTION DEVICES

The devices discussed above seek to remove plaque or thrombus from the target lesion, but it is increasingly clear that most, if not all, interventions (including balloon angioplasty and stent placement) tend to dislodge fragments of friable plaque or thrombus. Particle embolization, moreover, appears to be one of the main causes of no reflow and elevation of cardiac enzymes during saphenous vein graft intervention and primary PCI for acute MI (120,121), as well as the cause of ischemic stroke during carotid artery intervention (see Chapter 27). Various devices have been developed, undergone clinical trial evaluation, and gained regulatory approval to trap such embolic material and remove it from the circulation (Figs. 23.15, 23.16). It is likely that embolic protection will be used in combination with an ever-broader variety of interventional devices (such as thrombectomy and stent placement, Fig. 23.17) to protect the distal circulation from embolization and consequent no reflow and ischemic injury.

Distal Occlusion Systems (Guardwire)

The first FDA-approved device for distal embolic protection was an occlusion balloon and aspiration system, the PercuSurge Guardwire (Medtronic). The system consists of several elements: an angioplasty wire consisting of a 0.014-inch nitinol hypotube with a radiopaque, flexible tip; a 5.5-m-long elastometric balloon (mounted 3.5 cm from the tip of the wire) that can be inflated at low pressure (<2 atmospheres to a diameter of 3.5 to 5.0 mm); and a 135-cm-long side-hole monorail aspiration catheter (Export) used to remove particulate debris and blood after PCI and before deflation of the Guardwire balloon. Once the Guardwire has crossed the lesion and the balloon has been placed in the downstream vessel, the Guardwire

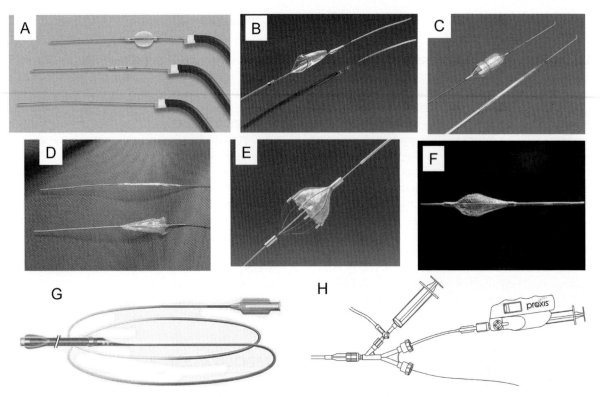

Figure 23.15 Embolus retrieval devices. **A.** The PercuSurge Guardwire shown at the tip of a guiding catheter in deflated and inflated states. **B.** BSC/EPI FilterWire in collapsed and deployed states. **C.** The MedNova filter device shown in collapsed and deployed states. **D.** The Rubicon filter device shown in collapsed and deployed states. **E.** The Cordis Angioguard filter shown in deployed state. **F.** The Medtronic Interceptor Filter shown in deployed state. **G.** The Proxis proximal protection catheter. **H.** The Proxis inflation device and catheter hub system.

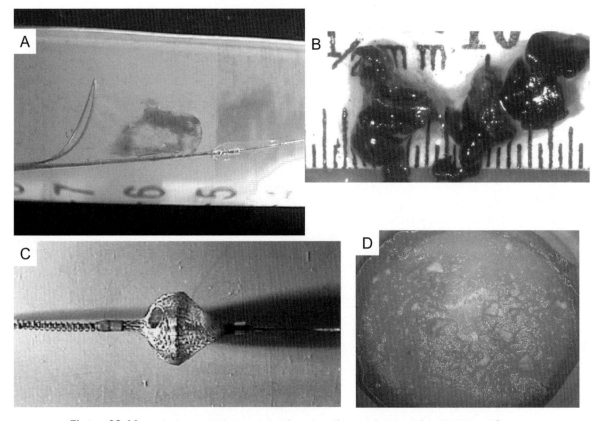

Figure 23.16 Embolic material retrieved with various devices during saphenous vein graft stenting procedures. **A.** EPI FilterWire. **B.** Aspirate during Guardwire occlusion. **C.** Interceptor filter. **D.** Aspirate during Proxis occlusion.

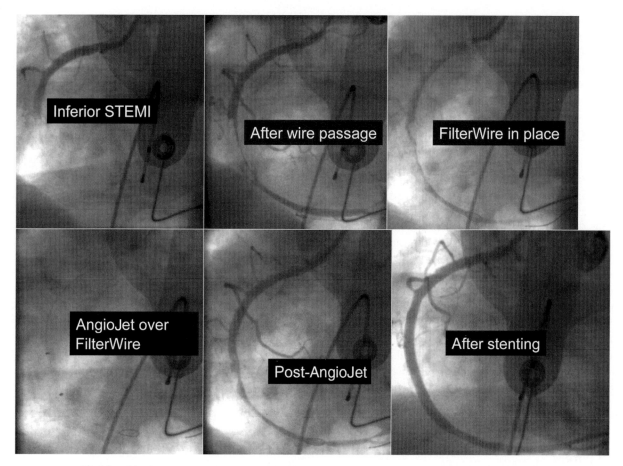

Figure 23.17 Combination of distal protection and Rheolytic thrombectomy. **Top left.** Thrombotic occlusion in the midsegment of the right coronary artery. **Top center.** Severe stenosis and bulky adherent thrombus is present after initial wire crossing. **Top right.** The EPI/BSC FilterWire has been passed into the distal vessel and deployed. **Bottom left.** Advancement of the AngioJet over the FilterWire. **Bottom center.** After removal of the thrombus, residual stenosis is evident. **Bottom right.** After stent placement, brisk flow is evident into the distal vessel.

balloon is inflated to interrupt antegrade flow while the PCI is carried out. All embolic material is trapped in the stagnant column of blood proximal to the balloon and aspirated with the Export catheter before the Guardwire balloon is deflated and antegrade flow is restored.

Strong evidence for distal embolization comes from the early use of this device. The phase I SAFE registry demonstrated safety of this device (122). Webb and colleagues (123) assessed the potential of distal protection by analyzing debris from 27 SVG interventions . The retrieved particles were 204 ± 57 μm in major axis and 83 ± 22 μm in minor axis and consisted of predominantly acellular atheromatous material found under the fibrous cap. Semiquantitative analysis of the plaque material suggested that more debris was released from balloon dilatation than from direct stenting.

The landmark SAFER (*S*aphenous *V*ein *G*raft *A*ngioplasty *F*ree of *E*mboli *R*andomized) trial was the first large randomized trial assessing the impact of embolic protection on clinical outcomes (124). The study assigned 801 patients with SVG lesions to intervention with either a standard guidewire

or a PercuSurge Guardwire. To allow adequate distal landing zone and to limit proximal reflux of debris during Guardwire inflation, lesions had to be >5 mm from the ostium and >20 mm from the distal anastomosis. The primary end point was 30-day MACE rate, defined as a composite of death, myocardial infarction (CK-MB greater than three times the upper limit of normal), emergent bypass surgery, or target vessel revascularization. Technical success with the Guardwire was achieved in 90.1 % of cases. There was a 6.9% absolute reduction (42% relative reduction) in the primary end point for the Guardwire ($P = 0.004$), which was owing primarily to a reduction in non–Q-wave myocardial infarctions. This benefit was seen independent of the use of platelet GP IIb/IIIa receptor blockers, for which enrollment was stratified. Patients treated with the Guardwire had higher rates of TIMI 3 flow and a less frequent no reflow.

Other Distal Occlusion Systems

A second-generation distal occlusion system has been developed and evaluated. The Kensey Nash Triactiv system incorporates a rapidly inflating and deflating CO_2-filled distal balloon and a selective infusion catheter to motivate suspended debris toward the tip of the guiding catheter, which is placed under suction. The randomized *PR*otection during Saphenous Vein Graft *I*ntervention to Prevent *D*istal *E*mbolization (PRIDE) trial was recently completed (124a), and demonstrated equivalence of this device with the Guardwire (30-day MACE rates of 10.2 and 11.2% in the Guardwire and Triactiv groups, respectively). A newer iteration in which the infusion and aspiration functions are combined in a single selective catheter is currently undergoing testing. The Possis GuardDOG (distal occlusion guidewire) also uses a CO_2-filled distal balloon, but uses the AngioJet catheter (see above) to macerate and remove any suspended debris. It is in preliminary clinical testing.

Strengths of all the distal occlusion system include the ability to remove all sizes of particulate debris and humoral factors, whereas weaknesses include the need to interrupt antegrade flow for 3 to 5 minutes during the intervention and aspiration cycles and the inability to inject contrast to visualize the target lesion during the interval. The former limitation can be overcome with careful procedural teamwork and planning, whereas the latter can be partially overcome by injecting contrast through the guiding catheter during balloon inflation and trapping it within the lesion.

Distal Filters

Because they do not interrupt flow, distal filters avoid procedural ischemia sometimes encountered with the Guardwire. Furthermore, they allow more precise positioning of stents and balloon inflations, since contrast puffs through the guiding catheter may be performed in the usual manner. There was initial concern, however, that filters might be less efficacious than distal occlusion, owing to incomplete capture of smaller particles or soluble mediators. Comparative trials, however, have shown that filters are generally as effective as distal occlusion.

FilterWire

The first filter to gain regulatory approval (in mid-2003) was the FilterWire EX. It consists of a conventional guidewire to which an elliptical, radiopaque, nitinol loop is attached. A polyurethane filter bag with 110-micron pores is suspended from the nitinol loop. The device can be used in vessels between 3.5 and 5.5 mm (smaller and larger diameter devices are in development). It is delivered in its collapsed state within a 3.2F (6F guide-compatible) delivery sheath, which is withdrawn to allow the filter to expand and the procedure to be performed over the guidewire shaft. At the end of the intervention, the filter is recollapsed and withdrawn with the aid of a retrieval sheath.

The FilterWire was studied in the initial phase I study (125) and then in the pivotal randomized FilterWire EX

Randomized Evaluation (FIRE) trial (126), which compared it with the Guardwire in saphenous vein graft stenting. This trial was the first to allow direct comparison of the relative efficacy and safety of filtering versus distal occlusion approaches for SVG stenting. The phase I portion treated 60 lesions in 48 patients, and the initial roll-in portion of the phase II study treated 248 lesions in 230 saphenous vein grafts. In combination, these two early experiences identified several technical aspects that were associated with adverse events (21.3% 30-day MACE) and were then addressed in the phase II study: (1) ensuring >2.5-cm distance between lesion and distal anastomosis; (2) placement of the FilterWire in a straight landing zone segment (>2 cm); (3) use of orthogonal angiographic views to document circumferential filter apposition to the vessel wall prior to stenting; (4) retracting only the proximal end of the debris-containing filter into the retrieval sheath. Incorporating these changes, the second phase of toll in patients in the FIRE trial showed a markedly lower 30-day MACE rate of 11.3%.

This favorable performance was continued in the randomized phase of the FIRE trial, which showed 30-day MACE rates with the FilterWire of 9.9%, compared with 11.6% with the GuardWire. The recently approved second-generation FilterWire (FilterWire EZ) has several improvements to the FilterWire EX device, including a mechanism to enhance filter centering even in curved segments and a lower profile peel-away delivery sheath. A small-vessel FilterWire intended for use in saphenous vein bypass grafts <3.0 mm in caliber and in native vessels is also under study.

Other Filters

The Angioguard (Cordis, J&J) is a filter integrated into a 0.014-inch stainless steel angioplasty wire. It has a nickel/titanium skeleton supporting a polyurethane membrane creating a collection basket with laser drilled 100 μm. The basket is delivered via a delivery sheath (2.5F). The MedNova Cardioshield is a distal protection filter consisting of a nonnitinol self-expanding system with a porous polymeric membrane mounted on a 0.014-inch guidewire. An important feature of this device is that it is free to rotate on the guidewire, perhaps enhancing apposition and limiting vascular injury. It was the subject of the randomized CAPTIVE trial, whose results just missed demonstration of noninferiority to the Guardwire ($P = 0.057$) by intent to treat analysis (126a). The Interceptor (Medtronic) is a nitinol basket affixed to a 0.014-inch guidewire. Its first generation required a delivery and retrieval sheath akin to the FilterWire, and initial clinical experience in saphenous vein bypass grafts was reported in the SECURE trial (127). Subsequent generations have incorporated opening and closing of the device from the proximal end of the wire without need for a delivery or retrieval sheath, thus lowering crossing profile and enhancing ease of use. This device is under more broad study in the pivotal randomized AMETHYST trial. Finally, the Rubicon filter (Rubicon, Inc.) is a filter incorporated directly into an 0.014-inch wire, making it the lowest profile filter yet. As with the Interceptor, it is deployed through proximal actuation without the need for a delivery sheath, although a sheath is required for retrieval at the conclusion of the procedure.

General Issues

Although there has been a concern with all filters regarding a lesser completeness of protection than might be afforded by occlusion balloons, several pieces of evidence argue against this. First, the FIRE trial provided reassurance that clinical events were no more common with a filter than with an occlusion balloon (126). Second, analysis of particulate retrieved from filters (first-generation Interceptor) or Guardwire has shown that the aggregate volume of particulate and the distribution of particle size are similar for the two approaches (128). Taken together, these two pieces of data suggest that filters will ensnare the same particulate as occlusion balloons and that soluble mediators do not contribute substantially to adverse events or no reflow. It is important to acknowledge, however, that adverse events still occur even with distal embolic protection. The 30-day MACE rates in the FIRE, SAFER, and PRIDE trial protection groups were all between 9.6 and 11.6%. Although the genesis of these events is not clear, possible contributors include (a) particles released during initial lesion crossing before filter or balloon deployment at the time of deployment of the protection device itself, (b) incomplete aspiration of particles (particularly those adherent to the device itself), (c) motion of the protection device during the procedure with transient loss of apposition and escape of particles, or (d) embolic fragments adherent to the stented site, not freely mobile, which embolize in the early postprocedure hours. Furthermore, it has been difficult to predict which diseased vein grafts will have the greatest risk for particle embolization. A recent analysis on the SAFER and FIRE trials has established two angiographic predictors of saphenous vein graft MACE—the degree of graft degeneration and estimated plaque volume in the lesion being treated (129). Although predicted risk varies between 10 and 50% based on these factors, there is protection against MACE at all levels of risk. In our practice, we therefore use embolic protection devices in essentially all saphenous vein graft interventions for which there is an adequate distal landing zone.

Proximal Occlusion Systems

In an attempt to provide more complete embolic protection (particularly during initial wire crossing), to allow choice of different conventional wire attributes during the procedure, and to permit protection even for lesions too distal to permit use of a distal filter or balloon, novel proximal occlusion systems have been developed. The Proxis device (Velocimed) is a highly flexible 6F balloon-tipped catheter advanced through a conventional 7 or 8F guide to a point proximal to the lesion. With the balloon inflated and distal flow interrupted, guidewires, balloon, and stents can be introduced. At any point during and at the conclusion of the intervention, the distal vascular bed is evacuated by simple aspiration and flow reversal through the guiding catheter. As such, this proximal protection system allows the establishment of protection before any contact with the lesion, including guidewire crossing. It also allows the theoretical protection of all side branches proximal to and distal to the lesion. Initial clinical experience in Europe in the FASTER trial (130) showed a 30-day MACE rate of 5.7% in a mixture of native coronaries and vein grafts, and the pivotal randomized PROXIMAL trial comparing outcomes to FilterWire or Guardwire is underway.

Native Coronary Artery Intervention

Although the initial test bed for embolic protection was the diseased saphenous vein graft, distal embolization during primary angioplasty for acute myocardial infarction is increasingly appreciated. In one report of 178 patients undergoing primary angioplasty, distal embolization was observed in 15.2% and was associated with reduced angiographic success. Myocardial blush scores, ST-T segment resolution, left ventricle ejection fraction, and long-term survival were impaired in patients with distal embolization. Moreover, preliminary reports of embolic protection using the Guardwire and the FilterWire have suggested possible benefit (131). However, randomized clinical trials have provided conflicting data. In the 501-patient enhanced myocardial efficacy and recovery by aspiration of liberalized debris (EMERALD) trial, ST-segment resolution and myocardial perfusion with Tc-99 sestamibi failed to show a benefit of the Guardwire over conventional stenting in patients with acute myocardial infarction (132). In contrast, the much smaller DIPLOMAT trial, which randomized only 60 patients to the Angioguard filter versus conventional stenting and used ST-segment resolution as a primary end point, showed better outcomes in the filter group (133). The ongoing FLAME trial will study the FilterWire in a much larger randomized trial of patients with acute ST-elevation myocardial infarction.

There are, however, several inherent limitations to the use of distal protection devices in native coronary settings. Most important, unlike with saphenous vein grafts, there is the potential for embolization of particulate into side branches that arise between the lesion and the distal protection device. Furthermore, any delay introduced by virtue of needing to prepare and insert the device will result in delay in reperfusion. Third, initial crossing and reperfusion of the occluded infarct-related artery with conventional techniques and in the absence of protection is required to establish a suitable landing zone for the distal protection device. These limitations may be overcome through proximal protection approaches (see above), which would allow establishment of protection before initial crossing even of an occluded vessel and would theoretically permit protection of all side branches as well, with reversal of flow evacuating all vessels in the distribution of the infarct. In summary, the place of embolic protection in native coronary interventions is far from proven, and ongoing clinical trials are assessing novel approaches to this challenging setting.

SUMMARY

Although they have proven no more effective than stenting for the treatment of routine lesions, mechanical and laser-based atherectomy techniques continue to play an important supporting adjunctive role in coronary intervention in certain complex lesion subsets such as ostial, bifurcation, calcified, fibrotic, or in-stent restenotic lesions. In general, they are more challenging to use than balloon and stent techniques and frequently carry a higher cost and an increased risk of some complications (such as per-procedure CK elevation, perforation, or dissection). They have survived as important parts of interventional cardiology, however, because they extend the range of lesions treatable by catheter-based therapy and when used with proper care, may make some procedures simpler and safer. The newer devices for thrombus removal and distal embolic protection also extend the range of treatable lesions and improve procedural results, particularly in saphenous vein bypass graft interventions. Further trials will be required to establish the correct role for these devices in the treatment of native coronary arteries and the peripheral vascular circulation.

REFERENCES

1. Simpson J, Selmon M, Robertson G, et al. Transluminal atherectomy for occlusive peripheral vascular disease. *Am J Cardiol* 1988;61:96G.
2. Simpson J. How atherectomy began: a personal history. *Am J Cardiol* 1993;72:3E.
3. Safian R. Clinical and angiographic results of transluminal extraction coronary atherectomy in saphenous vein bypass grafts. *Circulation* 1994;89:302.
4. Ahn S, Auth D, Marcus D, Moore W. Removal of focal atheromatous lesions by angioscopically guided high-speed rotary atherectomy. *J Vasc Surg* 1988;7:292.
5. Fourrier J. Percutaneous coronary rotational atherectomy in humans: preliminary report. *J Am Coll Cardiol* 1989;14:1278.
6. Bittl J. Clinical results with excimer laser coronary angioplasty. *Semin Intervent Cardiol* 1996;1:129–34.
7. Hinohara T, Selmon M, Robertson G, et al. Directional atherectomy. New approaches for treatment of obstructive coronary and peripheral vascular disease. *Circulation* 1990;81(suppl):IV79.
8. Baim D, et al. Results of directional coronary atherectomy during multicenter preapproval testing. *Am J Cardiol* 1993;72:6E.
9. Matar F, Mintz G, Farb A, et al. The contribution of tissue removal to the lumen improvement after directional coronary atherectomy. *Am J Cardiol* 1994;74:647–650.
10. Penny W, Schmidt D, Safian R, et al. Insights into the mechanism of luminal improvement after directional coronary atherectomy. *Am J Cardiol* 1991;67:435.
11. Lansky A, Mintz G, Popma J. Remodeling after directional coronary atherectomy (with and without percutaneous adjunct transluminal coronary angioplasty): a serial angiographic and intravascular ultrasound analysis from the Optimal Atherectomy Restenosis Study. *J Am Coll Cardiol* 1998;32:329.
12. Moussa I, Moses J, DiMario C, et al. Stenting after optimal lesion debulking (SOLD) registry. Angiographic and clinical outcome. *Circulation* 1998;98:1604.
13. Baim D, Cutlip D, Sharma S, et al. Final results of the Balloon vs Optimal Atherectomy Trial (BOAT). *Circulation* 1998;97:322.
14. Gordon P, Kugelmass AD, Cohen DJ, et al. Balloon postdilation can safely improve the results of successful (but suboptimal) directional coronary atherectomy. *Am J Cardiol* 1993;72:71E.
15. Simonton C, Leon M, Baim D, et al. "Optimal" directional coronary atherectomy: final results of the Optimal Atherectomy Restenosis Study (OARS). *Circulation* 1998;97:332.
16. Fishman R, Kuntz R, Carrozza J, et al. Long-term results of directional coronary atherectomy: predictors of restenosis. *J Am Coll Cardiol* 1992;20:1101.
17. Hinohara T, Rowe M, Robertson G, et al. Effect of lesion characteristics on outcome of directional coronary atherectomy. *J Am Coll Cardiol* 1991;17:1112.
18. Waksman R, Popma J, Kennard E, et al. Directional coronary atherectomy: a report from the NACI Registry. *Am J Cardiol* 1997;80:50K.
19. Topol E, Leya F, Pinkerton C, et al. A comparison of directional atherectomy with coronary angioplasty in patients with coronary artery disease. *N Engl J Med* 1993;329:221.
20. Adelman A, et al. A comparison of directional atherectomy with balloon angioplasty for lesions of the left anterior descending coronary artery. *N Engl J Med* 1993;329:228.
21. Suzuki T, Hosokawa H, Katoh O, et al. Effects of adjunctive balloon angioplasty after intravascular ultrasound-guided optimal directional atherectomy: the result of Adjunctive Balloon Angioplasty After Coronary Atherectomy Study (ABACAS). *J Am Coll Cardiol* 1999;34:1028.
22. Kiesz R, Rozek M, Mego D, et al. Acute directional coronary atherectomy prior to stenting in complex coronary lesions: ADAPTS Study. *Cathet Cardiovasc Diagn* 1998;45:105.
23. Stankovic G, Colombo A, Bersin R, et al. Comparison of directional coronary atherectomy and stenting versus stenting alone for the treatment of de novo and restenotic coronary artery narrowing. *Am J Cardiol* 2004;93:953–958.
24. Aizawa T, Tamai H, Asakura Y, et al. Clinical and angiographic results of the Debulking and Stenting in Restenosis Elimination (DESIRE) trial. *Circulation* 2001;104:II624.
25. Schnitt S, Safian R, Kuntz R, et al. Histologic findings in specimens obtained by percutaneous directional coronary atherectomy. *Hum Pathol* 1992;23:415.
26. Miller M, Kuntz R, Friedrich S, et al. Frequency and consequences of intimal hyperplasia in specimens retrieved by directional atherectomy of native primary coronary artery stenoses and subsequent restenoses. *Am J Cardiol* 1993;71:652.
27. Kuntz R, Hinohara T, Safian RD, et al. Restenosis following directional coronary atherectomy: the effects of luminal diameter and deep wall excision. *Circulation* 1992;86:1394.
28. Holmes DR Jr, Garratt K, Isner J, et al. Effect of subintimal resection on initial outcome and restenosis for native coronary lesions and saphenous vein graft disease treated by directional coronary atherectomy. A report from the CAVEAT I and II investigators. Coronary Angioplasty Versus Excisional Atherectomy Trial. *J Am Coll Cardiol* 1996;28:645.
29. Imai Y, Hara K, Yamasaki M, et al. Mid-term follow-up of coronary artery aneurysm after directional coronary atherectomy. *J Cardiol* 1999;33:201.
30. Bell M, Garratt K, Bresnahan J, et al. Relation of deep arterial resection and coronary artery aneurysms after directional coronary atherectomy. *J Am Coll Cardiol* 1992;20:1474.

31. Eisenhauer A, Clugston R, Ruiz C. Sequential directional atherectomy of coronary bifurcation lesions. *Cathet Cardiovasc Diagn* 1993;suppl 1:54.

32. Mansour M, Fishman R, Kuntz R, et al. Feasibility of directional atherectomy for the treatment of bifurcation lesions. *Coronary Artery Dis* 1992;3:761.

33. Safian R, Screiber T, Baim D. Specific indications for directional atherectomy: origin left anterior descending coronary artery and bifurcation lesions. *Am J Cardiol* 1993;72:35E.

34. Dauerman H, Baim D, Cutlip DE, et al. Mechanical debulking versus balloon angioplasty for the treatment of diffuse in-stent restenosis. *Am J Cardiol* 1998;82:277.

35. Koch K, vom Dahl JV, Kleinhans E, et al. Influence of platelet GP IIb/IIIa receptor antagonist on myocardial hypoperfusion during rotational atherectomy as assessed by myocardial Tc-99m sestamibi scintigraphy. *J Am Coll Cardiol* 1999;33:998.

36. Reisman M, Shuman B, Dillard D, et al. Analysis of low-speed rotational atherectomy for the reduction of platelet aggregation. *Cathet Cardiovasc Diagn* 1998;45:208.

37. Auth D. Angioplasty with high speed rotary ablation. In: PW Serruys, et al, eds. *Restenosis After Intervention With New Mechanical Devices*. New York: Kluwer, 1992:275–288.

38. Hansen D, et al. Rotational endarterectomy in normal canine coronary arteries. *J Am Coll Cardiol* 1988;11:1073.

39. Hansen D, et al. Rotational atherectomy in atherosclerotic rabbit iliac arteries. *Am Heart J* 1988;115:160.

40. Friedman H, et al. Mechanical rotary atherectomy: the effects of microparticle embolization on myocardial blood flow and function. *J Interven Cardiol* 1989;2:77.

41. Teirstein P, et al. High-speed rotational coronary atherectomy for patients with diffuse coronary artery disease. *J Am Coll Cardiol* 1991;18:1694.

42. Zotz R, et al. Analysis of high-frequency rotational angioplasty-induced echo contrast. *Cathet Cardiovasc Diagn* 1991;22:137.

43. O'Neill W. Mechanical rotational atherectomy. *Am J Cardiol* 1992;69:12F.

44. Bertrand M, et al. Percutaneous transluminal coronary rotary ablation with Rotablator (European experience). *Am J Cardiol* 1992;69:470.

45. Warth D, et al. Rotational atherectomy multicenter registry: acute results, complications and 6-month angiographic follow-up in 709 patients. *J Am Coll Cardiol* 1994;24:641.

46. Zacca N, et al. Rotational ablation of coronary artery lesions using single, large burrs. *Cathet Cardiovasc Diagn* 1992;26:92.

47. Safian R, et al. Detailed angiographic analysis of high-speed mechanical rotational atherectomy in human coronary arteries. *Circulation* 1993;88:961.

48. Stertzer S, et al. Coronary rotational ablation: initial experience in 302 procedures. *J Am Coll Cardiol* 1993;21:287.

49. Ellis S, et al. Relation of clinical presentation, stenosis morphology, and operator technique to the procedural results of rotational atherectomy and rotational atherectomy-facilitated angioplasty. *Circulation* 1994;89:882.

50. Reisman M, Buchbinder M, Harms V, et al. Quantitative angiography of coronary artery dimensions 24 hours after rotational atherectomy. *Am J Cardiol* 1998;81:1427.

51. Mintz G, et al. Intravascular ultrasound evaluation of the effect of rotational atherectomy in obstructive atherosclerotic coronary artery disease. *Circulation* 1992;86:1383.

52. Henneke K, Regar E, Konig A, et al. Impact of target lesion calcification on coronary stent expansion after rotational atherectomy. *Am Heart J* 1999;137:93.

53. Safian R, Freed M, Reddy V, et al. Do excimer laser angioplasty and rotational atherectomy facilitate balloon angioplasty? Implications for lesion-specific coronary intervention. *J Am Coll Cardiol* 1996;27:552.

54. Reifart N, Vandormael M, Krajcar M, et al. Randomized comparison of angioplasty of complex coronary lesions at a single center. Excimer Laser, Rotational Atherectomy, and Balloon Angioplasty Comparison (ERBAC) Study. *Circulation* 1997;96:91.

55. Whitlow PL, et al. STRATA–study to determine rotablator and transluminal angioplasty strategy. http://www.tctmd.com/clinical-trials/let2004/one.html?mic_id-2971, last referenced April 26, 2005.

56. Mauri L, Reisman M, Buchbinder M, et al. Comparison of rotational atherectomy with conventional balloon angioplasty in the prevention of restenosis of small coronary arteries: results of the Dilatation vs Ablation Revascularization Trial Targeting Restenosis (DART). *Am Heart J* 2003;145:847–854.

57. Hoffman R, Mintz G, Kent K, et al. Comparative early and nine-month results of rotational atherectomy, stents, and the combination of both for calcified lesions in large coronary arteries. *Am J Cardiol* 1998;81:552.

58. Buchbinder M, et al. Debulking prior to stenting–long-term clinical and angiographic results from the SPORT trial. *Circulation* 2000:II-663.

59. Zimarino M, et al. Rotational coronary atherectomy with adjunctive balloon angioplasty for the treatment of ostial lesions. *Cathet Cardiovasc Diagn* 1994;33:22.

60. Lopez J, Ho K, Stoler RC, et al. Percutaneous treatment of protected and protected left main coronary stenosis with new devices: immediate angiographic results and intermediate-term follow-up. *J Am Coll Cardiol* 1997;29:345.

61. Rihal C, Garratt K, Holmes DR Jr. Rotational atherectomy for bifurcation lesions of the coronary circulation: technique and initial experience. *Int J Cardiol* 1998;65:L1.

62. Rosenblum J, et al. Rotational ablation of balloon angioplasty failures. *J Invasive Cardiol* 1992;4:312.

63. Sharma S, Duvvuri S, Dangas G. Rotational atherectomy for in-stent restenosis: acute and long-term results of the first 100 cases. *J Am Coll Cardiol* 1998;32:1358.

64. Lee S, Lee C, Cheong S, et al. Immediate and long-term outcomes of rotational atherectomy versus balloon angioplasty alone for the treatment of diffuse in-stent restenosis. *Am J Cardiol* 1998;82:140.

65. vom Dahl J, Radke P, Haager P, et al. Clinical and angiographic predictors of recurrent restenosis after percutaneous transluminal rotational atherectomy for treatment of diffuse in-stent restenosis. *Am J Cardiol* 1999;83:862.

66. vom Dahl J, Dietz U, Haager P, et al. Rotational atherectomy does not reduce recurrent in-stent restenosis: results of the angioplasty versus rotational atherectomy for treatment of diffuse in-stent restenosis trial (ARTIST). *Circulation* 2002;105:583–588.

67. Linsker R, Srinivasan R, Wynne J, Alonso D. Far-ultraviolet laser ablation of atherosclerotic lesions. *Laser Surg Med* 1984;4:201.

68. Isner J, Rosenfield K, White C, et al. In vivo assessment of vascular pathology resulting from laser irradiation: analysis of 23 patients studied by directional atherectomy immediately after laser angioplasty. *Circulation* 1992;85:2185.

69. Clarke R, Isner J, Donaldson R, Jones G. Gas chromatography light microscopic correlation of excimer laser photoablation of cardiovascular tissues: evidence for a thermal mechanism. *Circ Res* 1987;60:429.

70. Bonner R, Smith P, Prevosti L, Leon M. New sources for laser angioplasty: Er:YAG, excimer lasers, and nonlaser hot-tip catheters. In: Vogel J, King SI, eds. *Interventional Cardiology: Future Directions*. St Louis, MO: Mosby, 1989:101–118.

71. Appelman Y, Piek J, Verhoofstad G, et al. Tissue ablation and gas formation of two excimer laser systems: an in vitro evaluation on porcine aorta. *Lasers Surg Med* 1996;18:197–205.

72. Stone G, Marchena E, Dageforde D, et al. Prospective, randomized, multicenter comparison of laser-facilitated balloon angioplasty versus stand-alone balloon angioplasty in patients with obstructive coronary artery disease. The Laser Angioplasty Versus Angioplasty (LAVA) Trial Investigators. *J Am Coll Cardiol* 1997; 30:1714.

73. Appelman Y, Koolen J, Piek J, et al. Excimer laser angioplasty versus balloon angioplasty in functional and total coronary occlusions. *Am J Cardiol* 1996;78:757–762.

74. Litvack F, Eigler N, Margolis J, et al. Percutaneous excimer laser coronary angioplasty: results in the first consecutive 3,000 patients. *J Am Coll Cardiol* 1994;23:323.

75. de Marchena E, Mallon S, Knopf W, et al. Effectiveness of holmium laser-assisted coronary angioplasty. *Am J Cardiol* 1994; 73:117.

76. Holmes DR Jr, Reeder G, Ghazzal Z, et al. Coronary perforation after excimer laser coronary angioplasty: The Excimer Laser

Coronary Angioplasty Registry experience. *J Am Coll Cardiol* 1994;23:330.

77. Baumbach A, Bittl J, Fleck E, et al. Acute complications of coronary excimer laser angioplasty: analysis of two multicenter registries. *J Am Coll Cardiol* 1994;23:1305.

78. Tcheng J, Wells L, Phillips H, Deckelbaum L, Golobic R. Development of a new technique for reducing pressure pulse generation during 308 nm excimer laser coronary angioplasty. *Cathet Cardiovasc Diagn* 1995;34:15.

79. Bittl J, Kuntz R, Estella P, et al. Analysis of late lumen narrowing after excimer laser-facilitated coronary angioplasty. *J Am Coll Cardiol* 1994;23:1314.

80. Bittl J, Sanborn T, Tcheng J, Watson L. Excimer laser-facilitated angioplasty for undilatable coronary lesions: results of a prospective, controlled study. *Circulation* 1993;88:I–23.

81. Holmes DJ, Forrester J, Litvack F, et al. Chronic total obstruction and short-term outcome: The excimer laser angioplasty registry experience. *Mayo Clin Proc* 1993;68:5.

82. Schofer J, Kresser J, Rau T, et al. Recanalization of chronic coronary artery occlusions using laser followed by balloon angioplasty. *Am J Cardiol* 1996;78:836.

83. Oesterle S, Bittl J, Leon M, et al. Laser wire for crossing chronic total occlusions: "learning phase" results from the U.S. TOTAL trial. Total Occlusion Trial with Angioplasty by using a Laser wire. *Cathet Cardiovasc Diag.* 1998;44:235–243.

84. Hamburger J, Gijsbers G, Ozaki Y, et al. Recanalization of chronic total coronary occlusions using a laser guide wire: a pilot study. *J Am Coll Cardiol* 1997;30:649.

85. Hamburger J, Serruys P, Scabra-Gomes R, et al. Recanalization of total coronary occlusions using a laser guidewire (the European TOTAL Surveillance Study). *Am J Cardiol* 1997;80:1419.

86. Cook S, Eigler N, Shefer A, et al. Percutaneous excimer laser coronary angioplasty of lesions not ideal for balloon angioplasty. *Circulation* 1991;84:632.

87. Koster R, Hamm C, Seabra-Gomes R, et al. Laser angioplasty of restenosed coronary stents: results of a multicenter surveillance trial. *J Am Coll Cardiol* 1999;34:25.

88. Mehran R, Mintz G, Satler LF, et al. Treatment of in-stent restenosis with excimer laser coronary angioplasty: mechanisms and results compared with PTCA alone. *Circulation* 1997;96:2183.

89. Mizuno K, Satomura K, Miyamoto A, et al. Angioscopic evaluation of coronary-artery thrombi in acute coronary syndromes. *N Engl J Med* 1992;326:287.

90. Sherman C, Litvack F, Grundfest W, et al. Coronary angioscopy in patients with unstable angina pectoris. *N Engl J Med* 1986; 315:913.

91. Ambrose J, Weinrauch M. Thrombosis in ischemic heart disease. *Arch Intern Med* 1996;156:1382.

92. Hartmann J, McKeever L, Stamato N, et al. Recanalization of chronically occluded aortocoronary saphenous vein bypass grafts by extended infusion of urokinase: initial results and short-term clinical follow-up. *J Am Coll Cardiol* 1991;18:1517.

93. Chapekis A, George B, Candela R. Rapid thrombus dissolution by continuous infusion of urokinase through an intracoronary perfusion wire prior to and following PTCA: results in native coronaries and patent saphenous vein grafts. *Cathet Cardiovasc Diagn* 1991;23:89.

94. Bell C, Kern M, Kaiser G. Sequential proximal and distal infusion of urokinase resulting in recanalization of acutely occluded aortocoronary bypass graft after coronary angioplasty. *Cathet Cardiovasc Diagn* 1992;26:224.

95. Hartmann J, McKeever L, et al. Recanalization of Chronically Occluded Aortocoronary Saphenous Vein Bypass Grafts With Long-Term, Low Dose Direct Infusion of Urokinase (ROBUST): a serial trial. *J Am Coll Cardiol* 1997;27:60.

96. Ambrose J, Almeida O, Sharma SK, et al. Adjunctive thrombolytic therapy during angioplasty for ischemic rest angina. Results of the TAUSA Trial. TAUSA Investigators. Thrombolysis and Angioplasty in Unstable Angina trial. *Circulation* 1994; 90:69.

97. McKay R, Fram D, et al. Treatment of intracoronary thrombus with local urokinase infusion using a new, site-specific drug delivery system: the Dispatch catheter. *Cathet Cardiovasc Diagn* 1994;33:181.

98. Glazier J, Kiernan F, et al. Treatment of thrombotic saphenous vein bypass grafts using local urokinase infusion therapy with the Dispatch catheter. *Cathet Cardiovasc Diagn* 1997;41:261.

99. Mitchel J, Azrin M, et al. Inhibition of platelet deposition and lysis of intracoronary thrombus during balloon angioplasty using urokinase-coated hydrogel balloons. *Circulation* 1994;90:1979.

100. Twidale N, Barth CW, Kipperman R, et al. Acute results and long-term outcome of transluminal extraction catheter atherectomy for saphenous vein graft stenoses. *Cathet Cardiovasc Diagn* 1994; 31:187.

101. Meany T, Leon M, Kramer B, et al. Transluminal extraction catheter for the treatment of diseased saphenous vein grafts: a multicenter experience. *Cathet Cardiovasc Diagn* 1995;34:112.

102. Sullebarger J, Dalton R, Tauth J, Matar F. One-year follow-up of recanalization of totally occluded aortocornary saphenous vein grafts using transluminal extraction atherectomy. *Am J Cardiol* 1998;81:636.

103. Dooris M, et al. Comparative results of transluminal extraction atherectomy in saphenous vein graft lesions with and without thrombus. *J Am Coll Cardio* 1995;25:1700.

104. Braden G, Xenopoulos N, Young T, et al. Transluminal extraction catheter atherectomy followed by immediate stenting in treatment of saphenous vein grafts. *J Am Coll Cardiol* 1997;30:657.

105. Stone G, Cox D, Low R, et al. Safety and efficacy of a novel device for treatment of thrombotic and atherosclerotic lesions in native coronary arteries and saphenous vein grafts: results from the multicenter X-Sizer for treatment of thrombus and atherosclerosis in coronary applications trial (X-TRACT) study. *Cathet Cardiovasc Intervent* 2003;58(4):419–427.

106. Rousseau H, Sapoval M, et al. Percutaneous recanalization of acutely thrombosed vessels by hydrodynamic thrombectomy (Hydrolyser). *Eur Radiol* 1997;7:935.

107. Overbosch E, Pattynama P, et al. Occluded hemodialysis shunts: Dutch multicenter experience with the Hydrolyser catheter. *Radiology* 1996;201:485.

108. van den Bos A, Ommen Vv, Corbeij H. A new thrombosuction catheter for coronary use: initial results with clinical and angiographic follow-up in seven patients. *Cathet Cardiovasc Diagn* 1997;40:192.

109. van Ommen V, Bos Avd, et al. Removal of thrombus from aortocoronary bypass grafts and coronary arteries using the 6Fr Hydrolyser. *Am J Cardiol* 1997;79:1012.

110. Drasler W, Jenson M, Wilson G, et al. Rheolytic catheter for percutaneous removal of thrombus. *Radiology* 1992;182:263.

111. Hamburger J, Serruys P. Treatment of thrombus containing lesions in diseased vein bypass grafts using the AngioJet Rapid Thrombectomy System. *Herz* 1997;22:318.

112. Whisenant B, Baim D, Kuntz R, et al. Rheolytic thrombectomy with the Possis AngioJet: technical considerations and initial clinical experience. *J Invas Cardiol* 1999;11:421.

113. Nakagawa Y, Matsuo S, Kiura T, et al. Thrombectomy with AngioJet catheter in native coronary arteries for patients with acute or recent myocardial infarction. *Am J Cardiol* 1999;83:994.

114. Popma J, Carrozza J, Ho K, et al. One-year outcomes for the Vein Graft AngioJet Study I (VeGAS I) pilot trial. *Circulation* 1997;96: 216-I–217-I.

115. Kuntz R, Baim D, Cutlip DE, et al. A trial comparing Rheolytic thrombectomy with intracoronary urokinase for coronary and vein graft thrombus (the Vein Graft AngioJet Study [VeGAS 2]). *Am J Cardiol* 2002;89:326–330.

115a. Ali A, et al. AngioJet rheolytic thrombectomy in patients undergoing primary angioplasty for acute myocardial infarction (AiMI Trial). Presented at Transcatheter Cardiovascular Therapeutics, September 30, 2004.

116. Rosenschein U, Roth A, Rassin T, Basan S, Laniado S, Miller HI. Analysis of coronary ultrasound thrombolysis endpoints in acute myocardial infarction (ACUTE trial). Results of the feasibility phase. *Circulation* 1997;95:1411.

117. Rosenschein U, Gaul G, Erbel R, et al. Percutaneous transluminal therapy of occluded saphenous vein grafts. *Circulation* 1999; 99:26.

118. Singh M, Rosenschein U, Ho K, Berger P, Kuntz R, Holmes DR Jr. Treatment of saphenous vein bypass grafts with ultrasound thrombolysis: a randomized study (ATLAS). *Circulation* 2003;107:2331–2336.

119. Rosenschein U, Furman V, Kerner E, Fabian I, Bernheim J, Eshel Y. Ultrasound imaging-guided noninvasive ultrasound thrombolysis: preclinical results. *Circulation* 2000;102: 238–245.

120. Piana R, Palik G, Moscucci M, et al. Incidence and treatment of "no-reflow" after percutaneous coronary intervention. *Circulation* 1994;89:2514–2518.

121. Resnic F, Wainstein M, Lee M, et al. No-reflow is an independent predictor of death and myocardial infarction after percutaneous coronary intervention. *Am Heart J* 2002;145:42–46.

122. Grube E, Schofer JJ, Webb J, et al. Evaluation of a balloon occlusion and aspiration system for protection from distal embolization during stenting in saphenous vein grafts. *Am J Cardiol* 2002;89: 941–945.

123. Webb JG, Carere RG, Virmani R, et al. Retrieval and analysis of particulate debris after saphenous vein graft intervention. *J Am Coll Cardiol* 1999;34:468–475.

124. Baim DS, Wahr D, George B, et al. Randomized trial of a distal embolic protection device during percutaneous intervention of saphenous vein aorto-coronary bypass grafts. *Circulations* 2002;105:1285–1290.

124a. Carrozza JP, et al. PRIDE-a multicenter randomized trial of protection during saphenous vein graft intervention to prevent distal embolization. Presented at *Transcatheter Cardiovascular Therapeutics*, September 30, 2004.

125. Stone GW, Rogers C, Ramee S, et al. Distal filter protection during saphenous vein graft stenting: technical and clinical correlates of efficacy. *J Am Coll Cardiol* 2002;40:1882–1888.

126. Stone GW, Rogers C, Hermiller J, et al. Randomized comparison of distal protection with a filter-based catheter and a balloon occlusion and aspiration system during percutaneous intervention of diseased saphenous vein aorto-coronary bypass grafts. *Circulation* 2003;108:548–553.

126a. Holmes DR, et al. CardioShield application protects during transluminal intervention of vein grafts by reducing emboli (CAPTIVE). Presented at *Transcatheter Cardiovascular Therapeutics*, September 30, 2004.

127. Schluter M, Chevalier B, Seth A, et al. Saphenous vein graft stenting using a novel filter device for distal protection. *Am J Cardiol* 2003;91:736–739.

128. Rogers C, Huynh R, Seifert P, et al. Embolic protection with filtering or occlusion balloons during saphenous vein graft stenting retrieve identical volumes and sizes of particulate debris. *Circulation* 2004;109:1735–1740.

129. Giugliano G, Kuntz R, MD J, Cutlip D, Baim D. Determinants of 30-day adverse events following saphenous vein graft intervention with and without a distal occlusion embolic protection device. *Am J Cardiol* 2005;95:173–7.

130. Seivert H, Wahr D, Schuler G, et al. Effectiveness and safety of the Proxis system in demonstrating retrograde coronary blood flow during proximal occlusion and in capturing embolic material. *Am J Cardiol* 2004;94:1134–1139.

131. Limbruno U, Micheli A, Carlo MD, et al. Mechanical prevention of distal embolization during primary angioplasty: safety, feasibility, and impact on myocardial reperfusion. *Circulation* 2003; 108:171–176.

132. Stone GW, Webb J, et al. For the Enhanced myocardial efficacy and recovery by aspiration of liberated debris (EMERALD) investigators. Distal microcirculatory protection during PCI in acute ST-elevation MI—a randomized controlled trial. *JAMA* 2005;293:1116–1118.

133. Lefèvre T, Guyon P, Reimers B, et al. Evaluation of a distal protection filter device in patients with acute myocardial infarction: final Results of the DIPLOMAT Study. *J Am Coll Cardiol* 2004;43:72A.

Coronary Stenting[a]

24

Gregg W. Stone

Stents are metallic scaffolds that are deployed within a diseased coronary artery segment to maintain wide luminal patency. Stent-assisted coronary intervention has now supplanted coronary artery bypass graft surgery as *the most common revascularization modality* in patients with coronary artery disease. The acute and late results of stent implantation, however, vary greatly depending on the clinical risk profile of the patient and the complexity of the coronary anatomy. A broad range of evidence is available from clinical trials, however, to guide appropriate stent usage in most situations. This chapter reviews the developmental history of the coronary stent, emphasizing the elements of stent design that impact procedural success and long-term outcomes, the optimal procedural technique and adjunct pharmacology, the key comparative studies, the breakthrough technology of drug-eluting stents, and patient- and lesion-specific issues in stent implantation.

HISTORICAL PERSPECTIVES

Limitations of Balloon Angioplasty

The mechanism of balloon angioplasty involves plaque fracture (dissection) into the deep media, with expansion of the external elastic lamina, as well as partial axial plaque redistribution along the length of the vessel (see Chapter 22). This acute benefit is eroded by various degrees of early elastic recoil, late neointimal hyperplasia (smooth muscle proliferation, migration, and extracellular matrix production), and chronic negative vascular remodeling at the treatment site, contributing to a 3% incidence of abrupt vessel closure and a 30% incidence of late restenosis. The coronary stent was devised as a permanent endoluminal prosthesis that could

seal dissections, create a predictably large initial lumen, and oppose early recoil and late vascular remodeling to improve both the early and late results of balloon angioplasty.

Development of the Coronary Stent

The term *stent* derives from a dental prosthesis developed by the London dentist Charles Stent (1807–1885) and is now used to indicate any device used for "extending, stretching, or fixing in an expanded state" (1). Alexis Carrel had described the concept of a *vascular* stent (actually a glass tube) to support the endoluminal surface of a canine thoracic aorta in 1912 (2), and in 1964 Charles Dotter had proposed and evaluated an endovascular metallic prosthesis to seal dissections and overcome elastic recoil (3). But the first attempts at percutaneous arterial stenting in man were by Maass and colleagues from Switzerland, who implanted a self-expanding helical coil stent in three patients with dissecting aortic aneurysm (4). Shortly thereafter, Rabkin and coworkers in Russia began using heat-expandable nitinol stents in peripheral and carotid arteries (5). The first stents were implanted in human coronary arteries in 1986 by Sigwart, Puel, and colleagues, who placed Wallstent sheathed self-expanding metallic mesh scaffolds in the peripheral and coronary arteries of eight patients (6). Their initial favorable reports were subsequently tempered by a multicenter study of the Wallstent that described high rates of thrombotic occlusion and late mortality (7). The patients who did not suffer from subacute thrombosis, however, had a 6-month angiographic restenosis rate of only 14%, suggesting for the first time that stenting might improve date clinical outcomes.

Contemporaneously, Cesare Gianturco and Gary Roubin developed a balloon-expandable coil stent consisting of a stainless steel wire wrapped in a serpiginous manner to form a clamshell shape (8; Fig. 24.1, left). In 1988, they began a phase II study using the Gianturco-Roubin stent to reverse postangioplasty acute or threatened vessel closure (9), which

---

[a]Some of the material included in this chapter was contributed by Donald Baim and Joseph Carrozza, Jr. in the prior edition.

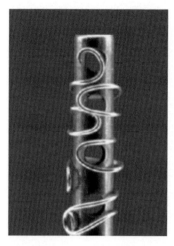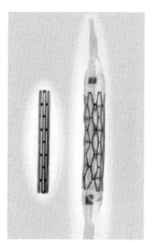

Figure 24.1 **Left.** In the original configuration for the Gianturco-Roubin stent, surgical stainless steel sutures were wound around a cylindrical rod using pegs to shape the wire, resulting in a clamshell design. **Right.** The original Palmaz 15-mm-long slotted tube stent (shown without the central articulation suggested by Richard Schatz).

ultimately led to Food and Drug Administration (FDA) approval of the device for this indication in June 1993 (Fig. 24.2). In 1984, Julio Palmaz designed a balloon-expandable slotted tube stainless steel stent in which rectangular slots were cut were cut into thin-walled stainless steel tubing and deformed into diamond-shaped windows during expansion by an underlying delivery balloon (10). The rigidity of this design made passage through bends in guiding catheters and tortuous vessels difficult, however, until Richard Schatz added a 1-mm central articulating bridge between two rigid 7-mm segments (11,12) to create the 15-mm long Palmaz-Schatz stent (Johnson and Johnson Interventional Systems, Warren, NJ; Fig. 24.1, right). The first coronary Palmaz-Schatz stent was placed by Eduardo Sousa in Sao Paulo, Brazil, in 1987, with a U.S. pilot study begun in 1988.

In 1989, enrollment commenced in two randomized multicenter studies (STRESS and BENESTENT) comparing balloon angioplasty to *elective* Palmaz-Schatz stenting with an end point of improved long-term outcomes (13,14). These studies each showed markedly improved

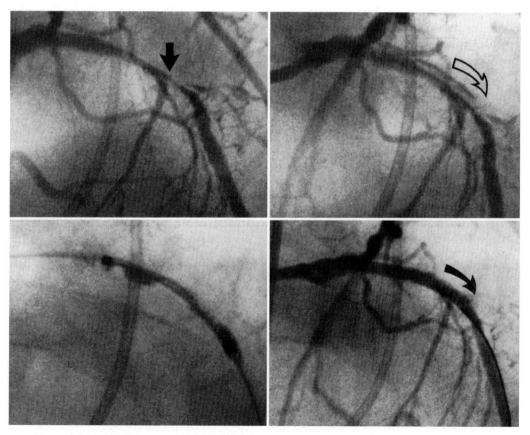

Figure 24.2 Early example of placement of a Gianturco-Roubin coil stent for threatened abrupt closure. A long lesion is present in the left anterior descending **(top left),** with a long dissection after angioplasty (*open arrow*, **upper right**), placement of a coil stent **(bottom left)** results in effacement of the dissection and elimination of the need for emergency bypass great surgery **(bottom right).**

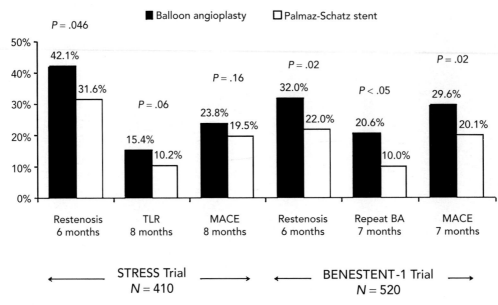

Figure 24.3   Results of the STRESS and BENESTENT-1 studies, which provided the evidence base for FDA approval of the Palmaz-Schatz stent for the prevention of restenosis in de novo lesions. BA, balloon angioplasty; TLR, target lesion revascularization; MACE, major adverse cardiac events.

initial angiographic results, with a larger postprocedural minimal luminal diameter, fewer residual dissections, a lower rate of subacute vessel closure, as well as a 20 to 30% reduction in clinical and angiographic restenosis compared with conventional balloon angioplasty (Fig. 24.3). This led to FDA approval of the Palmaz-Schatz Stent in 1994 for the elective treatment of focal de novo lesions in native coronary arteries with reference diameter 3 to 4 mm. Long-term follow-up to 5 years has subsequently demonstrated few late clinical or angiographic recurrences beyond 1 year after coronary stent implantation (15,16).

Overcoming Stent Limitations

Despite the impressive acute and long-term results with the Palmaz-Schatz stent, widespread adoption of this technology was hindered by the need for an intense anticoagulation regimen (consisting of aspirin, dextran, dipyridamole, heparin, and warfarin) to inhibit stent thrombosis (which nonetheless still occurred in approximately 3% of patients; see below). This profound degree of anticoagulation, however, resulted in a marked increase in hemorrhagic and vascular complications, prolonging the hospital stay and increasing costs compared with balloon angioplasty alone (14). In the early 1990s, Colombo and colleagues used intravascular ultrasound to demonstrate that most stents remained inadequately expanded despite an acceptable angiographic appearance (17). By routine high-pressure adjunctive dilatation (>14 atm), and the use of aspirin plus a second antiplatelet agent (the

thienopyridine, ticlopidine) in place of warfarin therapy, they reduced the incidence of stent thrombosis to approximately 1 to 2%, while markedly reducing bleeding and femoral arterial complications (18). Subsequently, four randomized trials have established the superiority of dual antiplatelet therapy (with aspirin and ticlopidine) over anticoagulation with warfarin for prevention of stent thrombosis (19–22; Fig. 24.4).

The combination of improved procedural technique, more effective antiplatelet regimens, expanding indications, and the introduction of more flexible and easily delivered second-generation stents made coronary stenting the default therapy for most patients with coronary artery disease (23). Even though slotted tube and multicellular stents inhibit chronic recoil, lumen renarrowing still occurs after bare metal stent implantation owing to neointimal hyperplasia that is often even greater than that seen after balloon angioplasty alone (24). But the larger acute lumen diameter (i.e., greater acute gain) provided by stenting usually still allows a larger late lumen and an overall lower rate of restenosis than balloon angioplasty, an example of the "bigger is better" principle (see Chapter 22; 25–27). More recently, the site-specific release of antiproliferative bioactive agents from drug-eluting stents has emerged as a safe and effective way to mitigate the amount of in-stent tissue that accumulates after stent implantation, further reducing (to 5 to 7%) the rates of clinical and angiographic restenosis (28,29). As a result, the coronary stent is certain to remain the mainstay of coronary intervention for the foreseeable future.

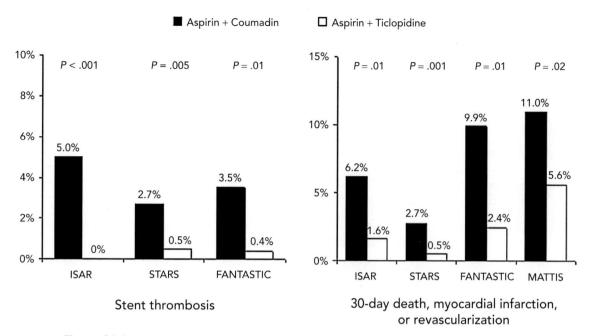

Figure 24.4 Results of four randomized trials comparing dual antiplatelet therapy (with aspirin and ticlopidine) with anticoagulation (with aspirin and warfarin) in patients undergoing elective stent placement, showing that dual antiplatelet therapy reduces both stent thrombosis and 30-day major adverse clinical events (death, myocardial infarction, or repeat revascularization).

STENT DESIGN: IMPACT ON PERFORMANCE AND CLINICAL OUTCOMES

Classification

Stents may be classified based on their *composition* (e.g., metallic or polymeric), *configuration* (e.g., slotted tube versus coiled wire), *mode of implantation* (e.g., self-expanding or balloon expandable), *bioabsorption* (inert/biostable or degradable/bioabsorbable), and *coating* (none, passive [such as covalent heparin or PTFE polymer], or bioactive [such as eluting sirolimus or paclitaxel]). In theory, a perfect coronary stent would be made of a nonthrombogenic material and have sufficient flexibility in its unexpanded state to allow passage through guiding catheters and tortuous vessels, and yet have an expanded configuration that provides uniform scaffolding of the vessel wall with low recoil and maximal radial strength while conforming to vessel bends. In addition, the stent should be sufficiently radiopaque to allow fluoroscopic visualization to guide accurate placement and management of in-stent restenosis, but not so opaque as to obscure important angiographic luminal details.

In recent years, the importance of the *stent delivery system* to device profile, flexibility, and trackability around tortuous and calcific coronary vessels has received increasing appreciation. The stent must be tightly crimped to the delivery balloon to avoid dislodgement, and the overhang of the balloon beyond the ends of the stent should be minimized (<1 mm) to avoid vessel trauma outside the stent margins. The balloon must be able to withstand high pressures (>18 atm) without rupture and should have low compliance to facilitate predictable sizing and avoid excessive growth outside the stent edges (see Chapter 22). By 2005, more than 50 stent designs have been implanted in the human coronary circulation, some of which are shown in Fig. 24.5. To date, none of these stent designs fully achieve all of the ideal characteristics described above, but they have nonetheless revolutionized the practice of percutaneous coronary intervention.

Stent Composition

Most clinically tested coronary stents to date are constructed from metallic alloys. The most widely used metal in *balloon-expandable* stents is 316L stainless steel (typically laser cut from a thin-walled hollow tube). Stainless steel is predominately composed of iron, which is biologically inert but also contains approximately 5% nickel, allergy to which may be linked to an increased risk of in-stent restenosis (30). Tantalum, cobalt/platinum alloys, and cobalt chromium alloys have been used instead of stainless steel to allow thinner stent struts (75 μm versus 100 to 150 μm in most stainless steel stents) without sacrificing strength or radiopacity (31,32). A chromium oxide surface

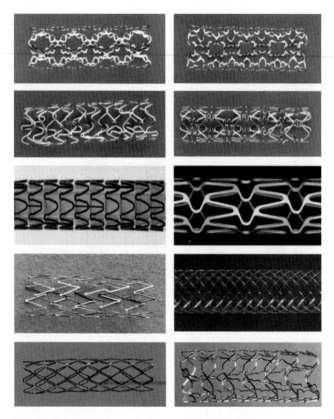

Figure 24.5 Eight early bare metal stent designs **Top row.** Crown Stent *(left)*, Minicrown Stent *(right)*. **Second row.** CrossFlex LC Stent *(left)*, BX Stent *(right)*. **Third row.** Duet Stent *(left)*, NIR Stent *(right)*. **Fourth row.** Radius Stent *(left)*, Wallstent *(right)*. **Bottom row.** GFX stent *(left)*, BeStent *(right)*.

thermal shape memory properties that allow it to be set into a particular expanded shape by baking at high temperature. The stent can then be squeezed down and constrained on the delivery system, able to return to that set shape when released in the coronary artery. Other than the well-documented adverse effect of gold, there is little evidence that thrombosis or restenosis rates vary with the specific stent metal, but surface finishing, smoothing, and purification or passivation may affect early thrombotic and late restenotic processes (35).

Recent interest has surfaced in *biodegradable stents*, which theoretically offer the advantages of increased flexibility (though usually with reduced radial force), compatibility with magnetic resonance imaging and multidetector computerized tomography (though most are fluoroscopically invisible, requiring markers to ensure accurate placement), and complete bioabsorption over a period of months (which may reduce the risk of late stent thrombosis and facilitate subsequent revascularization procedures). To date, only a single polymer-based completely bioabsorbable stent has undergone human testing (the Igaki-Tamai stent in Japan [36]); several other polymer-based bioabsorbable stents will be entering clinical investigation shortly. The Biotronik magnesium stent is also completely degradable (by rapid corrosion) and has been implanted in human peripheral and coronary vessels in Europe (37). Given the beneficial outcomes recently reported with paclitaxel-eluting and sirolimus-eluting stents, these biodegradable stents will likely also require drug-eluting capability to equal the results of the permanent counterparts.

Stent Configuration

Stents can be assigned to one of three subgroups, based on their construction. These are wire coils, slotted tubes, and modular designs.

layer may serve to reduce biological activity, but the use of gold surface coating has been uniformly found to increase restenosis compared with stainless steel alone (Table 24.1; 33,34). The material most widely used in *self-expanding* stents is nitinol, a nickel/titanium alloy that has superelastic and

TABLE 24.1
OUTCOMES OF CLINICAL TRIALS WITH GOLD-COATED STENTS

	Total *N* Randomized	Type of Gold Stent	6–12-Month Target Lesion Revascularization			6-Month Binary Angiographic Restenosis		
			Gold Stent (%)	Control Stent (%)	*P* Value	Gold Stent (%)	Control Stent (%)	*P* Value
vom Dahl et al.[a]	203	Inflow	3	0	NS	36	24	.13
Park et al.[b]	261	NIR	22.7	15.1	.15	46.7	26.4	<.05
Reifart et al. (34)	603	NIROYAL	—	—	—	37.7	20.6	<.001
Kastrati et al. (33)	731	Inflow	25.1	15.7	.002	49.7	38.1	.003

[a] vom Dahl J, Haager PK, Grube E, et al. Effects of gold coating of coronary stents on neointimal proliferation following stent implantation. *Am J Cardiol* 2002;89:801–805.
[b] Park SJ, Lee CW, Hong MK, et al. Comparison of gold-coated NIR stents with uncoated NIR stents in patients with coronary artery disease. *Am J Cardiol* 2002;89:872–875.

Wire Coils

The Gianturco-Roubin FlexStent (Cook Cardiology, Indiana-polis, IN) was the initial coil stent prototype, constructed by winding a 0.006-inch monofilament stainless steel wire into a serpiginous pattern of reversing loops and then fold-ing that pattern onto a compliant balloon to create an inter-digitating coil (Fig. 24.1, left). The mechanical deficiencies of this design (e.g., low axial and radial strength and a ten-dency for plaque to prolapse through large gaps between adjacent loops) largely limited its use to acute or threatened vessel closure (9). A second-generation Gianturco-Roubin II stent used a polymer-coated flat wire made from 0.006-inch 316L stainless steel with a longitudinal spine to enhance radial and axial strength and prevent foreshorten-ing. It was compared with the Palmaz-Schatz slotted tube stent in a 755-patient multicenter trial, demonstrating that the GR-II resulted in significantly greater acute recoil and plaque prolapse, more frequent edge dissections, a lower initial minimal luminal diameter, and a greater incidence of acute closure and late restenosis (38; Table 24.2). As a result, this stent (and the coil design in general) rapidly fell out of favor and is no longer used.

Slotted Tubes and Multicellular Stents

The original Palmaz stent design involved offset rows of rec-tangular slots, each of which was plastically deformed into a diamond shape during balloon expansion. This trusslike pattern made the stent relatively resistant to recoil and com-pression once expanded, but also made it relatively rigid during passage down the coronary artery. The initial rigidity of the stent was reduced by breaking the 15-mm rigid length into two 7-mm segments, joined by a 1-mm-long central articulation (Fig. 24.1, right). This Palmaz-Schatz stent was mounted on a balloon and covered by a protec-tive 5F delivery sheath to protect the stent from dislodge-ment during passage through tortuous and fibrocalcific anatomy. Although this design was used for the pivotal ran-domized trials of stenting and the commercial release in 1994, its relative inflexibility and bulky (5 French) delivery sheath, requiring large lumen (>0.084-inch) 8F guiding catheters, remained difficult to deliver through tortuous anatomy and was plagued by suboptimal scaffolding at the articulation site.

In an effort to preserve the radial strength and wall cov-erage of the tubular design but improve flexibility in their collapsed state, several generations of slotted tube and mul-ticellular stents have been introduced by various manufac-turers. Each is laser cut from a metallic tube into a unique pattern that increases the overall flexibility of the stent by distributing bending throughout the stent length with-out compromising radial strength or elastic recoil in the expanded state. The newer stents are manufactured in a broader range of stent lengths (8 to 38 mm) and diameters (2.25 to 6.0 mm) to facilitate stenting of long lesions, small vessels, saphenous vein grafts, and distal lesions. To elimi-nate the need for a protective sheath, various mechanical,

---

TABLE 24.2

RESULTS OF THE GR-II RANDOMIZED TRIAL

	Gianturco-Roubin II Stent (N = 380)	Palmaz-Schatz (N = 375)	P Value
30-day clinical results			
MACE	4.2%	1.3%	<.01
TLR	3.9%	0.5%	<.01
Stent thrombosis	3.9%	0.3%	.001
12-month clinical results			
MACE	29.8%	17.8%	<.001
TLR	27.4%	15.3%	<.001
Angiographic results			
Number stents per lesion	1.27 ± 0.57	1.47 ± 0.72	<.001
Total stent length	29.3 ± 15.1	22.0 ± 10.9	<.001
Stent to lesion length ratio	2.5	1.9	<.001
Stent to artery ratio	1.02 ± 0.12	1.06 ± 0.12	<.001
Balloon to artery ratio	1.16 ± 0.16	1.14 ± 0.17	.06
Stent recoil	17.9 ± 12.4%	11.2 ± 14.2%	<.001
ACC/AHA grade B dissections	18.2%	8.0%	<.001
MLD postprocedure (mm)	2.64 ± 0.41	2.83 ± 0.43	<.001
MLD at 9 months (mm)	1.48 ± 0.73	1.90 ± 0.74	<.001
Late loss (mm)	1.21 ± 0.69	0.92 ± 0.72	<.01
Binary restenosis	47.3%	20.6%	<.001

MLD, minimal luminal diameter; MACE, major adverse cardiac events: death, Q-wave myocardial infarc-tion, or TLR; TLR, target lesion revascularization; ACC/AHA, American College of Cardiology/American Heart Association.

balloon wrapping, and heat curing processes have been developed to tightly crimp the stent onto the balloon until it is deployed. This bare mounting onto the delivery balloon has reduced stent delivery profiles to <0.040 inch (1 mm), comparable with the best angioplasty balloons of the late 1990s, and has kept stent embolization rates below approximately 1 to 3 per 1,000 procedures).

Depending on the cellular configuration, multicellular stents can be broadly subclassified as either open cell or closed cell. *Open cell* designs tend to have varying cell sizes and shapes along the stent, and provide increased flexibility, deliverability, and side-branch access by staggering the cross-linking elements to provide radial strength. Open cell designs thus tend to conform better on bends, though the cell area may open excessively on the outer curve of an angulated segment. *Closed cell* designs typically incorporate a repeating unicellular element that provides more uniform wall coverage with less tendency for plaque prolapse, at the expense of reduced flexibility and side-branch access. Closed cell designs also tend to straighten vessel bends more than do open cell designs.

Modular stents

Despite their enhanced flexibility, even the latest-generation slotted tube stents are sometimes difficult to deliver through tortuous and noncompliant vessels. In an effort to enhance flexibility and deliverability without sacrificing the excellent scaffolding of the slotted tube stents, modular or hybrid stents have been created by flexibly joining multiple short repeating modules to each other. The initial modular stent was the Arterial Vascular Engineering MicroStent (subsequently purchased by Medtronic Corp., Santa Rosa, CA), which had a series of 4-mm-long rounded stainless steel corrugated ring subunits welded to each other. Subsequent designs have incorporated an elliptorectangular (rounded) strut profile and progressively reduced the length of the individual modules to 3 mm (Micro II), then to 2 mm (GFX), 1.5 mm (S670), and finally 1.0 mm (S7 and the cobalt chrome Driver), with progressive reductions in crossing profile and increased surface area coverage.

Stent Coatings

Various coatings have been used in an attempt to reduce the thrombogenicity or restenosis of metallic stents (Table 24.3). Experimental studies have demonstrated that coating stents with inert polymers may reduce surface reactivity and thrombosis (39), but most polymer coatings also provoked intense inflammatory reactions (40), possibly partly responsible for the poor results with the GR-II stent. Phosphorylcholine is a synthetic polymer that mimics the phosphatidylcholine head group present in the phospholipids of erythrocyte membranes. When used to coat stainless steel stents, it appears to be biocompatible, have less platelet activation and thrombus deposition (41),

TABLE 24.3
STENT COATINGS TO POTENTIALLY REDUCE THROMBOGENICITY

Heparin
- Carmeda BioActive Surface (CBAS) covalently heparin-bonded Palmaz-Schatz and Bx Velocity stents
- Medtronic Hepamed covalently heparin-coupled Wiktor and beStent
- Jomed corline heparin surface (CHS) heparin-coated Jostent

Phosphorylcholine
- Biocompatibles BiodivYsio stent
- Medtronic Endeavor stent
- Abbott Trimax and Zomaxx stents

Carbon
- Turbostratic (Sorin Carbostent)
- Silicon carbide (Biotronik Tensum stent)
- Diamond-like films (Phytis Diamond Flex and Global Therapeutics Freedom stents)

Abciximab and other glycoprotein IIb/IIIa inhibitors
Activated protein C
Hirudin and bivalirudin
Prostacyclin

and have similar long-term healing responses to a bare metal. Clinical studies have confirmed similar rates of stent thrombosis and restenosis with phosphorylcholine coated and uncoated bare metal stents (Fig. 24.5; 42–45). This polymer is currently being actively investigated as a drug delivery vehicle (46).

Heparin has proven utility as a coating for indwelling catheters, dialysis membranes, and extracorporeal circulation equipment, and has been evaluated for its potential to reduce stent thrombosis. Heparin may be covalently bonded to a priming layer applied to the stent surface. In both baboon arteriovenous shunt fistula and porcine models, the heparin-coated stent markedly reduces platelet deposition, thrombus accumulation and vessel thrombosis compared to uncoated stents (47,48). Several heparin-coated stents have been tested in humans (49–52). The clinical and angiographic outcomes with these stents have been similar to uncoated stents, with no differences in stent thrombosis, angiographic restenosis at 6 months, or clinical events at 1 year (Fig. 24.6).

A variety of carbon formulations (turbostratic carbon in the Sorin Carbostent, silicon carbide in the Biotronik Tensum stent, and diamondlike films in the Phytis Medical Devices Diamond Flex and Global Therapeutics Freedom stents) have been shown to have reduced thrombogenicity, platelet and/or complement activation, and foreign body reactions in animals. Comparative studies against bare metal stents have proven these devices to be safe but have not demonstrated clinical or angiographic benefits compared with uncoated bare metal stents (Table 24.4; 53–55). The physicochemical properties of carbon coatings may also be used for the site-specific elution of bioactive materials (56).

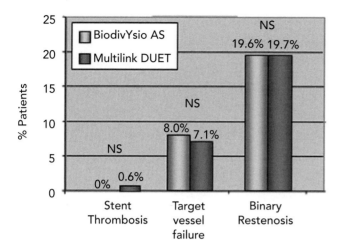

Figure 24.6 Six-month results of the DISTINCT trial in which 622 patients with de novo lesions 25 mm or less in length in 3- to 4-mm vessels were randomized to receive either a BiodivYsio phosphorylcholine-coated stent or a Multi-Link Duet stent. The results demonstrated short-term and late equivalency between the two devices. Of note, no BiodivYsio-assigned patient developed stent thrombosis (*P* = NS [not significant]).

Covered Stents

Metallic stents covered by a distensible microporous polytetrafluoroethylene (PTFE) membrane offer the potential to treat perforations, while theoretically decreasing periprocedural debris embolization, and reducing restenosis by acting as a mechanical barrier to neointimal hyperplasia (57). PTFE-covered stents for coronary and saphenous vein graft use have been developed by Boston Scientific (the Symbiot stent, consisting of a double layer of PTFE surrounding a modified self-expanding RADIUS-like nitinol stent), Jomed (the Jostent Coronary Stent Graft, consisting of a single PTFE layer sandwiched between two stents), and Cardiovasc (the Nuvasc Stent Graft, a stainless steel stent surrounded by PTFE coated with the synthetic peptide P-15, a cell adhesion protein to promote endothelialization; Fig. 24.7). PTFE-covered stents are of unquestioned clinical utility in treating life-threatening perforations and excluding giant aneurysms, pseudoaneurysms, or clinically significant fistulae (58–60; see Chapter 3), and early clinical studies suggested a favorable role in enhancing the early safety and late outcomes in saphenous vein grafts compared with bare metal stents (61,62). But four large, multicenter randomized trials comparing PTFE stent grafts and bare metal stents in degenerated saphenous vein grafts have shown that these stents do not improve clinical outcomes and may be associated with a *higher* incidence of restenosis and/or early thrombosis and late occlusion of the target vessel (Table 24.5; 63–66).

Balloon-Expandable Versus Self-Expanding Stents

Balloon-expandable stents are mounted onto a delivery balloon and delivered into the coronary artery in their collapsed

TABLE 24.4
RESULTS OF RANDOMIZED STUDIES OF CARBON-COATED AND BARE METAL STENTS

	Total N Randomized	Type of Carbon-Coated Stent	In-Hospital or 30-Day Major Adverse Cardiac Events			6–12-Month Target Lesion or Vessel Revascularization			6-Month Binary Angiographic Restenosis		
			Carbon-Coated Stent (%)	Control Stent (%)	P value	Carbon-Coated Stent (%)	Control Stent (%)	P Value	Carbon-Coated Stent (%)	Control Stent (%)	P Value
Haase et al. (58)	329	Sorin Carbostent	3.4	3.2	NS	16.4	21.5	0.31	18.1	20.6	.59
Sick et al.[b]	420	Sorin Carbostent	—	—	—	17.6	12.7	0.21	23.5	15.9	.07
Unverdorben et al.[c]	446	Tenax stent	3.2	2.8	NS	5.1	3.3	NS	21.3[a]	21.0[a]	1.0
Hamm et al.[d]	485	Tenax stent	0.4	0.4	1.0	13.9	15.8	0.78	23.9	23.7	1.0
Airoldi et al.[e]	347	Phytis Diamond Flex AS	2.8	4.5	0.29	25.9	26.1	0.59	31.8	35.9	.45

[a] At a mean time of 4.7 months.
[b] Sick PB, Gelbrich G, Kalnins U, et al. Comparison of early and late results of a Carbofilm-coated stent versus a pure high-grade stainless steel stent (the CarboStent Trial). *Am J Cardiol* 2004;93:1351–1356.
[c] Unverdorben M, Sattler K, Degenhardt R, et al. Comparison of a silicon carbide coated stent versus a noncoated stent in humans: the Tenax- versus Nir-Stent Study (TENISS). *J Intervent Cardiol* 2003;16:325–333.
[d] Hamm CW, Hugenholtz PG; TRUST Investigators. Silicon carbide-coated stents in patients with acute coronary syndrome. *Cathet Cardiovasc Intervent* 2003;60:375–381.
[e] Airoldi F, Colombo A, Tavano D, et al. Comparison of diamond-like carbon-coated stents versus uncoated stainless steel stents in coronary artery disease. *Am J Cardiol* 2004;93:474–477.

The Boston Scientific SYMBIOT Stent Graft   The Jomed JOSTENT Stent Graft

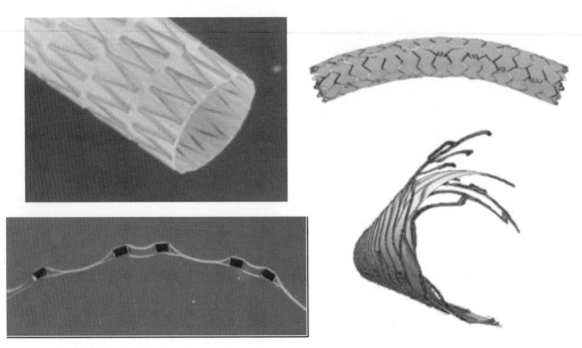

Figure 24.7   The two most widely investigated PTFE-coated stent grafts, the Boston Scientific SYMBIOT stent *(left)* and the Jomed JOSTENT *(right)*. Note that the PTFE membrane encapsulates the SYMBIOT stent struts, whereas it is sandwiched between an inner and an outer metal stent in the JOSTENT.

state. Once in the desired location, inflation of the delivery balloon expands the stent and imbeds it into the arterial wall, following which the stent delivery system is removed. A stent diameter chosen to be 1 to 1.1 times the reference arterial lumen, with a length several millimeters longer than the lesion, is implanted at ≥12 to 15 atm. Angiography is then performed, and a decision is made whether it is necessary to use a higher-pressure noncompliant and/or larger postdilatation balloon to achieve a residual stenosis as close to 0% as possible. More than 98% of all coronary stents used currently are of the balloon-expandable type.

Self-expanding stents incorporate either specific geometric designs or nitinol shape-retaining metal to achieve a preset diameter. The stent is mounted onto the delivery system in its collapsed state and constrained by a restraining membrane or sheath. Retraction of the membrane allows the stent to reassume its unconstrained (expanded) geometry. Self-expanding stents are typically selected to have an unconstrained diameter 0.5 to 1.0 mm greater than the adjacent reference segment to ensure contact with the vessel wall and adequate expansile force to resist vessel recoil. Still, final optimization of stent expansion usually requires additional dilatation within the stent using a high-pressure, noncompliant angioplasty balloon. Examples of self-expanding stents include the Boston Scientific Magic Wallstent, which incorporates a nonferrogmagnetic cobalt woven mesh wire frame with a platinum core (to increase radiopacity) and has the ability to readvance the delivery

sheath and recapture a partially deployed stent; and the Boston Scientific Radius stent, which is a self-expanding nitinol stent that shortens much less than the Wallstent during deployment. The two main advantages of self-expanding stents are as follows: The absence of a stent delivery balloon results in these devices being extremely flexible, allowing long stent lengths to be delivered through tortuous vessels; and the presence of a sheath reduces friction in fibrocalcific vessels, further enhancing stent delivery in complex anatomy and eliminating the risk of stent dislodgment. Although it was initially hoped that these stents would reduce vessel trauma and subsequent restenosis, this was shown not to be the case in controlled clinical trials (67). Moreover, difficulties relating to accurate sizing and precise placement of self-expanding stents necessitate a longer operator learning curve and render these devices unsuitable for treating ostial lesions or stenoses adjacent to side branches. These stents are still widely used in carotid and femoral stenting (see Chapter 26), where resistance to crushing of the stent by external pressure is important.

Comparison Among Stents: The Bare Metal Stent Versus Stent Trials

More than 20 randomized trials have been performed comparing one stent type versus another to investigate relative angiographic and/or clinical outcomes. In general, these

TABLE 24.5
RANDOMIZED STUDIES OF PTFE STENT GRAFTS VERSUS BARE METAL STENTS IN PATIENTS UNDERGOING PERCUTANEOUS CORONARY INTERVENTION IN SAPHENOUS VEIN GRAFTS

	Total N Randomized	PTFE-Coated Stent	In-hospital or 30-Day Major Adverse Cardiac Events			6–15-Month Target Lesion or Vessel Revascularization			6–9-Month Binary Angiographic Restenosis			6–9 month Angiographic Total Occlusion		
			PTFE-Coated Stent (%)	Bare Metal Control Stent (%)	P Value	PTFE-Coated Stent (%)	Bare Metal Control Stent (%)	P Value	PTFE-Coated Stent (%)	Bare Metal Control Stent (%)	P Value	PTFE-Coated Stent	Bare metal control stent	P value
Stankovic et al. (66)	301	Jomed Jostent	10.9	4.1	.047	9.6	8.3	.84	24.2	24.8	0.24	12.9%	12.0%	NS
Schachinger et al. (67)	211	Jomed Jostent	7.8	6.7	.76	20	24	.44	29	20	0.15	16%	7%	0.07
Buchbinder et al. (68)	400	Boston Scientific Symbiot	9.0	8.2	.86	23.5	15.6	.055	34.9	23.3	0.04	—	—	—
Stone et al. (69)	243	Jomed Jostent	10.5	7.0	.35	21.8	14.2	.15	39.2	27.9	0.14	20.3%	10.5%	0.09

PTFE, polytetrafluoroethylene.

trials can be broken down into two types: those sponsored by industry for the purpose of achieving approval by the U.S. FDA for marketing of a new stent (68–70) and those sponsored by investigators for academic purposes.

The FDA-approval trials were powered to demonstrate noninferiority of the new stent design to the predicate stent. All incorporated an angiographic follow-up substudy. Ten of the twelve industry sponsored approval trials used the Palmaz-Schatz stent as the control stent. For the most part, these trials involved stent implantation of a single de novo focal lesion in a native coronary artery (the type of simple stenosis amenable to treatment with the Palmaz-Schatz). As seen in Table 24.6, the trials conducted for FDA approval demonstrated noninferiority in all cases (except for the GR-II and PARAGON stents, which demonstrated statistically significantly greater rates of clinical and angiographic restenosis; 38,71). Once receiving FDA approval, newer, more advanced stent designs typically replaced earlier-generation stents in the marketplace because of enhanced deliverability and/or radiopacity, rather than because of any perception of improved acute or late outcomes.

In contrast to the FDA approval trials, the investigator-driven studies tended to enroll more complex real-world patients and lesions with fewer exclusion criteria. This is an important issue, as enrollment of complex lesions may be required to detect otherwise modest differences between stents (72). One trial randomized five stent types within the framework of the same study (73). Table 24.7 displays the results of the seven studies in which two stents were randomized in head-to-head fashion, generally demonstrating superior clinical and angiographic outcomes with thin strut stents. Thus, these clinical investigations collectively demonstrate that stent design may matter in more complex lesions, but the overwhelming superiority of drug-eluting stents dwarf any design-specific differences in bare metal stent design.

STENT IMPLANTATION TECHNIQUE

Achieving optimal stent outcomes requires operator skill in guide catheter, guidewire, and stent selection and usage (see Chapter 22). Understanding the utility of adjunctive imaging and physiologic lesion assessment catheters (e.g., intravascular ultrasound [IVUS], fractional flow reserve; see Chapters 18 and 19), lesion modification devices (e.g., atherectomy, thrombectomy), and distal protection devices (see Chapter 23) is also critical to optimizing stent results. Perhaps most important, however, intimate knowledge is required regarding the appropriate indications for stent implantation versus alternative medical therapy or surgical revascularization, identification and treatment of high-risk patients and lesions, appropriate use of adjunct pharmacotherapy, and the recognition and management of stent-related complications (see Chapters 3 and 22).

Technical Aspects of Coronary Stent Implantation

Guide Catheter and Guidewire Selection

Optimal guide catheter selection is critical for the successful completion of most stent procedures and requires the operator to consider *prior to the beginning of the case* the amount of backup support required and the luminal dimensions of the guide to accommodate the devices likely to be used. Stenting of noncomplex lesions is typically performed through 6 French guiding catheters. Smaller-diameter guides, however, provide reduced backup support, a disadvantage that may necessitate active guide catheter manipulation (deep guide intubation), a technique that is usually safe when performed by experienced operators, although it may occasionally result in proximal coronary dissection requiring placement of additional stents.

If significant guide catheter backup support is anticipated (e.g., fibrocalcific or tortuous vessels, distal lesions, or chronic total occlusions), or simultaneous delivery of multiple stents or use of atherectomy devices is planned, *larger-dimension guiding catheters* (typically 7F or 8F for greater passive support) or specialized shapes (e.g., Extra-Back Up or Voda shapes for the left coronary artery, and hockey stick or Amplatz shapes for the right coronary artery and saphenous vein grafts) should be chosen. Larger guiding catheters may also be required for stenting of bifurcation lesions (see below).

Floppy wires should be used for most stent implant procedures, although at least medium shaft support is required to advance most stents (see Chapter 22). A second parallel ("buddy") wire may be placed alongside the wire being used to deliver the stent when difficulty advancing the stent over an extra-support wire is still encountered.

Stent Selection and Techniques to Optimize Acute and Long-Term Outcomes

Optimal stent selection and implantation technique will minimize procedural complications, reduce the risk of stent thrombosis, and enhance long-term freedom from restenosis. Key issues include selection of the appropriate stent (including its diameter and length), implantation pressure, the decision whether to predilate versus direct stent, and whether to postdilate or implant additional stents to achieve an optimal result (Table 24.8). Balloon-expandable rather than self-expanding stents are almost universally used for coronary applications, given their simplicity and accuracy in positioning. Open cell designs are generally more trackable than closed cell stents and may be favored in tortuous vessels where conformability on bends is important or when stenting across bifurcation lesions (to reduce the risk of side-branch closure and preserve side-branch access). Closed cell designs, in contrast, may be desirable when uniform or optimal scaffolding is required, such as in ostial lesions.

TABLE 24.6
THE STAINLESS STEEL INDUSTRY SPONSORED STENT VERSUS STENT TRIALS (FOR FDA APPROVAL)

Trial	Stents Randomized A	Stents Randomized B	Total N Patients	Key Entry Criteria	Angiographic Follow-up	Restenosis Rate (%) A	Restenosis Rate (%) B	Clinical Follow-up	Death (%) A	Death (%) B	Myocardial Infarction (%) A	Myocardial Infarction (%) B	TLR or TVR (%) A	TLR or TVR (%) B	TVF or MACE, % A	TVF or MACE, % B
ASCENT (71)	Multi-Link (Guidant)	Palmaz-Schatz	1,040	*	9 months	16.0	22.1	9 months	1.4	2.5	4.2	5.2	10.6[2]	11.5[2]	15.1[3]	16.7[3]
NIRVANA (72)	NIR (Medinol)	Palmaz-Schatz	849	*	9 months	19.3	22.4	9 months	1.0	0.9	4.8	4.2	12.2[2]	13.4[2]	16.0[3]	17.2[3]
SMART (73)	Microstent II (AVE)	Palmaz-Schatz	661	**	6 months	25.2	22.1	6 months (9 months MACE)	2.1	1.2	5.8	3.9	13.6[1]	13.0[1]	17.3[4]	13.3[4]
PARAGON (74)	PARAGON (PAS)	Palmaz-Schatz	688	**	6 months	32.5	24.4	6 months	2.0	1.2	9.2[†]	3.7[†]	12.0[1][††]	5.9[1][††]	19.8[3][††]	11.2[3]
EXTRA	XT (Bard)	Palmaz-Schatz	795	*	6 months	35	27	12 months	—	—	—	—	8.5[1]	8.7[1]	20.0[3]	19.0[3]
SCORES (70)	Radius (Boston Scientific)	Palmaz-Schatz	1,096	**	6 months	24.2	18.7	9 months	1.5	1.1	2.4	2.7	13.9[2]	14.0[2]	19.3[3]	20.1[3]
GR-II randomized trial (38)	GR-II (Cook)	Palmaz-Schatz	755	*	9 months	47.3[††]	20.6[††]	12 months	2.7	2.7	15.0	12.0	27.4[1][††]	15.3[1][††]	29.8[4][††]	17.8[4][††]
WIN[a]	Magic Wallstent (Boston Scientific)	Balloon angioplasty	586	**	6 months	38	38	6 months	—	—	—	—	13[1]	15[1]	20[4]	20[4]
WINS[a]	Magic Wallstent (Boston Scientific)	Palmaz-Schatz	268	***	6 months	33	33	6 months	—	—	—	—	13[1]	12[1]	28[4]	23[4]
BEST[b]	BeStent (Medtronic)	Palmaz-Schatz	652	*	6 months	21.2	27.5	12 months	1.5	1.2	4.6	5.2	11.7[2][†]	19.9[2][†]	—	—
DISTINCT (48)	BiodivYsio (Biocompatibles)	Multi-Link Duet (Guidant)	622	*	6 months	19.6	19.7	6 months	—	—	—	—	—	—	8.0[3]	7.1[3]
CONSERVE	LP (IVT)	Multi-Link Duet or Tristar	1,003	*	6 months (registry in LP patients)	40.9	—	6 months	—	—	—	—	10.0[2]	7.8[2]	—	—

* Focal de novo native coronary lesion; ** Focal de novo or restenotic native coronary lesion; *** De novo or restenotic saphenous vein graft lesions.
† $P < .05$; †† $P < .01$.
[a] Safian RD, Freed MS, eds. The Manual of Interventional Cardiology, 3rd ed. Birmingham, MI: Physicians' Press, 2001:332, 543.
[b] Brinker JA. The BeStent BEST trial. http://www.tctmd.com/clinical-trials/tct2004/one.html?mic_id=2507
[c] Brener SJ, Midei MG, Nukta D, et al. A randomized multicenter trial comparing a new, low-pressure versus a conventional coronary stent: primary results from the CONSERVE trial. J Invasive Cardiol 2003;15:128–132.
[1]TLR, target lesion revascularization; [2]TVR, target vessel revascularization; [3]TVF, target vessel failure; [4]MACE, major adverse cardiac events.

TABLE 24.7
INVESTIGATOR-SPONSORED STAINLESS STEEL STENT VERSUS STENT TRIALS

Trial	Stents Randomized A	Stents Randomized B	Total N Patients	Key Entry Criteria	Angio-graphic Follow-up	Restenosis Rate (%) A	Restenosis Rate (%) B	Clinical Follow-up	Death (%) A	Death (%) B	Myocardial Infarction (%) A	Myocardial Infarction (%) B	TLR or TVR (%) A	TLR or TVR (%) B	TVF or MACE, % A	TVF or MACE, % B
ISAR-STEREO-1[a]	Multi-Link (Guidant)	Multi-Link Duet (Guidant)	651	Native vessels with RVD >2.8 mm	6 months	15.0††	25.8††	12 months	4.9	5.2	—	—	8.6²†	13.8²†	—	—
ISAR-STEREO-2[b]	Multi-Link (Guidant)	Bx Velocity (Cordis)	611	Native vessels	6 months	17.9††	31.4††	12 months	3.9	4.6	—	—	12.3²††	21.9²††	—	—
Mehilli et al.[c]	Jostent (Jomed)	Multi-Link (Guidant)	505	Native vessels with RVD >2.8 mm	6 months	24.2	25.2	12 months	4.0	4.3	—	—	13.9²	15.4²	21.0⁴	22.9⁴
DANSTENT[d]	NIR (Medinol)	Palmaz-Schatz	424	*	6 months	9.9	12.6	12 months	1.9	0.5	4.2	2.9	11.7¹	9.5¹	15.9⁴	11.9⁴
Yoshitomi et al.[e]	GFX (AVE)	Multi-Link (Guidant)	100	* With AMI within 6 hours	4 months	25.5††	4.0††	—	—	—	—	—	—	—	—	—
Miketic et al.[f]	Crown (Cordis)	NIR (Medinol)	203	No exclusions	6 months	18.4	22.0	—	—	—	—	—	—	—	—	—
RENEWAL[g]	Wallstent (Boston Scientific)	NIR (Medinol)	82	Native vessels, length >20 mm, RVD ≥3.0 mm	6 months	46.2	26.3	6 months	0	0	5.1	5.3	7.7¹	7.9¹	—	—

AMI, acute myocardial infarction; RVD, reference vessel diameter; abbreviations otherwise as in Table 24.6.

[a] Kastrati A, Mehilli J, Dirschinger J, et al. Intracoronary stenting and angiographic results: strut thickness effect on restenosis outcome (ISAR-STEREO) trial. *Circulation* 2001;103:2816–2821.

[b] Pache J, Kastrati A, Mehilli J, et al. Intracoronary stenting and angiographic results: strut thickness effect on restenosis outcome (ISAR-STEREO-2) trial. *J Am Coll Cardiol* 2003;41:1283–1288.

[c] Mehilli J, Kastrati A, Dirschinger J, et al. A randomized trial comparing the hand-mounted Jostent with the pre-mounted Multi-Link Duet stent in patients with coronary artery disease. *Cathet Cardiovasc Intervent* 2001;54:414–419.

[d] Jorgensen E, Kelbaek H, Helqvist S, et al. Low restenosis rate of the NIR coronary stent: results of the Danish multicenter stent study (DANSTENT)—a randomized trial comparing a first-generation stent with a second-generation stent. *Am Heart J* 2003;145:e5.

[e] Yoshitomi Y, Kojima S, Yano M, et al. Does stent design affect probability of restenosis? A randomized trial comparing Multilink stents with GFX stents. *Am Heart J* 2001;142:445–451.

[f] Miketic S, Carlsson J, Tebbe U. Randomized comparison of J&J Crown stent versus NIR stent after routine coronary angioplasty. *Am Heart J* 2001;142:E8.

[g] Nageh T, de Belder AJ, Thomas MR, Williams IL, Wainwright RJ. A randomised trial of endoluminal reconstruction comparing the NIR stent and the Wallstent in angioplasty of long segment coronary disease: results of the RENEWAL Study. *Am Heart J* 2001;141:971–976.

TABLE 24.8
GUIDELINES FOR OPTIMAL STENT SELECTION AND IMPLANTATION

1. Choose the optimal stent length.
   A. Ensure adequate lesion coverage while avoiding excessively long stents, as stent length is a risk factor for periprocedural myonecrosis, stent thrombosis, and restenosis (166–170).
   B. Implant the stent from normal reference to normal reference if possible (starting 2 mm before and after the lesion shoulder), which will avoid edge dissections (171). An edge dissection, unless mild, should be treated with an additional short (8–10 mm) overlapping stent (172).
   C. In diffusely diseased vessels, a normal reference segment often cannot be identified. The most severe atherosclerotic segments should be stented so there are no major inflow or outflow lesions to any stenosis. Spot stenting may be preferable to the "full metal jacket" with bare metal stents (173,174).
   D. For long lesions, use one long stent if possible. If multiple stents are required, they should overlap by ~3 mm to ensure complete lesion coverage, a technique that does not increase restenosis (175,176).
   E. Modification for drug-eluting stents: Stent and lesion length are not as critical for restenosis, so more liberal use of long stents is favored (62,63,177). Use 3–4-mm edge margins.
2. Choose the optimal stent diameter.
   A. Size the stent diameter with a ratio of 1.0–1.1:1 to the distal reference vessel diameter.
   B. If the vessel is tapering, a larger noncompliant balloon can then be used to more fully expand the proximal stent segments.
   C. Be aware that within the same stent line, different-sized stents exist for different-diameter vessels (e.g., the six-cell Cypher for 2.5–3.0-mm vessels, and the seven-cell Cypher for 3.5–4.0-mm vessels; 62). Oversizing stents designed for small vessels will lead to inadequate scaffolding and possibly strut fracture.
3. Predilatation vs. direct stenting.
   A. Direct stenting may be considered with bare metal or drug-eluting stents when guide catheter support is good to excellent. Lesions not generally amendable for direct stenting include those with excessive vessel or lesion tortuosity or calcification, diffuse disease or subtotal stenoses, bifurcations, acute myocardial infarction or chronic total occlusions (190–202).
   B. If direct stenting is not feasible, predilatation should be performed with balloons undersized to the reference diameter by 0.5 mm, and with length shorter than the lesion so as to not extend the length of stenosis requiring stenting. If this degree of predilatation does not allow stent passage, larger and/or higher-pressure balloon inflations may be required.
4. Implant the stent at adequate pressure.
   A. Most stents should be implanted at ≥12 atm.
   B. Higher routine implantation pressures (16–18 atm or greater) are preferred by many to optimize stent expansion and are required in fibrocalcific lesions.
   C. In diffusely diseased vessels, consider implanting the stent at 12–14 atm to avoid edge dissections, and then postdilate the stent at higher pressures using a short noncompliant balloon positioned within the stent margins.
5. Strive for an optimal angiographic stent result, defined as:
   A. A residual stenosis <10%
   B. No edge dissection greater than NHLBI type A
   C. TIMI grade 3 flow
   D. Patency of all side branches ≥2.0 mm in diameter
   E. Absence of distal thromboemboli, perforation, or other angiographic complications with associated chest pain, electrocardiographic changes, or hemodynamic instability

NHLBI, National Heart, Lung, and Blood Institute; TIMI, Thrombolysis in Myocardial Infarction.

The optimal pressure for stent implantation has been a matter of some debate. Colombo first demonstrated that high-pressure stent implantation techniques were important to achieve optimal stent expansion and appose the stent completely to the vessel wall. Although Colombo initially achieved these results with the use of adjunctive IVUS imaging (74), acceptable results were also demonstrated with moderate pressure implantation techniques without IVUS imaging (75). In a randomized trial of high (mean 16.9 atm) versus moderate (mean 11.1 atm) pressure for stent implantation in 934 patients, similar rates of stent thrombosis and restenosis were observed (76). In contrast, in a second randomized trial, routine high (17.0 atm) versus low (9.9 atm) pressure stent implantation resulted in greater initial and 6-month follow-up minimal stent cross-sectional areas (77).

Complete lesion coverage without edge dissections is also believed to be important, eliminating inflow and outflow stenoses, thereby resulting in optimal flow conditions and minimizing the risk of stent thrombosis. With optimal stent implantation technique, this complication should occur in no greater than 1% of patients (78). Implantation of additional short stents may be required to cover edge dissections and achieve optimal lumen dimensions, thereby minimizing the risk of stent thrombosis (79). Although routine high-pressure stent implantation and high balloon-to-artery ratios will result in greater stent expansion, and optimize late outcomes, care must be taken to avoid edge dissections and perforation.

Intravascular ultrasound (see Chapter 19) may be helpful in measuring true (media-to-media) vessel size prior to stent implantation and in evaluating how well the stent is expanded. It may allow stent implantation in vessels that otherwise appear too small and appropriate only for balloon angioplasty (80). Seven large studies (five randomized trials and two carefully controlled studies comparing outcomes in centers that used versus did not use IVUS) have been performed, collectively demonstrating improved outcomes with routine IVUS usage (Table 24.9; 81–87). Nonetheless, IVUS is currently used in <10% of patients undergoing stent implantation in the United States, a reflection of the learning curve this technique requires (compounded by frequently suboptimal image quality), difficulties in incorporating the information IVUS provides into treatment decisions, logistic issues, and lack of widespread reimbursement.

Like IVUS, physiologic lesion assessment (measurement of either coronary flow reserve or fractional flow reserve [FFR]) has utility during coronary stent implant procedures (see Chapter 19). It may identify hemodynamically significant borderline lesions by a fractional flow reserve of <0.75, and may also be used to determine the adequacy of stent implantation; an FFR of <0.95 correlates with an underdeployed stent by IVUS (88). In the FFR Post Stent Registry (89), FFR was >0.95 in 36% of patients, >0.90 to 0.95 in 32%, <0.90 in 32%, and <0.75 in 1.5% of patients. FFR may also be useful in provisional stenting to identify cases where the results of balloon angioplasty alone are suffi-

cient such that long-term outcomes will not be improved by bare metal stent implantation. This is no longer relevant, however, in the drug-eluting stent era.

Direct Stenting

Numerous randomized trials have been performed to determine the benefit of direct stent implantation (i.e., stenting without predilatation; 90–97). These studies have demonstrated that direct stenting is feasible in 28 to 72% of lesions, resulting in use of fewer balloons, less contrast, and lower fluoroscopy time, with equivalent early and late outcomes compared with stenting after predilatation. Preliminary data suggest that direct stenting does not impair the outcomes of either sirolimus- or paclitaxel-eluting stent implantation (98,99). Careful lesion selection is required, however, as direct stenting in severe stenoses (especially if angulated or calcific), may increase the risk of inappropriate stent positioning (from lack of visualization), and either vessel closure or stent embolization if the stenosis cannot be crossed (which may occur in as many as 10% of attempts). Excessive force should *never* be applied in trying to pass a stent across a rigid, nondilated lesion; such efforts are likely to be unsuccessful and increase the risk of stripping the stent from the balloon. If guide support is adequate and the stent doesn't easily pass across the lesion, it should be carefully withdrawn

TABLE 24.9

RESULTS OF CONTROLLED TRIALS OF INTRAVASCULAR ULTRASOUND VERSUS ANGIOGRAPHIC GUIDANCE OF BARE METAL STENT IMPLANTATION

	Total N Randomized/ Enrolled[a]	6–24-Month Target Lesion or Vessel Revascularization			6-Month Binary Angiographic Restenosis		
		IVUS Guided (%)	Control (%)	P Value	IVUS Guided (%)	Control (%)	P Value
CRUISE (84)	499	8.5	15.3	.02	—	—	—
SIPS (85)	269[b]	17	29	.02	29	35	.42
AVID (42)	759	8.1	12.0	.08[c]	—	—	—
OPTICUS (43)	550	5.5[d]	5.8[d]	NS	24.5	22.8	.68
RESIST (44)	155	—	—	—	22.5	28.8	.25
TULIP (86)	150	10	23	.018	23	46	.008

[a] CRUISE was a substudy of the STARS trial. Sites were assigned in nonrandomized fashion to no IVUS, documentary (blinded) IVUS, or guided IVUS. This table represents the results of the documentary and guided IVUS arms.
[b] In SIPS, patients could undergo balloon angioplasty with or without stenting; approximately 50% of patients in both groups received stents.
[c] Subgroup analyses demonstrated that IVUS guidance reduced the 12-month rates of target lesion revascularization in saphenous vein grafts (20.4% vs. 5.7%, P =.05), in vessels <3.25 mm in diameter (14.6% vs. 7.9%, P =.04), and in lesions with a baseline diameter stenosis of >70% preintervention (14.2% vs. 3.1%, P =.003).
[d] Hierarchical analysis, excluding patients with death or myocardial infarction during follow-up.
IVUS, intravascular ultrasound; CRUISE, Can Routine Intravascular Ultrasound Influence Stent Expansion?; SIPS, Strategy for Intracoronary ultrasound-guided PTCA and Stenting; AVID, Angiography Versus Intravascular ultrasound-Directed stent placement; OPTICUS, The OPTimization with ICUS to reduce restenosis; RESIST, REStenosis after IVUS-guided Stenting Trial; TULIP, Thrombocyte activity evaluation and effects of Ultrasound guidance in Long Intracoronary stent Placement.

back into the guide catheter under fluoroscopic visualization and the lesion predilated before an attempt to readvance the stent is made.

Role of Plaque Modification During Coronary Stent Implantation

Atherectomy Devices

The amount of plaque present prior to and after stent implantation has been shown to be a strong determinant of subsequent restenosis (100,101), leading to the hypothesis that plaque debulking prior to stenting would enhance event-free survival. Unfortunately, despite favorable pilot series (102–104), two randomized trials have been unable to demonstrate improved clinical or angiographic outcomes with directional atherectomy prior to stent implantation compared with stenting alone (105), although it may still be useful in selected cases of stenting in left main, ostial, or bifurcation lesions to reduce plaque shift and subsequent side-branch compromise (106,107; see Chapter 23).

Similarly, the circumferential extent of calcium is a strong determinant of inadequate stent expansion (108,109), and pilot studies initially demonstrated greater stent dimensions when stenting was preceded by high-speed rotational atherectomy (109,110; Fig. 24.8). However, in the randomized SPORT trial of rotational atherectomy followed by stenting versus stenting alone in >700 long and mildly calcified lesions, rotational atherectomy prior to stent implantation resulted in slightly larger acute gain and postprocedural minimal stent diameter, but failed to improve the 6-month target vessel revascularization and angiographic restenosis rates. Thus, rotational atherectomy prior to stenting is primarily reserved for heavily calcified lesions or those resistant to balloon crossing or predilatation. Similarly, the major contemporary role for excimer laser angioplasty is for recalcitrant lesions.

ADJUNCT PHARMACOTHERAPY

A thorough working knowledge of basic coagulation hematology and the appropriate use of adjunct pharmacologic regimens is essential to optimizing interventional outcomes with stenting (see Chapter 3). Adjunct pharmacology should be viewed as a means to an end, a critical component of the interventional procedure to safely allow stents to be implanted without periprocedural or late complications so they may provide long-term vessel patency and freedom from restenosis. This section will focus on the use of antiplatelet mediations before, during, and after the procedure. These agents must be given in addition to antithrombin drugs in any coronary intervention, but are particularly important in placement of a potentially thrombogenic metallic stent.

Aspirin and Thienopyridines

The necessity for aspirin in patients undergoing stent implantation has never been formally tested, but given the

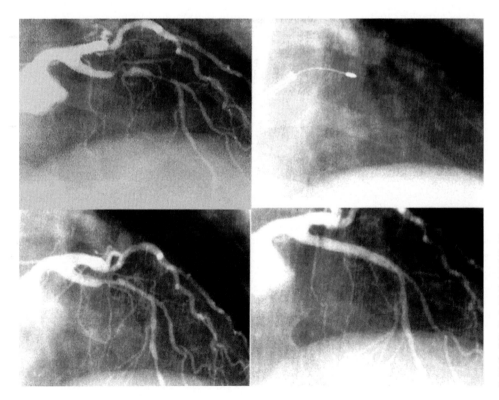

Figure 24.8 Rota-stenting. A long, calcified stenosis is present in the left anterior descending artery **(top left).** Following rotational atherectomy burr **(top right),** a smooth lumen with significant residual stenosis is present **(bottom left).** Following stent deployment, excellent expansion is observed **(bottom right).** Without rotational atherectomy pretreatment, stent passage and obtaining full stent expansion would have each been unlikely.

relative safety and track record of this inexpensive agent, its use is considered mandatory. Though no dose-ranging trials have been performed, expert consensus is that 325 mg of aspirin should be administered at least 24 hours prior to stent implantation, then daily indefinitely. There is some evidence that hemorrhagic complications during the follow-up period may be safely reduced by using an 81 mg per day dose after patient discharge, though this has never been validated in patients receiving drug-eluting stents.

The transition from the early anticoagulant-based stent regimen—prolonged heparin and warfarin—to a dual antiplatelet regimen consisting of aspirin and a thienopyridine (which inhibits adenosine diphosphate [ADP]-induced platelet activation) represents a seminal event in the history of interventional cardiology. Four randomized trials in large numbers of patients have definitively proven that compared with prolonged anticoagulation, aspirin and the thienopyridine agent ticlopidine results in reduced rates of major adverse cardiac events (including stent thrombosis and myocardial infarction), as well as hemorrhagic and vascular complications, thereby facilitating earlier discharge (Fig. 24.4; 111–114). Ticlopidine results in frequent side effects, however, including the development of neutropenia and thrombocytopenia (rarely thrombotic, thrombocytopenic purpura, which is often fatal), as well as rash and dyspepsia (115). *Clopidogrel* is a congener of ticlopidine which has a much lower incidence of side effects, and therefore does not require routine monitoring of hematologic indices, as does ticlopidine.

The relative safety and efficacy of ticlopidine and clopidogrel (with or without a loading dose) were compared in the Clopidogrel Aspirin Stent International Cooperative Study (CLASSICS) in 1,020 patients undergoing bare metal stent implantation (116). The primary endpoint, the composite occurrence of major peripheral or bleeding complications, neutropenia, thrombocytopenia, or early discontinuation of the study drug because of a noncardiac adverse event at 28 days occurred in 9.1% of patients in the ticlopidine group and 4.6% of patients in the clopidogrel group ($P < .005$). Overall rates of major adverse cardiac events were low and comparable between treatment groups (0.9% with ticlopidine versus 1.3% with clopidogrel, $P = $ NS). These results were confirmed in two other randomized comparative trials between the two agents (117,118). *As a result, clopidogrel has essentially replaced ticlopidine in patients undergoing stent implantation because of its convenience and more favorable side effect profile.* Loading doses of 600 mg of clopidogrel are also being used given a more rapid onset of action, especially in patients in whom percutaneous coronary intervention (PCI) will be performed within several hours of receiving the medication (119,120). The decision whether or not to use a clopidogrel loading dose in patients in whom the coronary anatomy is not known (and who therefore may be triaged to bypass graft surgery rather than PCI for revascularization) is not trivial, as clopidogrel usage within 7 days prior to surgery has been associated with

increased peri-operative bleeding requiring transfusion or re-operation, prolonged stays in the intensive care unit and increased costs (121). Finally, the weight of the evidence also suggests that long-term outcomes may be improved by a 9–12 month course of clopidogrel after stent implantation, especially in patients with acute coronary syndromes (122,123), though not all investigators believe that the long-term risk to benefit ratio of chronic clopidogrel use has been verified (124).

Glycoprotein IIb/IIIa Inhibitors

Glycoprotein IIb/IIIa receptor inhibitors bind to the integrin $\alpha_{2b}\beta_3$ receptor on the platelet surface, thereby preventing the cross-linking of platelets by fibrinogen and vWF (125). As such, glycoprotein IIb/IIIa receptor inhibitors block the final common pathway of platelet aggregation after their activation by a variety of agonists (thromboxanes, ADP, collagen, etc.). Three IIb/IIIa receptor antagonists are in clinical use: abciximab, which is a univalent monoclonal chimeric antibody to the integrin receptor, and the small-molecule agents tirofiban and eptifibatide, the former a peptidomimetic tyrosine derivative and the latter a cyclic heptapeptide. Two large-scale, prospective placebo-controlled randomized trials have demonstrated that both abciximab and double-bolus eptifibatide significantly reduce periprocedural myonecrosis in patients undergoing elective or urgent PCI with stent implantation (Fig. 24.9; 126,127), but failed to decrease restenosis (128).

In patients presenting with acute coronary syndromes (unstable angina and non–ST-segment elevation myocardial infarction), the upstream use of either tirofiban or eptifibatide, continuing though angiography and PCI when appropriate, has been found to be effective in reducing composite rates of death, myocardial infarction, and recurrent ischemia (129,130). Abciximab has also been tested extensively in patients with acute myocardial infarction as an adjunct to primary angioplasty and stenting, with variable results. In CADILLAC, a total of 2,082 patients with acute myocardial infarction were randomized to primary balloon angioplasty versus stenting, with or without abciximab (131). In patients receiving stents, abciximab reduced the early rate of stent thrombosis (from 1.0% to 0%, $P = .03$) and recurrent ischemia, with no impact on early or late rates of death, reinfarction, restenosis, infarct artery reocclusion, or myocardial recovery, and at the expense of modest increases in bleeding and thrombocytopenia (132).

COMPLICATIONS OF CORONARY STENTING

Stent Thrombosis

Subacute stent thrombosis is the most feared complication of contemporary PCI. It occurs suddenly without preceding

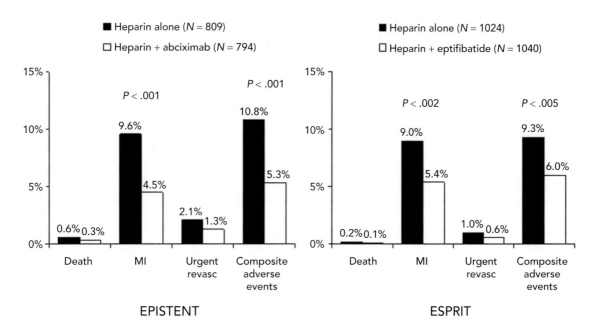

EPISTENT ESPRIT

Figure 24.9 Thirty-day results of the EPISTENT and ESPRIT trials, in which patients undergoing stent implantation were randomized to unfractionated heparin plus either a glycoprotein IIb/IIIa inhibitor or placebo. MI, myocardial infarction. Revasc, revascularization. Note the significant reduction in periprocedural myocardial infarction and the composite that includes myocardial infarction in both studies (see also Chapters 3 and 22).

angina, most commonly between 1 and 4 days postprocedure (Fig. 24.10). In reported series, almost all patients with stent thrombosis have sustained a myocardial infarction; 30-day mortality rates ranged from 15 to 48% (78,133,134). Risk factors for stent thrombosis include acute coronary syndrome presentation (and possibly thrombus), smaller postprocedural minimal luminal diameter, longer total

stent length, multivessel intervention, and persistent dissection. Late stent thrombosis (between 30 days and 2 years) may also occur in as many as 10% of patients who receive a new stent after being treated with vascular brachytherapy (135), and late thromboses have also been reported with drug-eluting stents after discontinuation of clopidogrel as long as 1 year after implantation (136).

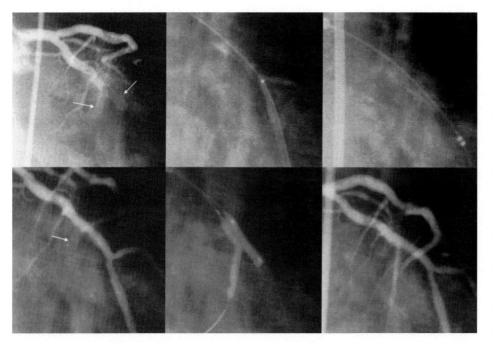

Figure 24.10 Subacute stent throm-bosis 10 days after T-stenting the bifurcation of the left circumflex and its obtuse marginal branch **(top left).** The lesion is crossed with a hydrophilic guidewire and an infusion catheter to establish extent of thrombus and exclude passage under stent struts **(top center).** The Possis AngioJet **(top right,** see Chapter 23) is positioned distal to the bifurcation. Following aspiration with the AngioJet, antegrade flow is restored and filling defects are no longer apparent **(bottom left).** However, flow is decreased in the AV groove portion of the bifurcation *(arrow).* Kissing balloon angioplasty is performed **(bottom center),** restoring normal flow in both branches **(bottom right).**

Fortunately, the incidence of stent thrombosis has markedly decreased as a function of improved stent design, implantation technique, and improved adjunctive pharmacologic regimens. Stent thrombosis with the first Palmaz-Schatz and Wallstent implants, using an antiplatelet and anticoagulant regimen of aspirin, dipyridamole, and low–molecular-weight dextran, occurred in as many as 16 to 20% of patients (6,7,12). This prompted the addition of warfarin therapy for 4 to 8 weeks, which reduced the incidence of stent thrombosis to 3% after elective Palmaz-Schatz implantation (12–14). High-pressure stent implantation, coupled with the conversion to a dual antiplatelet-based regimen (with aspirin and a thienopyridine; 19–22), resulted in stent thrombosis rates being further reduced, currently occurring in 0.5 to 1.0% of patients (78,133,134). Most stent thromboses occur within the first 30 days after stent implantation, but roughly a 0.25% incidence of later stent thrombosis can occur up to 1 year after stenting (particularly when dual antiplatelet therapy is discontinued). As discussed below, there has been some concern whether the incidence of early or late stent thrombosis is increased with drug-eluting compared to bare metal stents.

Stent thrombosis may be treated with emergency balloon angioplasty or rheolytic thrombectomy (see Chapter 23), often in conjunction with administration of a glycoprotein IIb/IIIa receptor antagonist (137). Intravascular ultrasound will often reveal a possible cause of stent thrombosis, such as stent underexpansion or malapposition, residual dissection, or significant inflow or outflow stenosis, and is thus recommended after interventional treatment (138). In the absence of a mechanical cause, hematologic evaluation should be performed to exclude a hypercoagulable state (including resistance to aspirin or clopidogrel) or thrombocytosis.

Restenosis

Restenosis is most commonly defined as renarrowing to a diameter stenosis >50%, either within the stent or within 5 mm proximal or distal to the stent margin. The frequency of restenosis after bare metal stent implantation is >20% overall, rising to >40% in certain subsets of patients. Three clinical and angiographic risk factors for restenosis that have been uniformly identified are small reference vessel diameter, long lesion (or stent) length, and medically treated diabetes mellitus (138). By IVUS imaging, a small minimal stent area is also a powerful independent determinant of restenosis (139–141).

Restenosis occurring within the stent is almost exclusively attributable to smooth muscle hyperplasia combined with elaboration of extracellular matrix. Although this proliferative response peaks at 8 weeks in animal models, serial angiographic and angioscopic studies in humans demonstrate that the greatest proliferation occurs between 1 and 6 months, with only a small fraction of stents exhibiting further narrowing between 6 and 12 months (142–144).

Thereafter, the proliferating smooth muscle cells are replaced by relatively inactive fibrosis, often with a slight increase in the minimal luminal diameter. This transformation of the neointima from active proliferation to a quiescent, fibrotic matrix also explains the extremely low incidence (<2%) of target site revascularization observed clinically after 1 year (16,145). The two exceptions when continuing late lumen loss, restenosis and target lesion revascularization may occur for years after the stent implantation are after vascular brachytherapy (wherein normal healing processes are impaired; 146), and possibly after stenting in saphenous vein grafts (147). Restenosis may also occur at the edges of the stent at the site of balloon injury, typically owing to negative vessel remodeling rather than to neointimal growth (148).

In contrast to stent thrombosis, restenosis presents most commonly as stable angina, though if ignored may progress to unstable angina or (rarely) acute myocardial infarction (149). More than half of patients with angiographic restenosis (usually those with a diameter stenosis of <70%) are asymptomatic (150). In the absence of spontaneous or exercise-induced ischemia, the prognosis of asymptomatic patients with silent in-stent restenosis managed medically may be excellent (151). Revascularization is indicated, however, when symptoms recur or ischemia is demonstrated.

The interventional management of bare metal stent restenosis typically consists of repeat balloon angioplasty, which has a high (>98%) procedural success rate and low risk of complications. Since the metallic struts are not typically re-exposed to blood elements, thienopyridine administration is not necessary. The rates of recurrent restenosis after balloon angioplasty for in-stent restenosis have ranged from <10% to >80%, depending on the length of the lesion. Mehran et al. described an angiographic classification of the pattern of bare metal in-stent restenosis, which has proven useful for predicting the response to treatment (152):

> Focal (≤10 mm long), 42% of cases
> Diffuse (>10 mm long, confined within the stent), 21%
> Proliferative (>10 mm long, extending beyond the margin), 30%
> Totally occlusive, 7%.

Following repeat PCI, the recurrent target lesion revascularization rates at 1 year rose progressively with the in-stent restenosis class (from 19% to 35% to 50% and to 83%, respectively). In-stent restenosis recurring within 3 months of the initial procedure also portends a high rate of subsequent restenosis after repeat angioplasty (153).

Treatment of in-stent restenosis with the cutting balloon or other force-focused device (see Chapter 22) may be useful in that it minimizes balloon slipping and affords a better initial angiographic result (requiring fewer balloons and less restenting), although long-term outcomes are similar compared with balloon angioplasty without cutting (154). Prior studies of debulking with directional or rotational atherectomy (155–157), laser angioplasty

TABLE 24.10

EFFICACY OF VASCULAR BRACHYTHERAPY IN REDUCING RECURRENT RESTENOSIS AFTER TREATMENT OF BARE METAL STENT IN-STENT RESTENOSIS

	Total N Randomized	Brachytherapy Source	Duration (months) of Clinical and Angiographic Follow-up	Target Lesion or Vessel Revascularization			Binary Angiographic Restenosis		
				Brachytherapy (%)	Control (%)	P Value	Brachytherapy (%)	Control (%)	P Value
SCRIPPS (163)	55	Gamma	12 and 6	15	48	.01	17	54	.01
GAMMA-1 (164)	252	Gamma	9 and 9	32.4	55.3	.01	31.3	46.3	.01
WRIST (165)	131	Gamma	12 and 6	33.8	67.6	<.001	22	60	.0001
Long WRIST (165[a])	120	Gamma	12 and 6	39.0	61.7	<.05	45	73	<.05
START (166)	476	Beta	8 and 8	17.0	26.8	.02	28.8	45.2	.001
INHIBIT[a]	332	Beta	9 and 9	20	37	.025	26	52	<.0001
BRITE-II[b]	423	Beta	9 and 9	25	43	.02	29.0	49.7	.002

[a] Waksman R, Raizner AE, Yeung AC, et al. Use of localised intracoronary beta radiation in treatment of in-stent restenosis: the INHIBIT randomised controlled trial. *Lancet* 2003;359:551–557.
[b] Waksman R, for the BRITE II Investigators. Balloon-based radiation for coronary in-stent restenosis: 9-month results from the BRITE II study. Presented at the meeting of the American College of Cardiology, Chicago, IL, 2003.

(158–161), or restenting with bare metal stents (162) have not yielded results clearly superior to balloon angioplasty alone (see Chapter 23).

The delivery of intracoronary radiation with either beta or gamma sources has been demonstrated to further reduce recurrent restenosis by an additional 30 to 70% after balloon angioplasty treatment of in-stent restenosis (163–166; Table 24.10). However, in addition to logistic complexities (the need for coordination with a radiation therapist, physicist, and safety officer), plus additional shielding and costs, new issues that have surfaced with this therapy include severe recurrent restenosis at the margins of the radiation field (the so-called edge effect, possibly owing to geographic miss; 167–169) and late stent thrombosis (which can usually be prevented by prolonged [1 year] clopidogrel use and avoiding implanting new stents into the fresh radiation field [170]). In the GAMMA-1 trial, all of the early benefit of vascular brachytherapy was lost by 4 years (171). *Thus, despite the fact that intracoronary radiation has been approved by the FDA for the treatment of bare metal stent restenosis (the only such therapy approved for this purpose), simpler, safer, and more effective approaches to this common problem are required.*

Drug-eluting stents may prove to be the optimal approach for bare metal stent restenosis. Both sirolimus-eluting and paclitaxel-eluting stents (see below) further reduced clinical and angiographic restenosis in patients with bare metal stent restenosis in a 300-patient single-center randomized trial (172). In a small study in which consecutive series of 44 and 43 patients with in-stent restenosis were treated with balloon angioplasty plus brachytherapy and sirolimus-eluting stents, respectively, the drug-eluting stent (DES) had similar safety and efficacy compared with intracoronary radiation therapy at 9 months

follow-up (173). Two pivotal randomized trials of sirolimus-eluting and paclitaxel-eluting stents compared with vascular brachytherapy in patients with restenosis of bare metal stents have recently been completed. No studies have yet been reported examining the outcomes following repeat PCI for restenosis in DES.

Other Complications of Coronary Stent Implantation

A review of all complications that can occur during or after PCI is beyond the scope of this chapter (see Chapters 3 and 22). However, several risks that are unique to or are increased in frequency with coronary stenting compared with balloon angioplasty should be appreciated.

Side-Branch Occlusion

Side-branch compromise after stent implantation most commonly results from the so-called snowplow phenomenon—shifting of plaque during stent deployment or high-pressure dilatation (though coronary spasm may contribute). The incidence of side-branch compromise after coronary stent implantation is greater than after balloon angioplasty (174–176). In the early experience with the Palmaz-Schatz stent, a 5% incidence of acute branch occlusion was noted when the stent was placed across a side branch >1 mm in diameter (174). This risk is increased to 20% or greater when both the parent vessel and side branch are involved (177). Stent-induced occlusion of a large side branch may result in significant myocardial ischemia and infarction, though in most patients the long-term prognosis is excellent, and most initially occluded side branches are patent at late angiographic follow-up (175,176).

Side-branch occlusion should be anticipated whenever a stent is placed across a bifurcation. If the side branch is large (≥3.0 mm in diameter), or is ≥2.5 mm in diameter and diseased at its ostium, it should be protected with a second guidewire prior to PCI. If the origin of the branch is narrowed, it should also be predilated prior to stent implantation in the main branch. Although this is most commonly performed with balloon angioplasty, alternatives include use of the cutting balloon or debulking techniques with atherectomy, though this approach has not been clearly shown to preserve side-branch patency beyond that achieved by balloon angioplasty alone. Once the side branch is protected with a second wire (and predilated if necessary), a stent may be placed in the main vessel across the branch origin, temporarily "jailing" the wire. This usually preserves patency of the side branch should occlusion otherwise occur and serves as a locator for the side-branch origin. If additional angioplasty is planned, a third wire should then be passed through the stent struts into the narrowed side branch, after which the jailed wire is removed. The likelihood of a jailed wire becoming "stuck" is rare if the parent vessel stent is implanted at ≤12 atm of pressure, but jailing a long segment of wire in the parent vessel should be avoided, and hydrophilic wires should be used cautiously because of the risk of stripping the polymer coating on its withdrawal. Alternatively, if there is minimal narrowing at the origin of the side branch at baseline or after balloon dilatation, a stent may be placed in the main vessel across the side-branch origin with the option of wiring it should it narrow after stent placement.

If the side branch significantly narrows after predilatation of either limb of the bifurcation, or the result is not acceptable after predilatation (which typically depends on the plaque burden, extent of calcification, and angle or origin of the side branch from the parent), a second stent should be implanted in the side branch using one of numerous techniques (178; see Bifurcation Lesions, below). With all these dual-stent techniques, however, the subacute thrombosis rate is increased compared with a single-stent approach, and the restenosis rate within the second stent at the side-branch origin is increased compared with the main branch (even with drug-eluting stents). As such, the single-stent strategy is preferable if an acceptable balloon-only result in the side branch cannot be obtained.

Stent Embolization

Stent embolization from the stent delivery system may occur during antegrade passage in a fibrocalcific or tortuous vessel, or upon withdrawal of the device after failure to cross a lesion (often when the edge of the stent snags on the tip of the guide catheter). Risk factors for stent embolization include heavy vessel calcification, pronounced vessel tortuosity, diffuse disease, and attempting to deliver a stent to a distal lesion through a previously implanted proximal

stent (179). When the original Palmaz-Schatz stent was hand-mounted on a conventional angioplasty balloon and no sheath was used, stent embolization occurred in 8.4% of patients (12). Over the years, the development of tighter stent-to-balloon crimping processes in concert with lower-profile, more flexible devices has resulted in the incidence of this complication decreasing to <1 to 2% (180–181). Stent embolization into the peripheral vasculature usually has no adverse clinical sequelae, but may rarely cause limb ischemia or a cerebrovascular event. Conversely, intracoronary stent embolization is associated with significant rates of coronary thrombosis, coronary artery occlusion, and subsequent myocardial infarction, with mortality rates as high as 17%. If the stent can be removed nonoperatively, survival has been reported in >96% of patients (180,183).

If the guidewire is still across the stent and has been maintained in the distal coronary artery, a low-profile balloon may be placed back through the stent, allowing it to be repositioned across the target lesion and expanded. If the stent cannot be repositioned, the balloon can be placed distal to the stent and inflated to trap the stent between the balloon and guiding catheter, withdrawing all components together into the femoral sheath. If guidewire position has been lost and the unexpanded stent is located in a proximal portion of the coronary artery or has embolized into a peripheral artery, it may be removed using a variety of forceps or snare devices. If displaced from the wire or more distal, a series of wires can be wrapped around it to ensnare it. Alternatively, a second stent may be expanded adjacent to the dislodged stent to trap it against the vessel wall, effectively excluding it from the lumen.

Success rates for percutaneous retrieval of lost stents from the coronary tree have been reported in 47 to 71% of patients in contemporary series (181–183). If the stent cannot be removed or effectively "excluded" from the coronary lumen, strong consideration should be given for coronary artery bypass surgery, though high mortality rates have been described in his situation.

Coronary Perforation

Although the routine use of high-pressure postdilatation improves stent expansion, the significant barotrauma imparted to the vessel may result in frank perforation (see Chapter 3; 184). In a retrospective analysis, Ellis and colleagues documented a 0.5% incidence of perforation among 12,900 procedures (185). From most contemporary series with stents, perforation has been reported in 0.2 to 1.0% of patients, though mild perforations are likely under-reported. Risk factors for perforation include female gender, advanced age, lesion calcification and angulation, chronic total occlusions, and adjunctive atherectomy use (185). Device oversizing is also a risk for perforation;

Colombo reported that the use of markedly oversized balloons (balloon-to-artery ratio >1.2 in the absence of IVUS guidance) has a risk of perforation and vessel rupture ranging from 1.2 to 3.0% (18).

An angiographic classification of the severity of coronary artery perforation has proven useful in determining prognosis and guiding treatment (185). A *type I* or concealed perforation is the most common type, and usually requires no specific therapy. As delayed tamponade may occasionally occur, however, observation for 24 hours is warranted. A *type II* or limited perforation usually appears as a stain or blush at the site of the arterial tear, and can usually be managed with prolonged balloon inflation with or without reversal of anticoagulation. Echocardiography postprocedure and 24 hours later to ensure the absence of a growing pericardial effusion is prudent in type II perforations. Patients with a history of prior bypass surgery usually have extensive mediastinal adhesions, and perforations are rarely greater than type II. *Type III* or freeflowing perforations typically appear with continuous jetlike dye extravasation and may rapidly result in hypotension and tamponade requiring emergency pericardiocentesis. When a type III perforation is visualized, the angioplasty balloon should urgently be passed across the coronary rupture to obtain immediate hemostasis.

Most small perforations can be sealed with prolonged balloon inflations and reversal of UFH anticoagulation with protamine, unless a platelet glycoprotein IIb/IIIa receptor antagonist has been given (186). If the perforation is not readily closed with these measures and is severe, deployment of PTFE-covered stents provides reliable sealing, usually obviating the need for emergency surgery (61,62). Given their porous nature, two overlapping PTFE-covered stent grafts may occasionally be required for hemostasis. If a stent graft is unable to be delivered to the site of the perforation, emergency surgery is usually required, though the associated rates of morbidity and mortality in this setting are high.

Infectious Endarteritis

Placement of a foreign body endovascular prosthesis carries the theoretical risk of bacterial endarteritis. In an experimental porcine model, following the induction of transient bacteremia, a significant number of recently placed coronary stents cultured positive for bacteria (187). The risk of suppurative endarteritis in stented coronary arteries is extremely rare, however, with only a handful of documented cases in the literature (188–190). Although periprocedural antibiotic therapy is thus not routinely recommended, antibiotic prophylaxis may be considered if sterile technique has been breached or if the patient requires invasive procedures associated with transient bacteremia during the first 4 weeks following stenting, though the utility of this approach has never been shown.

RESULTS OF STENTING COMPARED WITH SURGICAL REVASCULARIZATION

As seen in Table 24.11, nine randomized trials have been published in which 4,061 patients have been randomized to bare metal stent implantation versus coronary artery bypass graft surgery (191–202). Five of these trials compared multilesion stenting with surgery in patients with multivessel disease, whereas four examined the outcomes of stent implantation versus bypass with a left internal mammary artery in patients with isolated disease of the proximal left anterior descending coronary artery. Although the results of these trials varied slightly from study to study, there were no differences in the 6-month to 3-year rates of death, myocardial infarction, or stroke between the two approaches, though repeat revascularization procedures were more common with stent-supported PCI. In one study in which patients with isolated lesions in the proximal left anterior descending artery underwent repeat angiography 6 months after being randomized to stenting versus minimally invasive surgery, in-stent restenosis was present in 33% of stented patients whereas a diameter stenosis of >50% in a graft (usually a the distal anastomosis) was observed in 18% of bypassed patients ($P < .05$; 200). Quality of life measures during convalescence were similar with the two strategies, and long-term total costs were generally lower with stenting rather than surgery, despite the greater number of repeat procedures (194).

Thus, in most patients with either single or multivessel disease, bare metal stent implantation provides similar results to coronary artery bypass graft surgery in terms of freedom from death, myocardial infarction, and stroke, though recurrent angina and repeat revascularization procedures are more common with PCI. Long-term quality of life is similar, however, with the two approaches, and stenting is somewhat less expensive in the short and long term. Of note, however, these trials have excluded patients with left main disease and other highly complex lesions for PCI, severely depressed left ventricular function, and prior bypass surgery. Whether bypass graft surgery prolongs survival compared with PCI in patients with diabetes mellitus is still an open question. Several large-scale randomized trials of drug-eluting stents versus surgery are now underway to determine whether the enhanced freedom from restenosis with these bioactive devices translates into equivalent event-free survival with the two revascularization modalities.

DRUG-ELUTING STENTS

Bare metal stents eliminate acute and chronic vascular recoil and remodeling and also reduce restenosis compared with balloon angioplasty. However, bare metal stents

TABLE 24.11
RANDOMIZED TRIALS OF CORONARY STENT IMPLANTATION VERSUS BYPASS GRAFT SURGERY

Trial	Population	Total N Randomized	Duration of Follow-up	Mortality		Myocardial Infarction		Repeat Revascularization		Stroke		Comments
				Stent	CABG	Stent	CABG	Stent	CABG	Stent	CABG	
ARTS (192)	Multivessel disease	1,205	1 year	2.5%	2.8%	6.2%	4.8%	21.0%a	3.8%	1.7%	2.1%	Stenting less expensive at 1 year
SOS (193)	Multivessel disease	988	2 years	5%*	2%	5%*	8%	21%*	6%	1%	2%	Stenting less expensive at 1 year, with quality of life similar in both groups
AWESOME (195,196)	Refractory unstable angina with high risk features	454	5 years	22%	27%	—	—	—	—	—	—	54% stents in angioplasty group
ERACI-II (197)	Multivessel disease	450	1.5 years	3.1%*	7.5%	2.3%*	6.6%	16.8%*	4.8%	—	—	Total costs similar in both groups
MASS-II (198)	Multivessel disease	408	1 year	4.5%	4.0%	8.3%*	2.0%	13.3%*	0.5%	1.0%	1.5%	—
SIMA (199)	Proximal LAD	134	5 years	1.5%	1.5%	14.7%*	4.5%	38.2%*	9.1%	—	—	—
Driegler et al. (200)	Proximal LAD	220	6 months	0%	1.8%	2.8%	4.6%	28.7%*	8.3%	—	—	Minimally invasive surgery
Drenth et al. (201)	Proximal LAD	102	3 years	0%	3.9%	9.8%	12.0%	15.7%	3.9%	2.0%	0%	Minimally invasive surgery
Reeves et al. (202)	Proximal LAD	100	1 year	—	—	—	—	—	—	—	—	Minimally invasive surgery; MACE at 1 year 7.2% for stent vs. 9.1% for CABG (P = NS); stenting less expensive

* $P <.05$.
CABG, coronary artery bypass graft surgery; LAD, left anterior descending artery; MACE, major adverse cardiac events.

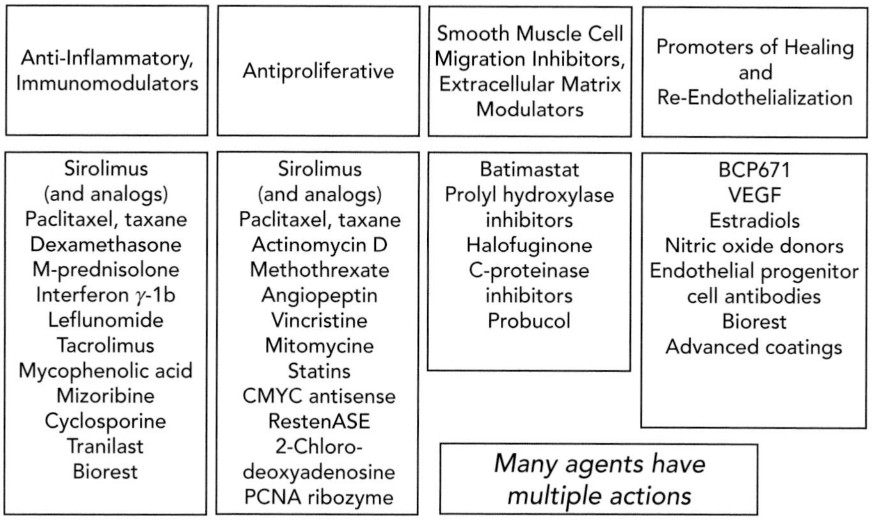

Anti-Inflammatory, Immunomodulators	Antiproliferative	Smooth Muscle Cell Migration Inhibitors, Extracellular Matrix Modulators	Promoters of Healing and Re-Endothelialization
Sirolimus (and analogs) Paclitaxel, taxane Dexamethasone M-prednisolone Interferon γ-1b Leflunomide Tacrolimus Mycophenolic acid Mizoribine Cyclosporine Tranilast Biorest	Sirolimus (and analogs) Paclitaxel, taxane Actinomycin D Methothrexate Angiopeptin Vincristine Mitomycine Statins CMYC antisense RestenASE 2-Chloro-deoxyadenosine PCNA ribozyme	Batimastat Prolyl hydroxylase inhibitors Halofuginone C-proteinase inhibitors Probucol	BCP671 VEGF Estradiols Nitric oxide donors Endothelial progenitor cell antibodies Biorest Advanced coatings

Many agents have multiple actions

Figure 24.11 Bioactive agents that have undergone preclinical evaluation for their antirestenotic properties for drug-eluting stents. Compounds may be roughly classified as possessing primarily anti-inflammatory or immunomodulatory properties, acting principally as an antiproliferative agent, inhibiting smooth muscle cell migration or extracellular matrix production, or promoting re-endothelialization and healing. Many compounds, however, overlap and have multiple functions. PCNA, proliferating cell nuclear antigen; VEGF, vascular endothelial growth factor.

induce more arterial injury and subsequently greater neointimal hyperplasia than balloon angioplasty. The concept of blunting the degree of neointimal hyperplasia by various intravenous or orally administered compounds was investigated for this purpose, but proved ineffective in humans despite promising results in preclinical animal models (203,204). This was likely due to the inability to achieve high enough local arterial drug concentrations without invoking excessive systemic toxicity. Thus the concept of the *local delivery* of bioactive agents was evaluated with a series of drugs delivered to the site of arterial injury after PCI, using a variety of porous angioplasty balloons (205). These attempts also failed to reduce neointimal hyperplasia, (206,207), owing to poor delivery or retention rates of the bioactive compound in the arterial wall (208) or excessive barotrauma-induced vascular injury (209). To overcome these limitations, drug-eluting stents emerged as a way to ensure the extended release of a high concentration of a biologic agent to the vessel wall during the critical 30-day initial healing period. The demonstration that drug-eluting stents can safely reduce angiographic and clinical restenosis compared with bare metal stents has radically altered treatment paradigms of patients with coronary artery disease, representing a true revolution in the field of medicine.

Components of a Drug-Eluting Stent

Drug-eluting stents consist of three components: a *bioactive agent* to reduce neointimal hyperplasia; a *drug carrier vehicle* designed to control the local dosing and delivery of the drug; and the *stent platform* to scaffold the lumen and physically deliver the drug to the vessel wall in an appropriate distribution. The optimization of each component and their integration are critical to ensure the safety and efficacy of these devices. Numerous drugs have been investigated for this purpose, which may broadly be classified as

anti-inflammatory and/or immunomodulatory agents, antiproliferative agents, inhibitors of smooth muscle cell migration or extracellular matrix production, or promoters of healing and re-endothelialization (Fig. 24.11). Many compounds have multiple mechanisms of action.

Various approaches to permit controlled drug elution have been developed and are undergoing investigation (Table 24.12). As described below, the two proven drug-eluting stents load and release their bioactive agents from encapsulated, elastomeric nonerodable biostable polymers. In many respects, formulating and optimizing the drug carrier vehicle has proven even more complex than identifying and evaluating the drug itself. Properties that must be considered for a controlled release vehicle include its biocompatability, solubility, diffusivity and porosity, molecular size, weight and distribution, elongation, functional requirements, degradation products, durability, relative hydrophobicity, purity, availability, adhesion, crystallinity, sterilization, solvent solubility, biostability, miscibility, bioabsorbable versus permanent nature, evaporation rate, thermal properties, resistance to

TABLE 24.12

POTENTIAL DRUG CARRIER VEHICLES

- Direct applications to the stent (surface modification)
- Nondegradable polymer sleeves
- Encapsulated, nonreactive, elastomeric nondegradable polymer
- Encapsulated, nonreactive, elastomeric bioabsorbable polymer (with or without polymer-drug conjugates)
- Phosphorylcholine coatings
- Ceramic and other novel coatings
- Polymers embedded within the stent geometry
- Stent grafts (e.g., PTFE)
- Polymer-based or metallic-erodable bioabsorbable stents

PTFE, polytetrafluoroethylene.

humidity and temperature extremes, compatibility with specific drugs, approval for implant use, processability (which relates to shelf life), and packaging requirements.

Finally, the stent itself is an essential component. Stent geometry must be optimized for homogeneous drug distribution (which involves considerations of closed versus open cell designs, interstrut distances, etc.). Circumferential stent to vessel wall contact must be ensured to ensure drug delivery. As a result, the stent must be conformable to angulated segments, while at the same time minimizing geometric distortion. The stent should also have sufficient radiopacity to facilitate precise lesion coverage (while avoiding excessive stent overlap or interstent gaps). Side-branch access should be maintained. The stent must be low profile, flexible, and deliverable to reach and treat complex anatomies.

Lessons from Failed Drug-Eluting Stent Programs

Several drug-eluting stent programs have failed or shown clinical results that were only marginally better than bare metal control stents. Valuable lessons have been learned from these unsuccessful attempts, three of which will be briefly reviewed here, including the consequences of using the *wrong drug*, the *wrong platform*, or the *wrong release kinetics*.

The first drug-eluting stent was the Quanam QuaDDS stent, consisting of the paclitaxel derivative 7-hexanoyl paclitaxel (QP2, or taxane), loaded onto multiple polymer sleeves mounted on the stainless steel QueST stent. A very large dose of taxane was loaded onto each stent (4,000 µg on a 17-mm stent), and the pivotal SCORE trial (210) was halted prematurely owing to markedly higher rates of myocardial infarction (11.9% versus 2.1%, P = .002) and stent thrombosis (3.2% versus 0%, P = .049) at 1 and 6 months compared with a bare metal control stent. At 1 year, patients receiving this stent had higher rates of cardiac death (4.0% versus 0%, P = .02), myocardial infarction (19.% versus 2.1%, P < .001), and stent thrombosis (10.3% versus 0.7%, P < .001), with similar rates of target vessel revascularization (19.8% versus 23.6%, P = .55). In retrospect, a combination of factors contributed to the untoward outcomes with this device, including the excessive vasculotoxic doses of taxane; the use of a proinflammatory polymer delivery vehicle; and the polymeric sleeves that physically covered side branches.

The Guidant Tetra-D stent eluting the cell cycle inhibitor actinomycin-D from a biostable polymer was evaluated in the multicenter, prospective ACTION trial (211). In this study, 357 patients were randomized to one of two actinomycin-D dose formulations (2.5 or 10 µg/cm^2) or a bare metal control stent. At a median angiographic follow-up time of 5.3 months, both the extent of late loss (mean 0.76 versus 1.01 and 0.93 mm, respectively) and binary restenosis (14% versus 26% and 28%, respectively) were *greater* in the two actinomycin-D arms. Similarly, major adverse cardiac events at 1 year were increased with actinomycin-D, driven by markedly increased rates of target lesion revascularization

with similar rates of death and myocardial infarction. In retrospect, the adverse clinical responses to this stent may have been predicted by the suboptimal results of preclinical porcine studies.

Even an effective drug may yield negative results with incorrect dosing or release kinetics. Paclitaxel has thus been applied directly to stainless steel stents using a proprietary surface modification process, and has been tested in a series of pilot and pivotal randomized trials (212–214). In the ELUTES trial, 190 patients were randomized to the Cook V-Flex Plus stent with escalating doses of paclitaxel (0, 0.2, 0.7, 1.4, and 2.7 µg/mm^2 stent surface area). Among these five groups, both the angiographic late loss (mean 0.73, 0.71, 0.47, 0.47, and 0.11%, respectively, P = .002) and binary restenosis rates (20.6, 20.6, 14.3, 13.5, and 3.2% respectively, P = .056) at 6 months decreased progressively, though there were no differences in target lesion revascularization or event-free survival (212). In the ASPECT trial, 178 patients with discrete coronary lesions underwent implantation of paclitaxel-eluting Cook Supra-G stents (low-dose, 1.3 µg/mm^2, or high-dose, 3.1 µg per mm^2) or control stents. Comparing the bare metal with the low- and high-dose formulations, there was a progressive reduction in binary angiographic restenosis at 6 months (27% versus 12% versus 4%, respectively, P < .001), late lumen loss (mean 1.04 versus 0.57 versus 0.29 mmm, respectively, p < 0.001), and intrastent neointimal volume determined by IVUS (mean 31 versus 18 versus 13 mm^3, P < 0.001) (213).

These promising angiographic results led to the pivotal DELIVER trial, in which 1,043 patients with focal de novo coronary lesions were randomized to paclitaxel-coated Guidant Penta stents (3.0 µg paclitaxel/mm^2 stent surface area applied using the Cook surface modification process) or bare metal control Penta stents, followed by aspirin for 1 year and clopidogrel for at least 3 months. At 8-month angiographic follow-up, only a modest reduction in in-stent late loss (mean 0.81 versus 0.98 mm, P = .0025), and only weak trends for binary angiographic restenosis (14.9% versus 20.6%, respectively, P = .076) and target lesion revascularization (8.1% versus 11.3%, respectively, P = .09) were present (214). No differences were present in the rates of cardiac death, myocardial infarction, or stent thrombosis between the two groups. Thus, although this stent was safe and exhibited mild antirestenotic properties, it was not nearly as effective as the TAXUS paclitaxel-eluting stent (29), which uses a durable polymer to ensure the consistency of dosing and release kinetics from the stent. These contrary results with two different drug-eluting stents using the same antiproliferative compound emphasize the importance of the control release vehicle.

Proven Drug-Eluting Stents I: Sirolimus Elution from a Durable Polymer

Sirolimus (rapamycin) is a highly lipophilic, naturally occurring macrocyclic lactone, which was first isolated from *Streptomyces hygroscopicus* found in a soil sample from Easter Island (also known as Rapa Nui) and was initially developed as an antifungal agent. Shortly thereafter, it became apparent that this agent also was a potent immunosuppressive, and was initially approved by the Food and Drug Administration (as Rapamune) for prevention of renal transplant rejection in 1999. Marx and colleagues noted that sirolimus inhibits smooth muscle cell proliferation and migration (215,216), resulting in its development as an antirestenotic agent (217). It works by binding to the intracellular cytosolic receptor FK-506-binding protein (FKBP12), with the sirolimus–FKBP12 complex interacting specifically with mTOR (the mammalian Target Of Rapamycin), to upregulate the cyclin-dependent kinase inhibitor p27[kip1] and other regulatory proteins, and thereby prevent cell cycle progression past the late G1 phase. By inhibiting smooth muscle cell migration and proliferation, sirolimus has been shown to reduce neointimal hyperplasia after mechanical injury in rats and porcine coronary arteries without evident toxicity. Chemical derivatives of rapamycin, including ABT-578 and everolimus, have all shown antirestenotic effect in human drug-eluting stent trials and are expected to enter clinical practice in the United States in 2007 or beyond. Given the limited current data and time to market release, the remainder of this section will focus on sirolimus.

The Cypher stent (Cordis Johnson & Johnson) consists of sirolimus (140 μg/cm^2) incorporated within an amalgam of two biostable polymers (thickness approximately 5 μm)

coated on the 316L stainless steel Bx Velocity stent. The fast-release Cypher stent elutes >80% of the drug within 15 days, but the clinical slow-release version includes a topcoat of polymer only without drug to act as a diffusion barrier, thus retarding drug elution (total polymer thickness approximately 10 um, >80% drug released over 28 days).

Human experience with the Cypher stent was first reported from the First-In-Man (FIM) study initiated in 1999 in 45 patients (218). Remarkable suppression of instent neointimal hyperplasia was observed with both the slow- and fast-release Cypher stent. Serial angiography and intravascular ultrasound has now been performed at 4 years, with continued vessel patency without further late loss (216; Figs. 24.12 and 24.13).

Six randomized trials have been performed to date comparing the slow-release Cypher stent to the bare metal Bx velocity control (Table 24.13; 28,220–227). Collectively, these trials demonstrate that the Cypher stent results in a near abolition of in-stent late loss (averaging approximately 0.15 mm across studies), with an approximate 70 to 80% reduction in angiographic restenosis and clinical recurrence (target lesion revascularization) rates within 1 year compared with the bare metal control stent. In addition, the Cypher stent proved safe, with similar rates of death, myocardial infarction, and stent thrombosis found in the control and treatment arms. In the SIRIUS trial, 1,058 patients with a single de novo nonoccluded coronary stenosis 15 to 30 mm long with reference vessel diameter of 2.5 to

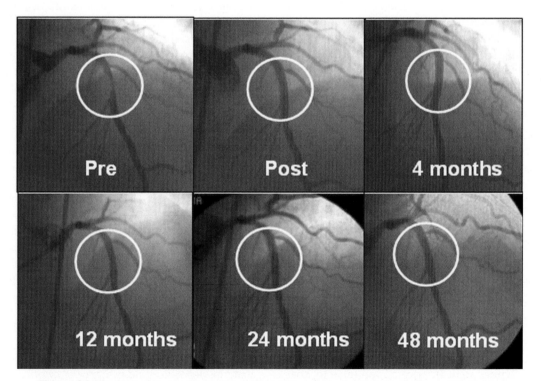

Figure 24.12   Long-term results from one of the first patients to receive a sirolimus-eluting stent in the early Sao Paulo experience. A high-grade stenosis in the proximal left anterior descending artery is stented with a single 3.0-mm sirolimus-eluting stent. Serial angiography shows sustained vessel patency with minimal late loss over a 4-year period.

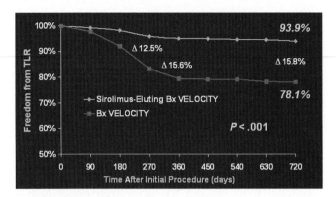

Figure 24.13 Two-year freedom from target lesion revascularization after randomization of 1,055 patients to either a sirolimus-eluting stent or bare metal Bx Velocity stent. The marked early benefit of the drug-eluting stent is maintained at 2 years, with no evidence of loss of effect with long-term follow-up.

3.5 mm were randomized to the Cypher or bare metal Bx Velocity stents (28,223,224), with 3 months of postprocedure clopidogrel. The primary end point of target vessel failure at 9 months was reduced with the Cypher from 21 to 8.6% ($P < .001$). Target lesion revascularization rates at 9 months were reduced from 16.6 to 4.1% ($P < .001$). Subacute stent thrombosis was rare and occurred with similar frequency in the two groups (0.4% with Cypher versus 0.8% with the Bx Velocity). Follow-up angiography at 8 months in 703 patients demonstrated marked reductions in in-stent late loss (from mean 1.00 to 0.17 mm, $P < .001$), in-segment late loss (mean 0.81 versus 0.24 mm, $P < .001$), and binary in-stent and in-segment restenosis (35.4% versus 3.2%, and 36.3% versus 8.9%, respectively, both $P < .001$). When restenosis did occur, the lesions were typically focal in nature (mean length 9.1 mm with Cypher versus 14.8 mm with Bx Velocity, $P < .001$; 221). Late coronary aneurysms were infrequent in both groups and not increased with sirolimus. By IVUS, the in-stent percent volumetric obstruction at 8 months was reduced from 33.4% with the Bx Velocity to 3.1% with the sirolimus-eluting stent ($P < .001$). However, IVUS showed late stent malapposition in 9.7% of Cypher patients versus 0% of Bx velocity patients ($P = .02$). Clinical and angiographic efficacy were present across a broad range of patient and lesion subtypes.

In April 2003, the Cypher became the first drug-eluting stent approved by the Food and Drug Administration in the United States. Follow-up thus far has been reported to 2 years, demonstrating sustained efficacy (Fig. 24.11), in contradistinction to the narrowing in event-free survival already seen with vascular brachytherapy during this time interval (171). Subsequent randomized trials performed in Europe (225) and Canada (226) reproduced or surpassed these results in smaller vessels. These trials have also shown that direct stenting (without predilatation) is feasible with the Cypher stent in selected lesions and does not adversely impact late outcomes. Moreover, in SIRIUS, questions arose whether the Cypher was somewhat less effective in patients with diabetes (especially insulin

requiring) compared with those without diabetes (228). Such concerns have diminished with the results of subsequent studies, however, including the recently reported dedicated DIABETES trial (229), in which the 9-month in-stent late loss was 0.66 mm with the Bx Velocity versus 0.08 mm with the Cypher ($P < .0001$).

Proven Drug-Eluting Stents II: Paclitaxel Elution from a Durable Polymer

Paclitaxel, a highly lipophilic diterpenoid compound, was first isolated in 1963 from the pacific yew tree (*Taxus brevifolius*) and developed for its potent antineoplastic properties. Its principal action is to interfere with microtubule dynamics, preventing their depolymerization. This leads to widespread dose-dependent multicellular activity: antiproliferative and anti-inflammatory properties, reduced smooth muscle migration, blocking of cytokine and growth factor release and activity, interference with secretory processes, antiangiogenic effects, and impaired signal transduction (230). At high doses, paclitaxel produces mitotic arrest in the G2/M phases of the cell cycle and promotes apoptosis. At low doses (similar to those in drug-eluting stent applications), however, paclitaxel affects the G0-G1 and G1-S phases (G1 arrest), resulting in cytostasis without cell death (probably via induction of p53/p21 tumor suppression genes; 230,231). Moreover, paclitaxel inhibits smooth muscle cell proliferation at 10% of the concentration required for endothelial cells (230).

The TAXUS stent (Boston Scientific) consists of paclitaxel contained within a polyolefin derivative biostable polymer coated originally on the NIR stent, but currently on the Express stent platform (soon to transition to the Liberté stent). Depending on the relative weight of paclitaxel to polymer, the stent may be formulated as slow release (SR; relatively more polymer to drug, coat thickness 18 μm, approximately 8% in vivo paclitaxel elution in 30 days), moderate release (MR; 7 μm coat thickness, approximately 22% paclitaxel elution in 30 days), or fast release (4 μm coat thickness, approximately 50% paclitaxel elution in 30 days). The paclitaxel concentration is 1 μg/mm^2 of stent surface (i.e., 108 μg on a 16-mm stent) for all formulations. The drug is eluted in a rapid-burst phase over the initial 48 hours, followed by a slow, sustained release for the next 10 to 30 days, with the remainder sequestered permanently in the bulk of the polymer matrix. In a series of porcine experiments at 30, 90, 180, and 360 days involving a total of 350 swine and 800 stents, both the slow and moderate rate release TAXUS stent formulations were shown to be vasculocompatible, with early development of a thin, mature neointima with low levels of inflammation, microthrombi. and peristent amorphous material deposition; no evidence of cytotoxicity; and with complete healing and endothelialization within 90 days, similar to both control bare metal or polymer-only coated stents (data on file, Boston Scientific).

TABLE 24.13

COMPLETED RANDOMIZED TRIALS OF THE CYPHER POLYMER-BASED SIROLIMUS-ELUTING STENT IN DE NOVO CORONARY LESIONS

	Total N (with angio follow-up)	Diabetes	RVD (mm)	LL (mm)	Clinical (angio) Follow-up (months)	Death (%)		Myocardial Infarction (%)		Target lesion Revascularization (%)		Major Adverse Cardiac Events (%)[c]		Stent Thrombosis (%)[d]		Binary Angiographic Restenosis (in-segment, %)	
						DES	BMS	DES	BMS	DES	BMS	DES	BMS	DES	BMS	DES	BMS
RAVEL (220–222)	238(211)	19%	2.62	9.6	12(6)	1.7%	1.7%	3.3%	4.2%	0%[b]	22.9%	5.9%[b]	29.1%	0%	0%	0%[b]	26.6
SIRIUS (28,223)	1,058(703)	26%	2.80	14.4	9(8)	0.9%	0.6%	2.8%	3.2%	4.1%[b]	16.6%	7.1%[b]	18.9%	0.4%	0.8%	8.9%[b]	36.3
E-SIRIUS (225)	352(308)	23%	2.55	15.0	9(8)	1.1%	0.6%	4.6%	2.3%	4.0%[b]	20.9%	8.0%[b]	22.6%	1.1%	0%	3.9%[b]	41.7%
C-SIRIUS (226)	100(88)	24%	2.63	13.6	9(8)	0%	0%	2.0%	4.0%	4.0%[b]	18.0%	4.0%[b]	18.0%	2.0%	2.0%	2.3%[b]	52.3
SES-SMART (227)	257(236)	25%	2.20	11.8	8(8)	0%	1.6%	1.6%[b]	7.8%	7.0%[b]	21.1%	9.3%[b]	31.3%	0.8%	3.1%	9.8%[b]	53.1
DIABETES[a]	160(~90%)	100%	2.34	14.9	12(9)	1.3%	2.5%	2.5%	6.2%	7.5%[b]	31.3%	11.3%[b]	36.3%	0%	0%	7.7%[b]	33.0

[a] Sabate M. The DIABETES Trial. Presented at TCT 2004, Washington DC, September 2004.
[b] P < .05.
[c] Includes death, myocardial infarction, or target lesion revascularization for all studies except RAVEL, which incorporates target vessel revascularization in the MACE endpoint, and SES-SMART, which incorporates stent thrombosis and stroke.
[d] Angiographically confirmed.
Angio, angiographic; RVD, reference vessel diameter; LL, lesion length; DES, drug-eluting stent (Cypher); BMS, bare metal stent control (Bx Velocity).

The clinical safety and efficacy of the TAXUS stent has been tested in seven randomized TAXUS trials (29,232–238). TAXUS I, II, and III evaluated the TAXUS stent on the NIR platform in focal lesions, whereas TAXUS IV, V, and VI investigated the TAXUS Express stent in more complex lesions with longer-term follow-up. The results of the completed randomized TAXUS trials enrolling patients with de novo lesions in native coronary arteries appear in Table 24.14. Collectively, these trials show a marked decrease of binary restenosis rates, an approximately 70 to 75% reduction in the need for target lesion revascularization compared with the bare metal control stents, with no increased risks of death, myocardial infarction, or stent thrombosis.

In the pivotal prospective, randomized, double-blind TAXUS IV study, 1,314 patients with single de novo lesions with visually estimated length of 10 to 28 mm in native coronary arteries with reference diameter 2.5 to 3.75 mm were assigned to either a TAXUS SR stent or bare metal Express stent control (29,238). Six months of postprocedure clopidogrel was prescribed to all patients.

At 9 months, the primary end point of target vessel revascularization was reduced with TAXUS from 12.0 to 4.7% ($P < .001$). Target lesion revascularization rates at 9 months were reduced from 11.3 to 3.0% ($P < .001$). Subacute thrombosis was rare and occurred with similar frequency in the two groups (0.6% with TAXUS versus 0.8% with the Express). Follow-up angiography at 9 months demonstrated marked reductions in in-stent and analysis segment late loss (from mean 0.92 to 0.39 mm, and 0.61 versus 0.23 mm, respectively, both $P < .001$), and binary in-stent and in-segment restenosis (24.4% versus 5.5%, and 26.6% versus 7.9%, respectively, both $P < .001$). Restenotic lesions were typically focal in nature with TAXUS (mean length 9.8 mm versus 15.3 mm with Express, $P < .001$). Late coronary aneurysms were infrequent in both groups and not increased with paclitaxel. By IVUS, the in-stent percent volumetric obstruction at 8 months was reduced from 29.4% with the bare metal Express to 12.2% with the paclitaxel-eluting stent ($P < .001$). Late stent malapposition at 9 months was present in 1.1% of TAXUS patients versus 2.2% of Express patients ($P = .62$). Clinical and angiographic efficacy was present across a broad range of patient and lesion subtypes, in particular, in patients with both insulin-requiring and oral-mediation-treated diabetes, in whom clinical and angiographic restenosis rates were similar to the nondiabetic population. In March 2004, the TAXUS SR stent became the second drug-eluting stent approved by the Food and Drug Administration in the United States. Follow-up thus far has been reported to 2 years, demonstrating sustained efficacy (Fig. 24.14).

Comparison of Cypher and TAXUS Stent Performance

The pivotal TAXUS IV and SIRIUS trials demonstrate that both TAXUS and Cypher stents are safe and markedly effective in reducing clinical and angiographic restenosis

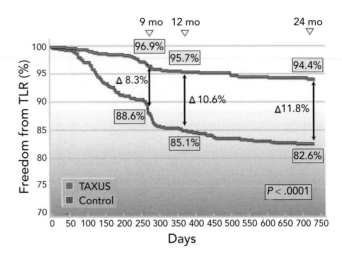

Figure 24.14 Two-year freedom from target lesion revascularization after randomization of 1,314 patients to either a paclitaxel-eluting stent or bare metal Express stent. The early clinical benefit achieved by 9 months is maintained late, and in fact is shown by a slight further spreading of the curves between 1 and 2 years.

compared with their bare metal counterparts. Though the TAXUS stent has slightly greater in-stent late loss than Cypher, in-segment segment late loss is similar between the two stents, with no major differences in target lesion revascularization rates. Similarly, though most studies have demonstrated greater rates of late incomplete stent apposition with Cypher than TAXUS, to date this observation does not seem to be of clinical consequence, though the numbers of patients studied with this phenomenon are too small to exclude low-frequency events. Only appropriately powered head-to-head trials can answer these questions. One small randomized trial (202 patients) in native coronary lesions found no difference in clinical outcomes between the two devices (239), whereas a second small trial in 200 patients with bare metal in-stent restenosis found enhanced results with the Cypher (172).

The REALITY trial randomized 1,386 patients (240) with 1911 native coronary de novo lesions >15 mm long and reference diameter 2.25 to 3.00 mm to receive either Cypher or TAXUS stents. Despite a lower in-lesion late loss with Cypher (0.04 versus 0.16 mm, $P < .001$), there was no significant difference in either binary angiographic restenosis (9.6% versus 11.1%, $P =$ NS) or clinically driven target lesion revascularization (TLR, 5.0% versus 5.4%). This trial did suggest a trend toward less stent thrombosis with the Cypher stent, but that pattern has not been borne out in other series or meta-analyses (see below).

Unsettled Issues: Drug-Eluting Stent Failure and Stent Thrombosis

Restenosis After Drug-Eluting Stent Implantation

Given the efficacy of drug-eluting stents, it is now somewhat surprising to see an in-stent restenosis (treatment of

TABLE 24.14

COMPLETED RANDOMIZED TRIALS OF THE TAXUS POLYMER-BASED PACLITAXEL-ELUTING STENT IN DE NOVO CORONARY LESIONS

	Total N (with angio follow-up)	Diabetes (%)	RVD (mm)	LL (mm)	Clinical (angio) Follow-up (months)	Death (%)		Myocardial Infarction (%)		Target Lesion Revascularization (%)		Major Adverse Cardiac Events (%)[c]		Stent Thrombosis (%)[d]		Binary Angiographic Restenosis (in-segment, %)	
						DES	BMS	DES	BMS	DES	BMS	DES	BMS	DES	BMS	DES	BMS
TAXUS I (SR) (232,233)	61(59)	18	2.97	11.3	12(6)	0	0	0	0	3.3	10.0	3.3	10.0	0	0	0	10.0
TAXUS II (SR) (234–236)	267(262)	14	2.80	10.6	12(6)	0	1.5	2.4	5.3	4.7[b]	12.9	10.9[b]	22.0	1.7	0	5.5[b]	20.1
TAXUS II (MR) (234–236)	268(258)	15	2.70	10.4	12(6)	0	0	3.8	5.4	3.8[b]	16.0	9.9[b]	21.4	0.7	0	8.6[b]	23.8
TAXUS IV (SR) (29,237)	1,314(559)	24	2.75	13.4	9(9)	1.4	1.1	3.5	3.7	3.0[b]	11.3	8.5[b]	15.0	0.6	0.0%	7.9[b]	26.6
TAXUS VI (MR)[a]	446(417)	20	2.79	20.6	9(9)	0	0.9	8.2	6.1	6.8[b]	18.9	16.4	22.5	1.3	05	12.4[b]	35.7

[a] Dawkins K, Grube E. The TAXUS-VI trial. Presented at the meeting of EuroPCR, Paris, May 2004.

[b] $P < .05.$ **

[c] The composite rate of death, myocardial infarction, or target vessel revascularization.

[d] Angiographically confirmed and presumed.

Angio, angiographic; RVD, reference vessel diameter; LL, lesion length; DES, drug-eluting stent (TAXUS); BMS, bare metal stent control (NIR in TAXUS I and II; Express in TAXUS IV and VI); SR, slow rate release formulation; MR, moderate rate release formulation (never commercialized).

which previously accounted for nearly 10% of interventional volume). It should be realized, however, that real-world performance of drug-eluting stents is not quite as impressive as what was seen in randomized trials that were largely restricted to de novo coronary lesions with moderate lesion length and visually estimated reference diameter between 2.5 and 3.75 mm. *In clinical practice, restenosis rates have been higher after implantation of drug-eluting stents in more complex lesions that were excluded from these trials, exceeding 10%.* In the RESEARCH registry, treatment of in-stent restenosis, ostial lesions, diabetes, longer stent length, smaller vessel reference diameter, and non–left anterior descending artery lesions were reported to be independent predictors of restenosis after sirolimus-eluting stents (241). In a large single-center experience with sirolimus-eluting stents in complex lesions from Milan, the only predictor of target vessel revascularization was diabetes (242). Restenosis is also increased after drug-eluting stent implantation when used in patients with prior restenosis of bare or drug-eluting stents, especially in the setting of prior brachytherapy (243,244).

The reasons why drug-eluting stents fail in some patients are unknown, but several possible explanations have been offered. Lack of full stent expansion continues to be a predictor of restenosis, even with drug-eluting stents (245,246). Moreover, some stents are not completely opposed, which intuitively might limit drug delivery to the vessel wall, especially at branch points or side-branch ostia (247,248). Calcification may theoretically impede penetration of an active proliferative agent directly, or by resulting in nonuniform strut distribution (249). Edge restenosis may occur due to incomplete lesion coverage, axial plaque translation, or balloon trauma outside the stented segment, with or without residual dissection. Sirolimus-resistant cells have been identified that may contribute to restenosis (250), as may Cypher strut fracture (251).

Doubtless multiple causative mechanisms contribute to restenosis after drug-eluting stent implantation in individual patients and lesions, and a greater understanding of these failures will be required to guide the development of more efficacious devices.

Few reports are available to guide further therapy when restenosis does occur in drug-eluting stents. In one series of 24 patients with 27 post-Cypher restenoses (focal in 93%), repeat intervention was performed with additional drug-eluting stents in 86% of patients (half Cypher and half TAXUS), 11% were treated with balloon angioplasty, and 3% with a bare metal stent (252). The recurrent restenosis rate was 42.9%, but was 18.2% in originally de novo lesions with a single Cypher restenosis, re-treated with drug-eluting stents. In 17 lesions re-treated with drug-eluting stents, the recurrent restenosis rate was 29.4%, with no significant differences between repeat sirolimus-eluting and paclitaxel-eluting stents (33.3% versus 25.0%, respectively, $P = 1.0$). Predictors of recurrent restenosis included hypercholesterolemia, previous angioplasty, failed brachytherapy, Cypher restenosis within 6 months, and treatment with balloon dilatation; restenotic lesion length, of interest, was not a predictor.

Practical recommendations for the treatment of drug-eluting stent restenosis are presented in Fig. 24.15. For focal restenotic lesions (the most common type), treatment with balloon angioplasty (preferably with the cutting balloon to reduce balloon slippage and the need to restent) or placement of an additional short drug-eluting stent is reasonable. IVUS can help exclude strut fracture, lack of expansion, incomplete apposition, or other mechanical causes of restenosis. If marked underexpansion is seen with little tissue proliferation, balloon angioplasty with a larger or higher-pressure balloon may be the most appropriate treatment. Whether diffuse, proliferative, or occlusive restenosis of a drug-eluting stent should be

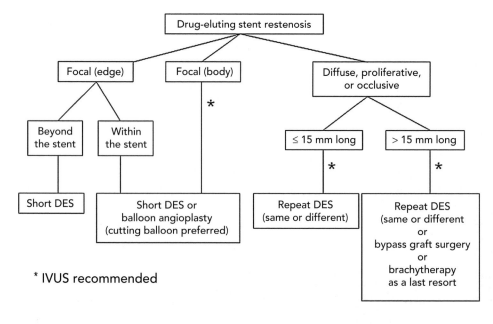

Figure 24.15 An algorithm for the treatment of restenosis after drug-eluting stent (DES) implantation. IVUS, intravascular ultrasound.

* IVUS recommended

treated with repeat drug-eluting stenting (with the same or a different stent), vascular brachytherapy, or surgery is unknown. It is unlikely, however, that balloon angioplasty alone will be effective in this situation.

Drug-Eluting Stent Thrombosis

Shortly after approval of the sirolimus-eluting stent in the United States, concerns arose regarding a potentially increased rate of stent thrombosis compared with bare metal stents, despite a 3-month course of clopidogrel (253). Although most episodes of stent thrombosis occurring shortly after the device approval could be ascribed to poor mismatch between vessel and lesion diameter and length (reflecting the initial uneven availability of the full range of stent lengths and sizes) and off-label device usage in complex anatomies (254), concern remains that drug-eluting stents may be slightly more thrombogenic than their bare metal counterparts. Though the carefully controlled randomized trials have found similar rates of stent thrombosis in the control and treatment arms (Tables 24.13 and 24.14), no study has been adequately sized and powered to appropriately address this issue with real-world applications of drug-eluting stents, with the additional risks of incomplete patient compliance with antiplatelet agents. Modest-sized registries of drug-eluting stent use outside of carefully controlled trials have reported short-term thrombosis rates of approximately 1%. In a series of 2,229 patients undergoing sirolimus- and paclitaxel-eluting stent implantation at two centers, the mean stent thrombosis rate at a mean time of 9.3 months was 1.3% (255). However, the stent thrombosis rate was significantly increased in several high-risk subsets, including thrombotic lesions (2.0%), diabetics (2.6%), bifurcation lesions treated with two stents (3.5%), unprotected left main disease (3.2%), in patients with renal insufficiency (5.5%), prior brachytherapy (8.7%), and those with left ventricular dysfunction.

Stent thrombosis may also occur many months after implantation of a drug-eluting stent. In patients with bare metal stents treated with a dual anti-platelet regime, thrombosis typically occurs within 2 weeks postprocedure and has rarely been described beyond 1 month (except after concomitant exposure to coronary irradiation; 135). In contrast, stent thrombosis after drug-eluting stent implantation has been reported to occur both intraprocedurally (256) and after 6 to 12 months with both Cypher and TAXUS stents (136). Patients may be especially at risk for early or late stent thrombosis following premature discontinuation of prescribed antiplatelet medications, especially following elective surgery (136,257). Thus, the optimal duration for dual antiplatelet therapy after drug-eluting stent implantation, weighing the benefits versus the costs and complications, is a matter of ongoing debate.

A propensity for increased stent thrombosis with drug-eluting compared with bare metal stents might be explained by thrombogenicity of the drug or the polymer (including localized hypersensitivity reactions), vascular toxicity or lack of vessel healing (including delayed endothelialization), or polymer webbing that serves as a nidus for platelet and thrombus deposition. Late stent malapposition, which is seen more commonly with the Cypher stent than with the TAXUS stent, has thus far not been related to stent thrombosis (222). Current large single-center studies and meta-analysis of published data, however, do not presently suggest a difference in stent thrombosis between Cypher versus Taxus stents (257a, 257b).

Nonetheless, a wide variety of stent designs, polymers, and drugs are now or will soon be tested to reduce the thrombogenicity of drug-eluting stents and the long-term reliance on thienopyridine therapy. These include the development of less toxic agents; drugs or other approaches to promote vascular healing (such as endothelial progenitor cell capture technology); the addition of thromboresistant drugs on the stent surface (such as heparin, bivalirudin, or glycoprotein IIb/IIIa inhibitors); the formulation of thromboresistant polymers; and the development of bioabsorbable polymers and stents. Until these approaches are proven, dual antiplatelet therapy for at least 3 to 6 months will remain an integral part of drug-eluting stent implantation.

CLINICAL OUTCOMES OF CORONARY STENTS: A PATIENT- AND LESION-SPECIFIC ANALYSIS

Stenting After Failed Balloon Angioplasty

Stents may be used either on a routine (planned) basis, selectively to improve a suboptimal angioplasty result (provisional stenting), or after failed balloon angioplasty for acute or threatened vessel closure (bailout stenting). One of the major benefits of stenting is the ability to prevent or definitively reverse abrupt closure owing to dissection and recoil, thus virtually eliminating the need for high-risk emergency bypass surgery (258; see Chapter 22). The outcomes of stent implantation in this emergent setting, however, may not be as favorable as with routine, planned stent implantation. In the 518-patient multicenter registry of the Gianturco-Roubin FlexStent as treatment for acute or threatened vessel closure (local dissection, reduced antegrade flow, or clinical evidence of ongoing ischemia) conducted from 1988 through 1991, although 95% of patients were successfully stented, 7.7% of patients with frank closure (and 2.7% of those with threatened closure) still required surgery, and there was an 8.7% incidence of stent thrombosis, particularly in smaller (≤2.5 mm) stents (9). Moreover, numerous randomized trials (as discussed below) have demonstrated that routine stent implantation provides superior acute results and greater event-free survival compared with balloon angioplasty in almost every patient and lesion subtype studied to date, relegating balloon dilation to the rare lesion that is too small (<2.25 mm) for stenting, to which a stent cannot be delivered because of excessive vessel tortuosity or calcification, or patients in whom thienopyridines are contraindicated.

Stenting has also been shown to be superior to repeat balloon angioplasty in patients who have developed restenosis after balloon angioplasty. PCI in these patient is associated with a higher restenosis than after a first-time intervention, even after correction for confounding factors such as diabetes mellitus or small reference vessel diameter that might have predisposed to the original restenosis (259). In the Restenosis Stent Study (REST), 383 patients with prior restenosis were randomized to either balloon angioplasty or implantation of the Palmaz-Schatz stent (260). The stent group demonstrated reductions in angiographic restenosis (18% versus 32%, $P = .03$) and subsequent target vessel revascularization (10% versus 27%, $P = .001$) compared with treatment with repeat balloon angioplasty.

Stress/Benestent Lesions

The utility of routine stent implantation as a modality to reduce acute vessel closure and late restenosis was first demonstrated in randomized trials that enrolled patients undergoing PCI of discrete, focal lesions. The two such pivotal trials that resulted in approval of the Palmaz-Schatz stent in the United States were the Stent Restenosis Study (STRESS; 14) and the Belgium Netherlands Stent (Benestent-I) study (13), and the stenoses studied in these investigations (discrete de novo lesions, with reference vessel diameter 3.0–4.0 mm, coverable by a single stent) have subsequently become known as *Stress/Benestent lesions* to differentiate them from more complex stenoses. Additional randomized trials of stenting versus balloon angioplasty for focal, discrete lesions have subsequently been published (261–269), and collectively these six trials have established beyond doubt that the implantation of bare metal stents provides superior acute angiographic outcomes, reduced long-term angiographic restenosis rates, and enhanced late event-free survival compared with balloon angioplasty, results that are sustained for at least 5 years (Table 24.15). These trials also confirmed that the incremental reduction in angiographic restenosis with stents was achieved consequent to the ability of the stent to provide a larger acute lumen than balloon angioplasty—the strongest predictor of freedom from restenosis was a large post-treatment lumen diameter, and once post-treatment lumen diameter was incorporated into the statistical model of restenosis, there was not any independent effect attributable to the stent itself (25,265). This paradigm has now been modified with the advent of drug-eluting stents, which compared with bare metal stents result in similar acute luminal dimensions but reduced late loss, further reducing angiographic and clinical restenosis even in the focal lesions in large vessels such as those enrolled in Stress and Benestent-I.

Real-World Stenting

The results of the Stress and Benestent studies resulted in global widespread usage of coronary stents (especially after the validation of the safety and efficacy of thienopyridine-based anticoagulant regimens), including the treatment of lesions not studied in the early randomized trials. Subsequent registries have demonstrated that only 7 to 20% of patients treated in the real world with coronary stents would have qualified for stent implantation in these early trials and that the clinical outcomes with bare metal stents in more complex lesions were inferior to those in Stress and Benestent trials (266). In particular, clinical and angiographic restenosis rates after bare metal stent implantation have been found to be increased in patients with diabetes mellitus and in those with small vessels and long lesions. Other lesion subtypes often associated with increased stent restenosis are chronic total occlusions, ostial lesions, and bifurcation stenoses. As reviewed below, randomized trials have now been performed comparing bare metal stents with balloon angioplasty in most complex lesion subsets, in almost all cases confirming distinct superiority of stent implantation. Moreover, data are now emerging that drug-eluting stents may further reduce clinical and angiographic restenosis in complex patients and lesion subtypes.

Stent Implantation in Small Vessels

Bare metal stents result in greater acute lumen gain than balloon angioplasty, but also greater late lumen loss (averaging 0.8 to 1.0 mm, an amount that is similar or increased in small compared with large vessels (267–268). As a result, restenosis rates are increased after stent implantation in small vessels, a function primarily of the smaller postprocedural minimal luminal diameter achieved. Thus, whereas stents reduce restenosis by approximately 25 to 30% in vessels ≥3.0 mm in diameter (Table 24.15), concern has been expressed that stenting in smaller vessels may not improve outcomes compared with balloon angioplasty.

To date, 13 randomized trials of stenting versus balloon angioplasty in 4,383 patients undergoing PCI of small vessels have been performed, with the outcomes summarized in a recent meta-analysis (269; Fig. 24.16). The mean reference vessel diameter was 2.32 mm and lesion length 10.1 mm. Diabetes mellitus was present in 28% of patients, and 35% had unstable angina. A bare metal stent was used in six trials, whereas a coated stent (heparin, silicon carbide, or phosphorylcholine) was used in seven trials. Among patients randomized to balloon angioplasty, crossover to stenting was performed in 22.2% of patients. Though the results of the individual trials varied somewhat, collectively these studies demonstrated that bare metal stents reduce angiographic restenosis and enhance event-free survival owing to greater freedom from repeat target lesion and target vessel revascularization compared with treatment with balloon angioplasty (Fig. 24.14). There is some debate, however, whether

TABLE 24.15

RANDOMIZED TRIALS OF STENT IMPLANTATION VERSUS BALLOON ANGIOPLASTY IN FOCAL, DE NOVO LESIONS OF NATIVE CORONARY ARTERIES

Trial	Stent	Total N	Enrollment Criteria	Early Clinical Follow-up Duration	MACE (%) B	MACE (%) S	Late Clinical Follow-up Duration	TLR (%) B	TLR (%) S	MACE (%) B	MACE (%) S	Angiographic Follow-up (N at xx months)	MLD Post-Procedure (mm) B	MLD Post-Procedure (mm) S	MLD Follow-up (mm) B	MLD Follow-up (mm) S	Binary Restenosis (%) B	Binary Restenosis (%) S
STRESS (14)	PS	410	Stable angina; LL<15 mm; RVD>3 mm; left main, ostial, SVG, CTO, thrombus excluded.	14 days	7.9	5.9	6 months	15.4[c]	10.2	23.8	19.5	336 at 6 months	1.99[b]	2.49	1.56[b]	1.74	42.1*	31.6
BENESTENT I (13)[a]	PS	520	Similar to STRESS	In-hospital	6.2	6.9	1 year	20.6[b]	10.0[d]	31.5[b]	23.2	477 at 6 months	2.05[b]	2.48	1.72	1.82	32*	22
BENESTENT II (261)	H-PS	827	Stable or unstable angina; LL <18 mm; otherwise similar to BENESTENT I	1 month	5.1	3.9	1 year	17.8[b]	11.9[d]	22.4[b]	15.7	416 at 6 months	2.13[b]	2.69	1.66	1.89	31	16
Versaci et al. (262)	PS	120	Proximal LAD; otherwise similar to	In-hospital	2.2	5.0	5 years	35[b]	15	47[b]	20	95 at 1 year	2.1[b]	2.8	1.4[b]	1.8	40*	19
START (263)	PS	452	Similar to BENESTENT II	—	—	—	4 years	24.6[b]	12.0	29.9[b]	16.9	397 at 6 months	2.25[b]	2.82	1.63[b]	1.98	37*	22*
AS (264)	PS	400	Similar to BENESTENT II, except RVD ≥2.5 mm	14 days	1.6	2.1	2 years	25.5[b]	17.2	27.6[b]	19.8	388 at 6 months	2.51[b]	3.05	2.00[b]	2.29	24.9**	18.2

[a] Macaya C, Serruys PW, Ruygrok P, et al. Continued benefit of coronary stenting versus balloon angioplasty: one-year clinical follow-up of Benestent trial. Benestent Study Group. *J Am Coll Cardiol* 1996;27:255–261.
[b] $P < .05$.
[c] $P = .06$.
[d] Repeat angioplasty of the target lesion.
MACE, major adverse cardiac events; TLR, target lesion revascularization; MLD, minimal luminal diameter; B, balloon angioplasty group; S, stent group; LL, lesion length (visually assessed); RVD, reference vessel diameter (visually assessed); SVG, saphenous vein graft; CTO, chronic total occlusion; LAD, left anterior descending artery; PS, Palmaz-Schatz stent; H-PS, heparin-coated Palmaz-Schatz stent.
STRESS, Stent REStenosis Study; BENESTENT, Belgium and The Netherlands Stent Trial; START, STent vs. Angioplasty Restenosis Trial; AS, Angioplasty or Stent.

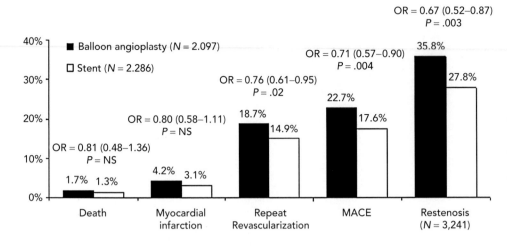

Figure 24.16 Results of a pooled analysis of 13 randomized trials of balloon angioplasty versus bare metal stent implantation in small vessels. Stenting resulted in modest reductions in clinical and angiographic restenosis, without significantly affecting rates of death or myocardial infarction. OR, odds ratio; NS, not significant; MACE, major adverse cardiac event.

these results apply to the smallest vessels studied (reference vessel diameter <2.25 mm; 270). Moreover, the results with balloon angioplasty were similar to stents when an optimal result was obtained (diameter stenosis <20%). Dedicated small vessel stents as diminutive as 2.0 mm in diameter have been developed with thinner struts and lower-profile delivery systems that may enhance stent delivery to distal lesions in small coronary arteries, though it is unclear whether the long-term outcomes are improved with these devices compared with alternative therapies (271,272).

Drug-eluting stents have further improved the outcomes of stent implantation in small vessels. In both the SIRIUS and TAXUS IV trials, absolute target lesion revascularization rates were reduced to the greatest extent in the tertile of patients with the smallest vessels (28,29; Fig. 24.17). In

the Sirolimus-Eluting Stent in the Prevention of Restenosis in Small Coronary Arteries (SES-SMART) trial (227), 257 patients undergoing stent implantation in lesions with reference vessel diameter <2.75 mm (mean 2.20 mm) were randomized to the Cypher stent versus the Bx Velocity. The sirolimus-eluting stent reduced the 8-month binary restenosis rates from 53.1% with the bare metal stent to 9.8% (P < .001) and reduced the rate of target lesion revascularization from 21.1% to 7.0% (P = .002). Thus, drug-eluting stents have become the treatment of choice for lesions in small vessels requiring PCI. The smallest drug-eluting stents currently available, however, are 2.5 mm in diameter, though 2.25-mm stents are undergoing clinical investigation, and 2.0 mm (and smaller) drug-eluting stents are under development.

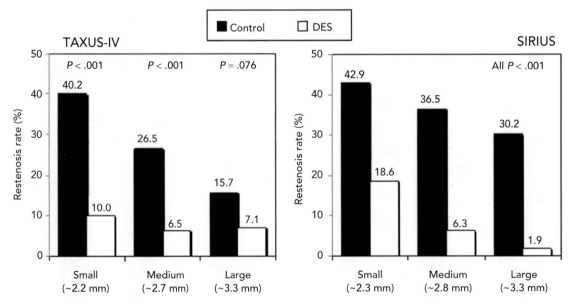

Figure 24.17 Both the paclitaxel-eluting and sirolimus-eluting stent improve outcomes in small as well as large vessels compared with bare metal stents, as seen in these subset analyses from the pivotal U.S. TAXUS-IV and SIRIUS trials, respectively.

Stent Implantation in Long Lesions

Lesion length and stent length have both been demonstrated to be independent predictors of restenosis after bare metal stent implantation (26,27,273,274); whether excessive stent length in the absence of underlying atherosclerotic disease further increases restenosis beyond the effect of lesion length is a matter of controversy. The impact of lesion and stent length on restenosis is particularly evident in small vessels (275). Cutlip and colleagues also found total stent length was independently associated with stent thrombosis, with an odds ratio of 1.2 for each additional 10 mm of stent placed (81).

Only one randomized trial has evaluated the relative efficacy of bare metal stent implantation versus balloon angioplasty in long lesions. In the Additional Value of NIR Stents for Treatment of Long Coronary Lesions (ADVANCE) trial, 288 patients undergoing PCI of a single coronary lesion 20 to 50 mm long (mean 27 mm) in a native coronary vessel 2.5 to 4.0 mm (mean 2.78 mm) in diameter, in whom balloon angioplasty resulted in a diameter stenosis <30% without significant dissection, were randomized to either stenting with NIR stents or no additional treatment (276). Routine stent implantation after optimal balloon angioplasty in long lesions resulted in similar rates of major adverse cardiac events at 30 days (3.4% versus 7.0%, $P = .17$) and at 300 days (23.4% versus 23.1%, $P = .98$), though the rate of angiographic restenosis was lower (27% versus 42%, $P = 0.02$).

The outcomes of stent implantation in long lesions may be improved by the routine use of IVUS. In the TULIP trial, 150 patients undergoing elective stent implantation for lesions >20 mm long were randomized to angiographic versus IVUS guidance (86). The angiographic minimal luminal diameter was larger in the IVUS-guided group immediately postprocedure (mean 3.01 versus 2.80 mm, $P = .008$) and at 6 months angiographic follow-up (mean 1.82 versus 1.51, $P = .04$), corresponding to a reduced binary angiographic restenosis rate (23% versus 46%, $P = .008$.). IVUS guidance also resulted in lower rates of target lesion revascularization and major adverse cardiac events at 12 months (10% versus 23%, $P = .018$, and 12% versus 27%, $P = .03$, respectively).

Fortunately, drug-eluting stents have markedly improved late outcomes in patients undergoing stent implantation of long lesions. Though lesion length remains a predictor of restenosis with both paclitaxel-eluting and sirolimus-eluting stents, the incremental increase in restenosis with additional stent length is markedly blunted with drug-eluting compared with bare metal stents (28). The only completed randomized study to date of drug-eluting stents specifically in long lesions is the TAXUS VI trial, in which 446 patients with lesions between 18 and 40 mm (mean 20.6 mm) long were randomized to the Express stent or the moderate-release TAXUS stent. At 9 months, the TAXUS stent reduced the rate of angiographic restenosis from 35.7% to 12.4 ($P < .0001$) and reduced target lesion revascularization rates from 18.9% to 6.8% ($P = .0001$).

Stent Implantation in Patients with Diabetes Mellitus

Along with smaller reference vessel diameter and longer lesions, the presence of diabetes mellitus (especially insulin-requiring diabetes) is unequivocally associated with increased clinical and angiographic restenosis rates after balloon angioplasty or bare metal stent implantation (27), related to smaller vessel size, greater negative remodeling, and increased neointimal hyperplasia in diabetic compared with nondiabetic vessels (277). The percent reduction of restenosis with bare metal stents compared with balloon angioplasty is similar in diabetic and nondiabetic patients (278), with further reduction by drug-eluting stents. In the TAXUS II, IV, and VI, trials, 458 patients had medically treated diabetes (including 154 requiring insulin) and 1,831 did not have diabetes (279). Among patients in whom bare metal stents were implanted, the 12-month target lesion revascularization rates in nondiabetic versus diabetic patients requiring oral hypoglycemic agents only to insulin-requiring diabetics was 14.2% versus 21.4% versus 19.3%, respectively ($P = .01$). In contrast, the 12-month rates of target lesion revascularization in the same three groups of patients receiving the TAXUS stent were 4.6% versus 6.2% versus 5.6% ($P = .67$). Both Cypher and TAXUS stents appear to be effective in reducing restenosis rates in patients with diabetes mellitus, and studies examining their relative efficacy in this challenging cohort are in progress.

Stent Implantation in Multivessel Disease

Multiple randomized trials have demonstrated that multivessel balloon angioplasty compared with coronary artery bypass graft surgery is associated with similar rates of survival (in all except possibly diabetic patients) and myocardial infarction, but a significantly higher incidence of recurrent angina and need for repeat revascularization within the first year (277; see also Chapter 22). As discussed above, multivessel stent implantation has narrowed but not eliminated this gap (Table 24.11). Multivessel implantation of drug-eluting stents holds promise to equalize the subsequent rates of revascularization after PCI and surgery. In the prospective, multicenter Arterial Revascularization Therapies Study II (ARTS-II), the outcomes of 607 patients with multivessel disease who received multiple sirolimus-eluting stents were compared with the bare metal stent and surgical groups from the 1,205-patient randomized ARTS-I trial (191,281). Though the ARTS-II cohort had significantly more extensive atherosclerosis than in ARTS-I, the long-term outcomes were significantly improved compared with the ARTS-I bare metal stent group and were similar to the ARTS-I surgery group (Table 24.16, Fig. 24.18).

TABLE 24.16

COMPARISON OF BARE METAL STENTS AND SURGERY IN ARTS-1 TO DRUG-ELUTING STENTS IN ARTS-II IN PATIENTS WITH MULTIVESSEL DISEASE

	ARTS-1 Bare Metal (Crown) Stent Implantation N = 600	ARTS-1 Coronary Artery Bypass Graft Surgery N = 605	ARTS-II Sirolimus-Eluting (Cypher) Stent Implantation N = 607
Diabetes	18.7%	15.9%	26.2%[a,b]
No. lesions per patient	2.8 ± 1.0	2.8 ± 1.0	3.6 ± 1.3[a,b]
Type C lesions	7.5%	7.9%	13.9%[a,b]
No. stented lesions or anastomosed segments	2.5 ± 1.0	2.6 ± 1.0	3.2 ± 1.1[a,b]
No. stents implanted	2.8 ± 1.3	—	3.7 ± 1.5[a]
Total stent length	48 ± 22	—	73 ± 32[a]
MACCE at 30 days	9.2%	6.3%	2.8%[a]
6-month outcomes			
Death	2.3%	1.8%	0.5%
Stroke	1.5%	1.2%	0.5%
Myocardial infarction	4.5%	3.5%	0.7%
(Re) surgery	3.8%	0.5%	1.6%
(Re)angioplasty	7.8%	2.0%	3.1%[a]
Repeat revascularization	15.3%	5.5%	2.7%[a]
MACCE	20.0%	9.0%	6.4%[a]

[a] $P < .05$ vs. ARTS-I stent implantation.
[b] $P < .05$ vs. ARTS-I surgery.
MACCE, major adverse cardiac or cerebrovascular events: the occurrence of death, stroke, myocardial infarction, angioplasty, or surgery.

Other studies, however, have not been as favorable. In contrast to the 6-month major adverse cardiac event rate after multivessel Cypher implantation of 6.4% in ARTS-II, Orlic et al. reported a 22.3% adverse event rate 6.5 months after

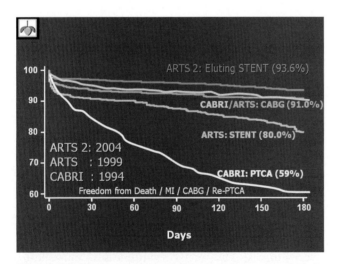

Figure 24.18 In a series of trials spanning a decade from 1994–2004, the 180-day event-free survival of bypass surgery has remained 91%. This was markedly superior to balloon coronary angioplasty in CABRI (32% absolute difference) owing to the effect of restenosis. In ARTS, this deficit improved to 11% with the use of bare metal stenting. In the ARTS 2 trial, the event-free survival of drug-eluting stents was actually superior to that of bypass by 2.6%. Although the patient groups are not exactly comparable, the significant improvement in repeat revascularization with the drug-eluting stents has shifted the balance further toward percutaneous coronary intervention.

implantation of a mean of 3.7 Cypher stents in a mean of 3.3 lesions in 155 patients (282). Target lesion revascularization was required in only 6.7% of lesions, but in 14.3% of patients. The higher adverse event rate in this study compared with ARTS-II may be related to enrollment of more complex patient and lesion cohorts. Two large-scale randomized trials comparing multivessel stenting with both Cypher and TAXUS stents with bypass graft surgery (one restricted to patients with diabetes mellitus) are currently ongoing.

Stent Implantation in Chronic Total Occlusions

Clinical and angiographic restenosis rates after both balloon angioplasty and stent implantation are increased following PCI of chronic total occlusions compared with nonoccluded stenoses, owing principally to an increased incidence of diabetes, greater lesion length, plaque mass, and calcification. Several randomized trials of bare metal stent placement compared with balloon angioplasty have been performed, which have uniformly demonstrated statistically significant reductions in angiographic restenosis and reocclusion, benefits that translate to improved freedom from the need for repeat target vessel revascularization for up to 6 years (Table 24.17; 283–287).

Nonetheless, restenosis rates remain high after bare metal stent implantation in chronic total occlusions (CTOs). Emerging nonrandomized data suggest that outcomes may also be strikingly improved in these lesions with drug-eluting stents. In a multicenter Asian registry in which 88 patients with successfully recanalized CTOs were

TABLE 24.17

RANDOMIZED TRIALS OF BARE METAL STENT IMPLANTATION VERSUS BALLOON ANGIOPLASTY FOR CHRONIC TOTAL CORONARY OCCLUSIONS

Trial	N	Reocclusion			Restenosis			Follow-up Duration	Target Lesion or Vessel Revascularization		
		BA	Stent	P Value	BA	Stent	P Value		BA	Stent	P Value
TOSCA (283)	410	20%	11%	0.02	70%	55%	<0.01	6 months	15%	8%	0.03
PRISON (284)	200	7%	8%	0.99	33%	22%	0.14	12 months	29%	13%	<0.0001
SICCO (285,286)	114	26%	16%	0.058	74%	32%	<0.001	33 months	53%	24%	0.002
GISSOC (287)	110	34%	8%	0.004	68%	32%	0.0008	6 years	36%	15%	0.02
SARECCO[a]	110	14%	2%	0.05	62%	26%	0.01	2 years	55%	24%	0.05
Mori et al[b]	96	11%	7%	0.04	57%	28%	0.005	6 months	49%	28%	<0.05
STOP[c]	96	17%	8%	NS	71%	42%	0.032	6 months	42%	25%	NS
SPACTO[d]	85	24%	3%	0.01	64%	32%	0.01	6 months	40%	25%	NS

[a] Sievert H, Rohde S, Utech A, et al. Stent or angioplasty after recanalization of chronic coronary occlusions? *Am J Cardiol* 1999;84:386–390.
[b] Mori M, Kurogane H, Hayashi T, et al. Comparison of results of intracoronary implantation of the Palmaz-Schatz stent with conventional balloon angioplasty in chronic total coronary arterial occlusion. *Am J Cardiol* 1996;78: 985–989.
[c] Lotan C, Rozenman Y, Hendler A, et al. Stents in total occlusion for restenosis prevention. *Eur Heart J* 2000;21: 1960–1966.
[d] Hoher M, Wohrle J, Grebe OC, et al. A randomized trial of elective stenting after balloon recanalization of chronic total occlusions. *J Am Coll Cardiol* 1999;34:722–729.
BA, balloon angioplasty; TOSCA, Total Occlusion Study of Canada; PRISON, Primary Stenting of Occluded Native Coronary Arteries; SICCO, Stenting in Chronic Coronary Occlusion; GISSOC, Gruppo Italiano di Studi sulla Stent nelle Occlusioni coronariche; SARECCO, Stent or Angioplasty after Recanalization of Chronic Coronary Occlusions; STOP, Stents in Total Occlusion for Restenosis Prevention; SPACTO, Stent vs. Percutaneous Angioplasty in Chronic Total Occlusion; NS, not significant.

treated with sirolimus-eluting stents, the 6-month major adverse cardiac event rate was only 4.5% (consisting of all repeat target vessel revascularizations), and the angiographic restenosis rate was 3.4% (288). Treatment of 48 chronic total occlusions with paclitaxel-eluting stents compared with a historical matched series with bare metal stents resulted in markedly reduced rates of angiographic restenosis and reocclusion at 6 months (8.3% versus 51.1%, $P < .001$, and 2.1% versus 23.4%, $P < .001$, respectively) and in major adverse cardiac events at 1 year (12.5% versus 47.9%, $P < .001$; 289).

Stent Implantation in Aorto-ostial Lesions

True aorto-ostial lesions extend proximal to the coronary ostia into aortic wall where abundant elastic fibers contribute to elastic recoil and poor outcome after balloon angioplasty (290). By resisting recoil, stents provide significantly larger lumens and lower the risk of restenosis in this lesion subset. Although randomized trials comparing stenting with balloon angioplasty or atherectomy techniques as treatment for aorto-ostial lesions have not been performed, comparative registry series have demonstrated greater acute gain and lower restenosis rates with stenting (291). Preliminary data suggest that the outcomes of aorto-ostial stenting may be further improved with drug-eluting stents (292). Iakovou and colleagues compared the outcomes of sirolimus-eluting stent implantation in 32 aorto-ostial lesions with bare metal stent implantation in 50 aorto-ostial

lesions (293). At 10-month follow-up, the sirolimus-eluting stent was associated with reduced rates of target lesion revascularization (6.3% versus 28.0%, $P = .01$) and binary angiographic restenosis (11% versus 51%, $P = .001$).

Stent Implantation in Bifurcation Lesions

Atherosclerosis develops frequently at branch points owing to turbulence resulting in high endothelial stress, and as a result bifurcation lesions are present in 20% or more of lesions undergoing angioplasty (178). PCI of lesions involving a bifurcation of a coronary artery is associated with increased procedural complications and poor long-term outcomes, owing to recoil and plaque shifting at the origin of the side branch.

When the side-branch ostium is not diseased, the likelihood of its narrowing after the main branch is stented is low, and the side branch can be rescued by kissing balloon inflation of the main vessel stent and side branch if it is compromised. For true bifurcation lesions (atherosclerotic involvement of both the parent and side branch), the major decision is whether to undertake a provisional or dual-stent strategy. With *provisional stenting*, the main vessel is stented (often after optimal predilatation of the side branch), and the side branch is dilated or stented only for a truly unacceptable result (typically a diameter stenosis >50% or severe dissection). This approach is usually preferred if the parent vessel is large and the side branch relatively small. Alternatively, when both the parent vessel and side branch

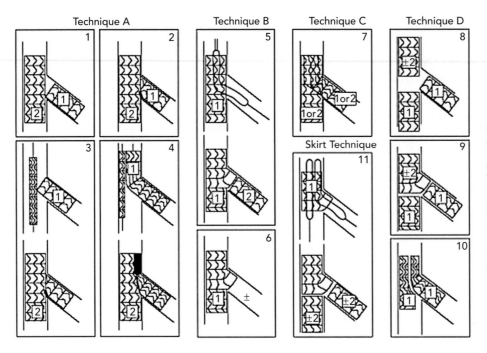

Figure 24.19 Classification of various approaches to bifurcation stenting. **1** and **2**. Classic T-stenting beginning with side branch stenting. **3**. Modified T-stenting. **4**. "Crush" technique. **5**. Classic T stenting beginning with main branch stenting. **6**. Provisional T stenting. **7**. "Culotte" or "trousers" technique. **8**. Touching stents completed or not as Y technique. **9**. "Trouser legs and seat" technique, a classic touching stents technique completed proximally by a "skirt" technique. **10**. Kissing stents technique. **11**. "Skirt" technique. (From Louvard Y, Lefevre T, Morice MC. Percutaneous coronary intervention for bifurcation coronary disease. *Heart* 2004;90:714.)

are large (≥2.5 mm), especially when the side branch arises at a shallow angle, planned stenting of both branches may be considered. Various approaches to dual stenting of bifurcation lesions have been developed (178; Fig. 24.19).

1. T-stent technique: A stent is deployed at the ostium of the side branch, followed by a second stent in the parent vessel. Unless the angle of origin of the side branch is 90°, however, the operator is faced with the dilemma of whether it is better to leave a portion of the ostial side-branch lesion unstented or risk having part of the stent protrude into the parent vessel (making subsequent advancement of the parent vessel stent difficult or impossible).

2. "Culotte" stent technique: A stent is deployed into the side branch with extension into the proximal aspect of the parent vessel. A wire is then passed through the side struts of this stent and into the distal parent vessel. After balloon dilatation, a second stent is passed through the side struts into the distal, so that the proximal ends of the first and second stents overlap in the proximal vessel. This technique is the most technically complex, but offers excellent scaffolding and coverage of the bifurcation.

3. Simultaneous kissing stents: Two stents are deployed simultaneously over separate guidewires—one in the parent vessel and one in the side branch. Both stents extend side by side in the main vessel proximal to the bifurcation. Although this technique offers the advantage of simplicity and control of both vessels, a new, more proximal carina is created in the center of the proximal parent vessel, which is unlikely to endothelialize fully. Also, placement of an additional stent is problematic should a proximal dissection occur.

4. "Crush" stent technique: After predilatation of both limbs, two stents are positioned simultaneously in the side branch and main branch. The side-branch stent extends into the proximal main vessel 2 to 3 mm; the parent branch stent extends at least several mm more proximally. The side-branch stent is inflated first, trapping the main-branch stent delivery system. After confirmation of patency without dissection in the side branch, the side-branch guidewire and stent delivery system are removed and the main-branch stent is implanted, "crushing" the side branch stent. Following this, the side-branch stent is rewired and simultaneous kissing balloon inflations are performed. Indeed, it is generally recommended that all bifurcation stent techniques be completed by this technique.

The crush technique is simpler than the culotte technique and affords excellent coverage of the carina. Recrossing the crushed side-branch stent with a guidewire and balloon can be challenging and time consuming, however, but is essential because late restenosis is significantly reduced following a simultaneous kissing balloon inflation with this technique (294).

A variation of this technique is the "reverse crush," applicable when side-branch stenting was not planned but becomes necessary because of failure of provisional balloon angioplasty of the side branch after main-branch stenting. In this case, a second stent is placed in the side branch extending several mm into the proximal parent vessel (within the previously placed stent), and a balloon angioplasty catheter is placed in the main vessel. The side-branch stent is then deployed, impinging on the balloon. After removal of the side-branch stent delivery system and wire, the main-branch balloon is then inflated to crush the proximal portion of the side-branch stent. A final simultaneous kissing balloon inflation is then recommended. The main difference between crush and reverse crush is that with the latter technique, several mm of side-branch stent are crushed against the main-branch stent *within the lumen*, rather than external to the parent stent struts.

All of these dual-stent techniques are technically complex, require use of a larger (7F or 8F) guiding catheter, and pose difficulty in accessing the parent vessel or side branch through overlapping metallic elements. Moreover, prior studies with bare metal stents have not demonstrated superior clinical or angiographic results compared with a simpler provisional stent approach (178). Long-term outcomes may be improved with the use of drug-eluting rather than bare metal stents in bifurcation lesions (295). Recently, however, two small randomized studies of provisional stenting versus routine dual-stent implantation (mostly T-stenting) using Cypher stents have been performed in true bifurcation lesions, with no obvious benefit to the routine two-stent approach (though the results were clearly improved compared with the historical use of bare metal stents, especially in the main vessel; 248,296). Though a randomized trial of provisional versus crush stenting with drug-eluting stents has not yet been performed, unpublished registry studies to date have not clearly demonstrated marked superiority of the crush technique compared with a provisional approach (291). Moreover, stent thrombosis rates appear to be approximately doubled when two drug-eluting stents rather than one are implanted in a bifurcation (296,255). At the present time, a provisional drug-eluting stent strategy is thus recommended except when the side-branch lesion is very long, calcified, tortuous, or arises at a very shallow angle (making it unlikely that an acceptable result will be obtained with balloon angioplasty only); in distal left main bifurcations involving both the artial left anterior descending and circumflex arteries; or in patients with depressed left ventricular function where the rapid achievement of a stable angiographic result is desirable.

Finally, several side-branch access stents have been developed and are under investigation in the United States to preserve side-branch patency or facilitate side-branch wiring and balloon crossing should ostial narrowing occur (297). Efforts are also underway to develop a true Y-limbed bifurcated drug-eluting stent, which theoretically would provide optimal coverage of the carina.

Stent Implantation in Unprotected Left Main Lesions

For many years coronary artery bypass graft surgery has been considered the therapy of choice for left main coronary artery disease as a result of small studies showing a significant survival benefit after surgery compared with medical therapy. Although PCI of protected left main coronary artery stenoses (a patent bypass graft present to either the left anterior descending or circumflex arteries) may be performed with a high rate of success and favorable long-term outcomes, early attempts at balloon angioplasty of unprotected left lesions resulted in a high rate of procedural complications owing to elastic recoil and dissections. Moreover,

restenosis occurred in as many as 50% of patients, often presenting as sudden death (see Chapter 22).

Several multicenter registries of *left main stenting* have been performed, clearly demonstrating that the results of PCI in patients with left main disease depend on the baseline clinical stability and left ventricular function of the patient. The prospective multicenter ULTIMA registry reported the early and late outcomes from 279 patients undergoing PCI of left main disease: 17% of patients were deemed inoperable, an additional 27% were considered to be high surgical risk, 28% had a left ventricular ejection fraction <40%, 33% had triple-vessel disease, and almost half required intra-aortic balloon counterpulsation. Stent implantation was performed in 69% of patients. In-hospital death occurred in 38 patients (13.7%). At 1 year, cardiac mortality occurred in 20.2% of patients, 9.8% had a myocardial infarction, and 9.4% required coronary bypass surgery. Independent correlates of all-cause mortality were left ventricular ejection fraction <30%, mitral regurgitation grade 3 or 4, presentation with myocardial infarction and shock, serum creatinine >2.0 mg/dL, and severe lesion calcification. Approximately one third of the patients were <65 years of age, had a left ventricular ejection fraction >30%, and were without baseline shock; in this most favorable group, the 1-year survival was 96.6% and only 2.3% developed a myocardial infarction, though 25% required repeat revisualization procedures (including 17% who ultimately required bypass graft surgery).

The results from a multicenter European registry of bare metal stenting of unprotected left main lesions in 92 patients also reported markedly lower 6-month mortality in patients who were versus were not candidates for bypass graft surgery (3.8% versus 20.5%, $P < .02$; 296). In a four-center Asian registry of patients with normal left ventricular function undergoing left main stenting, there were no in-hospital deaths and event-free survival was 77.7% at 3 years. Angiographic restenosis was documented in 21.1% of lesions (300).

Drug-eluting stents may significantly improve outcomes in patients with left main disease (301,302). In the largest published study to date, the results of elective PCI with sirolimus-eluting stents in 102 patients with left main disease (70% at the distal bifurcation) were compared with a 121-patient bare metal stent historical control cohort (301). Neither group had an in-hospital major adverse cardiac event. Angiographic restenosis at 6 months was 7% in the sirolimus stent group compared with 30% in the bare metal stent group ($P < .001$), which was associated with a marked improvement in 1-year event-free survival (98% versus 81.4%, $P = .0003$). In a second report of 85 patients with left main disease treated with sirolimus- or paclitaxel-eluting stents (88% at the distal bifurcation), major adverse cardiac events at 6 months were reduced to 24.7% from 42.1% in a 64-patient historical control group ($P = .03$), despite more frequent adverse characteristics in the drug-eluting stent cohort (302). Target vessel revascularization was also lower in the drug-eluting stent cohort (18.8% versus 30.6%, $P = .11$).

In summary, though drug-eluting stents have improved the outcomes for patients undergoing PCI of left main disease, management of disease at the distal left main bifurcation (the most common location) still carries a nontrivial incidence of restenosis, and consensus regarding the optimal technical approach has not been determined. Pending the results of a recently initiated large-scale multicenter randomized trial of bypass graft surgery versus paclitaxel-eluting stents, surgery still must be considered the standard of care for good operative candidates with left main disease.

Stent Implantation in Saphenous Vein Grafts

The most common cause of recurrent ischemia following coronary artery bypass surgery is atheromatous degeneration within the body of the saphenous vein graft. Following bypass graft surgery, approximately 5 to 10% of patients per year develop recurrent angina, and by 10 years, as many as 50% of saphenous vein grafts are occluded and 40% of the remainder are stenotic (see Chapter 22). Single-center and multicenter registries of stent implantation in saphenous vein grafts demonstrated high rates of procedural success and potentially improved event-free survival compared to either balloon angioplasty and atherectomy (303,304). Randomized trials comparing balloon angioplasty and stent implantation (using the Palmaz-Schatz and Wiktor I stents) in focal lesions in saphenous vein grafts have now been performed, collectively demonstrating that bare metal stents result in reduced angiographic restenosis and greater freedom from target lesion and vessel revascularization (Fig. 24.20; 305,306).

Drug-eluting stent implantation in saphenous vein grafts may further improve outcomes (307). It must be recognized however, that although repeat revascularization triggered by failure of the stented *site* may be relatively low, the incidence of clinical events approaches 50% by 5 years owing to progression of disease at nontarget sites within

the treated graft, as well as attrition of other grafts and progression of native coronary disease (145,308). Moreover, the event-free rate after bare metal stenting in either diffusely diseased or occluded saphenous vein grafts is poor; whether drug-eluting stents improve late graft patency and clinical outcomes in these high-risk cohorts has not been evaluated. Finally, all PCI procedures in deteriorated saphenous vein grafts result in frequent atheroembolism and periprocedural myonecrosis, which may contribute to late mortality, and is reduced but not eliminated by the use of distal protection devices (see Chapter 23).

Stent Implantation in Acute Myocardial Infarction

Twenty-three randomized trials have definitively proven that compared with thrombolytic therapy, balloon angioplasty reduces mortality, reinfarction, stroke, and intracranial bleeding (see Chapter 22). Balloon angioplasty in this setting, however, is associated with a relatively high rate of infarct artery restenosis (30 to 40%) and reocclusion (5 to 10%). Initial fears of a high rate of stent thrombosis given the prothrombotic milieu of acute myocardial infarction were allayed with the results of large multicenter trials demonstrating favorable early and late clinical outcomes after implantation of both bare metal and heparin-coated Palmaz-Schatz stents (309–311). Numerous prospective, randomized trials have now been performed comparing the results of balloon angioplasty and bare metal stent implantation during primary PCI (Table 24.18; 312–319). In a meta-analysis of these trials, primary stenting as compared with balloon angioplasty was associated with similar early and late mortality, but statistically significantly reduced rates of reinfarction (48% reduction at 30 days and 33% reduction at 12 months) and target vessel revascularization (54% and 42% reductions at 30 days and 12 months, respectively; 317).Though few studies have

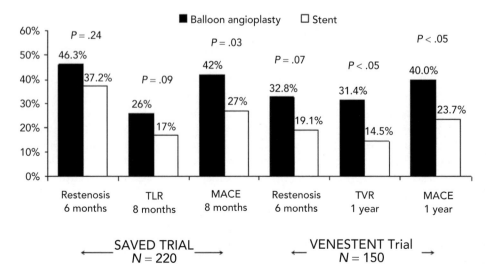

Figure 24.20 Compared with balloon angioplasty, bare metal stents have been shown to enhance event-free survival by reducing target lesion and vessel revascularization after intervention in primarily focal lesions in diseased saphenous vein grafts, as seen in the results of these two randomized trials. TLR, target lesion repeat; MACE, major adverse cardiac event; TVR, target vessel revascularization.

TABLE 24.18

RANDOMIZED TRIALS (WITH GREATER THAN 100 PATIENTS) OF BARE METAL STENT IMPLANTATION VERSUS BALLOON ANGIOPLASTY OF THE CULPRIT VESSEL IN ACUTE MYOCARDIAL INFARCTION

Trial	Stent	N	Infarct Artery Restenosis BA (%)	Stent (%)	P Value	Infarct Artery Reocclusion BA (%)	Stent (%)	P Value	Follow-up Duration	Target Lesion or Vessel Revascularization BA (%)	Stent (%)	P Value	Major Adverse Cardiac Events BA (%)	Stent (%)	P Value
CADILLAC (312)	ML	2,082	40.8	22.2	<.001	11.3	5.7	<.001	6 months	14.7	6.7	<.001	18.3	10.8	<.001
Stent PAMI (313)	H-PS	900	33.5	20.3	<.001	9.3	5.1	.03	6 months	17.0	7.7	<.001	20.1	12.6	<.01
Zwolle (314)	PS	227	—	—	—	—	—	—	6 months	17	4	.002	20	5	.001
STENTIM-2 (315)	Wiktor GX	211	39.6	25.3	.04	6.3	7.2	.79	1 year	28.2	17.8	.10	28.2	19.8	.16
FRESCO (316)	Mixed (63% GR-II)	150[a]	43	17	.001	—	—	—	6 months	25	7	.002	28	9	.003
PASTA (317)	PS	136	37.5	17.0	.02	17	3	.015	1 year	—	—	—	49	22	.001
GRAMI (318)	GR-II	104	—	—	—	—	—	—	1 year	20	14	.80	35	17	.002

[a] Randomized after successful balloon angioplasty.

BA, balloon angioplasty; ML, MultiLink; H-PS, heparin-coated Palmaz-Schatz; PS, Palmaz-Schatz; GR-II, Gianturco-Roubin II; CADILLAC, Controlled Abciximab and Device Investigation to Lower Late Angioplasty Complications; PAMI, Primary Angioplasty in Myocardial Infarction; FRESCO, Florence Randomized Elective Stenting in Acute Coronary Occlusions; GRAMI, Gianturco-Roubin in Acute Myocardial Infarction; STENTIM, STENTing In acute Myocardial infarction; PASTA, Primary Angioplasty vs. STent implantation in Acute myocardial infarction.

reported the rates of subacute vessel thrombosis, the CADILLAC trial observed subacute vessel thrombosis within 30 days in 1.4% of patients assigned to balloon angioplasty versus 0.5% after stenting (P = .03), demonstrating the safety of stent implantation in this condition (312). Primary stenting has been shown to be superior to balloon angioplasty even after an optimal angioplasty result was obtained (316,321), is cost-effective (322), and improves quality of life (323). Routine stent implantation compared with balloon angioplasty does not, however, improve indices of infarct artery reperfusion (324,325), reduce infarct size (312,326), or enhance survival (320).

Though the results of primary PCI in patients with evolving acute myocardial infarction are clearly improved with stenting compared with balloon angioplasty, restenosis and infarct artery reocclusion rates still remain high with bare metal stents. It is not known whether drug-eluting stents can safely improve outcomes in this setting. Lemos et al. compared the results of primary angioplasty performed with sirolimus-eluting stents in 186 consecutive patients with acute myocardial infarction with 183 patients treated with bare metal stents (327). At 30 days, the frequency of adverse events was similar in both the sirolimus and the bare metal stent groups (7.5% versus 10.4%, respectively; P = .4). At 300 days, the rate of repeat PCI was reduced in the drug-eluting stent group (1.1% versus 8.2%, P = .01), which drove a significant reduction in event-free survival (90.6% versus 83.0%, P = 0.02). Larger studies are required to demonstrate the safety of drug-eluting stents in a thrombotic environment, however. In this regard, a 4.7% stent thrombosis rate was recently reported in 171 patients undergoing PCI within 24 hours of acute myocardial infarction in the e-Cypher registry (328). A 3,000-patient 3:1 randomized trial of paclitaxel-eluting TAXUS stents versus bare metal control Express stents is now underway in patients with acute myocardial infarction within 12 hours of onset to examine the safety and efficacy of drug-eluting stents in this setting.

CURRENT PERSPECTIVES AND FUTURE DIRECTIONS

Over the past decade, coronary stenting has emerged as the dominant technology for catheter-based coronary revascularization. The availability of stents with excellent deliverability and scaffolding, the demonstration that stenting improves acute and long-term outcome in a wide variety of lesion types, the development of effective and better-tolerated regimens to prevent stent thrombosis, and now the marked suppression of restenosis with antiproliferative bioactive coatings, have facilitated the application of stenting to almost every patient and lesion subset. The potent reduction in restenosis with drug-eluting stents has already resulted in a marked shift from surgical referral to a percutaneous approach for all but the most complex anatomy,

placing even greater emphasis on technical skill and experience of the operator. Moreover, with the threat of restenosis gone, the threshold to treat borderline lesions is diminished, and active investigation is underway to diagnose and prophylactic treatment of vulnerable plaques (see Chapters 11 and 19). Future directions for the coronary stent will likely include the incorporation of thromboresistant polymers and agents and complete bioabsorbability of the endovascular frame. In any event, the coronary stent is certain to remain the foundation for the treatment of coronary atherosclerosis for the foreseeable future.

REFERENCES

1. Mulliken JB, Goldwyn RM. Impressions of Charles Stent. *Plast Reconstruct Surg* 1978;62:173–176.
2. Carrel A. Results of the permanent intubation of the thoracic aorta. *Surg Gyn Ob* 1912;15:245–248.
3. Dotter CT. Transluminally placed coil spring arterial tube grafts: long-term patency in canine popliteal artery. *Invest Radiol* 1969;4:329–332.
4. Maass D, Zollikofer CHL, Largiader F, et al. Radiological follow-up of transluminally inserted vascular endoprostheses: an experimental study using expanding spirals. *Radiology* 1984;152:659–663.
5. Rabkin I, Zaimovskii VA, Khmelevskaia I, Maksimovich IV, Rabkin DI. Experimental basis and first clinical trial of x-ray intravascular blood vessel prosthesis. *Vestn Rentgenol Radio.* 1984;4:59–64.
6. Sigwart U, Puel J, Mirkovitch V, Joffre F, Kappenberger L. Intravascular stents to prevent occlusion and restenosis after transluminal angioplasty. *N Engl J Med* 1987;316:701–706.
7. Serruys PW, Strauss BH, Beatt KJ, et al. Angiographic follow-up after placement of a self-expanding coronary artery stent. *N Engl J Med* 1991;324:13–17.
8. Roubin GS, Robinson KA, King SB III, et al. Early and late results of intracoronary arterial stenting after coronary angioplasty in dogs. *Circulation* 1987;76:891–897.
9. George BS, Voohees III WD, Roubin GS, et al. Multicenter investigation of coronary stenting to treat acute or threatened closure after percutaneous transluminal coronary angioplasty: clinical and angiographic outcomes. *J Am Coll Cardiol* 1993;22:135–143.
10. Palmaz JC, Sibbitt RR, Reuter SR, Tio FO, Rice WJ. Expandable intraluminal graft: a preliminary study. *Radiology* 1985;156:723–726.
11. Schatz RA. A view of vascular stents. *Circulation* 1989;79:445–457.
12. Schatz RA, Baim DS, Leon MB, et al. Clinical experience with the Palmaz-Schatz coronary stent. Initial results of a multicenter study. *Circulation* 1991;83:148–161.
13. Serruys PW, de Jaegere P, Kiemeneij F, et al. A comparison of balloon-expandable stent implantation with balloon angioplasty in patients with coronary artery disease. *N Engl J Med* 1994;331:489–495.
14. Fischman DL, Leon MB, Baim DS, et al. A randomized comparison of coronary stent placement and balloon angioplasty in the treatment of coronary artery disease. *N Engl J Med* 1994;331:496–501.
15. Kimura T, Abe K, Shizuta S, et al. Long-term clinical and angiographic follow-up after coronary stent placement in native coronary arteries. *N Engl J Med* 2002;105:2986–2991.
16. Cutlip DE, Chhabra AG, Baim DS, et al. Beyond restenosis: five-year clinical outcomes from second generation coronary stent trials. *Circulation* 2004;110:1226–1230.
17. Nakamura S, Colombo A, Gaglione A, et al. Intracoronary ultrasound observations during stent implantation. *Circulation* 1994;89:2026–2034.
18. Colombo A, Hall P, Nakamura S, et al. Intracoronary stenting without anticoagulation accomplished with intravascular ultrasound guidance. *Circulation* 1995;91:676–688.

19. Schomig A, Neumann F, Kastrati A, et al. A randomized comparison of antiplatelet and anticoagulant therapy after placement of coronary-artery stents. *N Engl J Med* 1996;334:1084–1089.

20. Leon MB, Baim DS, Popma JJ, et al. A clinical trial comparing three antithrombotic-drug regimens following coronary artery stenting. *N Engl J Med* 1998;339:1665–1671.

21. Bertrand ME, Legrand V, Boland J, et al. Randomized multicenter comparison of conventional anticoagulation versus antiplatelet therapy in unplanned and elective coronary stenting: the Full Anticoagulation Versus Aspirin and Ticlopidine (FANTASTIC) Study. *Circulation* 1998;98:1597–1603.

22. Urban P, Macaya C, Rupprecht H-J, et al. Randomized evaluation of anticoagulation versus antiplatelet therapy after coronary stent implantation in high-risk patients: the Multicenter Aspirin and Ticlopidine Trial after Intracoronary Stenting (MATTIS). *Circulation* 1998;98:2126–2132.

23. Holmes DR, Hirshfeld J, Faxon D, et al. ACC Expert Consensus Document on Coronary Artery Stents. *J Am Coll Cardiol* 1998;32:1471–1482.

24. Kuntz RE, Safian RD, Schmidt DA, et al. Novel approach to the analysis of restenosis after the use of three new coronary devices. *J Am Coll Cardiol* 1992;19:1493–1400.

25. Kuntz RE, Gibson CM, Nobuyoshi M. Baim DS. Generalized model of restenosis after conventional balloon angioplasty, stenting, and directional atherectomy. *J Am Coll Cardiol* 1993;21:15–25.

26. Ho KKL, Senerchia C, Rodriguez O, Chauhan MS, Kuntz RE. Predictors of angiographic restenosis after stenting: pooled analysis of 1197 patients with protocol-mandated angiographic follow-up from five randomized stent trials. *Circulation* 1998;98:362–368.

27. Cutlip DE, Chauhan MS, Baim DS, et al. Clinical restenosis after coronary stenting: perspectives from multicenter clinical trials. *J Am Coll Cardiol* 2002;40:2082–2089.

28. Moses JW, Leon MB, Popma JJ, Fitzgerald, et al. Sirolimus-eluting stents versus standard stents in patients with stenosis in a native coronary artery. *N Engl J Med* 2003;349:1315–1323.

29. Stone GW, Ellis SG, Cox DA, et al. A polymer-based paclitaxel-eluting stent in patients with coronary artery disease. *N Engl J Med* 2004;350:221–231.

30. Koster R, Vieluf D, Kiehn M, et al. Nickel and molybdenum contact allergies in patients with coronary in-stent restenosis. *Lancet* 2000;356:1895–1897.

31. Kereiakes DJ, Cox DA, Hermiller JB, et al. Usefulness of a cobalt chromium coronary stent alloy. *Am J Cardiol* 2003;92:463–466.

32. Sketch MH Jr, Ball M, Rutherford B, et al. Evaluation of the Medtronic (Driver) cobalt-chromium alloy coronary stent system. *Am J Cardiol* 2005;95:8–12.

33. Kastrati A, Schomig A, Dirschinger J, et al. Increased risk of restenosis after placement of gold-coated stents: results of a randomized trial comparing gold-coated with uncoated steel stents in patients with coronary artery disease. *Circulation* 2000;101:2478–2483.

34. Reifart N, Morice MC, Silber S, et al. The NUGGET study: NIR ultra gold-gilded equivalency trial. *Cathet Cardiovasc Intervent* 2004;62:18–25.

35. Hehrlein C., Zimmerman M, Metz J, et al. Influence of surface texture and charge on the biocompatiblity of endovascular stents. *Coronary Artery Dis* 1995;6:581–586.

36. Tamai H, Igaki K, Kyo E, et al. Initial and 6-month results of biodegradable poly-l-lactic acid coronary stents in humans. *Circulation* 2000;102:399–404.

37. Di Mario C, Griffiths H, Goktekin O, et al. Drug-eluting bioabsorbable magnesium stent. *J Intervent Cardiol* 2004;17:391–395.

38. Lansky AJ, Roubin GS, O'Shaughnessy CD, et al. Randomized comparison of GR-II stent and Palmaz-Schatz stent for elective treatment of coronary stenoses. *Circulation* 2000;102:1364–1368.

39. Rogers C, Edelman ER. Endovascular stent design dictates experimental restenosis and thrombosis. *Circulation* 1995;91:2995–3001.

40. van der Giessen WJ, Lincoff AM, Schwartz RS, et al. Marked inflammatory sequelae to implantation of biodegradable and nonbiodegradable polymers in porcine coronary arteries. *Circulation* 1996;94:1690–1697.

41. Atalar E, Haznedaroglu I, Aytemir K, et al. Effects of stent coating on platelets and endothelial cells after intracoronary stent implantation. *Clin Cardiol* 2001;24:159–164.

42. Lewis AL, Tolhurst LA, Strafford PW. Analysis of a phosphorylcholine-based polymer coating on a coronary stent pre- and post-implantation. *Biomaterials.* 2002;23:1697–706.

43. Malik N, Gunn J, Shepherd L, et al. Phosphorylcholine-coated stents in porcine coronary arteries: in vivo assessment of biocompatibility. *J Invasive Cardiol.* 2001;13:193–201.

44. Whelan DM, van der Glessen WJ, Krabbendam SC, et al. Biocompatibility of phosphorylcholine coated stents in normal porcine coronary arteries. *Heart* 2000;83:338–45.

45. Moses JW, Buller CEH, Nukta ED, et al. The first clinical trial comparing a coated versus a non-coated coronary stent: the Biocompatibles BiodivYsio stent in randomized controlled trial. *Circulation* 2000;102:II-664.

46. Palmer RR, Lewis AL, Kirkwood LC, et al. Biological evaluation and drug delivery application of cationically modified phospholipid polymers. *Biomaterials* 2004;25:4785–4796.

47. Hardhammar PA, van Beusekom HM, Emanuelsson HU, et al. Reduction in thrombotic events with heparin-coated Palmaz-Schatz stents in normal porcine coronary arteries. *Circulation* 1996;93:423–430.

48. Chronos NA, Robinson KA, King SB. Heparin coated Palmaz-Schatz stents are highly thromboresistant: a baboon A-V shunt study [abstract]. *J Am Coll Cardiol* 1996;27:904.

49. Serruys PW, Hout BV, Bonnier H, et al. Randomized comparison of implantation of heparin-coated stents with balloon angioplasty in selected patients with coronary artery disease (Benestent II). *Lancet* 1998;352:673–681.

50. Vrolix ME, Legrand VM, Reiber JH, et al. Heparin-coated Wiktor stents in human coronary arteries (MENTOR trial). *Am J Cardiol* 2000;86:385–389.

51. Legrand VM, Reiber JH. Moer R, Myreng Y, Mosltad P, et al. Stenting in small coronary arteries (SISCA) trial. A randomized comparison between balloon angioplasty and the heparin-coated beStent. *J Am Coll Cardiol* 2001;38:1598–1603.

52. Wöhrle J, Al-Khayer E, Grotzinger U, et al. Comparison of the heparin-coated vs. the uncoated Jostent. No influence on restenosis or clinical outcome. *Eur Heart J* 2001;22:1808–1816.

53. Monnink SH, van Boven AJ, Peels HO, et al. Silicon-carbide coated coronary stents have low platelet and leukocyte adhesion during platelet activation. *J Investig Med* 1999;47:304–310.

54. DeScheerder I, Szilard M, Yanming H, et al. Evaluation of the biocompatibility of two new diamond-like stent coatings (Dylyn) in a porcine coronary stent model. *J Invasive Cardiol* 2000;12:389–394.

55. Haase J, Storger H, Hofmann M, et al. Comparison of stainless steel stents coated with turbostratic carbon and uncoated stents for percutaneous coronary interventions. *J Invasive Cardiol* 2003;15:562–565.

56. Bartorelli AL, Trabattoni D, Fabbiocchi F, et al. Synergy of passive coating and targeted drug delivery: the tacrolimus-eluting Janus CarboStent. *J Intervent Cardiol* 2003;499–505.

57. Palmaz JC. Review of polymeric graft materials for endovascular applications. *J Vasc Intervent Radiol* 1998;9:7–13.

58. Briguori C, Nishida T, Anzuini A, et al. Emergency polytetrafluoroethylene-covered stent implantation to treat coronary ruptures. *Circulation* 2000;102:3028–3031.

59. Briguori C, Sarais C, Sivieri G, et al. Polytetrafluoroethylene-covered stent and coronary artery aneurysms. *Cathet Cardiovasc Intervent* 2002;55:326–330.

60. Abbott JD, Brennan JJ, Remetz MS. Treatment of a left internal mammary artery to pulmonary artery fistula with polytetrafluoroethylene covered stents. *Cardiovasc Intervent Radiol* 2004;27:74–76.

61. Baldus S, Köster R, Elsner M, et al. Treatment of aortocoronary vein graft lesion with membrane-covered stents: a multicenter surveillance trial. *Circulation* 2000;102:2024–2027.

62. Gercken U, Lansky AJ, Buellesfeld L, et al. Results of the Jostent coronary stent graft implantation in various clinical settings: procedural and follow-up results. *Cather Cardiovasc Intervent* 2002;56:353–360.

63. Stankovic G, Colombo A, Presbitero P, et al. Randomized evaluation of polytetrafluoroethylene-covered stent in saphenous vein grafts: the Randomized Evaluation of polytetrafluoroethylene COVERed stent in Saphenous vein grafts (RECOVERS) trial. *Circulation* 2003;108:37–42.

64. Schachinger V, Hamm CW, Munzel T, et al. A randomized trial of polytetrafluoroethylene-membrane-covered stents compared with conventional stents in aortocoronary saphenous vein grafts. *J Am Coll Cardiol* 2003;42:1360–1369.

65. Buchbinder M for the Symbiot III Investigators. Eight-month results from the Symbiot III randomized SVG trial. Presented at the meeting of Transcatheter Cardiovascular Therapies, Washington, DC, 2004.

66. Stone GW for the Barricade Investigators. A prospective, randomized U.S. trial of the PTFE covered Jostent for the treatment of diseased saphenous vein grafts [abstract]. *J Am Coll Cardiol* 2005;45:27A.

67. Han RO, Schwartz RS, Kobayashi Y, et al. Comparison of self-expanding and balloon-expandable stents for the reduction of restenosis. *Am J Cardiol* 2001;88:253–259.

68. Baim DS, Cutlip DE, Midei M, et al. Final results of a randomized trial comparing the MULTI-LINK stent with the Palmaz-Schatz stent for narrowings in native coronary arteries. *Am J Cardiol* 2001;87:157–162.

69. Baim DS, Cutlip DE, O'Shaughnessy CD, et al. Final results of a randomized trial comparing the NIR stent to the Palmaz-Schatz stent for narrowings in native coronary arteries. *Am J Cardiol* 2001;87:152–156.

70. Heuser R, Lopez A, Kuntz R, et al. SMART: the microstent's ability to limit restenosis trial. *Cathet Cardiovasc Intervent* 2001;52: 269–277.

71. Holmes DR Jr, Lansky A, Kuntz R, et al. The PARAGON stent study: a randomized trial of a new martensitic nitinol stent versus the Palmaz-Schatz stent for treatment of complex native coronary arterial lesions. *Am J Cardiol* 2000;86:1073–1079.

72. Hausleiter J, Kastrati A, Mehilli J, et al. Impact of lesion complexity on the capacity of a trial to detect differences in stent performance: results from the ISAR-STEREO trial. *Am Heart J* 2003; 146:882–886.

73. Kastrati A, Dirschinger J, Boekstegers P, et al. Influence of stent design on 1-year outcome after coronary stent placement: a randomized comparison of five stent types in 1,147 unselected patients. *Cathet Cardiovasc Intervent* 2000;50:290–297.

74. Colombo A, Hall P, Nakamura S, et al. Intracoronary stenting without anticoagulation accomplished with intravascular ultrasound guidance. *Circulation* 1995;91:1676–1688.

75. Karrillon GJ, Morice MC, Benveniste E, et al. Intracoronary stent implantation without ultrasound guidance and with replacement of conventional anticoagulation by antiplatelet therapy. 30-day clinical outcome of the French Multicenter Registry. *Circulation* 1996;94:1519–1527.

76. Dirschinger J, Kastrati A, Neumann FJ, et al. Influence of balloon pressure during stent placement in native coronary arteries on early and late angiographic and clinical outcome: a randomized evaluation of high-pressure inflation. *Circulation* 1999;100: 918–923.

77. Hoffmann R, Haager P, Mintz GS, et al. The impact of high pressure vs low pressure stent implantation on intimal hyperplasia and follow-up lumen dimensions; results of a randomized trial. *Eur Heart J* 2001;22:2015–2024.

78. Cutlip DE, Baim DS, Ho KK, et al. Stent thrombosis in the modern era: a pooled analysis of multicenter coronary stent clinical trials. *Circulation* 2001;103:1967–1971.

79. Moussa I, Di Mario C, Reimers B, et al. Subacute stent thrombosis in the era of intravascular ultrasound-guided coronary stenting without anticoagulation: frequency, predictors and clinical outcome. *J Am Coll Cardiol* 1997;29:6–12.

80. Okabe T, Asakura Y, Ishikawa S, et al. Determining appropriate small vessels for stenting by intravascular ultrasound. *J Invasive Cardiol* 2000;12:625–630.

81. Fitzgerald PJ, Oshima A, Hayase M, et al. Final results of the Can Routine Ultrasound Influence Stent Expansion (CRUISE) study. *Circulation* 2000;102:523–530.

82. Frey AW, Hodgson JM, Muller C, Bestehorn HP, Roskamm H. Ultrasound-guided strategy for provisional stenting with focal balloon combination catheter: results from the randomized Strategy for Intracoronary Ultrasound-guided PTCA and Stenting (SIPS) trial. *Circulation* 2000;102:2497–2502.

83. Russo RJ. Ultrasound-guided stent placement. *Cardiol Clin* 1997; 15:49–61.

84. Mudra H, di Mario C, de Jaegere P, et al. Randomized comparison of coronary stent implantation under ultrasound or angiographic guidance to reduce stent restenosis (OPTICUS Study). *Circulation* 2001;104:1343–1349.

85. Schiele F, Meneveau N, Vuillemenot A, et al. Impact of intravascular ultrasound guidance in stent deployment on 6-month restenosis rate: a multicenter, randomized study comparing two strategies—with and without intravascular ultrasound guidance. RESIST Study Group. REStenosis after Ivus guided STenting. *J Am Coll Cardiol* 1998;32:320–328.

86. Oemrawsingh PV, Mintz GS, Schalij MJ, et al. Intravascular ultrasound guidance improves angiographic and clinical outcome of stent implantation for long coronary artery stenoses: final results of a randomized comparison with angiographic guidance (TULIP Study). *Circulation* 2003;107:62–67.

87. Albiero R, Rau T, Schluter M, et al. Comparison of immediate and intermediate-term results of intravascular ultrasound versus angiography-guided Palmaz-Schatz stent implantation in matched lesions. *Circulation* 1997;96:2997–3005.

88. Hanekamp CEE, Koolen JJ, Pijls NHJ, et al. Comparison of Quantitative coronary angiography, intravascular ultrasound, and coronary pressure measurement to assess optimum stent deployment. *Circulation* 1999;99:1015–1021.

89. Pijls NHJ, Klauss V, Siebert U, et al. Coronary pressure after stenting predicts adverse events at follow-up. A multicenter registry. *Circulation* 2002;105:2950–2954.

90. Le Breton H, Boschat J, Commeau PH, et al. Randomized comparison of coronary stenting with and without balloon predilatation in selected patients. *Heart* 2001;84:302–308.

91. Baim DS, Flatley M, Caputo R, et al. Comparison of predilatation versus direct stenting in coronary treatment using the Medtronic S 670 coronary stent system (the PREDICT trial). *Am J Cardiol* 200;88:1364–1369.

92. Chevalier B, Stables R, Te Riele J, et al. Safety and feasibility of direct stenting strategy with the ACS Multilink Duet stent: results from the Slide randomized trial [abstract]. *Circulation* 2000; 102:II-730.

93. Ijsselmuiden AJ, Serruys PW, Scholte A, et al. Direct coronary stent implantation does not reduce the incidence of in-stent restenosis or major adverse cardiac events: six month results of a randomized trial. *Eur Heart J* 2003;24:421–449.

94. Serruys PW, Ijsselmuiden S, Hout B, et al. Direct stenting with the Bx VERLOCITY balloon-expandable stent mounted on the Raptor rapid exchange delivery system versus predilatation in a European randomized trial: the VELVET trial. *Int J Cardiovasc Intervent* 2003;5:17–26.

95. Miketic S, Carlsson J, Tebbe U. Clinical and angiographic outcome after conventional angioplasty with optional stent implantation compared with direct stenting without predilatation. *Heart* 2002;88:622–626.

96. Martinez-Elbal L, Ruiz-Nodar JM, Zueco J, et al. Direct coronary stenting versus stenting with balloon pre-dilation: immediate and follow-up results of a multicentre, prospective, randomized study. The DISCO trial. Direct Stenting of Coronary Arteries. *Eur Heart J* 2002;23:633–640.

97. Weber F, Schneider H, Warzok F, et al. Randomized comparison of direct and provisional stenting in de novo coronary artery lesions: the RADICAL study. *Z Kardiol* 2003;92: 173–181.

98. Silber S, Hamburger J, Grube E, et al. Direct stenting with TAXUS stents seems to be as safe and effective as with predilatation. A post hoc analysis of TAXUS II. *Herz* 2004;29:171–180.

99. Schluter M, Schofer J, Gershlick AH, et al. Direct stenting of native de novo coronary artery lesions with the sirolimus-eluting stent: a post hoc subanalysis of the pooled E- and C-SIRIUS trials. *J Am Coll Cardiol* 2005;45:10–13.

100. Prati F, DiMario C, Moussa I, et al. In-stent neointimal proliferation correlates with the amount of residual plaque burden outside the stent: an intravascular ultrasound study. *Circulation* 1999;99: 1011–1014.

101. Shiran A, Weissman NJ, Leiboff B, et al. Effect of preintervention plaque burden on subsequent intimal hyperplasia in stented coronary artery lesions. *Am J Cardiol* 2000;86: 1318–1321.

102. Moussa I, Moses J, Di Mario C, et al. Stenting after optimal lesion debulking (SOLD) registry. Angiographic and clinical outcome. *Circulation* 1998;98:1604–1609.

103. Kiesz RS, Rozek MM, Mego DM, et al. Acute directional coronary atherectomy prior to stenting in complex coronary lesions: ADAPTS Study. *Cathet Cardiovasc Diagn* 1998;45;105–112.

104. AtheroLink Study Group. A synergistic approach to optimal stenting: directional coronary atherectomy prior to coronary artery stent implantation—the AtheroLink Registry. *J Am Coll Cardiol* 2000;36:1853–1859.

105. Stankovic G, Colombo A, Bersin R, et al. Comparison of directional coronary atherectomy and stenting versus stenting alone for the treatment of de novo and restenotic coronary artery narrowing. *Am J Cardiol* 2004;93:953–958.

106. Karvouni E, Di Mario C, Nishida T, et al. Directional atherectomy prior to stenting in bifurcation lesions: a matched comparison study with stenting alone. *Cathet Cardiovasc Intervent* 2001;53:12–20.

107. Airoldi F, Di Mario C, Stankovic G, et al. Clinical and angiographic outcome of directional atherectomy followed by stent implantation in de novo lesions located at the ostium of the left anterior descending coronary artery. *Heart* 2003;89:1050–1054.

108. Hoffman R, Mintz GS, Popma JJ, et al. Treatment of calcified coronary lesions with Palmaz-Schatz stents. An intravascular ultrasound study. *Eur Heart J* 1998;19:1224–1231.

109. Henneke KH, Regar E, Konig A, et al. Impact of target lesion calcification on coronary stent expansion after rotational atherectomy. *Am Heart J* 1999;137:93–99.

110. Hoffmann R, Mintz GS, Kent KM, et al. Comparative early and nine-month results of rotational atherectomy, stents, and the combination of both for calcified lesions in large coronary arteries. *Am J Cardiol* 1998;81:552–557.

111. Schomig A, Neumann F, Kastrati A, et al. A randomized comparison of antiplatelet and anticoagulation therapy after placement of coronary-artery stents. *N Engl J Med* 1996;334:1084–1089.

112. Leon, MB, Baim DS, Popma JJ, et al. A clinical trial comparing three antithrombotic-drug regimens following coronary artery stenting. *N Engl J Med* 1998;339:1665–1671.

113. Bertrand ME, Legrand V, Boland J, et al. Randomized multicenter comparison of conventional anticoagulation versus antiplatelet therapy in unplanned and elective coronary stenting: the Full Anticoagulation Versus Aspirin and Ticlopidine (FANTASTIC) study. *Circulation* 1998;98:1597–1603.

114. Urban P, Macaya C, Rupprecht H-J, et al. Randomized evaluation of anticoagulation versus antiplatelet therapy after coronary stent implantation in high-risk patients: the Multicenter Aspirin and Ticlopidine Trial after Intracoronary Stenting (MATTIS). *Circulation* 1998;98:2126–2132.

115. Bennett CL, Weinberg PD, Rosenberg-Ben-Dror K, et al. Thrombotic thrombocytopenia purpura associated with ticlopidine: a review of 60 cases. *Ann Intern Med* 1998;128:541–544.

116. Bertrand ME, Ruppert HJ, Urban P, et al. Double-blind study of the safety of clopidogrel with and without a loading dose in combination with aspirin compared with ticlopidine in combination with aspirin after coronary stenting: the Clopidogrel Aspirin Stent International Cooperative Study (CLASSICS). *Circulation* 2000;102:624–629.

117. Muller C, Buttner HJ, Petersen J, Roskamm H. A randomized comparison of clopidogrel and aspirin versus ticlopidine and aspirin after the placement of coronary artery stents. *Circulation* 2000;101:590–593.

118. Taniuchi M, Kurz HI, Lasala JM. Randomized comparison of ticlopidine and clopidogrel after intracoronary stent implantation in a broad patient population. *Circulation* 2001;104:539–543.

119. Muller I, Seyfath M, Rudiger S, et al. Effect of a high loading dose of clopidogrel on platelet function in patients undergoing coronary angioplasty. *Heart* 2001;85:92–93.

120. Kastrati A, Mehilli J, Schühlen H, for the ISAR REACT investigators. A clinical trial of abciximab in elective percutaneous coronary intervention after pretreatment with clopidogrel. *N Engl J Med* 2004;350:232–238.

121. Hongo RH, Ley J, Dick SE, Yee RR. The effect of clopidogrel in combination with aspirin when given before coronary artery bypass grafting. *J Am Coll Cardiol* 2002;40:231–237.

122. Steinhubl SR, Berger PB, Mann JT III, et al. Early and sustained oral antiplatelet therapy following percutaneous coronary intervention. *JAMA* 2002;288:2411–2420.

123. Clopidogrel in Unstable Angina to Prevent Recurrent Events Trial Investigators. Effects of clopidogrel in addition to aspirin in patients with acute coronary syndromes without ST-segment elevation. *N Engl J Med* 2001;345:494–502.

124. Eriksson P. Long-term clopidogrel therapy after percutaneous coronary intervention in PCI-CURE and CREDO: the "Emperor's New Clothes" revisited. *Eur Heart J* 2004;25:720–722.

125. Coller BS, Folts, JD, Smith SR, Scudder LE, Jordan R. Abolition of in vivo platelet thrombus formation in primates with monoclonal antibodies to the platelet GPllb/llla receptor. Correlation with bleeding time, platelet aggregation, and blockade of GPllb/IIIa receptors. *Circulation* 1989;80:1766–1774.

126. The EPISTENT Investigators. Randomised placebo-controlled and balloon-angioplasty-controlled trial to assess safety of coronary stenting with use of platelet glycoprotein llb/llla blockade. Evaluation of Platelet llb/llla Inhibitor for Stenting. *Lancet* 1998;352:87–92.

127. The ESPRIT investigators. Novel dosing regimen of eptifibatide in planned coronary stent implantation (ESPRIT): a randomised, placebo-controlled trial. *Lancet* 2000;356:2037–2044.

128. The ERASER Investigators. Acute platelet inhibition wtih abciximab does not reduce in-stent restenosis (ERASER study). *Circulation* 1999;100:799–806.

129. Inhibition of the platelet glycoprotein llb/llla receptor with tirofiban in unstable angina and non-Q-wave myocardial infarction. Platelet Receptor Inhibition in Ischemic Syndrome Management in Patients Limited by Unstable Signs and Symptoms (PRISM-PLUS) Study Investigators. *N Engl J Med* 1998;338:1488–1497.

130. The PURSUIT Trial Investigators. Inhibition of platelet glycoprotein llb/llla with eptifibatide in patients with acute coronary syndromes. *N Engl J Med* 1998;339:436–443.

131. Stone GW, Grines CL, Cox DA, et al. Controlled Abciximab and Device Investigation to Lower Late Angioplasty Complications (CADILLAC) Investigators. Comparison of angioplasty with stenting, with or without abciximab, in acute myocardial infarction. *N Engl J Med* 2002;346:957–966.

132. Tcheng JE, Kandzari DE, Grines CL, et al. Benefits and risks of abciximab use in primary angioplasty for acute myocardial infarction: the Controlled Abciximab and Device Investigation to Lower Late Angioplasty Complications (CADILLAC) trial. *Circulation* 2003;108:1316–1323.

133. Orford JL, Lennon R, Melby S. Frequency and correlates of coronary stent thrombosis in the modern era: analysis of a single center registry. *J Am Coll Cardiol* 2002;40:1567–1572.

134. Reynolds MR, Rinaldi MJ, Pinto DS, Cohen DJ. Current clinical characteristics and economic impact of subacute stent thrombosis. *J Invasive Cardiol* 2002;14:364–368.

135. Costa MA, Sabate M, van der Giessen WJ, et al. Late coronary occlusion after intracoronary brachytherapy. *Circulation* 1999;100:789–792.

136. Ong ATL, et al. Late angiographic stent thrombosis (LAST) events with drug eluting stents. *J Am Coll Cardiol* 2005 (in press).

137. Rinfret S, Cutlip DE, Katsiyiannis PT, et al. Rheolytic thrombectomy and platelet glycoprotein llb/llla blockade for stent thrombosis. *Cathet Cardiovasc Intervent* 2002;57:24–30.

138. Ho KKL, Senerchia C, Rodriquez O, Chauhan MS, Kuntz RE. Predictors of angiographic restenosis after stenting: pooled analysis of 1197 patients with protocol-mandated angiographic follow-up from five randomized stent trials. *Circulation* 1998;98:362–368.

139. Kasaoka S, Tobis JM, Akiyama T, et al. Angiographic and intravascular ultrasound predictors of in-stent restenosis. *J Am Coll Cardiol* 1998;32:1630–1635.

140. Morino Y, Honda Y, Okura H, et al. An optimal diagnostic threshold for minimal stent area to predict target lesion revascularization following stent implantation in native coronary lesions. *Am J Cardiol* 2001;88:301–303.

141. de Feyter PJ, Kay P, Disco C, Serruys PW. Reference chart derived from post-stent-implantation intravascular ultrasound predictors of 6-month expected restenosis on quantitative coronary angiography. *Circulation* 1999;100:1777–1783.

142. Asakura M, Ueda Y, Nanto S, et al. Remodeling of in-stent neointima, which became thinner and transparent over 3 years: Serial angiographic and angioscopic follow-up. *Circulation* 1998;97:2003–2006.

143. Kimura T, Nosaka H, Yokoi H, Iwabuchi M, Nobuyoshi M. Serial angiography follow-up after Palmaz-Schatz stent implantation: comparison with conventional balloon angioplasty. *J Am Coll Cardiol* 1993;21:1557–1563.

144. Farb A, Sangiorgi G, Carter AJ, et al. Pathology of acute and chronic coronary stenting in humans. *Circulation* 1999;99: 44–52.

145. Laham RJ, Carrozza JP, Berger C, et al. Long-term (4–6 year) outcome of Palmaz-Schatz stenting: paucity of late clinical stent-related problems. *J Am Coll Cardiol* 1996;28:820–826.

146. Teirstein PS, Massullo V, Jani S, et al. Three-year clinical and angiographic follow-up after intracoronary radiation: results of a randomized clinical trial. *Circulation* 2000;101:360–365.

147. Hong MK, Mehran R, Dangas G, et al. Comparison of time course of target lesion revascularization following successful saphenous vein graft angioplasty versus successful native coronary angioplasty. *Am J Cardiol* 2000;85:256–258.

148. Hoffmann R, Mintz GS, Dussaillant GR, et al. Patterns and mechanisms of in-stent restenosis. A serial intravascular ultrasound study. *Circulation* 1996;94:1247–1254.

149. Walters DL, Harding SA, Walsh CR, Wong P, Pomerantsev E, Jang IK. Acute coronary syndrome is a common clinical presentation of in-stent restenosis. *Am J Cardiol* 2002;89:491–494.

150. Cutlip DE, Chauhan MS, Baim DS, et al. Clinical restenosis after coronary stenting: perspectives from multicenter clinical trials. *J Am Coll Cardiol* 2002;40:2082–2089.

151. Gordon PC, Friedrich SP, Piana RN, et al. Is 40% to 70% diameter narrowing at the site of previous stenting or directional coronary atherectomy clinically significant? *Am J Cardiol* 1994;74:26–32.

152. Mehran R, Dangas G, Abizaid AS, et al. Angiographic patterns of in-stent restenosis: classification and implications for long-term outcome. *Circulation* 1999;100:1872–1878.

153. Mercado N, et al. Clinical and quantitative coronary angiographic predictors of coronary restenosis: a comparative analysis from the balloon-to-stent era. *J Am Coll Cardiol* 2001;38:645–652.

154. Albiero R, Silber S, Di Mario C, et al. RESCUT Investigators. Cutting balloon versus conventional balloon angioplasty for the treatment of in-stent restenosis: results of the restenosis cutting balloon evaluation trial (RESCUT). *J Am Coll Cardiol* 2004;43:943–949.

155. Mahdi NA, Pathan AZ, Harrell L, et al. Directional coronary atherectomy for the treatment of Palmaz-Schatz in-stent restenosis. *Am J Cardiol* 1998;82:1345–1351.

156. Mehran R, Dangas G, Mintz GS, et al. Treatment of in-stent restenosis with excimer laser coronary angioplasty versus rotational atherectomy: comparative mechanisms and results. *Circulation* 2000;101:2484–2489.

157. vom Dahl J, Dietz U, Haager PK, et al. Rotational atherectomy does not reduce recurrent in-stent restenosis: results of the angioplasty versus rotational atherectomy for treatment of diffuse in-stent restenosis trial (ARTIST). *Circulation* 2002;105:583–588.

158. Mehran R, Mintz GS, Satler LF, et al. Treatment of in-stent restenosis with excimer laser coronary angioplasty: mechanisms and results compared with PTCA alone. *Circulation* 1997;96:2183–2189.

159. Giri S, Ito S, Lansky AJ, et al. Clinical and angiographic outcome in the laser angioplasty for restenotic stents (LARS) multicenter registry. *Cathet Cardiovasc Intervent* 2001;52:24–34.

160. Hamburger JN, Foley DP, de Feyter PJ, Wardeh AJ, Serruys PW. Six-month outcome after excimer laser coronary angioplasty for diffuse in-stent restenosis in native coronary arteries. *Am J Cardiol* 2000;86:390–394.

161. Koster R, Kahler J, Terres W, et al. Six-month clinical and angiographic outcome after successful excimer laser angioplasty for in-stent restenosis. *J Am Coll Cardiol* 2000;36:69–74.

162. Alfonso F, Zueco J, Cequier A, et al. A randomized comparison of repeat stenting with balloon angioplasty in patients with in-stent restenosis. *J Am Coll Cardiol* 2003;42:796–805.

163. Teirstein PS, Massulo V, Jani S, et al. Catheter-based radiotherapy to inhibit restenosis after coronary stenting. *N Engl J Med* 1997;336:1697–1703.

164. Leon MB, Teirstein PS, Moses JW, et al. Localized intracoronary gamma-radiation therapy to inhibit the recurrence of restenosis after stenting. *N Engl J Med* 2001;344:250–256.

165. Waksman R, White LR, Chan RC, et al. Washington Radiation for In-Stent Restenosis Trial (WRIST) Investigators. Intracoronary gamma-radiation therapy after angioplasty inhibits recurrence in patients with in-stent restenosis. *Circulation* 2000;101:2165–2171.

165a. Waksman R, Cheneau E, Ajani AE, et al. Intracoronary radiation therapy improves the clinical and angiographic outcomes of diffuse in-stent restenotic lesions: results of the Washington Radiation for In-Stent Restenosis Trial for Long Lesions (Long WRIST) studies. *Circulation* 2003;107:1744–1749.

166. Popma J. Late clinical and angiographic outcomes after use of 90Sr/90Y beta radiation for the treatment of in-stent restenosis: results from the 90Sr Treatment of Angiographic Restenosis (START) Trial. *J Am Coll Cardiol* 2000;36:311–312.

167. Kim HS, Waksman R, Cottin Y, et al. Edge stenosis and geographical miss following intracoronary gamma radiation therapy for in-stent restenosis. *J Am Coll Cardiol* 2001;37:1026–1030.

168. Sianos G, Kay IP, Costa MA, et al. Geographical miss during catheter-based intracoronary beta-radiation: incidence and implications in the BRIE study. Beta-Radiation In Europe. *J Am Coll Cardiol* 2001;38:415–420.

169. Sabate M, Costa MA, Kozuma K, et al. Geographic miss: a cause of treatment failure in radio-oncology applied to intracoronary radiation therapy. *Circulation* 2000;101:2467–2471.

170. Waksman R, Ajani AE, White RL, et al. Prolonged antiplatelet therapy to prevent late thrombosis after intracoronary gamma-radiation in patients with in-stent restenosis: Washington Radiation for In-Stent Restenosis Trial plus 6 months of clopidogrel (WRIST PLUS). *Circulation* 2001;103:2332–2335.

171. Leon MB, Teirstein PS, Moses JW, et al. Declining long-term efficacy of vascular brachytherapy for in-stent restenosis: 5-year follow-up from the GAMMA-1 Randomized trial [abstract]. *Circulation* 2004;110:III-405.

172. Kastrati A, Mehilli J, von Beckerath N, et al. Sirolimus-eluting stent or paclitaxel-eluting stent vs balloon angioplasty for prevention of recurrences in patients with coronary in-stent restenosis. *JAMA* 2005;293:165–171.

173. Saia F, Lemos PA, Hoye A, et al. Clinical outcomes for sirolimus-eluting stent implantation and vascular brachytherapy for the treatment of in-stent restenosis. *Cathet Cardiovasc Intervent* 2004;62:283–288.

174. Fischman DL, Savage MP, Leon MB, et al. Fate of lesion-related side branches after coronary artery stenting. *J Am Coll Cardiol* 1993;22:1641–1666.

175. Aliabadi D, Tilli FV, Bowers TR, et al. Incidence and angiographic predictors of side branch occlusion following high-pressure intracoronary stenting. *Am J Cardiol* 1997;80:994–997.

176. Poerner TC, Kralev S, Voelker W, et al. Natural history of small and medium side branches after coronary stent implantation. *Am Heart J* 2002;143:627–635.

177. Lefévre T, Louvard Y, Morice MC, et al. Stenting of bifurcation lesions: classification, treatment, and results. *Cathet Cardiovasc Intervent* 2000;49:274–283.

178. Louvard Y, Lefevre T, Morice MC. Percutaneous coronary intervention for bifurcation coronary disease. *Heart* 2004;90:713–722.

179. Holmes DR Jr, Garratt KN, Popma JJ. Stent complications. *J Invasive Cardiol* 1998;10:385–395.

180. Bolte J, Neumann U, Pfafferott C, et al. Incidence, management, and outcome of stent loss during intracoronary stenting. *Am J Cardiol* 2001;88:565–567.

181. Kozman H, Wiseman AH, Cook JR. Long-term outcome following coronary stent embolization or misdeployment. *Am J Cardiol* 2001;88:630–634.

182. Alfonso F, Martinez D, Hernandez R, et al. Stent embolization during intracoronary stenting. *Am J Cardiol* 1996;78:833–835.

183. Eggebrecht H, Haude M, von Birgelen C, et al. Nonsurgical retrieval of embolized coronary stents. *Cathet Cardiovasc Intervent* 2000;51:432–440.

184. Alfonso F, Goicolea J, Hernandez R, et al. Arterial perforation during optimization of coronary stents using high-pressure balloon inflations. *Am J Cardiol* 1996;78:1169–1172.

185. Ellis SG, Ajluni S, Arnold AZ, et al. Increased coronary perforation in the new device era. Incidence, classification, management, and outcome. *Circulation* 1994;90:2725–2730.

186. Dippel EJ, Kereiakes DJ, Tramuta DA, et al. Coronary perforation during percutaneous coronary intervention in the era of abciximab platelet glycoprotein IIb/IIIa blockade: an algorithm for percutaneous management. *Cathet Cardiovasc Intervent* 2001;52: 279–286.

187. Thibodeaux LC, James KV, Lohr JM, et al. Infection of endovascular stents in a swine model. *Am J Surg* 1996;172:151.

188. Leroy O, Martin E, Prat A, et al. Fatal infection of coronary stent implantation. *Cathet Cardiovasc Diagn* 1996;39:168–170.

189. Dieter RS. Coronary artery stent infection. *Clin Cardiol* 2000;23: 808–810.

190. Liu JC, Cziperle DJ, Kleinman B, Loeb H. Coronary abscess: a complication of stenting. *Cathet Cardiovasc Intervent* 2003;58: 69–71.

191. Serruys PW, Unger F, Sousa JE, et al. Comparison of coronary-artery bypass surgery and stenting for the treatment of multivessel disease. *N Engl J Med* 2001;344:1117–1124.

192. Legrand VM, Serruys PW, Unger F, et al. Three-year outcome after coronary stenting versus bypass surgery for the treatment of multivessel disease. *Circulation* 2004;109:1114–1120.

193. SOS Investigators. Coronary artery bypass surgery versus percutaneous coronary intervention with stent implantation in patients with multivessel coronary artery disease (the Stent or Surgery trial): a randomised controlled trial. *Lancet* 2002;360: 965–970.

194. Weintraub WS, Mahoney EM, Zhang Z, et al. One year comparison of costs of coronary surgery versus percutaneous coronary intervention in the stent or surgery trial. *Heart* 2004;90:782–788.

195. Morrison DA, Sethi G, Sacks J, et al. Percutaneous coronary intervention versus coronary artery bypass graft surgery for patients with medically refractory myocardial ischemia and risk factors for adverse outcomes with bypass: a multicenter, randomized trial. Investigators of the Department of Veterans Affairs Cooperative Study #385, the Angina With Extremely Serious Operative Mortality Evaluation (AWESOME). *J Am Coll Cardiol* 2001;38: 143–149.

196. Rumsfeld JS, Magid DJ, Plomondon ME, et al. Health-related quality of life after percutaneous coronary intervention versus coronary bypass surgery in high-risk patients with medically refractory ischemia. *J Am Coll Cardiol* 2003;41:1732–1738.

197. Rodriguez A, Bernardi V, Navia J, Baldi, et al. Argentine randomized study: coronary angioplasty with stenting versus coronary bypass surgery in patients with multiple-vessel disease (ERACI II): 30-day and one-year follow-up results. ERACI II Investigators. *J Am Coll Cardiol* 2001;37:51–58.

198. Hueb W, Soares PR, Gersh BJ, et al. The medicine, angioplasty, or surgery study (MASS-II): a randomized, controlled clinical trial of three therapeutic strategies for multivessel coronary artery disease: one-year results. *J Am Coll Cardiol* 2004;43: 1743–1751.

199. Goy JJ, Eeckhout E, Moret C, et al. Five-year outcome in patients with isolated proximal left anterior descending coronary artery stenosis treated by angioplasty or left internal mammary artery grafting. A prospective trial. *Circulation* 1999;99: 3255–3259.

200. Diegeler A, Thiele H, Falk V, et al. Comparison of stenting with minimally invasive bypass surgery for stenosis of the left anterior descending coronary artery. *N Engl J Med* 2002;347: 561–566.

201. Drenth DJ, Veeger NJ, Winter JB, et al. A prospective randomized trial comparing stenting with off-pump coronary surgery for high-grade stenosis in the proximal left anterior descending coronary artery: three-year follow-up. *J Am Coll Cardiol* 2002;40: 1955–1960.

202. Reeves BC, Angelini GD, Bryan AJ, et al. A multi-centre randomised controlled trial of minimally invasive direct coronary bypass grafting versus percutaneous transluminal coronary angioplasty with stenting for proximal stenosis of the left anterior descending coronary artery. *Health Technol Assess* 2004; 8:1–43.

203. Lefkovits J, Topol EJ. Pharmacological approaches for the prevention of restenosis after percutaneous coronary intervention. *Prog Cardiovasc Dis* 1997;40:141–158.

204. Chan A, Chew D, Lincoff A. Update on pharmacology for restenosis. *Curr Intervent Cardiol Rep* 2001;3:149–155.

205. Gonschior P, Pahl C, Huehns TY, et al. Comparison of local intravascular drug-delivery catheter systems. *Am Heart J* 1995; 130:1174–1181.

206. Wilensky RL, Tanguay JF, Ito S, et al. Heparin infusion prior to stenting (HIPS) trial: final results of a prospective, randomized, controlled trial evaluating the effects of local vascular delivery on intimal hyperplasia. *Am Heart J* 2000;139:1061–1070.

207. Kutryk MJB, Foley DP, van den Brand M, et al. Local intracoronary administration of antisense oligonucleotide against c-myc for the prevention of in-stent restenosis. *J Am Coll Cardiol* 2002; 39:281–287.

208. Camenzind E, Bakker WH, Ambroos R, et al. Site-specific intracoronary heparin delivery in man after balloon angioplasty: a radioisotopic assessment of regional pharmacokinetics. *Circulation* 1997;96:154–165.

209. Kim WH, Hong MK, Kornowski R, Tio FO, Leon MB. Saline infusion via local drug delivery catheters is associated with increased neointimal hyperplasia in a porcine coronary in-stent restenosis model. *Coronary Artery Dis* 1999;10:629–632.

210. Grube E, Lansky A, Hauptmann KE, et al. High-dose 7-hexanoyltaxol-eluting stent with polymer sleeves for coronary revascularization: one-year results from the SCORE randomized trial. *J Am Coll Cardiol* 2004;44:1368–1372.

211. Serruys PW, Ormiston JA, Sianos G, et al. Actinomycin-eluting stent for coronary revascularization: a randomized feasibility and safety study: the ACTION trial. *J Am Coll Cardiol* 2004;44: 1363–1367.

212. Gershlick A, DeScheerder I, Chevalier B, et al. Inhibition of restenosis with a paclitaxel-eluting, polymer-free coronary stent: the European evaLUation of pacliTaxel Eluting Stent (ELUTES) trial. *Circulation* 2004;109:487–493.

213. Park SJ, Shim WH, Ho DS, et al. A paclitaxel-eluting stent for the prevention of coronary restenosis. *N Engl J Med* 2003;348:1537–1545.

214. Lansky AJ, Costa RA, Mintz GS, et al. Non–polymer-based paclitaxel-coated coronary stents for the treatment of patients with de novo coronary lesions. Angiographic follow-up of the DELIVER clinical trial. *Circulation* 2004;109:1948–1954.

215. Marx SO, et al. Rapamycin-FKBP inhibits cell cycle regulators of proliferation in vascular smooth muscle cells. *Circ Res* 1995;76: 412–417.

216. Poon M, et al. Rapamycin inhibits vascular smooth muscle cell migration. *J Clin Invest* 1996;98:2277–2283.

217. Marx SO, Marks AR. Bench to bedside: the development of rapamycin and its application to stent restenosis. *Circulation* 2001;104:852–855.

218. Sousa JE, Costa MA, Abizaid A, et al. Lack of neointimal proliferation after implantation of sirolimus-coated stents in human coronary arteries: a quantitative coronary angiography and three-dimensional intravascular ultrasound study. *Circulation* 2001;103:192–195.

219. Sousa JE, Costa MA, Sousa AG, et al. Two-year angiographic and intravascular ultrasound follow-up after implantation of sirolimus-eluting stents in human coronary arteries. *Circulation* 2003;107:381–383.

220. Morice M-C, Serruys PW, Sousa JE, et al. A randomized comparison of a sirolimus eluting stent with a standard stent for coronary revascularization. *N Engl J Med* 2002;346:1773–1780.

221. Regar E, Serruys PW, Bode C, et al. Angiographic findings of the multicenter Randomized Study With the Sirolimus-Eluting Bx Velocity Balloon-Expandable Stent (RAVEL): sirolimus-eluting stents inhibit restenosis irrespective of the vessel size. *Circulation* 2002;106:1949–1956.

222. Serruys PW, Degertekin M, Tanabe K, et al. Intravascular ultrasound findings in the multicenter, randomized, double-blind RAVEL (RAndomized study with the sirolimus-eluting VElocity balloon-expandable stent in the treatment of patients with de novo native coronary artery Lesions) trial. *Circulation* 2002;106: 798–803.

223. Holmes DR Jr, Leon MB, Moses JW, et al. Analysis of 1-year clinical outcomes in the SIRIUS trial: a randomized trial of a sirolimus-eluting stent versus a standard stent in patients at high risk for coronary restenosis. *Circulation* 2004;109:634–640.

224. Popma JJ, Leon MB, Moses JW, et al. Quantitative assessment of angiographic restenosis after sirolimus-eluting stent implantation in native coronary arteries. *Circulation* 2004;110:3773–3780.

225. Schofer J, Schluter M, Gershlick AH, et al. Sirolimus-eluting stents for treatment of patients with long atherosclerotic lesions in small coronary arteries: double-blind, randomised controlled trial (E-SIRIUS). *Lancet* 2003;362:1093–1099.

226. Schampaert E, Cohen EA, Schluter M, et al. The Canadian study of the sirolimus-eluting stent in the treatment of patients with long de novo lesions in small native coronary arteries (C-SIRIUS). *J Am Coll Cardiol* 2004;43:1110–1115.

227. Ardissino D, Cavallini C, Bramucci E, et al. Sirolimus-eluting vs uncoated stents for prevention of restenosis in small coronary arteries: a randomized trial. *JAMA* 2004;292:2727–2734.

228. Schluter M, Schofer J, Gershlick AH, et al. Direct stenting of native de novo coronary artery lesions with the sirolimus-eluting stent: a post hoc subanalysis of the pooled E- and C-SIRIUS trials. *J Am Coll Cardiol* 2005;45:10–13.

229. Sabate M. The DIABETES trial. Presented at the meeting of Transcatheter Cardiovascular Therapies, 2004, Washington, DC September 2004.

230. Axel DI, Kunert W, Göggelmann C, et al. Paclitaxel inhibits arterial smooth muscle cell proliferation and migration in vitro and in vivo using local drug delivery. *Circulation* 1997;96:636–645.

231. Giannakakou P, Robey R, Fojo T, Blagosklonny MV. Low concentrations of paclitaxel induce cell type-dependent p53, p21 and G1/G2 arrest instead of mitotic arrest: molecular determinants of paclitaxel-induced cytotoxicity. *Oncogene* 2001;20;3806–3813.

232. Grube E, Silber S, Hauptmann KE, et al. TAXUS I: six- and twelve-month results from a randomized, double-blind trial on a slow-release paclitaxel-eluting stent for de novo coronary lesions. *Circulation* 2003;107:38–42.

233. Bullesfeld L, Gerckens U, Muller R, Grube E. Long-term evaluation of paclitaxel-coated stents for treatment of native coronary lesions. First results of both the clinical and angiographic 18 month follow-up of TAXUS I. *Z Kardiol* 2003;92:825–832.

234. Colombo A, Drzewiecki J, Banning A, et al. Randomized study to assess the effectiveness of slow- and moderate-release polymer-based paclitaxel-eluting stents for coronary artery lesions. *Circulation* 2003;108:788–794.

235. Serruys PW, Degertekin M, Tanabe K, et al. Vascular responses at proximal and distal edges of paclitaxel-eluting stents: serial intravascular ultrasound analysis from the TAXUS II trial. *Circulation* 2004;109:627–633.

236. Tanabe K, Serruys PW, Degertekin M, et al. Chronic arterial responses to polymer-controlled paclitaxel-eluting stents: comparison with bare metal stents by serial intravascular ultrasound analyses: data from the randomized TAXUS-II trial. *Circulation* 2004;109:196–200.

237. Tanabe K, Serruys PW, Grube E, et al. TAXUS III Trial: in-stent restenosis treated with stent-based delivery of paclitaxel incorporated in a slow-release polymer formulation. *Circulation* 2003;107:559–564.

238. Stone GW, Ellis SG, Cox DA, et al. One-year clinical results with the slow-release, polymer-based, paclitaxel-eluting TAXUS stent: the TAXUS-IV trial. *Circulation* 2004;109:1942–1947.

239. Goy JJ, Stauffer JC, Siegenthaler M, Benoit A, Seydoux C. A prospective randomized comparison between paclitaxel and sirolimus stents in the real world of interventional cardiology: the TAXi trial. *J Am Coll Cardiol* 2005;45:308–311.

240. Morice MC for the REALITY investigators. A prospective randomized, multicenter comparison study of the sirolimus-eluting and TAXUS paclitaxel-eluting stent systems. Presented at the meeting of the American College of Cardiology, Orlando, FL, March 2005.

241. Lemos PA, Hoye A, Goedhart D, et al. Clinical, angiographic, and procedural predictors of angiographic restenosis after sirolimus-eluting stent implantation in complex patients: an evaluation from the Rapamycin-Eluting Stent Evaluated At Rotterdam Cardiology Hospital (RESEARCH) study. *Circulation* 2004;109:1366–1370.

242. Mikhail GW, Airoldi F, Tavano D, et al. The use of drug eluting stents in single and multivessel disease: results from a single centre experience. *Heart* 2004;90:990–994.

243. Teirstein PS, Dangas GD, Moussa I, et al. Sirolimus-eluting stents for failed brachytherapy: update from the SECURE registry [abstract]. *Circulation* 2004;110:III-405.

244. Saia F, Lemos PA, Arampatzis CA, et al. Routine sirolimus eluting stent implantation for unselected in-stent restenosis: insights from the rapamycin eluting stent evaluated at Rotterdam Cardiology Hospital (RESEARCH) registry. *Heart* 2004;90:1183–1138.

245. Sonoda S, Morino Y, Ako J, et al. Impact of final stent dimensions on long-term results following sirolimus-eluting stent implantation: serial intravascular ultrasound analysis from the Sirius trial. *J Am Coll Cardiol* 2004;43:1959–1963.

246. Fujii K, Mintz GS, Kobayashi Y, et al. Contribution of stent underexpansion to recurrence after sirolimus-eluting stent implantation for in-stent restenosis. *Circulation* 2004;109:1085–1088.

247. Colombo A, Moses JW, Morice MC, et al. Randomized study to evaluate sirolimus-eluting stents implanted at coronary bifurcation lesions. *Circulation* 2004;109:1244–1249.

248. Pan M, Suarez de Lezo J, Medina A, et al. Rapamycin-eluting stents for the treatment of bifurcated coronary lesions: a randomized comparison of a simple versus complex strategy. *Am Heart J* 2004;148:857–864.

249. Takebayashi H, Mintz GS, Carlier SG, et al. Nonuniform strut distribution correlates with more neointimal hyperplasia after sirolimus-eluting stent implantation. *Circulation* 2004;110:3430–3434.

250. Luo Y, Marx SO, Kiyokawa H, Koff A, Massague J, Marks AR. Rapamycin resistance tied to defective regulation of p27Kip1. *Mol Cell Biol* 1996;16:6744–6751.

251. Sianos G, Hofma S, Ligthart JM, et al. Stent fracture and restenosis in the drug-eluting stent era. *Cathet Cardiovasc Intervent* 2004;6:111–116.

252. Lemos PA, van Mieghem CA, Arampatzis CA, et al. Post-sirolimus-eluting stent restenosis treated with repeat percutaneous intervention: late angiographic and clinical outcomes. *Circulation* 2004;109:2500–2502.

253. Muni NI, Gross TP. Problems with drug-eluting coronary stents. The FDA perspective. *N Engl J Med* 2004;351:1593–1595.

254. Kereiakes DJ, Choo JK, Young JJ, Broderick TM. Thrombosis and drug-eluting stents: a critical appraisal. *Rev Cardiovasc Med* 2004;5:9–15.

255. Iakovou I, Sangiorgi G, Schmidt T, et al. Incidence and predictors of stent thrombosis after paclitaxel and sirolimus-eluting stent implantation in the "real world" [abstract]. *Circulation* 2004;110:III-688.

256. Chieffo A, Bonizzoni E, Orlic D, et al. Intraprocedural stent thrombosis during implantation of sirolimus-eluting stents. *Circulation* 2004;109:2732–2736.

257. McFadden EP, Stabile E, Regar E, et al. Late thrombosis in drug-eluting coronary stents after discontinuation of antiplatelet therapy. *Lancet* 2004;364:1519–1521.

257a. Ong AT, et al. Thirty-day and six month clinical outcome of thrombotic stent occlusion after bare-metal, sirolimus, pr paclitaxel stent implantation. *J Am Coll Cardiol* 2005;45:947–953.

257b. Moreno R, et al. Drug-eluting stent thrombosis—results from a pooled analysis including 10 randomized studies. *J Am coll Cardiol* 2005;45:954–959.

258. Schomig A, Kastrati A, Mudra H, et al. Four-year experience with Palmaz-Schatz stenting in coronary angioplasty complicated by dissection with threatened or present vessel closure. Circulation. 1994;90:2716–24.

259. Moscucci M, Piana RN, Kuntz RE, et al. Effect of prior coronary restenosis on the risk of subsequent restenosis after stent placement or directional atherectomy. *Am J Cardiol* 1994;73:1147–1153.

260. Erbel R, Haude M, Hopp HW, et al. Coronary-artery stenting compared with balloon angioplasty for restenosis after initial balloon angioplasty. Restenosis Stent Study Group. *N Engl J Med* 1998;339:1672–1678.

261. Serruys PW, van Hout B, Bonnier H, et al. Randomised comparison of implantation of heparin-coated stents with balloon angioplasty in selected patients with coronary artery disease (Benestent II). *Lancet* 1998;352:673–681.

262. Versaci F, Gaspardone A, Tomai F, et al. A comparison of coronary artery stenting with angioplasty for isolated stenosis of the proximal left anterior descending coronary artery: five year clinical follow up. *Heart* 2004;90:672–675.

263. Betriu A, Masotti M, Serra A, et al. Randomized comparison of coronary stent implantation and balloon angioplasty in the treatment of de novo coronary artery lesions (START): a four-year follow-up. *J Am Coll Cardiol* 1999;34:1498–1506.

264. Witkowski A, Ruzyllo W, Gil R, et al. A randomized comparison of elective high-pressure stenting with balloon angioplasty: six-month angiographic and two-year clinical follow-up. On behalf of AS (Angioplasty or Stent) trial investigators. *Am Heart J* 2000;140:264–271.

265. Serruys PW, Kay P, Disco C, et al. Procedural quantitative coronary angiography after Palmaz-Schatz stent implantation predicts restenosis rate at six months. *J Am Coll Cardiol* 1999;34:1067–1074.

266. Antoniucci D, Valenti R, Santoro GM, et al. Restenosis after coronary stenting in current clinical practice. *Am Heart J* 1998;135: 510–518.

267. Hoffmann R, Mintz GS, Pichard AD, et al. Intimal hyperplasia thickness at follow-up is independent of stent size: a serial intravascular ultrasound study. *Am J Cardiol* 1998;82:1168–1172.

268. Foley DP, Melkert R, Serruys PW. Influence of coronary vessel size on renarrowing process and late angiographic outcome after successful balloon angioplasty. *Circulation* 1994;90:1239–1251.

269. Agostoni P, Biondi-Zoccai GG, Gasparini GL, et al. Is bare-metal stenting superior to balloon angioplasty for small vessel coronary artery disease? Evidence from a meta-analysis of randomized trials. *Eur Heart J* 2005 Jan 28 [Epub ahead of print].

270. Moreno R, Fernandez C, Alfonso F, et al. Coronary stenting versus balloon angioplasty in small vessels: a meta-analysis from 11 randomized studies. *J Am Coll Cardiol* 2004;43:1964–1972.

271. Casella G, Prati F. Stenting small coronary arteries: The Multi-Link PIXEL Multicenter Italian Registry. *J Invasive Cardiol* 2003; 15:371–376.

272. Grenadier E, Roguin A, Hertz I, et al. Stenting very small coronary narrowings (<2 mm) using the biocompatible phosphorylcholine-coated coronary stent. *Cathet Cardiovasc Intervent* 2002;55:303–308.

273. Kastrati A, Elezi S, Dirschinger J, et al. Influence of lesion length on restenosis after coronary stent placement. *Am J Cardiol* 1999; 83:1617–1622.

274. Kobayashi Y, De Gregorio J, Kobayashi N, et al. Stented segment length as an independent predictor of restenosis. *J Am Coll Cardiol* 1999;34:651–659.

275. Kornowski R, Mehran R, Hong MK, et al. Procedural results and late clinical outcomes after placement of three or more stents in single coronary lesions. *Circulation* 1998;97:1355–1361.

276. Serruys PW, Foley DP, Suttorp MJ, et al. A randomized comparison of the value of additional stenting after optimal balloon angioplasty for long coronary lesions: final results of the additional value of NIR stents for treatment of long coronary lesions (ADVANCE) study. *J Am Coll Cardiol* 2002;39:393–399.

277. Kornowski R, Mintz GS, Kent KM, et al. Increased restenosis in diabetes mellitus after coronary interventions is due to exaggerated intimal hyperplasia. A serial intravascular ultrasound study. *Circulation* 1997;95:1366–1369.

278. Van Belle E, Perie M, Braune D, et al. Effects of coronary stenting on vessel patency and long-term clinical outcome after percutaneous coronary revascularization in diabetic patients. *J Am Coll Cardiol* 2002;40:410–417.

279. Stone GW. TAXUS II, IV, and VI meta-analysis. Presented at the meeting of Transcatheter Cardiovascular Therapies, 2004, Washington, DC September, 2004.

280. Hoffman SN, TenBrook JA, Wolf MP, et al. A meta-analysis of randomized controlled trials comparing coronary artery bypass graft with percutaneous transluminal coronary angioplasty: one-to eight-year outcomes. *J Am Coll Cardiol* 2003;41:1293–1304.

281. Serruys PW. Arterial Revascularization Therapies Study, Part II of the Sirolimus-Eluting Stent in the Treatment of Patients with Multivessel De novo Coronary Artery Lesions. Presented at the meeting of Transcatheter Cardiovascular Therapies, 2004, Washington, DC September 2004.

282. Orlic D, Bonizzoni E, Stankovic G, et al. Treatment of multivessel coronary artery disease with sirolimus-eluting stent implantation: immediate and mid-term results. *J Am Coll Cardiol* 2004;43:1154–1160.

283. Buller CE, Dzavik V, Carere RG, et al. Primary stenting versus balloon angioplasty in occluded coronary arteries: the Total Occlusion Study of Canada (TOSCA). *Circulation* 1999;100:236–242.

284. Rahel BM, Suttorp MJ, Laarman GJ, et al. Primary stenting of occluded native coronary arteries: final results of the Primary Stenting of Occluded Native Coronary Arteries (PRISON) study. *Am Heart J* 2004;147:e22.

285. Sirnes PA, Golf S, Myreng Y, et al. Stenting in Chronic Coronary Occlusion (SICCO): a randomized, controlled trial of adding stent implantation after successful angioplasty. *J Am Coll Cardiol* 1996;28:1444–1451.

286. Sirnes PA, Golf S, Myreng Y, et al. Sustained benefit of stenting chronic coronary occlusion: long-term clinical follow-up of the Stenting in Chronic Coronary Occlusion (SICCO) study. *J Am Coll Cardiol* 1998;32:305–310.

287. Rubartelli P, Verna E, Niccoli L, et al. Coronary stent implantation is superior to balloon angioplasty for chronic coronary occlusions: six-year clinical follow-up of the GISSOC trial. *J Am Coll Cardiol* 2003;41:1488–1492.

288. Nakamura S, Muthusamy TS, Bae JH, et al. Impact of sirolimus-eluting stent on the outcome of patients with chronic total occlusions. *Am J Cardiol* 2005;95:161–166.

289. Werner GS, Krack A, Schwarz G, et al. Prevention of lesion recurrence in chronic total coronary occlusions by paclitaxel-eluting stents. *J Am Coll Cardiol* 2004;44:2301–2306.

290. Kereiakes DJ. Percutaneous transcatheter therapy of aorto-ostial stenoses. *Cathet Cardiovasc Diagn* 1996;38:292–300.

291. Jain SP, Liu MW, Dean LS, et al. Comparison of balloon angioplasty versus debulking devices versus stenting in right coronary ostial lesions. *Am J Cardiol* 1997;79:1334–1338.

292. Vijayakumar M, Alfredo Rodriguez Granillo GA, Lemos PA, et al. Sirolimus-eluting stents for the treatment of atherosclerotic ostial lesions. *J Invasive Cardiol* 2005;17:10–12.

293. Iakovou I, Ge L, Michev I, Sangiorgi GM, et al. Clinical and angiographic outcome after sirolimus-eluting stent implantation in aorto-ostial lesions. *J Am Coll Cardiol* 2004;44: 967–971.

294. Airoldi F, Colombo A, Michev I, et al. Sirolimus eluting stent implantation in bifurcational coronary artery lesions utilizing the crush technique: immediate and mid term outcomes [abstract]. *J Am Coll Cardiol* 2005;45:47A.

295. Tanabe K, Hoye A, Lemos PA, et al. Restenosis rates following bifurcation stenting with sirolimus-eluting stents for de novo narrowings. *Am J Cardiol* 2004;94:115–118.

296. Colombo A, Moses JW, Morice MC, et al. Randomized study to evaluate sirolimus-eluting stents implanted at coronary bifurcation lesions *Circulation*. 2004;109:1244–1249.

297. Cervinka P, Foley DP, Sabate M, et al. Coronary bifurcation stenting using dedicated bifurcation stents. *Cathet Cardiovasc Intervent* 2000;49:105–111.

298. Tan WA, Tamai H, Park SJ, et al. Long-term clinical outcomes after unprotected left main trunk percutaneous revascularization in 279 patients. *Circulation* 2001;104:1609–1614.

299. Black A Jr, Cortina R, Bossi I, et al. Unprotected left main coronary artery stenting. Correlates of midterm survival and impact of patient selection. *J Am Coll Cardiol* 2001;37:832–838.

300. Park SJ, Park SW, Hong MK, et al. Long-term (three-year) outcomes after stenting of unprotected left main coronary artery stenosis in patients with normal left ventricular function. *Am J Cardiol* 2003;91:12–16.

301. Park SJ, Kim YH, Lee BK, et al. Sirolimus-eluting stent implantation for unprotected left main coronary artery stenosis Comparison with bare metal stent implantation. *J Am Coll Cardiol* 2005;45:351–356.

302. Chieffo A, Stankovic G, Bonizzoni E, et al. Early and mid-term results of drug-eluting stent implantation in unprotected left main. *Circulation* 2005;111:791–795 [Epub 2005 Feb 7].

303. Piana RN, Moscucci M, Cohen DJ, et al. Palmaz-Schatz stenting for treatment of focal vein graft stenosis: immediate results and longterm outcome. *J Am Coll Cardiol* 1994;23:1296–1304.

304. Wong SC, Popma JJ, Pichard AD, et al. Comparison of clinical and angiographic outcomes after saphenous vein graft angioplasty using coronary versus biliary tubular slotted stents. *Circulation* 1995;91:339–346.

305. Savage MP, Douglas JS Jr, Fischman DL, et al. Stent placement compared with balloon angioplasty for obstructed coronary bypass grafts. *N Engl J Med* 1997;337:740–747.

306. Hanekamp CE, Koolen JJ, Den Heijer P, et al. Randomized study to compare balloon angioplasty and elective stent implantation in venous bypass grafts: the Venestent study. *Cathet Cardiovasc Intervent* 2003;60:452–457.

307. Hoye A, Lemos PA, Arampatzis CA, et al. Effectiveness of the sirolimus-eluting stent in the treatment of saphenous vein graft disease. *J Invasive Cardiol* 2004;16:230–233.

308. Glaser R, Selzer F, Faxon DP, et al. Clinical progression of incidental, asymptomatic lesions discovered during culprit vessel coronary intervention. *Circulation* 2005;11:143–149.

309. Stone GW, Brodie BR, Griffin JJ, et al. A prospective, multicenter study of the safety and feasibility of primary stenting in acute myocardial infarction: in-hospital and 30 day results of the PAMI Stent Pilot Trial. *J Am Coll Cardiol* 1998;31:23–30.

310. Stone GW, Brodie BR, Griffin JJ, et al. Clinical and angiographic follow-up after primary stenting in acute myocardial infarction: the Primary Angioplasty in Myocardial Infarction (PAMI) stent pilot trial. *Circulation* 1999;99:1548–1554.

311. Serruys PW, Grines CL, Stone GW, et al. Stent implantation in acute myocardial infarction using a heparin-coated stent: a pilot study as a preamble to a randomized trial comparing balloon angioplasty and stenting. *J Intervent Cardiovasc Intervent* 1998;1:19–27.

312. Stone GW, Grines CL, Cox DA, et al. Comparison of angioplasty with stenting, with or without abciximab, in acute myocardial infarction. *N Engl J Med* 2002;346:957–966.

313. Grines CL, Cox DA, Stone GW, et al. Coronary angioplasty with or without stent implantation for acute myocardial infarction. Stent Primary Angioplasty in Myocardial Infarction Study Group. *N Engl J Med* 1999;341:1949–1956.

314. Suryapranata H, van't Hof AW, Hoorntje JC, de Boer MJ, Zijlstra F. Randomized comparison of coronary stenting with balloon angioplasty in selected patients with acute myocardial infarction. *Circulation* 1998;97:2502–2505.

315. Maillard L, Hamon M, Khalife K, et al. A comparison of systematic stenting and conventional balloon angioplasty during primary percutaneous transluminal coronary angioplasty for acute myocardial infarction. STENTIM-2 Investigators. *J Am Coll Cardiol* 2000;35:1729–1736.

316. Antoniucci D, Santoro GM, Bolognese L, et al. A clinical trial comparing primary stenting of the infarct-related artery with optimal primary angioplasty for acute myocardial infarction: results from the Florence Randomized Elective Stenting in Acute Coronary Occlusions (FRESCO) trial. *J Am Coll Cardiol* 1998;31:1234–1239.

317. Saito S, Hosokawa G, Tanaka S, Nakamura S. Primary stent implantation is superior to balloon angioplasty in acute myocardial infarction: final results of the primary angioplasty versus stent implantation in acute myocardial infarction (PASTA) trial. PASTA Trial Investigators. *Cathet Cardiovasc Intervent* 1999;48:262–268.

318. Rodriguez A, Bernardi V, Fernandez M, et al. In-hospital and late results of coronary stents versus conventional balloon angioplasty in acute myocardial infarction (GRAMI trial). Gianturco-Roubin in Acute Myocardial Infarction. *Am J Cardiol* 1998;81:1286–1291.

319. Scheller B, Hennen B, Severin-Kneib S, et al. Long-term follow-up of a randomized study of primary stenting versus angioplasty in acute myocardial infarction. *Am J Med* 2001;110:1–6.

320. Nordmann AJ, Hengstler P, Harr T, Young J, Bucher HC. Clinical outcomes of primary stenting versus balloon angioplasty in patients with myocardial infarction: a meta-analysis of randomized controlled trials. *Am J Med* 2004;116:253–262.

321. Cox DA, Stone GW, Grines CL, et al. Outcomes of optimal or "stent-like" balloon angioplasty in acute myocardial infarction: the CADILLAC trial. *J Am Coll Cardiol* 2003;42:971–977.

322. Cohen DJ, Taira DA, Berezin R, et al. Cost-effectiveness of coronary stenting in acute myocardial infarction: results from the stent primary angioplasty in myocardial infarction (stent-PAMI) trial. *Circulation* 2001;104:3039–3045.

323. Rinfret S, Grines CL, Cosgrove RS, et al. Quality of life after balloon angioplasty or stenting for acute myocardial infarction. One-year results from the Stent-PAMI trial. *J Am Coll Cardiol* 2001;38:1614–1621.

324. Costantini CO, Stone GW, Mehran R, et al. Frequency, correlates, and clinical implications of myocardial perfusion after primary angioplasty and stenting, with and without glycoprotein IIb/IIIa inhibition, in acute myocardial infarction. *J Am Coll Cardiol* 2004;44:305–312.

325. McLaughlin MG, Stone GW, Aymong E, et al. Prognostic utility of comparative methods for assessment of ST-segment resolution after primary angioplasty for acute myocardial infarction: the Controlled Abciximab and Device Investigation to Lower Late Angioplasty Complications (CADILLAC) trial. *J Am Coll Cardiol* 2004;44:1215–1223.

326. Kastrati A, Mehilli J, Nekolla S, et al. A randomized trial comparing myocardial salvage achieved by coronary stenting versus balloon angioplasty in patients with acute myocardial infarction considered ineligible for reperfusion therapy. *J Am Coll Cardiol* 2004;43:734–741.

327. Lemos PA, Saia F, Hofma SH, et al. Short- and long-term clinical benefit of sirolimus-eluting stents compared to conventional bare stents for patients with acute myocardial infarction. *J Am Coll Cardiol* 2004;43:704–708.

328. Berger PB, Costa MA, Cohen S, et al. Six month clinical outcomes using sirolimus eluting stents in clinical practice: results from the US post marketing surveillance registry (the e-Cypher study) [abstract]. *J Am Coll Cardiol* 2005;45:73A.

Percutaneous Therapies for Valvular Heart Disease[a]

25

Ted Feldman

Although percutaneous intervention began with coronary angioplasty and other interventional tools (see Chapters 22 through 24), the concept of treating diseased heart valves began soon thereafter. The initial thrust was to open stenotic pulmonic, mitral, and aortic valves via balloon valvuloplasty for which the basic techniques and equipment have changed little over the last two decades. More recently, there has been a renewed interest in this area as exciting new therapies for percutaneous treatment of mitral regurgitation and percutaneous replacement of pulmonic and aortic valves have entered clinical testing. This chapter will review the mechanisms, indications, techniques, and clinical results of balloon valvuloplasty of the mitral, pulmonic, and aortic valves and describe the novel catheter-based approaches for valve repair and replacement now being attempted.

PERCUTANEOUS BALLOON MITRAL VALVULOPLASTY

Percutaneous mitral valvuloplasty is an important therapeutic tool in treating rheumatic mitral stenosis. Although the prevalence of rheumatic heart disease has declined significantly in the United States, this procedure still remains an important therapeutic option for the symptomatic patient with mitral stenosis. In third world or developing countries where rheumatic heart disease remains prevalent, percutaneous mitral valvuloplasty is the treatment of choice for treating patients with mitral stenosis (1–3).

Mechanisms

Percutaneous mitral valvuloplasty is more appropriately called percutaneous mitral *commissurotomy* because the balloon dilatation improves the valve orifice by separating the fused mitral commissures. As shown by echocardiographic, fluoroscopic, and anatomic studies, the expanding balloon splits fused commissures in the same manner as a surgical commissurotomy (4,5).

Patient Selection

Patients should be selected for percutaneous mitral valvuloplasty based on both clinical and anatomic factors. In most cases they should be symptomatic, and mitral valve area as measured by echocardiography and hemodynamics should be <1.5 cm^2. Unlike for valve surgery, the presence of pulmonary hypertension or abnormal left ventricular function is not a contraindication. Patients with anatomically suitable valves who have developed restenosis (commissural refusion) after prior surgical or balloon commissurotomy can also undergo percutaneous mitral valvuloplasty with results almost as good as previously untreated patients (6,7). Although the procedure can be performed in patients of almost any age, the best clinical results are observed in younger patients, with less predictable long-term results

[a]Some of the material in this chapter was contributed by Thomas Ports and William Grossman, MD, in previous editions.

occurring in patients older than 70 years, who are more likely to have deformed and calcified valves. Percutaneous mitral valvuloplasty is a particularly valuable tool in treating the symptomatic pregnant woman with critical mitral stenosis. It can also be a lifesaving emergency procedure in the patient with mitral stenosis and refractory pulmonary edema or cardiogenic shock (8).

Asymptomatic patients should be considered for percutaneous mitral commissurotomy when they develop pulmonary hypertension or new-onset atrial fibrillation (9). A pulmonary artery peak systolic pressure >50 mm Hg at rest or 60 mm Hg with exercise in an otherwise asymptomatic patient represents disease severity that has reached the point where percutaneous commissurotomy should be considered (9). New atrial fibrillation is less clear an indication but should be considered, especially in patients with mitral valve morphology well suited for percutaneous commissurotomy.

Contraindications

Although the procedure can be performed at higher risk with thrombus localized to the left atrial appendage, thrombus within the left atrium itself is a contraindication to this procedure (10). Moderate or severe (≥2+ on a scale of 0 to 4, determined angiographically) mitral regurgitation is also a contraindication to percutaneous mitral valvuloplasty. Patients with mitral stenosis and aortic or tricuspid valve lesions that require cardiac surgery should be referred for surgery. Concomitant coronary disease can be treated with PCI in conjunction with valvuloplasty when the coronary anatomy is suitable. This can be done in one session or staged, with the more clinically severe lesion treated first.

Anatomic Factors in Patient Selection for Balloon Mitral Valvuloplasty

High-quality transthoracic and transesophageal echocardiography (TEE) is an essential part of proper patient selection. TEE prior to the planned valvuloplasty procedure excludes the presence of left atrial thrombus and moderate or greater mitral regurgitation. In addition to ensuring that there are no anatomic contraindications, echocardiography provides valuable information that helps the interventional cardiologist select patients and predict results (11). The ideal patient has pliable, noncalcified mitral leaflets and mild subvalvular disease. As the degree of subvalvular disease increases, the quality of the result with percutaneous mitral valvuloplasty decreases. Similarly, increasing degrees of calcification of the mitral valve diminish the effectiveness of mitral valve dilatation and increase the complication rate. Dilating mitral valves with commissural calcification may lead to leaflet tearing along noncommissural lines and is associated with a higher incidence of procedure related mitral regurgitation (12). Heavy calcification of the valve and/or bicommissural calcification are

also associated with poorer acute and long term outcomes. When commissural fusion is symmetric, even in the presence of calcification, bicommissural splitting is more likely than when commissural fusion is asymmetric (13,14).

Valve deformity increases substantially with age. Older patients who present with mitral stenosis often have valves poorly suited for percutaneous mitral commissurotomy. In these cases, the goals of therapy must be considered individually for patient selection. Patients who are excellent candidates for mitral valve replacement, or those who have associated multivalve or complex coronary disease, may be better served by surgery. The very elderly, or patients with multiple comorbid conditions or prior median sternotomy, may have excellent palliation from percutaneous mitral commissurotomy despite a high degree of valve and subvalvular deformity and calcification. A prototypic example is the octogenarian patient with prior aortic valve replacement and coronary bypass surgery who presents with a heavily calcified mitral valve and severe symptomatic mitral stenosis. The results of percutaneous commissurotomy in these patients are clearly less good than in younger patients with pliable valves, but the value of palliative therapy is substantial.

Many find the echocardiographic scoring system of Wilkins et al. (15) useful in assessing patients for percutaneous mitral valvuloplasty. This echocardiographic classification system is shown in Table 25.1. Points are given for

TABLE 25.1
ECHOCARDIOGRAPHIC SCORING SYSTEM[a]

Leaflet mobility
1 Highly mobile valve with restriction of only the leaflet tips
2 Midportion and base of leaflets have reduced mobility
3 Valve leaflets move forward in diastole mainly at the base
4 No or minimal forward movement of the leaflets in diastole

Valvular thickening
1 Leaflets near normal (4–5 mm)
2 Midleaflet thickening, marked thickening of the margins
3 Thickening extends through the entire leaflets (5–8 mm)
4 Marked thickening of all leaflet tissue (>8–10 mm)

Subvalvular Thickening
1 Minimal thickening of chordal structures just below the valve
2 Thickening of chordae extending up to one third of chordal length
3 Thickening extending to the distal third of the chordae
4 Extensive thickening and shortening of all chordae extending down to the papillary muscle

Valvular Calcification
1 A single area of increased echo brightness
2 Scattered areas of brightness confined to leaflet margins
3 Brightness extending into the midportion of leaflets
4 Extensive brightness through most of the leaflet tissue

[a]Adding each of the components determines final score (maximum, 16 points).
From Wilkins GT, Weyman AE, Abascal VM, et al. Percutaneous balloon dilatation of the mitral valve: an analysis of echocardiographic variables related to outcome and the mechanism of dilatation. *Br Heart J* 1988;60:299.

leaflet mobility, valve thickening, subvalvular thickening, and valvular calcification. The final score is determined by adding up the points from each category. Higher scores indicate more severe anatomic disease and a lower likelihood of a successful procedure. The maximum score is 16, and percutaneous mitral commissurotomy results are generally excellent in patients with an echo score of ≤8, indicating favorable anatomy, i.e., pliable leaflets, mild or moderate subvalvular disease, and mild or absent valve calcification. A review of over 1,500 patients undergoing balloon mitral valvuloplasty was carried out using a logistic model to improve patient selection (16). As expected, younger patients with echocardiographic evidence of less severe disease had a better outcome.

Patients with significant valve deformity and echocardiographic scores >8 should not be excluded a priori from consideration for percutaneous mitral valvuloplasty. There is no absolute contraindication to percutaneous mitral valvuloplasty in patients with higher echocardiographic scores, but patients with echocardiographic scores >8 require an individualized approach. The duration of palliation may be less than in patients with ideal valve morphology, and the acute procedure success rate is lower. When valve deformity is associated with other clear indications for open heart surgery, the decision is relatively simple. This includes patients with associated significant aortic stenosis or insufficiency, multivessel coronary artery disease, or those with severe tricuspid regurgitation in need of repair. When none of these indications are present or clear, percutaneous commissurotomy in patients with significant valve deformity can be a successful palliative therapy. This is an especially useful strategy in patients with borderline aortic insufficiency or stenosis, in whom a waiting period after mitral commissurotomy may allow for a more timely decision for double-valve replacement at a later date.

Technique

Several basic techniques of percutaneous mitral valvuloplasty (PMV) are in use. Retrograde transarterial techniques, used alone or in combination with antegrade (trans-septal puncture) techniques, have been used in some centers for single- and double-balloon PMV (17). They offer the advantage of not requiring trans-septal puncture or using only minimal dilatation of the intra-atrial septum. Disadvantages of these techniques include the opportunity for arterial injury because of the larger balloons used. In addition, the procedures can be technically difficult and time consuming.

The most commonly used approaches are transvenous antegrade (i.e., trans-septal) techniques, using either a double balloon or the Inoue balloon system (2,3). The Inoue balloon is the only device approved specifically for percutaneous mitral valvuloplasty in the United States and is the most commonly used device worldwide. Alternatively, a double-balloon technique can be used with two balloons advanced over separate guidewires from the femoral vein to the left atrium, across the mitral valve into the left ventricle (18). The two balloons are then inflated simultaneously across the mitral valve. Figure 25.1 illustrates the two-balloon technique. In this patient, the mitral valve was first dilated with a single balloon, after which double balloons were used to achieve the desired hemodynamic result. When properly performed, the double-balloon technique results in excellent improvement in mitral valve area (19,20). Multiple studies have shown no significant difference in hemodynamic results (mitral valve gradient or mitral valve area) postprocedure between the double-balloon technique and the Inoue balloon system (21).

An adaptation of the double-balloon technique uses a monorail approach to deliver two balloons across the mitral valve over a single guidewire (22). The first valvuloplasty balloon with a short monorail segment is passed over the wire across the mitral valve, followed by a second conventional balloon that is then passed over the wire until it is parallel with the first balloon. There are no substantial differences in the mechanism of delivery of force by two balloons using this approach compared with conventional double-wire, double-balloon technique.

In the early surgical era of closed heart mitral commissurotomy, a metallic dilator, or commissurotome, was used via a left ventricular apical incision. Cribier et al. (23) have adapted this established surgical technique for percutaneous use. A 19F metallic commissurotome can be passed across the interatrial septum over a guidewire and used to accomplish mitral commissurotomy. There has been some evidence that bicommissural splitting can be accomplished more frequently with the metal commissurotome. Randomized comparisons of the Inoue balloon and metallic commissurotome have not demonstrated significant differences in long-term outcome (24).

However, the Inoue balloon technique is faster and less cumbersome and generally requires less fluoroscopy time than these other approaches (25). The Inoue balloon allows simple progressive upsizing of the balloon without withdrawing the balloon from the left atrium—an important advantage if larger balloon sizes are needed. The Inoue balloon system may, however, result in a slightly higher incidence of mitral regurgitation (26).

Inoue Balloon Technique

All antegrade approaches begin with the crucial first step of successful trans-septal catheterization. This technique, which is described in Chapter 4, not only requires successful access to the left atrium, but must also be through the proper part of the atrial septum to allow easy access to the mitral valve. After successful placement of a Mullins-type dilator and sheath into the left atrium and confirmation of its position by a hand injection of contrast, the patient is anticoagulated with heparin. Baseline hemodynamics are

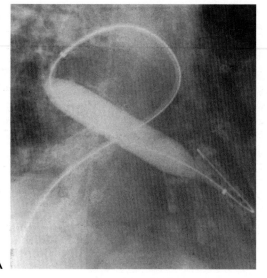

A

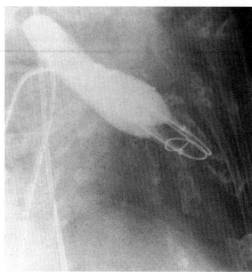

B

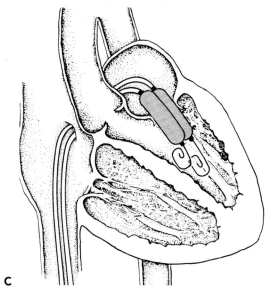

C

Figure 25.1 Mitral balloon valvuloplasty in a 72-year-old woman who presented with progressive dyspnea on exertion. Her hemodynamic evaluation showed a mean mitral valve gradient of 22 mm Hg. This was reduced to 10 mm Hg after single-balloon valvuloplasty **(A)** and 4 mm Hg after double-balloon dilatation **(B)**. Figure 25.1C is a schematic drawing showing the anatomic path and catheter positions for double-balloon mitral valvuloplasty.

then recorded, confirming the appropriate degree of mitral stenosis. Subsequently, a special solid-core coiled 0.025-inch guidewire is introduced into the left atrium, and the Mullins sheath dilator system is removed. The femoral vein and interatrial septum are then dilated with a long 14F dilator over the coiled guidewire within the left atrium. The previously prepared, tested, and now slenderized Inoue balloon is then introduced over the guidewire into the left atrium. The Inoue balloon (Fig. 25.2) is made of nylon and rubber micromesh. Owing to the variable elasticity along its length, the balloon inflates in three distinct stages as illustrated in Fig. 25.2. This allows for stable positioning of the balloon catheter across the mitral valve, as described below.

After the slenderized balloon has been positioned within the left atrium, the stretching tube is removed, and a preshaped "J" stylet is introduced into the Inoue balloon. The distal portion of the balloon is inflated slightly to aid in crossing the valve and to prevent intrachordal passage. By maneuvering the balloon catheter while rotating and withdrawing the stylet, the balloon tip will move anteriorly and inferiorly toward the mitral orifice. After the balloon catheter is across the mitral orifice, the distal portion of the balloon is inflated more fully and the catheter is pulled back gently to confirm that the inflated distal portion of the balloon is secure across the mitral valve. As further volume is added to the balloon, the proximal end inflates to lock the valve between the proximal and distal balloon. Inflation to precalibrated volume then dilates the valve orifice to the corresponding preset size. Figure 25.3 illustrates the sequential filling and positioning of the Inoue balloon. It is then allowed to deflate passively before it is withdrawn into the left atrium.

The pressure gradient across the mitral valve is measured after each balloon dilatation, and echocardiography may be used to assess the mitral valve area, leaflet mobility,

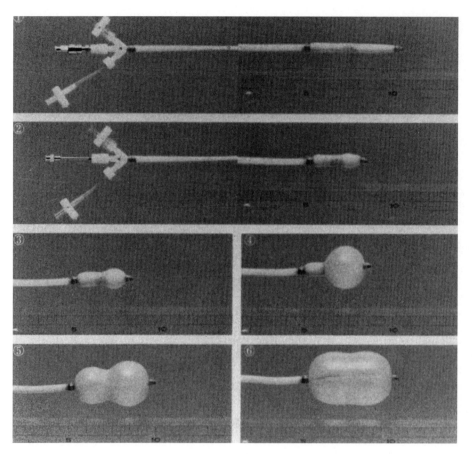

Figure 25.2 The figure shows the Inoue balloon catheter. The top panel shows the length of the catheter. On the far left, at the hub, the stretching metal-tube has been fully advanced, resulting in stretching and elongation of the balloon catheter, seen on the right side of the figure. This results in a minimized profile to facilitate passage through a femoral venous sheath or directly through the skin. In the second panel, the stretching metal tube on the far left has been pulled back, allowing the balloon to shorten and fatten. The stretching tube is puled back in this manner after the balloon is passed across the atrial septal puncture. This is seen on the right side of the second panel. Panels 3 through 6 show the step-wise inflation characteristics of the balloon. In panel 3, the balloon is un-inflated. In panel 4, the distal portion has been inflated. This portion of the balloon can be "floated" or manipulated across the mitral valve from the left atrium to the left ventricle in a manner analogous to crossing the tricuspid valve with a right heart balloon floatation catheter. In panel 5, the balloon in further inflated to create a "dog bone" configuration. This allows the balloon to self-position within the mitral valve. Upon final inflation, as seen in panel 6, the waist of the balloon is fully expanded, ultimately resulting in commisural splitting.

and the degree of mitral regurgitation. If the first inflation has not resulted in a satisfactory increase in the mitral valve area, and the degree of mitral regurgitation has not increased, the balloon is then readvanced across the mitral valve and inflation repeated with the balloon diameter increased by 1 or 2 mm by delivery of slightly more of the precalibrated syringe volume in a stepwise dilatation process that is repeated until the desired result is achieved.

The Inoue balloon comes in four sizes—24, 26, 28, and 30 mm, referring to the fully inflated maximal balloon diameter. However, since actual balloon size is dependent on the volume used for inflation, the actual diameter can be varied over a range from 6 mm less than nominal up to the full rated diameter, as required. We generally estimate the expected maximal inflated balloon catheter diameter using an empiric formula based on the height of the patient (one-tenth the height in cm plus 10 mm). It is important to start with a smaller balloon diameter, especially for valves that are very thickened or rigid or have moderate amounts of subvalvular disease, to minimize the development of mitral regurgitation, which can develop suddenly with as little as a 1- to 2-mm increase in diameter of inflation size.

The Inoue balloon is fundamentally different than conventional balloons, being volume driven. The balloon is precalibrated so that inflation with volumes labeled on the inflation syringe result in corresponding balloon-inflated

diameters. The pressure that the balloon is inflated to is thus different for different inflation volumes. A smaller maximal-size balloon when inflated to its maximal size, such as 26 mm, will be at a higher pressure than a balloon that has a larger capacity, such as a 30-mm balloon inflated to the same 26 mm. The Inoue balloon has a low-pressure zone encompassing the first two thirds of its range of inflation. The balloon pressure at this point is typically approximately two or three atmospheres. As the balloon is inflated to its last couple of millimeters of diameter with increasing inflation volumes, the balloon pressure rises toward four atmospheres of pressure. Randomized trials have examined the effects of using balloons in the low-pressure zone compared with the high-pressure zone (27,28). With similar maximal inflated diameters, inflations in the low-pressure zone result in less mitral regurgitation than inflations in the high-pressure zone. Thus, using a 30-mm balloon inflated to a maximum diameter of 28 mm will overall result in causing less mitral regurgitation than using a maximal nominal 28-mm balloon inflated to 28 mm (in the high-pressure zone).

It is important to assess for increases in mitral regurgitation after each inflation before proceeding to the next inflation diameter. After each balloon inflation, the mean left atrial pressure should be expected to decrease in conjunction with a decrease in the transmitral pressure gradient. When the left atrial pressure remains unchanged both

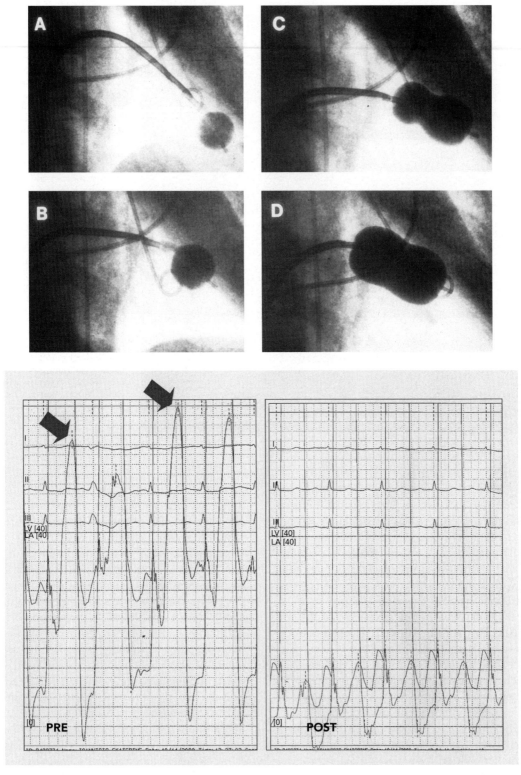

Figure 25.3   Balloon mitral valvuloplasty in a 42-year-old man who presented with dyspnea on exertion. **A.** Distal tip of the Inoue balloon has crossed the mitral valve. **B.** With the distal tip of the balloon filled, the catheter was withdrawn to straddle the mitral valve. **C.** Partial filling of the balloon. **D.** Complete filling of the Inoue balloon across the mitral valve. Following this dilation, the mitral valve gradient was reduced from 18 mm Hg to 2 mm Hg. **E.** A large V wave is seen prior to percutaneous mitral valvuloplasty. There is a large diastolic transmitral valve gradient. The *filled arrows* denote the peak of the V waves. No mitral regurgitation was noted at this point by either echocardiography or left ventriculography. **F.** Post mitral valvuloplasty, the transmitral gradient has been dramatically reduced, as has the V wave. Ventriculography and Doppler echocardiography at this point show no mitral regurgitation. (From Syed Z, Salinger MH, Feldman T. Alterations in left atrial pressure and compliance during balloon mitral valvuloplasty. *Cathet Cardiovasc Intervent* 2004;61:577.)

in magnitude and morphology of the waveform after balloon inflation, it is likely that no progress has been made. If a persistent gradient is present, an additional inflation is warranted. The evaluation is more difficult when the left atrial pressure rises after a balloon inflation, or when the waveform changes with an increase in the V wave. Decision making is all the more complicated because the presence and size of V waves in the left atrial pressure tracing is often misleading.

A V wave in the left atrial pressure tracing is dynamic. Large V waves are frequently seen in the left atrium in patients with mitral valve disease in the absence of mitral regurgitation reflecting alterations in left atrial compliance, so that V waves are neither sensitive nor specific for the presence or importance of mitral regurgitation. In percutaneous commissurotomy, it is common to see a V wave diminish during the course of successive successful balloon inflations, reflecting left atrial decompression with improved left atrial compliance (Fig. 25.3; 29). Changes in the V wave must be assessed carefully during percutaneous commissurotomy procedures, but additional information such as Doppler echocardiography or repeat left ventriculography is necessary to fully interpret these findings.

Following successful mitral valve dilatation, the Inoue balloon is then reslenderized by first reintroducing the guidewire and then the stretching tube. The slenderized balloon is subsequently withdrawn from the body over a guidewire. If no sheath has been used, a 10F sheath is inserted into the femoral vein over the guidewire before removal of the wire. It is useful to leave the guidewire across the atrial septal puncture in the left atrium for 3 to 5 minutes after completion of the procedure, while monitoring the systemic arterial pressure. In rare cases, the trans-septal puncture can be made low in the right atrium, and rather than going through the atrial septum, the needle may tra-verse the right atrial wall, the transverse pericardial sinus, and then enter the inferior border of the left atrium. In this situation, a satisfactory left atrial pressure waveform is obtained through the tip of the trans-septal needle, and the path of the puncture through the pericardial space is not apparent until devices are removed at the conclusion of the procedure. If a wire is left in place at the end of the procedure and the blood pressure drops precipitously after a couple of minutes, with the wire in place, a small balloon catheter can be passed back across the puncture site and inflated to stabilize the patient while pericardial centesis is performed and plans for further management are made. This is a rare occurrence, but catastrophic when it does occur. This small step of leaving the wire across the puncture for just a few moments can be lifesaving in that situation.

Immediate Results

Immediate results of mitral valvuloplasty are assessed by a combination of echo Doppler measurements and hemodynamics. Repeat evaluation of mitral valve area during the procedure by hemodynamic measurements can be performed with reasonable degrees of accuracy in catheterization laboratories equipped with systems with computer analysis. There is some inaccuracy to the Gorlin formula in the presence of an atrial shunt or mitral regurgitation (30). Nevertheless, in successful procedures, the mitral valve gradient will be observed to be substantially reduced.

Figure 25.4 illustrates a typical reduction in left atrial pressure and transmitral gradient immediately after balloon mitral valvuloplasty. The mitral valve orifice area will generally be increased by >1 cm^2/m^2 body surface area, or by $>80\%$. By echocardiographic assessment in the laboratory, particularly planimetry of the mitral valve orifice image in the two-dimensional echocardiogram short-axis

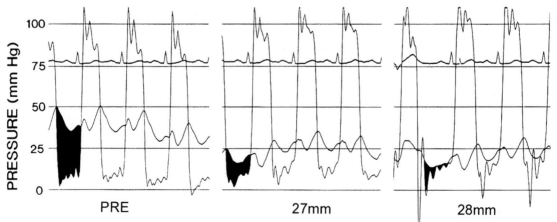

Figure 25.4 Before valvuloplasty, there is a large transmitral valve pressure gradient, filled in black in the first diastolic period in the prevalvuloplasty tracing. After a 27-mm balloon inflation, the transmitral valve pressure gradient is significantly reduced, and following a 28-mm diameter balloon inflation, the gradient is nearly resolved. (From Feldman T, Carroll JD, Herrmann HC, et al. Effect of balloon size and stepwise inflation technique on the results of Inoue mitral commissurotomy. *Cathet Cardiovasc Diagn* 1993;28:200.)

view, another confirmation of improvement of mitral valve orifice area can be measured. The accuracy of Doppler measurements during valvuloplasty can be variable, but color Doppler assessment is the method of choice for sequential evaluation of the degree of mitral regurgitation (31). When Doppler echocardiography is not available in the catheterization lab, serial left ventriculograms can be done to evaluate the degree of mitral regurgitation. The new appearance of mitral regurgitation or an increase greater than one grade on the 0 to 4 classification of pre-existing mitral regurgitation in general signals an end point of the procedure. Additionally, if the mitral valve area has increased to >2 cm^2, or if the mean gradient has been reduced to <5 mm Hg without a decrease in cardiac output, the procedure has been completed successfully.

In some cases, a single commissure is split during one of the first balloon inflations. This is often the result of asymmetric commissural fusion or calcification. But splitting of a single commissure often makes it difficult to split the second commissure, since the inflated balloon will be displaced into the already opened side of the valve. This typically results in an adequate rather than an excellent postprocedure valve area. With the Inoue balloon, single commissural splitting typically results in a valve area between 1.6 cm^2 and 1.8 cm^2. When both commissures are split, the valve area is more frequently 1.8 cm^2 or greater and frequently >2.0 cm^2. However, the clinical circumstances and anatomic factors of each patient must be considered carefully in determining the end point of the procedure.

Long-Term Hemodynamic Results

Numerous studies have demonstrated the effectiveness of balloon valvuloplasty in increasing mitral valve area (1,16). There is almost always a near doubling of effective mitral valve area, a decrease in left atrial pressure, and usually a slight increase in cardiac output. Over time, there is a gradual decrease in pulmonary artery pressure and pulmonary vascular resistance (32). Longer-term follow-ups of >5 years are now available. These studies show quite satisfactory results for this technique. Table 25.2 looks at the 4- and 5-year

follow-up in patients from four series (33–36). In a fifth series, the National Heart, Lung, and Blood Institute (NHLBI) Balloon Valvuloplasty Registry reported multicenter results in 736 patients older than 18 years who were followed for 4 years (37). The actuarial survival rates at 1, 2, 3, and 4 years were 93%, 90%, 87%, and 84%, respectively. The event-free survival (freedom from death, mitral valve surgery, or repeat balloon valvuloplasty) at 1, 2, 3, and 4 years was 80%, 71%, 66%, and 62%, respectively. Multivariate predictions of mortality were New York Heart Association (NYHA) functional class IV, echocardiographic mitral valve score >12, systolic pulmonary artery pressure >40 mm Hg postprocedure, and left ventricular end-diastolic pressure >15 mm Hg.

Comparison of Percutaneous Balloon Mitral Valvuloplasty and Surgery

Randomized comparisons of percutaneous balloon valvuloplasty with surgical commissurotomy have demonstrated similar acute and long-term results. The equivalence of the various percutaneous commissurotomy approaches with each other, and of percutaneous commissurotomy with surgical commissurotomy, suggest that commissurotomy by any method yields comparable results (38).

Two prospective randomized studies of young patients in India and South Africa compared the clinical and hemodynamic results of percutaneous balloon valvuloplasty with closed surgical valvotomy (39,40). The valvuloplasty results compared favorably with those obtained surgically. In one study, better functional and hemodynamic results occurred in the patients treated with percutaneous balloon valvuloplasty (40). An additional trial looked at 60 patients randomized prospectively to percutaneous balloon valvuloplasty or open surgical commissurotomy (41). Initial mitral valve area increased from a mean of 0.9 to 2.1 cm^2 in the balloon valvuloplasty group and from 0.9 to 2.0 cm^2 in the surgical patients. However, after 3 years the patients treated with balloon valvuloplasty had a higher average mitral valve area (2.4 versus 1.8 cm^2) and a greater likelihood of NYHA class I status (72% versus 57%).

TABLE 25.2

LONG-TERM RESULTS OF BALLOON MITRAL VALVULOPLASTY FOR MITRAL STENOSIS

Author (Reference)	No. of Patients	Mean Age (Years)	Follow-Up (Months)	Survival (%)	Freedom From Operation (%)	NYHA Class I–II and Freedom from Operation
Palacios (33)	327	54	48	90	79	66
Cohen (34)	146	59	60	76	51	—
Pan (35)	350	46	60	94	91	85
Iung (36)	606	46	60	94	74	66

NYHA, New York Heart Association.

Open surgical commissurotomy, closed surgical commissurotomy, and percutaneous balloon valvuloplasty were compared in a trial of 90 patients (42). Short- and long-term (7-year) outcomes were not as good with closed surgical commissurotomy. Mitral valve area was greater after percutaneous balloon valvuloplasty (0.9 to 2.2 cm^2) and open commissurotomy (0.9 to 2.0 cm^2) than closed commissurotomy (0.6 to 1.6 cm^2). Early and late mortality and thromboembolism were similar among the three groups. At 7 years follow-up, NYHA class I was present in 87%, 90%, and 33% of patients for balloon valvuloplasty, open commissurotomy, and closed commissurotomy, respectively. Freedom from repeat intervention at 7 years for the balloon valvuloplasty, open commissurotomy, and closed surgical commissurotomy patients was 90%, 93%, and 53%, respectively.

Complications

In skilled hands, the failure rate of the procedure should be <5%. Failure usually results from the inability to safely puncture the interatrial septum because of anatomic difficulties or, in some cases, to position the balloon catheter successfully across the mitral valve. The procedural mortality rate varies from 0 to 3% in most series (16,43). Hemopericardium related to trans-septal catheterization, atrial puncture, or, rarely, left ventricular apical perforation by the balloon or wires varies in incidence from 0.5 to 10%. Systemic embolization has been encountered in 0.5 to 5% of cases. These complications diminish with increasing operator experience.

Severe mitral regurgitation is fortunately uncommon, ranging in incidence from 2 to 9%, and is related to noncommissural leaflet tearing or chordal rupture. Leaflet tears are largely unpredictable and unpreventable, but chordal rupture can be minimized by careful technique (44). Usually, in these circumstances one or both of the mitral commissures were too tightly fused to be split successfully by the balloon, and the leaflets have torn along noncommissural lines. Most cases of severe mitral regurgitation occur in patients with unfavorable mitral valve anatomy. Same-day surgical mitral valve replacement is necessary in 2 to 3%. Usually even severe mitral regurgitation is well tolerated for a time by the patient, and in the acute setting is usually responsive to intravenous nitroglycerin or nitroprusside. In general, elective surgical replacement rather than repair of the valve will be necessary when severe mitral regurgitation occurs because of the severity of the underlying valvular and subvalvular disease (45).

PULMONIC VALVULOPLASTY

Pulmonary valve stenosis is a relatively common congenital defect. Mild to moderate pulmonary stenosis in children has generally a benign clinical course, with a high rate of survival into adulthood. Therefore, the adult interventional cardiologist will encounter previously undetected and untreated patients who are candidates for balloon valvuloplasty.

Pathophysiology

The typical patient with valvular pulmonic stenosis has a trileaflet valve, with varying degrees of fibrous thickening and fusion of the commissures. These restricted valve leaflets have a characteristic domed-shaped, or conical, appearance during systole on angiography or echocardiography. Bicuspid pulmonic valves are uncommon (<20%), and heavy calcification of the stenotic valve is rare. These features make the stenotic pulmonary valve well suited for balloon valvuloplasty. Other forms of congenital pulmonic stenosis not well suited for valvuloplasty include dysplastic valves (Noonan Syndrome; 46) and patients with primary fibromuscular subvalvular narrowing.

Balloon valvuloplasty evolved from a long surgical experience with mechanical valve dilatation, valvulotomies (Brock procedure), bougies, and finally, under cardiopulmonary bypass, direct incision of fused pulmonic valve commissures. Since the initial balloon valvuloplasty of the pulmonary valve in 1979 with an angiographic balloon catheter, larger-diameter, longer polyethylene balloon catheters have been developed to allow this procedure to be performed successfully and safely in children and adults (47,48). The Inoue balloon may be used as well. The proposed mechanism for successful balloon valvuloplasty is predominantly mechanical separation of congenitally fused commissures. Also, there appears to be in some patients minor tearing of valve leaflets and occasionally avulsion of the cusps.

Patients with moderate pulmonic stenosis and a gradient of 50 to 100 mm Hg who have symptoms of exercise intolerance will probably benefit from balloon valvuloplasty (9). Patients with severe pulmonic stenosis, defined as a gradient >100 mm Hg or those with evidence of right ventricular dysfunction may benefit from balloon valvuloplasty even in the absence of symptoms, because of the significant afterload that the obstructive pulmonary valve places on the right ventricle (49).

Technique

After selection of a symptomatic patient with a moderate or severe gradient across the pulmonary valve by echocardiographic and Doppler evaluation, successful pulmonary valvuloplasty begins with a careful measurement of the pulmonic valve annulus diameter on echo for balloon sizing. A right heart catheterization is done to document the pulmonary valve gradient and to exclude a significant supravalvular or subvalvular component. A 5F sheath may be placed in the left femoral artery for pressure monitoring, and the procedure is performed from the right femoral vein after the introduction of an 8F sheath. A right ventricular angiogram is done in the anteroposterior and lateral projections to determine the exact location of the pulmonary valve and to confirm sizing of the pulmonary annulus. In the lateral projection, right ventriculography demonstrates the morphology of the outflow tract. Subvalvular hypertrophy typically accompanies pulmonic stenosis. In some cases, a secondary subvalvular stenosis results. If on prevalvuloplasty right ventriculography the subvalvular hypertrophy causes near obstruction, relief of the pulmonic stenosis with afterload reduction may allow for muscular obstruction to be accentuated after valvuloplasty. It is important to appreciate this preprocedure, since severe hypotension may result after successful pulmonary valvuloplasty as a consequence of subvalvular dynamic obstruction. This has been referred to as "suicide right ventricle."

For sizing, we generally use a pigtail catheter with markers spaced a centimeter apart to facilitate assessment using quantitative coronary angiography. Single-balloon, double-balloon, and Inoue balloon techniques may be used. For the dual-balloon technique in adult patients, balloon sizes approximating the diameter of the annulus, and then increasing in size are chosen, if necessary, to abolish the gradient. It is often necessary to oversize the calculated annulus diameter by as much as 25%. Both balloons may be inserted via a single femoral vein, which necessitates a sheathless approach. Bilateral venous cannulation allows the use of sheaths. The Inoue balloon is large enough to use a single balloon in most adult patients, with a target inflated diameter 1.2 times larger than the pulmonic annulus.

Following the angiographic localization of the pulmonary valve, the valve is crossed with a dual-lumen balloon flotation catheter. This catheter is useful for measuring the gradient from its end-hole lumen, as well as its side-hole lumen, 5 cm from the tip. Pressure gradients can be measured by this catheter before and after balloon dilatation. Both lumens are passed distally into the pulmonary artery, and for the double-balloon technique two 0.038-inch heavy-duty exchange-length guidewires are passed into the distal pulmonary artery, one through the end-hole lumen and one through the side-hole lumen. The catheter is then removed, leaving the wires in place in the pulmonary artery exiting the body through the femoral vein. The pulmonary valvuloplasty balloons, having been previously purged of air and filled with diluted radiographic contrast, are then inserted one after the other in tandem into the femoral vein. They are then positioned one at a time with the aid of both the external markers and the balloon markers so that the midportion of the valvuloplasty balloon is straddling the pulmonary valve. When both balloon catheters are in place, they are rapidly and simultaneously filled with the dilute radiographic contrast. The balloons are filled until the "waist" is seen to disappear on fluoroscopy. The balloon catheters are emptied and then withdrawn from the body sequentially over the two heavy-duty

J wires. A 12F sheath is introduced into the femoral vein over the guidewires, and the dual-lumen catheter is reintroduced through the sheath and positioned across the pulmonary valve over one of the wires. That guidewire is then removed, and a careful determination made of the residual valvular gradient, if any.

In a successful balloon pulmonic valvuloplasty, the valvular gradient is almost always nearly abolished. However, on occasion the operator will encounter a previously undetected sub-valvular gradient, after the valvular gradient has been eliminated (so-called suicidal right ventricle). When the subvalvular gradient is severe enough to cause hypotension, beta-blockade and volume expansion must be rapidly instituted. This subvalvular gradient will usually diminish and disappear over the ensuing weeks, with regression of the right ventricular hypertrophy. Repeat dilatation of the pulmonary valve should be performed with larger balloons only when there is a persistent and significant *valvular* gradient. Repeat dilatation of the pulmonary valve for a subvalvular gradient is contraindicated.

Clinical Results and Complications

The impressive acute and long-term results of this procedure in adolescents and adults make balloon valvuloplasty the treatment of choice for valvular pulmonic stenosis. A pooled analysis involving 784 patients of all ages showed that the clinical success was achieved with balloon valvuloplasty in 98% of patients (50). Procedural mortality was <0.5%, and the average peak valve gradient fell from 85 mm Hg to 33 mm Hg. Several series have looked at the long-term efficacy of balloon valvuloplasty. Chen and colleagues (51) reported a series of 53 adolescent and adult patients, age 13 to 55, treated between 1985 and 1995. The systolic pressure gradient across the pulmonary valve fell from 91 ± 46 to 38 ± 32 mm Hg after the procedure. On late follow-up (average of 7 years), the gradient had fallen further. Seven of 53 patients developed pulmonary insufficiency immediately after the valvuloplasty, but none had this complication at late follow-up evaluation.

Procedural complications are rare during the procedure. Pulmonic valvuloplasty is generally planned as an outpatient procedure. Patients may have arrhythmias and occasional hypotension during balloon inflation. Transient right bundle branch block has been observed. Despite the use of large balloon catheters, bleeding and vascular complications are infrequent because this procedure is done through the femoral vein.

BALLOON AORTIC VALVULOPLASTY

Dilatation of the stenotic aortic valve, whether by surgical technique or percutaneous balloon, has not enjoyed the same level of success as balloon therapy for the pulmonic and mitral valves. Surgical mechanical dilatation of the stenotic adult aortic valve has been attempted since the 1950s, but the various valvulotomy approaches have failed to provide a significant solution for the problem of calcific aortic stenosis and have largely been abandoned in favor of aortic valve replacement in acceptable surgical candidates.

Noncalcific Aortic Stenosis

Percutaneous balloon aortic valvuloplasty was first performed in children and young adults by Lababidi (52) in 1984. Balloon dilatation resulted in a significant decrease in peak aortic valve gradient. Considerable experience exists using balloon valvuloplasty in children and adolescents with noncalcified congenital stenotic aortic valves, with excellent short-term and satisfactory long-term results (53–55). The predominantly fibrotic nature of these congenitally stenotic valves makes them well suited for balloon valvuloplasty (9). The procedure is effective 80 to 90% of the time with a mortality of approximately 0.7%. Survival at 8 years has been reported at 95% with a need for repeat intervention of 25% at 4 years and 50% at 8 years (56). There may be a role for balloon valvuloplasty in the young adult without significant valve calcification. One study of young adults ages 17 to 40 (mean age 23) with congenital aortic stenosis showed that balloon aortic valvuloplasty produced a significant reduction in the gradient across the aortic valve and an increase in the aortic valve area (57). In this series, there were no deaths or embolic cerebrovascular events. Intermediate follow-up at 38 months showed that 50% of patients required no further intervention. The absence of significant valve calcification is an important predictor of a good short- and long-term result.

Calcific Aortic Stenosis

The more typical patient encountered by the adult cardiologist is the elderly patient with acquired calcific aortic stenosis. Although experience with successful balloon valvuloplasty for this condition dates back to 1986 (58,59), the procedure has a limited role at present because of limited durability owing to the high rate of recurrence or restenosis. Virtually all symptomatic patients with calcific aortic stenosis should undergo aortic valve replacement as the treatment of choice. There are, however, certain settings where balloon valvuloplasty may play an important palliative role in patients who are poor candidates for immediate valve replacement. These are listed in Table 25.3. Balloon aortic valvuloplasty is useful in the patient presenting with cardiogenic shock owing to aortic stenosis and can serve as a successful bridge to definitive surgery in these hemodynamically unstable patients (60). It may also be used for palliation in patients with serious comorbid conditions. The technique is also used in patients with critical aortic stenosis who require urgent noncardiac surgery, if it is felt that more conservative medical therapy presents excessive risk. Typical examples include patients undergoing hemicolectomy for colon cancer or

operations of a similar magnitude. Last, valvuloplasty may be useful as a diagnostic tool. Patients with low gradient, low cardiac output, and markedly depressed ejection fraction do poorly with surgical valve replacement. Balloon valvuloplasty may be used to assess the potential for improvement in left ventricular function: those patients who do not improve represent a group who have underlying cardiomyopathy, while those who do improve after balloon dilatation generally have a good outcome with subsequent aortic valve replacement.

Mechanism of Improved Aortic Orifice Area

Postmortem and intraoperative dilatations have demonstrated how balloon aortic valvuloplasty improves the adult aortic valve with calcific degenerative aortic stenosis (61). Balloon dilatation increases the mobility of leaflets, thus enlarging the aortic valve orifice. The mechanism of dilatation appears predominantly to be fracturing of the calcific aortic valve nodules (61). In addition, in some elderly patients there is rheumatic disease with superimposed calcification, and there may be separation of postinflammatory fused commissures that contributes to the results of dilatation. The likely mechanism of restenosis is fusion of the cracks or crevices in calcific nodules on the aortic leaflets. The balloon dilatation process rarely dislodges the amorphus calcific deposits, and embolization is rare. The fractured calcific nodules may heal with fibrosis, which is probably the most common occurrence, and in some cases even with ossification and true bone formation (62).

Technique

The retrograde aortic technique for balloon aortic valvuloplasty is the one most commonly used. One or both femoral arteries may be used. A 5F pigtail catheter is inserted from the left femoral artery and positioned in the ascending aorta for pressure monitoring and gradient determination. Right heart catheterization is done from the left femoral vein. A balloon flotation thermodilution catheter is placed in the pulmonary artery and remains there throughout the procedure to allow

---

TABLE 25.3

INDICATIONS FOR BALLOON AORTIC VALVULOPLASTY IN ADULTS

Cardiogenic shock
Bridge to aortic valve surgery
Symptomatic critical aortic stenosis requiring emergent
   noncardiac surgery
Poor surgical risk, age >90 years
Diagnostic test in low-gradient/low-output setting
Congenital aortic stenosis
Rheumatic aortic stenosis

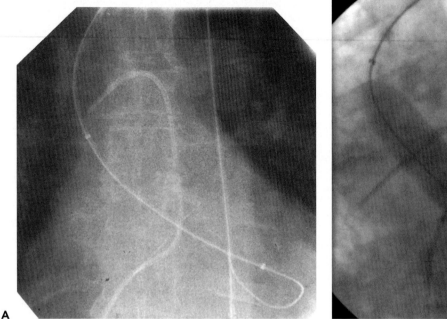

A

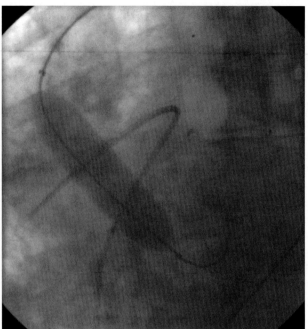

B

Figure 25.5 **A.** Anteroposterior projection shows passage of the deflated aortic valvuloplasty balloon across a stenotic aortic valve. Balloon markers are positioned so that the balloon straddles the calcified aortic valve. **B.** Anteroposterior projection showing an inflated aortic valvuloplasty balloon across the stenotic aortic valve. The tip of the guidewire has been formed into a concentric curve to minimize the potential for left ventricular apical trauma.

determination of the cardiac output. Using the right femoral artery, an 8F sheath is introduced to allow left heart catheterization to be performed. A 0.035-inch or 0.038-inch straight-tipped guidewire is used to cross the aortic valve, advanced through an angled pigtail catheter, a left Amplatz catheter, or a specialized catheter designed to cross the aortic valve (63). The aortic valve gradient is measured and aortic valve area determined using the Gorlin formula. Patients may be heparinized prior to any attempt to cross the aortic valve.

Following these prevalvuloplasty measurements, a heavy-duty 0.038-inch exchange-length (300-cm) guidewire, shaped with a pigtail or ram's horn curve at its tip, is inserted into the left ventricle. The wire tip is shaped by pulling the wire between a finger and the edge of a hemostat, and helps it lie benignly in the left ventricular apex (without perforation or undue ventricular arrhythmia). The previously placed left ventricular catheter is removed, and a 12F sheath is placed over this wire into the femoral artery. It is important that the groin be anesthetized adequately to avoid discomfort and possible vagal reaction during sheath exchange. Through the sheath, the previously prepared dilatation balloon is advanced over the guidewire. To keep its profile minimal, the balloon (purged of air) is kept completely deflated by constant negative pressure from a syringe and is introduced into the sheath with rotation.

Under fluoroscopy, using two operators, the heavy-duty guidewire is kept in the left ventricle as the balloon valvuloplasty catheter is advanced and positioned to straddle the aortic valve. Using the proximal and distal markers of the balloon, the operator attempts to place the midballoon at the level of the calcific aortic valve. Figure 25.5 illustrates the unfilled balloon straddling the aortic valve.

In most normal-sized adults with an adequate aortic valve annulus, we begin with a 20 or 22-mm-diameter/4- to 6-cm-long balloon. In very small or frail patients, the operator can start with an 18-mm balloon or (very rarely) a 15-mm balloon. The balloon is filled with diluted contrast media using either a very large syringe or angioplasty end-deflator-type device. Care must be taken to maintain balloon position within the valve orifice to achieve an effective dilatation. The balloon catheter may tend to jump either forward or backward with the force of ventricular systole. To achieve a stable balloon position, the balloon is filled slowly as its position is fixed. If still in good position, the balloon is filled rapidly to its maximum diameter. A brief burst of rapid ventricular pacing (180–220 bpm) may also be used to reduce balloon movement by temporarily minimizing left ventricular ejection. We constantly monitor the ECG for arrhythmia and ischemia, as well as aortic pressure. If tolerated clinically, the balloon can be left inflated for 15 to 20 seconds. It is then withdrawn into the aorta as it begins to deflate, maintaining guidewire position in the left ventricle. Pulling the balloon back immediately after full inflation is reached minimizes the duration of hypotension caused by obstruction of the aortic valve. A period of stabilization to allow blood pressure and ECG changes to return to baseline should be allowed before further dilatations.

It is often necessary to exert considerable force on these balloons to expand them fully and relieve the "waist" caused by the stenotic aortic valve, and it is difficult to achieve full inflation of these large balloons using the 20-mL syringe that is needed to provide adequate volume. If the balloon is connected to the larger syringe with a short pressure tubing and a high-pressure stopcock, the side arm of the stopcock can be attached to a 10-mL syringe filled with dilute contrast to boost the inflation after the larger syringe has been used to its maximal volume (64). This maneuver of adding additional contrast to the balloon through the side arm of the three-way stopcock, however, can easily result in balloon rupture. A first balloon inflation with the large syringe only to test the patient's response to balloon inflation, followed by second or third inflations boosted to a maximum balloon diameter, is a careful approach to achieving optimal use of each size balloon. After several dilatations with a single balloon or after balloon rupture (a frequent occurrence), the balloon then is withdrawn through the sheath, leaving the exchange-length, heavy-duty wire in place. It is frequently necessary to remove the 12F sheath along with the deflated valvuloplasty balloon, since valvuloplasty balloons do not always rewrap adequately to allow removal through the 12F sheath. A 12.5F sheath makes balloon withdrawal easier.

A pigtail catheter is then reintroduced over the guidewire back into the left ventricle, and measurements of the pressure gradient and cardiac output are repeated. The aortic valve area is calculated. Our usual goal is to increase the aortic valve area by >100% and to achieve a valve area of at least 1 cm^2. If a desirable result has not been achieved, we then change to a 23-mm-diameter balloon and repeat the procedure (a 14F sheath is usually necessary to accommodate a 23–24-mm balloon). If an adequate result is still not achieved, a dual balloon technique (using a pair of 15- or 18-mm balloons if aortic annulus size permits) can be attempted, although this requires accessing the contralateral femoral artery for introduction of the second balloon. Pressure is monitored through the side arm of the 12F sheaths during the procedure. Figure 25.6 illustrates the dual balloon technique, and Fig. 25.7 shows the progressive reduction in gradient with single-, followed by dual-, balloon valvuloplasty.

Following a successful procedure, patients are placed in a recovery area or in the coronary care unit for continued observation. The femoral artery sheaths are removed using suture closure devices, or when the coagulation parameters are in range, with hemostasis maintained by a Fem-Stop device. Since prolonged compression is needed, rigid clamps should be avoided.

An alternative approach is to use an antegrade trans-septal route (65, 65a). After right femoral venous and trans-septal access, a balloon flotation catheter is used to pass through the left atrium, left ventricle, and into the aorta (Fig. 25.6B). A wire is exchanged into the descending aorta (Fig. 25.6C). An extra-support guidewire is passed into the descending aorta and snared from the arterial side for stability (Fig. 25.6D).

The valvuloplasty balloon catheter is then maneuvered over the guidewire antegrade and inflated in the aortic valve.

The technique is more complex than the retrograde approach. After transseptal access is accomplished via a 14F venous sheath, a single-lumen balloon flotation catheter is passed across the mitral valve into the left ventricle. With the balloon inflated, preshaped curved guidewires can be introduced to encourage the balloon to make a curve around the left ventricular apex and take a course upward toward the aortic valve. The valve is crossed antegrade, sometimes with the balloon deflated to facilitate passage across the stenotic valve. Once in the ascending aorta, a guidewire can be advanced through the aortic arch into the descending aorta. Via a 6F or 7F arterial sheath, a 10-mm gooseneck snare is used to grasp the wire in the descending aorta. The wire can be either exteriorized and clamped on the arterial side or left within the snare to tightly fix the wire in the descending aorta. The balloon catheter and Mullins sheath are withdrawn over the wire through the 14F femoral sheath. It is possible to advance an Inoue balloon catheter (stretched into the left atrium, and then unstretched as it is advanced through the left atrium, across the mitral valve, around the left ventricular apex, and into the aortic valve). The balloon is inflated and deflated rapidly (Fig. 25.6E). After between one and three balloon inflations, the balloon can be withdrawn and a pigtail catheter replaced in the left ventricle over the wire to determine the final hemodynamic results. Special care must be taken to remove the transcirculatory guidewire sheathed within a diagnostic catheter, at least into the aortic arch and ideally into the descending aorta. If the wire is pulled without the protective covering of a plastic catheter, tremendous friction will be encountered, which may cause damage to the aortic or mitral valves!

Advantages of the antegrade approach include the use of a large-caliber venous (rather than arterial) puncture with subsequently much easier puncture management. The venous puncture may be "preclosed" with a percutaneous suture closure device (see Chapter 4). A 6F closer is adequate for this purpose. Also, a relatively larger balloon can be introduced in this manner compared with the retrograde approach. The Inoue balloon can be inflated to 24 to 26 mm diameter without having to exchange balloons. The inflate/deflate cycle of the Inoue balloon is also more rapid than a conventional large balloon and thus results in a shorter period of hemodynamic instability during balloon inflations. The transcirculatory wire, however, can prop open the mitral or aortic valves in some patients, causing regurgitation with slowly progressive hypotension. In this situation, the technique must be abandoned and the retrograde approach used. Another advantage of the antegrade approach is lack of dependence on the arterial circulation for passage of catheters in a population where diffuse arterial disease is relatively common. Even so, some patients will have a progressive decline or lack of recovery of systolic pressure after balloon inflations using either the antegrade or retrograde techniques, and it may then be wise to accept

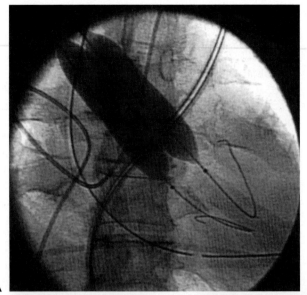

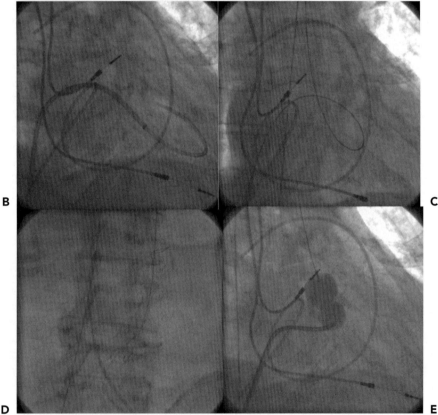

Figure 25.6 A. Balloon aortic valvuloplasty using the double-balloon technique in a 94-year-old woman who presented with syncope and failure. Full inflation of two 18-mm-diameter, 5.5-cm-long Scimed balloons across the stenotic aortic valve. **B.** A Mullins sheath has been passed through the left atrium across the mitral valve. The tip marker can be seen in the left ventricular inflow. Through the Mullins sheath, a 7F single-lumen balloon catheter has been advanced into the left ventricle and looped in the apex to point upward toward the aortic valve. The silhouette of the inflated balloon at the tip of the catheter can be noted just within the curve of the pulmonary artery catheter. **C.** A wire has been passed through the 7F balloon tip catheter, traversing the left ventricle and passing into the aortic arch and then the descending aorta. **D.** The proximal part of a 0.032-inch wire can be seen passing through a 14F sheath in the inferior vena cava *(left)*. The J curve of the wire can be seen in the descending aorta *(right)*. A microsnare has been passed over the distal end of the wire in the descending aorta. The snare will be anchored on the wire and left in place in the descending aorta to stabilize the wire for balloon passage through the left ventricle into the aortic valve. **E.** The inflated Inoue balloon is seen in the calcified aortic valve leaflets. The wire loop has been straightened in the left ventricle during inflation. After balloon deflation, the balloon will be pulled back into the left atrium and the loop re-established in the left ventricle.

the result of the first balloon inflation. Larger valve areas have been obtained with the antegrade approach, possibly because larger balloons can be used or because the shape of the Inoue balloon conforms better to the sinus of Valsalva.

Clinical Results and Complications

In the large Mansfield balloon aortic valve registry, data were collected from 27 clinical centers across the United States and Europe from 6,742 patients with calcific aortic

stenosis undergoing balloon aortic valvuloplasty between 1986 and 1987 (66). Balloon aortic valvuloplasty resulted in an increase in aortic valve area from 0.5 ± 0.18 to 0.81 ± 0.18 cm^2, and a decrease in mean aortic valve pressure gradient from 60 ± 24 to 30 ± 14 mm Hg. There was also an accompanying increase in cardiac output from 3.86 ± 0.55 to 4.01 ± 0.51 L/minute. Complications were experienced in 22.6% of patients, including a procedural death rate of 4.9%, death within 7 days of 2.6%, emboli 2.2%, ventricular perforation 1.4 %, and emergency aortic

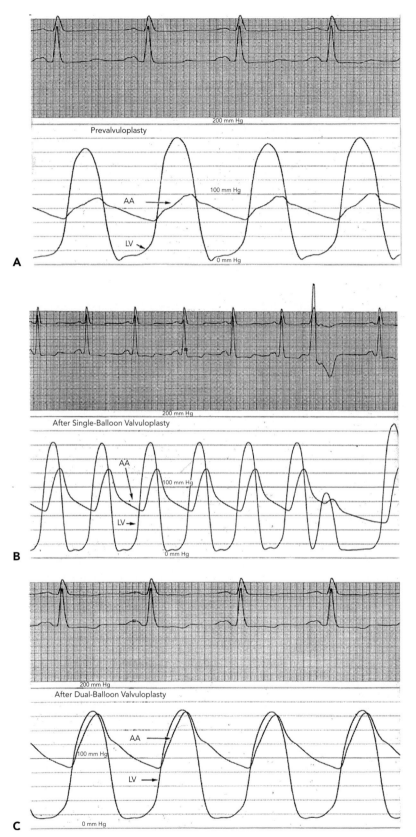

Figure 25.7 Balloon aortic valvuloplasty in an elderly patient with severe calcific aortic stenosis. **A.** Baseline pressure gradient across the stenotic aortic valve measured with one catheter in the left ventricle (LV) and a separate pigtail catheter in the ascending aorta (AA). There is a 58-mm Hg mean gradient and an 80-mm Hg peak-to-peak gradient across the valve. **B.** A reduction in the aortic valve gradient after a series of progressive single-balloon dilatations of the aortic valve. **C.** A marked reduction in aortic valve gradient after dual-balloon valvuloplasty.

valve replacement 1.2%. The NHLBI balloon valvuloplasty registry enrolled patients from 1987 to 1989 at 24 clinical centers (67). Similar results were obtained, with balloon aortic valvuloplasty increasing aortic valve area from 0.5 ± 2 to $0.8 \pm .5$ cm^2, decreasing aortic valve pressure gradient from 57 ± 30 to 29 ± 13 mm Hg, and increasing cardiac output from 3.9 ± 1.2 to 4.1 ± 1.2 L/minute.

The most common complication was local vascular injury, requiring surgical repair in 5.7% of patients (68). The requirement for transfusions has been significantly diminished by the use of percutaneous suture closure for management of the large-caliber arterial puncture necessary for retrograde aortic valvuloplasty. Perclose devices must be preplaced after arterial access is obtained (69,70). After placing a 6F or 8F sheath in the femoral artery, the sheath is exchanged for a Perclose device, whose sutures are deployed but not tied. A wire is replaced in the Perclose device, and an exchange is made for a 12F or 14F sheath for valvuloplasty. At the conclusion of the procedure, a wire is replaced in the sheath so that vascular access can be protected while the Perclose knots are tied. If hemostasis is secure, the wire is removed and the knots tightened. If hemostasis with Perclose fails, the sheath can be replaced and a compression device can be used. In one report, this approach decreased the need for transfusions after aortic valvuloplasty from 23% to 0% of patients (70). Preclosure techniques may also be used in the same manner for large-bore venous punctures for antegrade aortic valvuloplasty, mitral valvuloplasty, or pulmonic valvuloplasty.

Overall complications include procedural death (2%), cardiac arrest (5%), emergency aortic valve replacement (1%), left ventricular perforation (2%), embolic stroke and systemic emboli (1%). Ventricular arrhythmias and left bundle branch block are very commonly induced during the procedure; however, both are usually transient. In patients with underlying bundle branch block, it is useful to place a temporary right ventricular pacemaker for aortic valvuloplasty procedures.

Long-Term Results

Restenosis with recurrent symptoms is common in the first year following balloon valvuloplasty in the adult with calcific aortic stenosis (71–73). The mean duration of relief of symptoms is about 1 year. In the NHLBI-sponsored balloon valvuloplasty registry, the survival at 1, 2, and 3 years was 55%, 35%, and 23%, respectively, in the 674 patients undergoing balloon aortic valvuloplasty (67). The 1-year survival rate in the Mansfield registry of 492 patients was 64%, with an event-free survival rate of 43% (66,74). Therefore, it must be emphasized that, when at all feasible, definitive aortic valve replacement is the technique of choice for managing the adult patient with severe calcific aortic stenosis.

Short-term clinical improvements associated with balloon aortic valvuloplasty may be accompanied by improve-

ment in systolic and diastolic left ventricular function in some patients (75). Patients with significantly depressed left ventricular function undergoing this procedure have a very poor long-term prognosis (76). In the patient with cardiogenic shock who has been stabilized with successful balloon aortic valvuloplasty, cardiac surgery with definitive aortic valve replacement should be undertaken soon after the patient stabilizes (60,77).

PERCUTANEOUS VALVE REPLACEMENT AND REPAIR

Surgical valve replacement and repair has been the gold standard for valve disease for several decades. Recently, however, great progress has been made in adapting these surgical approaches to the percutaneous arena. Recently, both pulmonic and aortic valve replacement have been accomplished using catheter techniques (78–81). Bioprosthetic valve leaflets are mounted on balloon-expandable or self-expanding stents and delivered within the diseased valve using modifications of standard angioplasty and valvuloplasty techniques.

Percutaneous prosthetic treatment for pulmonic stenosis has been pioneered in children with congenital heart disease who have been previously treated with Fontan conduits in the pulmonary circulation. These conduits contain a porcine prosthetic valve that degenerates as the children age. Reoperation for degeneration of the pulmonic prosthetic is frequently necessary in patients who have already undergone two or three prior surgical procedures for their congenital heart disease. As a non-surgical alternative, Bonhoeffer et al. have adapted a bovine jugular venous valve prosthesis for stent delivery (78,79). Successful placement of the bioprosthetic valve has been performed consistently in more than 80 patients with excellent hemodynamic and angiographic results. The durability of the prosthesis will become better known as time passes.

Aortic stenosis has also been successfully treated with percutaneous prosthetic valve therapy. Cribier et al. have used equine pericardial leaflets placed in a balloon-expandable stent to treat aortic stenosis in elderly patients deemed nonsurgical or poor surgical candidates (80,81). Both antegrade and retrograde techniques have been utilized for delivery of the aortic valve prosthesis. Each approach has benefits and limitations. The profile of the aortic valve prosthesis was 24F in its initial iterations, which made use of the antegrade transvenous approach attractive, although delivery of a large prosthesis through the turns involved in traversing the left atrium and left ventricular apex en route to the aortic valve may be difficult. The retrograde approach requires this large 24F arterial sheath, and, in some cases, the large profile of the valve may not be able to cross the native aortic valve in the retrograde direction, necessitating either implantation in the descending aorta or removal of the prosthesis surgically. More recently, a second percutaneous aortic valve replacement utilizing pericardial leaflets mounted on a self-expanding stent (CoreValve, Irvine CA) has entered clinical investigation, and several more percutaneous aortic valve replacement devices are under development.

It is clear that the development of percutaneous valve prosthetic devices will move rapidly and that improvement in the profile of the devices and delivery systems will occur incrementally. The durability of valve prostheses that have been crimped on a balloon and then compressed by a relatively high-pressure balloon expansion may not be assumed to be similar to surgically implanted tissue valves, and experience with the long-term results of these patients will take a great deal of time to develop.

Although we have already discussed the success of balloon valvuloplasty for the treatment of mitral stenosis, mitral regurgitation previously has been treatable only by surgical methods (placement of an annuloplasty ring or the edge-to-edge Alfieri stitch repair). Percutaneous approaches to mitral valve repair have now been used successfully, and both annuloplasty and edge-to-edge repair approaches in active investigation. Annuloplasty may be accomplished via the coronary sinus, whose course parallels the mitral annulus, by placing devices that tension or reshape the coronary sinus to cause contraction of the mitral annulus, with displacement of the posterior mitral annulus toward the septum. Several of these devices have shown efficacy in preclinical experience and are now entering clinical trials. Some of the challenges involved with this approach include the variability of the coronary sinus in its anatomic relation to the mitral valve annulus, the course of the circumflex coronary artery and its branches over or under the coronary sinus, and the potential for injury to the thin-walled sinus. To overcome those limitations, trans-ventricular approaches are also under development, which involve plication of the mitral annulus percutaneously via annular sutures placed by a retrograde approach (across the aortic valve and into the space between the posterior leaflet and the lateral left ventricular wall).

Another surgical approach for mitral valve repair involves the plication of the free edges of the two mitral leaflets using a suture or pledget, with a resultant bow tie or double-orifice mitral valve. This edge-to-edge technique was pioneered by Alfieri in the early 1990s (82). A percutaneous method to deliver a clip to the mitral leaflets via a trans-septal approach has been used successfully in a 40-patient Phase 1 trial (83). The resultant double-orifice repair is similar to the surgical repair, ultimately being maintained by fibrosis of the clip with a tissue bridge. The procedure is done using transesophageal echocardiographic guidance so the results of clip placement can be evaluated during the procedure, in a manner analogous to the evaluation of the results of surgical repair on the operating table. In the event that adequate control of the mitral regurgitation is not achieved, a second clip may be used, or the clip may be withdrawn with no apparent harm to the mitral leaflets. The randomized trial comparing percutaneous edge-to-edge mitral repair to surgical mitral repair is now underway.

From the above discussion, it is clear that percutaneous treatments for valvular heart disease (84) are poised for major technical and clinical growth over the next decade. In some cases, the percutaneous approach may be a treatment for patients with critical valve disease and no (or probability of high risk) surgical option, a treatment for patients with regurgitant lesions at an earlier point in their natural history (before surgical repair would typically be employed, in an effort to prevent progressive ventricular dysfunction), or perhaps as a true alternative to surgical valve correction (akin to what percutaneous coronary intervention now offers relative to bypass surgery). Issues regarding optimal device design, indications, safety, and efficacy still need to be worked out, however, before the position of these exciting new catheter-based therapies can be established relative to conventional medical and surgical treatments.

REFERENCES

1. Carroll JD, Feldman T. Percutaneous mitral balloon valvotomy and the new demographics of mitral stenosis. *JAMA* 1993;207:1731.
2. Inoue K, Owaki T, Nakamura T, et al. Clinical application of transvenous mitral commissurotomy by a new balloon catheter. *J Thorac Cardiovasc Surg* 1984;87:394.
3. Lock JE, Kalilullah M, Shrivastava S, et al. Percutaneous catheter commissurotomy in rheumatic mitral stenosis. *N Engl J Med* 1985;313:1515.
4. Inoue K, Feldman T. Percutaneous transvenous mitral commissurotomy using Inoue balloon catheter. *Cathet Cardiovasc Diagn* 1993;28:119.
5. McKay RG, Lock JE, Safian RD, et al. Balloon dilatation of mitral stenosis in adult patients: postmortem and percutaneous mitral valvuloplasty studies. *J Am Coll Cardiol* 1987;9:723–731.
6. Lau KW, Ding ZP, Gao W, et al. Percutaneous balloon mitral valvuloplasty in patients with mitral restenosis after previous surgical commissurotomy. *Eur Heart J* 1996;17:1367.
7. Gupta S, Vora A, Lokhandwalla Y, et al. Percutaneous balloon mitral valvotomy in mitral restenosis. *Eur Heart J* 1996;17:1560.
8. Lokhandwalla YY, Banker D, Vora AM, et al. Emergent balloon mitral valvotomy in patients presenting with cardiac arrest, cardiogenic shock or refractory pulmonary edema. *J Am Coll Cardiol* 1998;32:154.
9. ACC/AHA guidelines for the management of patients with valvular heart disease. A report of the American College of Cardiology/ American Heart Association. Task Force on Practice Guidelines (Committee on Management of Patients with Valvular Heart Disease). *J Am Coll Cardiol* 1998;32:1486–1588.
10. Tessier P, Mercier LA, Burelle D, Bonan R. Results of percutaneous mitral commissurotomy in patients with a left atrial appendage thrombus detected by transesophageal echocardiography. *J Am Soc Echocardiogr* 1994;7:394–399.
11. Padial LR, Freitas N, Sagie A, et al. Echocardiography can predict which patients will develop severe mitral regurgitation after percutaneous mitral valvulotomy. *J Am Coll Cardiol* 1996;27:1225.
12. Cannan CR, Nishimura RA, Reeder GS, et al. Echocardiographic assessment of commissural calcium: a simple predictor of outcome after percutaneous mitral balloon valvotomy. *J Am Coll Cardiol* 1997;29:175.
13. Fatkin D, Roy P, Morgan JJ, Feneley MP. Percutaneous balloon mitral valvotomy with the Inoue single-balloon catheter: commissural morphology as a determinant of outcome. *J Am Coll Cardiol* 1993;21:390–397.
14. Levin TN, Feldman T, Bednarz J, Carroll JD, Lang RM. Transesophageal echocardiographic evaluation of mitral valve

morphology to predict outcome after balloon mitral valvotomy. *Am J Cardiol* 1994;73:707–710.

15. Wilkins GT, Weyman AE, Abascal VM, et al. Percutaneous balloon dilatation of the mitral valve: an analysis of echocardiographic variables related to outcome and the mechanism of dilatation. *Br Heart J* 1988;60:299.

16. Iung B, Cormier B, Ducimetiere P, et al. Immediate results of percutaneous mitral commissurotomy. A predictive model on a series of 1,514 patients. *Circulation* 1996;94:2124.

17. Stefanadis CI, Stratos CG, Lambrou SG, et al. Retrograde non-transseptal balloon mitral valvuloplasty: immediate results and intermediate long-term outcome in 441 cases—a multicenter experience. *J Am Coll Cardiol* 1998;32:1009–1016.

18. al Zaibag M, Ribeiro PA, al Kasab S, et al. Percutaneous double balloon mitral valvotomy for rheumatic mitral valve stenosis. *Lancet* 1986;1:757–761.

19. Vahanian A, Michel PL, Cormier B, et al. Results of percutaneous mitral commissurotomy in 200 patients. *Am J Cardiol* 1989;63:847–852.

20. Tuzcu EM, Block PC, Palacios IF, et al. Comparison of early versus late experience with percutaneous mitral balloon valvuloplasty. *J Am Coll Cardiol* 1991;17:1121–1124.

21. Rihal CS, Holmes DR. Percutaneous balloon mitral valvuloplasty: issues involved in comparing techniques. *Cathet Cardiovasc Diagn* 1994;2:8–15.

22. Bonhoeffer P, Piechaud JF, Sidi D, et al. Mitral dilatation with the Multi-Track system: an alternative approach. *Cathet Cardiovasc Diagn* 1995;36:189–193.

23. Cribier A, Rath PC, Letac B. Percutaneous mitral valvotomy with a metal dilatator [letter]. *Lancet* 1997;349:1967.

24. Zaki AM, Kasem HH, Bakhoum S, et al. Comparison of early results of percutaneous metallic mitral commissurotome with Inoue balloon technique in patients with high mitral echocardiographic scores. *Catheter Cardiovasc Intervent* 2002;57:312–317.

25. Feldman T, Herrmann HC, Inoue K. Technique of percutaneous transvenous mitral commissurotomy using the Inoue balloon catheter. *Cathet Cardiovasc Diagn* 1994;2:26–34.

26. Roth BR, Block PC, Palacios IF. Predictors of increased mitral regurgitation after percutaneous mitral balloon valvotomy. *Cathet Cardiovasc Diagn* 1990;20:17–21.

27. Yamabe T, Nagata S, Ishikura F, Kimura K, Miyatake K. Influence of intraballoon pressure on development of severe mitral regurgitation after percutaneous transvenous mitral commissurotomy. *Cathet Cardiovasc Diagn* 1994;31:270–276.

28. Goel PK, Garg N, Sinha N. Pressure zone used and the occurrence of mitral regurgitation in Inoue balloon mitral commissurotomy. *Cathet Cardiovasc Diagn* 1998;43:141–146.

29. Syed, Z, Salinger MH, Feldman T. Alterations in left atrial pressure and compliance during balloon mitral valvuloplasty. *Cathet Cardiovasc Intervent* 2004;61:571–579.

30. Levin TN, Feldman T, Carroll JD. Effect of atrial septal occlusion on mitral area after Inoue balloon valvotomy. *Cathet Cardiovasc Diagn* 1994;33:308–314.

31. Otto CM, Davies KB, Holmes DR, et al. Methodologic issues in clinical evaluation of stenosis severity in adults undergoing aortic or mitral balloon valvuloplasty. *Am J Cardiol* 1992;69:1607.

32. Levine MJ, Weinstein JS, Diver DJ, et al. Progressive improvement in pulmonary vascular resistance following percutaneous mitral valvuloplasty. *Circulation* 1989;79:1061–1067.

33. Palacios IF, Tuzcu ME, Weyman AE, et al. Clinical follow-up of patients undergoing percutaneous mitral balloon valvotomy. *Circulation* 1995;91:671–676.

34. Cohen DJ, Kuntz RE, Gordon SPF, et al. Predictors of long-term outcome after percutaneous balloon mitral valvuloplasty. *N Engl J Med* 1992;327:1329–1335.

35. Pan M, Medina A, Lezo JJ, et al. Factors determining late success after mitral balloon valvulotomy. *Am J Cardiol* 1993;71:1181–1186.

36. Iung B, Cormier B, Ducimetiere P, et al. Functional results 5 years after successful percutaneous mitral commissurotomy in a series of 528 patients and analysis of predictive factors. *J Am Coll Cardiol* 1996;27:407–414.

37. Dean LS, Mickel M, Bonan R, et al. Four-year follow-up of patients undergoing percutaneous balloon mitral commissurotomy. A report from the National Heart, Lung, and Blood Institute Balloon Valvuloplasty Registry. *J Am Coll Cardiol* 1996; 28:1452.

38. Kang DH, Park SW, Song JK, et al. Long-term clinical and echocardiographic outcome of percutaneous mitral valvuloplasty: randomized comparison of Inoue and double-balloon techniques. *J Am Coll Cardiol* 2000;35:169–175.

39. Turi ZG, Reyes VP, Raju BS, et al. Percutaneous balloon versus closed commissurotomy for mitral restenosis: a prospective, randomized trial. *Circulation* 1991;83:1179.

40. Patel JJ, Shama D, Mitha AS, et al. Balloon valvuloplasty versus closed commissurotomy for pliable mitral stenosis: a prospective hemodynamic study. *J Am Coll Cardiol* 1991;18:1318.

41. Reyes VP, Raju BS, Wynne J, et al. Percutaneous balloon valvuloplasty compared with open surgical commissurotomy for mitral stenosis. *N Engl J Med* 1994;331:961.

42. Farhat MB, Ayari M, Maatoul F, et al. Percutaneous balloon versus surgical closed and open mitral commissurotomy: Seven-year follow-up results of a randomized trial. *Circulation* 1998;97:245.

43. The National Heart, Lung, and Blood Institute Balloon Valvuloplasty Registry. Complications and mortality of percutaneous balloon mitral commissurotomy. *Circulation* 1992;85:2014–2024.

44. Chern MS, Chang HJ, Lin FC, Wu D. String-plucking as a mechanism of chordal rupture during balloon mitral valvuloplasty using Inoue balloon catheter [see comment]. *Cathet Cardiovasc Intervent* 1999;47:213–217.

45. Acar C, Jebara VA, Grare PH, et al. Traumatic mitral insufficiency following percutaneous mitral dilation of anatomic lesions and surgical implications. *Eur J Cardiothorac Surg* 1992; 6:660–664.

46. Carter JE, Feldman T, Carroll JD. Sustained reversal of right-to-left ASD flow after pulmonic valvuloplasty in an adult. *Eur Heart J* 1994;15:575–576.

47. Semb BKH, Tjonneland S, Stake G, Aabyholm G. Balloon valvulotomy of congenital pulmonary valve stenosis with tricuspid insufficiency. *Cardiovasc Radiol* 1979;2:239.

48. Kan J, White RI, Mitchell SE, Gardner TJ. Percutaneous balloon valvuloplasty: a new method for treating congenital pulmonary valve stenosis. *N Engl J Med* 1982;307:540.

49. Johnson LW, Grossman W, Dalen JE, et al. Pulmonic stenosis in the adult: long-term follow-up results. *N Engl J Med* 1972;287:1159.

50. Stanger P, Cassidy SC, Girod DA, et al. Balloon pulmonary valvuloplasty: results of the Valvuloplasty and Angioplasty of Congenital Anomalies Registry. *Am J Cardiol* 1990;65:775.

51. Chen C-R, Cheng TO, Huant T, et al. Percutaneous balloon valvuloplasty for pulmonic stenosis in adolescents and adults. *N Engl J Med* 1996;335:21.

52. Lababidi Z, Wu JR, Walls JT. Percutaneous balloon aortic valvuloplasty: results in 23 patients. *Am J Cardiol* 1984;53:194.

53. Rocchini AP, Beekman RH, Shachar GB, et al. Balloon aortic valvuloplasty: results of the valvuloplasty and angioplasty of congenital anomalies registry. *Am J Cardiol* 1990;65:784.

54. Rao PS, Thapar MK, Wilson AD, et al. Intermediate-term follow-up results of balloon aortic valvuloplasty in infants and children with special reference to causes of restenosis. *Am J Cardiol* 1989; 64:1356.

55. O'Connor BK, Beekman RB, Rocchini AP, Rosenthal A. Intermediate-term effectiveness of balloon valvuloplasty for congenital aortic stenosis. *Circulation* 1991;84:732.

56. Moore P, Egito E, Mowrey H, et al. Midterm results of balloon dilation of congenital aortic stenosis: predictors of success. *J Am Coll Cardiol* 1996;27:1257.

57. Rosenfeld HM, Landzberg MJ, Perry SB, et al. Balloon aortic valvuloplasty in the young adult with congenital aortic stenosis. *Am J Cardiol* 1994;73:1112.

58. McKay RG, Safian RD, Lock JE, et al. Balloon dilatation of calcific aortic stenosis in elderly patients: post-mortem, intra-operative and percutaneous valvuloplasty studies. *Circulation* 1986;74:119–125.

59. Cribier A, Savin T, Berland J, et al. Percutaneous transluminal balloon valvuloplasty of adult aortic stenosis: report of 92 cases. *J Am Coll Cardiol* 1987;9:381.

60. Smedira NG, Ports TA, Merrick SH, Rankin JS. Balloon aortic valvuloplasty as a bridge to aortic valve replacement in critically ill patients. *Ann Thorac Surg* 1993;55:914–916.

61. Safian RD, Mandell VS, Thurer RE, et al. Post-mortem and intra-operative balloon valvuloplasty of calcific aortic stenosis in elderly patients: mechanisms of successful dilatation. *J Am Coll Cardiol* 1987;9:665–670.

62. Feldman T, Glagov S, Carroll JD: Restenosis following successful balloon valvuloplasty; bone formation in aortic valve leaflets. *Cathet Cardiovasc Diagn* 1993;29:1–7.

63. Feldman T, Carroll JD, Chiu YC. An improved catheter for crossing stenosed aortic valves. *Cathet Cardiovasc Diagn* 1989;16:279–283.

64. Feldman T, Chiu YC, Carroll JD. Single balloon aortic valvuloplasty: increased valve areas with improved technique. *J Invasive Cardiol* 1989;1:295–300.

65. Eisenhauer AC, Hadjipetrou P, Piemonte TC. Balloon aortic valvuloplasty revisited: the role of the Inoue balloon and transseptal antegrade approach. *Cathet Cardiovasc Intervent* 2000; 50:484–491.

65a. Sakata Y, Sayed Y, Salinger MH, Feldman T: Percutaneous balloon aortic valvuloplasty: antegrade transseptal vs. conventional retrograde transarterial approach. *Cathet Cardiovasc Intervent* 2005; 64:314–321.

66. O'Neill WW. Predictors of long-term survival after percutaneous aortic valvuloplasty: report of the Mansfield Valvuloplasty Registry. *J Am Coll Cardiol* 1991;17:193–198.

67. NHLBI Balloon Valvuloplasty Registry Participants. Percutaneous balloon aortic valvuloplasty. Acute and 30-day follow-up results in 674 patients from the NHLBI Balloon Valvuloplasty Registry. *Circulation* 1991;84:2383.

68. Holmes DR Jr, Nishimura RA, Reeder GS. In-hospital mortality after balloon aortic valvuloplasty: frequency and associated factors. *J Am Coll Cardiol* 1991;17:189–192.

69. Feldman T. Percutaneous suture closure for management of large French size arterial and venous puncture. *J Intervent Cardiol* 2000;13:237–242.

70. Solomon LW, Fusman B, Jolly N, Kim A, Feldman T. Percutaneous suture closure for management of large French size arterial puncture in aortic valvuloplasty. *J Invasive Cardiol* 2001;13:592–596.

71. Safian RD, Berman AD, Diver DJ, et al. Balloon aortic valvuloplasty in 170 consecutive patients. *N Engl J Med* 1988;319:125–130.

72. Lieberman EB, Bashore TM, Hermiller JB, et al. Balloon aortic valvuloplasty in adults: failure of procedure to improve long-term survival. *J Am Coll Cardiol* 1995;26:1522–1528.

73. Otto CM, Mickel MC, Kennedy W, et al. Three-year outcome after balloon aortic valvuloplasty: insights into prognosis of valvular aortic stenosis. *Circulation* 1994;89:642–650.

74. Bashore TM, Davidson CJ. Follow-up recatheterization after balloon aortic valvuloplasty. Mansfield Scientific Aortic Valvuloplasty Registry Investigators. *J Am Coll Cardiol* 1991;17:1188–1195.

75. McKay RG, Safian RD, Lock JE, et al. Assessment of left ventricular and aortic valve function after balloon valvuloplasty in adult patients with aortic stenosis. *Circulation* 1987;75:192–203.

76. Davidson CJ, Harrison JK, Leithe ME, et al. Failure of aortic balloon valvuloplasty to result in sustained clinical improvement in patients with depressed left ventricular function. *Am J Cardiol* 1990;65:72–77.

77. Moreno PR, Jang IK, Newell JB, Block PC, Palacios IF. The role of percutaneous aortic balloon valvuloplasty in patients with cardiogenic shock and critical aortic stenosis. *J Am Coll Cardiol* 1994;23:1071–1075.

78. Bonhoeffer P, Boudjemline Y, Qureshi SA, et al. Percutaneous insertion of the pulmonary valve. *J Am Coll Cardiol* 2002;39:1664–1669.

79. Bonhoeffer P, Boudjemline Y, Saliba Z, et al. Percutaneous replacement of pulmonary valve in a right-ventricle to pulmonary-artery prosthetic conduit with valve dysfunction. *Lancet* 2000;356: 1403–1405.

80. Cribier A, Eltchaninoff H, Bash A, et al. Percutaneous transcatheter implantation of an aortic valve prosthesis for calcific aortic stenosis: first human case description. *Circulation* 2002;106:3006–3008.

81. Cribier A, Eltchaninoff H, Tron C, et al. Early experience with percutaneous transcatheter implantation of heart valve prosthesis for the treatment of end-stage inoperable patients with calcific aortic stenosis. *J Am Coll Cardiol* 2004;43:698–703.

82. Maisano F, Torracca L, Oppizzi M, et al. The edge-to-edge technique: a simplified method to correct mitral insufficiency. *Eur J Cardiothorac Surg* 1998;13:240–245.

83. St Goar FG, Fann JI, Komtebedde J, et al. Endovascular edge-to-edge mitral valve repair: short-term results in a porcine model. *Circulation* 2003;108:1990–1993.

84. Vahanian A, Palacios, IF. Percutaneous approaches to valvular disease. *Circulation* 2004;109:1572–1579.

Peripheral Intervention

26

Briain MacNeill   Kenneth Rosenfield

Although the primary focus of cardiovascular specialists remains the diagnosis and treatment of cardiac disorders, they are increasingly adopting a strategy of global vascular management that also involves treating the noncoronary manifestations of atherosclerosis. This is appropriate, given that peripheral arterial disease (PAD) and coronary artery disease (CAD) share the same etiology and risk factors, coexist in the same patients, and may each cause disabling or life-threatening symptoms (stroke, renal ischemia, claudication, or limb loss). Furthermore, treatment of one may be influenced by the other. For example, patients requiring vascular surgery generally have an increased cardiac risk because of the increased prevalence of CAD, patients with severe carotid artery disease have increased incidence of stroke during coronary bypass surgery; and patients with severe renal artery disease and associated hypertension are liable to worsening of underlying cardiac conditions and an increased risk for contrast-induced renal dysfunction during coronary intervention.

With that background, invasive and interventional cardiologists are increasingly undergoing the additional training required to understand the natural history, noninvasive workup, angiography, and therapeutic alternatives (medical, surgical, and catheter based) that are relevant to the management of these conditions. This chapter is one of three on peripheral vascular disease included in this book. The main focus of this chapter is on catheter-based interventional techniques; the reader is also referred to Chapter 14 for additional information on angiography of the aorta and peripheral arteries and to Chapter 34 for integration of clinical, diagnostic, and therapeutic aspects in real-life case profiles, organized in the same head-to-foot sequence of regional techniques.

GENERAL CONSIDERATIONS

The pathophysiologic basis of atherosclerosis of the peripheral arteries is identical to that in coronary arteries and is associated with the same risk factors—positive family history, tobacco smoking, diabetes mellitus, hypertension, hyperlipidemia, advanced age, and inactivity. The estimated prevalence of PAD in people older than 65 years of age is approximately 20%, likely underestimated by the large number of patients whose peripheral vascular disease (PVD) symptoms are overlooked or falsely attributed to other causes (deconditioning, arthritis, sciatica). As is the case in CAD, symptoms related to PAD generally do not occur until the atherosclerotic process has narrowed the vessel diameter by at least 50%; similarly, the mere presence of a lesion ≥50% does not imply that the patient will be symptomatic (i.e., if an ample collateral supply is present).

The range of symptoms depends on the vascular territory involved. In the limbs, the most common symptom is intermittent claudication, described variably as pain, tightness, aching, soreness, hardness, or heaviness that occurs in the calf, buttock, hip, or arch of the foot during ambulation and resolves with rest, similar to the pattern of exertional angina in CAD. This may range from mild lower extremity discomfort during intense exercise to severe symptoms on minimal exertion or even at rest. More advanced ischemia leads to tissue necrosis, manifested as painful ulceration or frank gangrene. In the cerebral circulation, the dominant symptom is transient neurologic dysfunction owing to embolic events or post-stenotic ischemia from underperfusion, or permanent cerebral damage owing to occlusion (stroke). In mesenteric vessels, the extensive collateral circulation generally prevents symptoms from developing until

TABLE 26.1

FACTORS INFLUENCING DECISIONS REGARDING INVASIVE THERAPY FOR PERIPHERAL VASCULAR DISEASE

1. Natural history of the disease (likelihood of progression/ regression)
2. Degree of ischemia (Rutherford category)
3. Current effect of the disease on mortality, morbidity, and lifestyle
4. Anticipated benefit of interventional therapy
5. Anticipated cost
6. Potential for complications
7. Patient preference

several major vessels are occluded or critically narrowed, at which point abdominal angina or bowel infarction may ensue. Renal artery stenosis, in contrast, may cause progressive loss in renal mass and function or severe arterial hypertension via activation of the renin-angiotensin system, since collateral supply is limited. The cardiovascular disease specialist must be familiar with the range of symptoms and findings related to vascular disease in each arterial territory, the natural history, the indications for intervention, and the therapeutic alternatives.

As indicated in Chapter 14, approximately 70% of PAD patients will remain unchanged or even become less symptomatic after 5 to 10 years—with <30% progressing to require intervention and <10% needing amputation. The slow progression of symptoms should thus temper aggressive recommendations for invasive therapy in PAD, except in two unique subgroups: patients with diabetes mellitus (who have a higher likelihood of developing critical limb ischemia and seven times greater chance of progressing to amputation), and patients who develop acute limb ischemia (ALI; 1,2). ALI most commonly occurs as a result of embolic arterial occlusion (usually from a cardiac source such as atrial fibrillation), in situ thrombosis of a diseased native extremity vessel or bypass graft, or spontaneous thrombosis as the result of a hypercoagulable state. The

clinical presentation of acute limb ischemia is typically a dramatic one; there is the acute onset of severe pain, followed shortly thereafter by paresthesia, and ultimately, motor dysfunction (i.e., paralysis). On examination, the extremity is cool, pale, and pulseless. Rutherford and colleagues (3) have described a series of clinical categories of limb ischemia (Table 26.1) with well-defined diagnostic criteria that help determine whether the affected limb is viable, in imminent jeopardy (e.g., threatened), or already irreversibly damaged. These are analogous to the Rutherford criteria for chronic limb ischemia (Table 26.2). (Paradoxically, it is the patient with less underlying atherosclerotic PVD and poorly developed collateral circulation—e.g., the patient with atrial fibrillation who develops sudden embolic occlusion of a normal common femoral or popliteal artery—who develops the most acute ischemia.)

Once the indications for invasive therapy are clear (Table 26.3), and the anatomic substrate has been defined, the choice must be made between conventional surgery and catheter-based techniques. The details of surgical therapy are beyond the scope of this chapter, but typically involve either plaque removal (endarterectomy) or placement of natural (saphenous vein) or prosthetic (Dacron or PTFE) materials to bypass or substitute for the diseased native artery. In some situations, such as the carotid artery, surgical removal of the obstructing atheroma (i.e., carotid endarterectomy) is preferred over bypass. In general, these operations are undertaken using general anesthesia, with significant potential blood loss and fluid shifts, in patients who may have profound involvement of other critical organ supply (e.g., extensive coronary artery disease). When it is possible to provide a similar level of correction and durability of benefit with catheter-based (e.g., endovascular) treatments, risk and disability may be minimized.

Endovascular therapy—the subject of this chapter—shares the same heritage as coronary intervention (see Chapter 24), through the pioneering work of Dotter, Judkins, Gruntzig, and others (4–7). In fact, most of the techniques now used in the coronaries (balloon dilatation,

TABLE 26.2

CLINICAL CATEGORIES OF ACUTE LIMB ISCHEMIA

Category	Description	Capillary Return	Muscle Weakness	Sensory Loss	Doppler Signals	
					Arterial	Venous
Viable	Not immediately threatened	Intact	None	None	Audible (ankle pressure >30 mm Hg)	Audible
Threatened	Salvageable if promptly treated	Intact, slow	Mild, partial	Mild, incomplete	Inaudible	Audible
Irreversible	Major tissue loss, amputation regardless of treatment	Absent (marbling)	Profound, paralysis	Profound, anesthetic	Inaudible	Inaudible

Adapted from Rutherford RB, Flanigan DP, Guptka, SK. Suggested standards for reports with lower extremity ischemia. *J Vasc Surg* 1986;4:80.

TABLE 26.3

CLINICAL CATEGORIES OF CHRONIC LIMB ISCHEMIA

Grade	Category	Clinical Description	Objective Criteria
0	0	Asymptomatic	Normal treadmill/stress test
	1	Mild claudication	Completes treadmill exercise[a], ankle pressure after exercise <50 mm Hg but >25 mm Hg less than brachial
I	2	Moderate claudication	Between categories 1 and 3
	3	Severe claudication	Cannot complete treadmill exercise and ankle pressure after exercise <50 mm Hg
II	4	Ischemic rest pain	Resting ankle pressure <60 mm Hg, ankle or metatarsal pulse volume recording flat or barely pulsatile; toe pressure <40 mm Hg
	5	Minor tissue loss—nonhealing ulcer, focal gangrene with diffuse pedal ischemia	Resting ankle pressure <40 mm Hg, flat or barely pulsatile ankle or metatarsal pulse volume recording; toe pressure <30 mm Hg
III	6	Major tissue loss—extending above transmetatarsal level, functional foot no longer salvageable	Same as category 5

[a] Five minutes at 2 mph on a 12% incline. Adapted from Rutherford RB, Flanigan DP, Guptka SK. Suggested standards for reports dealing with lower extremity ischemia. *J Vasc Surg* 1986;4:80.

stenting, atherectomy) were first used in the peripheral circulation. Recent innovations that have made such therapies safer and more effective include lower-profile catheters, lubricious guidewire coating, debulking techniques, and endovascular stents (Fig. 26.1; 8–10). Outcomes have also been improved by innovations and improvements in imaging techniques, such as digital enhancement of conventional contrast images (see Chapter 14) and intravascular ultrasound (IVUS; See Chapter 19). The latter provides a cross-sectional view of the vessel similar to a histologic section and better comprehension of the mechanisms responsible for successful angioplasty (11–15).

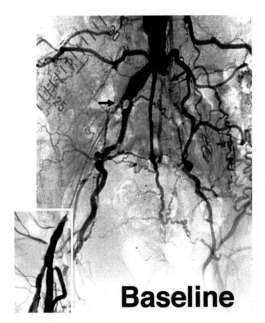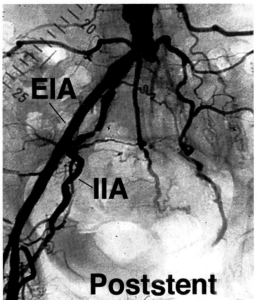

Figure 26.1 Percutaneous revascularization in 84-year-old female, whose ability to live independently is compromised owing to bilateral iliac artery occlusion and resulting severe (Rutherford class III) claudication. Lubricious, hydrophilic guidewire (Glidewire) facilitates traversal of lengthy, chronic iliac occlusion, low-profile high-pressure balloon provides effective dilation, and stenting enables result superior to balloon angioplasty alone. Availability of these technologies enhances outcome and lowers threshold for intervention in such high-risk patients, who would not meet the higher threshold required for major surgical bypass. In this patient, anticipated fem-fem grafting was cancelled, since symptoms improved enough to resume independent living after balloon angioplasty (PTA)/stent.

When catheter-based therapy is possible, it is attractive to patients, providers, and insurers, since it can usually be performed as a cost-saving same-day procedure with low morbidity and rapid convalescence. Even in instances where the degree of revascularization is not as complete or where symptomatic improvement may not be as durable, the reduced morbidity of a catheter-based therapy may make it attractive in high-risk patients (such as those with both severe CAD and limb-threatening ischemic ulceration owing to infrapopliteal disease, where restoration of ante-grade flow is required for ulcer healing and long-term limb salvage; 16). Lower-risk, partial revascularization by percu-taneous means may thus be preferable to higher-risk attempts at complete surgical revascularization, particu-larly in high-risk patients with advanced age or other cardiovascular disease. The availability of effective less invasive percutaneous options for revascularization has also led to a re-evaluation and reduction of the threshold for intervention. For example, a patient whose claudication is not severe enough to warrant major surgical bypass may nonetheless be appropriate for percutaneous transluminal angioplasty (PTA; Fig. 26.1). Indeed, the less invasive endovascular approach is increasingly preferred for initial therapy, as cardiologists and vascular surgeons acquire endovascular skills and reserve surgery for the occasional failed intervention (Fig. 26.2).

The current recommendations for revascularization at various peripheral sites are summarized in Table 26.4. Since therapy for many sites is evolving rapidly, vascular specialists must have a comprehensive understanding of all aspects of a given revascularization procedure including: (a) the indications for intervention, (b) the therapeutic

alternatives available and their expected outcomes, (c) the techniques used during an intervention, and (d) the poten-tial complications. In the remainder of this chapter, we will review the various percutaneous treatments available for disorders in each region of the body, progressing from the thorax to the lower extremities.

THORACIC AORTA

Disorders of the thoracic aorta requiring correction include coarctation, dissection, aneurysm, and patent ductus arte-riosis (see Chapter 14). Until recently, surgery—often high risk—was the only option available for intervention at this level. The introduction of very large, low-profile balloons and oversized stents married to prosthetic graft material (stent grafts), has enabled the endovascular repair of many thoracic aortic disorders, particularly in patients with other comorbid conditions that may have previously excluded them from complex surgical correction.

Coarctation of Thoracic Aorta

Coarctation in Infancy

Coarctation of the thoracic aorta is a rare congenital disor-der that typically presents early in life (younger than 5 years). Although it may be isolated or idiopathic, it is more commonly associated with various congenital cardiac dis-orders, including bicuspid aortic valve, hypoplastic left heart syndrome, or ventricular septal defect (VSD). For severe cases, correction is typically required during the first year of life to prevent complications such as coronary heart failure (CHF), severe hypertension, and cardiomyopathy (see also Chapters 27, 33, and 34).

Adult Coarctation

De novo coarctation can also present in adulthood. Although there is not universal agreement about the treat-ment of these patients, a consensus is developing that balloon angioplasty should be used as the initial treatment modality, although others have recommended its restric-tion to patients with recurrent coarctation after surgery (Fig. 26.3; 17–20). In a series of 970 patients, the acute and long-term results of PTA for native and recurrent coarcta-tion were found to be equivalent or slightly better in the native group (17). The treatment may be further improved by stenting, including the use of covered stent grafts for treatment for the pseudoaneurysm or aneurysm that may occur as a delayed complication of balloon angioplasty or surgical therapy of thoracic coarctation (18,20,21). To min-imize dissection and recoil, and to reduce the relatively high incidence of restenosis (up to 44%), some interven-tionalists believe that primary stenting is appropriate (21,22).

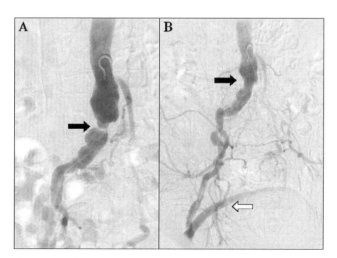

Figure 26.2 **A.** Aortography demonstrating an occluded left common iliac and a high-grade right common iliac lesion *(arrow)*. **B.** Follow up angiography demonstrating a hybrid treatment with endovascular treatment of the right common iliac stenosis with a balloon-expandable stent *(black arrow)* combined with a fem-fem bypass seen distally *(white arrow)* to vascularize the left lower limb. (Compliments of Dr. D. Drachman, Massachusetts General Hospital, Boston, MA.)

TABLE 26.4

REVASCULARIZATION STRATEGY FOR VARIOUS LOCATIONS (AS OF 2005)

Arterial Site and Lesion Type	Revascularization Strategy					Clinical Indication (e.g. Rutherford category/other)[a]	
	Percutaneous						
	Balloon Angioplasty (PTA)	Adjunctive Therapy			Surgery	Percutaneous	Surgery
		Stent	Thrombolysis	Other			
Iliac and infrarenal aorta							
Stenosis or occlusion	Approved, but many feel acute results not as favorable and restenosis more likely than with stents.	Approved for suboptimal PTA result. Most useful for complex stenosis or occlusion. Primary stenting likely improves results and reduces restenosis.	Essential for Rx of recent occlusion (<1 month). Also may be used for chronic occlusions.	Preliminary experience with early covered stents not better than bare metal, but more recent studies may show benefit.	Reserved for cases of severe, diffuse disease or lengthy occlusions; deemed inappropriate for PTA/stent.	≥2/3	≥3
Aneurysm		Endografts approved as first line of therapy for high-risk surgical candidates with anatomically suitable AAA.		Coils and occlusion devices required to eliminate internal iliac and branch flow in some instances of AAA endografting.	Remains current accepted gold standard for conventional-risk patients.	AAA ≥ 5 cm diameter and/or rapidly expanding in high-risk surgical patient; AAA causing thromboembolism.	AAA ≥ 5 cm and/or rapidly expanding; AAA causing thromboembolism.
Common femoral	Reserved for patients with severe fibrosis owing to previous surgery. Some reports of PTA as first line of therapy in selected patients.	Not approved. Flexible self-expanding stents may be used under certain "salvage" situations.			Preferred treatment (endarterectomy with or without patch), especially if in association with proximal/distal bypass.	≥2/3	≥2/3
Profunda femoris	Reserved for cases of at least moderately severe ischemia. Stakes high if SFA occluded already.	Not approved, but anecdotal success.			Preferred treatment for proximal disease (endarterectomy with or without patch). Mid/distal vessel not easily accessed.	≥4	≥3

TABLE 26.4

(continued)

Arterial Site and Lesion Type	Revascularization Strategy					Clinical Indication (e.g. Rutherford category/other)[a]	
	Percutaneous						
	Balloon Angioplasty (PTA)	Adjunctive Therapy			Surgery	Percutaneous	Surgery
		Stent	Thrombolysis	Other			
SFA/ popliteal							
Stenosis	Treatment of choice for short lesions. Can be used in lengthy lesions as initial treatment: long-term results less favorable, but risk is less than surgery.	Self-expanding stents approved for use where PTA results suboptimal. Recent reports of favorable results with strategy of primary stenting compared with PTA alone.	Useful only if nonocclusive thrombus present.	Atherectomy (Fox Hollow, Rotablator, Excimer laser) may be useful to debulk, but no clear-cut long-term improvement over PTA alone. Covered stents show some promise, but not widely accepted.	Reserved for cases of diffuse disease deemed inappropriate for PTA	≥2/3	≥3
Occlusion	Treatment of choice for short (<7 cm) occlusion.	Self-expanding stents approved for use in suboptimal PTA results. Many believe should be used routinely for occlusive lesions to enhance patency.	Use highly recommended for recent (<1 month) thrombosis/ occlusion. Few operators also prefer for chronic occlusion. May convert short or long occlusion into focal or segmental stenosis, facilitating treatment.		Previously, treatment of choice for lengthy (e.g., >10 cm) occlusion. Practice evolving as stent use more widespread and results acceptable with less associated cardiovascular risk compared with surgery.		
Infra-popliteal	Appropriate choice for treatment of discrete stenosis or focal occlusion.	Not approved. Useful for salvaging failed PTA.	Useful for recent thrombosis or thromboembolism.	Rotational or Fox Hollow atherectomy may be useful for debulking calcified lesions. Excimer laser useful for debulking. Positive anecdotal experience with DES.	Treatment of choice for lengthy diffuse disease/long occlusion(s), and not suitable or high-risk for percutaneous Rx.	≥3/4	≥4

(continued)

TABLE 26.4
(continued)

Arterial Site and Lesion Type	Revascularization Strategy — Percutaneous — Balloon Angioplasty (PTA)	Adjunctive Therapy — Stent	Adjunctive Therapy — Thrombolysis	Adjunctive Therapy — Other	Surgery	Clinical Indication (e.g. Rutherford category/other)[a] — Percutaneous	Clinical Indication — Surgery
Subclavian stenosis/ occlusion	Initial treatment for stenosis. Successful in most occlusions.	Many prefer as definitive therapy. Choice of balloon expandable or self-expanding depends on anatomical location and potential for stent compression.	Indicated for recent occlusion (<1 month). May facilitate PTA in chronic occlusion, but little published experience.	Distal protection of the ipsilateral vertebra may be advisable depending on the angiographic appearance and the position of the stenosis.	Reserved for patients unsuitable for PTA and stenting.	Moderate arm claudication, subclavian steal syndrome, coronary steal syndrome, or coronary steal via internal mammary artery.	Severe arm claudication and/or subclavian steal syndrome, not amenable to percutaneous therapy.
Vertebral and basilar	Preferred treatment for proximal or midvessel stenosis.	Not approved, but useful or preferred for optimal result, especially proximal vertebral, where recoil is common.	Useful and potentially lifesaving in acute/sub-acute thrombosis.		Reserved for PTA failures and symptomatic occlusions.	Unequivocal symptoms of VBI: visual/ vestibular disturbance, posterior circulation TIA. For basilar-acute occlusion/severe stenosis with uncontrolled side effects	Severe symptoms of VBI; PTA impossible or unsuccessful.
Carotid Innominate and common carotid (intrathoracic)	Preferred therapy (with stents to prevent recoil) for lesions in this location, which are inaccessible for CEA	Adjunct stenting preferred, owing to high incidence of recoil and heavily calcified lesions at origins of CCA/innominate	No published data.	Distal protection advisable, although may be technically challenging for ostial CCA lesions.	Many surgeons prefer (e.g., subclavian to carotid bypass) as first line therapy for symptomatic patients. No definitive comparison with CAS. Surgery definitely appropriate if poor PTA candidate, e.g., hostile aortic arch.	Mild-to-severe symptoms, or asymptomatic with stenosis >80 or 85%. Possible role preop before CABG.	Moderate-to-severe symptoms.

TABLE 26.4

(continued)

Arterial Site and Lesion Type	Revascularization Strategy					Clinical Indication (e.g. Rutherford category/other)[a]	
	Percutaneous						
	Balloon Angioplasty (PTA)	Adjunctive Therapy			Surgery	Percutaneous	Surgery
		Stent	Thrombolysis	Other			
Bifurcation and proximal ICA	Experimental but favorable results in recent, nonrandomized clinical trials (if performed with stenting).	Carotid artery stenting (CAS) at least equivalent to and probably superior to CEA for high-risk patient groups, as defined by the SAPPHIRE study. Multiple prospective studies underway comparing CAS with CEA for lower-risk symptomatic patients and asymptomatic patients.	Anecdotal reports of successful use in conjunction with PTA and stent for active or acute lesion.	Embolic protection recommended. IIB/IIIA inhibitors rarely used on individual case basis.	Accepted gold standard for lesions amenable to CEA.	Symptomatic or critical asymptomatic stenosis, if CEA not feasible; possibly for high-risk CEA patients.	Fulfill NASCET or ACAS criteria.
Renal FMD	Treatment of choice.	Not approved. Useful for lesions with recoil or restenosis.			Reserved for branch stenosis or aneurysmal disease not amenable to PTRA.	Moderate HTN; accelerated or refractory HTN; renal insufficiency.	Accelerated or refractory HTN; not amenable to PTA.
Atherosclerotic (ostial or nonostial)	Some prefer as sole treatment for nonostial lesions. For ostial lesions, incidence of recoil and restenosis high.	Treatment of choice for ostial and proximal lesions. Most prefer for all atherosclerotic lesions.	Reserved for acute thrombosis, an infrequent event.	Embolic protection devices show promise in reducing atheroemboli and may help prevent renal deterioration. Studies underway.	Effectively replaced by stenting as gold standard for atherosclerotic RAS. Reserved for RAS arising within aortic aneurysm, inaccessible for PTRA/stent, and for occlusions requiring revascularization.	HTN refractory or resistant to med Rx; accelerated HTN; progressive renal dysfunction; CHF; angina. No benefit yet demonstrated when creatinine normal and HTN easily controlled by med. Rx.	Same indications for PTRA, when PTRA technically not feasible.

(continued)

TABLE 26.4
(continued)

Arterial and Site Lesion Type	Revascularization Strategy					Clinical Indication (e.g. Rutherford category/other)[a]	
	Percutaneous						
	Balloon Angioplasty (PTA)	Adjunctive Therapy			Surgery	Percutaneous	Surgery
		Stent	Thrombolysis	Other			
Mesenteric	Reasonable first line of therapy, but untested. Compared with surgery.	Treatment of choice for ostial lesions. May be less favorable for lengthy lesions, thrombotic lesions, and occlusions.			Previously accepted standard but PTA/stent likely equal with less risk, if lesion favorable.	Significant clinical evidence of mesenteric ischemia.	Clearcut evidence of mesenteric ischemia and PTA/stent not feasible.

[a] Indications vary widely depending on risk–benefit ratio of a given procedure in a given patient. These are intended as general guidelines only.
AAA, Abdominal aortic aneurysm; CABG, Coronary artery bypass grafting; CEA, Carotid endarterectomy; CHF, congestive heart failure; DA, directional atherectomy; DES, Drug eluding stent; FMD, fibromuscular dysplasia; HTN, hypertension; Med Rx, medical therapy; NA, not applicable; PTA, percutaneous transluminal angioplasty; POBA, plain old balloon angioplasty; PTRA, percutaneous transluminal renal angioplasty; RAS, renal artery stenosis; Rx, treatment; SFA, superficial femoral artery; VBI, vertibo-basilar insufficiency.

Technique

Access to the coarctation is largely dependent on its location. Most lesions are at the isthmus, adjacent to the ligamentum arteriosum and just distal to the subclavian artery.

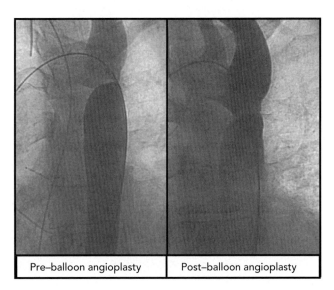

Pre–balloon angioplasty | Post–balloon angioplasty

Figure 26.3 A. Aortography demonstrating aortic coarctation with dilatation of the greater vessels of the neck. **B.** Post balloon angioplasty aortography demonstrates improvement of the coarctation. (Compliments of Dr. I. Inglessis, Massachusetts General Hospital, Boston, MA.)

The retrograde femoral approach is preferred. Prograde access via the left subclavian or innominate artery (brachial approach) is possible, although the large profile of the balloons/stents required for treatment may present an increased risk for brachial artery injury. A pull-through technique, using combined femoral and brachial (or transseptal) access, enables control of both ends of a single (0.035-inch) guidewire to help counteract the forceful jet of aortic blood flow and thereby facilitate accurate stent or stent–graft placement.

Balloon diameter should not exceed 1.1 times the size of the adjacent isthmus or descending aorta; sizing to the diameter of the post-stenotic dilation may lead to aortic rupture or dissection particularly in the thin-walled post-stenotic segment. Sizing should therefore be conservative, as complications can be catastrophic. The pressure gradient need not be completely eliminated to achieve a successful hemodynamic and clinical outcome. Intravascular ultrasound may be very useful for assessing vessel size and the result of intervention. Finally, in the current era, large stent grafts and aortic occlusion balloons should be available, and operators should be familiar with their us in the event of potentially catastrophic rupture or dissection complicating dilatation of an aortic coarctation. For operators without familiarity with stent grafts or balloon occlusion, collaboration with vascular surgery and/or radiology colleagues is appropriate.

Thoracic Aortic Aneurysm

Considerable controversy exists regarding the indications and threshold for repair of thoracic aortic aneurysms (TAAs; 23–25). The relative infrequency (compared with abdominal aortic aneurysm), lack of associated symptoms, and the perception that conventional surgical repair is associated with significant risk of spinal cord ischemia and paralysis limits enthusiasm for aggressive diagnosis and referrals for repair. Despite the tendency to ignore or treat medically, available data suggest that the natural history of TAA may be similar to that of abdominal aortic aneurysm (AAA): both can be expected to progress and potentially rupture, particularly if the diameter is ≥5 cm or there is associated dissection (see Chapter 14). For patients selected for surgery, significant morbidity or mortality in the hands of even the most experienced surgeons remains in the range of ≥10%. The advent of stent grafts has provided a catheter-based alternative treatment, especially for high-risk patients. In a landmark report, Dake and colleagues (26) described the first series of patients undergoing endovascular TAA repair using stent grafts (see Chapter 34). Although this study was not controlled or randomized, updated preliminary results from the same group show a 6.8% 30-day mortality, which is superior to surgical series of TAA repairs (27).

Subsequent studies have proven endovascular repair of thoracic aortic aneurysms to be attractive options, particularly in high-risk cases. Anatomically favorable TAAs are those that do not involve the great vessels of the aortic arch, have a 1- to 2-cm neck of aorta (beyond the subclavian origin) to anchor the stent, and have suitable distal aortoiliac vessels to enable access with the large (22 to 28 French) sheath. The etiology and extent of the aneurysm and coexisting distal disease thus must be clearly defined (by chest radiograph, spiral computed tomography [CT] scan with three-dimensional reconstruction, magnetic resonance imaging [MRA], and formal angiography) prior to undertaking stent grafting (28–31). A strategic approach must be developed in advance to ensure optimal stent deployment and avoid potential adverse events like graft migration by systolic flow. A number of purpose-specific newer stent–graft designs are being developed for treatment of TAA, to replace the homemade devices used in early clinical experience. Some, for example, incorporate side limbs for the greater vessels to enable more proximal anchoring. Hybrid strategies involving a combination of surgical and endovascular techniques are also feasible, including carotid to subclavian bypass combined with stent grafting across the subclavian origin (used for aneurysms that involve the left subclavian origin). As is the case with stent grafts placed at other sites, collaboration among specialists (surgeons and endovascular specialists) is essential for the successful completion of these procedures.

Aortic Dissection

Acute dissection of the aorta is a catastrophic illness. Although the incidence is relatively low (approximately two cases per 100,000 of population), the consequences are frequently devastating. The International Registry of Acute Aortic Dissection (IRAD) reported a 28% in-hospital mortality of aortic dissection (32,33). Untreated dissections of the ascending aorta (DeBakey type I or II/Stanford type A) carry a 90% 3-month mortality, owing to extension with cardiac tamponade, aortic regurgitation, myocardial infarction, and stroke. Although dissection limited to the descending aorta (DeBakey type III/Stanford type B) carries a more favorable outcome, its manifestations include ischemic complications in up to 30% of cases and late rupture in up to 20% of patients over their lifetimes (34). In the past, asymptomatic dissections were treated simply with antihypertensive therapy, but it is now apparent that 30 to 40% of these patients will ultimately suffer an aortic-related death or require urgent aortic surgery (35). The mortality for surgical repair in the setting of end organ ischemia approaches 50%, particularly in patients with ongoing visceral infarction or hemodynamic instability (25,36,37). Consequently, novel interventional approaches for management of both acute and chronic aortic dissection have been sought. There are currently three interventional approaches for treating acute and chronic aortic dissection—aortic stent grafting of the dissection entry site, balloon fenestration, and prophylactic stenting of the visceral arteries.

The most common acute complication is peripheral or visceral ischemia, typically arising owing to one of two causes (38,39). The first results from a proximal dissection plane without distal communication, allowing flow into a false lumen that progressively expands and compresses the true aortic lumen. The second is visceral or lower limb ischemia arising from extension of the dissection plane across the origin of branching vessels, occluding their blood supply by thrombus formation or mechanical obstruction arising from the dissection flap. Because the pathophysiology of aortic dissection frequently involves more than one of these processes occurring simultaneously, the interventional strategy for a given patient is unique, involving careful evaluation and a multidisciplinary approach. Each of the interventional strategies is designed to address or palliate a specific cause. The choice of therapy must take into consideration the degree of true lumen compression, the extent and patency of the false lumen, compromise of major branch vessels, presence of multiple proximal and distal natural fenestrations, and the ability to precisely image the origin of the dissection and the origin of the branch vessels. Equally important in deciding on appropriate therapy is the clinical status of the patient, especially the pulse examinations, symptoms, and serum markers indicative of ischemia that allow appropriate treatment and its timing to prevent end organ tissue loss.

The most dramatic interventional procedure recently introduced for this condition is endovascular stenting of the proximal portion of the origin or "in-flow" of the dissection plane. The aim is to direct flow away from or to occlude the origin of the dissection, resulting in false lumen thrombosis and subsequent absorption of the intramural hematoma. A complicating issue with this intervention is the fact that the false lumen pressure usually exceeds the true lumen pressure, thereby requiring high stent deployment pressures to adequately compress or occlude the false lumen. These pressures may exceed the

strength of an already diseased aorta. In such cases, Dake and Kato have described endovascular repair of the primary entry tear using stent grafts in the descending thoracic aorta (40,41).

Endovascular fenestration (Fig. 26.4) is a technique designed to minimize extension of the dissection plane or progressive compression of the true lumen. Its effect is most dramatic when there is minimal distal communication between the true and false lumens and in the presence of end organ ischemia. It functions by creating a channel between the true and the false lumens (a) to equalize their

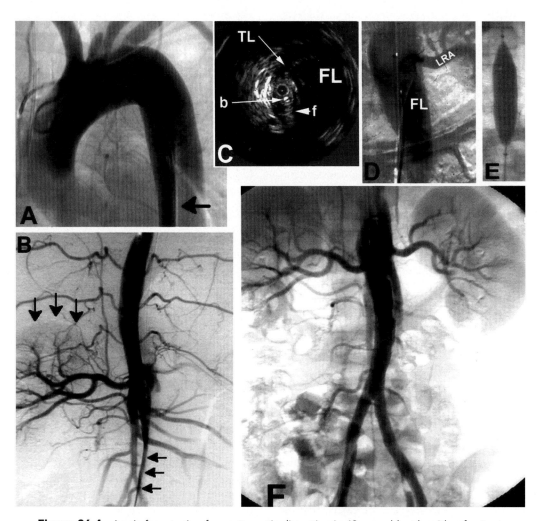

Figure 26.4 Aortic fenestration for acute aortic dissection in 42-year-old male with refractory severe hypertension (HTN), persistent pain owing to extending dissection, and ongoing lower extremity ischemia and acidosis. Considering hemodynamic instability and anticipated difficult recovery from surgery owing to partial spinal cord paralysis, fenestration was performed after diagnostic angiography. Bilateral femoral access required. **A.** Angiography shows classic flap *(arrow)* in thoracic aorta. **B.** Compression by false lumen obliterates descending aortic true lumen below renal arteries. Nephrogram seen on right *(arrows)*, but not on left; underperfusion of left kidney is responsible for refractory HTN. **C.** Intravascular ultrasound shows false lumen (FL) compressing true lumen (TL) and directs Brockenbrough needle (b) toward aortic flap (f). **D.** After fenestration, injection through Mullins dilator shows contrast in false lumen and left renal artery. **E.** Large balloon enlarges fenestration. **F.** Final angiogram after fenestration and stenting of distal abdominal aorta and common iliac arteries shows simultaneous filling of both renal arteries, restoration of outflow, and scaffolding of dissection flap. Patient's hemodynamic status corrected instantaneously and recovery/rehabilitation were greatly accelerated by absence of surgical incision and general anesthetics. Patient walking and stable 2 years postfenestration. Aortic size unchanged.

internal pressure, (b) to improve blood flow to vessels arising from the false channel, and (c) to limit the forces responsible for distal propagation of the dissection (42,43). Creating an egress for blood thus depressurizes the false channel and may, in theory, reduce the aneurysmal dilatation.

Type I and II (Stanford type A) dissections are more challenging for percutaneous techniques. Standard therapy for these dissections is surgical reconstruction of the aortic arch, which should be performed early to prevent the sudden and devastating consequences of retrograde dissection into the pericardium, right coronary artery, and cerebral vessels. The surgeon typically completes the repair of the aortic arch, but does not address the remaining portion of the dissection flap, which extends into the descending and sometimes abdominal aortic segments. Early results using stent grafts, either in conjunction with surgery or later to complete the repair of the dissected aorta, have been encouraging (41).

Treatment Considerations and Technique

Experience with percutaneous aortic fenestration is limited to select centers. Time is of the essence in making decisions regarding best treatment. Noninvasive imaging (with TEE, CT, or MRI) must be performed to identify the primary entry site and Stanford type of the dissection. Stanford type A dissections are currently treated with surgical repair. Stanford type B dissections that are stable and asymptomatic can be medically managed while more extensive evaluation is performed. Development of visceral or lower limb ischemia in the presence of an adequate or moderately compromised true lumen is optimally treated with branch vessel stenting with or without fenestration of the dissection flap. Severe compromise of the true lumen usually requires a combination of endograft stenting of the proximal dissection plane in addition to endovascular fenestration, and possibly, branch vessel stenting.

Treatment requires bilateral femoral access, carefully advancing guidewires to retain their position within the true lumen. Complete aortography (starting with the left anterior oblique [LAO] projection) from the aortic arch down to the abdominal aorta and iliac arteries should be performed prior to endovascular manipulation. On occasion, natural fenestrations may have occurred at sites where the native vessels are shorn off from the true lumen; these may be traversed and used as a starting point for balloon dilation. In most instances, however, the intimal flap will need to be punctured with a trans-septal (or similar) needle under intravascular ultrasound guidance, followed by balloon dilatation and stenting of the intimal flap below the fenestration site. The recently developed CrossPoint TransAccess catheter system (Medtronic Inc., Minneapolis, MN), which integrates phased array IVUS imaging with a needle delivery system, may be advantageous for this indication. The fenestration creates a new

egress for blood flow from the false channel and improves organ and limb perfusion by resolving compression of the true lumen (Fig. 26.4). Similar to treatment of coarctation, large balloons/stenting and extensive peripheral vascular skills are required for the treatment of dissection.

VESSELS OF THE AORTIC ARCH

Subclavian and Innominate Arteries

The vast majority of disease in these vessels is owing to atherosclerosis, although giant cell arteritis (Takayasu) and fibromuscular disease (FMD) can also cause clinically relevant disease (see Chapter 14; 44). Clinical indications for subclavian revascularization are listed in Table 26.5 (see also Fig. 26.5). Routine examination (measurement of cuff pressure and palpation of pulses in both upper extremities, plus auscultation over the supraclavicular and subclavicular areas) will uncover a substantial number of patients with asymptomatic subclavian disease. Asymptomatic patients do not require treatment initially, but should be followed closely for the development of related symptoms, such as those related to subclavian steal or upper limb ischemia. If coronary bypass surgery has or will likely be performed to prevent coronary to subclavian steal and resultant myocardial ischemia, preservation of the antegrade flow to the internal mammary conduit is important.

Subclavian and innominate PTA was first performed in 1980 and is now considered to be the treatment of choice over surgical options for subclavian disease (carotid-subclavian, aortosubclavian, or axilloaxillary bypass or endarterectomy; 45). Most published series of subclavian PTA report technical success and complication rates consistently >90% and <10%, respectively (46–48). Primary stenting may further improve these results (49).

TABLE 26.5

INDICATIONS FOR SUBCLAVIAN OR INNOMINATE ARTERY REVASCULARIZATION

Symptomatic ischemia of the posterior fossa (e.g., vertebral-basilar insufficiency)
Symptomatic subclavian steal syndrome
Disabling upper extremity claudication
Preservation of flow to LIMA/RIMA
    Preop coronary bypass surgery, where LIMA/RIMA will be used
    Postop CABG LIMA/RIMA with ischemia (with or without coronary-subclavian steal syndrome)
Preservation of inflow to axillary graft or dialysis conduit
"Blue-digit" syndrome (embolization to fingers)
Inability to measure blood pressure
Progressive stenosis or thromboembolus threatening cerebral blood supply

---

CABG, coronary artery bypass graft; LIMA, left internal mammary artery; RIMA, right internal mammary artery.

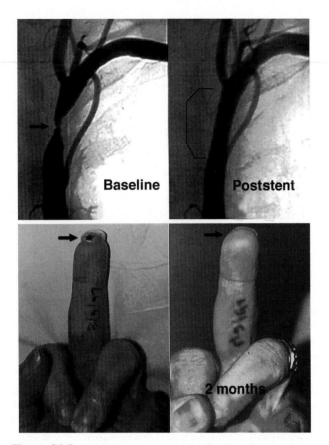

Figure 26.5 Subclavian artery stenting for blue digit syndrome. **Top left.** Severe irregular stenosis in left subclavian, associated with 60-mm Hg reduction in left brachial cuff pressure and **(bottom left)** painful embolic ulcer at fingertip. **Top right.** Balloon angioplasty (PTA)/stenting (Palmaz P-204) performed via femoral approach using 85-cm-long 7F sheath. Care used to avoid stenting over vertebral origin. **Bottom right.** Healed ulcer 2 months poststent.

Complications are generally minor and infrequent, but may include problems at the femoral or brachial access site, as well as inadvertent "jailing," dissection, or embolization of the vertebral or left internal mammary artery (LIMA), which may resolve after lytic therapy. Alternatively, these complications may be prevented using embolic protection of the vertebral or internal mammary arteries (see Chapter 23). Recurrence rates are generally low (5 to 10%; 50).

Direct comparison between surgery and PTA for subclavian disease is hampered by the absence of randomized controlled studies. Hadjipetrou et al. (51), in a multicenter analysis, compared the results of primary subclavian stenting in 108 patients with those of 2,496 surgical patients reported in 52 papers from the literature (1966 and 1998). The surgical series had complications of stroke in 3%, mortality in 2%, and overall complications in 13% of patients; the stent series had 0% stroke, 0% death, and 6% overall complications. Recurrence rate was 12% for surgical series and 3% for stent series, although follow-up was shorter in the latter. These data, however, mostly relate to stenotic disease rather than occlusive disease, which has a lower chance of success (50 to 75%) and an increased risk of

embolization of thrombus or atheroma into the cerebral, upper extremity, or coronary circulation.

Treatment Considerations and Technique

Preprocedure
Thorough evaluation of the patient prior to undertaking subclavian or angioplasty is essential. Noninvasive testing should include duplex evaluation, with determination of the direction of flow in the vertebral arteries (antegrade or retrograde, the latter indicating the presence of a steal phenomenon) and documentation of associated carotid disease. If there is a clinical suggestion of vasculitis, an erythrocyte sedimentation rate (ESR) or C-reactive protein (CRP) should be measured. Premedication with aspirin is standard, with optional addition of clopidogrel. In cases of subclavian occlusion, because nascent thrombus may potentially lie in the segment immediately beyond the occlusion, patients may benefit from anticoagulation for a period of several weeks prior to revascularization.

Access
The femoral approach is used most commonly, but requires careful catheter manipulation in the diseased aortic arch to avoid atheroembolic complications. The brachial approach may be useful and is preferred by some, particularly for total occlusions that are flush with the aorta. Embolization to the brachial artery can be controlled with this approach, particularly if it is done via a cutdown, although the current ability to deliver stents through 5F and 6F sheaths usually makes percutaneous access preferable.

Catheters and Guidewires
A nonselective aortic arch angiogram, using a multiple-side-hole catheter (i.e., a pigtail) should be obtained to provide a "roadmap" prior to gaining selective access into the subclavian or innominate artery. It may be possible to steer a guidewire directly across a stenosis from the sheath, but crossing a high-grade stenosis or total occlusion requires prior selective cannulation of the subclavian with a diagnostic catheter (JR4, Cobra, Simmons, etc.) and advancement of the guidewire through the catheter. The diagnostic catheter may then be advanced over the wire and across the stenosis, where it is used to measure a baseline pressure gradient and place a longer or heavier guidewire, if necessary, to allow exchange of the diagnostic catheter for either a long sheath (5F or 6F, 80 to 90 cm) or a 7F to 8F coronary multipurpose or right Judkins guiding catheter. Although previously 0.035-inch balloon and stent systems were dominant, 0.014- and 0.018-inch systems are now preferred because of their lower profile and the ability to reduce access size. The reduction of device profile enables subclavian revascularization to be performed in a fashion analogous to coronary intervention, placing a 6F to 7F guide in the vessel origin, wire placement, and device delivery.

Balloons and Stents

Predilation is performed with an undersized (usually 4 to 5 mm in diameter) balloon, which can be used to select final stent/balloon length and dimension. The guiding catheter or sheath may be advanced over the balloon into the distal vessel to facilitate passage of the stent, although this is required less frequently with current low-profile stents. A stent of appropriate size and length to cover the lesion should be selected. Both balloon-expandable stainless steel and cobalt-chromium and self-expanding nitinol stents have been used, but no stent has yet received specific FDA approval for use in the subclavian artery.

If the lesion is adjacent to the origins of the vertebral and/or IMA, attempts should be made to avoid placing these vessels into "stent jail." Most left subclavian lesions are located proximal to the vertebral artery, where use of either balloon-expandable or self-expanding stents is reasonable. For lesions located beyond the internal mammary artery, self-expanding stents should be used to avoid the potential for late stent compression by extravascular structures at the thoracic outlet. When stenting the brachiocephalic (innominate artery), care should be taken to avoid impinging on the origin of the right common carotid artery with a stent. Stents should be postdilated to match the size of the subclavian artery (generally between 5 and 8 mm). Overdilation should be avoided to minimize the risk of dissection that might extend into the vertebral artery or internal mammary artery. If such dissections do occur, they can often be salvaged by placement of a stent within the origin of the affected branch vessel, although distal extension of the dissection within the branch vessel may render attempts at salvage futile. Following postdilatation, pressure gradients may be repeated to demonstrate complete elimination of the gradient.

Follow-up

No data exist regarding the use of clopidogrel, though many maintain this regimen for 4 weeks postprocedure. During clinical follow-up, the resolution of symptoms should be documented, equalization of blood pressures in both upper extremities should be confirmed, and the duplex study should show triphasic brachial waveforms with restoration of normal antegrade flow in the vertebral arteries. Restenosis within subclavian arteries occurs in 10 to 20% of patients and may be treated by stenting (if not stented initially) or balloon angioplasty (for in-stent restenosis). Use of brachytherapy or drug-eluting stents has not been studied. Stent compression should be treated by balloon re-expansion and placement of a self-expanding stent within the old balloon-expandable stent.

Vertebral and Basilar Arteries

Vertebral artery stenosis is a common finding in patients undergoing arch or subclavian angiography. Although the vertebral artery is usually easy to access, revascularization is

TABLE 26.6

SYMPTOMS OF VERTEBRAL-BASILAR INSUFFICIENCY (VBI)

Visual disturbance	Diplopia
Language/speech disturbance	Global aphasia, dysarthria
Altered state of consciousness	Confusion, syncope
Vestibular dysfunction	Dizziness, vertigo

indicated only in patients with indisputable symptoms of vertebral basilar insufficiency (VBI; Table 26.6). In rare instances, a patient with a previously obstructed carotid may present with classic carotid, as opposed to vertebral, symptoms. In such cases, if the stenotic vertebral gives rise to collaterals to the anterior circulation (via the posterior communicating artery and the circle of Willis), then PTA of the stenotic vertebral lesion may be justified (Fig. 26.6). The significant downside of failed or complicated vertebral PTA (including potentially fatal or disabling brainstem cerebrovascular accident [CVA]) makes case selection critical. Before undertaking vertebral intervention, therefore, it is important to define the pattern of intracerebral blood flow and collateral circulation (with MRA or four-vessel angiography).

Intervention in the basilar artery is considered to be even more dangerous than in the vertebral, as it is a terminal vessel that is responsible alone for perfusion to a number of critical areas in the brainstem. Accordingly, basilar artery PTA is reserved for the rare instances in which patients present with symptoms unequivocally related to a critical stenosis or acute occlusion. Revascularization in the latter case often requires use of thrombolytic therapy and can produce dramatic recovery of patients who were previously near death (52–55). Given the high stakes involved in vertebral-basilar instrumentation, consultations with neurology and neuroradiology are advisable when making decisions regarding therapy for the posterior cerebral circulation.

Treatment Considerations and Technique

The technique of vertebral angioplasty is similar to that for subclavian (or ostial coronary) PTA. The femoral approach is generally used, and a coronary guiding catheter or long sheath (Fig. 26.6) is advanced into the proximal subclavian artery over an introducing catheter or dilation to avoid scraping any proximal plaque. The vertebral artery stenosis is crossed with 0.014-inch or 0.018-inch wire, over which a coronary or small-vessel balloon (2.5 to 4.5 mm) is advanced to dilate the vessel. Careful neurologic evaluation should be performed during and after the balloon inflation. Intra-arterial nitroglycerin should be administered in cases of distal spasm, to be distinguished from pleating or pseudostenosis caused by guidewires straightening a

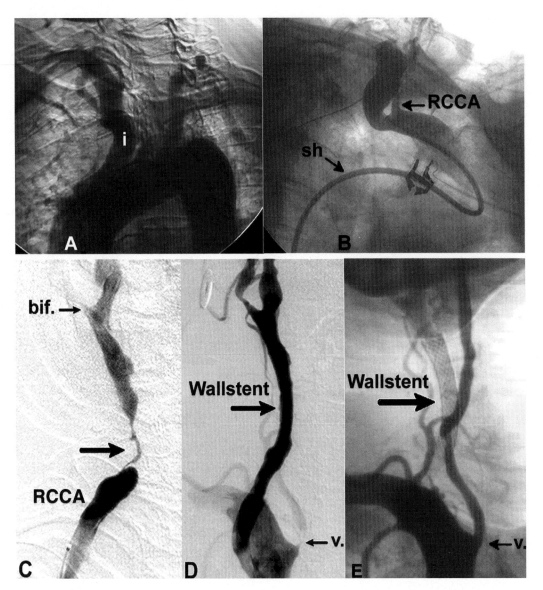

Figure 26.6 Right carotid and vertebral stenting in 65-year-old male with prior radical neck dissection and irradiation for laryngeal CA (residual tracheostomy, prior left hemispheric cardiovascular accident [CVA] owing to left internal carotid artery [ICA] occlusion, left vertebral occlusion, and recurrent syncopal episodes from global cerebral ischemia. **A.** Initial attempt to obtain guiding catheter or sheath access in extremely tortuous right innominate (i) failed. **B.** Second attempt succeeded using 8F ArrowFlex sheath (sh), which provided adequate support for carotid/vertebral angiography and stenting. Flow pattern to CNS is via collaterals (thyrocervical to external carotid, then retrograde in external carotid artery [ECA] to bifurcation [bif.] and antegrade up ICA). Right ICA then cross-fills to left ICA. **C.** Critical RCCA stenosis *(arrow)* at baseline. **D.** Status post PTA/Wallstent RCCA. Antegrade flow restored to ECA; however, vertebral artery origin (v.) severely narrowed. **E.** Vertebral patent status post coronary stent (Multilink). Symptoms completely resolved. Stents patent at 6-month follow-up angiography.

tortuous vessel. Patients should be well heparinized, and extreme caution should be applied to prevent air embolism. Unlike many other vascular sites, routinely crossing the dilated site with the guiding catheter is not recommended, to reduce the potential for additional disruption of the lesion and plaque embolization. For stenting ostial lesions, stents should be placed either flush with the origin or protruding 0.5 to 1.0 mm into the subclavian artery. Use of embolic protection devices has not been formally tested

in this setting but may be appropriate in some of these procedures. Completion angiography with intracerebral views and postprocedure neurology re-evaluation are both useful.

Carotid Arteries

Stroke remains a leading cause of morbidity and mortality, with 600,000 strokes occurring annually in the United

States alone (56)—approximately 20% as the direct result of carotid atherosclerosis. The natural history of untreated carotid artery disease can be seen in the control arms of carotid endarterectomy studies in which the incidence of ipsilateral stroke was 26% at 2 years in symptomatic patients with a >70% stenosis and 5% at 2 years in asymptomatic patients with a >60% stenosis (57,58). Furthermore, the presence of carotid artery disease is a significant marker of cardiovascular risk, highlighting the importance of risk factor modification and preventive strategies in this high-risk patient population (59).

Carotid endarterectomy (CEA) has long been considered the gold standard for carotid artery intervention. During the more than 50 years since CEA was initially reported, significant technical improvements have improved morbidity, mortality, cost, and patient inconvenience (60,61). It was only after 40 years of widespread application of CEA, however, that definitive proof of its benefit was obtained. The landmark North American Symptomatic Carotid Endarterectomy Trial (NASCET) and Asymptomatic Carotid Atherosclerosis Study (ACAS) investigations thus demonstrated that surgical endarterectomy, when performed for carotid bifurcation disease by experienced vascular surgeons on appropriately selected patients, effectively reduced the likelihood of ipsilateral stroke compared with standard medical therapy (57,58,62,63).

In the NASCET study of symptomatic carotid artery disease, CEA was associated with a 60% relative reduction in ipsilateral stroke over a 2-year period (9% for CEA versus 26% for medical therapy; 57). In the ACAS study of asymptomatic carotid stenosis >60%, CEA resulted in a 53% reduction in the 5-year stroke rate (5.1% for CEA versus 11% for medical therapy; 58), although it is important to note that best medical therapy has improved significantly since these studies were performed (64–68). It has been suggested that these improved medical outcomes merit revaluation compared with revascularization, particularly for asymptomatic patient populations.

The entry criteria for the early CEA studies were for low-risk patients, making it difficult to extrapolate these dramatic results to higher-risk groups such as elderly patients (>79 years), those with concomitant cardiovascular disease, and those with higher-risk lesions (specifically restenotic lesions following prior CEA, radiation-induced stenosis, following radical neck surgery, or difficult surgical access). Although carotid atherosclerotic occurs predominantly at the carotid bifurcation, a site that is convenient for CEA, it may extend beyond the bifurcation or involve the origin or proximal aspect of the common carotid artery, which is more complex to treat surgically and may require thoracotomy or subclavian-carotid bypass.

It is against this background that percutaneous carotid intervention has been compared (Fig. 26.6). Although carotid balloon angioplasty (CPTA) was performed as early as 1983, the widespread application of CEA, coupled

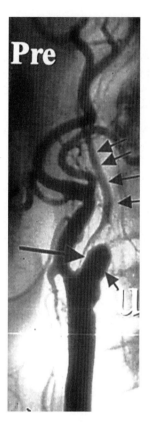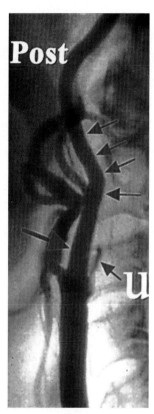

Figure 26.7 Carotid balloon angioplasty (CPTA)/stent deployment in 77-year-old male with unstable angina on intravenous nitroglycerin, awaiting CABG. **Left.** Contralateral internal carotid artery (ICA) is occluded, and ipsilateral is critically narrowed (*large arrow*). Distal ICA (*small arrow*) is atretic owing to underperfusion. Large ulcer (u) is located at ICA origin. Surgeon reluctant to do coronary artery bypass graft (CABG) until carotid revascularized. CPTA/stent performed via 7F Cook Shuttle catheter placed in CCA. Atraumatic 0.014-inch coronary guidewire used to cross lesion, predilation performed with 3.5-mm coronary balloon, then Wallstent placed, extending back into CCA. **Right.** Poststent, distal ICA restored to normal caliber, ulcer (u) is compressed and was absent on 6-month follow-up angiogram. Patient had uneventful CABG and remains asymptomatic at 3 years.

with concerns of distal embolization (69) and vessel recoil or thrombosis, relegated CPTA to single-center, anecdotal reports (70–72). In the 1990s, work by Roubin, Iyer, Yadav, Vitek, and others advanced this technique and demonstrated superior results for primary (as opposed to provisional) stenting in carotid arteries (73–77). The apparent benefits resulted from more complete effacement of the plaque and associated ulcerations (Fig. 26.7), reduction in elastic recoil, and restoration of laminar flow with resultant reduction in thrombus formation and subsequent embolization of thrombus or plaque. But no single issue in cardiovascular medicine (perhaps since the advent of balloon angioplasty) has raised as much controversy as the subject of carotid angioplasty and stenting (78–82).

In most institutions, percutaneous treatment of carotid arteries remained reserved for those circumstances wherein

TABLE 26.7

PROPOSED CURRENT CLASSIFICATION AND STRATEGY FOR PATIENTS IN WHOM CAROTID REVASCULARIZATION IS APPROPRIATE FOR PURPOSES OF STROKE PREVENTION

Category A: Surgery difficult, very high risk, or not feasible
Anatomy/morphology
- Lesion location inaccessible for standard CEA
  - Intracranial
  - Distal cervical (C2 or above)
  - Aorto-ostial or proximal CCA
- Previous radical neck dissection
- Previous neck irradiation
Strategy: Carotid stent with embolic protection is first-line therapy.

Category B: Surgery feasible, but with somewhat greater risk than NASCET/ACAS
Anatomy/morphology
- CEA restenosis lesion
- Contralateral ICA occlusion
- High lesion
Medical condition
- Severe CAD or unstable angina
- Coexisting need for CABG
- Recent acute MI
- CHF (class III or IV)
- Severe COPD
- Contralateral laryngeal nerve palsy
Strategy: Carotid stent with embolic protection is considered equivalent to CEA; choice of therapy based on patient preference and experience/availability of surgeon and interventionalist.

Category C: Conventional risk for surgery
- NASCET/ACAS eligible
- Uncomplicated surgical access
Strategy: CEA is treatment of choice. Subject of ongoing investigation as of 2005.

Category D: Carotid stent very high risk or not feasible
- Vessel or lesion inaccessible via catheter-based approach
- Unfavorable aortic arch (e.g., shaggy aorta)
- Pedunculated thrombus in vessel
- Allergy to stainless steel or nitinol
Strategy: If revascularization warranted, CEA is treatment of choice.

ACAS, Asymptomatic Carotid Atherosclerosis Study; CAD, Coronary Artery Disease; CCA, Common carotid artery; CEA, Carotid endarterectomy; CHF, Congestive Heart Failure; CABG, Coronary artery bypass grafting; COPD, Chronic obstructive pulmonary disease; ICA, Internal carotid artery; NASCET, North American Symptomatic Carotid Endarterectomy Study.

the surgical risk was prohibitive (Table 26.7; 74,76,83). In 2001, Roubin published a 5-year single-center follow-up of 528 consecutive patients undergoing carotid stenting, with a 98% success rate, a 1.6% mortality, and a combined end point of death and stroke of 7.4% at 30-day follow-up (84). Of note, the rate of stroke decreased significantly over the 5-year time frame of the study, from 7.1% within the first year to 3.1% in the fifth year. This was felt to reflect improvements in technique, interventional devices, and also pharmacotherapy. The seminal work of Roubin and colleagues demonstrated that the results of carotid stenting could be comparable with CEA and highlighted the need

for randomized controlled studies to determine the optimal treatment strategy.

The first such randomized controlled trial was the Carotid and Vertebral Artery Transluminal Angioplasty Study (CAVATAS) trial (85). The angioplasty procedure included stent insertion in only 26% of cases, the remainder performed with balloon angioplasty alone. Distal protection was not available. Despite these limitations, the immediate and long-term results of angioplasty and endarterectomy were equivalent. Subsequently, smaller studies confirmed the benefits of carotid stenting, although the potential for distal embolization and consequent stroke remained a limiting factor.

To address this concern, distal protection devices were developed to minimize or prevent distal embolization. The first randomized trial comparing carotid stenting with emboli protection to carotid endarterectomy was the Stenting and Angioplasty with Protection in Patients at High Risk for Endarterectomy (SAPPHIRE) trial (86). The SAPPHIRE study randomized 307 patients from 29 American centers to either carotid artery stenting (CAS) with distal protection or carotid endarterectomy. Entry criteria included asymptomatic carotid stenosis (>80% by ultrasound) or symptomatic stenosis (>50%), plus at least one feature putting the patient at higher risk for surgical endarterectomy. These features included age older than 80 years, the presence of congestive heart failure, severe chronic obstructive pulmonary disease (COPD), previous endarterectomy with restenosis, previous radiation therapy or radical neck surgery, or lesions distal or proximal to the usual cervical location. Patients were screened by a team including a vascular surgeon, an interventionalist, and a neurologist. Consensus that the patient was a good candidate for both procedures was required before randomization; those rejected as surgical candidates underwent stenting and were included in a separate stent registry; whereas those rejected as candidates for intervention underwent surgery and were included in a surgical registry. At 30 days, the major adverse clinical events (MACE) were reduced by more than 50% by the interventional procedure as compared with surgery (5.8% for CAS, 12.6% for CEA, $P = .047$). Interestingly, 408 patients in the SAPPHIRE study were deemed inappropriate for CEA and were therefore enrolled in the stent arm. Only seven patients were deemed inappropriate for carotid stenting (86). In these registry data, the 30-day MACE rate was 7.8% in the stenting registry (32/409) and 14.3% (1/7) in the surgery registry.

Two subsequent prospective multicenter trials, the Acculink for Revascularization of Carotids in High Risk Patient (ARCHeR; 87) and the Registry Study to evaluate the NeuroShield Bare-Wire Cerebral Protection System and X-Act Stent in patients at high risk for Carotid Endarterectomy (SECuRITY; 88) have demonstrated equally impressive results with the combination of purpose-designed stents and distal protection devices. Further studies are underway to evaluate newer designs of protection devices and stents designed specifically for carotid revascularization.

TABLE 26.8

TREATMENT CONSIDERATIONS AND TECHNIQUE FOR EXTRACRANIAL CAROTID PTA/STENTING

Programmatic issues
- Multidisciplinary team should be in place (Neurology, Vascular Surgery, Neuroradiology, Cardiology or Vascular Interventional Service, Vascular Non Invasive Lab, and Techs/nurses in Interventional Suite)
- Hospital infrastructure (quality assurance mechanisms and privileging criteria defined)

Preprocedure
- Complete evaluation by multispecialty group
- Neuro exam/NIH Stroke Scale by qualified individual
- Complete vascular exam (access issues, cardiac issues, etc.)
- Noninvasive studies (duplex, EKG, echo)
- Diagnostic angiography: aortic arch in LAO projection; selective 2/4-vessel study; lesion measurement using NASCET criteria
- Careful review/consideration of options (CEA; med Rx; carotid stenting) with patient and family; complete informed consent
- Full loading dose of ASA/Plavix before instrumenting; hydration preintervention

Procedure
- Access femoral artery ± vein
- Anticoagulate to ACT 250–300 (no IIb/IIIa inhibitor, unless special circumstances warrant)
- Mild conscious sedation; constant neurologic monitoring throughout procedure
- Access carotid with soft, diagnostic catheter (VITEK or other)
- Anchor 0.038/0.035" glidewire or Wholey in common or external carotid; advance diagnostic catheter into common or external carotid artery
- Advance 6F sheath/guide or 8F guide catheter over wire and diagnostic catheter into CCA
- Perform selective angiograms including baseline intracranial views
- Cross lesion with embolic protection device and deploy it
- Predilate with 3.5–4.0 mm diameter coronary-type balloon
- Advance stent delivery system and deploy self-expanding noncompressible stent
- Postdilate to size of reference site, or slightly less, using low/nominal pressure
- Monitor hemodynamic status closely; administer atropine for bradycardia, fluid and pressors for hypotension, IV NTG for hypertension
- Obtain final angiograms after removal of embolic protection device. Include orthogonal carotid views and lateral and AP (e.g., Townes) intracranial views

Postprocedure in hospital
- Close monitoring in immediate 8–12 hours postprocedure
- Neurologic exam and NIHSS day 1

Follow-up
- ASA lifelong/Plavix X 4 weeks minimum
- Office at 1 month and 1 year (at minimum) for neuro exam/NIHSS/Duplex
- Repeat angio for recurrent symptoms or stenosis >70% by Duplex

NIH, National Institute of Health; LAO, Left anterior oblique; NASCET, North American Symptomatic Carotid Endarterectomy Study; ACT, Activated clotting time; CCA, Common carotid artery; IV NTG, Intravenous nitroglycerin; AP, Anteroposterior; NIHSS, National Institute of Health stroke scale.

Treatment Considerations and Technique (Table 26.8)

Preprocedure Evaluation

Prior to undertaking carotid stenting in an individual patient, a complete neurologic examination should be performed by an individual certified in the NIH stroke scale and capable of performing a comprehensive examination. A baseline carotid duplex, and ideally a CT or MRI of the head, should be obtained. Complete informed consent should be obtained from the patient, with participation by the family. Premedication should include aspirin 325 once or twice daily, clopidogrel (at least 300 mg prior to intervention with sufficient time to achieve efficacy), and prehydration to minimize hypotension. Baseline angiographic information should include nonselective angiography of the aortic arch (LAO projection) with selective two-vessel (or four-vessel if indicated) cerebral study. Formal mea-surements must be made of the target lesion using the NASCET criteria (57). Intracranial angiography should be performed at baseline to rule out intracerebral arterial abnormalities and to establish the baseline arterial anatomy. Of particular importance is the configuration of the aortic arch and the carotid anatomy, the lesion morphology and the presence of collateral flow, patency of the circle of Willis, and the dominance of the intracerebral arterial supply.

Carotid Angioplasty Procedure

Representative equipment required for CPTA/stenting is listed in Table 26.9. Access is typically obtained via the femoral approach. Most of the devices currently used are 6F compatible, allowing the use of an 85-cm-long nonkink-able sheath (i.e., Cook Shuttle, Pinnacle, or ArrowFlex sheaths). Long sheaths minimize the size of the puncture and tend to lie more coaxially within the common carotid

TABLE 26.9

REPRESENTATIVE EQUIPMENT TO HAVE AVAILABLE FOR CAROTID STENTING (2005)

Guidewires	0.035 (stiff)/0.038	Angled glidewire
(exchange-	0.035/0.038	Amplatz extra-support w/1-cm tip
length 300 cm)	0.035	Wholey, Supracore, Rosen
	0.018	V-18, Roadrunner, Steelcore
	0.014	Extra-support coronary wires
Embolic Protection Devices (some remain investigational)		
	Balloon occlusion device	
	Guardwire	
	Filter devices	
	Accunet	
	Angioguard	
	NeuroShield	
	Spider	
	Interceptor	
	FilterWire	
	Proximal balloon with flow reversal	
Diagnostic	5 F	Vitek (125 cm)
catheters	5 F	JB2 (125 cm)
	5/6 F	Berenstein (100/125 cm)
	5 F	Simmons 1, 2, and 3 (100 cm)
	5 F	Davis (100/125 cm)
	5/6 F	JR4 (100/125 cm)
	5 F	Glide cath: Simmons 1/2, JB1, others (100 cm)
	5 F	HN1/HN2/HN3 (100 cm)
Sheaths (adapted	6/7/8 F	Cook Shuttle (85 cm)
for Tuohy-Borst)	6/7/8 F	ArrowFlex (85 cm)
	6/7/8 F	Destination (85 cm)
Guiding catheters	8/9 F	Multipurpose/hockey stick/JR4/others
Balloons	0.014	Coronary balloons; 3.0–5.5 mm diameter $\times$ 15/20/30/40 mm
Stents	Variety of nitinol self-expanding stents or stainless steel stents; tapered/ nontapered configuration	
Temporary pacing wire and box		

artery; but may be more difficult to manipulate and require fastidious attention to flushing. Extreme angulation of the takeoff of the carotid renders selective cannulation challenging, but can usually be identified by baseline arch aortography in the LAO projection to allow the selection of specifically designed catheters (Vitek, JB2, or Simmons) for carotid engagement. Once selectively engaged in the common carotid, a stiffer guidewire is passed into the distal external carotid artery to support advancement of the guiding catheter into the common carotid over a smaller catheter or inner dilator. If the distal common carotid artery has a severe stenosis, this site should be avoided by maintaining guidewire position proximal to the stenosis.

There are certain principles to which one must always adhere when treating carotid or cerebral vessels: First, catheters should always be bled back to avoid any air or cholesterol/plaque embolization. Second, anticoagulation and antiplatelet therapy should commence prior to advanc-

ing any catheters into the carotid system. Third, less time in the carotid system is better. Although one should be cautious and deliberate in the performance of these procedures, the number of complications increases with additional intra-arterial time. Fourth, catheter advancement should always be over a wire, and larger catheters should be transitioned in a stepwise, coaxial fashion over smaller catheters. Fifth, only atraumatic guidewires should be advanced into the internal carotid artery to minimize the risk of spasm or dissection. Sixth, predilation is recommended to confirm the ability to adequately dilate the stenosis. Seventh, the use of self-expanding stents is preferred for the carotid bifurcation and other compressible sites (89,90). Balloon-expandable stents should be used only for aorto-ostial carotid lesions and distal (e.g., intracranial) internal carotid artery lesions. Eighth, when encountering resistance during advancement of balloons or stent delivery systems, removal and redilation with lower profile devices is appropriate. If a self-expanding stent will not easily cross a predilated lesion, it should not be forced. If redilation and readvancement are unsuccessful, placement of a short balloon-expandable stent to "scaffold" the plaque may facilitate subsequent placement of a self-expanding stent. Ninth, careful periprocedural hemodynamic monitoring is essential. Manipulation within the area of the carotid sinus can cause both acute and prolonged hypotension and/or bradycardia (91), requiring fluid resuscitation, atropine or α-adrenergic agents. Pacing is rarely needed but should be readily available (92). Postprocedure hypertension must also be avoided, so as to minimize the chances of hyperperfusion syndrome, a potentially devastating entity that is occasionally seen following revascularization, particularly in elderly patients with previous near-occlusion and underperfused CNS. Tenth, postdilation should be performed to relatively low or nominal pressure. It is not necessary to completely eliminate the stenosis to achieve an excellent result (93). Indeed, attempts to reduce the stenosis to 0% relative to the reference segment may lead to distal embolization, dissection, or resistant hypotension relating to carotid body stimulation or compression.

Stent Selection

The optimal stent design for use in the carotid arteries remains uncertain. Balloon-expandable Palmaz biliary stents were used initially by many groups, with excellent results reported by Wholey, Dietrich, and Satler (75,94).

However, the infrequent but troublesome occurrence of external stent compression has led most investigators to favor self-expanding stents (such as the Wallstent) at the carotid bifurcation (89,90). There is now more extensive experience with the newer nitinol stents (Cordis Smart, Bard Memotherm, Guidant Acculink, etc.), all of which have undergone feasibility trials in the United States. Most investigators agree that the future of carotid stenting will use nitinol, self-expanding stents that are lower profile, 0.014/0.018-inch based, and able to be placed accurately and allow use of distal protection.

Distal Protection

The combination of carotid stenting with distal protection has revolutionized carotid intervention (Fig. 26.8). The first trial demonstrating this benefit was the SAPPHIRE (86) study and was quickly followed by the ARCHeR (87) and SECuRITY (88) studies. Several further protection devices and stent/filter combinations are currently under trial with similarly impressive early results. In general, the available distal protection devices function either by filtering atheromatous debris out of the flowing blood or by occluding antegrade flow to allow removal of atheromatous debris at the completion of the procedure. Each design has relative merits and potential disadvantages (see also Chapter 23). The filtering devices allow for continuous visualization and precise stent placement, as antegrade blood flow is unobstructed. The current filter pore size ranges from 80 to 150 microns, raising the

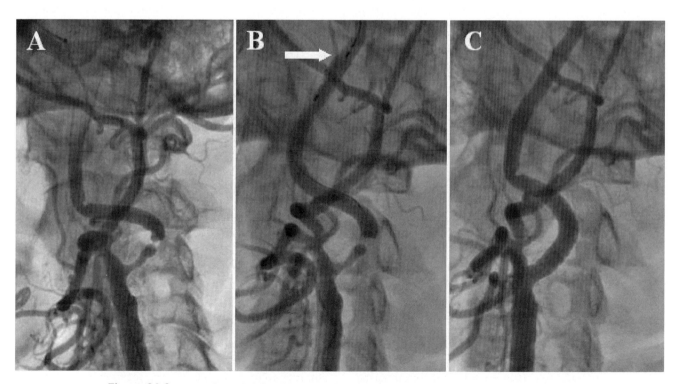

Figure 26.8   A. High-grade left internal carotid artery stenosis with slow flow in comparison with the external carotid. **B.** Flowing placement of a distal protection device in the distal internal carotid artery (*arrow*). **C.** Postplacement of a self-expanding stent (40 × 8.0 mm), dilated with a 6.0-mm balloon and retrieval of the distal protection.

question of what diameter of atheromatous debris is required to cause neurologic sequelae. The occluding devices, by design, limit visualization and, in the absence of adequate collateral circulation, prolong cerebral ischemia. Retrograde embolization to the aortic arch may occur if aggressive injection is performed. However, occluding devices offer the theoretical advantage of protecting against a wider range of particulate sizes. The optimal protection device or combination of protection device and stent remains unclear and is a source of intense clinical investigation.

ABDOMINAL AORTA

Abdominal Aortic Aneurysm

The endovascular repair of abdominal aortic aneurysms using stent grafts represents one of the most dramatic advances in the less invasive treatment of vascular disease. Although this field is still in its infancy, great strides have been made with the devices and technology so that most patients with abdominal aortic aneurysmal disease requiring repair would qualify anatomically for one of the available devices. Nonetheless, the current gold standard for treatment of this disorder remains open surgical repair, and any proposed alternative must be compared against that standard.

The indications for repair of abdominal aortic aneurysms (AAAs) have been discussed previously (see Chapter 14). But a substantial number of patients who have aneurysms greater than 5 cm in diameter are deemed not to be candidates for surgery owing to unsuitable anatomy or the presence of other comorbid conditions. Left untreated, the prognosis is grim, as described by Perko et al. (95). Of the 170 patients deemed inoperable, 132 patients (78%) died during the period of the study; including 78 patients (59% of the 132) who died specifically from rupture. For those who are surgical candidates, the operative mortality of aneurysm resection is between 1.4 and 7.6%, but increases substantially for those whose aneurysms are symptomatic (96). The possibility that endovascular stent grafts might lower the morbidity and mortality in these high-risk or inoperable patients has provided the most compelling reason to pursue the development of these devices.

The first stent-graft in a human was placed by Parodi (97) in Argentina and consisted of a straight Dacron tube graft affixed at its proximal end to a large balloon-expandable Palmaz stent. A distal stent was subsequently added to the device to control retrograde flow into the aneurysm sac (endoleak). Several more elaborate stent grafts have since been developed and subjected to clinical trials: Guidant EVT, Boston Scientific Vanguard, Medtronic AVE AneuRx, Medtronic AVE Talent, Cook Zenith, Corvita Endograft, and Gore Prograft. Two (the AneuRx and EVT devices) received FDA approval in 1999 and are commercially available. To address the fact that the abdominal aortic pathology frequently extends into the iliac vessels, most

abdominal endografts are now bifurcated or aortomonoiliac devices at their distal end to extend into the distal vasculature and thereby achieve a more complete seal (with an aortomonoiliac device, the contralateral iliac artery may be perfused via a fem-fem bypass graft).

Thousands of stent–graft procedures have been performed worldwide for abdominal aortic aneurysm exclusion. D'Ayala, Hollier, and Marin (98) summarized the results in 767 patients: success rate 74 to 100%, persistent endoleaks in 14% (one-third of which closed spontaneously), and 4% mortality. More recently published series describe the multicenter prospective experience with the AneuRx stent graft and the Boston Scientific Vanguard devices (98,99). Both demonstrate success rates approaching 90%, endoleaks in approximately 10%, and reduction in morbidity compared with conventional repair, but they have a steep learning curve that entails mastering device and patient selection issues. Aneurysms with a short or absent proximal neck (distance between the lower border of the renal artery and the beginning of the aneurysm) are more difficult to treat, although some device iterations now incorporate additional bare stent material designed to be deployed proximally overlying the renal vessels, with the graft material beginning just below the renal arteries. Other issues remain, such as the obligatory sacrifice of one or both of the internal iliac arteries (which sometimes potentially has deleterious consequences) and the large caliber of current devices (12F to 28F). Technical advances promise to address both of these issues. As in the case with endovascular treatment of other vascular sites, most successful endovascular stent–graft programs are based on spirited collaboration between vascular surgeons and endovascular specialists in cardiology and/or radiology.

Renal Arteries

Renal artery stenosis (RAS) is a common manifestation of generalized atherosclerosis whose clinical importance is increasingly being recognized. The interaction between coronary and renal atherosclerosis is complex, sharing common risk factors and a similarly insidious progression. Coronary disease and its treatment frequently exacerbate renal function, whereas renal disease accelerates coronary atherosclerosis and causes resistant hypertension by stimulating the rennin-angiotensin system. RAS thus represents the most common cause of secondary hypertension, affecting at least 5% of the general population (100) and as many as 39% of patients undergoing cardiac catheterization (101). It results in deteriorating renal function and progressive renal atrophy, and is the underlying pathology for 12 to 14% of patients with dialysis-dependent renal failure (102).

The goals of renal artery revascularization are to improve control of hypertension, preserve or restore renal function, and/or treat other potential adverse physiologic effects of severe renal artery stenosis (congestive heart failure, recurrent flash pulmonary edema, and angina; 103).

The options available for renal artery revascularization include surgery (endarterectomy, aortorenal bypass, or extra-anatomic bypass using hepatorenal, splenorenal, ileorenal, or superior mesenteric artery [SMA]–renal anastomosis) and PTA, with or without stent deployment. Balloon angioplasty of the renal arteries was first performed by Gruntzig in 1978, but as in other vascular beds, the results of stenting are superior to stand-alone angioplasty (see Chapter 24). With the widespread use of renal artery stenting, this procedure has gradually superseded surgery as the treatment of choice for most patients with renal vascular disease (6). When analyzing indications and results, it is important to distinguish between the two major causes of renal artery stenosis: fibromuscular dysplasia (FMD) and the more common atherosclerotic disease.

Fibromuscular Dysplasia

Fibromuscular dysplasia (FMD) is a nonatherosclerotic, noninflammatory disorder of unknown etiology that constitutes the second most common cause of RAS (104). It typically affects women from 15 to 50 years of age and is more common in first-degree relatives and in the presence of the ACE-I allele (105,106). FMD can also involve carotid and peripheral arteries, although renal artery involvement is seen in 60% of cases of FMD, with frequent bilateral involvement (104). Progressive renal stenosis is seen in 37% of cases and loss of renal mass in 63% (107,108). Fibromuscular dysplasia has a distinctive angiographic appearance, with a beaded, aneurysmal pattern (Fig. 26.9). Although medical management of hypertension is frequently successful, the high rates of procedural success, elimination of hypertension, and low recurrence rate (10%) of percutaneous intervention have resulted in a low threshold for intervening in these patients (109). FMD localized within the main renal artery or its primary branches can be treated quite effectively with balloon angioplasty alone, with stenting reserved for failure or complications of balloon angioplasty (see Fig. 34.11.) FMD that involves multiple branch vessels and/or aneurysmal disease, however, is usually better treated surgically, potentially using the technique of "bench" (i.e., extracorporeal) reconstruction of the branch vessels. Occasional cases may be treated with advanced stenting and coiling techniques (see Fig. 34.13A).

Atherosclerotic Renal Artery Stenosis

Percutaneous treatment of atherosclerotic renal artery stenosis (ARAS), which causes the vast majority of renal artery narrowing, has been less gratifying than that of FMD. During the 1980s, balloon angioplasty proved to be a safe and effective modality, but had an unacceptably high restenosis rate approaching 70% at 6 to 12 months. As a result, the gold standard of treatment remained surgical revascularization, despite a surgical mortality of 2 to 17%,

even in appropriately selected patients (110). In the 1990s, however, numerous investigators demonstrated better amelioration of the stenosis and trans-stenotic pressure gradient following stent deployment in aorto-ostial lesions compared with balloon angioplasty alone, followed by a lower restenosis rate. Palmaz (103) summarized the results of stenting in 349 patients from eight series followed for a mean duration of 10.9 months. Hypertension was improved in 56% and cured in 10%; renal function improved in 27% and stabilized (e.g., no further deterioration) in 38%. Restenosis occurred in approximately 16% of patients with major complications in 4.9%, but these were reduced in the more recent series.

Following these results, the Dutch Renal Artery Stenosis Intervention Cooperative Study (DRASTIC) randomized 106 patients treated with RAS to either balloon angioplasty or medical therapy (111). It found no difference between treatment arms, but had several limitations. First, most interventional strategies involved balloon angioplasty alone, with stenting reserved as a bailout (despite substantial evidence of the immediate and long-term superiority of stenting). Second, 44% of the medically treated cohort crossed over to intervention within 3 months owing to uncontrolled hypertension, thus jeopardizing the validity of an "intention to treat" analysis. Finally, progression of RAS to complete occlusion was seen in 16% of the medically treated arm, but did not occur in the interventional group. Therefore, 60% of the medical group either failed medical therapy or had progression of RAS to occlusion (111).

In contrast to DRASTIC, subsequent studies have confirmed the benefits of stenting for ARAS. A multicenter registry-based study reported the outcome of 1,058 patients, demonstrating improved hypertensive control, fewer antihypertensive agents, and a fall in serum creatinine concentration from 1.7 to 1.3 mg/dL over a 4-year period (112). Similarly, a meta-analysis of 10 studies demonstrated that renal function improved in 26%, remained stable in 48%, and deteriorated in 26% of cases (113). Promising results were also reported by Watson et al. (114), who demonstrated that, in patients with bilateral RAS, renal stenting successfully reversed or reduced the progression of renal insufficiency.

In general, the current indications for renal artery PTA and stenting are threefold: (1) control of hypertension, (2) elimination of congestive heart failure/flash pulmonary edema, and (3) preservation or salvage of renal function (Fig. 26.10 and Table 26.10). A common finding in studies to date, however, is that some patients fail to demonstrate any significant clinical response. Therefore, an important clinical challenge is to select the patients who are likely to benefit. Several clinical factors have been shown to be predictive of a successful outcome for control of hypertension: (a) rapid acceleration of hypertension over the prior weeks or months, (b) presence of "malignant" hypertension (e.g., end organ effect), (c) hypertension in association with flash pulmonary edema, (d) contemporaneous rise in

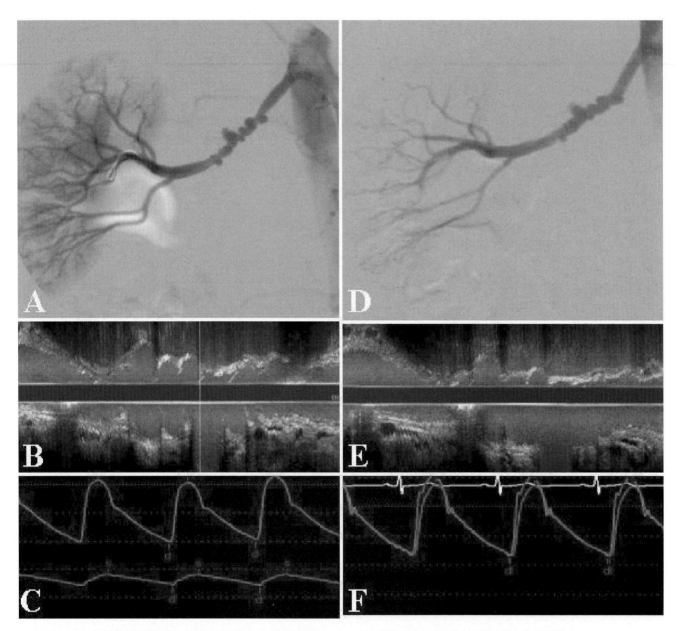

Figure 26.9   **A.** Classic "string of beads" appearance of fibromuscular dysplasia. **B.** Intravascular ultrasound (IVUS) with a 40-MHz catheter demonstrating multiple fine fibrous bands and foci of interband aneurysmal dilatation. **C.** Translesional gradient measured between a 6F guide catheter placed in the aorta and a 4F glide catheter placed in the distal renal artery. A 60-mm Hg resting gradient is demonstrated. **D.** Post–balloon angioplasty with a 4.5-mm-diameter balloon demonstrating improvement in the angiographic appearance, which is confirmed by the postangioplasty IVUS shown in **(E)**. Postprocedure IVUS demonstrates fracture of the fibrous bands, resulting in resolution of the gradient seen before the procedure **(F)**.

serum creatinine, and (e) development of azotemia in response to ACE inhibitors administered for control of hypertension. Predictors of successful salvage or preservation of renal function are similar and include (a) recent rapid rise in creatinine, unexplained by other factors; (b) azotemia resulting from ACE inhibitors; (c) absence of diabetes or other cause of intrinsic kidney disease; and (d) the presence of global renal ischemia, wherein the entire functioning renal mass is subtended by bilateral critically narrowed renal arteries or a vessel supplying a solitary kidney.

Conversely, predictors of poor functional renal recovery following ARAS stenting include (1) renal atrophy demonstrated by kidney length <7.5 cm on ultrasound, (2) high renal resistance index detected by duplex ultrasound, (3) proteinuria >1 gm/day, (4) hyperuricemia, and finally, (5) creatinine clearance <40 mL/minute. None of these, however, constitute an absolute contraindication, as individual patient responses are unpredictable.

It is important to note that the clinical spectrum of ARAS is very wide, and not every patient with ARAS needs

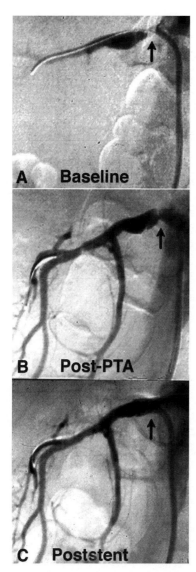

Figure 26.10 Reversal of renal failure with stenting. A 74-year-old male with baseline renal insufficiency (creatinine 2.8), who developed acute anuric renal failure following coronary artery bypass graft (CABG). **A.** After doing poorly on dialysis for 3 weeks, angiogram was repeated, showing critical stenosis to solitary kidney. **B.** Suboptimal result after balloon angioplasty (PTA), owing to recoil/plaque fracture. **C.** After stent, patient no longer required dialysis and remains off dialysis at 3-year follow-up.

TABLE 26.10
INDICATIONS FOR REVASCULARIZATION OF RAS

"Clear" indications
Preservation of renal function in progressive renal failure
1. Control of malignant or resistant hypertension
2. Treatment of recurrent flash pulmonary edema or unstable angina in association with severe renal artery stenosis (RAS)
3. RAS to a solitary kidney with non–dialysis-dependent renal failure
"Not-so-clear" indications
1. Hypertension that is difficult to control in patient with unilateral RAS, with or without renal insufficiency

---

and the interventionalist. Although the approach of delayed intervention allows instigation of comprehensive antihypertensive therapy and risk factor modification, there is mounting evidence that earlier RAS intervention yields greater preservation of renal function, better control of renovascular hypertension, and reduced cardiovascular morbidity. This hypothesis will be tested in an NIH-sponsored clinical trial (CORAL) examining cardiovascular mortality after randomization between medical therapy and stenting for RAS.

Finally, RAS should always be excluded in patients who present with flash pulmonary edema or unstable angina. Flash pulmonary edema is particularly prevalent in patients with bilateral RAS or unilateral RAS supplying a solitary functional kidney and is generally refractory to medical therapy. Among these patients, however, renal revascularization has been shown to effectively alleviate pulmonary edema and unstable angina.

Treatment Considerations and Technique

Access
Renal artery angioplasty and stenting are usually performed via the retrograde femoral approach. Because the proximal renal artery segment initially courses inferiorly and posteriorly, some interventionalists prefer the brachial approach to allow more coaxial alignment. However, the greater incidence of vascular entry site complications causes us to avoid the brachial approach except when the aorta is occluded distally or the renal artery takeoff is so severely angulated as to preclude stent delivery from below.

Diagnostic Angiography
These techniques are described in Chapter 14. Nonselective arteriography is recommended prior to selective cannulation to identify the location of the renal ostia and the configuration of the aorta and to minimize the need for catheter manipulation in a diseased, atherogenic aorta. It may also identify accessory renal arteries, which are present in roughly 25% of patients. Once the ostia are

to be stented. On one extreme is the patient with unilateral RAS, normal renal function, and mild or moderate hypertension well controlled medically, who would derive little immediate benefit and should probably be followed longitudinally, with serial re-evaluation of renal function, kidney size, and control of blood pressure. At the other extreme is the patient with long-standing severe baseline renal insufficiency secondary to nephrosclerosis (e.g., diabetic nephropathy) with superimposed RAS or ultrasound findings suggestive of atrophy, in which intervention is unlikely to procure any benefit. Determining the optimum timing for intervention within this spectrum is complex, often requiring close interaction between the nephrologist identified, then selective cannulation may be performed using any of several catheter shapes (IMA, J Judkins right, hockey stick, renal double curve, or Sos-Omni). A suitable guidewire is passed across the lesion, over which a diagnostic catheter can be advanced to measure a baseline pressure gradient. By convention, a significant pressure gradient is anything >10 mm Hg mean and/or 20 mm Hg peak, measured through a 4F or 5F catheter placed beyond the stenosis. Below this level of gradient, a patient is unlikely to benefit dramatically with respect to blood pressure control or renal function, although an argument could be made to treat to prevent progression.

Balloon Inflation and Stent Deployment

Following diagnostic measurements, the diagnostic catheter is exchanged over the guidewire for a guiding catheter (renal double curve, hockey stick, IMA or other), advanced with the nose of the predilatation balloon protruding. Classically, predilatation with a slightly undersized (e.g., 4-mm) balloon is recommended, which assesses vessel size, minimizes initial trauma, and allows the guiding catheter to be advanced into the midrenal artery over the deflating balloon. This then allows stent advancement across the lesion within the guiding catheter, which is in turn withdrawn slightly to expose the stent for expansion. The current availability of 0.014- and 0.018-inch balloons with flexible premounted stents (including monorail systems) has enabled modification of this technique. Specifically, smaller guide catheters, wires, and sheaths are now required, and the need to cross the lesion with the guide catheter before desheathing the stent to facilitate safe delivery is now much lower.

After confirmation of appropriate stent position, taking into account any expected foreshortening of the stent and the need for the stent to extend slightly (0.5 to 2 mm) into the aorta to cover true ostial lesions, the stent is deployed. Postdilation to high pressure (10 to 14 atmospheres) is performed, with care to avoid overdilation (heralded by severe discomfort) or dissection of the distal, nonstented vessel. The O-ring on the guiding catheter or sheath should be loosened during inflation to allow the dilating balloon to assume an orientation in line with the proximal renal artery rather than pulling the renal ostium down during inflation. Final angiography, pressures measurement, and intravascular ultrasound (IVUS) can be used to assess the outcome, especially if there remains a question regarding stent apposition or lumen size (Fig. 26.11). The guiding catheter is then removed over the wire.

Periprocedural Care

Fluids should be administered liberally prior to, during, and following the procedure, with diuretics held in reserve to prevent volume overload. Postprocedure monitoring of the hemodynamic state is mandatory—some patients with global renal ischemia may experience a significant fall in blood pressure as the high renin state abates, particularly if they have been allowed to become volume depleted. Blood pressure medications are thus reduced by half in anticipation of this response, but complete withdrawal of all antihypertensive medications is ill advised in patients with coexisting coronary artery disease. Since the full clinical response to renal artery revascularization may not occur until 1 to 2 weeks after the intervention, blood pressure, creatinine, and medications should be re-evaluated at 2 to 4 weeks follow-up.

Complications

Complications related to balloon angioplasty and/or stenting of renal arteries occur in <10% of patients and most commonly involve the access site. The most feared complication, however, is that of atheroembolism either into the renal or peripheral vascular bed. This is more likely to occur with aggressive manipulation of the diagnostic and/or guiding catheters; aortic wall contact can be minimized through identification of the renal ostia on a nonselective angiogram prior to selective cannulation with a soft, atraumatic diagnostic catheter. Distal embolization to the renal artery may be partially preventable using distal protection devices described above (see also Chapter 23). Peripheral embolization of atheromatous debris, termed *cholesterol embolization*, is more sinister. The signs of cholesterol embolization include persistent hypertension despite successful renal artery revascularization, gradual rise in creatinine over the succeeding weeks, the presence of livido reticularis on the abdominal wall or in the lower extremities, and the presence of eosinophilia on a peripheral blood smear. There is no known effective treatment for the manifestations of cholesterol embolization once it occurs, although some have reported the effective resolution of ischemic lower extremity rest pain and ulceration using intravenous prostaglandin (115). Other complications of percutaneous renal revascularization include dissection of the renal artery or the wall of the aorta, acute or delayed thrombosis, infection, rupture of the renal artery, or renal perforation by a distally placed guidewire.

Mesenteric Arteries

Indications for Treatment and Results

Stenosis of the mesenteric vessels is a frequent finding during routine angiography, although ischemic symptoms or consequences are rare. This is largely the result of the redundant blood supply emanating from the three visceral arteries, the superior mesenteric, the inferior mesenteric and the celiac artery, in combination with a rich source of potential collaterals. These collaterals allow communication between the inferior and superior mesenteric arteries either via the meandering mesenteric artery that courses deep in the colonic mesentery or via the arc of Riolan. The celiac and superior mesenteric territories are connected by the pancreaticoduodenal arteries; the inferior mesenteric territory may be collateralized by sigmoidal and

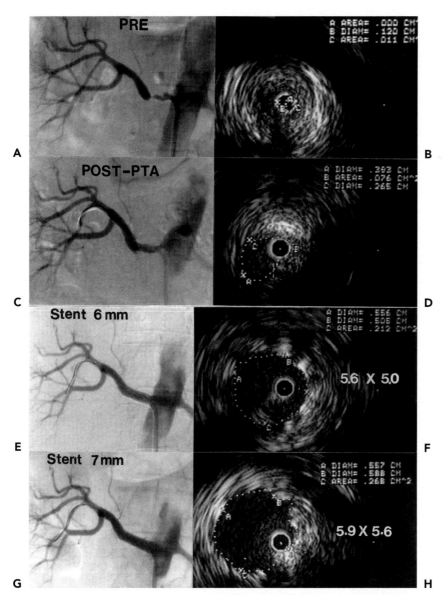

Figure 26.11 Balloon angioplasty (PTA) of proximal renal artery lesion, guided by intravascular ultrasound (IVUS). **A.** Baseline angiogram depicts severe proximal renal artery stenosis. **B.** Corresponding IVUS image shows plaque abutting catheter circumferentially. **C.** Post-PTA, irregular lumen with plaque fracture and residual stenosis. **D.** IVUS post-PTA shows only modest enlargement of lumen. **E.** Deployment and dilation of Palmaz stent with 6-mm balloon; angiographic result much improved over PTA alone. **F.** IVUS shows doubling in lumen diameter over PTA alone. However, in spite of excellent angiographic appearance, IVUS shows that diameter of treated segment is still less than reference segment. **G.** After inflation with 7-mm balloon, the angiographic result is slightly better. **H.** IVUS now shows size of stented vessel is equal to that of reference segment. This case highlights utility of IVUS in renal angioplasty.

hemorrhoidal arteries from the external iliac artery. As a result, true chronic mesenteric ischemia is uncommon. As with coronary atherosclerosis, an imbalance of the arterial supply and demand results in development of symptoms. Intestinal arterial demand is greatest following a large meal. Classically, postprandial symptoms of abdominal pain, gas, diarrhea, food avoidance, and ultimately weight loss indicate severe global compromise of mesenteric blood supply (such as occlusion of two out of three mesenteric vessels and a critical stenosis in the third). With less profound ischemia, symptoms can be vague, including nonspecific postprandial discomfort, fullness or bloating, prompting multiple investigations. Although vague, symptoms progress insidiously, resulting in "food fear" and ultimately profound weight loss; the median weight loss in one series was 28 lb (range, 3 to 100 lb). The angiographic diagnosis can be also be ambiguous as the mesenteric vessels originate and project anteriorly from the aorta and are inadequately visualized during conventional anteroposterior (AP) angiography. Therefore, extremely angulated and/or lateral views are required to define aorto-ostial and proximal lesions in these vessels.

As is the case with many other vascular sites, the standard of therapy for mesenteric disease has (until recently) been surgical (endarterectomy or bypass), with a mortality rate that approaches 6% (116,117). Balloon angioplasty can be effective in restoring acute patency, although restenosis rates are 50% or more owing to the ostial location of these lesions. Adjunctive stenting improves procedural success, reduces acute recoil and achieves long-term patency, although formal randomized studies have yet to be performed (see Chapter 34). The biggest dilemma in patients with mesenteric disease is deciding who is and is not likely to benefit. Decisions to intervene should clearly be symptom driven. Certainly, the incidental findings of a stenotic mesenteric vessel during routine angiography does not necessarily indicate the need for treatment. But the ability to effectively treat mesenteric ischemia has led to intervention in patients with more modest mesenteric ischemic syndromes, such as postprandial bloating, than profound weight loss and cachexia. At the other extreme, percutaneous treatment is also ill advised in patients with acute mesenteric ischemia in whom bowel infarction has already taken place, where surgical repair and intestinal resection is preferred.

Treatment Considerations and Technique

Aorto-ostial mesenteric disease is similar in most respects to aorto-ostial renal artery disease. Therefore, the approach to balloon angioplasty and stenting is identical. Thus far, there are no controlled trials nor any large series reported using stents in mesenteric arteries. Despite similar results and techniques, three factors distinguish the mesenteric vessels from the renals: First, the celiac and superior mesenteric arteries both tend to arise off the aorta at more of a downward angle than the renal arteries, making access from below somewhat more difficult. Second, visualization of the target lesion may be more difficult in these vessels than for the renal arteries; use of the lateral projection is often required. Third, the complications related to failure and/or embolization may include bowel infarction, sepsis, and death, highlighting the extreme caution and careful technique required.

Aortoiliac Obstructive Disease

Most infrarenal abdominal aorta and iliac arteries disease is atherosclerotic in origin. Treatment of atherosclerotic lesions within the distal aorta and iliac arteries is similar, and therefore will be considered together. Leriche first recognized the effects of impaired inflow at the level of the terminal aorta and iliac arteries in his classic 1923 publication (119,120). Surgical revascularization began with endarterectomy in the 1940s, and bypass surgery in the 1950s. In 1979, Gruntzig and Kumpe described their

experience with balloon angioplasty of iliac lesions, which yielded a 2-year patency rate of 87% (7). While balloon dilatation has been applied to atherosclerotic disease at every site in the body, nowhere have the results been superior to those achieved in the aortoiliac vessels.

Indications for Intervention and Results

Aortoiliac revascularization is currently recommended for three indications:

1. Relief of symptomatic lower extremity ischemia, including claudication, rest pain, ulceration or gangrene, or embolization causing blue toe syndrome (Fig. 26.1; Chapter 34)
2. Restoration and/or preservation of inflow to the lower extremity in the setting of pre-existing or anticipated distal bypass (Fig. 26.2)
3. Procurement of access to more proximal vascular beds for anticipated invasive procedures (e.g., cardiac catheterization/PTCA, intra-aortic balloon insertion; see Chapter 34). Occasionally, revascularization is indicated to rescue flow-limiting dissection complicating access for other invasive procedures (Fig. 26.12).

Aortobifemoral bypass has a long-term patency of 90% at 1 year, 75 to 80% at 5 years, and 60 to 70% at 10 years, but carries a mortality between 2 and 3%. Accordingly, surgical intervention has been reserved for patients with critical limb ischemia or advanced degrees of disability (Rutherford category 3 or above). Because percutaneous angioplasty is less invasive, generally has fewer complications, and is lower in cost, the threshold at which intervention is offered to patients with aortoiliac disease may be lower (Fig. 26.1; 1).

There are relatively few studies examining the outcome of PTA in isolated aortic segments (Fig. 26.13), owing to the relatively uncommon occurrence of this entity (compared with combined aortoiliac disease). Most atherosclerotic aortic disease is more diffuse and thus extends into the iliac arteries, requiring treatment of both territories.

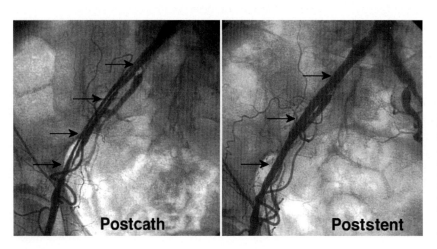

Figure 26.12 An 84-year-old female complaining of increasing right leg pain and coolness during cardiac catheterization. Following cath, iliac angiogram demonstrates flow-limiting, lengthy spiral dissection (arrows). Flow restored after treatment with Wallstent and balloon angioplasty (PTA). Severe left iliac disease is also noted. When encountering new symptoms of lower extremity ischemia during cath, angiographic delineation of the cause is preferable to removing the sheath and hoping for restoration of flow.

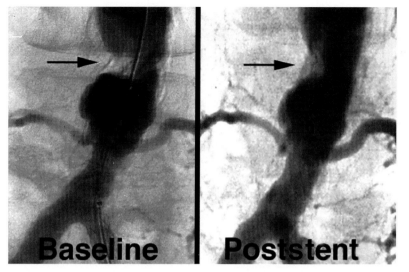

Figure 26.13 Balloon angioplasty (PTA)/stent of isolated infrarenal aortic stenosis, causing Rutherford category II claudication in 63-year-old female. Long (35-cm) 8F sheath is used to protect Palmaz P-308 stent until delivered to site. To minimize profile and optimize positioning, initial deployment is with 9-mm balloon. After dilation to 12 mm, lumen size is improved; in the aorta, there is no indication (and there may be contraindication) to enlarge stent to size of adjacent (ectatic) vessel. However, subsequent guidewire passage must be performed cautiously, as stent struts may be nonapposed.

In fact, revascularization at the aortic bifurcation commonly uses either kissing balloons or kissing stents. (See Chapter 34; 121). Considerable controversy remains in some circles concerning the optimal treatment, but increasingly both surgeons and interventionalists support angioplasty and stenting as the initial approach to revascularization, with aortobifemoral bypass reserved for occlusive disease or those not amenable to PTA or stenting (122,123).

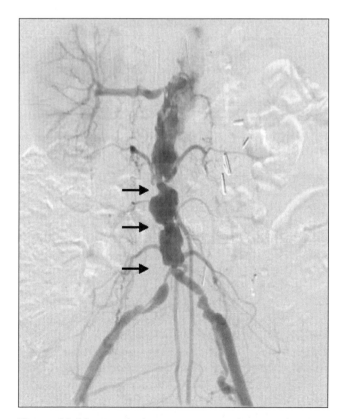

Figure 26.14 Digital subtraction angiography (DSA) depicting severe sequential infrarenal aortic stenosis extending into the aortoiliac bifurcation.

The results of balloon angioplasty alone for iliac stenoses, particularly focal lesions, is excellent, with acute technical and clinical success >90% across a large number of reports (124,125). Patency rates for 1, 3, and 5 years range from approximately 75 to 95%, 60 to 90%, and 55 to 85%, respectively. The wide disparity of these results is a reflection of multiple factors, including variations in selection criteria, discrepancies in measurements of outcome, and the evolution of technique over time. Factors associated with good results include short, focal lesion; large vessel size; common iliac (as opposed to external iliac); single lesion (as opposed to multiple serial lesions); male gender; lesser Rutherford category (claudication as opposed to critical limb ischemia); and presence of good runoff. The results in patients with diffuse disease, smaller vessels, diabetes mellitus, female gender, critical limb ischemia, and poor runoff are less favorable. The results for aortoiliac occlusions are also less favorable.

Stents for Aortoiliac Disease

In 1993, the FDA approved the use of Palmaz balloon-expandable stents (P-308 series, 30 mm long and 8 mm in diameter) for iliac arteries. Specific indications were for failed PTA (defined as a residual mean gradient of ≥5 mm, residual stenosis of >30%, or presence of a flow-limiting dissection; 126). The self-expanding Wallstent prosthesis was approved for similar indications in 1996 (127). The favorable acute results, relative ease of use, and paucity of complications encountered during aortoiliac stenting, however, has led to expanded use of these devices to reduce recoil and improve on the immediate hemodynamic and angiographic result of PTA. Using stents, acute technical success is in the range of 90 to 100%, with average 1-year patency of 90% and average 3-year patency of 75% (128). Because of these superior cosmetic and hemodynamic results, a strategy of primary stent deployment for aortoiliac vessels has been adopted by many, although others reserve stenting only for suboptimal angioplasty results.

Tetteroo and colleagues (124) published a randomized trial between balloon angioplasty and primary stenting, showing no difference in the primary end point when balloon angioplasty patients were allow to cross over to stenting for a residual stenosis of 50% or a residual gradient ≥10 mm mean (43% of provisional patients did so). If analyzed on a per protocol basis, stenting was far superior. Clinical and hemodynamic success rates were approximately 77 and 85%, respectively, at 24 months, comparable with many surgical series of aortobifemoral bypass. Even more compelling is the meta-analysis performed by Bosch et al. (125) on 14 recent studies (all published after 1990) involving more than 2,100 patients undergoing aortoiliac PTA. This meta-analysis showed a superior immediate success rate for stents than for PTA alone (96 versus 91%) with a subsequent 4-year primary patency rate for stenotic lesions of 77% for stenting versus 65% for PTA alone. For occlusions, 4-year patency rates were 61% for stents and 54% for PTA.

Treatment Considerations and Technique

Prior to undertaking aortoiliac PTA, careful consideration should be given to the issue of arterial access. Baseline angiographic and/or noninvasive studies form the basis of decisions regarding access. When treating unilateral disease that ends above the common femoral artery, we prefer ipsilateral retrograde access, which provides the most direct approach to the stenotic (or occlusive) lesion and facilitates stent deployment. The contralateral approach using crossover sheaths and guiding catheters is preferred when the target lesion is located near the common femoral artery or the femoral head, when the groin below the target is either scarred or the common femoral artery heavily calcified, or when there is particular concern about impeding the outflow during sheath removal following revascularization of an iliac lesion. The contralateral approach is also used when more distal revascularization is to be pursued in the same sitting, but is more challenging in cases of acutely angulated aortic bifurcations or stenosis at the origin of the common iliac artery. For iliac occlusions, either retrograde or contralateral access is appropriate, and frequently both are required to successfully recanalize occluded segments. For lesions involving the aortic bifurcation, a bilateral retrograde femoral approach is recommended to enable placement of kissing stents. Both balloon-expandable (BE) and self-expanding (SE) stents can be used in the aortoiliac region. Although SE stents are increasingly accurate in their deployment, BE stents remain superior where precise stent positioning is critical and by virtue of their greater radial strength. On the other hand, SE stents may be preferred in the external iliac artery as one approaches the flexion point at the femoral head (a BE stent at this site might be permanently deformed by compression).

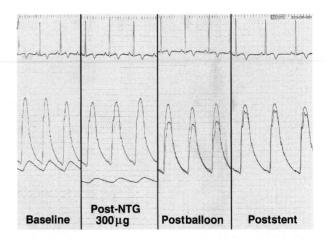

Figure 26.15 Pressure gradients obtained during revascularization of iliac occlusion from patient in Fig. 26.1. **A.** Baseline gradient. **B.** Gradient after distal administration of nitroglycerin (NTG). **C.** Postballoon, significant resting gradient remains, even without provocation . **D.** Gradient eliminated after stenting, demonstrating superior hemodynamic result.

Role of Pressure Gradients and Intravascular Ultrasound

Pressure gradients are routinely measured across iliac and aortic lesions (Fig. 26.15), but there are few objective data regarding what constitutes a significant hemodynamic stenosis. By convention, a 5 mm Hg mean resting pressure gradient is taken as indicative of a significant residual stenosis. If the resting gradient is borderline, a persistent (e.g., >60-sec) mean pressure gradient of >15 mm Hg after administration of a vasodilator (200 to 300 μg of nitroglycerin) is considered significant. Intravascular ultrasound (IVUS) is superior to contrast angiography in demonstrating detailed vessel anatomy and can be very useful during aortoiliac angioplasty by measuring the dimensions of the reference site, the degree of narrowing, and the characteristics of the vessel wall (calcium, etc.; 11,12).

Thrombolytic Therapy

The utility of thrombolytic therapy in iliac occlusions is controversial. For occlusions in peripheral vessels, catheter-directed thrombolysis is much more effective than systemic fibrinolysis. The technical aspects of use vary among investigators. There is agreement that the catheter must penetrate into the occlusion for the lytic agent to have any effect. Some prefer going one step farther and crossing the occlusion, primarily to "lace" the lytic agent throughout the occlusion and enhance the efficiency of thrombolysis. Others prefer crossing the occlusion and administering the lytic in pulsed spray fashion. This technique may accelerate clot dissolution, but is associated with a slightly higher incidence of distal embolization. Urokinase is no longer available, and thus t-PA and Retavase are the current agents of choice (129). These can be combined with rheolytic thrombectomy to augment clot removal (see Chapter 23).

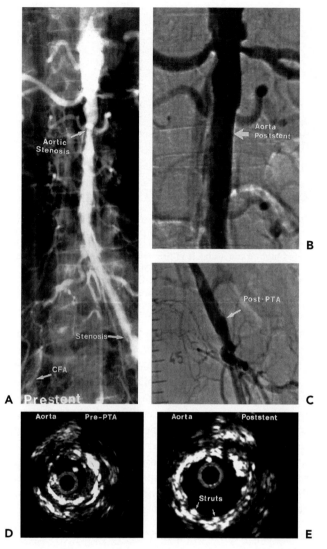

Figure 26.16 Balloon angioplasty (PTA) of aorta and common iliac artery in nonischemic (left) side in preparation for cross-femoral graft leads to unexpected resolution of ischemic pain. Patient is a 62-year-old woman, a poor surgical candidate, with rest pain and severe claudication in right leg. Occlusion of right common iliac artery and stenoses in infrarenal aorta and left common iliac artery pre-PTA **(A)**. Initial strategy was to dilate the stenotic sites, then graft from left to right common femoral artery (CFA). Following **(B)** PTA/stent of aorta, and **(C)** PTA alone of iliac artery, patient's right (contralateral) leg symptoms disappeared, presumably owing to increased left to right collateral flow via internal iliac artery tributaries. Planned cross-femoral bypass surgery was therefore canceled. PTA was guided by intravascular ultrasound (IVUS), which demonstrates marked improvement in lumen cross-sectional area of aortic lesion from pre-PTA **(D)** to poststent **(E)**.

Use of Aortoiliac PTA in Conjunction with Surgery

Many patients with aortoiliac disease also have infrainguinal disease. In such cases, the aortoiliac disease is treated first to improve inflow, which often obviates the need for reconstruction more distally (Fig. 26.16). In some instances, PTA of the "donor" iliac may be performed to preserve inflow to a planned cross-femoral graft (Fig. 26.2). The same strategy underlies the preparatory role of iliac angioplasty in patients undergoing surgical revascularization for treatment of distal disease. For example, common femoral artery cutdown, intraoperative balloon angioplasty, and iliac stent deployment may be followed by fem-pop or fem-fem bypass in the same sitting. Likewise, revascularization may be staged with proximal PTA first, followed by surgery some 3 to 4 weeks later. These approaches constitute a natural extension of the use of endovascular techniques to minimize morbidity and mortality and maximize the benefit for the patient.

In summary, percutaneous therapy has now become the first line of therapy for aortoiliac obstructive disease. With the exception of patients with very extensive disease, PTA with stent deployment is associated with a highly successful acute and long-term outcome. If this strategy fails, subsequent surgical intervention remains feasible. The guidelines published by the AHA in 1994 (1) list four categories of iliac disease: Category 1 includes stenoses <3 cm long, concentric and noncalcified, for which PTA is recommended. Category 2 includes stenoses 3 to 5 cm long or calcified, or eccentric stenoses <3 cm long, for which PTA was also felt to be well suited. Category 3 lesions consist of stenoses 5 to 10 cm long or occlusions <5 cm long, in which PTA could be performed, although the initial chance of technical success or long-term benefit might not be as good as with bypass surgery; however, PTA might be indicated, depending on the patient risk factor profile. Category 4 lesions include stenoses >10 cm long, occlusions >5 cm long, extensive bilateral aortoiliac atherosclerosis, or lesions in association with abdominal aortic aneurysm or other lesion requiring surgical repair, for which the percutaneous approach was not recommended. These guidelines are evolving, as the benefits of stenting have become manifest and the limits of percutaneous therapy are being extended.

Complications

Complications are relatively infrequent with aortoiliac angioplasty (<6% based on multiple series). Most common are access site complications, including local or retroperitoneal bleeding, pseudoaneurysm, and atrioventricular (AV) fistula (see Chapters 3 and 4) . Thrombotic occlusion at the site of angioplasty is extremely rare, as is rupture (which, however, can have devastating consequences). Arterial rupture must be recognized promptly and controlled by inflation of a balloon within the lesion (balloon tamponade), reversal of anticoagulation, and volume resuscitation. Surgery may be required infrequently, but stent grafts are increasingly being used to treat this complication. Other complications include distal embolization, which was said to occur with alarming frequency in early studies of recanalized total iliac occlusion. More recent studies indicate an incidence of <5% (129a). Systemic complications, such as contrast or atheroembolic induced renal failure, myocardial infarction, CVA, and death, all occur with an incidence of <0.5%. Complications requiring surgical repair are also relatively infrequent, in the range of 2%.

LOWER EXTREMITY

Common Femoral Artery

Revascularization of this vessel has previously been considered the exclusive purview of the vascular surgeon, whose approach through a local incision (often under local anesthesia) allows endarterectomy and/or patch angioplasty with outstanding results. Concerns about elastic recoil, mechanical compression of stents, and the possibility of dissection or thrombosis at the inflow to the entire leg have raised concerns about catheter-based intervention in this region. Lesion characteristics play a significant role in determining the success of femoral PTA, with the best results in lesions that are focal, concentric or bandlike, without extensive plaque burden or calcium. More complex lesions, including those with "cauliflower" calcified plaque and those with a large plaque burden that extends into the origins of the superficial femoral and profunda tend not to respond as well to balloon dilatation. However, the availability of plaque debulking devices (e.g., directional atherectomy, Fox Hollow atherectomy, laser atherectomy) facilitate recanalization in some instances (see Chapter 23).

Treatment Considerations and Technique

The common femoral artery can be approached either contralateral approach using a cross-over guiding catheter or sheath or from the brachial approach. In occasional instances, the lesion will be far enough from the sheath insertion site that ipsilateral access is possible, though more challenging technically. We occasionally use the ipsilateral approach using atherectomy (Fig. 26.17), but typically

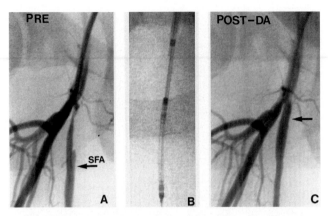

Figure 26.17 Directional atherectomy (DA) of right superficial femoral artery (SFA) via antegrade puncture. **A.** Angiography via antegrade puncture into right common femoral artery demonstrates high-grade stenosis in proximal SFA, not favorable for balloon angioplasty owing to ostial location/eccentricity. **B.** An 8F directional atherectomy catheter introduced via sheath, which is then pulled back to common femoral artery. **C.** Angiography following DA demonstrates excellent result.

perform balloon angioplasty via the contralateral approach (Fig. 26.18). When the lesion involves the bifurcation of the common femoral into profunda and superficial femoral artery (SFA) branches, kissing balloons must occasionally be used. The biggest limitation of common femoral artery angioplasty, however, is restenosis, which is generally accepted to be >50%. Nonetheless, patients often may experience persistent relief of critical symptoms, even in the face of moderately severe restenosis. Stenting the common femoral artery risks stent compression or fracture, renders subsequent surgical repair much more complicated, and should be avoided or reserved for exceptional circumstances.

Profunda Femoris Artery

The deep femoral artery is the main source of collaterals to the lower extremity. In the face of occlusion of the SFA or of a fem-pop bypass graft, the profunda alone becomes responsible for maintaining viability of the lower extremity. Surgery

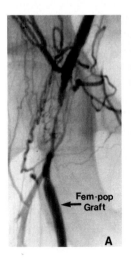
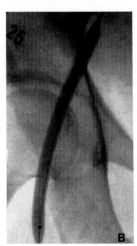
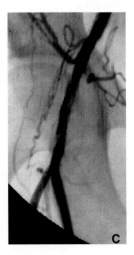

Figure 26.18 Balloon angioplasty (PTA) of common femoral artery in a patient with multiple previous right leg surgical interventions, resulting in severe scarring of right groin. **A.** High-grade, diffuse stenosis in right common femoral artery, with extensive collateral flow, supplying profunda and femoropopliteal (fem-pop). **B.** Balloon angioplasty (PTA) via contralateral approach. Balloon inflated to 15 atm. **C.** Post-PTA angiogram demonstrates mild plaque fracture, with excellent patency. Patient's claudication symptoms resolved, and he continues to be minimally symptomatic 4 years later.

for disease involving the ostia of the SFA and profunda involves endarterectomy and patch angioplasty. Balloon angioplasty has been reserved for situations in which severe ischemia is present (Rutherford category 4, 5, or 6) and surgery is absolutely contraindicated, or when critical lesions involve the mid or distal portions of the descending branch of the profunda that are less accessible to the surgeon. Technically satisfactory results of profunda PTA have been described and suggest that this is a relatively safe procedure. (See Chapter 34.) However, because of the potential for producing limb-threatening ischemia or limb loss if the vessel occludes, treatment of this site should generally be reserved for patients with rest pain or critical limb ischemia in whom no good surgical options are available.

Treatment Considerations and Technique

Angioplasty of the profunda, similar to that for the common femoral artery, is often most easily performed from the contralateral side. Antegrade access is sometimes appropriate, depending on the location of the stenosis and the condition of the common femoral artery. If the lesion is immediately adjacent to the common femoral, it may be problematic to treat. Directional atherectomy may be performed in an antegrade fashion at this site. Since the profunda is the vessel of last resort for maintaining blood flow to the lower extremity, a conservative posture should be maintained with respect to balloon size and inflation pressure. The outcome of stenting in the profunda is unknown, so that stenting should be reserved for cases of flow-limiting dissection or severe residual stenosis after balloon angioplasty, wherein patency of the vessel and viability of the limb might be threatened without maintaining an open vessel. Debulking devices (directional atherectomy, Fox Hollow Atherectomy, laser atherectomy) or novel balloon techniques (cutting balloon angioplasty or cryoplasty) may be used here and in the common femoral artery. However, systematic analysis of results with these devices has yet to be performed.

Superficial Femoral and Popliteal Arteries

The frequency of symptomatic femoral-popliteal disease is more than twice that of iliac disease and tends to occur in older patients who have a greater incidence of concomitant coronary artery disease. Despite a mean vessel diameter between 5 and 6 mm, restenosis is nearly twice (40 to 60%) that for coronary interventions. Enthusiasm for revascularization must thus be tempered by the lower likelihood of long-term success with either surgical or percutaneous approaches.

Patients with superficial femoral-popliteal disease usually present with claudication or (less commonly) with critical limb ischemia. The presence of the profunda femoris as a major source of collaterals to the lower limb protects most patients with SFA occlusion from the dire conse-

quences of critical limb ischemia, so that even patients with proximal SFA occlusion may have only mild claudication, or no claudication at all. Decisions regarding intervention, whether surgery or PTA, for infrainguinal disease must take into account the degree to which the patient is disabled, the presence of comorbid factors, and the anticipated short- and long-term outcome. In general, patients with mild, non-disabling claudication should be placed on conservative treatment with an exercise program to augment collateral flow rather than undergoing interventional therapy for SFA disease. Fewer than one-fourth of these patients will progress to the point of developing more disabling symptoms or a threatened limb, which mandate therapy.

Considerable controversy remains as to the relative role of percutaneous therapy versus surgery. The results of balloon angioplasty in the SFA have improved over time. Murray and colleagues (130) noted that the technical success improved from 70 to 91% between 1980 and 1989, with excellent acute and long-term efficacy even for lesions >10 cm long. Similarly, the success rate in crossing occluded segments of the SFA and popliteal have improved dramatically as a consequence of technical advances. Foremost among these is the use of hydrophilic guidewires. Among eight large series of patients undergoing PTA of femoral-popliteal stenoses and occlusions, most of whom were claudicants, the acute technical success ranged between 82 and 96% (130–136). Primary patency rates at 1, 3, and 5 years averaged 60%, 50%, and 45%. Several factors influence long-term outcome following SFA-pop angioplasty. Patients with intermittent claudication (versus tissue loss), a more severe lesion at baseline, and lower post-treatment residual stenosis tend to have a better outcome at 1 year, whereas those with diabetes, threatened limb loss, or diffuse atherosclerotic vascular disease with zero to one vessel runoff have a worse outcome. The analysis of Hunink and colleagues (137) examined the relative benefit and cost effectiveness of PTA versus bypass surgery for 5-year outcomes in approximately 4,800 PTA and 4,500 bypass procedures performed since 1995. Their conclusion was that, for patients with disabling claudication owing to femoral-popliteal stenosis or occlusion, PTA is the preferred initial treatment, whereas for patients with chronic critical ischemia owing to femoral-popliteal occlusion, bypass surgery is the preferred treatment (if feasible). The excellent acute results that can be obtained from percutaneous techniques in the current era, and the fact that subsequent surgical bypass is still possible if needed, has led some to support a strategy of initial endovascular therapy, including for the treatment of critical limb ischemia (138).

Adjunct Therapies

For stenoses of the SFA and popliteal, the standard approach is that of balloon angioplasty. Various technologies, including stents, directional atherectomy, rotational atherectomy, and laser angioplasty have been investigated as means of improving long-term patency and reducing restenosis in the SFA. In contrast with the documented benefits achieved by use of endovascular stents for iliac PTA, experience thus far in the SFA has been less favorable. Results with nitinol SE stents are conflicting: In some studies, the restenosis rate has been prohibitively high (139); yet in other studies, complex SFA disease treated with stenting has yielded exceptional long-term results (140). Recent revelations that stent strut fractures are occurring routinely in devices placed for SFA/popliteal stenosis has led to intensive analysis of the unique forces (stretching, twisting, bending) at play in these vessels. It is hoped that this scrutiny will result in development of devices more suitable for this venue. Preliminary results with drug-eluting stents in the SFA/popliteal circulation have not been as favorable as in the coronary circulation. Nonetheless, there is optimism that with appropriate dosing, delivery profiles, and stent platforms, the results will improve. Neither directional (Fig. 26.19) nor rotational atherectomy has thus far been demonstrated to have an advantage for SFA/pop revascularization, save for those rare patients in whom the extent of calcific deposits renders the lesion refractory to alternative techniques. Laser angioplasty has been used effectively in SFA/pop revascularization, and the recent approval of large catheters may enhance debulking. Nonetheless, no study thus far has demonstrated definitive benefit of this device.

For occluded femoral-popliteal arteries, whether or not to use thrombolytic therapy in advance of PTA is controversial. Lytic therapy can be successful in some patients with even chronic total occlusion, because the occlusion in lower extremity arteries is often characterized by a lengthy, gelatin-like thrombus superimposed on a high-grade atherosclerotic lesion. Lytic therapy thus can convert a long occlusion to one that is either shorter or nonocclusive, which may respond better to PTA. Despite the theoretical benefit, most interventionalists opt for direct revascularization with PTA, followed by use of SE stents for extensive recoil.

Some promising strategies lie on the horizon for treating the vexing problem of SFA restenosis: it is hoped that drug-eluting stents, covered stents, or local drug delivery might reduce the incidence of restenosis. For cases where the vessel is not amenable to revascularization, various strategies to increase blood flow by triggering growth of new collaterals, termed *therapeutic angiogenesis*, are being tested. Preliminary results have been encouraging (141–143).

Treatment Considerations and Technique

Access

There are four potential routes of access to the SFA and popliteal: antegrade common femoral artery puncture, contralateral retrograde access over the aortic bifurcation, retrograde popliteal artery access, and brachial access. The most common route of access has been the antegrade approach, which is more challenging than retrograde common femoral puncture. Familiarity with the local anatomy at the level of the common femoral artery is essential (see Chapter 14). As new catheters have been developed to facilitate contralateral access, that approach has become increasingly popular, especially among cardiovascular specialists who are more familiar with use of the retrograde approach. The use of a kink-resistant sheath is critical to maintaining access around the bifurcation of the aorta, especially in the case of the acutely angulated bifurcation. Any number of curved (Cobra, LIMA) or retroflexed (Omni, Simmons) catheters can be used to obtain access to the contralateral common iliac artery. The advantages to this approach include the ability to image the common femoral and its bifurcation and the ability to treat iliac and infrainguinal disease in the same sitting. The disadvantage is that of working from a distance with exchange-length wires and balloons. In addition, traversal of critically narrowed or occluded sites can be problematic because of lack of support. The third approach, retrograde popliteal, is reserved for rare cases where the antegrade or contralateral approach fails to traverse an occluded segment, or in the event that a subintimal channel has been created. Complications associated with this approach are more frequent, owing to the vital structures in the popliteal fossa, the small size of the vessel, and the lack of familiarity with this access. The brachial approach has the advantage of providing better radiation protection, since one is working

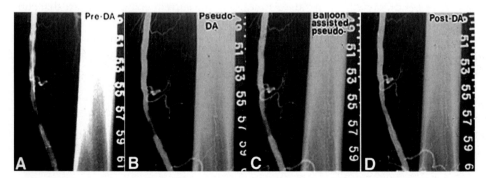

Figure 26.19 Incremental luminal patency resulting from individual components of directional atherectomy (DA). **A.** Angiogram shows high-grade stenosis in superficial femoral artery (SFA) pre-DA. **B.** Angiogram shows improved luminal patency resulting from Dotter effect of advancing DA catheter through lesion (no balloon inflation, no atherectomy). **C.** Angiogram shows further improvement in luminal patency resulting from balloon inflation (2 atm) without activating cutter. **D.** Angiogram shows final result accomplished by activating cutter.

far from the actual target site, but requires the use of lengthy wires and devices.

When considering choice of access, it is important to use all of the information at one's disposal, including prior angiographic examination, duplex study, and physical findings of disease along the planned access route. For example, if the contralateral iliac artery is severely diseased or occluded, contralateral access may be excluded. In the case of an aortic aneurysm, one might wish to avoid brachial access. If duplex shows severe calcification and diffuse disease in the popliteal artery, then that access site should be avoided. Likewise, if the common femoral artery has severe and diffuse disease, or if the origin of the SFA is the target lesion site, then access other than ipsilateral antegrade should be considered. In the current era, the detailed and complex imaging that is available by computed tomographic angiography (CTA) and magnetic resonance arteriography (MRA) allow the interventionalist to select the approach and interventional strategy preprocedurally (see Chapter 14).

Infrapopliteal Arteries

Dotter and Judkins (4), in their original description of peripheral angioplasty in 1964, included two cases of angioplasty of infrapopliteal vessels. Since their original report, the development of techniques and delineation of indications for intervention below the knee have evolved more slowly than for larger, more proximal vessels. Published clinical experience involving PTA of the anterior tibial, tibioperoneal trunk, posterior tibial, and peroneal arteries, although increasing, has been more limited than that described for aortoiliac and SFA/pop sites and reflects multiple issues: The relatively small size of these vessels (1.5 to 3.5 mm) and their distal location limits both access and success, and it is rare for claudication to be owing to isolated disease in one or two infrapopliteal arteries; knee-to-foot patency of only one of the three major branches is regarded as sufficient to prevent lower limb ischemia or claudication. Restenosis rates in infrapopliteal vessels appear to be considerably higher than those for more proximal sites, and disease in the infrapopliteal vessels is often occlusive, diffuse, and/or complicated by the presence of heavy calcific deposits. Furthermore, many patients with infrapopliteal disease have diabetes, which is associated with atretic and diffusely calcified vessels that respond poorly to balloon dilation.

As technological advances have been made, including the development of low-profile balloons and atraumatic coronary guidewires, the ability to treat infrapopliteal disease has improved. Over the past decade and a half since Schwarten and colleagues (144) reported the first sizable series of patients undergoing infrapopliteal revascularization, the application of these techniques has become more widespread. Infrapopliteal stenoses and occlusions can be revascularized percutaneously with remarkably low risk

and technical success rates in the range of 80 to 95%. In a large series reported by Dorros et al. (145), success was achieved in 406 out of 417 patients (96%); the success rate in stenoses (98%) was superior to that in occlusions (76%). In-hospital complications were extremely low. The vast majority of patients with critical limb ischemia (95%) improved following revascularization. Such improvement does not necessarily imply ongoing patency. Restoration of flow through only one of the three major vessels to the foot may be sufficient to heal a distal ischemic lesion. Once healed, most patients will do well even in the face of documented reocclusion or restenosis.

For patients with claudication, infrapopliteal disease usually coexists with more proximal disease, revascularization of which alone is often sufficient to achieve symptomatic relief. This differs from patients with ischemic ulceration, in whom restoration of uninterrupted patency to the foot is generally required to heal the lesion. There is a subset of patients who claudicate owing solely to infrapopliteal disease, in whom there is an increasing body of experience treating with percutaneous therapy. Such a strategy should be reserved, at least for the present, for patients who have severe symptoms (Rutherford category 3). Infrapopliteal PTA may also be justified in claudicants who undergo proximal revascularization (either with surgery or PTA) in whom the runoff is severely impaired. Indeed, data presented previously show that outflow is the principle determinant of long-term patency for fem-pop PTA. By recanalizing the outflow vessels, it is conceivable that the proximal PTA site or the bypass graft may be more likely to remain patent. This theory has not been formally tested in peripheral vessels, although it seems to be the case in coronary arteries.

Many of the patients treated with infrapopliteal angioplasty to date have been those who were too high risk or otherwise unqualified for bypass surgery (16). The latter is still considered to be the standard of care for patients with critical limb ischemia owing to infrapopliteal disease. Regardless of the conduit (reversed vein, in situ vein, or prosthetic material), patency rates are nonetheless inferior to those of more proximal reconstruction. It is conceivable that the long-term clinical outcome of percutaneous therapy may ultimately equal that of distal bypass grafting. A controlled trial will be required to address this issue. It is also conceivable that both of these revascularization strategies could be replaced or augmented in many instances by the strategy of therapeutic angiogenesis (146). If the body can be stimulated to create its own new microcirculation, then the issues of restenosis, reocclusion, and graft closure become moot.

Techniques

The technical aspects of infrapopliteal angioplasty are similar to those for coronary vessels. Antegrade common femoral access is preferred, so as to optimize the ability to manipulate catheters in the vessels below the knee. Selective injection via catheter placed at the level of the knee is advised to optimally visualize the distal vascular pattern. Digital subtraction is preferred. Not infrequently, anatomic variants will be present, such as the anterior tibial arising above the knee joint. Also, it is not unusual to mistake one of the small side branches or collaterals for the main arterial trunk. Adequate anticoagulation is critical, and administration of vasodilator therapy (nitroglycerin or papaverine) may be useful. Initial attempts to cross stenoses or occlusions should use small, coronary-type guidewires (0.014 or 0.018 inch), although 0.035-inch hydrophilic-type wires can also be used if necessary to cross complex occlusions. Confirmation of a luminal position in the distal vessel should be obtained prior to dilating, by removing the wire from the catheter and injecting a small amount of dilute contrast through the guidewire lumen into the distal vessel.

When performing infrapopliteal PTA, particular care should be taken to be sure that subsequent surgical options are not compromised. For example, overdilation and disruption of a previously uncompromised distal vessel may prohibit subsequent bypass to that site.

Rotational atherectomy, Fox Hollow atherectomy, cryoplasty, or excimer laser angioplasty (Figs. 26.20 and 26.21) can be useful as adjunctive therapy. Specifically, lesions that have unfavorable morphology, such as total occlusions, heavy calcification, and ostial disease, may benefit from these niche devices (8,147). Previous studies with rotational atherectomy have shown it to be useful acutely, although data on long-term follow-up does not suggest a benefit over balloon angioplasty alone. The use of stents—including drug-eluting stents—is currently under active investigation (Fig. 26.22). To summarize, the percutaneous therapy of infrapopliteal vessels is still in evolution, and indications are expanding. It is not unreasonable, especially for patients with threatened limbs who are high-risk surgical candidates, for experienced operators to attempt percutaneous revascularization of offending infrapopliteal lesions before committing the patient to surgery. Although the restenosis/reocclusion rates are high, long-term limb salvage can nonetheless be successfully achieved. For the rare patients who have severe intermittent claudication on the basis of infrapopliteal disease alone, PTA may be a reasonable option. Finally, when SFA/popliteal disease occurs in conjunction with infrapopliteal lesions, revascularization below the knee may be reasonable to increase the outflow following recanalization of the proximal vessel.

Lower Extremity Bypass Grafts

Stenosis in a lower extremity bypass graft can threaten the patency of the graft and shorten its life. The etiology of bypass graft stenoses is variable. Stenoses that occur within the first few weeks or months of graft placement usually

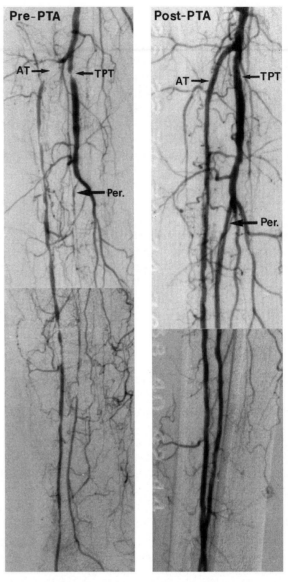

Figure 26.20 Balloon angioplasty (PTA) of occluded anterior tibial artery, tibioperoneal trunk, and peroneal artery in elderly patient with foot ulceration and threatened limb loss. **A.** Baseline angiogram demonstrates 2-cm occlusion of anterior tibial artery (AT), high-grade stenosis of tibioperoneal trunk (TPT), and lengthy occlusion of peroneal artery (per.). All three segments were recanalized with Glidewire, followed by excimer-laser angioplasty and PTA. **B.** Final angiogram post-PTA demonstrates widely patent anterior tibial, tibioperoneal trunk, peroneal artery.

indicate a technical problem that is best treated by repeat surgery and graft revision. Graft failure within a later time frame (several months to years) can be owing to myointimal hyperplasia, atherosclerosis, or progressive fibrosis of a poor venous conduit. Several other factors may contribute to graft failure, including the presence of poor inflow or outflow, low cardiac output, a hypercoagulable state, compromise of the graft owing to patients crossing their legs, or external compression of the graft by sclerosis and fibrosis (for example, from a scarred groin). Prosthetic conduits are more likely to present with abrupt occlusion, whereas

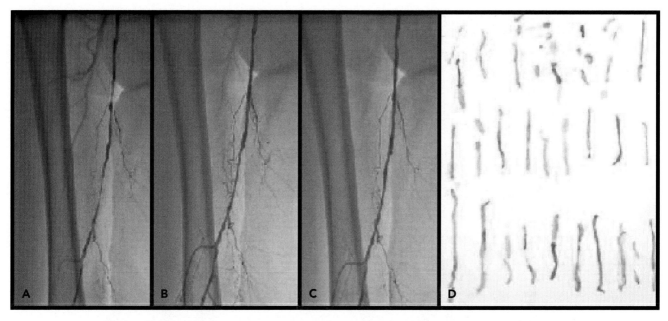

Figure 26.21 **A.** Diffuse right superficial femoral artery disease causing exertional claudication. **B.** Following initial treatment with Fox Hollow atherectomy demonstrating improvement in lesion severity but significant residual stenosis. **C.** Final angiographic result demonstrating a satisfactory atherectomy result. **D.** Atherectomy strips obtained following (B) and (C). The longest strip measures 4 cm.

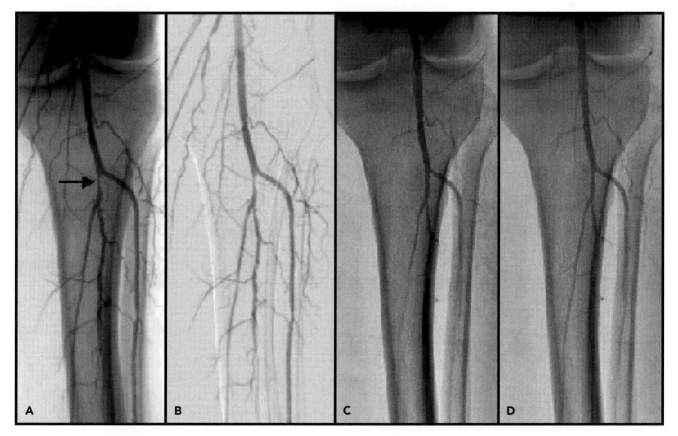

Figure 26.22 Infrapopliteal stenosis (**A**, *arrow*) causing lifestyle-limiting claudication. The lesion was treated successfully with balloon angioplasty, resulting in a 20% residual; however, recurrence of symptoms resulted in repeat angiography, which demonstrated significant restenosis at the site of balloon angioplasty (**B**). This was treated with a Taxus drug-eluting stent (2.75 × 12 mm **C**), which was widely patent at 6-month repeat angiography performed for progression of other disease (**D**).

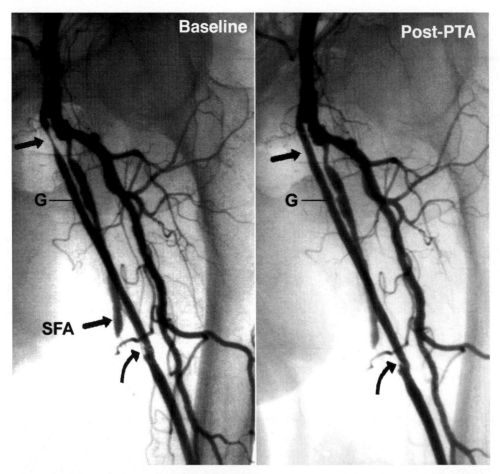

Figure 26.23 Right anterior oblique view of critical stenosis *(straight arrow)* at origin of fem-pop graft (G) and moderate irregular lesion *(curved arrow)* at distal end of jump-graft placed during previous graft revision. Superficial femoral artery (SFA) is occluded proximally. Lesions were detected during routine surveillance (patient asymptomatic). Because of proximity of lesions to ipsilateral common femoral artery, contralateral access may be preferred. Post–balloon angioplasty (PTA), stenoses eliminated, but regular surveillance will be essential to prevent graft failure.

native venous conduits tend to present with a progressive downhill course. Of course, even in the case of the latter, abrupt thrombosis and acute limb ischemia can occur.

Frank or impending graft failure is often not heralded by increasing clinical symptoms. Accordingly, a strategy of regular graft surveillance using duplex ultrasonography is recommended to preserve and extend the life of the graft. For impending graft failure, either detected by duplex ultrasonography or increasing symptoms, immediate arteriography is recommended, followed by either surgical or percutaneous revascularization. As stated in the AHA task force guidelines in 1994, focal lesions of the distal anastomosis of a fem-pop or fem-tib graft are amenable to PTA (Fig. 26.23; 1). Other lesions that may be amenable include focal stenoses of proximal graft anastomoses or short-segment lesions (3 cm or less) occurring within the bypass graft. Lengthy lesions (especially >10 cm) and stenoses associated with anastomotic aneurysms are recommended to undergo surgical revision.

Patients presenting with acute or subacute graft thromboses (<14 days) are best treated with catheter-directed thrombolysis (Fig. 26.24; 148,149). An alternative is balloon embolectomy, although the latter strategy may be associated with a higher morbidity and mortality over the ensuing year (149). The one exception to this is the recently placed graft that fails almost immediately, which should return immediately to the operating room for surgical thrombectomy and revision. For patients with longstanding grafts that fail, determination of the factors responsible may require re-establishing enough flow to visualize the graft angiographically. In cases of early graft failure, examination of angiographic studies may provide clues previously overlooked, such as stenosis of an inflow vessel, poor or inadequate distal runoff, or the presence of a venous side branch that was not sutured.

Technique

For patients presenting with impending graft failure based on a duplex study, access should be obtained so as to optimize the therapeutic alternatives. For example, after angiography documents the presence of a proximal or

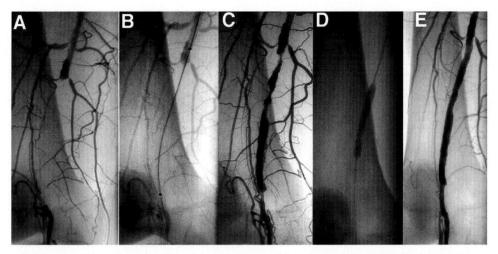

Figure 26.24 Thrombolysis, rheolytic thrombectomy, and balloon angioplasty (PTA) for subacute thrombosis of superficial femoral artery (SFA)-to-popliteal Dacron graft. **A.** Distal SFA occluded at proximal graft anastomosis; popliteal reconstituted by collaterals, so limb not imminently in jeopardy. **B.** Infusion catheter placed across thrombosed graft, after traversing with hydrophilic wire; t-PA administered for 6 hours at 3 mg/hour. Residual hazy filling defect treated with Possis AngioJet. **C.** Postlysis and Possis, underlying inflow and outflow stenoses (caused by pseudointima) and responsible for flow compromise and graft thrombosis, were identified and **(D).** dilated. **E.** Final result shows restoration of normal flow/caliber.

distal anastomotic lesion, it is conceivable that the lesion may be resistant to balloon dilation alone. In these cases, directional atherectomy may prove useful for salvaging the graft. The results using directional atherectomy appear to be comparable with those of surgical revision, although direct head-to-head comparison has not been carried out. Likewise, although stents have been advocated by some for use in failing vein grafts, their utility has not been studied in any formal trials to date.

TRAINING AND CREDENTIALING

Percutaneous intervention for treatment of peripheral vascular disease has been adopted by multiple specialties, including interventional cardiology, vascular surgery, interventional radiology, and others. Such widespread application necessitates development of standardized guidelines for physician training and credentialing to ensure that patients will receive optimum care. Accepted guidelines regarding the minimal requirements necessary to care for patients with PAD and perform peripheral vascular procedures have been described in the multidisciplinary Clinical Competence Statement on vascular medicine and catheter-based peripheral vascular interventions (150). More specific recommendations apply to carotid interventions and have recently been ratified by the cardiology, vascular surgery, and vascular medicine communities, with a view to establishing a common set of criteria for training and credentialing to facilitate safe and orderly dissemination of this new therapy into clinical practice (151).

Cardiologists, whether still in fellowship or established in practice, who wish to care for patients with PAD and perform peripheral interventions must prepare properly to provide their patients optimal care. Until the cognitive, clinical, and procedural skills are incorporated routinely into formal cardiology fellowship programs, additional training is necessary. In particular, carotid revascularization involves interventional skills, equipment, and clinical management skills that differ significantly from that used in other vascular distributions. Moreover, it involves treatment of a uniquely sensitive organ system, wherein minor errors or complications can have catastrophic effects. Given the high-risk nature of carotid revascularization and the availability of alternative treatment modalities, decisions regarding optimal therapy require a comprehensive knowledge base of the disease and its ramifications to properly assess the risk—benefit ratio of each therapeutic option. Experienced operators have been shown to have improved outcomes in carotid stenting.

As a result of these considerations, a joint committee including the societies of each specialty involved have proposed minimal training requirements that cover proficiency in the cognitive, technical, and clinical skills necessary to safely perform carotid stenting. The cognitive requirements include comprehensive understanding of the risk factors, epidemiology, pathology, pathophysiology, natural history, clinical presentation, and therapeutic alternatives for patients with carotid artery disease to allow appropriate decision-making regarding indications, limitations, and complications of the procedure.

REFERENCES

1. Pentecost MJ, Criqui MH, Dorros G, et al. Guidelines for peripheral percutaneous transluminal angioplasty of the abdominal aorta and lower extremity vessels. A statement for health professionals from a special writing group of the Councils on Cardiovascular Radiology, Arteriosclerosis, Cardio-Thoracic and Vascular Surgery, Clinical Cardiology, and Epidemiology and Prevention, the American Heart Association. *Circulation* 1994; 89:511–531.

2. Weitz JI, Byrne J, Clagett GP, et al. Diagnosis and treatment of chronic arterial insufficiency of the lower extremities: a critical review. *Circulation* 1996;94:3026–3049.

3. Rutherford RB, Becker GJ. Standards for evaluating and reporting the results of surgical and percutaneous therapy for peripheral arterial disease. *J Vasc Intervent Radiol* 1991;2:169–174.

4. Dotter CT, Judkins MP. Transluminal treatment of arteriosclerotic obstruction. Description of a new technique and a preliminary report of its application. *Circulation* 1964;30:654–670.

5. Gruntzig AR. Transluminal dilatation of coronary artery stenosis [letter to the editor]. *Lancet* 1978;1:263.

6. Gruntzig A, Kuhlmann U, Vetter W, Lutolf U, Meier B, Siegenthaler W. Treatment of renovascular hypertension with percutaneous transluminal dilatation of a renal-artery stenosis. *Lancet* 1978;1:801–802.

7. Gruntzig A, Kumpe DA. Technique of percutaneous transluminal angioplasty with the Gruntzig balloon catheter. *Am J Roentgenol* 1979;132:547–552.

8. Isner JM, Rosenfield K. Redefining the treatment of peripheral artery disease. Role of percutaneous revascularization. *Circulation* 1993;88(Pt 1):1534–1557.

9. Blum U, Krumme B, Flugel P, et al. Treatment of ostial renal-artery stenoses with vascular endoprostheses after unsuccessful balloon angioplasty. *N Engl J Med* 1997;336:459–465.

10. Dorros G, Jaff M, Mathiak L, et al. Four-year follow-up of Palmaz-Schatz stent revascularization as treatment for atherosclerotic renal artery stenosis. *Circulation* 1998;98:642–647.

11. Isner JM, Rosenfield K, Losordo DW, et al. Percutaneous intravascular US as adjunct to catheter-based interventions: preliminary experience in patients with peripheral vascular disease. *Radiology* 1990;175:61–70.

12. Rosenfield K, Kaufman J, Pieczek AM, et al. Human coronary and peripheral arteries: on-line three-dimensional reconstruction from two-dimensional intravascular US scans. Work in progress. *Radiology* 1992;184:823–832.

13. Mecley M, Rosenfield K, Kaufman J, Langevin RE Jr, Razvi S, Isner JM. Atherosclerotic plaque hemorrhage and rupture associated with crescendo claudication. *Ann Intern Med* 1992;117: 663–666.

14. Rosenfield K, Losordo DW, Ramaswamy K, et al. Three-dimensional reconstruction of human coronary and peripheral arteries from images recorded during two-dimensional intravascular ultrasound examination. *Circulation* 1991;84:1938–1956.

15. Isner JM, Rosenfield K, Losordo DW, et al. Combination balloon-ultrasound imaging catheter for percutaneous transluminal angioplasty. Validation of imaging, analysis of recoil, and identification of plaque fracture. *Circulation* 1991;84:739–754.

16. Isner JM, Pieczek A, Rosenfield K. Images in cardiovascular medicine. Untreated gangrene in patients with peripheral artery disease. *Circulation* 1994;89:482–483.

17. McCrindle BW, Jones TK, Morrow WR, et al. Acute results of balloon angioplasty of native coarctation versus recurrent aortic obstruction are equivalent. Valvuloplasty and Angioplasty of Congenital Anomalies (VACA) Registry Investigators. *J Am Coll Cardiol* 1996;28:1810–1817.

18. deGiovanni JV, Lip GY, Osman K, et al. Percutaneous balloon dilatation of aortic coarctation in adults. *Am J Cardiol* 1996;77: 435–439.

19. Storey GS, Marks MP, Dake M, Norbash AM, Steinberg GK. Vertebral artery stenting following percutaneous transluminal angioplasty. Technical note. *J Neurosurg* 1996;84:883–887.

20. Lababidi Z. Percutaneous balloon coarctation angioplasty: long-term results. *J Intervent Cardiol* 1992;5:57–62.

21. Rao PS. Stents in treatment of aortic coarctation. *J Am Coll Cardiol* 1997;30:1853–1855.

22. Zellers TM. Balloon angioplasty for recurrent coarctation of the aorta in patients following staged palliation for hypoplastic left heart syndrome. *Am J Cardiol* 1999;84:231–233.

23. Crawford ES, Hess KR, Cohen ES, Coselli JS, Safi HJ. Ruptured aneurysm of the descending thoracic and thoracoabdominal aorta. Analysis according to size and treatment. *Ann Surg* 1991; 213:417–425.

24. Cambria RA, Gloviczki P, Stanson AW, et al. Outcome and expansion rate of 57 thoracoabdominal aortic aneurysms managed nonoperatively. *Am J Surg* 1995;170:213–217.

25. Ergin MA, Phillips RA, Galla JD, et al. Significance of distal false lumen after type A dissection repair. *Ann Thorac Surg* 1994;57: 820–824.

26. Dake MD, Miller DC, Semba CP, Mitchell RS, Walker PJ, Liddell RP. Transluminal placement of endovascular stent-grafts for the treatment of descending thoracic aortic aneurysms. *N Engl J Med* 1994;331:1729–1734.

27. Mitchell RS, Dake MD, Sembra CP, et al. Endovascular stent-graft repair of thoracic aortic aneurysms. *J Thorac Cardiovasc Surg* 1996;111:1054–1062.

28. Dake MD, Miller DC, Mitchell RS, Semba CP, Moore KA, Sakai T. The "first generation" of endovascular stent-grafts for patients with aneurysms of the descending thoracic aorta. *J Thorac Cardiovasc Surg* 1998;116:689–703.

29. Ehrlich M, Grabenwoeger M, Cartes-Zumelzu F, et al. Endovascular stent graft repair for aneurysms on the descending thoracic aorta. *Ann Thorac Surg* 1998;66:19–24.

30. Nienaber CA, Fattori R, Lund G, et al. Nonsurgical reconstruction of thoracic aortic dissection by stent-graft placement [see comment]. *N Engl J Med* 1999;340:1539–1545.

31. Bortone AS, De Cillis E, D'Agostino D, de Luca Tupputi Schinosa L. Endovascular treatment of thoracic aortic disease: four years of experience. *Circulation* 2004;11:262–267.

32. Hagan PG, Nienaber CA, Isselbacher EM, et al. The International Registry of Acute Aortic Dissection (IRAD): new insights into an old disease. *JAMA* 2000;283:897–903.

33. Mehta RH, Suzuki T, Hagan PG, et al. Predicting death in patients with acute type A aortic dissection. *Circulation* 2002; 105:200–206.

34. Cambria RP, Brewster DC, Gertler J, et al. Vascular complications associated with spontaneous aortic dissection. *J Vasc Surg* 1988; 7:199–209.

35. DeBakey ME, McCollum CH, Crawford ES, et al. Dissection and dissecting aneurysms of the aorta: twenty-year follow-up of five hundred twenty-seven patients treated surgically. *Surgery* 1982; 92:1118–1134.

36. Miller DC, Mitchell RS, Oyer PE, Stinson EB, Jamieson SW, Shumway NE. Independent determinants of operative mortality for patients with aortic dissections. *Circulation* 1984;70(Pt 2): 153–164.

37. Crawford ES, Svensson LG, Coselli JS, Safi HJ, Hess KR. Aortic dissection and dissecting aortic aneurysms. *Ann Surg* 1988;208: 254–273.

38. Chung JW, Elkins C, Sakai T, et al. True-lumen collapse in aortic dissection. I: evaluation of causative factors in phantoms with pulsatile flow. *Radiology* 2000;214:87–98.

39. Greenberg R, Khwaja J, Haulon S, Fulton G. Aortic dissections: new perspectives and treatment paradigms. *Eur J Vasc Endovasc Surg* 2003;26:579–586.

40. Dake MD, Kato N, Mitchell RS, et al. Endovascular stent-graft placement for the treatment of acute aortic dissection. *N Engl J Med* 1999;340:1546–1552.

41. Kato M, Matsuda T, Kaneko M, et al. Outcomes of stent-graft treatment of false lumen in aortic dissection. *Circulation* 1998; 98(suppl):305–311.

42. Slonim SM, Nyman UR, Semba CP, Miller DC, Mitchell RS, Dake MD. True lumen obliteration in complicated aortic dissection: endovascular treatment. *Radiology* 1996;201:161–166.

43. Williams DM, Lee DY, Hamilton BH, et al. The dissected aorta: percutaneous treatment of ischemic complications—principles and results. *J Vasc Intervent Radiol* 1997;8:605–625.

44. Arend WP, Michel BA, Bloch DA, et al. The American College of Rheumatology 1990 criteria for the classification of Takayasu arteritis. *Arthritis Rheum* 1990;33:1129–1134.

45. Bachman DM, Kim RM. Transluminal dilatation for subclavian steal syndrome. *Am J Roentgenol* 1980;135:995–996.

46. Millaire A, Trinca M, Marache P, de Groote P, Jabinet JL, Ducloux G. Subclavian angioplasty: immediate and late results in 50 patients. *Cathet Cardiovasc Diagn* 1993;29:8–17.

47. Dorros G, Lewin RF, Jamnadas P, Mathiak LM. Peripheral transluminal angioplasty of the subclavian and innominate arteries utilizing the brachial approach: acute outcome and follow-up. *Cathet Cardiovasc Diagn* 1990;19:71–76.

48. Duber C, Klose KJ, Kopp H, Schmiedt W. Percutaneous transluminal angioplasty for occlusion of the subclavian artery: short- and long-term results. *Cardiovasc Intervent Radiol* 1992;15: 205–210.

49. Kumar K, Dorros G, Bates MC, Palmer L, Mathiak L, Dufek C. Primary stent deployment in occlusive subclavian artery disease. *Cathet Cardiovasc Diagn* 1995;34:281–285.

50. Sullivan TM, Gray BH, Bacharach JM, et al. Angioplasty and primary stenting of the subclavian, innominate, and common carotid arteries in 83 patients. *J Vasc Surg* 1998;28:1059–1065.

51. Hadjipetrou P, Cox S, Piemonte T, Eisenhauer A. Percutaneous revascularization of atherosclerotic obstruction of aortic arch vessels. *J Am Coll Cardiol* 1999;33:1238–1245.

52. Becker KJ, Purcell LL, Hacke W, Hanley DF. Vertebrobasilar thrombosis: diagnosis, management, and the use of intra-arterial thrombolytics. *Crit Care Med* 1996;24:1729–1742.

53. Cross DT 3rd, Moran CJ, Angtuaco EE, Diringer MN. Relationship between clot location and outcome after basilar artery thrombolysis. *Am J Neuroradiol* 1997;18:1221–1228.

54. Brandt T, von Kummer R, Muller-Kuppers M, Hacke W. Thrombolytic therapy of acute basilar artery occlusion. Variables affecting recanalization and outcome. *Stroke* 1996; 27:875–881.

55. Hacke W, Zeumer H, Ferbert A, Bruckmann H, del Zoppo GJ. Intra-arterial thrombolytic therapy improves outcome in patients with acute vertebrobasilar occlusive disease. *Stroke* 1988;19:1216–1222.

56. American Heart Association. *2002 Heart and Stroke Statistical Update.* Dallas, TX: American Heart Association; 2001.

57. Beneficial effect of carotid endarterectomy in symptomatic patients with high-grade carotid stenosis. North American Symptomatic Carotid Endarterectomy Trial Collaborators. *N Engl J Med* 1991;325:445–453.

58. Endarterectomy for asymptomatic carotid artery stenosis. Executive Committee for the Asymptomatic Carotid Atherosclerosis Study. *JAMA* 1995;273:1421–1428.

59. Wang TJ, Nam BH, D'Agostino RB, et al. Carotid intima-media thickness is associated with premature parental coronary heart disease: the Framingham Heart Study. *Circulation* 2003;108: 572–576.

60. DeBakey ME. Successful carotid endarterectomy for cerebrovascular insufficiency. Nineteen-year follow-up. *JAMA* 1975;233: 1083–1085.

61. Eastcott HH, Pickering GW, Rob CG. Reconstruction of internal carotid artery in a patient with intermittent attacks of hemiplegia. *Lancet* 1954;267:994–996.

62. MRC European Carotid Surgery Trial: interim results for symptomatic patients with severe (70–99%) or with mild (0–29%) carotid stenosis. European Carotid Surgery Trialists' Collaborative Group. *Lancet* 1991;337:1235–1243.

63. Mayberg MR, Wilson SE, Yatsu F, et al. Carotid endarterectomy and prevention of cerebral ischemia in symptomatic carotid stenosis. Veterans Affairs Cooperative Studies Program 309 Trialist Group. *JAMA* 1991;266:3289–3294.

64. Randomised trial of cholesterol lowering in 4444 patients with coronary heart disease: the Scandinavian Simvastatin Survival Study (4S). *Lancet* 1994;344:1383–1389.

65. Pfeffer MA, Sacks FM, Moye LA, et al. Cholesterol and Recurrent Events: a secondary prevention trial for normolipidemic patients. CARE Investigators. *Am J Cardiol* 1995;76:98–106.

66. Yusuf S, Sleight P, Pogue J, Bosch J, Davies R, Dagenais G. Effects of an angiotensin-converting-enzyme inhibitor, ramipril, on cardiovascular events in high-risk patients. The Heart Outcomes Prevention Evaluation Study Investigators. *N Engl J Med* 2000; 342:145–153.

67. Collins R, Peto R, MacMahon S, et al. Blood pressure, stroke, and coronary heart disease. Part 2: short-term reductions in blood pressure: overview of randomised drug trials in their epidemiological context. *Lancet* 1990;335:827–838.

68. A randomised, blinded, trial of clopidogrel versus aspirin in patients at risk of ischaemic events (CAPRIE). CAPRIE Steering Committee. *Lancet* 1996;348:1329–1339.

69. Ohki T, Marin ML, Lyon RT, et al. Ex vivo human carotid artery bifurcation stenting: correlation of lesion characteristics with embolic potential. *J Vasc Surg* 1998;27:463–471.

70. Kachel R, Endert G, Basche S, Grossmann K, Glaser FH. Percutaneous transluminal angioplasty (dilatation) of carotid, vertebral, and innominate artery stenoses. *Cardiovasc Intervent Radiol* 1987;10:142–146.

71. Dublin AB, Baltaxe HA, Cobb CA 3rd. Percutaneous transluminal carotid angioplasty in fibromuscular dysplasia. Case report. *J Neurosurg* 1983;59:162–165.

72. Theron J, Raymond J, Casasco A, Courtheoux F. Percutaneous angioplasty of atherosclerotic and postsurgical stenosis of carotid arteries. *AJNR Am J Neuroradiol* 1987;8(3):495–500.

73. Roubin GS, Yadav S, Iyer SS, Vitek J. Carotid stent-supported angioplasty: a neurovascular intervention to prevent stroke. *Am J Cardiol* 1996;78:8–12.

74. Yadav JS, Roubin GS, King P, Iyer S, Vitek J. Angioplasty and stenting for restenosis after carotid endarterectomy. Initial experience. *Stroke* 1996;27:2075–2079.

75. Diethrich EB, Ndiaye M, Reid DB. Stenting in the carotid artery: initial experience in 110 patients. *J Endovasc Surg* 1996;3:42–62.

76. Guterman LR, Budny JL, Gibbons KJ, Hopkins LN. Thrombolysis of the cervical internal carotid artery before balloon angioplasty and stent placement: report of two cases. *Neurosurgery* 1996;38:620–623.

77. Mathur A, Roubin GS, Iyer SS, et al. Predictors of stroke complicating carotid artery stenting. *Circulation* 1998;97:1239–1245.

78. Beebe HG, Archie JP, Baker WH, et al. Concern about safety of carotid angioplasty. *Stroke* 1996;27:197–198.

79. Bettmann MA, Katzen BT, Whisnant J, et al. Carotid stenting and angioplasty: a statement for healthcare professionals from the Councils on Cardiovascular Radiology, Stroke, Cardio-Thoracic and Vascular Surgery, Epidemiology and Prevention, and Clinical Cardiology, American Heart Association. *Stroke* 1998; 29:336–338.

80. Hobson RW 2nd, Brott T, Ferguson R, et al. Regarding "Statement regarding carotid angioplasty and stenting". *J Vasc Surg* 1997;25:1117.

81. LaMuraglia GM, Brewster DC, Moncure AC, et al. Carotid endarterectomy at the millennium: what interventional therapy must match. *Ann Surg* 2004;240:535–544.

82. Brott TG, Brown RD Jr, Meyer FB, Miller DA, Cloft HJ, Sullivan TM. Carotid revascularization for prevention of stroke: carotid endarterectomy and carotid artery stenting. *Mayo Clin Proc* 2004;79:1197–1208.

83. Waigand J, Gross CM, Uhlich F, et al. Elective stenting of carotid artery stenosis in patients with severe coronary artery disease. *Eur Heart J* 1998;19:1365–1370.

84. Roubin GS, New G, Iyer SS, et al. Immediate and late clinical outcomes of carotid artery stenting in patients with symptomatic and asymptomatic carotid artery stenosis: a 5-year prospective analysis. *Circulation* 2001;103:532–537.

85. Endovascular versus surgical treatment in patients with carotid stenosis in the Carotid and Vertebral Artery Transluminal Angioplasty Study (CAVATAS): a randomised trial. *Lancet* 2001; 357:1729–1737.

86. Yadav JS, Wholey MH, Kuntz RE, et al. Protected carotid-artery stenting versus endarterectomy in high-risk patients. *N Engl J Med* 2004;351:1493–1501.

87. Wholey MH, and the Investigators for ARCHeR. The ARCHeR trial: prospective clinical trial for carotid stenting in high surgical risk patients: preliminary thirty-day results. *J Am Coll Cardiol* 2003 Mar 19;41 (6 Suppl A):1A-685A.

88. Whitlow P. A registry study to evaluate the neuro shield bare wire cerebral protection system and X.act stent in patients at

high risk for carotid endarterectomy (abstract). *Am J Cardiol* 2003 Sep 15–17;92(6A):1L-252L.

89. Rosenfield K, Schainfeld R, Pieczek A, Haley L, Isner JM. Restenosis of endovascular stents from stent compression. *J Am Coll Cardiol* 1997;29:328–338.

90. Mathur A, Dorros G, Iyer SS, Vitek JJ, Yadav SS, Roubin GS. Palmaz stent compression in patients following carotid artery stenting. *Cathet Cardiovasc Diagn* 1997;41:137–140.

91. Dorros G. Complications associated with extracranial carotid artery interventions. *J Endovasc Surg* 1996;3:166–170.

92. Mendelsohn FO, Weissman NJ, Lederman RJ, et al. Acute hemodynamic changes during carotid artery stenting. *Am J Cardiol* 1998;82:1077–1081.

93. Piamsomboon C, Roubin GS, Liu MW, et al. Relationship between oversizing of self-expanding stents and late loss index in carotid stenting. *Cathet Cardiovasc Diagn* 1998;45: 139–143.

94. Vozzi CR, Rodriguez AO, Paolantonio D, Smith JA, Wholey MH. Extracranial carotid angioplasty and stenting. Initial results and short-term follow-up. *Tex Heart Inst J* 1997;24:167–172.

95. Perko MJ, Norgaard M, Herzog TM, Olsen PS, Schroeder TV, Pettersson G. Unoperated aortic aneurysm: a survey of 170 patients. *Ann Thorac Surg* 1995;59:1204–1209.

96. Blum U, Voshage G, Lammer J, et al. Endoluminal stent-grafts for infrarenal abdominal aortic aneurysms. *N Engl J Med* 1997; 336:13–20.

97. Parodi JC, Criado FJ, Barone HD, Schonholz C, Queral LA. Endoluminal aortic aneurysm repair using a balloon-expandable stent-graft device: a progress report. *Ann Vasc Surg* 1994;8:523–529.

98. D'Ayala M, Hollier LH, Marin ML. Endovascular grafting for abdominal aortic aneurysms. *Surg Clin North Am* 1998;78:845–862.

99. Zarins CK, White RA, Schwarten D, et al. AneuRx stent graft versus open surgical repair of abdominal aortic aneurysms: multicenter prospective clinical trial. *J Vasc Surg* 1999;29:292–305; discussion 306–308.

100. Simon N, Franklin SS, Bleifer KH, Maxwell MH. Clinical characteristics of renovascular hypertension. *JAMA* 1972;220:1209–1218.

101. Buller C, Nogareda J, Ramanathan K, et al. The profile of cardiac patients with renal artery stenosis. *J Am Coll Cardiol* 2004;43: 1606–1613.

102. Incidence and prevalence of ESRD. USRDS. United States Renal Data System. *Am J Kidney Dis* 1997;30(suppl 1):40–53.

103. Palmaz JC. The current status of vascular intervention in ischemic nephropathy. *J Vasc Intervent Radiol* 1998;9:539–543.

104. Slovut DP, Olin JW. Fibromuscular dysplasia. *N Engl J Med* 2004;350:1862–1871.

105. Pannier-Moreau I, Grimbert P, Fiquet-Kempf B, et al. Possible familial origin of multifocal renal artery fibromuscular dysplasia. *J Hypertens* 1997;15(pt 2):1797–1801.

106. Bofinger A, Hawley C, Fisher P, Daunt N, Stowasser M, Gordon R. Polymorphisms of the renin-angiotensin system in patients with multifocal renal arterial fibromuscular dysplasia. *J Hum Hypertens* 2001;15:185–190.

107. Kincaid OW, Davis GD, Hallermann FJ, Hunt JC. Fibromuscular dysplasia of the renal arteries. Arteriographic features, classification, and observations on natural history of the disease. *Am J Roentgenol Radium Ther Nucl Med* 1968;104:271–282.

108. Goncharenko V, Gerlock AJ Jr, Shaff MI, Hollifield JW. Progression of renal artery fibromuscular dysplasia in 42 patients as seen on angiography. *Radiology* 1981;139:45–51.

109. Surowiec SM, Sivamurthy N, Rhodes JM, et al. Percutaneous therapy for renal artery fibromuscular dysplasia. *Ann Vasc Surg* 2003;17:650–655.

110. Rimmer JM, Gennari FJ. Atherosclerotic renovascular disease and progressive renal failure. *Ann Intern Med* 1993;118: 712–719.

111. van Jaarsveld BC, Krijnen P, Pieterman H, et al. The effect of balloon angioplasty on hypertension in atherosclerotic renal-artery stenosis. Dutch Renal Artery Stenosis Intervention Cooperative Study Group. *N Engl J Med* 2000;342:1007–1014.

112. Dorros G, Jaff M, Mathiak L, He T, Multicenter Registry Participants. Multicenter Palmaz stent renal artery stenosis revascularization registry report: four-year follow-up of 1,058 successful patients. *Cathet Cardiovasc Intervent* 2002;55:182–188.

113. Isles CG, Robertson S, Hill D. Management of renovascular disease: a review of renal artery stenting in ten studies. *QJM* 1999; 92:159–167.

114. Watson PS, Hadjipetrou P, Cox SV, Piemonte TC, Eisenhauer AC. Effect of renal artery stenting on renal function and size in patients with atherosclerotic renovascular disease. *Circulation* 2000;102:1671–1677.

115. Dormandy JA. Prostanoid drug therapy for peripheral arterial occlusive disease—the European experience. *Vasc Med* 1996;1: 155–158.

116. Johnston KW, Lindsay TF, Walker PM, Kalman PG. Mesenteric arterial bypass grafts: early and late results and suggested surgical approach for chronic and acute mesenteric ischemia. *Surgery* 1995;118:1–7.

117. Harward TR, Brooks DL, Flynn TC, Seeger JM. Multiple organ dysfunction after mesenteric artery revascularization. *J Vasc Surg* 1993;18:459–467.

118. Matsumoto AH, Angle JF, Spinosa DJ, et al. Percutaneous transluminal angioplasty and stenting in the treatment of chronic mesenteric ischemia: results and longterm followup. *J Am Coll Surg* 2002;194(suppl):S22–31.

119. Leriche R. Des oblitérations artérielles hautes comme cause des insuffisances circulatoires des membres inférieurs. *Bull Mem Soc Chir* 1923:1404–1406.

120. Leriche R, Morel A. The syndrome of thrombotic obliteration of the aortic bifurcation. *Ann Surg* 1948;127:193.

121. Mendelsohn FO, Santos RM, Crowley JJ, et al. Kissing stents in the aortic bifurcation. *Am Heart J* 1998;136(pt 1):600–605.

122. Brewster DC. Current controversies in the management of aortoiliac occlusive disease. *J Vasc Surg* 1997;25:365–379.

123. Sullivan TM, Childs MB, Bacharach JM, Gray BH, Piedmonte MR. Percutaneous transluminal angioplasty and primary stenting of the iliac arteries in 288 patients. *J Vasc Surg* 1997;25: 829–838.

124. Tetteroo E, van der Graaf Y, Bosch JL, et al. Randomised comparison of primary stent placement versus primary angioplasty followed by selective stent placement in patients with iliac-artery occlusive disease. Dutch Iliac Stent Trial Study Group. *Lancet* 1998;351:1153–1159.

125. Bosch JL, Hunink MG. Meta-analysis of the results of percutaneous transluminal angioplasty and stent placement for aortoiliac occlusive disease. *Radiology* 1997;204:87–96.

126. Palmaz JC, Garcia OJ, Schatz RA, et al. Placement of balloon-expandable intraluminal stents in iliac arteries: first 171 procedures. *Radiology* 1990;174(pt 2):969–975.

127. Martin EC, Katzen BT, Benenati JF, et al. Multicenter trial of the Wallstent in the iliac and femoral arteries. *J Vasc Intervent Radiol* 1995;6:843–849.

128. Dormandy JA, Rutherford RB. Management of peripheral arterial disease (PAD). TASC Working Group. TransAtlantic Inter-Society Concensus (TASC). *J Vasc Surg* 2000;31(pt 2):1–296.

129. Weaver FA, Comerota AJ, Youngblood M, Froehlich J, Hosking JD, Papanicolaou G. Surgical revascularization versus thrombolysis for nonembolic lower extremity native artery occlusions: results of a prospective randomized trial. The STILE Investigators. Surgery versus Thrombolysis for Ischemia of the Lower Extremity. *J Vasc Surg* 1996;24:513–521.

129a. Galaria II, G, Davies M. Percutaneous transluminal revascularization for Iliac occlusive disease: long-term outcomes in transAtlantic inter-society consensus A and B lesions. *Ann Vasc Surg* 2005; published online Apr 6.

130. Murray JG, Apthorp LA, Wilkins RA. Long-segment (> or = 10 cm) femoropopliteal angioplasty: improved technical success and long-term patency. *Radiology* 1995;195:158–162.

131. Gallino A, Mahler F, Probst P, Nachbur B. Percutaneous transluminal angioplasty of the arteries of the lower limbs: a 5 year follow-up. *Circulation* 1984;70:619–623.

132. Krepel VM, van Andel GJ, van Erp WF, Breslau PJ. Percutaneous transluminal angioplasty of the femoropopliteal artery: initial and long-term results. *Radiology* 1985;156:325–328.

133. Capek P, McLean GK, Berkowitz HD. Femoropopliteal angioplasty. Factors influencing long-term success. *Circulation* 1991; 83(suppl):I70–80.

134. Jeans WD, Armstrong S, Cole SE, Horrocks M, Baird RN. Fate of patients undergoing transluminal angioplasty for lower-limb ischemia. *Radiology* 1990;177:559–564.

135. Johnston KW. Femoral and popliteal arteries: reanalysis of results of balloon angioplasty. *Radiology* 1992;183:767–771.

136. Matsi PJ, Manninen HI, Vanninen RL, et al. Femoropopliteal angioplasty in patients with claudication: primary and secondary patency in 140 limbs with 1-3-year follow-up. *Radiology* 1994;191:727–733.

137. Hunink MG, Wong JB, Donaldson MC, Meyerovitz MF, de Vries J, Harrington DP. Revascularization for femoropopliteal disease. A decision and cost-effectiveness analysis. *JAMA* 1995;274:165–171.

138. Ansel GM, Botti CF, Silver Barry SGMJ, George BS. Why endovascular therapy should be utilized before surgical bypass for femoropopliteal occlusive disease. *J Invasive Cardiol* 2001;13: 608–610.

139. Gray BH, Olin JW. Limitations of percutaneous transluminal angioplasty with stenting for femoropopliteal arterial occlusive disease. *Seminars in Vascular Surgery* 1997;10:8–16.

140. Jahnke T, Andresen R, Muller-Hulsbeck S, et al. Hemobahn stent-grafts for treatment of femoropopliteal arterial obstructions: midterm results of a prospective trial. *J Vasc Intervent Radiol* 2003;14:41–51.

141. Isner JM, Pieczek A, Schainfeld R, et al. Clinical evidence of angiogenesis after arterial gene transfer of phVEGF165 in patient with ischaemic limb. *Lancet* 1996;348:370–374.

142. Isner JM, Asahara T. Angiogenesis and vasculogenesis as therapeutic strategies for postnatal neovascularization. *J Clin Invest* 1999;103:1231–1236.

143. Isner JM, Walsh K, Rosenfield K, et al. Arterial gene therapy for restenosis. *Hum Gene Ther* 1996;7:989–1011.

144. Schwarten DE, Cutcliff WB. Arterial occlusive disease below the knee: treatment with percutaneous transluminal angioplasty performed with low-profile catheters and steerable guide wires. *Radiology* 1988;169:71–74.

145. Dorros G, Jaff MR, Murphy KJ, Mathiak L. The acute outcome of tibioperoneal vessel angioplasty in 417 cases with claudication and critical limb ischemia. *Cathet Cardiovasc Diagn* 1998;45: 251–256.

146. Baumgartner I, Pieczek A, Manor O, et al. Constitutive expression of phVEGF165 after intramuscular gene transfer promotes collateral vessel development in patients with critical limb ischemia. *Circulation* 1998;97:1114–1123.

147. Henry M, Amor M, Ethevenot G, Henry I, Allaoui M. Percutaneous peripheral atherectomy using the rotablator: a single-center experience. *J Endovasc Surg* 1995;2:51–66.

148. Results of a prospective randomized trial evaluating surgery versus thrombolysis for ischemia of the lower extremity. The STILE trial. *Ann Surg* 1994;220:251–266.

149. Ouriel K, Shortell CK, DeWeese JA, et al. A comparison of thrombolytic therapy with operative revascularization in the initial treatment of acute peripheral arterial ischemia. *J Vasc Surg* 1994; 19:1021–1030.

150. Creager MA, Goldstone J, Hirshfeld JW Jr, et al. ACC/ ACP/ SCAI/SVMB/SVS Clinical Competence Statement on vascular medicine and catheter-based peripheral vascular interventions: a report of the American College of Cardiology/ American Heart Association/American College of Physicians Task Force on Clinical Competence (ACC/ACP/SCAI/SVMB/SVS Writing Committee to develop a clinical competence statement on peripheral vascular disease). *J Am Coll Cardiol* 2004;44: 941–957.

151. Rosenfield K, Babb J, Cates C, et al. Clinical competence statement on carotid stenting: training and credentialing for carotid stenting—multispecialty consensus recommendations: a report of the SCAI/SVMB/SVS Writing Committee to develop a clinical competence statement on carotid interventions. *J Am Coll Cardiol* 2005;45:165–174.

Intervention for Pediatric and Adult Congenital Heart Disease

27

Robert J. Sommer

The catheter-based treatment of congenital heart disease has been the traditional domain of Pediatric interventional cardiologists. But the successes of both pediatric cardiac medicine and pediatric cardiac surgery over the past 40 years have resulted in a growing population of adults with corrected congenital cardiac lesions that few adult cardiologists are prepared to manage. Concurrently, structural and congenital cardiac disease have become increasingly important issues in adult cardiology as the clinical significance of lesions such as patent foramen ovale are recognized and new catheter devices and procedures for their correction are introduced. Most adult interventional cardiologists, however, have little training in the evaluation and repair of these congenital lesions, whereas pediatric interventional cardiologists have little training in the common superimposed "adult" cardiology issues (such as hypertension, obesity, and coronary artery disease) or the differences in symptoms and indications for intervention compared with those in children with the same lesion. To help bridge this gap, this chapter will focus on a series of interventions for congenital heart disease that apply to *both* the pediatric and the adult population, noting procedural modifications that are required to accommodate a baby or an adult patient. Since knowledge of the physiologic and hemodynamic consequences of these lesions is at least as critical as knowing the steps of the procedures, a brief review of the underlying pathophysiology is also included in each section (see also Chapters 6 and 33).

THE CONGENITAL CATH LAB

Catheterization laboratories that perform procedures on patients with congenital heart disease differ from those treating mostly coronary disease. Many congenital procedures are best done in a biplane cath lab, as finding holes and complex surgically constructed pathways requires three-dimensional imaging, case times are usually longer than those of coronary cases, and the spectrum of equipment required for congenital cases is quite different. Because of the wide variety of congenital lesions and patient sizes, as well as the uncertainty as to when a particular catheter or device might be needed, a large number of items must be stocked. The laboratory administration thus must be willing to accept having some equipment expire unused rather than risk not having the critical catheter or wire available when it is needed.

In contrast to the early days of congenital catheterization, it is currently uncommon to perform purely diagnostic procedures. Echocardiography (transthoracic in children, transesophageal in adults), and now cardiac magnetic resonance imaging (MRI), are powerful noninvasive imaging modalities that allow the definition of the anatomy and assessment of both simple and complex physiology (including shunts, valvar dysfunction, and obstructions within the circulatory pathways). Instead, cardiac catheterization has become the preferred and minimally invasive way to perform repairs and palliations of straightforward congenital heart defects whose correction was previously limited to the operating room.

CONGENITAL OBSTRUCTIVE LESIONS

Obstructive Lesions of the Right Ventricular Outflow Tract

Obstruction to pulmonary blood flow is one of the most common and important abnormalities associated with congenital heart disease, and congenital interventions therefore frequently involve relief of this problem. Congenital obstruction of the right ventricular outflow tract can occur at the subvalvar level (muscular obstruction), at the valvar level, at the supravalvar level, or at the level of the branch pulmonary arteries. Although the level of obstruction can usually be determined echocardiographically, each lesion has a unique hemodynamic pattern and angiographic appearance (Fig. 27.1A–C). They have in common, however, increased afterload on the right ventricle (RV) myocardium, resulting in right ventricular hypertrophy and reduced diastolic compliance of the ventricle as a receiving chamber with a corresponding increase in right atrial filling pressures. The clinical symptoms associated with this lesion depend both on the degree of obstruction and the age of the patient.

Subvalvar Pulmonary Stenosis

Subvalvar obstruction is usually muscular in nature and is not generally amenable to catheter intervention (Fig. 27.1A). Residual or recurrent infundibular obstruction is most commonly found in patients who have undergone repair of tetralogy of Fallot. Double-chambered right ventricle (DCRV) also features hypertrophy of the infundibular muscle, causing it to closely appose the free wall of the RV in systole and narrow the outflow tract below the pulmonary valve. In children, this lesion may be associated with small membranous ventricular septal defects or membranous subaortic obstruction. Over time, the membranous ventricular septal defect may close spontaneously as the infundibular obstruction progresses, so that DCRV may present in the adult as an apparent isolated subvalvar obstruction. Pulmonary valve annular hypoplasia may also present in the setting of significant right ventricular outflow obstruction and can be found in patients as residua of surgically corrected coronary heart disease (CHD). This lesion is not generally amenable to transcatheter intervention owing to the fibrous ring of the hypoplastic annulus that resists balloon dilation.

Supravalvar Pulmonary Stenosis

Except when scarring from previous surgical interventions produces narrowing of the main pulmonary artery (MPA; i.e., following arterial reconstruction in neonatal transposition of the great arteries, or tetralogy of Fallot), supravalvar obstruction occurs at the sinotubular junction and is con- genital. Supravalvar stenosis at the sinotubular junction can be confused echocardiographically with valvar disease, because the normal leaflets are limited in their forward motion by the distal ridge of muscular tissue (Fig. 27.1B), appear to dome, and exhibit turbulent flow at the leaflet tips on Doppler, just as is seen in valvar pulmonary stenosis (PS). Balloon dilation of supravalvar obstructions is largely unsuccessful owing to the muscular/elastic nature of the arterial wall in the MPA. Stents have been placed successfully to relieve obstruction in the supravalvar region, but risk stenting open the pulmonary valve and causing severe insufficiency, most often a poor trade-off for moderate PS.

Valvar Pulmonary Stenosis

Valvar PS is a common congenital lesion. Similar in nature to congenital aortic stenosis, it is caused by commissural fusion that precludes the leaflets separating fully (Fig. 27.1C). The result is a diminished valve orifice/valve area resulting in increased RV afterload.

The natural history studies of isolated valvar pulmonary stenosis in children indicate that a pressure gradient >50 mm Hg is associated with poor long-term outcomes, including RV myocardial dysfunction, ventricular arrhythmia, and sudden death (1–3), whereas pressure gradients <30 mm Hg are not associated with symptoms, changes in lifestyle, or life expectancy. As treatment has shifted from surgical to catheter-based therapy, the indications for intervention have changed somewhat. *Currently, any patient with a valvar gradient ≥40 mm Hg should undergo balloon valvuloplasty.*

Neonatal Critical PS

Critical PS, or valvar pulmonary atresia in the neonate, presents with cyanosis. Desaturated blood returning to the right atrium (RA) can either enter the severely hypertrophied, sometimes diminutive RV chamber or flow right to left across the patent foramen ovale (PFO), as it did throughout fetal life. This shunt adds desaturated blood to the pulmonary venous return on the left side of the heart, accounting for the cyanosis. If the atrial level shunt is large enough, the patient may be dependent on the coexistence of a patent ductus arteriosus (PDA) to provide pulmonary blood flow. When the PDA begins to close (12 to 48 hours), the child becomes progressively hypoxemic, requiring prostaglandin E1 (PGE1) to reopen and to maintain ductal patency until an appropriate intervention can be performed.

Even after successful balloon intervention (see below), the hypertrophied RV continues to present a diastolic impediment to forward flow, allowing systemic venous blood to cross the PFO to the LA, causing ongoing systemic desaturation. However, as long as the infant can maintain an oxygen saturations greater than 70% and does not develop acidosis, PGE1 can be discontinued, however. Over a course of weeks

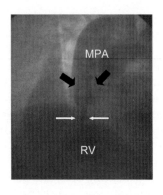

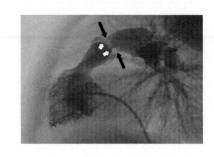

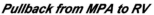

Pullback from MPA to RV

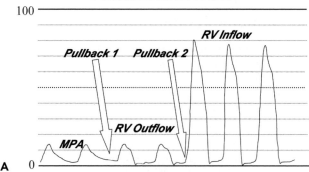

A

Pullback from MPA to RV

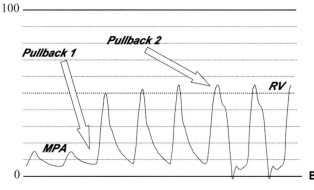

B

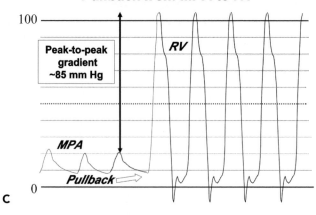

Pullback from MPA to RV

Peak-to-peak gradient ~85 mm Hg

C

Figure 27.1 **A.** *Top.* Subvalvar pulmonary stenosis (PS). Severe muscular dynamic narrowing of the RV outflow tract *(white arrows)*, well below the level of the valve leaflets *(black arrows)*. *Bottom.* Systolic pressure remains unchanged (pullback 1) as diastolic pressure falls indicating transition into the ventricle. On further withdrawal of the catheter (pullback 2), there is a large systolic gradient with no change in diastole, consistent with an intraventricular obstruction. MPA, main pulmonary artery; RV, right ventricle. **B.** *Top.* Supravalvar PS. The thickened pulmonary valve leaflets *(white arrows)* abut the supravalvar muscular ridge at the sinotubular junction *(black arrows)*, not allowing full leaflet excursion. *Bottom.* There is a jump in the systolic pressure on pullback, but no fall in the diastolic pressure, indicating that the catheter remains in the PA, distal to the valve. A second pullback reveals no further systolic gradient coming back into the ventricle. **C.** *Top.* Valvar PS. Doming valve leaflets *(black arrows)* are fused and cannot open fully. Jet of contrast through valve orifice is well profiled. *Bottom.* Systolic pressure gradient occurs at same site/time where diastolic pressure falls, indicating transition through the valve from artery to ventricle.

to months, after elimination of the right ventricular afterload, the right ventricular myocardium thins and becomes more compliant so that right-to-left shunting diminishes and the patient's oxygen saturation normalizes. Rarely, ongoing RV noncompliance, often in combination with right ventricular and tricuspid valve hypoplasia, may result in persistent desaturation in the absence of significant residual PS, requiring closure of the PFO to eliminate the right-to-left shunt.

PS in Children

In most children, PS presents as an asymptomatic heart murmur. Gradients are followed noninvasively with Doppler echocardiography. It is important to note that the peak instantaneous echo gradient usually overestimates the peak-to-peak gradient measured in the cath lab (Fig. 27.2) when considering the timing of the intervention in a child. Severe obstruction is associated with surprisingly few symptoms in young children, who often maintain patency of the PFO to allow for right-to-left shunt at times of peak exercise (exercise-induced cyanosis). In patients who are cyanotic at rest, it is important to recognize that neither the echo nor catheter estimates of valve gradient accurately reflect the degree of obstruction, since only part of the cardiac output is traversing the valve.

Adolescents/Adult Patients

Valvar PS is one of the most common congenital valve lesions in the adolescent and adult population, since the lack of symptoms in the pediatric age group may delay early recognition. The most common presentation in adulthood is exercise intolerance, breathlessness, and

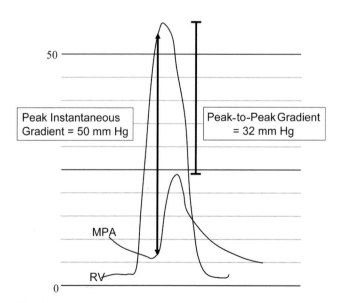

Figure 27.2 Simultaneous right ventricle (RV) and main pulmonary artery (MPA) tracings in a patient with pulmonary stenosis. The bracket demonstrates the peak-to-peak gradient as measured in the cath lab. The arrow shows the peak instantaneous pressure difference, which corresponds to the peak velocity as measured by Doppler echocardiography. In general, the echo overestimates the degree of obstruction found in the cath lab.

fatigue. Classic signs of right heart failure—peripheral edema, jugular venous distension, and ascites—are rare until a nearly premorbid state. But the excessive right ventricular afterload limits RV systolic performance, and thereby diminishes left ventricle (LV) preload and cardiac output during exertion. Adult PS patients thus tend to be more symptomatic than children with similar gradients, but we have seen patients in their eighth and ninth decades of life with very high gradients (80 to >100 mm Hg) and few or no symptoms.

Valvar PS in the adult may also be acquired as part of carcinoid heart disease (4). These valves become thickened and dense and more closely resemble the dysplastic neonatal valves, whose resistance to flow is not related to valve leaflet fusion, but rather to the force required to push open the thickened leaflets. These thickened valves are much less responsive to balloon valvuloplasty.

Percutaneous Balloon Pulmonary Valvuloplasty

Percutaneous pulmonary valvuloplasty in children was first reported by Semb et al. (5) in 1979. However, the static balloon technique, reported by Kan et al. (6) in 1982, was the first to be applied widely. Results have demonstrated the safety and effectiveness (7–10) of this technique and have established it as the treatment of choice for children and adults with isolated pulmonary valve stenosis (see Chapter 25).

Pediatric Technique

Echocardiographic evaluation is critical to successful outcome prior to intervention. It defines the degree of obstruction as well as the valve morphology, allows extremely accurate measurement of the pulmonary annulus, and rules out any associated defects. With advancing engineering and material technology, balloon dilation catheters are now available on catheters as small as 3F, allowing us to perform pulmonary balloon valvuloplasty in premature infants under 2 kg.

After intravenous sedation, femoral venous access is obtained and a balloon-tipped angiographic or end-hole catheter is used to perform right heart catheterization. In the absence of associated defects, the pulmonary artery (PA) saturation is used to estimate predilation cardiac index (Fick calculation). In most cases, femoral arterial access is not required, as complications from arterial access probably far outweigh the complications of the valvuloplasty in children under 10 kg. After administration of heparin in a dose of 50 to 100 U/kg, the right heart catheter is advanced across the valve to the branch pulmonary artery and a pressure pullback is performed (Fig. 27.1C). The peak-to-peak gradient across the pulmonary outflow is measured. A right ventricular angiogram is then performed using both lateral and cranial-angled AP projections (biplane) to localize the valve and confirm the echocardiographic annulus size by measuring across the outflow tract at the level of the valve hinge points. A balloon diameter 1.2 to 1.4 times that of the annulus is selected, since the use of oversized balloons in pulmonary valvuloplasty has been shown to produce optimal results in children (11). In larger patients, with an annulus size >20 mm, modifications in technique are required (see Adult Patients below). A balloon length of 2 to 3 cm is adequate in most children and avoids some of the potential complications of right ventricular outflow tract trauma and injury of the tricuspid valve.

A balloon end-hole catheter is floated to the distal right or left pulmonary artery (angled, torquable catheters may also be used), and a stiff exchange-length guidewire is placed in the branch PA. The sheath and catheter are removed, and the desired valvuloplasty balloon is introduced over the guidewire. Although introduction of "naked" balloon catheters have been advocated by some, we prefer the use of a short venous sheath large enough to accommodate the appropriately sized balloon. Once the balloon catheter is centered on the pulmonary valve, the position can be adjusted quickly using a series of very-low-pressure partial inflations to look for the valve "waist." When in the appropriate position, the balloon is inflated rapidly until the waist disappears, then immediately deflated. Ideally, the balloon, with mild traction, will remain centered on the valve, and with increasing radial pressure will "pop" open the valve. This popping sensation probably relates to the tearing of the stenotic valve commissures.

After successful opening of the valve, the balloon will jump forward with forward flow, which must be distinguished from the forward "squirting" of a balloon that has been positioned too far into the PA, since the latter means that the valve has not been effectively dilated. In patients with dysplastic or thickened pulmonary valves, there will be no pop as the balloon is inflated to full pressure, but only a gradual resolution of the waist with increasing balloon pressure and a return of the waist as balloon pressures fall—these valves are rarely amenable to balloon valvuloplasty.

If a suboptimal result is obtained, repositioning and immediate reinflation may help. A larger-lumen catheter (i.e., a guiding catheter) can be advanced over the guidewire into a branch PA, using a Y adapter (Tuohy-Borst valve) to measure pressure from the side arm as the catheter is withdrawn slowly across the dilated valve. In this way, residual pressure gradients can be measured and accurately localized to either the valvar or infundibular level (see Complications below). Residual valvar gradients of more than 20 to 30 mm Hg are unusual and suggest suboptimal balloon size or position and warrant repeat dilation with advancement of a suitable dilation catheter over the guidewire that is still in place in the PA.

Pediatric Modifications of the Procedure

In neonates, access for the procedure can be obtained at the umbilical vein, provided that the ductus venosus in the liver has not closed. This access route is readily accessible and avoids injury/obstruction of the femoral vein. In older patients, internal jugular and subclavian approaches are also acceptable for the procedure. Percutaneous transhepatic access has also been used.

With severe PS, the catheter across the tiny valve lumen may completely or virtually completely obstruct flow. In this setting, we prefer to perform the RV angiogram prior to crossing the valve to minimize hemodynamic compromise. Once the valve is crossed, the catheter is removed quickly, leaving only the guidewire to minimize obstruction to flow. In neonates, it is almost never possible to pass a balloon-tipped catheter through the valve, making our catheter of choice a torquable 4 or 5 French end-hole catheter with a multipurpose or Berenstein curve. This catheter is manipulated through the tricuspid valve and flipped up into the RV outflow tract, and a 0.014-inch torque-control guidewire is used to probe for the valve orifice. Once the valve is crossed, the wire is positioned either in a branch pulmonary artery or through the ductus arteriosus into the descending aorta where it can be snared from the descending aorta to stabilize the position further (12). Most often, we will first use a smaller balloon on a smaller catheter shaft to predilate the valve, followed by an oversized balloon to finish the procedure.

Valvar pulmonary atresia also presents with cyanosis in the neonate and requires patency of the ductus arteriosus to provide pulmonary blood flow. In some cases, the pulmonary valve annulus, the RV chamber volume, and the tricuspid valve annulus may be sufficient to allow handling of the normal pulmonary blood flow. In these patients, several techniques have been used to perforate the atretic valve, including stiff guidewires, trans-septal needles, or radiofrequency ablation (13,14). Once the valve is perforated and a wire advanced into one of the branches or down the descending aorta (through the PDA), balloon dilation proceeds as if for critical neonatal PS.

Adolescent/Adult Technique

Percutaneous balloon valvuloplasty in adults is discussed extensively in Chapter 25 and is similar to what we describe for younger children. The principle difference is that the valve annulus is larger, and owing to balloon diameter oversizing by 20 to 40% compared with the annulus, balloons of 25 mm or larger are often required. There are three solutions to this size issue.

1. Custom balloons are available in sizes up to 30 mm. No real differences are therefore required in the technique, but these balloons require longer inflation times, longer deflation times, lower burst pressures, and larger sheath sizes.

2. Double balloon technique. A second venous access is obtained and a balloon-tipped end-hole catheter is passed to the distal PA. A second stiff exchange-length guidewire is placed across the valve. The perimeter of the combined

balloons is selected to be 20 to 40% larger than the measured annulus (15), and the balloons are inflated simultaneously. The double balloon technique allows the use of two smaller sheaths but requires additional venous access and additional personnel; it also has increased technical difficulties of accurately positioning two balloons during inflation.

3. We prefer the use of an Inoue balloon for adolescent/adult pulmonary valvuloplasty (16). After hemodynamic evaluation and RV angiography, a 14 French sheath is exchanged over a wire and a 0.032-inch stiff exchange guidewire is positioned in the branch pulmonary artery. An Inoue Balloon is selected with a diameter 1.2 times the valve annulus, stretched/slenderized, and passed over the wire to the right atrium. At that point, the balloon is softened by retraction of the metal slenderizing rod, and the distal portion of the balloon is inflated slightly to help float the catheter through the valve. If there is difficulty in manipulating the Inoue balloon through the RV to the PA, a long 14 French Mullins sheath can be passed over a wire into the PA, and the Inoue can be advanced through the long sheath (the sheath may need to be cut shorter to accommodate the Inoue length). Once positioned in the main pulmonary artery, the valvuloplasty is performed exactly as a mitral valvuloplasty (see Chapter 25). A Y adapter can be attached directly to the back of the Inoue, and a pressure can be measured from the sidepost during pullback, over the wire. Advantages of the Inoue technique include providing variability in balloon size and minimizing the risk of tricuspid valve or branch pulmonary artery injury owing to the short length and positional accuracy of the balloon. Disadvantages are the large sheath size required and the higher cost of the Inoue compared with other balloon dilation catheters.

Complications

Acute Subvalvar (Infundibular) Obstruction

With severe valvar PS, particularly in older children and adults, concentric right ventricular hypertrophy is present universally. When the afterload at the valve is acutely removed, a hypercontractile RV outflow tract may create dynamic subvalvar muscular obstruction, which has been termed the "suicidal right ventricle." *The total gradient across the outflow tract may actually be higher than it was prior to the balloon dilation. It is critical to recognize the difference between residual valvar obstruction and resulting subvalvar reactive obstruction, so as not to perform unnecessary additional valve dilations.* A careful pullback pressure recording performed over a wire (as outlined above) is the best way to determine the level of residual obstruction. If the subvalvar obstruction is severe enough, cardiac output may fall acutely. The treatment of these patients is much like that with left-sided hypertrophic obstructive cardiomyopathy. Volume loading should be combined with beta- and/or calcium channel blockers to reduce myocardial contractility. But the hypertrophy of the outflow tract muscle generally

recedes over a course of several weeks to months (17) with elimination of the subvalvar gradient.

Other complications are extremely rare and include tricuspid valve injury, as a result of wire tension on the tricuspid valve leaflet during inflation or in pulling the partially deflated balloon back through the TV. Pulmonary insufficiency can be seen after successful dilation, but is usually well tolerated acutely. Long-standing valvar regurgitation, however, may lead to RV dilation and dysfunction in adults. In children, long balloons may rarely injure/rupture the curved RV outflow tract as the balloon straightens, and a long balloon advanced or propelled too far into one of the branch PAs may cause injury at that site. Finally, the wire tracking through the tricuspid valve can pinch or damage the AV node, resulting in high-degree AV block. At our center, however, more than 94% of pulmonary valve procedures in all age groups were uncomplicated.

Current Status

Over more than two decades, pulmonary balloon valvuloplasty has been shown to be an extremely safe and effective therapy in all age groups. Acute and long-term gradient reductions are comparable to surgical interventions, whereas complications, including pulmonary regurgitation, are less prevalent than after surgery (18). Balloon valvuloplasty is a curative procedure for most patients and should be considered the procedure of choice for valvar pulmonary stenosis with a transvalvar gradient of >40 mmHg at any age, in symptomatic adults with gradients >30 mm Hg, and in neonates with critical pulmonary stenosis.

Over the last 5 years, much research has been devoted to the development of transcatheter semilunar valve replacement therapy. Because pulmonary artery surgery is such a central part of the repair of CHD, Bonhoeffer's group has focused on the replacement of the pulmonary valve. Their work, with a bovine jugular valve sewn inside a balloon-dilatable stent, has yielded excellent bench, animal, and now early human results (19–21; see Chapter 25).

Branch Pulmonary Artery Stenosis

Branch pulmonary artery stenosis or hypoplasia may be acquired (e.g., at sites of prior surgery) or may be congenital (i.e., tetralogy of Fallot). Numerous systemic congenital syndromes are also associated with branch PA stenosis/hypoplasia (Williams, congenital rubella, Alagille, etc.). Branch PA stenosis is typically a hemodynamic burden that must be dealt with in children, but can be seen in adults as residua of earlier congenital heart surgery or rarely as an isolated congenital lesion (22).

Anatomy ranges from single stenotic areas to multiple stenoses to diffuse hypoplasia of the vessel. In contrast with other right-sided obstructive lesions, the branch PA stenosis not only increases RV afterload, but also results in hypoperfusion of one lung or selected lung segments, with overcirculation to others because of the parallel pathways available to the pulmonary blood flow. Indications for angioplasty include elevated right ventricular systolic pressure (greater than one-half of aortic systolic pressure), hypertension in unaffected portions of the vascular bed, marked decrease in flow to an affected portion, and/or symptoms.

Quantitative lung perfusion scans have been extremely useful in the preoperative assessment of these patients (23). Unlike most other imaging modalities, flow to each individual lobe can be quantified, yielding information about relative severity of the individual stenotic lesions. This can help direct therapy prior to arrival in the cath lab and avoid unnecessary catheter/wire manipulation during what are often lengthy procedures. Cardiac MRI is also now being used to assess flow volumes in this setting.

Balloon angioplasty for hemodynamically important branch pulmonary artery lesions can be accomplished with various small peripheral vascular balloon catheters. Specially designed high-pressure balloon catheters or bladed cutting balloons may be used for more resistant lesions. Placement of intravascular stents has become the treatment of choice in older children and adults who have completed or nearly completed their growth. Particularly in the proximal, more muscular branches of the pulmonary tree, stents more reliably improve vessel size, overcoming the recoil of these elastic vessels, and reduce the need for oversized balloons. With increased experience demonstrating that later stent re-expansion is possible/safe, stents are now being used in even the youngest patients in critical situations.

Balloon Angioplasty for Branch PA Stenosis

Technique

Pulmonary arteries are most commonly dilated from the femoral veins, but can be dilated from the subclavian or internal jugular vein or from the femoral arteries in patients with systemic-to-pulmonary artery shunts. Though less commonly used, the subclavian or internal jugular approach is easier in many patients owing to the support afforded to the catheter course at the right atrial floor. After heparinization, and the optional placement of a small arterial catheter for blood pressure monitoring, right heart hemodynamics are measured, and the magnitude and location of gradients in the pulmonary arteries are determined. In patients with symptoms of right ventricular failure, creation of an atrial septal defect prior to dilation may decrease morbidity and mortality. Pulmonary angiograms should include selective injections (anteroposterior [AP] and lateral) in each lung and in affected lobes or segments (see Chapter 13). Selective catheterization of the lung segments is best accomplished using a steerable end-hole catheter and a floppy-tipped torque wire. Once satisfactory wire position is attained, a cutoff pigtail with a side-arm adapter may be exchanged over the guidewire, or one of the newer angiographic monorail catheters may be used. Either technique allows pressure measurements, angiograms, and dilations

to be performed without losing wire position. Lower-volume, selective injections in the affected lobes almost always yield superior images compared with injections to both lungs. Prior to dilation, a stiffer exchange-length wire should be passed to the largest vessel distal to the stenosis to minimize the risk of aneurysm formation with overdilation of small distal vessels.

The ideal balloon has a low profile, a short distal tip, and a high maximal inflation pressure. The balloon diameter is chosen to be two to four times the diameter of the lesion but not more than two times the diameter of the normal vessel on either side (24,25). The balloon is inflated until the waist disappears or until maximum inflation pressure is reached. Inflation times range from 10 to 60 seconds, depending on the response of the waist and how well the cardiac output is maintained. Unlike dilation of the semilunar valves, in which all output from the ventricle is eliminated during inflation, perfusion of the other lung/lobes will maintain cardiac output and will allow longer inflation times. Like with coronary angioplasty (Chapter 22), successful dilation generally results in tearing of the intima and media (26).

Following dilation, the balloon catheter is exchanged over the guidewire for a cutoff pigtail or monorail catheter, and the lesion is reassessed hemodynamically and angiographically. Successful dilation usually is accompanied by an increase in pressure distal to the angioplasty site, and usually results in both a decrease in proximal pressures and a decrease in the gradient across the area. Angiograms are repeated to measure the diameter of the stenosis and to look carefully for tears and aneurysms that may preclude further balloon dilation. For this reason, distal lesions are dilated prior to proximal lesions, and more severe stenoses are dilated prior to milder ones.

Results

The criteria for successful dilation have been arbitrarily defined as an increase in diameter of >50%, an increase in flow in the affected segment of >20%, and/or a decrease of >20% in the systolic right ventricular-to-aortic pressure ratio. Using these criteria, the success rate using low-pressure balloons was approximately 60% (27,28). The use of high-pressure balloons with inflation pressures as high as 21 atmospheres increased the success rate to 75% (29). The success rate for postoperative stenoses is higher than for congenital stenoses. The incidence of restenosis following balloon angioplasty is approximately 15%. Complications have included death in approximately 1% of patients secondary to pulmonary artery rupture or pulmonary edema. Aneurysms occur in 3% of dilations and are most common in small vessels distal to the stenosis. Although the success rate using low-pressure balloons has changed little over the years, the complication rate has decreased owing primarily to improved technique. The use of high-pressure balloons does not seem to have significantly altered the complication rate. Balloon angioplasty at surgical sites should be used with caution in patients less than 4 to 6 weeks after surgery to minimize the risk of vessel rupture.

Use of Bladed Cutting Balloons

Early work with bladed cutting balloon catheters has shown significant promise for the treatment of what were previously considered undilatable lesions. Small studies, under compassionate use protocols, have shown significant improvement in vessel size using oversized cutting balloons that cut through intimal and medial layers (30,31). After cutting-balloon inflation, subsequent use of high-pressure balloons and/or intravascular stents has further improved outcome with success rates reported in up to 92% of vessels (32). Clinical trials are underway.

Use of Intravascular Stents

Intravascular stents were first used for resistant branch pulmonary arteries in 1989 (33–35) and this use is now the most common use of stents in CHD. Although balloon angioplasty remains the treatment of choice in peripheral lesions, in lesions at branch points, and in infants/small children (growth issues), stent implantation in the pulmonary artery bed has become first-line therapy for proximal obstructions, lesions owing to surgical distortion, external compression, inadequate results of balloon angioplasty, and obstructive intimal flaps following angioplasty. Infants who undergo surgical repairs such as the arterial switch for transposition of the great arteries, repair of tetralogy of Fallot with branch PA plasty, and palliations such as shunts or PA banding may have acute postoperative obstructions that create hemodynamic instability or place the obstructed lung at risk of long term hypoperfusion. Stent usage in the immediate postoperative period, as an alternative to repeat surgical intervention, can be lifesaving and is usually safer (smaller balloons) and more effective than balloon angioplasty. Since early stent use in the branch PAs, technology has improved both in the stents themselves and in the delivery balloons. The use of stents has improved the success rate of branch pulmonary artery interventions to >90% (36).

Most experience with stent implantation in branch PAs is with the Palmaz stent (Johnson & Johnson, New Brunswick, NJ), though newer stents may have significant advantages including trackability, conformability to vessel course, reduction in balloon and vessel damage owing to smoother device edges, diminished stent shortening with expansion, and improved visibility with alternative materials. Innovations in balloon design include a marked reduction in catheter shaft diameter and slip-/scratch-resistant balloon surfaces (to reduce the incidence of the stent slipping off or puncturing the balloon). A balloon-in-a-balloon catheter (Nu-Med, Hopkinton, NY), is being used for a number of indications and helps minimize the risks of stent malposition.

Heparinization and prophylactic antibiotic use is important in these often-long procedures. Predilation with a balloon is optional but is not necessary for most branch PA lesions. Stent and balloon sizes are selected for the individual lesion. The stent is crimped onto the balloon and can be delivered using one of two techniques. With a standard approach, a long sheath or guiding catheter is passed over an extra-stiff exchange-length guidewire (with a short floppy tip), such that the sheath tip is distal to the lesion to be stented. The balloon/stent combination is then advanced over the guidewire through the sheath to the implantation site. Alternatively, the front-loading technique involves passing the balloon catheter fully through the sheath outside the body, crimping the stent onto the balloon, and pulling it back into the front of the sheath before introducing this assembly over the wire. Hybrid techniques are also used in which the long sheath is advanced over the wire to the inferior vena cava, the stent then mounted on the balloon and advanced over the wire to the tip of the sheath *prior* to advancing the entire system over the wire to the target lesion. The stent is deployed as described in Chapter 24. Anticoagulation is indicated for a period of 3 to 6 months to prevent stent thrombosis, prior to endothelialization. For patients with normal pulsatile flow in the PAs, aspirin alone should be sufficient. For patients with nonpulsatile flow (bidirectional Glenn shunt or Fontan), warfarin is probably warranted. There is a very low rate of restenosis in the branch PAs except the relative stenosis that develops owing to the lack of change in stent diameter as the patient grows (37).

Stents in Extracardiac Conduits

Stents may also be used to extend the life of surgical conduits inserted between the heart and the branch pulmonary arteries (37a). With rapid growth of the infant, the conduit may kink, developing intraluminal obstruction. Balloon angioplasty alone in this setting has been largely unsuccessful because the conduit will reassume its kinked course on balloon deflation. In several patients, we have been able to hold off conduit replacement for several years using this approach, removing the stent with the explanted conduit at later surgery.

OBSTRUCTION OF THE LEFT VENTRICULAR OUTFLOW TRACT

Anatomy/Physiology

Similar to obstructions of the right ventricular outflow tract, congenital obstruction of the left ventricular outflow tract can occur at the subvalvar level, at the valvar level, at the supravalvar level, or in the aortic arch itself (coarctation of the aorta). The increased afterload on the LV myocardium results in concentric left ventricular hypertrophy and reduced diastolic compliance of the ventricle as a receiving chamber with a corresponding increase in pulmonary venous pressures. The degree of patient symptoms relates to the elevation of left ventricular filling pressures. Patients may present with dyspnea on exertion when symptoms are mild and with orthopnea, syncope, or sudden death with increasing cardiac dysfunction. Most children tolerate large degrees of valvar obstruction without symptoms, presenting with a murmur alone, but symptoms become more common in the older child and adult.

Transcatheter Therapy for Left-Sided Obstruction

Subaortic stenosis encompasses a spectrum of disorders ranging from simple membranous obstructions of the subaortic area, to fibromuscular tunnel obstructions, to the more familiar hypertrophic cardiomyopathy. Like subvalvar lesions of the right side, subaortic obstructions are primarily a surgical issue. Membranous obstructions of the left ventricular outflow were treated with balloon angioplasty early in the interventional era (38,39), but with limited success and routine recurrence of obstruction.

Fibromuscular tunnel obstructions are generally not amenable to catheter intervention. Stents have been used in a few patients with critical postoperative obstructions, with very limited success, high morbidity, and a significant incidence of stent failure. These should be considered only in life-threatening situations where surgical intervention is not possible.

For the more common hypertrophic cardiomyopathy with muscular subaortic obstruction, alcohol ablation of septal tissue in adults has been widely adopted as an alternative to surgical muscle resection (see Chapter 31). There is no significant experience with this technique in children and adolescents, because septal hypertrophy is rarely clinically apparent before puberty and continues to develop during adolescence and young adulthood. Dual-chamber pacing has been reported to alleviate the degree of obstruction in younger patients, but with comparative studies now seems less effective in adults than either surgery or alcohol ablation (40).

Supravalvar aortic stenosis may occur at the sinotubular junction, as a congenital lesion. This is the pathognomonic lesion for Williams syndrome and genetic deletion syndrome associated with developmental delay, abnormalities of calcium metabolism, and a diffuse arteriopathy. This lesion should also be treated surgically because the elastic properties of the tissue at that site make balloon angioplasty ineffective, and the use of a stent in this position risks entrapping aortic valve leaflets with resulting aortic regurgitation.

Valvar Aortic Stenosis

Balloon aortic valvuloplasty for congenital aortic stenosis (AS) in a child was first reported in 1983 (41). It has been performed subsequently in large numbers of patients with both congenital and acquired stenoses (41–46). In acquired calcific valve stenosis, acute relief of gradient is possible (see Chapter 25). However, the rapid rate of restenosis along with modest degrees of obstruction relief has left balloon valvuloplasty for calcified valves as an emergency option only. Most adult centers now prefer valve replacement, reserving balloon valvuloplasty for patients who are high-risk surgical candidates. In children, adolescents, and young adults with congenital valvar AS, however, balloon valvuloplasty remains an excellent alternative to surgical valvotomy or to valve replacement, since the pathology involves more commissural fusion and less the leaflet rigidity seen in adult patients with senescent and densely calcified aortic valves.

Neonatal Critical Aortic Stenosis

Physiologically, critical aortic stenosis is a different entity than severe aortic stenosis in older children, since the valve may be virtually atretic and the left ventricular cavity may be moderately to severely hypoplastic. Unlike hypoplasia of the *right* ventricle in critical PS (in which right atrial blood may cross the PFO to maintain LV preload and cardiac output), the size of the *left* ventricle has a direct impact on survival. LV hypoplasia, reduced LV compliance, and reduced emptying in the face of extraordinary afterload, lead to increased left atrial and pulmonary venous pressures. Any blood that shunts left to right through the PFO reduces both LV preload and cardiac output. Low cardiac output and pulmonary venous congestion may be incompatible with life. If LV hypoplasia is a concern, the alternative is to assign these patients to a stage I palliation for hypoplastic left heart syndrome. A retrospective analysis of a group of patients with critical aortic stenosis undergoing surgical valvotomy or balloon dilation at Boston Children's Hospital led to a scoring system (based on echocardiographic measurement of left-sided structures) that can be used to triage such patients (47).

The neonate with critical AS may be largely asymptomatic after birth because of the normal remnants of the fetal circulation. Left atrial return crosses the patent foramen ovale to the right atrium, rather than entering the LV. The volume-loaded RV ejects blood into the MPA, where flow is distributed between the lungs and the systemic circulation via the ductus arteriosus, based on the relative resistance of each pathway. If a normal blood volume reaches the aorta, there are no clinical problems. However, as pulmonary resistance falls and as the ductus arteriosus starts to close, blood is preferentially shunted to the lungs. A corresponding fall in systemic flow results in diminished tissue oxygen delivery, anaerobic respiration at the cellular level, and profound metabolic acidosis. Re-establishing and maximizing systemic flow is the key to resuscitating the acidotic newborn. Prostaglandin is required to reopen the ductus, and elevation of pulmonary vascular resistance is desirable (minimize FiO_2, allow pCO_2 to rise). When most of the systemic flow arises from the ductus arteriosus, rather than the LV, the measured valvar pressure gradient is not a meaningful number, as the output across the valve can approach zero and critical AS is manifest by right-to-left systolic flow at the ductus arteriosus with equal systemic arterial desaturation in all extremities.

Pediatric Technique

Using routine sedation, a femoral vein and artery are entered percutaneously and the patient heparinized. The venous catheter is used to measure right heart pressures and cardiac output (when no shunts are present) before and after dilation. In older patients, aortic valves can be dilated from the femoral vein using a trans-septal approach, but the retrograde approach from the femoral artery remains the most common technique. We start with a pigtail catheter of an appropriate size to perform left ventriculography and measure a valvar gradient. An aortogram is done to define the anatomic landmarks if the time for crossing becomes prolonged. We do not routinely do a baseline aortic angiogram, as the amount of aortic regurgitation should have been documented by echo as part of the precath evaluation.

The typical method for crossing the stenotic aortic valve from the aorta is to advance the soft end of a straight wire out of a pigtail catheter and use it to probe for the valve orifice (see Chapter 4). We will often use a hydrophilic guidewire, as the reduced friction of its surface allows for more rapid in-and-out movements, but probing must be done gently to avoid perforating a cusp or damaging the coronary arteries. When the left ventricle is entered, a transvalvar gradient is measured by simultaneously recording pressure from the pigtail and femoral sheath. A left ventriculogram is performed and the aortic annulus measured at the hinge points of the valve.

In contrast to the pulmonary valvuloplasty, the balloon diameter is chosen to be only 75 to 90% of the annulus diameter. Animal and clinical studies demonstrate that aortic valvuloplasty with a balloon/annulus ratio greater than 1.0 is more likely to be associated with aortic regurgitation (48,49). A double-balloon technique may be used when the annulus is large. The pigtail catheter is exchanged for the dilation catheter, which is centered across the valve, inflated and deflated rapidly, and pulled back to the descending aorta. The gradient and the cardiac output are remeasured following dilation, and an aortogram is performed to look for aortic regurgitation. If the residual gradient is >55 mm Hg and an aortogram shows no or only mild regurgitation, a larger balloon is used. It is far better, however, to leave a residual gradient than to cause significant aortic insufficiency in the small child, as surgical backout options are limited (Ross procedure).

It can often be difficult to keep the balloon positioned in the valve during inflation, against the force of left ventricular ejection. A stiff catheter shaft, long balloon, and extra-stiff exchange wire will help stabilize the position, or the balloon can be advanced so that it lies along the top of the aortic arch rather than around the underside of the arch. The double-balloon technique, which does not totally obstruct flow, may make it easier to maintain balloon position. We have also begun to use the technique of Cribier (50), who uses a transvenous pacing catheter positioned in the RV to rapidly pace the ventricle during the dilation to reduce ventricular ejection and provide a more stable balloon position.

Technique for Critical Neonatal AS

Before the catheterization begins, the baby's hemodynamic status must be optimized. We generally perform this procedure with the baby intubated and paralyzed. The FiO_2 is turned down to 21%, and PCO_2 is allowed to rise to the mid-40s to increase pulmonary vascular resistance and maximize systemic flow across the PDA. Body temperature is carefully monitored.

The umbilical artery can usually be used in the first week of life. Catheter manipulation is more difficult from the umbilical artery owing to the inferoposterior loop in its course before entering the descending aorta, but its use avoids damage to the femoral artery in these very small infants. A number of centers have used a surgical cutdown at the carotid artery for catheter access, an approach that simplifies crossing the valve (51) because of the straight path to the valve from the neck. As with older patients, a trans-septal approach can be used from either the femoral or umbilical vein, with no puncture required since all neonates have a patent foramen ovale. But this approach is rarely used, since it carries a much higher risk of mitral valve injury than in the older population.

Results/Complications

As congenital valvar aortic stenosis is a relatively uncommon diagnosis, there are few large series in the literature (52–54). However, all of the studies concur: Balloon valvuloplasty for congenital aortic stenosis is an effective palliation with excellent gradient reduction and increase in valve area, but is complicated by the development of significant aortic regurgitation in 10 to 30% either immediately or within weeks of the procedure (inversely related to balloon/annulus ratio; 53) femoral arterial complications in 30 to 40% (inversely related to the size of the patient), and restenosis. Survival with freedom from reintervention was seen in only 50% of patients at 14.4 years in one cohort of 269 patients (53) and in 60% at 12 years in a group of 74 patients (52). Transient left bundle branch block occurred in 15% and ventricular arrhythmias requiring cardioversion in 3% (53). Death is rare in non-neonatal patients.

Neonates as a group have significantly different results and complications (55). Eleven of 27 neonates with critical aortic stenosis at Boston Children's Hospital (unpublished data) were considered unsuccessful, resulting in death ($N = 9$) or the need for a stage I palliation for hypoplastic left heart syndrome ($N = 2$). New valvar regurgitation occurred in 11 of 27. In eight survivors, there was mild aortic regurgitation. In three nonsurvivors, AR was deemed severe. Analysis of this group is difficult, as no selection was made for aortic annulus size, ventricular volume, or ventricular function, many of whom in retrospect should have been referred for a stage 1 hypoplastic left heart operation as a first choice. Patient selection based on echo criteria and improved catheter technology are improving outcomes in this difficult group. We currently recommend balloon dilation of congenitally stenotic aortic valves in patients with transvalvar gradients >55 mmHg and no more than mild aortic regurgitation and in neonates with critical aortic stenosis who have adequate left heart size.

COARCTATION OF THE AORTA

The location of the obstruction in a patient with coarctation of the aorta (just distal to the takeoff of the left subclavian artery) creates not only an increase in left ventricular afterload, but also differential hypertension, with high pressures proximal to the obstruction and low to normal pressures distal (Fig. 27.3A). As a result, the natural history of untreated coarctation includes risks of developing premature coronary artery disease and cerebral aneurysm formation/rupture. Unlike patients with systemic hypertension, however, patients with coarctation of the aorta cannot be treated pharmacologically since reducing descending aortic pressure can cause increased claudication with exercise, abdominal cramping with splanchnic hypoperfusion, and renal dysfunction (prerenal azotemia). Intervention on the coarctation is thus required to achieve normotension in this population.

Percutaneous balloon angioplasty of coarctation was first described in 1982 (56) as an alternative to surgery and has been used since in numerous patients with both native (unoperated) coarctation as well as with recurrent (postoperative) coarctation (57–66). A study of experimental coarctation in lambs (67) demonstrated that relief of obstruction occurs by tearing the intima and media, similar to other angioplasty procedures. Short- and long-term complications seen in that study, including perforation/rupture resulting in death, dissection, and late aneurysm formation have now also been described in patients. Surgical aortic arch reconstructions have become routine at major pediatric heart centers as part of the stage I palliation of hypoplastic left heart syndrome. As a result, many such centers continue to send coarctation patients for surgical interventions as a primary therapy, reserving balloon angioplasty for recurrent postoperative obstruction. There is general consensus that surgical intervention is preferable in the neonatal patients (68).

Pediatric Technique

Under routine sedation, femoral venous and arterial access is obtained percutaneously. The patient is heparinized to an activated clotting time (ACT) >200 seconds. Coarctation is almost always best approached from a retrograde femoral arterial approach, though transvenous, trans-septal, and antegrade approaches have been reported (when residual aortic arch obstruction must be addressed following stage I surgical palliation of single ventricles, a venous approach is commonly used). Right and left heart hemodynamics are measured (including cardiac output), and pullbacks are performed with an end-hole catheter from the left ventricle back through the aortic valve and through the area of the coarctation. *Multiple levels of obstruction are possible—a bicuspid aortic valve is associated with coarctation of the aorta in >70% of patients.* Biplane aortography is best performed with right and left anterior oblique (RAO and LAO) projections. The diameters of the narrowest area of coarctation and of the normal proximal and distal aorta are measured.

For postoperative recurrent coarctation, the balloon is chosen to be 2.5 to 3 times the narrowest area but not greater than 1.5 times the normal proximal or distal aorta. For native obstructions, the balloon is commonly chosen to be equal to the diameter of the aorta at the isthmus. The balloon dilation catheter is centered across the coarctation, inflated until the waist disappears, and deflated. The balloon catheter is exchanged for a smaller pigtail catheter to allow simultaneous measurement of the ascending aortic pressure with the pigtail in comparison with the distal pressure from the side arm of the existing sheath. The dilated area should not be recrossed without a guidewire because of the danger of perforating a weakened portion of the arterial wall. A repeat aortogram should be performed following dilation to determine the angiographic effect of the inflation and to detect tears, ruptures, or dissections. If significant obstruction remains despite disappearance of the balloon waist during inflation, a larger balloon can be used. Although chest pain may be quite significant during balloon inflation, persistent pain after balloon deflation suggests aortic rupture or dissection.

Results

Of the first 64 angioplasties at Boston Children's Hospital (unpublished data) in 62 patients ranging in age from 3 days to 67 years, 5 had native and 59 recurrent coarctation. In that series, procedures were considered successful if the gradient was reduced >50% and the diameter was increased >30%. Based on those criteria, 83% of procedures were successful. The balloon-to-lesion ratio was 3.0 for the successful group and 1.6 for the failures. The most consistent predictor of failure, in this and in others' experience, is the patient with "mild" coarctation: lower pressure gradients and larger minimal coarctation diameters prior to intervention. Balloons substantially larger than the native aorta are necessary in this group, risking injury to the normal aorta (69). This group is probably best addressed with a stent angioplasty technique (see below). Transverse aortic arch hypoplasia is another consistent predictor of suboptimal outcome (70).

The most common complication in children is loss of the arterial pulse secondary to large catheter/artery size ratio. Iliac artery rupture and a retroperitoneal hemorrhage resulting in death have been reported in infants. The incidence of femoral artery injury has decreased with the availability of lower-profile balloons. During follow-up in the Boston series, three patients were found to have small asymptomatic aneurysms at the angioplasty site (two recurrent and one native coarctation). Aneurysm formation following dilation of both native and recurrent coarctation has been reported by several groups. There appears to be little difference in the incidence of aortic injury between the two groups in published data (70) with an incidence of <10% in either group.

Coarctation of the Aorta in the Adult

The technique as outlined above is also applicable to adult patients, and several series have reported excellent out-comes in adult patients with <10% rupture, dissection, aneurysm formation, or restenosis rate (71–73). *In the adult population, some of the severe complications result from trying to normalize the diameter of a very small aortic segment.* Some interventionalists have suggested that the area be enlarged by no more than five times the initial vessel diameter, and that further dilation will be possible once healing occurs at the site of dilation. In this way, as in many congenital diseases, staging the repair may reduce morbidity.

Stent Angioplasty

Primary stent implantation is now the procedure of choice in many labs for either native or recurrent coarctation in the adolescent and adult patient (Fig. 27.3B). It was first reported in patients in 1995 (74,75). Stent implantation eliminates elastic recoil of the aortic tissue and allows the use of substantially smaller balloons. This may result ultimately in a smaller number of aortic injuries, though acute dissections and aortic rupture have been reported with stenting (76). Again, some of these complications may be reduced by staging the stent dilation.

Stent implantation has several other decided advantages in terms of lower residual gradients and reduced restenosis.

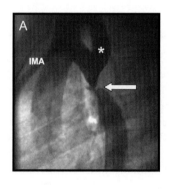

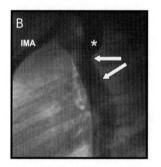

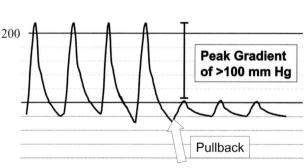

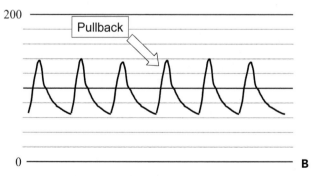

Figure 27.3 **A.** *Top.* Pre–stent implant. *Arrow* denotes coarctation site distal to left subclavian artery (*). The dilated internal mammary artery (IMA) acts as a collateral between ascending and descending aorta. *Bottom.* Pullback tracing from ascending to descending aorta. Large systolic gradient present, descending aorta with damped tracing. **B.** Post–stent implant. *Top.* S/p stent angioplasty of coarctation site. IMA and left subclavian (*) remain marked. The stent margins are demonstrated by the *arrows. Bottom.* Pullback tracings from ascending to descending aorta. Post–stent implantation, there remains no pressure gradient through the aorta. Systolic pressures in the ascending aorta have fallen, and the damped tracing of the descending aorta has normalized.

Stent angioplasty is markedly more effective in the patient with mild native or recurrent coarctation. Stent malposition is rare and usually results from balloon puncture by the partially inflated stent. In all cases, the stent can be safely re-expanded lower in the aorta, avoiding coverage of side branches. One other issue with stent placement is the tendency of the balloon/stent to be pushed distally by the systolic force of the forward aortic flow, particularly with milder coarctation. We have begun to use a technique of rapid ventricular pacing to minimize balloon motion during inflation (see aortic stenosis), whereas others have used balloon-in-balloon technology to set the stent in place before expanding it more fully.

Coarctation of the aorta is the fastest growing indication for stent implantation in patients with congenital heart disease. Longer-term follow-up of stent implantation for adult coarctation, as an alternative to balloon angioplasty alone, is required before definitive recommendations can be made. Younger children are generally excluded from stent implantations owing to growth issues.

Congenital Mitral Stenosis

Congenital mitral stenosis usually involves abnormalities of the chordae tendineae, with either shortened chordal attachments or abnormal attachments, such as in the "parachute" mitral valve. Unlike patients with acquired rheumatic mitral valve stenosis (see Chapter 25), congenital mitral stenosis is generally not suited to balloon valvuloplasty. In young children, the morbidity and mortality rate make this a treatment of last resort.

CONGENITAL LESIONS ASSOCIATED WITH SHUNTS

Clinically important left-to-right as well as right-to-left shunts can result from congenital defects of the cardiac septa or anomalous vascular connections outside the heart. The degree of shunting and the patient's tolerance of that shunt depend on the defect size, the resistance of each of the alternate paths of flow, and to a large degree on ventricular compliance (see Chapter 9). Since left ventricular compliance diminishes as part of the normal aging process, many shunt lesions that have been well tolerated through childhood can become hemodynamically burdensome for patients later in life, similar to chronic aortic or mitral regurgitation.

INTRACARDIAC SHUNT LESIONS

Atrial Level Communications: Anatomy of the Atrial Septum

The fetal circulation requires a right-to-left shunt at the atrial level (via the foramen ovale). The formation of the atrial septum involves a complex embryologic process whereby two independent crescent-shaped tissue membranes (septum primum and septum secundum) form the elements of the septum and grow to overlap one another centrally. The compliant septum primum is situated to the right of the more rigid septum secundum and acts as a one-way flap valve that allows ongoing right-to-left flow during fetal life. After birth, left atrial pressure rises, the flap valve of the foramen ovale closes, and the septum primum and secundum then fuse to one another (in 80 to 85% of the population) to complete septation of the atrial chambers. The remaining 15 to 20%, however, have a persistent flap valve—a patent foramen ovale (PFO)—with the potential for ongoing or intermittent right-to-left flow.

Other failures in the normal development of the septum primum and septum secundum can result in true holes in the septal wall, known as *atrial septal defects (ASDs)*. These defects are named for their location in the septum and include septum primum ASDs at the crux of the heart, adjacent to the semilunar valves; secundum ASDs located centrally in the fossa ovale; and sinus venosus ASDs, most commonly at the superior margin of the septum between superior vena cava and right pulmonary venous return. *Shunting defects of the atrial septum are by far the most common congenital heart disease discovered de novo in adults.*

Pathophysiology of Patent Foramen Ovale

Since LA mean pressure exceeds RA mean pressure due to the differences in left and right ventricular compliance (diastolic filling properties), the flap valve of the PFO remains closed under normal physiologic conditions. With a Valsalva maneuver, however, the right atrial pressure rises, the PFO opens, and right-to-left flow across the atrial septum may ensue. The volume of blood shunted across the PFO is too small under most conditions to have any physiologic or hemodynamic effect, and patients are asymptomatic unless a paradoxical embolization of thrombotic material occurs to cause stroke, transient ischemic attacks, or obstruction of other systemic arteries. We have seen strokes in patients as young as 9 years, and a patient with documented myocardial infarction at 18 years, due to paradoxical embolization via a PFO. Alternatively, poor RV compliance, owing to either RV myocardial hypertrophy or RV infarction, may raise right atrial pressure so that it exceeds LA pressure throughout the cardiac cycle, and a continuous flow from right to left across the PFO may develop. If flow is large enough, patients may become hypoxemic, either continuously or only when in an upright position—orthodeoxia-platypnea (77,78). Migraine headaches, particularly those associated with preceding visual aura, have now been linked to PFO, perhaps by allowing vasoactive agents such as serotonin that are normally cleared during passage through the lungs to reach the cerebral circulation (79,80). Early observational studies indicate that closure of the PFO can reduce the severity of, or eliminate, migraines in some patients. Recurrent decompression illness in scuba divers has also been linked to PFO, presumably related to paradoxical embolization of venous air bubbles (81).

Pathophysiology of Atrial Septal Defect

When an atrial septal defect (ASD) is present, there is left-to-right flow across the defect throughout the cardiac cycle. In diastole, the more compliant RV fills more easily than the stiffer LV, resulting in RV volume loading. This RV volume traverses the lungs, overloads the LA, and is the driving force of left-to-right shunting when the AV valves are closed.

Because of the ability of the RV to maintain its systolic performance in a dilated state, children are virtually never symptomatic with atrial septal defects. Physiologic parameters change with maturation, as the relatively thin compliant LV walls begin to hypertrophy as afterload increases (part of the normal aging process). This often results in increasing left-to-right shunt across the ASD, so that patients become symptomatic only in the third to fifth decades of life. ASDs in adults typically present in one of three ways: new-onset progressive exercise intolerance (inability to sufficiently raise cardiac output with exertion owing to left-to-right shunting at the atrial level and reduction of LV preload), atrial arrhythmia (secondary to RA volume overload and stretch), or paradoxical embolization. Similar to PFO patients, cyanosis can be present with RV noncompliance, with or without pulmonary hypertension. Frequently, ASDs are discovered incidentally on echocardiograms performed for another indication.

Transcatheter Closure of Patent Foramen Ovale

Four double-disk occluder devices currently share the bulk of the world market: CardioSEAL and STARFlex by NMT Medical (Boston, MA), Amplatzer PFO Occluder by AGA Medical (Golden Valley, MN), and the PFO Star by Cardia (Burnsville, MN). In addition to the implantable devices, other technologies are being investigated including transcatheter suturing techniques, radiofrequency ablation techniques, and glue techniques, but are not yet in use in human subjects. The United States' FDA has currently defined patients as eligible for device closure only if they have had recurrent stroke while on adequate levels of anticoagulants. Two nationwide studies are underway (CLOSURE I, RESPECT) to try to define the comparative safety and efficacy of device closure and medical therapy (aspirin or warfarin) following a first stroke or transient ischemic attack (TIA).

The first consideration in PFO closure is the form of echocardiographic guidance to be used. In adults and children >30 kg, we prefer intracardiac echocardiography (82,83; Acuson International, Mountain View, CA), which

requires intravenous sedation and local lidocaine infiltration only. Transesophageal echo (TEE) is the more traditional approach (84) and can be performed with either conscious sedation or general anesthesia, although general anesthesia with a laryngeal/mask airway technique is usually preferred. Some catheterizers perform PFO closure without echo guidance, using fluoroscopic images alone (85)—but this increases the risk of device malposition or embolization in all but the most experienced hands. It also increases the chance that small additional fenestrations of the atrial septum primum may go unnoticed, negating the purpose of the intervention to eliminate the pathway(s) for potential paradoxical embolization.

Imaging with Intracardiac Echocardiography

With minimal sedation and local lidocaine infiltration, the intracardiac echo catheter is passed from a femoral venous access to the RA–inferior vena cava (IVC) junction. With the catheter in a neutral position, the catheter is rotated until the imaging surface is facing to the patient's left. It is then advanced in and out until the aorta valve is imaged in cross section, with the tricuspid valve in the same plane of imaging. From this position, the tip of the catheter is retroflexed by about 30° toward the right atrial free wall. With slight clockwise rotation, the imaging surface is turned posteriorly and brings into image the atrial septum primum and septum secundum overlapping in a horizontal plane, with the thicker septum secundum adjacent to the aorta (Fig. 27.4A). With slight rotation and left-right deflection of the catheter, the image is fine-tuned to show the plane of opening of the PFO. Rarely, because of the anatomic relationships of the cardiac structures, this view may be difficult to obtain. An alternative view is to angle the imaging surface to the RA free wall, well into the RA, and retroflex the catheter back over the tricuspid valve annulus, looking straight up the septum. From this view, the septum primum comes down from the top of the screen and the septum secundum is on the bottom (Fig. 27.4B). Once an acceptable plane of imaging is obtained, the catheter is left in that position for the remainder of the case.

TEE Technique

The patient receives a bolus of propofol, with or without a short-acting muscle relaxant. The TEE probe is passed to the midesophagus. The laryngeal/mask airway is then positioned over the larynx to create a seal around the echo probe. Patients can be bagged as needed, but will breathe spontaneously throughout the case. When the airway is secured, the TEE probe is rotated until the atrial septum is identified. The biggest advantage with TEE is the enormous number of imaging planes that are possible with an omniplane probe. Two views are most helpful: first, the 45° angle (Fig. 27.4C) shows the aortic valve in cross section,

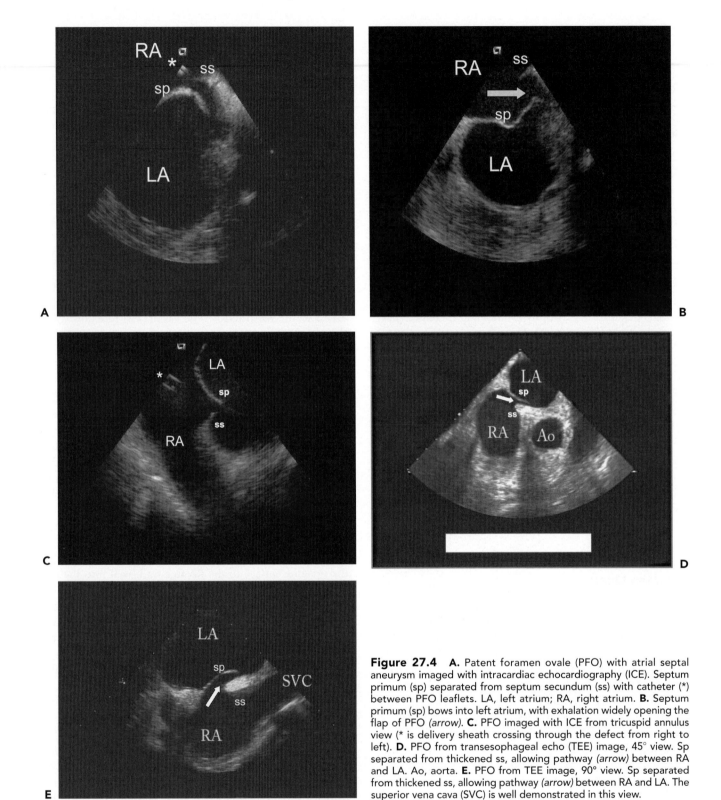

Figure 27.4 **A.** Patent foramen ovale (PFO) with atrial septal aneurysm imaged with intracardiac echocardiography (ICE). Septum primum (sp) separated from septum secundum (ss) with catheter (*) between PFO leaflets. LA, left atrium; RA, right atrium. **B.** Septum primum (sp) bows into left atrium, with exhalation widely opening the flap of PFO *(arrow)*. **C.** PFO imaged with ICE from tricuspid annulus view (* is delivery sheath crossing through the defect from right to left). **D.** PFO from transesophageal echo (TEE) image, 45° view. Sp separated from thickened ss, allowing pathway *(arrow)* between RA and LA. Ao, aorta. **E.** PFO from TEE image, 90° view. Sp separated from thickened ss, allowing pathway *(arrow)* between RA and LA. The superior vena cava (SVC) is well demonstrated in this view.

with the atrial septum displayed with the septum primum originating from the top right of the screen to overlap the septum secundum just posterior and inferior to the aortic valve; second, the 90° view opens the superior vena cava (SVC) and displays the septum in a horizontal plane with septum primum to the left and septum secundum to the right adjacent to the SVC (Fig. 27.4C and D). With a PFO, the optimal plane of imaging is usually somewhere between these two angles, but is different and must be adjusted for each patient.

PFO Closure Technique

Once an echo image is obtained, we assess the defect for separation of septum primum and septum secundum, floppiness/rigidity of septum primum, length of PFO tunnel (septal overlap in plane of maximum separation), thickness of septum secundum, and amount of right-to-left shunting based on an agitated saline injection. These features may affect the delivery method or the size of the device selected for implantation.

The techniques for placing any of the double-disk occluders are similar, regardless of the specific device used. Femoral venous access is obtained. After a right heart pressure assessment, a 6 or 7 French multipurpose catheter with an A-2 curve is passed to the superior vena cava. The catheter is then withdrawn slowly, aiming the tip toward the patient's left shoulder, until it "jumps" into the fossa ovale. The catheter may then be advanced into the LA or may require a slight clockwise (posterior) rotation to follow the PFO tunnel. Echo can be quite helpful in crossing the smallest PFOs. In rare cases, a floppy-tipped guidewire can be used to cross the defect via a multipurpose guiding catheter positioned in the fossa ovale. Once through the defect, the catheter is manipulated to the left upper pulmonary vein, and a stiff exchange-length guidewire is advanced to the PV. The catheter is withdrawn, and balloon sizing of the defect can be performed. Although the manufacturers recommend a device size of twice the stretched diameter of the defect, the PFO can be stretched to almost any size with enough balloon pressure, making this data less useful. However, inflation of the sizing balloon within the PFO tunnel gives important anatomic information about the length and compliance of the PFO tunnel.

A long sheath is advanced over the wire to the LA and carefully debubbled. The closure device is folded into the sheath and advanced to the end of the sheath. The left atrial occluder is opened and pulled back firmly against the septum under echo guidance. When the device is firmly against the septum, the right atrial occluder is opened. If the device position is suboptimal prior to release, transcatheter retrieval is possible with all of the devices, but is less straightforward with the NMT devices than the others. When the position is appropriate, the device is released (Figs. 27.5 and 27.6), and a follow-up injection of agitated saline is performed.

Special Techniques

1. Additional fenestrations: In some patients there will be additional fenestrations of the septum primum. If these defects are clustered in the fossa ovale as is usually the case, a large single-occlusion device can be used. Rarely, the distance between these defects is too great for closure with a single device, and we have placed additional devices during the same procedure. To ensure that the first device does not partially cover the distal defects and make subsequent

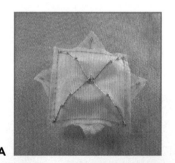

A

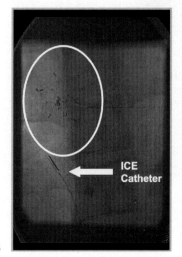

B

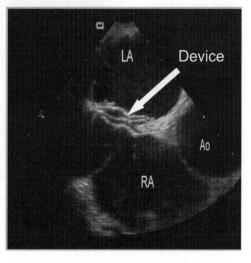

C

Figure 27.5 **A.** CardioSEAL Septal Occluder (NMT Medical, Boston, MA). **B.** Postimplant fluoroscopy showing device *(circle)*. Intracardiac echo image catheter noted by *arrow*. **C.** Postimplant transesophageal echo image, showing device in good position in septum. LA, left atrium; RA, right atrium; Ao, aorta.

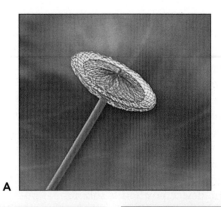

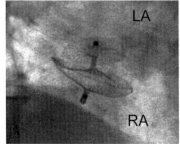

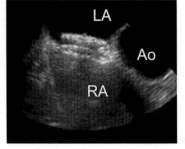

Figure 27.6 A. Amplatzer PFO Occluder (AGA Medical, Golden Valley, MN). **B.** Postimplant fluoroscopy. **C.** Postimplant transesophageal echo image, showing device in good position in septum. LA, left atrium; RA, right atrium; Ao, aorta.

crossing more difficult, we sometimes place an additional femoral venous access and cross both the PFO and the most distal defect with separate catheters and wires. With the wire in place through the distal defect, the PFO is closed using the usual technique. A second sheath is then advanced over the wire through the additional fenestration, and a second device is placed (Fig. 27.7).

2. Long, rigid PFO tunnel: Rarely, if the septum primum is relatively inflexible and the overlap of septum primum and septum secundum is long (>1 cm), it may be difficult to withdraw the closure device far enough into the tunnel to successfully open the right atrial occluder. This may leave a partially opened RA occluder or extra traction on the LA occluder that may back it into the tun-

nel in a partially collapsed position. There are two techniques for dealing with this unusual situation after removal of the first device.

a. Trans-septal puncture technique: Instead of crossing the septum through the PFO, a standard Brockenbrough trans-septal puncture can be performed under echo guidance (86). The septum primum is punctured just at the overlap site of the septum secundum (Fig. 27.8). Once across the septum, the wires are exchanged to

Figure 27.7 Side-by-side CardioSEAL devices for closure of PFO with additional distant fenestrations (20° right anterior oblique view).

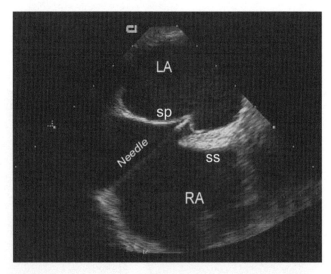

Figure 27.8 Trans-septal puncture under transesophageal echo guidance, target site just below the overlap of septum primum and septum secundum. Septum "tents" as needle pushes it toward the left atrium. LA, left atrium; RA, right atrium; sp, septum primum; ss, septum secundum.

place the superstiff guidewire in the left upper pulmonary vein as above. Echo guidance is critical here, as it is imperative that the puncture be performed as close to the overlap as possible, and that the puncture position be checked from orthogonal angles prior to device placement. We have performed more than 100 such deliveries over the past 3½ years with excellent results.

b. Balloon eversion technique: Once the wire is through the PFO to the pulmonary vein, a balloon wedge catheter can be advanced over the wire to the LA. The balloon is inflated and slowly but forcefully pulled back against the septum, pulling the septum primum from the LA side of the defect to the RA side. This shortens tunnel length, flattens the LA septal surface, and allows for the usual delivery of the device (87).

3. Rarely, femoral venous access to the heart will be unavailable, owing to previous instrumentation, venous thrombosis, or an IVC filter that will not allow passage of the necessary catheters. In these cases, an alternative access will be required. For those experienced with transhepatic access, this is the first choice, because the catheter course from the IVC to the flap valve of the PFO is maintained. For others, a right internal jugular (RIJ) approach or right subclavian approach is possible. However, because of the orientation of the PFO's flap valve, the catheter from the SVC impacts the septum on the wrong angle to cross the defect. We have used a technique with a JR4 or JR5 catheter advanced from the RIJ to the floor of the RA. The curve of the catheter will then direct a guidewire toward the PFO as if it had come up the IVC. If sufficient wire length can be advanced into the left heart, the wire will support the catheter traversing the defect. We will pass a 4 or 5 French hydrophilic catheter over the wire into the LA, and then into the LV. A stiff, looped exchange-length guidewire is then advanced into the LV apex to provide the straightest wire course to traverse the septum with the delivery sheath. The device is then delivered in the usual fashion.

Results/Complications

Between March 2000 and December 2003, 456 PFO closures were done by the author in five institutions. A CardioSEAL Septal Occluder was implanted successfully in all 456 cases, 94 with the trans-septal puncture technique (65% of which occurred in the first 18 months of the study period). There were eight device retrievals acutely in the cath lab, for poor device position, and seven patients who developed sustained atrial arrhythmia (two supraventricular tachycardia, five atrial fibrillation) and were successfully cardioverted. A large hematoma at the catheter insertion site was noted in six patients, and there were two cardiac perforations (one of the left atrial appendage as a complication of a trans-septal puncture and one laceration of the left pulmonary artery as a complication of retrieving an embolized device). There were two clinically detectable air embolisms, two patients with unexplained fever, one

patient with transient complete heart block as a result of catheter manipulation in the RV, and one patient who required a cutdown to remove a device that became lodged in the femoral vein during retrieval.

In the first month following device implantation, 87 of 456 patients developed atrial arrhythmia that brought them to attention. Seventy-one of 87 patients with arrhythmia had only premature atrial contractions, whereas 16 of 81 patients had sustained atrial arrhythmia. Twelve patients developed clinically significant migraine headaches after the procedure, which were largely resolved by 3 months after implantation. Four patients had new transient ischemic attacks, and three had recurrent stroke at an average follow-up of 18 months. Two patients had unexplained shortness of breath, and one had symptomatic bradycardia that required a pacemaker. There was one death at 4 months as a complication of another cardiac procedure unrelated to the PFO device. There was one large thrombus detected on a device and one surgical removal (at 13 months) for persistent shunt and poor device position. At 6 months, by transthoracic echo with agitated saline injection, a residual shunt was detected in only six of 371 patients.

Transcatheter Closure of an ASD

Closure of ASD has been shown to significantly increase exercise capacity (88,89). Right ventricular volume usually returns to normal or near normal levels (90), but the right atrium may remain enlarged even after device closure. This may account for the early observation that closing an atrial septal defect in adults may not eliminate the increased long-term risk of developing atrial fibrillation seen with atrial septal defects (91). Closure eliminates the risk of paradoxical embolization. Severe pulmonary hypertension, with right-to-left shunt at the defect resulting in systemic desaturation, is a contraindication to defect closure (92).

In 1975, the first transcatheter ASD closure was performed by Mills and King in a 17-year-old female patient (93). Lock's original Clamshell Device was the first device to be used in a widespread clinical trial, but was removed from use owing to a >80% incidence of device arm fracture (94). From the late 1980s through the mid 1990s, the button device (95) and the ASDOS device (96) were used extensively in Europe. In the mid 1990s, Das developed Angel Wings, the first self-centering device (97). But transcatheter closure of ASD has become a routine clinical procedure. Both ASDOS and Angel Wings are out of clinical use because of the increased risk of cardiac perforation. Currently, the Amplatzer Septal Occluder (98), the STARFlex Septal Occluder (99), and the Helex device (100) are the most frequently used devices worldwide. New technologies and concepts for nonsurgical ASD closure continue to be developed.

The technical aspects of ASD closure are identical in concept to the PFO closure. Although there are a number

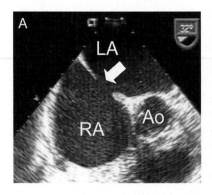

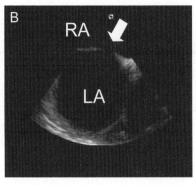

Figure 27.9   Secundum atrial septal defect (ASD) denoted by *arrow*. **A.** Transesophageal echo image. **B.** Intracardiac echo image. RA, right atrium; LA, left atrium; Ao, aorta.

of devices available, the Amplatzer Septal Occluder is the only approved device in the United States and has by far the largest market share in Europe. For echo guidance, we again prefer intracardiac to transesophageal echo (Fig. 27.9), although TEE does provide additional angles on the implanted device to assess position prior to release. We do balloon sizing in all ASD closures. The tissue surrounding a defect is often quite flimsy and may not support the device well enough to preclude embolization; balloon sizing will push the softest tissue out of the way and yield a balloon diameter that corresponds to a margin of tissue substantial enough to hold the device. In addition, the balloon will stretch the defect, making it round regardless of its initial shape. On echo, if all flow across the defect has stopped, one can be confident that the round Amplatzer Septal Occluder, of the same or slightly larger dimension, will also occlude the defect. As with PFO closure, the device is opened in the left atrium and pulled

back toward the septal defect, where the middle waist of the device and the right atrial occluder are delivered, leaving the device straddling the septum (Fig. 27.10).

Results/Complications

In the period March 2000 through December 2003, 251 patients came to our labs for transcatheter closure of an ASD. Prior to the approval of the Amplatzer Septal Occluder, we used only the CardioSEAL Septal Occluder ($N = 58$). Subsequently, we have used primarily the Amplatzer Septal Occluder ($N = 187$). In six patients, we were unable to implant a device (in four, the ASD was too large; in two, the ASD had insufficient tissue rims). Five of the six failed implants occurred prior to use of the Amplatzer device. In our primarily adult congenital practice, patients ranged in age from 2.1 to 83.9 years (median age, 37.7 years). Acutely, there were two device retrievals in

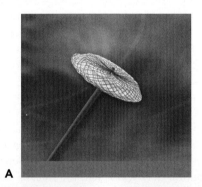

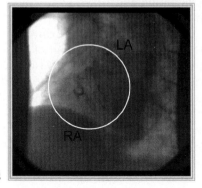

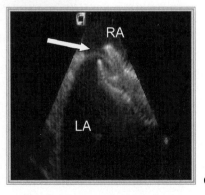

Figure 27.10   **A.** Amplatzer Septal Occluder (AGA Medical, Golden Valley, MN). **B.** Postimplant fluoroscopy (device in circle). **C.** Postimplant intracardiac echo image, showing device entrapping thin septum primum *(arrow)*. LA, left atrium; RA, right atrium.

the cath lab for device embolization (both with the CardioSEAL Septal Occluder, in the first 25 patients). One of these patients developed ventricular fibrillation (and was successfully defibrillated) when the device embolized to the right ventricle. There were no embolizations in the Amplatzer group. Three patients developed sustained atrial arrhythmia (atrial fibrillation in one and SVT in one) and were electrically cardioverted in the cath lab. A large hematoma at the catheter insertion site was noted in three patients. In one child, the Amplatzer Septal Occluder was opened entirely on the left atrial side of the septum. When the device was retracted into the sheath for repositioning, septal tissue became entrapped with the device and a 1.5-cm piece of septal tissue was removed from the body with the device. Despite hemodynamic stability and no pericardial effusion, by echo, the child was sent for urgent surgical intervention to inspect the heart and repair the ASD. There was one air embolization with transient ST segment elevation.

In the first month following device implantation, 17 of 245 patients developed atrial arrhythmia that brought them to attention. Ten of the 12 had only premature atrial contractions, whereas two developed atrial fibrillation. Six patients developed clinically significant migraine headaches after the procedure, which had resolved by 6 months after implantation. One patient had an Amplatzer Septal Occluder erode through the left atrial roof 6 months after an uneventful implantation and survived emergent open heart surgery to relieve cardiac tamponade and to repair/reinforce the area damaged by the device. Another patient had an unexplained small pericardial effusion at 6 weeks after implantation of an Amplatzer Septal Occluder, which was treated successfully with anti-inflammatory medication. There was complete closure by color flow Doppler at 6 months in all but one patient. There were no thromboembolic events and no late deaths in this group.

Several important issues remain with the currently approved devices for atrial septal repair. Based on reporting to the U.S. Food and Drug Administration's Medical Device Complication web site (101), the most commonly reported complication related to the CardioSEAL device (NMT Medical, Boston, MA) is thrombus formation on the device in the first few months (101–103), whereas device erosion (cardiac perforation) is the most commonly reported complication with the Amplatzer devices (AGA Medical, Golden Valley, MN). Thrombus formation has been reported with the Amplatzer device as well (104,105). There is no consensus yet on the appropriate degree of anticoagulation after device implantation. Aspirin alone has been used in many centers with combination of aspirin, Plavix, and warfarin being used by others. We generally treat our patients with aspirin 325 mg daily for 6 months and Plavix 75 mg for 3 months. Amplatzer Septal Occluder erosion with pericardial tamponade has been reported in a number of patients, as late as 3 years after implantation (101). The actual occurrence rate of these complications is unknown, but is quite low in our experience. Antibiotic prophylaxis is indicated for dental work or other minor surgical procedures for 6 to 12 months from the time of device implantation.

Ventricular Septal Defects

Like atrial septal defects, congenital deficiencies in the ventricular septum are varied in anatomy. The most common ventricular septal defects (VSDs) occur in the membranous and the muscular portion of the septum. Left-to-right shunts at the ventricular level result in pulmonary overcirculation, with a concomitant left ventricular volume overload. As a result of LV volume loading, patients may present with the classic symptoms of congestive heart failure in infancy (if the defect is large enough) or with an asymptomatic dilated left ventricle (moderate defect), or they may become symptomatic only later in life when LV compliance changes result in higher LA filling pressures and pulmonary venous congestion. Patients with unrestrictive defects, who do not undergo repair in the first 2–3 years of life, risk the development of irreversible pulmonary vascular disease.

Transcatheter Closure of VSDs

Anatomically, the design of devices to close *membranous* VSDs was quite challenging, as the aortic valve, the tricuspid valve, and the conduction system all abut in this portion of the septum. The device suffers from many of the problems of other primarily pediatric therapies: The potential population for this device is quite limited. There are significant patient selection issues, as well as technical issues related to patient size. Severe congestive heart failure is the norm with large defects in patients as young as 2 to 3 months of age. Catheter manipulation is prohibitively risky in patients of that size. Older patients will have either developed pulmonary vascular disease or will have defects that are very small and probably need not be addressed. A new Amplatzer device is currently in trial to close membranous defects (106). Early, unpublished results demonstrate a moderate risk of conduction system disturbance at the atrioventricular node similar to other series of transcatheter VSD closure, with some cases of complete heart block. Outcome data will need to be compared, in controlled clinical trials, with surgical VSD closures.

Although much less common than membranous VSDs, large *muscular* VSDs, which may occur anywhere in the muscular portion of the septum, present a difficult challenge for the surgeon. Apical and anterior defects may be impossible to visualize and repair through the tricuspid valve. Right ventricular septal trabeculations make identification from the RV septal surface difficult. The traditional surgical approach has been from a left ventriculotomy. However, long-term follow-up of these patients revealed a high rate of LV aneurysms and an equally disturbing number of patients with global LV dysfunction (Boston Children's Hospital, unpublished data).

The need for successful transcatheter therapy has therefore been more acute in patients with muscular rather than with the membranous defects. Reports of successful transcatheter closures have appeared since the early 1990s (107–109). The procedure remains technically challenging in small children, but has been used, in combination with surgical intervention, to stage a repair. Pulmonary artery banding, to limit pulmonary flow and reduce symptoms of congestive heart failure, can be accomplished off bypass. Subsequent growth of the child and transcatheter defect closure can be followed with surgical band removal (also a closed procedure), as an alternative to an open repair of the defect through a left ventriculotomy.

Numerous devices have been used for closing muscular VSDs including the original Clamshell Device, the CardioSEAL Septal Occluder, and the STARFlex devices. Amplatzer has developed a device designed specifically for muscular VSD closure, which is under clinical trial at the time of this publication. Transcatheter closure of inlet (endocardial cushion-type) VSD and supracristal VSDs are not yet possible based on the intimate relationship of these defects to defects of the atrioventricular and semilunar valves, respectively.

Technique of Muscular VSD Closure

There are several approaches possible for delivering the VSD device. After a complete echocardiographic assessment (TEE in the cath lab is helpful in most cases), and a left and right heart hemodynamic assessment, an LV angiogram is performed to best profile the defect (Fig. 27.11). The defect

size and distances to critical surrounding structures are measured best with TEE, to help in device selection. In all techniques, the defect is crossed from the left ventricular septal surface, with a steerable catheter introduced via the retrograde or trans-septal approach.

A soft extension-length guidewire is passed through the defect to the PA, where it is captured with a gooseneck snare device from either the femoral or internal jugular vein (depending on the location of the muscular VSD). With midmuscular and apical VSD positions, the jugular approach can yield the straightest catheter course to the defect. This minimizes the tendency of the delivery sheath to kink. Anterior muscular VSDs are best approached from a femoral access. Capturing the wire in the PA avoids the risk of having the wire become entangled in the tricuspid valve. The wire is then exteriorized at the venous sheath. The largest dimension of the defect may then be confirmed with balloon sizing (the balloon introduced over wire to straddle the defect—see ASD closure above). The device is then chosen to exceed the defect size by 1.6 to 2.0 times when a double-umbrella device is used, or by 3 mm when an Amplatzer VSD Occluder is selected.

Next the appropriate-size delivery system is advanced from the venous access, over the snared wire to the RA, RV, and through the defect to the LV. Echocardiography and hand injections through the sheath will confirm its position. The wire is then removed, and the device is delivered in the usual fashion. The LV occluder is opened and pulled back against the septum. Resistance will be felt as the device is pulled into the defect. Echo and angiographic injections will confirm LV septal position, and the RV septal occluder is then delivered. When angiographic and/or echo images confirm the position of the device on both sides of the septum, the device is released.

Results

Between February 1989 and July 1998, 148 VSDs were closed at Boston Children's Hospital (double-umbrella device) with no deaths or late morbidity (unpublished data). Echocardiographic follow-up showed that 83% of the defects were either closed or had trivial residual leaks. Several patients had additional devices placed in the presence of multiple defects. Owing to the complexity and extent of the catheter manipulation involved in these procedures, transient arrhythmias and hemodynamic compromise are not uncommon during these procedures (110). Other complications have included asymptomatic hemothorax in one patient and a case in which the umbrella compromised the septal leaflet of the tricuspid valve. Preliminary results with the Amplatzer device suggest significantly higher closure rates than with the double-umbrella devices, with lower rates of complications (111).

The Amplatzer device seems better suited to this indication than the double-umbrella devices, having been designed specifically for this purpose with a longer central

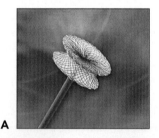
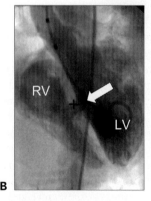
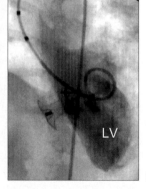

Figure 27.11   **A.** Amplatzer Muscular VSD Occluder. **B.** Left ventricle (LV) angiogram showing left-to-right shunt across a midmuscular VSD *(arrow)*, filling the right ventricle (RV). **C.** Defect closed with Amplatzer Muscular VSD Occluder. (Images courtesy of Z. Hijazi.)

waist than its ASD counterpart to account for the septal thickness. In addition, significantly smaller sheaths are used with the Amplatzer than with the double-umbrella devices. This facilitates advancing the delivery sheath through the defect over the wire. Ongoing investigation will determine the efficacy of each device.

One additional area of interest for interventionalists treating adult patients is postinfarction ventricular septal rupture. These defects are always muscular in location and nearly always occur more distally in the distribution of the LAD, yielding mid and apical muscular VSDs. Similar to infants with membranous VSDs, it is difficult to find large numbers of patients who are appropriate for this intervention. Large defects are nearly always fatal, as a large left-to-right shunt, pulmonary overcirculation, pulmonary hypertension, and left ventricular volume overload are superimposed on a severely compromised pump. Tiny defects are interesting from a diagnostic perspective, but do not impose a significant hemodynamic burden. Thus, only patients with moderate-size defects, who have large shunts, but who have been stabilized medically can be considered for either surgical or transcatheter repair. Interestingly, with ongoing tissue necrosis, the defect can become more hemodynamically important over a period of several weeks. Acute surgical intervention is difficult, because the surgeon has little reliable tissue in the margins of the defect in which to place his/her sutures. Similarly, following transcatheter closure, ongoing necrosis of surrounding tissue can lead to sizable residual shunts and device instability after early implantation. A recent surgical series of 65 such patients had a 30-day mortality of 23%, with marked improvement with concomitant grafting of the coronary arteries at the time of VSD repair (112).

The Amplatzer muscular VSD device was used in 18 patients in a U.S. registry between 2000 and 2003 (113). Thirteen of 18 underwent closure between 14 and 95 days after the infarction. A device was deployed in 16 of 18. The 30-day mortality was 28%, comparable with surgical survival. Eleven patients are alive and have been followed for a mean of 332 days, with two complete closures, two secondary device implants for residual shunts, six trivial or small residual shunts, and two moderate residual shunts. A new Amplatzer device, specifically for post–myocardial infarction VSDs, is in development.

Transcatheter Embolization of Extracardiac Shunts

Left-to-right shunts outside the heart occur when a congenitally abnormal connection between an arterial source and a venous or cardiac site exists. These shunts are associated with pulmonary overcirculation and a reduction in systemic perfusion, owing to the difference in resistance between the normal arteriolar bed and the low-resistance runoff site. The most common example is a persistently patent ductus arteriosus.

Right-to-left shunting can also occur through abnormal connections outside the heart. In patients with a Fontan or bidirectional Glenn, where systemic veins drain directly to the pulmonary arteries, systemic venous pressure is elevated. Venous collaterals may develop from the high-pressure veins to low-pressure systemic veins, to low-pressure cardiac veins, or to the pulmonary veins. The runoff acts as a steal from the pulmonary flow, and causes systemic hypoxemia.

PATENT DUCTUS ARTERIOSUS

The ductus arteriosus is a normal fetal arterial connection between the aorta and the pulmonary artery, which in the presence of high pulmonary resistance (as in the fetus), allows right ventricular outflow to return via the aorta to the placenta.

With the baby's first breath, pulmonary vascular resistance drops as the lungs aerate, and systemic resistance rises as the low resistance of the placenta is removed from the circulation. These physiologic changes induce an acute increase in pulmonary blood flow. Rapidly rising systemic oxygen levels trigger the smooth muscle layer in the ductal tissue, through a prostaglandin-mediated pathway, to contract. Within 48 to 72 hours of life, >95% of infants have a closed ductus arteriosus, completing the conversion of blood flow to the normal postnatal circulation. In some infants, the ductus does not close or remains partially open and is then termed a patent ductus arteriosus (PDA).

As the lungs mature over the first few weeks of life, pulmonary resistance continues to fall both absolutely and relative to systemic resistance. When a PDA is present, the aortic flow has an alternative, low-pressure runoff into the pulmonary circulation. With a large PDA, there is pulmonary overcirculation, systemic undercirculation, and the usual symptoms of congestive heart failure (CHF) within weeks of birth. Surgical correction remains the treatment of choice for most newborns with CHF secondary to a PDA. The development of the Amplatzer Duct Occluder (see below), which can be delivered via the venous circulation through small sheaths with good occlusion results (see below), is making some impact now in the smaller infants (114).

In most children, the PDA is small, a tiny fraction of its initial prenatal diameter. Resistance to flow through this small tube is high, and the resulting volume of the left-to-right shunt is small. The LV is not significantly volume loaded, and symptoms are uncommon. Most of these children are diagnosed when a cardiac murmur is identified, or when the PDA is discovered incidentally at echocardiogram. In this setting, the principle risk is that of endocarditis (endarteritis) at the ductus or at the site of the high-velocity jet's impact on the PA wall. Closure of the PDA has been recommended routinely in children, to eliminate both the volume load and the risk of infection, since the first successful litigation of a PDA by Gross in 1938.

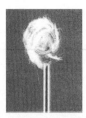
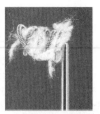
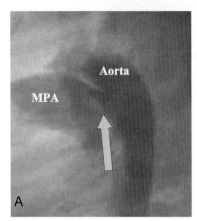
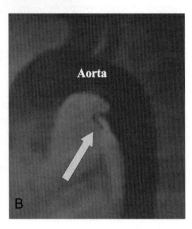

Figure 27.12 **Top.** Gianturco embolization coils. **A.** Aortogram in child with small patent ductus arteriosus (PDA). Pigtail catheter fills aorta and main pulmonary artery (MPA) via the PDA *(arrow)*. **B.** Following coil embolization; the coil is seen protruding into the MPA. The MPA is no longer visualized, as all flow through the PDA is occluded.

PDA is a relatively uncommon finding in adult patients. Most frequently, the defect is discovered incidentally during an echocardiogram, following an episode of endarteritis or when a murmur is present. In the older adult, other symptoms may occur. With decreasing LV compliance, the additional LV volume load from left to right shunting is less well tolerated, resulting in increased filling pressures and pulmonary venous congestion. Shortness of breath with exertion may develop in a patient who has tolerated the PDA for decades. Similarly, increased systemic vascular resistance, associated with adult onset hypertension, may drive more blood across the defect into the pulmonary circulation, increasing the shunt and bringing on symptoms of exercise intolerance for the first time.

We have treated several adult patients with PDA who develop frank angina on exertion in the setting of very mild coronary artery disease. ECG changes on stress tests, or hypoperfusion on a stress thallium examination, may be positive in the absence of significant coronary lesions by angiography, because the low-resistance runoff from the aorta produces a diastolic steal phenomenon.

Transcatheter Closure of PDA

Over the past two decades, successes with transcatheter closure techniques have all but eliminated surgical repair of small PDAs (115). The first device to gain widespread popularity was developed by Dr. William Rashkind (116). Although never achieving FDA approval in the United States, this double-umbrella device was used throughout the world and in clinical trials in the United States until the early 1990s.

In 1992, with the Rashkind device unavailable for closure of PDA, Dr. John Moore's group first described the technique of closing a PDA with a Gianturco coil (117; Fig. 27.12), a device that had been in use for other vascular occlusion procedures since 1972. Although the Rashkind devices were available only to physicians at selected study sites, the coil occlusion procedure brought PDA closure into the mainstream of pediatric interventional catheterization.

The principle of the coil closure is similar to that of the Rashkind umbrella device and the ASD devices. Coil loops, larger than the minimum diameter of the PDA, are delivered to straddle the PDA, with loops on both the aortic and pulmonary artery end of the PDA. The springlike characteristics of the coil loops hold the device in position while the Dacron fibers imbedded in the device attract platelets and promote thrombus formation, eliminating flow through the PDA. Within weeks to months the device is endothelialized.

In contrast with the Rashkind device, the coil can be delivered through catheters as small as 4 French, making it a viable alternative to surgery even in small children. Various techniques were developed to deliver the coils, including the original single-catheter, transarterial approach of Moore (118), a single-catheter transvenous approach (118), the snare-assisted technique (119,120), detachable coils (121), and the Latson catheter technique (122). The single most important factor in procedural efficacy seemed to be not the delivery technique selected, but the experience of the operator and the anatomy of the defect. Larger PDAs, particularly those with little length, were problematic for closure with a coil technique. Because complete closure was always the goal, other techniques emerged to deal with these larger defects, including the use of multiple coils, the use of 0.052-inch-thickness coils (123), and the placement of coils within a nylon sack inside the PDA (Grifka-Gianturco Sack; 124). More recently, the Amplatzer Duct Occluder has been approved for use in the United States. Because of the ease of using this system, and its history of safety and efficacy, the Amplatzer Duct Occluder has replaced coil embolization techniques in many labs for all but the smallest PDA.

All of the above techniques are applicable to the adult patient diagnosed with a PDA. We have used the coil occlusion technique in adults up to 76 years of age, but now prefer the Amplatzer device for all adult patients.

Technique of PDA Closure: Coil Occlusion

Arterial and venous sheaths are placed, under routine sedation. Following complete right and left heart pressure measurements and a shunt calculation, an aortic angiogram is performed with the holes of the pigtail just distal to the takeoff of the left subclavian artery. The minimum dimension of the PDA is measured. A catheter with a JR4 or Berenstein curve is advanced from the femoral artery to the level of the PDA. A floppy-tipped torque wire is passed through the PDA to the MPA. We continue to use the snare-assisted delivery technique for coil delivery in defects with a minimum dimension of <2 mm—a preformed gooseneck snare catheter is advanced from the femoral vein to the main pulmonary artery and used to "grab" the catheter coming through the PDA. In cases where a very small PDA is difficult to cross, the snare can be placed in the MPA to act as a target for the probing wire. In cases where the catheter will not easily follow the wire through the PDA, the snare can be used to stabilize the wire position in the MPA or RV. Once the catheter is snared on the MPA side, the wire is removed, and the coil is advanced through the catheter to the tip. We use 0.038-inch-thickness coils most often, and push approximately one-fourth of a coil loop out the end of the catheter. The snare is loosened and slowly withdrawn off the end of the catheter, falling onto the protruding coil loop, where it is retightened. The rest of the coil is then delivered into the aortic ampulla. Some traction is placed on the device to pull at least three-fourths of a coil loop into the MPA to stabilize its position. The snare is then opened and advanced into one of the branch PAs, unhooking it from the coil. A repeat aortic angiogram is performed. Additional coils may be placed for residual shunts.

Technique of PDA Closure: Amplatzer Duct Occluder

An aortic angiogram is performed with the holes of the pigtail just distal to the takeoff of the left subclavian artery. Both the minimum dimension of the PDA and the length of the ductus are measured. The Amplatzer Duct Occluder is selected based on these measurements, with the pulmonary end of the device selected to be approximately 2 mm larger than the minimum angiographic dimension. An end-hole catheter is manipulated to the MPA (we usually start with a multipurpose curve) and used as a guide to probe for the opening of the PDA with a floppy-tipped torque wire. In some circumstances, when the PDA could not be located from the PA side of the defect, we will cross the PDA from the aortic side with an exchange-length guidewire, snare the wire, and exteriorize it through the femoral vein. The long delivery sheath of the Amplatzer Duct Occluder can then be delivered over the wire from the venous approach. The sheath tip is positioned well down the descending aorta and carefully debubbled. The device is then loaded into the sheath. The large aortic retention disk is opened in the descending aorta and withdrawn into the ampulla of the PDA. The pulmonary artery end of the device is then delivered. A repeat aortic angiogram can be performed prior to release to ensure proper position (Fig. 27.13). In many cases, there may be substantial residual shunt for the first few minutes after initial implantation. This will resolve over a period of 10 to 15 minutes.

Results/Complications

Since 1994, we have performed over 500 PDA closures, of which only 15 recent cases involved use of the Amplatzer device (since FDA approval in 2003). At 6 months, there was no residual shunt seen by color flow Doppler in >97% of all patients. Risk factors for residual shunts were short ductal length (type B of Krichenko; 125); use of single coil in PDA dimension >2.5 mm; older age, particularly with calcified PDA (related both to poor angiographic imaging of residual shunts as well as to diminished PDA conformability to the coil); and procedure done early in our experience (prior to the use of the Amplatzer device or multiple coil implantation). Patients with residual shunts were recatheterized and one or more additional coils were placed. This has resulted in complete occlusion of all residual shunts.

Complications are rare, but are most often related to vascular injury in the small infant, to sedation-related respiratory compromise, and to hypothermia in small babies. One coil embolization occurred to the pulmonary artery, requiring surgical retrieval, and led to the development of the snare-assisted technique. There have been no subsequent coil embolizations. There have been no embolizations of the Amplatzer device. There were three patients who developed sustained SVT requiring therapy (adenosine in two, electrical cardioversion in one) from catheter manipulation. Three patients had retroperitoneal bleeding, one of whom required transfusion. In one patient during retrieval of a missized coil, the coil became lodged in the femoral vein, requiring surgical cutdown. One patient had an angiogram performed with the holes of the pigtail in the PDA itself, and had a minimal dissection without sequelae. As has been described by others (126), two of our patients with a small residual shunts developed hemolysis the

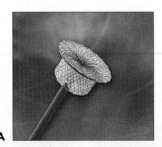

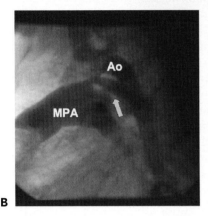

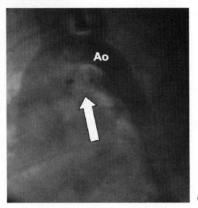

Figure 27.13 A. Amplatz Duct Occluder. **B.** Patent ductus arteriosus (PDA) as demonstrated on an aortic angiogram. A pigtail catheter in the aorta (Ao) fills the Ao, the PDA *(arrow)*, and main pulmonary artery (MPA). **C.** After implantation, the PDA is closed. The device is seen in the PDA, and the MPA no longer fills with contrast.

night of the procedure and presented with gross hematuria. One patient was recatheterized, and a second coil eliminated the residual shunt. No further hemolysis was seen. In the other patient, hemolysis resolved spontaneously with no further therapy.

Transcatheter closure of PDA is the treatment of choice for all asymptomatic children with small PDA. We use coil embolization techniques for PDA with a minimum dimension of <2 mm and the newer Amplatzer Duct Occluder for larger PDA and for adult patients.

OTHER EXTRACARDIAC SHUNTS

Various fistulous connections can have significant hemodynamic effects.

Systemic AV Fistulas

Fistulous connections between a systemic artery and a systemic vein may create a sizable left-to-right shunt, with symptoms of exercise intolerance or frank congestive heart failure. The vein provides a lower-resistance runoff for the blood in the involved arterial branch. Unlike other left-to-right shunt lesions, systemic AV fistulas create a volume load for both ventricles. These fistulas may be congenital, but may be acquired through trauma or complications from surgery or catheterization.

Coronary Fistulas

Coronary fistulas are hemodynamically similar to other systemic fistulas. Drainage is most commonly to the coro-

nary sinus or directly to the RA, RV, or PA. In addition to the usual symptoms of exercise intolerance and shortness of breath, these patients may present with a coronary steal, in which the low-resistance runoff to the fistula will reverse diastolic flow in the normal coronary artery branches. With diminished forward flow, ischemia may occur with exertion (see Chapter 11).

Aortopulmonary (Bronchial) Collaterals

Aortopulmonary collaterals may be congenital or may develop in children who undergo single ventricle repairs involving venous supply of pulmonary blood flow (Glenn shunt, Fontan operation). These vessels most often arise from the thoracic aorta, the internal mammary arteries, and other branches of the subclavia. The left-to-right shunt creates a volume load on the left ventricle, similar to a patent ductus arteriosus.

In patients who have undergone previous congenital surgical palliations, another lesion that may present as a collateral connection between the aorta and pulmonary artery is an old Blalock-Taussig or other surgical shunt that either recanalized or was never taken down at later surgical stages. When this connection is no longer needed, it also creates a left ventricular volume load.

Pulmonary Fistulas

These unusual defects connect pulmonary arterioles, proximal to the air containing spaces, to pulmonary venules, resulting in the return of unoxygenated blood to the left atrium (Fig. 27.14). If a defect is large enough, or if there

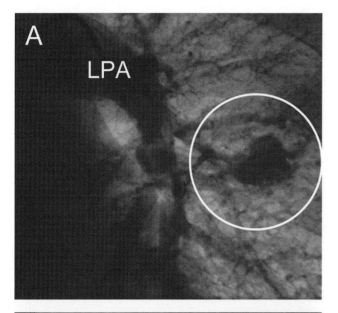

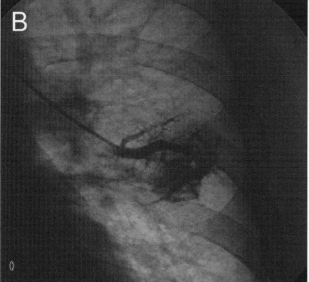

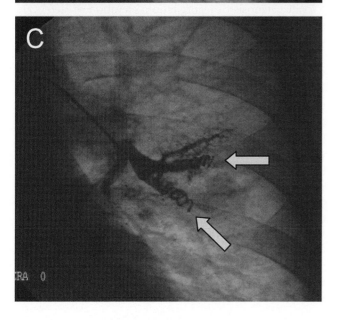

are multiple defects present (Osler-Weber-Rendu syndrome), patients may be quite cyanotic. These defects have been a source of paradoxical thromboembolization in some patients who were erroneously diagnosed with PFO.

Venovenous Collaterals

In patients with single ventricle repairs where the systemic veins bypass the right heart and connect directly to the pulmonary arteries, a pressure difference exist between those veins that lead to the lungs and those that return to the heart. This differential will result in rerouting blood flow away from the lungs to return via the lower-resistance pathway back to the atrium. In the patient dependent on venous flow to the lungs, these venous connections result in diminished pulmonary flow and cyanosis.

Technique of Device Embolization

All types of extracardiac vascular anomalies can be treated with catheter-based embolization techniques. These techniques are largely the same, regardless of the vessel designated for closure or the device chosen for the task. We generally prefer the use of Gianturco coils owing to the low cost, the long safety history, the ease of implantation, and the variety of delivery catheters that can be used. Special considerations must be taken for large vessels, which are discussed below.

The vessel to be embolized is identified angiographically. Regional as well as selective injection in the vessel is essential, as some defects have multiple feeding sources (i.e., pulmonary fistula, Fig. 27.14), all of which must be occluded for a successful intervention; and some target vessels supply normal structures as well as the fistulous connection (i.e., coronary fistula), making the positioning of the occlusion device more critical. We prefer to use a multipurpose catheter with distal side holes for the selective injections. Once the vessel has been acceptably imaged, a site for placement of the embolic device should be selected. Optimal locations include native narrowings, turns in vessel course, or bifurcation points. In some cases, the anatomy will preclude the use of one of these optimal sites and a straight tubular portion of the defect will offer the best site. The target vessel is measured at the desired embolization site. For coil embolization, a device diameter 1 to 2 mm larger than the site diameter is selected. The delivery catheter is an end-hole catheter of a shape that approximates the wire course for stability of the catheter

Figure 27.14 **A.** Large isolated pulmonary atrioventricular malformation (AVM) in left lower lobe *(circle)* in a patient with Osler-Weber-Rendu syndrome. LPA, left pulmonary artery. **B.** Selective injection in one of two arterial feeding vessels filling the AVM. **C.** Following coil embolization of the two feeding vessels *(arrows)*, there is no further filling of the AVM, with a concurrent increase in systemic saturation from 89% to 94% on room air.

position. The delivery catheter is exchanged over a wire and advanced past the desired site of implantation. The coil is then introduced to the catheter and pushed to the tip of the catheter (with a guidewire of a diameter approximating the inner lumen dimension), just distal to the site of implantation. The first loop of coil is delivered just distal to the optimal site by advancing the guidewire as the delivery catheter is withdrawn slightly. The remainder of the coil can be delivered in one of two ways: by fixing the delivery catheter and advancing the guidewire into the catheter to push out the coil; or the guidewire can be fixed in place, and the catheter withdrawn over the wire, exposing the coil. A repeat angiogram is performed, and additional coils may be placed behind the initial coil to complete the occlusion. Antibiotic prophylaxis is recommended for a period of 3 to 6 months to allow for complete endothelialization. MRI scanning will put significant stress on the implanted coil. We recommend that the device be allowed to endothelialize completely before exposing the patient to the magnetic field.

The use of coils has limitations, particularly for larger vessels. Other technologies such as the Grifka-Gianturco Sack (124) and detachable balloons (127) have been used in these settings. A newly approved device by Amplatzer, the Vascular Plug, is an excellent alternative for large vessels. The device is cylindrical and is delivered through small-caliber catheters as are the rest of the Amplatzer devices. It remains attached to its delivery cable until the operator wishes to release it, making it completely retrievable. It will conform its shape to the size/shape of the target vessel.

Results/Complications

Embolization techniques are straightforward and are limited only by the operator's ability to achieve a stable catheter position in the vessel to be occluded. Once such a position is achieved, the procedure should be successful in 100% of cases. Complications related to coil embolization include device embolization and potential obstruction of nearby side branches. Coil embolization occurs most frequently in arterial structures with high flow states when the coil selected is not large enough, or when the coil selected is too large, does not coil appropriately in the target vessel, and pushes the delivery catheter back out of the target vessel. Embolized coils can usually be retrieved with a snare technique. Hemolysis has been seen with incomplete closure of high flow defects.

CARDIAC CATHETERIZATION IN ADULT PATIENTS WITH FONTAN PHYSIOLOGY

Perhaps the greatest accomplishment in congenital heart disease in the last generation has been the combined surgical/interventional management of patients with functional single ventricles. In these patients, the systemic venous return is rerouted directly to the pulmonary arteries, no longer returning to the heart, leaving only the pulmonary venous return filling the single ventricle and being pumped to the aorta. Since Fontan described this approach to bypassing the right side of the heart over 40 years ago (128), the concept has been applied to all congenital lesions in which the heart cannot be fully septated.

Currently, the Fontan is performed between 2 and 4 years of age as the final step in a staged surgical approach. Acute management of these patients remains a largely pediatric issue. However, for the first time, a significant number of patients are reaching adulthood with Fontan physiology, presenting difficulties for adult cath labs that are not used to dealing with this physiology on a regular basis.

Fontan Physiology

In two-ventricle circulation, pulmonary venous return is pumped by the left ventricle to the systemic circulation with sufficient energy to traverse the systemic vascular bed (overcoming systemic vascular resistance). The blood then returns through the systemic veins to the right ventricle, which adds enough additional energy to the blood to traverse the pulmonary vascular bed (overcoming pulmonary resistance). In a Fontan circulation, the one functional ventricle must generate enough energy to traverse both systemic and pulmonary vascular beds in series.

Since there is no additional energy added after crossing through the systemic vascular bed, flow to the lungs is a passive flow system, where the blood from the SVC and IVC flows "downhill" through the pulmonary artery, pulmonary veins, left atrium, and then into the single ventricle. It is clear, therefore, that any derangements of pulmonary vasculature, including elevated pulmonary vascular resistance, competitive flow (aortopulmonary collaterals), AV valve stenosis or regurgitation, elevation of (left) ventricular end diastolic pressure, or even rhythm disturbances with loss of AV synchrony will impede forward flow in this circulation and create higher systemic venous pressures. When systemic venous pressures exceed 15 to 20 mm Hg, venous stasis/pooling will occur. The result is diminished pulmonary flow, diminished left atrial return, and inadequate left ventricular preload, resulting in low cardiac output. Patients with a failing Fontan physiology typically present with classic right heart failure: fluid retention, peripheral edema, ascites, and low output.

In some children, a small Fontan "fenestration" may be created at the time of surgery. This communication between the systemic venous Fontan pathway and the pulmonary venous atrium allows a limited right-to-left shunt at the atrial level. This technique has been shown to improve outcomes of the surgery by better maintaining cardiac output in the perioperative period, at the expense of mild cyanosis (129,130). Secondary Fontan fenestration creation may be helpful later in the patient with a failing Fontan circulation, and has been performed both in the operating room (131) and in the cath lab as an interventional procedure (132).

Other issues are common in a failing Fontan patient: *Protein-losing enteropathy* is a syndrome seen in some Fontan patients (133), in which serum proteins are lost through the stool. The exact mechanism for these losses is unknown, but in some cases may be related to bowel edema as a result of high venous pressures. These protein losses include albumin, which results in lower serum oncotic pressure, worsening the patient's fluid retention. Antithrombotic factors, such as antithrombin III, may also be lost, promoting hypercoagulable states.

Atrial arrhythmias, owing to stretching of the atria or to extensive atrial surgery, may be the chief presentation of a failing Fontan or may be one of the underlying causes of the physiologic derangement. *Ventricular dysfunction* is a common endpoint for Fontan patients. The mechanism of ventricular failure is unknown, but is probably related to the amount of time prior to the Fontan, when the LV myocardium was both stretched owing to volume overload and oxygen starved as the coronaries carried cyanotic blood. Interestingly, Fontan patients cannot develop pulmonary venous congestion like other patients with poor left ventricular function. Mean left atrial/pulmonary artery pressures cannot get high enough to cause pulmonary edema before systemic venous stasis occurs. These patients will present with "right heart failure" long before they develop typical symptoms of left heart failure. Because Fontan patients have begun to reach adult age in significant quantity, careful invasive assessment of the Fontan physiology will be required in the adult cath lab.

Hemodynamic Evaluation

Right and left heart hemodynamics should be obtained with particular focus on mechanical obstructions in the Fontan pathway. Ventricular end-diastolic pressure and PA wedge pressures should be compared to rule out pulmonary vein or AV valve obstruction. Pullbacks through both branch PAs should be done, looking for pressure gradients. Surgical anastomoses should be a site of particular attention. Cardiac output should be assessed using the Fick calculation. Saturations should be obtained in the central and distal PAs to rule out competitive aortopulmonary collateral flow.

Angiographically, all of the limbs of the Fontan pathway should be imaged, particularly because of the difficulties in imaging these branches using echocardiography. Venous collaterals draining to the heart or via a pulmonary vein directly to the atrium and via the coronary sinus should be ruled out, particularly in a patient who has issues of systemic desaturation. An aortogram should be performed at the distal arch to rule out aortopulmonary collaterals providing competitive flow and to exclude aortic arch obstructions

that may be affecting ventricular afterload. Atrial pacing can be performed to assess its effect on cardiac output and on atrial filling pressures for patients in nonsinus rhythm.

The interventions that may be required to improve Fontan physiology include a virtual manual of the procedures outlined in this chapter. Branch pulmonary artery stenosis should be ballooned or stented to relieve any pathway obstruction. Venous pathways, and surgical anastomoses may also require enlargement/angioplasty. Collaterals should be aggressively embolized. Fontan fenestrations may need to be occluded in a patient who is excessively cyanotic. The devices for atrial septal closure can be used for this purpose. In some patients, when there is little other relief available, the cath lab creation of a secondary Fontan fenestration has been shown to improve the symptoms of protein-losing enteropathy in some and to improve cardiac output in all (131–133). Pulmonary AV malformations may be present in patients who previously underwent a Glenn shunt and may need to be embolized.

SUMMARY

The above discussion covers only a few of the large array of interventional procedures performed in a catheterization laboratory that manages congenital heart disease. As important as familiarity with the procedures themselves is the need for a thorough understanding of the underlying anatomy and physiology. Like other expanding areas of interventional cardiology, existing specialists in congenital heart disease should play an important educational and collaborative role in training future specialists in adult congenital and structural heart disease.

REFERENCES

1. Gersony WM, et al. Second natural history study of congenital heart defects. Quality of life of patients with aortic stenosis, pulmonary stenosis, or ventricular septal defect. *Circulation* 1993; 87(suppl):I52–65.
2. Hayes CJ, et al. Second natural history study of congenital heart defects. Results of treatment of patients with pulmonary valvar stenosis. *Circulation* 1993;87(suppl):I28–37.
3. Wolfe RR, et al. Arrhythmias in patients with valvar aortic stenosis, valvar pulmonary stenosis, and ventricular septal defect. Results of 24-hour ECG monitoring. *Circulation* 1993;87 (suppl): I89–101.
4. Moyssakis IE, et al. Incidence and evolution of carcinoid syndrome in the heart. *J Heart Valve Dis* 1997;6:625–630.
5. Semb BKH, et al. Balloon valvulotomy of congenital pulmonary valve stenosis with tricuspid valve insufficiency. *Cardiovasc Radiol* 1979;2:239.
6. Kan JS, et al. Percutaneous balloon valvuloplasty: a new method for treating congenital pulmonary valve stenosis. *N Engl J Med* 1982;307:540.
7. Radkte W, et al. Percutaneous balloon valvotomy of congenital pulmonary stenosis using oversized balloons. *J Am Coll Cardiol* 1986;8:909.
8. Ali Khan MA, et al. Percutaneous transluminal balloon pulmonary valvuloplasty for the relief of pulmonary valve stenosis with special reference to double-balloon technique. *Am Heart J* 1986;112:158.

9. Stanger P, et al. Balloon pulmonary valvuloplasty: results of the valvuloplasty and angioplasty of congenital anomalies registry. *Am J Cardiol* 1990;65:775.

10. Perry SB, Keane JF, Lock JE. Interventional catheterization in pediatric congenital and acquired heart disease. *Am J Cardiol* 1988;61:109G.

11. Helgason H, et al. Balloon dilation of the aortic valve: studies in normal lambs and in children with aortic stenosis. *J Am Coll Cardiol* 1987;9:816.

12. Weber HS, Cyran SE. Effectiveness of an umbilical artery "snare assisted" approach for critical pulmonary valve stenosis or atresia in the neonate. *Am J Cardiol* 1997;80:1502–1505.

13. Humpl T, et al. Percutaneous balloon valvotomy in pulmonary atresia with intact ventricular septum: impact on patient care. *Circulation* 2003;108:826–832. Epub 2003 Jul 28.

14. Alwi M, et al. Pulmonary atresia with intact ventricular septum: percutaneous radiofrequency-assisted valvotomy and balloon dilation versus surgical valvotomy and Blalock Taussig shunt. *J Am Coll Cardiol* 2000;35:468–476.

15. Yeager S. Balloon selection for double balloon valvotomy. *J Am Coll Cardiol* 1987;9:467.

16. Chen CR, et al. Percutaneous balloon valvuloplasty for pulmonic stenosis in adolescents and adults. *N Engl J Med* 1996;335:21–25.

17. Thapar MK, Rao PS. Significance of infundibular obstruction following balloon valvuloplasty for valvar pulmonic stenosis. *Am Heart J* 1989;118:99–103.

18. O'Connor BK, et al. Intermediate-term outcome after pulmonary balloon valvuloplasty: comparison with a matched surgical control group. *J Am Coll Cardiol* 1992;20:169–173.

19. Bonhoeffer P, et al. Transcatheter implantation of a bovine valve in pulmonary position: a lamb study. *Circulation* 2000;102: 813–816.

20. Bonhoeffer P, et al Percutaneous insertion of the pulmonary valve. *J Am Coll Cardiol* 2002;39:1664–1669.

21. Boudjemline Y, et al. Percutaneous pulmonary valve replacement in a large right ventricular outflow tract: an experimental study. *J Am Coll Cardiol* 2004;43:1082–1087.

22. Kreutzer J, et al. Isolated peripheral pulmonary artery stenoses in the adult. *Circulation* 1996;93:1417–1423.

23. Kim JH, et al. Quantitative lung perfusion scintigraphy in postoperative evaluation of congenital right ventricular outflow obstructive lesions. *Clin Nucl Med* 1996;21:471–476.

24. Rao PS, Galal O, Smith PA, et al. Five to nine year follow up results of balloon angioplasty of native aortic coarctation in infants and children. *J Am Coll Cardiol* 1996;27:462.

25. Shaddy RE, Boucek MM, Sturtevant JE, et al. Comparison of angioplasty and surgery for unoperated coarctation of the aorta. *Circulation* 1993;87:793.

26. Edwards BS, et al. Morphologic changes in the pulmonary arteries after percutaneous balloon angioplasty for pulmonary arterial stenosis. *Circulation* 1985;71:195.

27. Rothman A, Perry SB, Keane JF, Lock JE. Early results and follow-up of balloon angioplasty for branch pulmonary artery stenosis. *J Am Coll Cardiol* 1990;15:1109.

28. Kan JS, Marvin WJ, Bass JL, Muster AJ, Murphy J. Balloon angioplasty—Branch pulmonary artery stenosis: results from the Valvuloplasty and Angioplasty of Congenital Anomalies Registry. *Am J Cardiol* 1990;65:798.

29. Gentles TL, Lock JE, Perry SB. High pressure balloon angioplasty for branch pulmonary artery stenosis: early experience. *J Am Coll Cardiol* 1993;22:867.

30. Rhodes JF, et al. Cutting balloon angioplasty for children with small-vessel pulmonary artery stenoses. *Cathet Cardiovasc Intervent* 2002;55:73–77.

31. Sugiyama H, et al. Bladed balloon angioplasty for peripheral pulmonary artery stenosis. *Cathet Cardiovasc Intervent* 2004;62: 71–77.

32. Bergersen LJ, Perry SB, Lock JE. Effect of cutting balloon angioplasty on resistant pulmonary artery stenosis. *Am J Cardiol* 2003;91:185–189.

33. O'Laughlin MP, Perry SB, Lock JE, Mullins CE. Use of endovascular stents in congenital heart disease. *Circulation* 1991;83: 1923.

34. O'Laughlin MP, et al. Implantation and intermediate-term follow-up of stents in congenital heart disease. *Circulation* 1993;88: 605.

35. Fogelman R, et al. Endovascular stents in the pulmonary circulation. Clinical impact on management and medium term follow-up. *Circulation* 1995;92:88.

36. Bacha EA, Kreutzer J. Comprehensive management of branch pulmonary artery stenosis. *J Intervent Cardiol* 2001;14:367–375.

37. Shaffer KM, Mullins et al. Intravascular stents in congenital heart odisease: short and long term results from a large single-center. *J Am Coll Cardiol* 1998;311:661.

37a. Ovaert C, et al. Endovascular stent implantation for the management of post-operative right ventricular outflow tract obstruction: clinical efficacy. *J Thorac Cardiovasc Surg* 1999;118: 886–893.

38. Jacob JL, et al. Treatment of membranous subaortic stenosis with balloon dilatation. *Arq Bras Cardiol* 1998;70:25–28.

39. Moskowitz WB, Schieken RM. Balloon dilation of discrete subaortic stenosis associated with other cardiac defects in children. *J Invasive Cardiol* 1999;11:116–120.

40. Dimitrow PP, et al. Comparison of dual-chamber pacing with nonsurgical septal reduction effect in patients with hypertrophic obstructive cardiomyopathy. *Int J Cardiol* 2004;94:31–34.

41. Lababidi Z. Aortic balloon valvuloplasty. *Am Heart J* 1983;106:751.

42. Sholler GF, et al. Balloon dilation of aortic stenosis: results and influence of technical and morphological features on outcome. *Circulation* 1988;78:351.

43. Rocchini AP, et al. Balloon aortic valvuloplasty: results of the valvuloplasty and angioplasty of congenital anomalies registry. *Am J Cardiol* 1990;65:784.

44. Cribier A, Savin T, Berland J, et al. Percutaneous transluminal balloon valvuloplasty of adult aortic stenosis: report of 92 cases. *J Am Coll Cardiol* 1987;9:381.

45. Rosenfeld HM, et al. Balloon aortic valvuloplasty in the young adult with congenital aortic stenosis. *Am J Cardiol* 1994;73:1112.

46. Moore P, et al. Midterm results of balloon dilation of congenital aortic stenosis: predictors of success. *J Am Coll Cardiol* 1996; 27:1257.

47. Rhodes LA, et al. Predictors of survival in neonates with critical aortic stenosis. *Circulation* 1991;84:2325.

48. Helgason H, et al. Balloon dilation of the aortic valve: studies in normal lambs and in children with aortic stenosis. *J Am Coll Cardiol* 1987;9:816.

49. Waller BF, Girod DA, Dillon JC. Transverse aortic wall tears in infants after balloon angioplasty for aortic valve stenosis: relation of aortic wall damage to diameter of inflated angioplasty balloon and aortic lumen in 7 necropsy cases. *J Am Coll Cardiol* 1984;4:1235.

50. Eltchaninoff H, Tron C, Cribier A. Percutaneous implantation of aortic valve prosthesis in patients with calcific aortic stenosis: technical aspects. *J Intervent Cardiol* 2003;16:515–521.

51. Weber HS, Mart CR, Myers JL. Transcarotid balloon valvuloplasty for critical aortic valve stenosis at the bedside via continuous transesophageal echocardiographic guidance. *Cathet Cardiovasc Intervent* 2000;50:326–329.

52. Jindal RC, et al. Long-term results of balloon aortic valvulotomy for congenital aortic stenosis in children and adolescents. *J Heart Valve Dis* 2000;9:623–628.

53. Reich O, et al. Long term results of percutaneous balloon valvoplasty of congenital aortic stenosis: independent predictors of outcome. *Heart* 2004;90:70–76.

54. Balmer C, et al. Balloon aortic valvoplasty in paediatric patients: progressive aortic regurgitation is common. *Heart* 2004;90:77–81.

55. Egito ES, et al. Transvascular balloon dilation for neonatal critical aortic stenosis: early and midterm results. *J Am Coll Cardiol* 1997;29:442.

56. Singer MI, Rowen M, Dorsey TJ. Transluminal aortic balloon angioplasty for coarctation of the aorta in the newborn. *Am Heart J* 1982;103:131.

57. Saul JP, Keane JF, Fellows KE, Lock JE. Balloon dilation angioplasty of postoperative aortic obstructions. *Am J Cardiol* 1987; 59:943.

58. Morrow WR, et al. Balloon dilation of unoperated coarctation of the aorta: short- and intermediate-term results. *J Am Coll Cardiol* 1988;11:133.

59. Beekman RH, Rocchini AP, Dick M. Percutaneous balloon angioplasty for native coarctation of the aorta. *J Am Coll Cardiol* 1987; 10:1078.

60. Tynan M, et al. Balloon angioplasty for the treatment of native coarctation: results of the valvuloplasty and angioplasty of congenital anomalies registry. *Am J Cardiol* 1990;65:790.

61. Hellenbrand WE, et al. Balloon angioplasty for aortic recoarctation: results of the valvuloplasty and angioplasty of congenital anomalies registry. *Am J Cardiol* 1990;65:793.

62. Rao PS, et al. Five to nine year follow up results of balloon angioplasty of native aortic coarctation in infants and children. *J Am Coll Cardiol* 1996;27:462.

63. Shaddy RE, et al. Comparison of angioplasty and surgery for unoperated coarctation of the aorta. *Circulation* 1993;87:793.

64. McCrindle BW, et al. Acute results of balloon angioplasty of native coarctation versus recurrent aortic obstruction are equivalent. *J Am Coll Cardiol* 1996;28:1810.

65. De Giovanni JV, et al. Percutaneous balloon dilatation of aortic coarctation in adults. *Am J Cardiol* 1996;77:435.

66. Fletcher SE, Nihill MR, Grifka RG, O'laughlin MP, Mullins CE. Balloon angioplasty of native coarctation of the aorta: midterm follow-up and prognostic factors. *J Am Coll Cardiol* 1995;25:730.

67. Lock JE, Niemi T, Burke B, Einzig S, Castaneda-Zuniga W. Transcutaneous angioplasty of experimental aortic coarctation. *Circulation* 1982;66:1280.

68. Fletcher SE, Nihill MR, Grifka RG, O'Laughlin MP, Mullins CE. Balloon angioplasty of native coarctation of the aorta: midterm follow-up and prognostic factors. *J Am Coll Cardiol* 1995;25:730–734.

69. Perry SB, Zeevi B, Keane JF, Lock JE. Interventional catheterization of left heart lesions, including aortic and mitral valve stenosis and coarctation of the aorta. *Cardiol Clin* 1989;7:341.

70. Hornung TS, Benson LN, McLaughlin PR. Interventions for aortic coarctation. *Cardiol Rev* 2002;10:139–148.

71. Fawzy ME, et al. Long-term outcome (up to 15 years) of balloon angioplasty of discrete native coarctation of the aorta in adolescents and adults. *J Am Coll Cardiol* 2004;43:1062–1067.

72. Paddon AJ, Nicholson AA, Ettles DF, Travis SJ, Dyet JF. Long-term follow-up of percutaneous balloon angioplasty in adult aortic coarctation. *Cardiovasc Intervent Radiol* 2000;23:364–367.

73. Zabal C, Attie F, Rosas M, Buendia-Hernandez A, Garcia-Montes JA. The adult patient with native coarctation of the aorta: balloon angioplasty or primary stenting? *Heart* 2003;89:77–83.

74. Suarez de Lezo J, et al. Balloon-expandable stent repair of severe coarctation of aorta. *Am Heart J* 1995;129:1002–1008.

75. Bulbul ZR, et al. Implantation of balloon-expandable stents for coarctation of the aorta: implantation data and short-term results. *Cathet Cardiovasc Diagn* 1996;39:36–42.

76. Korkola SJ, Tchervenkov CI, Shum-Tim D, Roy N. Aortic rupture after stenting of a native coarctation in an adult. *Ann Thorac Surg* 2002;74:936.

77. Landzberg MJ, et al. Orthodeoxia-platypnea due to intracardiac shunting—relief with transcatheter double umbrella closure. *Cathet Cardiovasc Diagn* 1995;36:247–250.

78. Rao PS, Palacios IF, Bach RG, Bitar SR, Sideris EB. Platypnea-orthodeoxia: management by transcatheter buttoned device implantation. *Cathet Cardiovasc Intervent* 2001;54:77–82.

79. Post MC, Thijs V, Herroelen L, Budts WI. Closure of a patent foramen ovale is associated with a decrease in prevalence of migraine. *Neurology* 2004 27;62:1439–1440.

80. Schwerzmann M, et al. Percutaneous closure of patent foramen ovale reduces the frequency of migraine attacks. *Neurology* 2004; 62:1399–1401.

81. Torti SR, et al. Risk of decompression illness among 230 divers in relation to the presence and size of patent foramen ovale. *Eur Heart J* 2004;25:1014–1020.

82. Earing MG, et al. Intracardiac echocardiographic guidance during transcatheter device closure of atrial septal defect and patent foramen ovale. *Mayo Clin Proc* 2004;79:24–34.

83. Koenig P, et al. Role of intracardiac echocardiographic guidance in transcatheter closure of atrial septal defects and patent foramen ovale using the Amplatzer device. *J Intervent Cardiol* 2003;16:51–62.

84. Hellenbrand W, et al Transesophageal echocardiographic guidance of transcatheter closure of atrial septal defect. *Am J Cardiol* 1990;66:207.

85. Meier B. Pacman sign during device closure of the patent foramen ovale. *Cathet Cardiovasc Intervent* 2003;60:221–223.

86. Ruiz CE, Alboliras ET, Pophal SG. The puncture technique: a new method for transcatheter closure of patent foramen ovale. *Cathet Cardiovasc Intervent* 2001;53:369–372.

87. Chintala K, et al Use of balloon pull-through technique to assist in CardioSEAL device closure of patent foramen ovale. *Cathet Cardiovasc Intervent* 2003;60:101–106.

88. Brochu MC, et al. Improvement in exercise capacity in asymptomatic and mildly symptomatic adults after atrial septal defect percutaneous closure. *Circulation* 2002;106:1821–1826.

89. Giardini A, et al. Determinants of cardiopulmonary functional improvement after transcatheter atrial septal defect closure in asymptomatic adults. *J Am Coll Cardiol* 2004;43:1886–1891.

90. Kort HW, Balzer DT, Johnson MC. Resolution of right heart enlargement after closure of secundum atrial septal defect with transcatheter technique. *J Am Coll Cardiol* 2001;38:1528–1532.

91. Konstantinides S, et al. A comparison of surgical and medical therapy for atrial septal defect in adults. *N Engl J Med* 1995;333:469–473.

92. Steele PM, Fuster V, Cohen M, Ritter DG, McGoon DC. Isolated atrial septal defect with pulmonary vascular obstructive disease—long-term follow-up and prediction of outcome after surgical correction. *Circulation* 1987; 76:1037–1042.

93. King TD, Thompson SL, Steiner C, Mills NL. Secundum atrial septal defect. Nonoperative closure during cardiac catheterization. *JAMA* 1976;235:2506–2509.

94. Prieto LR, Foreman CK, Cheatham JP, Latson LA. Intermediate-term outcome of transcatheter secundum atrial septal defect closure using the Bard Clamshell Septal Umbrella. *Am J Cardiol* 1996;78:1310–1312.

95. Sideris E, et al. Transvenous atrial septal occlusion in piglets using a "buttoned" double disc device. *Circulation* 1990;81:312.

96. Hansdorf G, et al. Transcatheter closure of secundum atrial septal defects with the atrial septal occlusion system (ASDOS): initial experience in children. *Heart* 1996;75:83.

97. Das G, et al. Experimental atrial septal defect closure with a new, transcatheter, self-centering device. *Circulation* 1993;88(pt 1):1754–1764.

98. Masura J, et al. US/International Multicenter trial of atrial septal catheter closure using the Amplatzer Septal Occluder: initial results. *J Am Coll Cardiol* 1998;31(suppl A):57A.

99. Carminati M, et al Transcatheter closure of atrial septal defects with the STARFlex device: early results and follow-up. *J Intervent Cardiol* 2001;14:319–324.

100. Latson LA, Zahn EM, Wilson N. Helex septal occluder for closure of atrial septal defects. *Curr Intervent Cardiol Rep* 2000;2:268–273.

101. FDA Website: http://www.accessdata.fda.gov/scripts/cdrh/cfdocs/cfMAUDE/search.CFM

102. Anzai H, et al. Incidence of thrombus formation on the Cardio SEAL and the Amplatzer interatrial closure devices. *Am J Cardiol* 2004;93:426–431.

103. Krumsdorf U, et al. Incidence and clinical course of thrombus formation on atrial septal defect and patient foramen ovale closure devices in 1,000 consecutive patients. *J Am Coll Cardiol* 2004;43:302–309.

104. Willcoxson FE, Thomson JD, Gibbs JL. Successful treatment of left atrial disk thrombus on an Amplatzer atrial septal defect occluder with abciximab and heparin. *Heart* 2004;90:e30.

105. Acar P, Aggoun Y, Abdel-Massih T. Images in cardiology: thrombus after transcatheter closure of ASD with an Amplatzer septal occluder assessed by three dimensional echocardiographic reconstruction. *Heart* 2002;88:52.

106. Bass JL, et al. Initial human experience with the Amplatzer perimembranous ventricular septal occluder device. *Cathet Cardiovasc Intervent* 2003;58:238–245.

107. Bridges ND, et al. Preoperative transcatheter closure of congenital muscular ventricular septal defects. *N Engl J Med* 1991;324:1312–1317.

108. Perry SB, et al. Transcatheter closure of atrial and ventricular septal defects. *Herz* 1993;18:135–142.

109. Arora R, et al. Transcatheter closure of congenital muscular ventricular septal defect. *J Intervent Cardiol* 2004;17:109–115.

110. Laussen P, et al. Transcatheter closure of ventricular septal defects: hemodynamic instability and anesthetic management. *Anesth Analg* 1995;80:1076.

111. Arora R, et al. Transcatheter closure of congenital ventricular septal defects: experience with various devices. *J Intervent Cardiol* 2003;16:83–91.

112. Barker TA, et al. Repair of post-infarct ventricular septal defect with or without coronary artery bypass grafting in the northwest of England: a 5-year multi-institutional experience. *Eur J Cardiothorac Surg* 2003;24:940–946.

113. Holtzer R, et al. Amplatzer Muscular Ventricular Septal Defect Investigators. Device closure of muscular ventricular septal defects using the Amplatzer muscular ventricular septal defect occluder: immediate and mid-term results of a U.S. registry. *J Am Coll Cardiol* 2004;43:1257–1263.

114. Ebeid MR, Masura J, Hijazi ZM. Early experience with the Amplatzer ductal occluder for closure of the persistently patent ductus arteriosus. *J Intervent Cardiol* 2001;14:33–36.

115. Portsmann W, et al Catheter closure of patent ductus arteriosus: 62 cases treated without thoracotomy. *Radiol Clin North Am* 1971;9:203.

116. Rashkind WJ, Miller WW. Creation of an atrial septal defect without thoracotomy: palliative approach to complete transposition of the great arteries. *JAMA* 1966;196:991.

117. Hijazi ZM, Geggel RL. Transcatheter closure of large patent ductus arteriosus (> or = 4 mm) with multiple Gianturco coils: immediate and mid-term results. *Heart* 1996;76:536–540.

118. Cambier PA, Kirby WC, Wortham DC, Moore JW. Percutaneous closure of small (<2.5 mm) patent ductus arteriosus using coil embolization. *Am J Cardiol* 1992;69:815.

119. Sommer RJ, Gutierrez A, Lai WW, Parness IA. Use of preformed nitinol snare to improve transcatheter coil delivery in occlusion of patent ductus arteriosus. *Am J Cardiol* 1994;74:836–839.

120. Ing FF, Sommer RJ. The snare-assisted technique for transcatheter coil occlusion of moderate to large patent ductus arteriosus: immediate and intermediate results. *J Am Coll Cardiol* 1999; 33:1710–1718.

121. Tometzki AJ, et al. Transcatheter occlusion of the patent ductus arteriosus with Cook detachable coils. *Heart* 1996;76:531–535.

122. Kuhn MA, Latson LA. Transcatheter embolization coil closure of patent ductus arteriosus—modified delivery for enhanced control during coil positioning. *Cathet Cardiovasc Diagn* 1995;36: 288–290.

123. Owada CY, Teitel DF, Moore P. Evaluation of Gianturco coils for closure of large (> or = 3.5 mm) patent ductus arteriosus. *J Am Coll Cardiol* 1997;30:1856–1862.

124. Grifka RG, Vincent JA, Nihill MR, Ing FF, Mullins CE. Transcatheter patent ductus arteriosus closure in an infant using the Gianturco-Grifka Vascular Occlusion Device. *Am J Cardiol* 1996;78:721–723.

125. Krichenko A, et al. Angiographic classification of the isolated, persistently patent ductus arteriosus and implications for percutaneous occlusion. *Am J Cardiol* 1989;63:877–880.

126. Anil SR, et al. Clinical course and management strategies for hemolysis after transcatheter closure of patent arterial ducts. *Cathet Cardiovasc Intervent* 2003;59:538–543. Review.

127. Barth KH, et al. Embolotherapy of pulmonary arteriovenous malformations with detachable balloons. *Radiology* 1982;142: 599.

128. Fontan F, Baudet E. Surgical repair of tricuspid atresia. *Thorax* 1971;26:240–248.

129. Bridges ND, et al. Effect of baffle fenestration on outcome of the modified Fontan operation. *Circulation* 1992;86:1762–1769.

130. Laks H, et al. Partial Fontan: advantages of an adjustable interatrial communication. *Ann Thorac Surg* 1991;52:1084–1094; discussion 1094–1095.

131. Rychik J, Rome JJ, Jacobs ML. Late surgical fenestration for complications after the Fontan operation. *Circulation* 1997;96: 33–36.

132. Kreutzer J, Lock JE, Jonas RA, Keane JF. Transcatheter fenestration dilation and/or creation in post-operative Fontan patients. *Am J Cardiol* 1997;79:228–232.

133. Mertens L, et al. Protein-losing enteropathy after the Fontan operation: an international multicenter study. PLE study group. *J Thorac Cardiovasc Surg* 1998;115:1063–1073.

Profiles of Specific Disorders

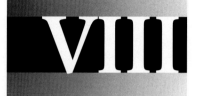

Profiles in Valvular Heart Disease

28

Ted Feldman   William Grossman

The cardiac valves function to maintain unidirectional flow, thus ensuring that the energy released during myocardial contraction is transformed efficiently into the circulation of blood around the body. When the valves become diseased (either by restriction [stenosis] or insufficiency [regurgitation]), efficient unidirectional flow is compromised and various compensatory mechanisms are brought into play to help the circulation meet the metabolic needs of the body. These mechanisms—chiefly dilatation and hypertrophy—have their own clinical costs, which are responsible for the major manifestations of valvular heart disease.

Valvular heart disease may be considered to impose two different types of stress on the cardiac chamber proximal to the lesion. These are either pressure overload (increased afterload) or volume overload (increased preload). The former is generally the result of valvular stenosis and the latter of valvular insufficiency. Both pressure overload and volume overload serve as stimuli for compensatory mechanisms, chiefly hypertrophy (which allows the generation of greater systolic force and at the same time tends to normalize wall stress by increasing wall thickness) and dilatation (which enables increased strength and extent of shortening by the Frank-Starling mechanism). These mechanisms preserve the circulation at the cost of increased myocardial oxygen needs and elevated ventricular filling pressures, leading to clinical evidence of ischemia and congestive heart failure.

This chapter will illustrate the hemodynamic and angiographic findings seen in patients with valvular heart disease. It is useful to apply the general physiologic principles discussed above in the interpretation of catheterization data obtained in patients with disordered valve function, and this approach generally will enable the physician to unravel even the most complicated of problems.

MITRAL STENOSIS

The orifice area of the normal mitral valve is about 4.5 cm^2. As a result of chronic rheumatic heart disease, the orifice becomes progressively smaller, and this leads to at least two distinct and important circulatory changes (1). The first is the development of a pressure gradient across the mitral valve, the left ventricular mean diastolic pressure remaining at its normal level of about 5 mm Hg and the left atrial mean pressure rising progressively, reaching about 25 mm Hg when the orifice of the mitral valve is reduced to approximately 1.0 cm^2 (Fig. 28.1). A second major circulatory change is reduction of blood flow across the mitral valve, i.e., reduction of the cardiac output. The normal resting cardiac output of 3.0 L/minute per m^2 usually falls to about 2.5 L/minute per m^2 when the valve size is 1.0 cm^2. A rise in left atrial pressure necessitates a similar rise in pressure in pulmonary veins and capillaries, and pulmonary edema occurs when the pulmonary capillary pressure exceeds the oncotic pressure of normal plasma, which is about 25 mm Hg.

Reactive pulmonary hypertension practically never occurs in mitral stenosis until the mitral valve area approaches 1.0 cm^2, i.e., when the resting left atrial pressure approaches 25 mm Hg. After this point, reactive changes in the pulmonary arteriolar bed develop frequently, resulting in progressive obstruction to blood flow through the lungs.

As pulmonary vascular obstruction becomes increasingly severe, the pulmonary arterial pressure rises and occasionally may exceed the systemic arterial pressure. In the extreme, the pulmonary vascular resistance can rise to 25 or 30 times normal. Despite substantial hypertrophy, the right ventricle cannot cope with the enormous pressure load imposed on it, and it dilates and fails.

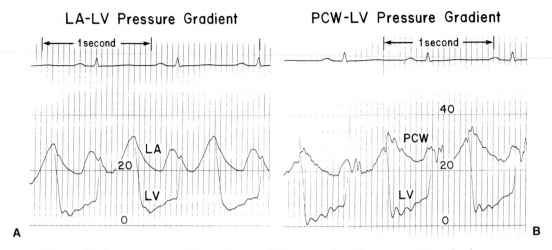

Figure 28.1 Simultaneous left atrial (LA) and left ventricular (LV) pressures **(A)** and pulmonary capillary wedge (PCW) and LV pressures **(B)** in a patient with tight mitral stenosis and a mean PCW pressure of approximately 25 mm Hg. LV end-diastolic pressure is normal at 10 mm Hg. Note the presence of *a* waves in the LA and PCW trace, which are not transmitted to the LV because of the damping effect of the stenotic mitral valve. (Reproduced from Lange RA, et al. Use of pulmonary capillary wedge pressure to assess severity of mitral stenosis: is true left atrial pressure needed in this condition? *J Am Coll Cardiol* 1989;13:825, with permission.)

The Second Stenosis

Thus, in mitral stenosis, two stenoses eventuate—first at the mitral valve and second in the arterioles of the lung. The hemodynamic findings in patients with tight mitral stenoses with and without major pulmonary vascular disease are illustrated in Fig. 28.2. As can be seen, the second stenosis (Fig. 28.2, bottom) has resulted in a 70-mm Hg mean pressure gradient across the lungs, giving a pul-monary vascular resistance of 1,866 dyn · sec · cm^{-5}. Workup of the patient with mitral stenosis should include an assessment of both these obstructions.

Catheterization Protocol

The usual indication for cardiac catheterization in patients with mitral stenosis is that the patient is being considered

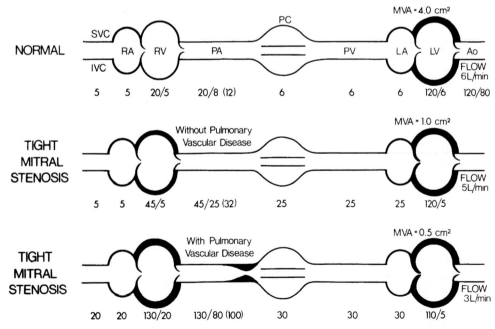

Figure 28.2 Diagrammatic representation of the circulation in patients with normal hemodynamics *(top)*, tight mitral stenosis *(center)*, and tight mitral stenosis with pulmonary vascular disease and the development of a second stenosis at the pulmonary arteriolar level *(bottom)*. See text for discussion.

for either balloon mitral valvuloplasty or corrective surgery. Catheterization should be a combined right and left heart procedure in which the following measurements and calculations are made:

1. Simultaneous left ventricular diastolic pressure, left atrial (or pulmonary capillary wedge) diastolic pressure, heart rate, diastolic filling period, and cardiac output. From these, the size of the mitral valve orifice may be calculated (see Chapter 10 for details of the orifice area calculation).

2. If the transmitral pressure gradient is <5 mm Hg, the error in calculation of the mitral valve orifice area is appreciable. The circulatory measurements should be repeated under circumstances of stress (exercise, reversible increase in preload resulting from passive elevation of the patient's legs, tachycardia induced by pacing) to increase the pressure gradient across the mitral valve.

3. Simultaneously, or in close order, pulmonary arterial mean pressure, left atrial (or pulmonary capillary wedge) mean pressure, and cardiac output for the calculation of pulmonary vascular resistance.

4. Right ventricular systolic and diastolic pressures for assessment of right ventricular function.

5. If other lesions are suspected (e.g., mitral regurgitation, aortic valve disease, left atrial myxoma), they too must be evaluated. In this regard, it should be pointed out that certain lesions tend to occur in combination with mitral stenosis. Many (if not most) patients with severe mitral stenosis have some degree of aortic regurgitation. Also, although it is rare, tricuspid stenosis always should be looked for in the patient with severe mitral stenosis, because it is seen only in association with this condition. Another condition that may be associated with mitral stenosis is atrial septal defect with left-to-right shunt. The combination of mitral stenosis and atrial septal defect is known as Lutembacher syndrome. Thus, as with standard right heart catheterization, described in Chapters 4 through 6, the operator should obtain screening blood samples from the superior vena cava and pulmonary artery for oximetry determination. This has taken on added importance in the present era when balloon mitral valvuloplasty (see Chapter 25) has become a standard treatment for mitral stenosis. Balloon mitral valvuloplasty generally requires trans-septal catheterization and involves limited dilatation of the interatrial septum; thus the procedure may create an atrial septal defect, thereby producing iatrogenic Lutembacher syndrome (2).

The following case studies illustrate the different clinical and hemodynamic syndromes seen in patients with mitral stenosis. The first is a typical example of a symptomatic patient with tight mitral stenosis, normal pulmonary vascular resistance, and a normal-sized heart (stage II, Fig. 28.3). The second is an example of a relatively asymptomatic patient with more severe mitral stenosis, a fivefold to tenfold increase of pulmonary vascular resistance, and an enlarged heart caused principally by enlargement of the right ventricle (stage III, Fig. 28.3). The third represents terminal mitral stenosis with an extreme degree of pul-

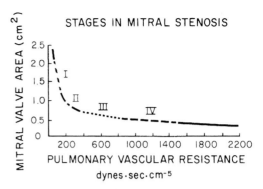

Figure 28.3 Stages in the natural history of mitral stenosis. As the mitral orifice progressively narrows, pulmonary vascular resistance increases. This increase is slow at first, but when the mitral valve area becomes "critical" (<1 cm^2), the increase is rapid, reflecting the development of a second stenosis at the level of the precapillary pulmonary arterioles. Clinical correlations are discussed in the text.

monary vascular resistance, pulmonary hypertension, and right ventricular failure (stage IV, Fig. 28.3).

Case 1: Tight Mitral Stenosis with Normal Pulmonary Vascular Resistance. A.R., a 35-year-old woman, had chorea as a child and was asymptomatic thereafter until age 33, when she noted the onset of exertional dyspnea. This progressed to the point of her having to stop after climbing one flight of stairs slowly. She had had one recent episode of hemoptysis. Her most troublesome symptom at the time of presentation had been paroxysmal atrial fibrillation over a period of several months. She had had orthopnea and one episode of paroxysmal nocturnal dyspnea.

On physical examination, she was in no apparent distress. Blood pressure was 130/70 mm Hg, and pulse rate was 80 beats per minute and regular. There was no jugular venous distension, lungs were normal, and the point of maximal impulse was in the fifth interspace in the midclavicular line. S$_1$ was accentuated. At the apex, there was a grade 1/6 holosystolic murmur, an opening snap, and a grade 2 diastolic rumble with presystolic accentuation. The liver edge was at the costal margin, and there was no edema. The ECG was within normal limits. The chest roentgenogram showed a normal-sized heart, an enlarged left atrium, a mild degree of pulmonary vascular redistribution, no calcification in the region of the mitral valve, and was otherwise normal.

Cardiac catheterization revealed the following:

Body surface area, m^2	1.78
O$_2$ consumption, mL/min	180
A-V O$_2$ difference, mL/L	40
Cardiac output, L/min	4.5
Heart rate, beats/min	76, NSR
Pressures, mm Hg	
Brachial artery	130/70, $\overline{90}$
Left ventricle	130/8
Diastolic mean	6

Diastolic filling period, sec/beat	0.42
Pulmonary capillary wedge	
Mean	24
Diastolic mean	20
Pulmonary artery	40/22, $\overline{28}$
Right ventricle	40/6
Right atrium, mean	4
Pulmonary vascular resistance,	
dyn·sec·cm^{-5}	71
Calculated mitral valve area, cm^2	1.0

Cineangiography of the left ventricle revealed no mitral regurgitation.

Interpretation. This patient was symptomatic because of her increased left atrial pressure and atrial arrhythmia. She had not yet developed the second stenosis, discussed previously, at the precapillary pulmonary arteriolar level. Thus her pulmonary artery pressure elevation was purely a consequence of the increased left atrial and pulmonary venous pressures, and the pulmonary vascular resistance was normal (<120 dyn·sec·cm^{-5}). In the spectrum of patients with mitral stenosis, she would fall into stage II of Fig. 28.3. Appropriate therapy might be balloon mitral valvuloplasty or surgical valve replacement, depending on the degree of valve deformity seen on echocardiography. Without relief of the mitral stenosis, her paroxysmal atrial fibrillation will likely become continuous.

Case 2: Severe Mitral Stenosis, Moderately Elevated Pulmonary Vascular Resistance, Few Symptoms, Fatigue Syndrome. E.C., a 42-year-old woman, had no history of acute rheumatic fever. She was asymptomatic until she was 19 years old, when during the last month of her first pregnancy, at which time she was quite anemic, she developed pulmonary congestion. She responded well to therapy and remained asymptomatic thereafter, even during three subsequent pregnancies. However, during her fifth pregnancy at age 37, dyspnea, orthopnea, paroxysmal nocturnal dyspnea, and one episode of hemoptysis of pure red blood occurred at the seventh month, necessitating hospitalization through term. Thereafter she improved, but became progressively tired with loss of energy and drive. She became less thorough in her housework and in her attention to the children's clothes and lost her previous meticulousness. If she pushed herself, she would become somewhat short of breath on a flight of stairs, but it was fatigue more than breathlessness that bothered her.

On examination, she was well nourished and had a malar flush. Her blood pressure was 115/70 mm Hg; her pulse, 90 beats per minute and irregularly irregular. Respirations were 15 per minute. There was no pulmonary or peripheral congestion. The neck veins were just visible at the clavicles with the patient sitting upright. The point of maximal impulse was in the fifth interspace just outside the midclavicular line. The impulse was normal. A prominent parasternal heave was present. S$_1$ was accentuated. No apical systolic murmur was present. There was an opening snap and a grade 2 apical diastolic rumble. The ECG showed right ventricular hypertrophy and atrial fibrillation. Chest radiographs showed the heart to be moderately enlarged because of enlargement of the left atrium and right ventricle. The pulmonary arteries were prominent, and there was a moderate degree of pulmonary vascular redistribution.

The findings at cardiac catheterization were as follows:

Body surface area, m^2	1.41
O$_2$ consumption, mL/min	188
A-V O$_2$ difference, mL/L	51
Cardiac output, L/min	3.7
Heart rate, beats/min	85, AF
Pressures, mm Hg	
Brachial artery	120/62, $\overline{84}$
Left ventricle	120/7
Diastolic mean	5
Diastolic filling period, sec/beat	0.38
Pulmonary capillary wedge	
Mean	27
Diastolic mean	23
Pulmonary artery	82/32,$\overline{51}$
Right ventricle	82/10
Right atrium, mean	8
Pulmonary vascular resistance, dyn·sec·cm^{-5}	520
Calculated mitral valve area, cm^2	0.7

Interpretation. This patient's symptoms were caused initially by elevated left atrial pressure when, during her fifth pregnancy, she developed hemoptysis, orthopnea, and paroxysmal nocturnal dyspnea. Subsequently, however, her major symptom was fatigue, associated with a reduced cardiac output and an increased arteriovenous O$_2$ difference. The orthopnea and paroxysmal dyspnea had receded somewhat despite the fact that her pulmonary capillary pressure was at the pulmonary edema level. This is a common, although poorly understood, phenomenon in patients with mitral stenosis when pulmonary vascular disease begins to occur. Thus, this patient was beginning to develop the second stenosis discussed previously, and this is apparent from the elevated pulmonary vascular resistance (520 dyn·sec·cm^{-5}). In the spectrum of patients with mitral stenosis, she would be representative of stage III of Fig. 28.3. As was true for the patient just discussed (case 1), appropriate therapy would be either balloon mitral valvuloplasty or surgical valve replacement.

Case 3: Terminal Mitral Stenosis with Severe Pulmonary Hypertension. C.A., a 47-year-old woman, had had acute rheumatic fever at 8 years of age and a murmur ever since. She did well thereafter until age 42, when she noticed exertional dyspnea and paroxysmal nocturnal dyspnea. At age 43, these symptoms worsened. Orthopnea and ankle edema appeared. Her symptoms then improved for nearly 2 years, only to return 2 months prior to admission. Since then, despite a good cardiac regimen, she had had to lead a bed-chair-bathroom existence.

On examination, she was cachectic, dyspneic, and orthopneic. Acrocyanosis was evident. Blood pressure was 96/72 mm Hg; pulse rate was 90 beats per minute and irregularly irregular; respirations were 32 per minute. Neck veins were distended to the angle of the jaw, v waves were prominent, and there were bibasilar rales over the lung fields. The point of maximal impulse was in the anterior axillary line. The apex impulse was normal, but a parasternal heave was present. S_1 was loud. Systole was silent. An opening snap was present, and there was a barely audible mitral diastolic murmur with appreciable presystolic accentuation. The pulmonary component of S_2 was loud and palpable. The liver was two fingerbreadths below the right costal margin and was tender. There was considerable pitting edema to the knees. The ECG showed atrial fibrillation, right-axis deviation, and right ventricular hypertrophy. Chest roentgenogram showed a large heart with prominent left atrium, right ventricle, pulmonary arteries, pulmonary vasculature, and Kerley B lines.

Cardiac catheterization revealed the following:

Body surface area, m^2	1.4
O_2 consumption, mL/min	201
A-V O_2 difference, mL/L	110
Cardiac output, L/min	1.8
Pulse rate, beats/min	92, AF
Pressures, mm Hg	
Brachial artery	108/70
Left ventricle	108/12
Diastolic mean	10
Diastolic filling period, sec/ beat	0.36
Pulmonary capillary wedge	
Mean	33
Diastolic mean	31
Pulmonary artery	125/65, $\overline{75}$
Right ventricle	125/20
Right atrium, mean	19
Pulmonary vascular resistance, dyn·sec·cm^{-5}	1,838
Calculated mitral valve area, cm^2	0.3

Interpretation. This patient had symptoms of left atrial hypertension 5 years before her catheterization, suggesting that she was in stage II (see Fig. 28.3) of mitral stenosis at that time. At the time of presentation to us, she had evidence of advanced right heart failure and pulmonary hypertension. This woman has two stenoses, and both are severe: The mitral orifice area is less than one-tenth normal at 0.3 cm^2, and the pulmonary vascular resistance is approximately 18 times normal at 1,838 dyn·sec·cm^{-5}. She is in late stage IV of mitral stenosis, as diagrammed in Fig. 28.3. Even at this stage in their course, patients can respond dramatically to correction of their mitral stenosis. As pointed out in Chapter 8, pulmonary vascular resistance

gradually returns toward normal in patients with advanced mitral stenosis (stage III or IV, Fig. 28.3) after successful balloon valvuloplasty or surgical commissurotomy/valve replacement.

MITRAL REGURGITATION

Mitral incompetence, failure of the valve to prevent regurgitation of blood from the left ventricle to the left atrium during ventricular systole, may be caused by functional or anatomic inadequacy of any one of the components of the mitral valve apparatus, which consists of two valve leaflets, two papillary muscles with their chordae tendineae, and the valve ring or annulus.

Mitral regurgitation may occur when there is destruction or deformation of the valve leaflets as a result of rheumatic fever or bacterial endocarditis. In patients with mitral regurgitation resulting from either of these conditions, mitral regurgitation begins during "isometric" ventricular contraction and continues throughout systole, thus giving rise to a holosystolic murmur. A fibromyxomatous process in the mitral valve leaflets and chordae tendineae may give rise to mitral prolapse and the floppy valve syndrome. In such patients, regurgitation usually does not begin until ventricular ejection has led to a reduction in left ventricular chamber size, so that the regurgitation and accompanying murmur occur in middle or late systole. There may or may not be evidence of Marfan syndrome in these patients. The papillary muscles are usually normal, but there is a marked redundancy of the valve leaflets and chordae with resulting prolapse into the left atrium during systole and accompanying regurgitation.

The papillary muscles are particularly vulnerable to ischemia from coronary artery disease as well as to damage from viral myocarditis. The posterior papillary muscle derives its blood supply from the right coronary and left circumflex arteries. Ischemic dysfunction of this muscle may occur in association with either an inferior or posterolateral myocardial infarction. Less frequently, ischemic involvement of the anterior papillary muscle in an anterior or anterolateral infarction produces mitral regurgitation. Papillary-chordal integrity is maintained to a point when the left ventricle dilates. The common occurrence of a mitral regurgitant murmur in patients with large left ventricles, however, may reflect a simple anatomic loss of this integrity, an involvement of the papillary muscle with the same disease that causes the left ventricle to dilate, or an abnormality of contraction of the mitral annulus.

Physiology

Mitral regurgitation from whatever cause implies a double outlet to the left ventricle: During systole, blood exits the left ventricle through both aortic and mitral valves. Although total left ventricular output rises, that going into the aorta may fall. The left ventricular "output" regurgitating through the mitral valve depends on at least five factors: the size of the regurgitant orifice, left atrial compliance, the systolic mean pressure difference between the left ventricle and the left atrium, the duration of systole, and the resistance to forward ejection of blood through the aortic valve and into the aorta (e.g., aortic stenosis or peripheral vasoconstriction exacerbate mitral regurgitation). Although hypertension aggravates and lowering of blood pressure lessens mitral regurgitation, the most important factor is probably the size of the regurgitant orifice. In normal subjects and most other valve lesions, the left ventricular mass-to-volume ratio is >1.0. There is proportionately less left ventricular mass in mitral regurgitation with a mass-to-volume ratio <1. Thus, the radius-to-thickness ratio is high and, despite the usual assumption that the left ventricle is unloaded into the left atrium, systolic wall stress is actually greater than normal.

In patients with mitral regurgitation, cardiac catheterization is important to provide a complete hemodynamic and angiographic assessment of the severity of the valvular lesion.

Hemodynamic Assessment

First, it is important to assess the hemodynamic consequences of the mitral regurgitation by measuring cardiac output and right and left heart pressures (3–8).

Interpretation of *v* Waves in the Pulmonary Capillary Wedge Tracing

With acute mitral regurgitation (e.g., ruptured chordae tendineae), giant *v* waves will be seen in the left atrial or pulmonary artery pressure tracing (Fig. 28.4). In this regard, our Fellows and Residents have often been asked, "How large must a *v* wave be to be diagnostic of severe mitral regurgitation?" In my experience, *v* waves up to twice the mean left atrial pressure can be seen in the absence of any mitral regurgitation. The patient with left ventricular failure from any cause may have a distended, noncompliant left atrium, and the normal *v* wave (which is owing to left atrial filling from the pulmonary veins during left ventricular systole) will be prominent in this circumstance (7). When pulmonary blood flow is increased, the normal *v* wave increases in prominence correspondingly; this is particularly striking in acute ventricular septal defect complicating myocardial infarction, in which enormous *v* waves (>50 mm Hg) can be seen in the absence of any mitral regurgitation (9).

A *v* wave greater than twice the mean left atrial (or pulmonary capillary wedge) pressure is suggestive of severe mitral regurgitation, and when the height of the *v* wave is three times the mean pulmonary capillary wedge or left

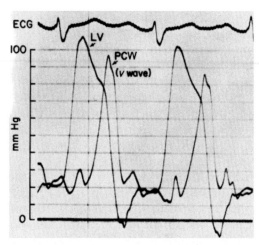

Figure 28.4   Left ventricular (LV) and pulmonary capillary wedge (PCW) pressure tracings taken in a patient with ruptured chordae tendineae and acute mitral insufficiency. The giant *v* wave results from regurgitation of blood into a relatively small and noncompliant left atrium. Electrocardiogram (ECG) illustrates the timing of the PC *v* wave, whose peak follows ventricular repolarization, as manifested by the T wave of the ECG.

atrial pressure, a diagnosis of severe mitral regurgitation is virtually certain (see Fig. 28.4). We hasten to point out, however, that the absence of a prominent *v* wave by no means rules out severe mitral regurgitation. Slowly developing chronic mitral regurgitation commonly leads to marked left atrial enlargement, and the dilated left atrium can accept an enormous regurgitant volume per beat without any increase in mean pressure or height of the *v* wave (10). Also, the level of afterload, as determined by systemic vascular resistance, may greatly affect the height of the regurgitant or *v* wave in patients with mitral regurgitation (4). As seen in Figure 28.5A, a patient with severe mitral regurgitation had a *v* wave of 48 mm Hg when left ventricular (LV) systolic pressure was approximately 140 mm Hg. With sodium nitroprusside (right), the LV systolic pressure came down to 120 mm Hg, and the *v* wave was essentially abolished (11). Although this patient's regurgitant fraction was reduced with sodium nitroprusside (from 80 to 64%), it still remained in the range of severe mitral regurgitation (see below). As summarized in a study by Snyder et al. (12) and more recently by Syed (9), prominent *v* waves in the pulmonary capillary wedge (PCW) tracing are insensitive and have a poor positive predictive value in identifying moderate or severe mitral regurgitation.

Exercise Hemodynamics

Another important hemodynamic parameter in the assessment of mitral regurgitation is the forward cardiac output. Low cardiac output is common in advanced mitral regurgitation and may account for much of the clinical picture. If resting cardiac output is near normal, and if the patient's primary symptoms are related to exertion (i.e., easy fatigability and dyspnea on exertion), dynamic exercise during

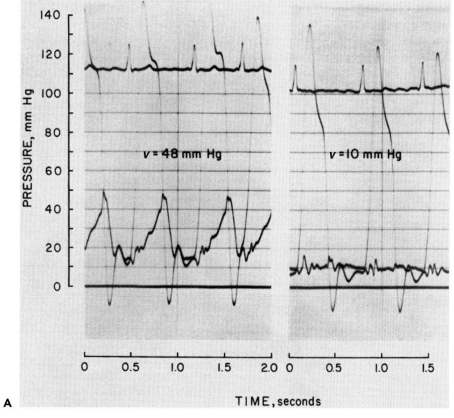

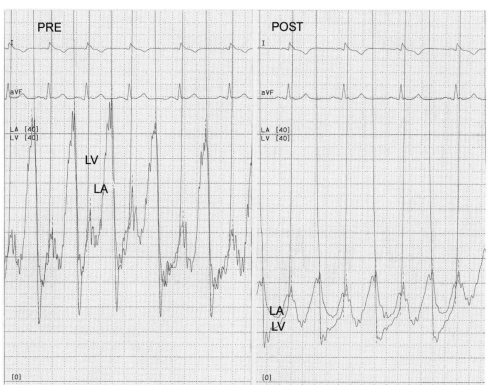

Figure 28.5 **A.** Left ventricular and pulmonary capillary wedge pressures before *(left)* and during *(right)* an infusion of sodium nitroprusside in a patient with severe mitral regurgitation and atrial fibrillation. This illustrates the sensitivity of the *v* wave height to LV afterload in patients with mitral regurgitation. See text for discussion. (From Harshaw CW, et al. Reduced systemic vascular resistance as therapy for severe mitral regurgitation of valvular origin. *Ann Intern Med* 1975;83:312.) **B.** Simultaneous left ventricular (LV) and left atrial (LA) pressures before and after percutaneous mitral repair. Prerepair, there is 4+ mitral regurgitation, but the peak of the *v* wave exceeds 40 mm Hg, which is less than twice the mean LA pressure. Following repair, the LA waveform has normalized with a dramatic change in the *v* wave morphology.

cardiac catheterization may be revealing. If the symptoms are cardiac in origin, the patient usually fails to increase cardiac output appropriately with exercise; i.e., the increase in cardiac output will be <80% of predicted (see formula for prediction of cardiac output increase with exercise in Chapter 15). In addition, pulmonary capillary wedge or left atrial mean pressure will rise with exercise, commonly reaching levels >35 mm Hg by 4 to 5 minutes of supine bicycle exercise, even if the control value was nearly normal.

Angiographic Assessment

The second objective of cardiac catheterization in patients with mitral regurgitation is the angiographic assessment of the severity of the regurgitation by left ventriculography. The assessment may be qualitative, by noting the degree of opacification of the left atrium owing to regurgitation back through the incompetent valve, using a scale of 1+ (mild), 2+ (moderate), 3+ (moderately severe), and 4+ (severe) regurgitation. Although these grades are subjective, certain criteria can be used to enhance consistency of their usage. Regurgitation that is 1+ essentially clears with each beat and never opacifies the entire left atrium. When regurgitation is 2+ (moderate), it does not clear with one beat and generally does opacify the entire left atrium (albeit faintly) after several beats; however, opacification of the left atrium does not equal that of the left ventricle. In 3+ regurgitation (moderately severe), the left atrium is completely opacified and achieves equal opacification with the left ventricle. In 4+ regurgitation (severe), opacification of the entire left atrium occurs within one beat, the opacification becomes progressively more dense with each beat, and contrast material can be seen refluxing into the pulmonary veins during left ventricular systole.

Regurgitant Fraction

The angiographic assessment of severity of mitral regurgitation also may be made more quantitative by calculation of the regurgitant fraction. This entails measurement of total left ventricular stroke volume (TSV) from the left ventriculogram and the amount that goes forward by way of the aorta to the body (the forward stroke volume, FSV) by Fick or indicator-dilution technique. The TSV is calculated as the difference between end-diastolic and end-systolic left ventricular volumes (EDV − ESV = TSV), as described in Chapter 16. Regurgitant stroke volume (RSV, regurgitant volume per beat) is then given as RSV = TSV − FSV. Regurgitant fraction (RF) is then calculated as RF = RSV/TSV.

The accuracy of these calculations depends on many factors. Because FSV is calculated by dividing cardiac output by heart rate at the time of the Fick (or other) cardiac output determination, it is an average stroke volume. The particular beat chosen from the left ventriculogram for volume determination must therefore be an average or representative beat; alternatively, volumes from multiple beats may be calculated and averaged. Thus, in patients with atrial fibrillation or extrasystoles during ventriculography, the regurgitant stroke volume and regurgitant fraction may be highly inaccurate and should not be calculated in such patients. It also should be obvious that the accuracy of the regurgitant fraction depends on a similar physiologic state prevailing between the cardiac output and angiographic phases of the catheterization procedure. An increase in arterial blood pressure may substantially increase the mitral regurgitation and decrease forward output. Therefore, if blood pressure or other hemodynamic variables change significantly between the time of cardiac output determination and left ventriculography, it is pointless to calculate regurgitant fraction. Finally, regurgitant fraction quantifies, at best, the total amount of regurgitation. Thus, if a patient has both mitral and aortic regurgitation, the regurgitant fraction gives an assessment of the regurgitation owing to both lesions combined.

A study from the Mayo Clinic used left ventricular cineangiography to calibrate Doppler echocardiographic techniques for quantification of mitral regurgitation in 180 patients with isolated, pure mitral regurgitation (13). Patients had left ventricular cineangiography to quantify mitral regurgitation, using a grading scale of I to IV, much as just described. They found that grade I angiographic mitral regurgitation corresponded to a Doppler measured regurgitant fraction of 28 ± 9%, grade II angiographic mitral regurgitation to a regurgitant fraction of 38 ± 9%, grade III mitral regurgitation to a regurgitant fraction of 44 ± 10%, and grade IV mitral regurgitation to a regurgitant fraction of 59 ± 12%. The finding that grade I angiographic mitral regurgitation corresponded to a regurgitant fraction of 28 ± 9% is surprising, and probably reflects the sensitivity of the Doppler technique in detecting mitral regurgitation. Using angiographic methods for quantifying left ventricular volumes and regurgitant fraction, grade I (mild) angiographic mitral regurgitation probably corresponds to a regurgitant fraction of <20%, grade II (moderate) mitral regurgitation to a regurgitant fraction of 20 to 40%, grade III (moderately severe) angiographic regurgitation to a regurgitant fraction of 41 to 60%, and grade IV (severe) angiographic mitral regurgitation to a regurgitant fraction of >60%, although greater precision is limited by contrast injection technique, arrhythmia, and variations in left atrial size (14; see Chapter 12).

A third objective of cardiac catheterization in patients with mitral regurgitation is the assessment of left ventricular function by measuring the left ventricular diastolic pressure and, more important, by measuring the left ventricular ejection fraction and end-systolic volume. As others have emphasized, the nearer the preoperative ejection fraction is to normal, the greater is the degree of postoperative restoration to full activity. Specific parameters of left ventricular function are discussed in Chapters 16 and 17.

Catheterization Protocol

1. Right heart catheterization for evaluation of right atrial pressure (to detect possible tricuspid valve disease or right ventricular failure), pulmonary artery pressure (degree of pulmonary hypertension), and wedge pressure (v wave height). In severe, acute mitral regurgitation, a v wave may actually be seen in the pulmonary artery as a second or late systolic hump in the pressure waveform (8).

2. Left heart catheterization for measurement of left ventricular end-diastolic pressure (LVEDP) and assessment of gradients (if any) across mitral or aortic valves. A characteristic of severe mitral regurgitation is that the LVEDP is usually much lower than the left atrial (LA) or PCW mean pressure. In contrast, in LV failure owing to cardiomyopathy or coronary artery disease, LVEDP is usually close or equal to the PCW mean pressure, whereas in aortic regurgitation or LV aneurysm, LVEDP is usually much higher than PCW mean pressure.

3. Cardiac output by Fick or indicator-dilution technique. This measures the fraction of blood going out by way of the aorta to the body and by itself yields no information about regurgitant flow. The response of forward cardiac output to dynamic exercise may provide useful information, however, because patients with severe mitral regurgitation are generally incapable of increasing forward output commensurate with the needs of the body, as estimated by the increased oxygen consumption (see Chapter 15).

4. Left ventriculography is the definitive method for evaluating mitral regurgitation. By this method, it is possible to measure left ventricular volumes and regurgitant fraction, as discussed previously. Coronary angiography usually is carried out as well, to assess the need for revascularization at the time of valve repair/replacement surgery, should that prove necessary.

5. Pharmacologic intervention. An infusion of sodium nitroprusside (see Fig. 28.5A) often has a dramatic and salutary effect on the hemodynamic abnormalities in mitral regurgitation and may have both diagnostic and therapeutic value. Although TSV may not change, RSV decreases and FSV increases, leading to increased cardiac output.

Case 4: Mitral Regurgitation. G.A. was a 59-year-old woman with no history of rheumatic fever in childhood. She was healthy and active until 6 months before admission, when she noticed both dyspnea and lower chest discomfort on mild exertion but no other symptoms of heart failure. There was no past history of bacterial endocarditis.

On physical examination, she had normal body habitus. Blood pressure was 130/70 mm Hg; pulse was 80 beats per minute and regular. The jugular veins were not distended, the carotid pulsations were normal, and the lungs were clear. The apical impulse was diffuse; S_1 was diminished. There was a grade 3/6 apical pansystolic murmur transmitted to the axilla. No opening snap, S_3, or diastolic murmurs were heard. There were no aortic murmurs. The ECG showed normal sinus rhythm, complete right bundle branch block, and left-axis deviation. Chest roentgenogram showed enlargement of the left ventricle and left atrium. No valvular calcification was seen.

Cardiac catheterization, left ventriculography, and coronary angiography were performed with the following findings:

Body surface area, m^2	1.95
O_2 consumption, mL/min	200
A-V O_2 difference, mL/L	52
Cardiac output, L/min	
Total left ventricular output (angiographic)	10.4
Forward flow (Fick)	3.9
Regurgitant flow	6.5
Heart rate, beats/min	67
Stroke volume, mL/beat	
End-diastolic LV volume, mL (angiography)	197
End-systolic LV volume, mL (angiography)	42
Total LV stroke volume, mL (angiography)	155
Forward stroke volume, mL (Fick)	58
Regurgitant stroke volume, mL	97
Ejection fraction (155 ÷ 197)	0.79
Regurgitant fraction (97 ÷ 155)	0.63
Pressures, mm Hg	
Brachial artery	140/84, $\overline{105}$
Left ventricle	140/14
Systolic mean	112
Systolic ejection period, sec/beat	0.28
Pulmonary capillary wedge, mean	12
V wave	24
Pulmonary artery	30/14, $\overline{19}$
Right ventricle	30/6
Right atrium, mean	4
Pulmonary vascular resistance	143
Systemic vascular resistance, dyn·sec·cm^{-5}	2,071

Left ventriculography showed excellent and uniform contraction of the left ventricle and a large regurgitant jet into the left atrium, which was filled completely within one beat. The mitral valve did not prolapse into the left atrium. Coronary angiography revealed normal epicardial vasculature, no irregularities or narrowings, and normal runoff.

Interpretation. Mitral regurgitation was identified and quantified. There were no other valvular lesions. Although the left ventricular end-diastolic pressure and volume were above normal, the left ventricle contracted uniformly and vigorously, as judged by cineangiography. The ejection fraction of 0.79 and the end-systolic volume were normal.

The slight elevation of pulmonary vascular resistance was mainly related to the low pulmonary blood flow (forward cardiac output) of 3.9 L/minute (cardiac index = 2.0 L/minute per m^2).

Systemic vascular resistance was substantially increased, perhaps representing excessive vasoconstriction in response to the decreased forward cardiac output. The increased systemic vascular resistance presented an augmented afterload to the left ventricle, thereby worsening this patient's mitral regurgitation. Reduced systemic vascular resistance, induced by vasodilator therapy with a converting-enzyme inhibitor, an angiotensin receptor antagonist, an α-adrenergic blocker, or hydralazine would probably improve this patient's cardiac output and her symptoms of dyspnea on exertion.

Case 5: Mitral Regurgitation with Degenerative Etiology, Amenable to Percutaneous Repair. H.M., an 84-year-old woman with a long-standing history of chronic obstructive pulmonary disease, was hospitalized 2 months prior to diagnostic catheterization with worsening dyspnea on exertion and orthopnea. Chest radiograph and computed tomography (CT) scan both showed bilateral pleural effusions. The brain natriuretic peptide (BNP) was elevated at 605. No evidence for myocardial infarction was noted.

An echocardiogram demonstrated left ventricular systolic function at the lower limits of normal with an estimated ejection fraction of 50%. There were no regional wall motion abnormalities. There was mild concentric left ventricular hypertrophy. The left atrium was moderately enlarged. Doppler examination across the mitral valve showed laterally and posteriorly directed mitral regurgitant jets reaching all the way to the posterior left atrial wall. Transesophageal echo exam showed moderate left atrial enlargement and Doppler findings of a posterolateral directed mitral regurgitant jet reaching in the left upper pulmonary vein. Systolic flow reversal was noted in the pulmonary vein.

Her symptoms have been progressively worsening over the last 6 months. At present, she cannot walk half a block without stopping several times to catch her breath and is incapable of ascending stairs. She is able to perform light household chores.

Coronary arteriography showed no significant coronary disease in the left main, right coronary, or circumflex. A 60% stenosis proximal to the first diagonal is noted in the left anterior descending, and 50 to 60% stenosis was noted in the left anterior descending distal to the first diagonal. An adenosine/thallium myocardial perfusion scan did not reveal any evidence for ischemia.

More detailed review of the transesophageal echo study showed significant mitral valve prolapse with prominent prolapse of the posterior leaflet and evidence of a small flail segment. The regurgitant jet originated from the central portion of the line of coaptation of the mitral leaflets, despite its eccentric course over the leaflets into the left atrium. It was felt that percutaneous mitral valve repair

would be a likely successful strategy for management of the mitral regurgitation.

A second procedure was planned 2 weeks following the diagnostic study to perform percutaneous mitral leaflet repair. Under general anesthesia, and using transesophageal echocardiographic guidance, trans-septal puncture was performed and hemodynamic assessments repeated, which revealed the following:

	Rest	Post MV Repair
Body surface area, m^2	1.71	1.71
Cardiac output, L/min	4.02	5.72
Heart rate, beats/min	91	83
Ejection fraction	65%	63%
Mitral regurgitation	4+	1+
Pressures, mm Hg		
Aorta, sys/dias/mean	147/63/96	97/36/59
Left ventricle, sys/dias/ED	140/7/13	98/9/9
Left atrium, a/v/mean	7/11/7	14/13/9
Pulmonary artery, sys/dias/mean	59/21/36	55/22/33
Right atrium, mean	4	5
Pulmonary vascular resistance, dyn·sec·cm^{-5}	576	335
Systemic vascular resistance, dyn·sec·cm^{-5}	1,829	756

Interpretation. A 24 French guide catheter was exchanged for the Mullins sheath into the left atrium through the echocardiographically guided trans-septal puncture site. The guide catheter was positioned above the mitral valve. An Evalve clip delivery system was used to place a mitral repair clip into the left atrium. The clip was manipulated into the center of the valve orifice, and the orientation of the clip arms were adjusted to be perpendicular to the line of mitral valve coaptation.

The clip arms were opened to about 180° and advanced across the mitral valve into the left ventricle. A quick withdrawal of the clip device from the left ventricular cavity back toward the left atrium resulted in grasping of the anterior and posterior mitral leaflets. The gripping arms were lowered and the clip closed. The mitral regurgitation was reassessed and noted to be dramatically attenuated. After further evaluation, complete normalization of pulmonary vein flow was seen using Doppler exam. The clip was released and mitral regurgitation assessed finally with Doppler echocardiography and left ventriculography. Hemodynamic tracings showing simultaneous left atrial and left ventricular pressures are shown in Fig. 28.5B. Prepair there is an elevated mean LA pressure and a prominent *v* wave. It is notable that the *v* wave height is not more than twice the mean LA wave height, despite the clear presence of severe mitral regurgitation.

The 24 French trans-septal catheter was removed using percutaneous suture closure, using a preclosure approach with a 10 French suture close device (15,16). The left femoral arterial and venous cannulae were removed using manual compression. After recovery from general anesthesia, the patient was discharged on the first postprocedure morning, with clearly dramatically improved symptoms.

A number of observations can be made regarding the changes in hemodynamics before and after percutaneous mitral valve repair. Cardiac output has risen substantially. Although this may reflect a diminished mitral regurgitant volume and an increase in forward stroke volume, it is as easily owing to shunting across the atrial septum from the passage of a 24F catheter after trans-septal puncture, and also possibly owing to diminished systemic resistance associated with general anesthesia necessary for the procedure. Note that the systemic vascular resistance has declined from almost 2,000 dyn·sec·cm^{-5} to 750 dyn·sec·cm^{-5}. The ejection fraction has not changed significantly. A decrease in EF may result from loss of the retrograde afterload reduction that is eliminated by improvement in the mitral regurgitation, the degree of which has diminished dramatically.

AORTIC STENOSIS

Aortic stenosis may be valvular, subvalvular, or supravalvular. Valvular aortic stenosis is most often of the acquired calcific type, which develops on the substrate of a congenitally deformed (e.g., bicuspid) aortic valve. Valvular aortic stenosis also may be present from birth (congenital aortic stenosis) or may develop as a consequence of rheumatic fever. Subaortic stenosis is of various types. Supravalvular stenosis is rare. All types of aortic stenosis can result in a significant systolic pressure difference between the left ventricle and the aorta. In subaortic stenosis, the gradient is between the main portion of the left ventricle and its outflow tract, although in tunnel subaortic stenosis there may be no discrete subvalvular chamber. In supravalvular stenosis, the gradient is just beyond the aortic valve, between the initial segment of the proximal aorta (just beyond the aortic valve) and the main segment of the ascending aorta. To facilitate surgical intervention, it is important to identify the site and nature of the obstruction in each instance. This is determined by both hemodynamics and angiography. In addition, left ventricular function and the presence or absence of aortic and mitral regurgitation should be evaluated. The left ventricle becomes progressively hypertrophied in aortic stenosis. The cardiac output is well maintained until the left ventricle dilates and fails; it then becomes progressively reduced. The following discussion will focus on valvular aortic stenosis in the adult.

The cardinal indications for cardiac catheterization in anticipation of surgery for all three types of aortic stenosis are left ventricular failure, angina pectoris, or syncope. Coronary angiography should be performed in essentially all adults being studied for evaluation of hemodynamically significant aortic stenosis.

TABLE 28.1

CORRELATION BETWEEN CLINICAL SEVERITY OF ACQUIRED AORTIC STENOSIS IN ADULTS AND AORTIC VALVE AREA

Aortic Valve Area	Clinical Severity
≥1.0 cm^2	Mild: symptoms rare in absence of other heart disease (coronary disease, other valve lesions)
0.7 to 1.0 cm^2	Moderate: symptoms with unusual stress, such as vigorous exercise, rapid atrial fibrillation, influenza
0.5 to 0.7 cm^2	Moderately severe: symptoms with ordinary activities of daily living
≤0.5 cm^2	Severe: symptoms at rest or minimal exertion, biventricular failure

Hemodynamic Assessment

In the hemodynamic assessment of valvular aortic stenosis, primary importance should be placed on obtaining simultaneous measurement of pressure and flow across the aortic valve. As discussed in Chapter 10, this permits calculation of the aortic orifice or valve area (AVA). In the typical adult with symptomatic aortic stenosis, AVA is reduced to ≤0.7 cm^2. Occasionally, a valve of 0.8 to 0.9 cm^2 results in a symptomatic presentation, especially when there is concomitant coronary artery disease or hypertension or when the absolute value of cardiac output is high (e.g., a large patient, anemia, fever, or thyrotoxicosis). When AVA is ≤0.5 cm^2, severe aortic stenosis is present and cardiac reserve is minimal or absent.

For the typical adult patient with acquired aortic stenosis, correlation between clinical severity and aortic valve area calculated by the Gorlin equation (see Chapter 10) is summarized in Table 28.1. If other cardiac disease is present (e.g., coronary disease, other valve disease, cardiomyopathy), the correlations listed in Table 28.1 will not be applicable.

Most patients with aortic stenosis, particularly those with the clinical presentation of angina and/or syncope, have a normal cardiac output/index, normal right heart and PCW mean pressures, and normal LV ejection fraction. The LVEDP is usually increased, reflecting a stiff LV chamber, and there is a prominent A wave in PCW, LA, and LV pressure tracings (Fig. 28.6). In more advanced cases, LV ejection fraction and cardiac output are depressed, and right heart and PCW mean pressures are elevated. Severe pulmonary hypertension with right heart failure, ascites, and edema may eventually dominate the picture. In these patients, the low-output state may lead to a reduction in the

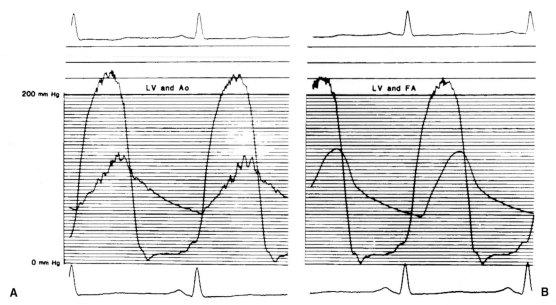

Figure 28.6 Pressure recordings in a patient with aortic stenosis. **A.** Left ventricular (LV) and central aortic (Ao) pressures recorded simultaneously. **B.** LV and femoral arterial (FA) pressures. The FA pressure is out of phase and exhibits distortion (a higher systolic peak and lower end-diastolic pressure) characteristic of peripheral arterial pressures. (From Blitz LR, Kolansky DM, Hirshfeld JW Jr. Valve function, stenosis and insufficiency. In Pepine CJ, Hill JA, Lambert CR, eds. *Diagnostic and Therapeutic Cardiac Catheterization*, 3rd ed. Baltimore: Williams & Wilkins, 1998.)

intensity of the characteristic systolic murmur, obscuring the diagnosis.

Carabello Sign

An interesting hemodynamic finding, described by Carabello and coworkers (17), is a rise in arterial blood

pressure during left heart catheter pullback in patients with severe aortic stenosis (Fig. 28.7). Catheter pullback (withdrawal from the LV to the central aorta of a catheter that had been placed in the LV by retrograde technique) showed increases in peripheral arterial pressure of 5 mm Hg in 15 of 42 patients. Fifteen of 20 patients (75%) with AVA of 0.6 cm^2 demonstrated this phenomenon, but none of 22

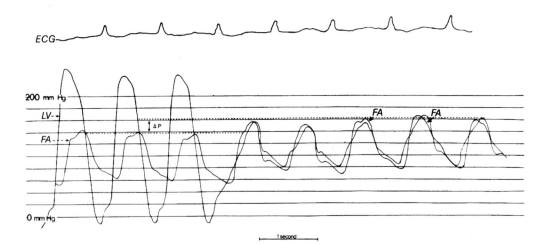

Figure 28.7 Left ventricular (LV) and femoral artery (FA) pressure tracings in a patient with severe aortic stenosis (aortic valve area 0.4 cm^2). During pullback of the retrograde catheter from LV to ascending aorta, the peak systolic femoral artery pressure can be seen to increase (ΔP) by approximately 20 mm Hg. This sign is seen only in patients with aortic valve areas <0.6 cm^2. The mechanism of this phenomenon is believed to be partial obstruction of an already narrowed aortic orifice by the retrograde catheter and relief of this obstruction with catheter withdrawal. (From Carabello BA, et al. Changes in arterial pressure during left heart pullback in patients with aortic stenosis. *Am J Cardiol* 1979;44:424.)

patients with AVA of 0.7 cm² showed such an increase. It was concluded that a rise in peak arterial pressure during LV catheter withdrawal is an ancillary hemodynamic finding of critical aortic stenosis (see Fig. 28.7). The mechanism of this phenomenon is most likely related to partial obstruction of an already narrowed aortic orifice by the retrograde catheter and relief of this obstruction when the catheter is withdrawn.

Angiographic Assessment

In patients with aortic stenosis, left ventriculography can yield important information, and we believe that it generally should be part of the catheterization procedure. It must be emphasized, however, that patients with LV failure and high PCW pressures owing to aortic stenosis may not tolerate the radiographic contrast load of left ventriculography. Adequate preparation (e.g., intravenous furosemide, morphine, or oxygen) before ventriculography and use of nonionic or low-osmolality contrast agents are mandatory in such patients, and ventriculography should not be done in such patients without careful consideration of risk versus benefit. The value to be obtained from left ventriculography includes assessment of the mitral valve (is there significant mitral regurgitation?), detection of regional wall motion abnormalities or LV aneurysm indicative of major coronary disease, and overall assessment of LV function. In addition, wall thickness and LV mass may be measured from the ventriculogram. Often this information can be obtained from echocardiography, and contrast left ventriculography can be avoided.

Aortography is generally not required in the patient with aortic stenosis, unless the gradient is small and the aortic pulse pressure is wide. Selective coronary arteriography should be done in most patients with acquired calcific aortic stenosis, especially if chest pain is present.

Catheterization Protocol

1. Right heart catheterization for measurement of right heart pressures and cardiac output.

2. Left heart catheterization for measurement of pressure gradient across aortic valve and LVEDP and assessment of the presence or absence of a transmitral gradient (concomitant mitral stenosis). Retrograde crossing of a tight aortic valve may be difficult. From the brachial approach, many operators have been successful in crossing a tight aortic valve using a Sones catheter. The Cordis polyurethane Sones catheter has high torque control and tapers to a 5.5F tip, which often can be negotiated across a stenotic aortic valve without the aid of a guidewire. A multipurpose catheter is more commonly used from the brachial or radial approach. When a guidewire is required, a 0.35-inch-diameter straight wire passes easily through the catheter and can help in crossing the aortic valve.

With a femoral approach, a pigtail catheter together with a straight guidewire protruded a short distance beyond the catheter tip is a widely used first approach to retrograde

catheterization of the left ventricle in the patient with aortic stenosis; this method is illustrated in Chapter 4. On occasion, a right or left Judkins coronary catheter used together with a straight guidewire is successful in crossing a tight aortic valve in a patient with aortic stenosis. In one patient with calcific aortic stenosis and a very eccentric aortic valve orifice in whom all these approaches failed, a left L2 Amplatz catheter with a straight guidewire was introduced successfully in retrograde catheterization of the left ventricle.

An improved catheter design for crossing stenosed aortic valves has been developed by Feldman and coworkers (18). Using this catheter (Cook, Inc., Feldman A1 catheter), the authors found that the median time to cross the aortic valve retrograde was 30 to 40 seconds in a group of 17 patients with a mean aortic valve area of 0.75 cm².

If these approaches are not successful (or are not desirable in a particular patient), a trans-septal approach may be used. In some laboratories, the trans-septal approach is the primary technique for patients with aortic stenosis (19). Retrograde crossing of the aortic valve results in clinically silent cerebral embolic lesions in some patients (20). The trans-septal approach presumably decreases this risk.

In patients with aortic stenosis, it is highly desirable to measure transvalvular gradients as close as possible to the site of obstruction. Thus, as seen in Fig. 28.6, the transaortic gradient measured with a catheter in the left ventricle and another catheter in the central aorta may differ from that obtained when arterial pressure is measured in the femoral artery. This problem is discussed in greater detail in Chapter 10. Double-lumen pigtail catheters (e.g., Cook Instruments) make it possible to measure left ventricular and central aortic pressures with a single catheter, avoiding the need for a separate arterial entry site. The central aortic pressure may also be compared with the left ventricular cavity pressure by passing a diagnostic catheter into the left ventricle, and then placing a 0.014-inch pressure wire (RADI Incorporated, Uppsala, Sweden) through the diagnostic catheter. The diagnostic catheter may then be withdrawn into the aortic root just above the valve, yielding simultaneous measurement of the central aortic and left ventricular pressures. This method produces tracings of sufficient quality to mimic high-fidelity micromanometer pressure recordings (19).

Another potentially important source of error in pressure measurement in patients with aortic stenosis can result from incomplete entry of a multiple-side-hole catheter into the left ventricular chamber. Figure 28.8 illustrates this problem, with a pigtail catheter partially (A) or completely (B) within the left ventricular chamber. The partial entry pressures lead to a gross underestimation of the severity of the aortic stenosis.

3. Angiography following the guidelines just discussed.

Left ventriculography demonstrates the stenotic orifice of the valve during systole as outlined by a jet of contrast material ejected into the aorta. The valve cusps may appear irregular, their mobility may be reduced, and often the

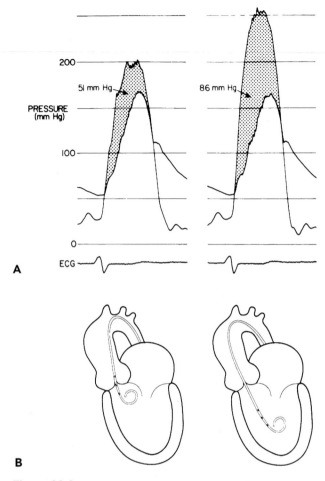

A

B

Figure 28.8 Pressure recordings in a patient with aortic stenosis **(A)**, illustrating the artifacts that can result when a multiple-side-hole pigtail catheter is incompletely advanced into the left ventricular chamber **(B)**. See text for details. (From Blitz LR, Kolansky DM, Hirshfeld JW Jr. Valve function, stenosis and insufficiency. In Pepine CJ, Hill JA, Lambert CR, eds. *Diagnostic and Therapeutic Cardiac Catheterization*, 3rd ed. Baltimore: Williams and Wilkins, 1998.)

number of cusps can be identified. In congenital aortic stenosis, the valve may form a funnel during systole. The ascending aorta is dilated (poststenotic dilatation), but the subvalvular area is widely patent. A subaortic membrane, with a small central orifice, or a subvalvular muscular ring may be seen. The characteristic changes of idiopathic hypertrophic subaortic stenosis may be observed. In supravalvular stenosis, the narrowing of the proximal aorta can be seen.

Aortography also can be helpful in evaluation of the patient with aortic stenosis. In "pure" aortic stenosis (no concomitant aortic regurgitation), aortography often demonstrates a negative jet of radiolucent blood exiting focally from the left ventricle. In congenital aortic stenosis, there may be upward doming of the aortic valve leaflets, which together with the central negative jet gives the so-called Prussian helmet sign (Fig. 28.8). In the patient with aortic stenosis who also has some aortic regurgitation, aor-

tography permits a rough quantitation of the severity of the regurgitation. If interventional catheter techniques (e.g., balloon aortic valvuloplasty) are under consideration, determination of the extent of associated aortic regurgitation may become important in clinical decision making.

Hemodynamic assessment often can detect the presence of mixed significant aortic stenosis and regurgitation, as illustrated by the patient whose pressure tracings are shown in Figure 28.9A. This 78-year-old man had the unusual combination of hemodynamically significant aortic stenosis (70 mm Hg gradient) and significant aortic regurgitation (3+, regurgitant fraction 48%).

Case 6: Aortic Stenosis without Appreciable Cardiomegaly. L.C. was a 48-year-old married woman with a history of rheumatic fever in childhood. Six months before admission, she noted increasing exertional dyspnea and decreased effort tolerance. She had had dizziness but no syncope or angina.

Physical examination was normal except for the heart. There was a forceful apex impulse in the midclavicular line in the fifth interspace. Rhythm was regular. S_1 and S_2 were normal. The only murmur was a grade 2/6 ejection-type systolic murmur, maximal along the left sternal border and transmitted to the apex and into the carotids. No thrill was detected. The carotid pulsations exhibited a slow upstroke but were of normal amplitude. The ECG revealed left ventricular hypertrophy and strain. Chest radiographs showed a heart of normal overall size. There was a little rounding in the region of the left ventricle. The other cardiac chambers appeared normal, as did the lungs. At fluoroscopy, there was calcification in the region of the aortic valve.

The findings at cardiac catheterization were as follows:

Body surface area, m²	1.87
O$_2$ consumption, mL/min	225
A-V O$_2$ difference, mL/L	40
Cardiac output, L/min	5.6
Heart rate, beats/min	70
Pressures, mm Hg	
Brachial artery	100/66
Systolic mean	84
Left ventricle	176/16
Systolic mean	140
Systolic ejection period, sec/beat	0.35
Pulmonary capillary wedge, mean	10
Pulmonary artery	25/11, $\overline{15}$
Right ventricle	25/5
Right atrium, mean	5
Pulmonary vascular resistance, dyn·sec·cm⁻⁵	72
Calculated aortic valve area, cm²	0.7
Ejection fraction	0.69

Left ventriculography showed a vigorously contracting normal-sized left ventricle and a calcified aortic valve with three cusps. The valve leaflets were almost immobile. A jet

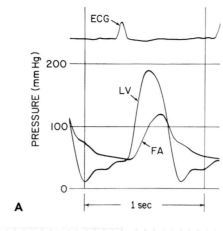

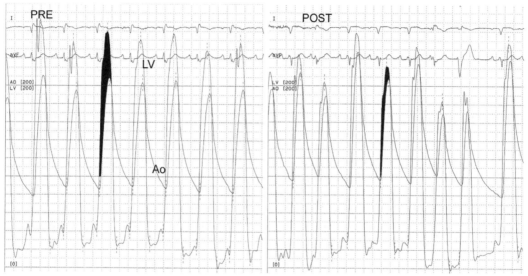

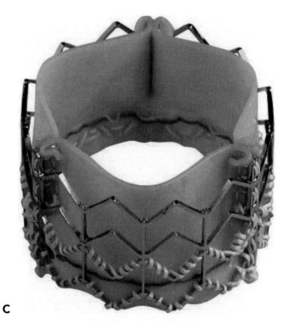

Figure 28.9 **A.** Left ventricular (LV) and femoral artery (FA) pressure tracings in a 78-year-old man with increasing dyspnea on exertion and one episode of pulmonary edema. In this case, femoral artery and central aortic pressures were nearly superimposable. There is a 70-mm Hg peak-to-peak systolic gradient, but there is also unusually rapid aortic diastolic runoff with equilibration (diastasis) of end-diastolic LV and FA pressures. This latter finding suggested significant aortic regurgitation, which was confirmed by aortography. **B.** Simultaneous recordings of LV and aortic (Ao) pressures. The prevalvuloplasty transaortic valve pressure gradient is shaded in black *(left).* After valvuloplasty, there is a marked reduction in the transvalvular gradient *(right).* It is notable that the left ventricular peak systolic pressure has decreased and the aortic peak systolic pressure has increased as a function of the relief of valve stenosis. **C.** Percutaneous heart valve prosthesis for the aortic valve position (Edwards Lifesciences, Irvine, California). Equine pericardial leaflet tissue has been mounted in a specially designed stainless steel stent. The stent is robust, with thick struts and reinforcement at the commissural lines.

was seen passing through the valve that almost immediately became obscured by the radiopacity of the aorta. There was a rather discrete poststenotic dilation of the ascending aorta just above the aortic valve.

Interpretation. The moderately severe calcific aortic stenosis in this woman was probably rheumatic in origin. The left ventricle contracted well, as indicated by an ejection fraction of 0.69 and a normal cardiac output. The elevated LVEDP at rest was compatible with a decreased chamber distensibility from hypertrophy.

Case 7: Aortic Stenosis with Appreciable Cardiomegaly. A.H., a 77-year-old man, was well until 3 years before admission, when exertional dyspnea, orthopnea, fatigue, and peripheral edema appeared. Despite therapy, these symptoms increased progressively to the point of invalidism. He had mild angina and had had two syncopal episodes.

On physical examination, the blood pressure was 110/80 mm Hg; the pulse was 78 beats per minute and regular; respirations were 24 per minute. The carotids were of small volume with slow upstroke. Neck veins were moderately distended. There were basilar rales audible over both lungs. The point of maximal impulse was in the sixth interspace 2 cm within the anterior axillary line, diffuse and forceful. There was no parasternal heave. A grade 2/6 aortic systolic ejection murmur was heard all along the left sternal border and over both carotid arteries. The liver was two palpable fingerbreadths below the right costal margin. There was slight pitting edema of both lower legs. The ECG showed left ventricular hypertrophy and strain pattern. Chest roentgenogram showed enlargement of the left ventricle, calcification in the region of the aortic valve, moderate redistribution of vascular markings to the upper lobes of the lungs, and a small amount of pleural fluid on the right.

Cardiac catheterization yielded the following results:

Body surface area, m^2	1.76
O$_2$ consumption, mL/min	218
A-V O$_2$ difference, mL/L	81
Cardiac output, L/min	2.7
Heart rate, beats/min	90
Pressures, mm Hg	
Brachial artery	135/78
Systolic mean	100
Left ventricle	184/35
Systolic mean	140
Systolic ejection period, sec/beat	0.27
Pulmonary capillary wedge, mean	29
Pulmonary artery	75/40, $\overline{52}$
Right ventricle	75/12
Right atrium, mean	10
Pulmonary vascular resistance, dyn · sec · cm^{-5}	683
Aortic valve area, cm^2	0.4
Ejection fraction	0.30

Left ventriculography was performed only after pretreatment with intravenous furosemide and showed a large dilated left ventricle with uniformly poor contractions in systole. There was no mitral or aortic regurgitation. The aortic valve had two leaflets that appeared ragged and were heavily calcified. There was considerable dilation of the ascending aorta. Left ventriculography was tolerated well, and coronary angiography (two injections of the left coronary artery and one injection of the right coronary artery) revealed the absence of significant coronary artery obstruction.

Interpretation. There was severe calcific aortic stenosis, as indicated by a calculated valve area of 0.4 cm^2. Severe left ventricular failure was present, as indicated by left ventricular dilatation, high left ventricular end-diastolic pressure (35 mm Hg), uniformly poor contraction by cineangiography, an ejection fraction of only 0.30, and a very low cardiac output. The aortic obstruction was severe, and the left ventricle was so decompensated that it generated a peak systolic pressure of only 184 mm Hg (instead of 250 to 300 mm Hg, as would be expected with a normal cardiac output), and the mean transaortic pressure gradient was only 40 mm Hg.

The pulmonary capillary wedge pressure of 29 mm Hg explained the rales heard at both lung bases as well as the patient's shortness of breath. The pulmonary hypertension was owing in part to the elevated left ventricular diastolic pressure (passive rise) and in part to reactive pulmonary hypertension, as revealed by the finding of a pulmonary vascular resistance of 683 dyn · sec · cm^{-5}, more than five times normal.

The pressure load on the right ventricle resulted in its decompensation, as indicated by a mild elevation of the right ventricular diastolic and right atrial pressures. The clinical counterpart was slight distension of the neck veins, an enlarged liver, and peripheral edema.

Case 8: Symptomatic Aortic Stenosis in a Poor Candidate for Aortic Valve Replacement. FH, an 87-year-old man with a history of coronary artery disease and prior bypass surgery, was admitted to the hospital with worsening heart failure and aortic stenosis. He had undergone coronary bypass graft surgery 6 years prior to admission and was not noted to have aortic stenosis at the time.

Over the past year, he has had increasingly frequent admissions for congestive heart failure. His clinical picture is complicated by chronic obstructive pulmonary disease requiring home oxygen and chronic renal failure with a creatinine that has been stable for over 6 months at a level of 2.6 mg/dL.

Echocardiographic examination demonstrated a poor left ventricle with an estimated ejection fraction of 35% and an estimated aortic valve area of 0.7 cm^2, with a mean gradient of 27 mm Hg. In addition to heart failure, he complains of postprandial chest pain that responds to sublingual nitroglycerin, usually after breakfast and occurring a few times each week.

Diagnostic catheterization demonstrated a patent left mammary graft to the LAD, but no other angiographic images were obtained to conserve contrast. The aortic valve area was estimated to be 0.8 cm^2 with a 30-mm transaortic valve mean pressure gradient. He was referred for evaluation for aortic valvuloplasty owing to his high risk for reoperation in the face of multiple comorbidities.

After bilateral local femoral anesthesia, a 6 French sheath was placed in the right femoral artery. Iliofemoral angiography was performed on the right side and demonstrated moderate diffuse disease in the femoral artery, but adequate for insertion of an 11 French sheath for retrograde valvuloplasty. Right femoral 8 French venous access was obtained as well. A balloon-tipped catheter was used for right heart pressure measurement and cardiac output. The aortic valve was crossed with a 5F aortic stenosis catheter (Cook, Inc., Bloomington, IN) and a straight movable core guidewire (18). The central aortic and femoral arterial sheath pressures were verified to match and recorded.

After initial catheterization, the following hemodynamic values were obtained:

	Rest	Post BAV
Body surface area, m^2	2.09	
Cardiac output, L/min	5.59	5.63
Heart rate, beats/min	79	88
Pressures, mm Hg		
Aorta, sys/dias/mean	211/95/140	207/95/136
Left ventricle, sys/dias/ED	264/11/28	214/16/22
Left atrium, a/v/mean	32/15/21	
Pulmonary artery, sys/dias/mean	45/29/35	46/32/36
Right atrium, mean	16	14
Transaortic valve gradient, mean	46	18
Aortic valve area, cm^2	0.8	1.3
Systemic vascular resistance, dyn·sec·cm^{-5}	1,731	1,903

After pressure measurements were made, a 260-cm extra-stiff guidewire was exchanged through the 5F catheter into the left ventricle and the catheter removed. A 20-mm-diameter by 6-cm-long balloon was passed retrograde across the aortic valve and inflated three times. The balloon never locked into the valve, but "watermelon seeded" back and forth, indicating that it was not sized adequately to achieve expansion of the aortic valve leaflets. Since the femoral arterial disease precluded insertion of a 14 French arterial sheath for a larger retrograde balloon, the procedure was converted to an antegrade valvuloplasty approach.

The right femoral venous access was upsized to 14F, and trans-septal puncture performed using a standard Mullins sheath and trans-septal needle. A 7 French single-lumen balloon catheter was passed through the Mullins sheath into the left atrium and then into the left ventricle. The balloon catheter was then passed antegrade across the stenotic aortic valve into the arch and then into the descending aorta. A 0.032-inch stiff guidewire was passed through the balloon-tipped catheter and snared with a 10-mm goose-

neck snare from the left femoral artery in the descending aorta. The snare and wire were left in the descending aorta. The Mullins sheath was removed, and a 14 French rigid dilator passed across the atrial septum and removed. An Inoue 26-mm-diameter balloon catheter was passed via the left atrium and positioned in the aortic valve. The balloon was inflated first to 24 mm and then to 26 mm diameter to accomplish aortic valve dilatation. The hemodynamic measurements were repeated (Fig. 28.9B). The catheters were ultimately removed and the femoral sheaths removed using preplaced suture closure.

Interpretation. The hemodynamic results of balloon valvuloplasty are illustrated in Fig. 28.9B. The mean transvalvular pressure gradient has been reduced from 46 mm to 18 mm. It is important to note that the peak left ventricular systolic pressure has declined, and the peak aortic systolic pressure has risen with relief of aortic valve obstruction. The rise in peak aortic systolic pressure is an excellent indicator of the hemodynamic success of balloon valvuloplasty. It is also notable that the aortic diastolic pressure has not decreased following dilatation of the valve, indicating that if aortic regurgitation has been caused, it is not hemodynamically important. Similarly, the left ventricular end-diastolic pressure has declined from nearly 30 mm Hg to 22 mm Hg, indicating relief of obstruction with acute improvement in the filling pressures.

An emerging approach that would also be suitable for a patient like this, with advanced age, prior sternotomy, and multiple comorbid factors causing increased surgical risk, would be percutaneous aortic valve replacement (21,22). Stent-mounted pericardial tissue valves are in development for percutaneous delivery into the aortic valve (Fig. 28.9C). After obtaining either antegrade or retrograde access, balloon valvuloplasty is performed to predilate the valve. Using a large-caliber sheath for delivery, the stent-mounted prosthetic (percutaneous heart valve, PHV) is crimped on a noncompliant 23-mm balloon catheter and delivered into the aortic valve. Right ventricular pacing at 200 to 220 beats per minute is used to effectively stop left ventricular ejection so that the prosthesis may be positioned carefully in the aortic annulus. The balloon is inflated, expanding the stent. Aortography is used to document free flow into the coronary arteries, since coronary obstruction is one of the greatest risks of placing a prosthesis in the aortic annulus in this manner. Initial experience with this approach shows excellent hemodynamic results with no residual transaortic valve pressure gradients and valve areas typically about 1.7 cm^2. Further trials will be necessary to demonstrate the appropriate target population, and, importantly, the durability of these prostheses over time.

AORTIC REGURGITATION

The dynamic effects of aortic regurgitation are caused by regurgitation of blood from the aorta to the left ventricle in diastole. The magnitude of the regurgitation depends on the size of the regurgitant orifice, the pressure difference between the aorta and the left ventricle in diastole, and the duration of diastole. The regurgitant aperture may be as large as 1.0 cm², but regurgitation is generally severe when the aperture is >0.5 cm². The total left ventricular stroke volume increases and equals that which supplies the body (forward flow) plus that which is regurgitated. The amount of blood regurgitated may be as much as 60% of the systolic discharge. The regurgitation usually occurs in early diastole.

Hemodynamic Assessment

The large stroke volume entering the aorta with systole produces an elevated systolic pressure, whereas the regurgitation produces a lowered aortic diastolic pressure (Fig. 28.10). Left ventricular workload increases progressively with the magnitude of regurgitation. This is owing not only to the raised stroke volume and to the rise of systolic pressure but also to the high left ventricular wall stress that develops when a dilated left ventricle contracts to produce a given pressure (Laplace's law). Dilatation and hypertrophy of the left ventricle are invariable consequences of aortic regurgitation. The heart may become the largest encountered in cardiac pathology—the so-called cor bovinum. Up to a point, the forward cardiac output is well maintained. The addition of blood regurgitated to the normal inflow from the left atrium increases the diastolic volume of the left ventricle, leading to a more forceful contraction (Starling's law). With time, the fraction of end-diastolic volume ejected per beat (ejection fraction) becomes diminished, reflecting impaired myocardial function. Furthermore, the left ventricle may operate with an excessive end-systolic volume—another index of left ventricular dysfunction.

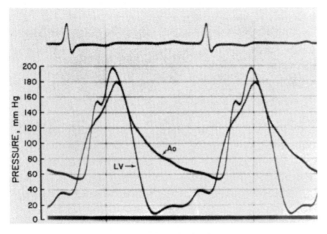

Figure 28.10 Left ventricular (LV) and aortic (Ao) pressure tracings in a patient with severe aortic insufficiency secondary to rheumatic heart disease. In this condition, the aortic and left ventricular pressures may equalize in late diastole, a phenomenon occasionally termed diastasis.

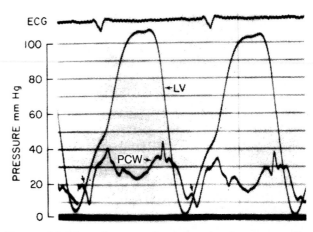

Figure 28.11 Left ventricular (LV) and pulmonary capillary wedge (PCW) pressures in a patient with acute aortic regurgitation owing to infective endocarditis. Note the unusual waveform of the LV pressure with its striking late diastolic rise, loss of clear *a* wave, and high elevation of LV end-diastolic pressure (approximately 45 to 50 mm Hg). LV diastolic pressure rises in late diastole to exceed left atrial and pulmonary wedge pressures *(arrow)*, forcing premature closure of the mitral valve. (From Mann T, et al. Assessing the hemodynamic severity of acute aortic regurgitation due to infective endocarditis. *N Engl J Med* 1975;293:108.)

Premature Mitral Valve Closure

The reflux of blood from the aorta into the left ventricle in diastole added to the blood streaming through the mitral valve from the left atrium results in a rapid rise in left ventricular pressure early in diastole. The mitral valve may close prematurely because the regurgitating blood may raise the left ventricular diastolic pressure to exceed that in the left atrium. This is particularly common in acute aortic regurgitation, where the sudden onset of severe regurgitation into a normal-sized left ventricle leads to striking elevations in LV diastolic pressure (Fig. 28.11). In the case illustrated in Fig. 28.11, LVEDP approaches 50 mm Hg, and LV diastolic pressure exceeds left atrial (or wedge) pressure for nearly half of diastole. This reversal of pressures is associated with premature mitral valve closure, which may be seen on the echocardiogram.

Another example of premature closure of the mitral valve in association with severe aortic regurgitation is shown in Fig. 28.12. These tracings were recorded during cardiac catheterization of a 71-year-old man who had previously undergone aortic valve replacement for aortic stenosis. After doing extremely well for more than 5 years, he suddenly developed marked shortness of breath and a new murmur of aortic regurgitation. Pressure recordings (see Fig. 28.12) show that left ventricular diastolic pressure exceeds left atrial (pulmonary capillary wedge pressure) by the end of the first third of the diastolic filling period. Also, complete diastasis of aortic and left ventricular pressures occurs by mid-diastole, at which point aortic regurgitation ceases because there is no longer any gradient driving the regurgitant flow. As expected, this patient's diastolic murmur was blowing in quality, decrescendo, and ended by mid-diastole.

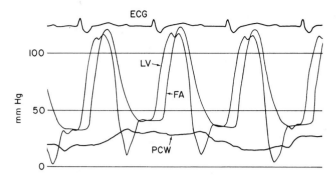

Figure 28.12 Severe aortic regurgitation developing in a 71-year-old man with a prosthetic aortic valve. There is diastasis between left ventricle (LV) and aorta. Also, LV diastolic pressure exceeds pulmonary capillary wedge (PCW) pressure early in diastole. FA, femoral artery. See text for details.

Acute Versus Chronic Aortic Regurgitation

The typical hemodynamic findings in acute versus chronic aortic regurgitation have been reported by Mann et al. (23) and are presented in Table 28.2. As can be seen, widened pulse pressure is characteristic only of chronic aortic regurgitation, reflecting both the enormous stroke volume associated with this condition and the tachycardia commonly seen in patients with acute aortic regurgitation. This may give rise to a situation in which there exists a high end-diastolic pressure in the noncompliant left ventricle in the presence of little if any elevation of the mean pressure in the left atrium. With time and with the severity of the leak, the mean diastolic pressure of the left ventricle rises, and

when this happens, left atrial and pulmonary capillary wedge pressures rise.

Another hemodynamic finding in aortic regurgitation is the amplification of peak systolic pressure in peripheral arteries (especially the femoral and popliteal) so that peak systolic femoral artery pressure may exceed central aortic pressure by 20 to 50 mm Hg. This is essentially an exaggeration of a normal phenomenon (see Chapter 7) but emphasizes the importance of central aortic pressure measurement in aortic regurgitation.

Angiographic Assessment

Aortic cineangiography (aortography) yields a graphic demonstration of the severity and dynamics of the regurgitation. Qualitative assessment is subjective, as for mitral regurgitation. A scale of 1+ to 4+ may be used, using the following definitions to aid discrimination of these four degrees of regurgitation. In 1+ regurgitation (mild), a small amount of contrast material enters the left ventricle in diastole; it is essentially cleared with each beat and never fills the ventricular chamber. More contrast material enters with each diastole in 2+ (moderate) regurgitation, and faint opacification of the entire chamber occurs. With moderately severe (3+) regurgitation, the LV chamber is well opacified and equal in density with the ascending aorta. Severe (4+) aortic regurgitation is characterized by complete, dense opacification of the LV chamber in one beat, and the left ventricle appears more densely opacified than the ascending aorta.

Quantitative assessment of aortic regurgitation involves calculation of the regurgitant fraction (RF), as described in

TABLE 28.2

COMPARISON OF HEMODYNAMIC AND ANGIOGRAPHIC FINDINGS IN ACUTE AND CHRONIC AORTIC REGURGITATION (MEAN ± SD)

Parameter	Acute AR	Chronic AR	P Value
Age (yr)	33 ± 14	40 ± 15	NS
Regurgitant fraction	0.6 ± 0.1	0.7 ± 0.1	NS
LVEDP (mm Hg)	41 ± 12	36 ± 13	NS
Ejection fraction	0.6 ± 0.1	0.6 ± 0.1	NS
Heart rate (bpm)	108 ± 15	71 ± 14	<0.01
LV volumes (mL/m^2)			
EDV	146 ± 28	264 ± 64	<0.01
ESV	57 ± 23	101 ± 42	<0.02
TSV	89 ± 22	163 ± 57	<0.01
Aortic pressure (mm Hg)			
Systolic	110 ± 14	155 ± 26	<0.01
Diastolic	56 ± 11	50 ± 6	NS
Mean	78 ± 12	90 ± 8	<0.02
Pulse pressure (mm Hg)	55 ± 7	105 ± 22	<0.01
Systemic vascular resistance (dyn·sec·cm^{-5})	1326 ± 372	1341 ± 461	NS

EDV, ESV, and TSV, left ventricular end-diastolic, end-systolic and total stroke volumes, respectively; AR, aortic regurgitation; LVEDP, left ventricular end-diastolic pressure; NS, not significant.
Modified from Mann JT, et al. Assessing the hemodynamic severity of acute aortic regurgitation due to infective endocarditis. *N Engl J Med* 1975;293:108.

Chapter 16. The same scale of interpretation holds as for mitral regurgitation with RF <20% corresponding to mild regurgitation; 20 to 40%, moderate; 40 to 60%, moderately severe; and >60%, severe aortic regurgitation.

Part of the angiographic assessment of aortic regurgitation involves assessment of the aortic valve leaflets (mobility, calcification, number of leaflets), the ascending aorta (extent and type of dilatation), and possible associated abnormalities (e.g., coronary lesions, sinus of Valsalva aneurysm, dissecting aneurysm of the aorta, and ventricular septal defect). All these aspects are best evaluated in the LAO view.

Catheterization Protocol

1. Right heart catheterization for measurement of right heart pressures and cardiac output.
2. Left heart catheterization for measurement of central aortic pulse pressure and LVEDP detection of transvalvular gradients (if any), of diastasis between LV and aorta, if this is present (see Fig. 28.12), and of relative height of LVEDP compared with PCW or LA mean pressure.
3. Angiography, including left ventriculography, aortography, and possibly coronary angiography (if indicated clinically).
4. If resting hemodynamics are normal, consider stress intervention, such as dynamic exercise.

TRICUSPID REGURGITATION

Tricuspid regurgitation can be functional or organic. Functional tricuspid regurgitation is thought to be owing to right ventricular dilatation and failure as a result of excessive right ventricular afterload. Most commonly, this is caused by pulmonary hypertension from mitral stenosis, cardiomyopathy, primary pulmonary hypertension, cor pulmonale, or pulmonary embolism.

Organic tricuspid regurgitation implies disease of the tricuspid valve or its supporting apparatus and is seen most commonly with bacterial endocarditis, rheumatic heart disease or right ventricular infarction.

Hemodynamic Assessment

In tricuspid regurgitation, either organic or functional, the primary hemodynamic finding is a large systolic wave in the right atrial pressure tracing. Tracings of jugular venous pulsations show *a*, *c*, and *v* waves in the normal subject; in the patient with moderate tricuspid regurgitation, there is a fourth pulsation, the *s* wave. This systolic wave precedes and blends with the normal venous filling (*v*) wave, and in severe tricuspid regurgitation, the *s* and *v* waves form a single regurgitant systolic wave (Fig. 28.13). As can be seen in Fig. 28.13, the right atrial pressure tracing in severe tricus-

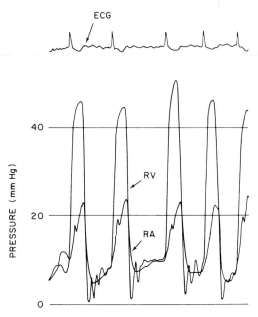

Figure 28.13   Right atrial (RA) and right ventricular (RV) pressures in a 75-year-old woman with rheumatic heart disease. There is severe organic tricuspid regurgitation with RA waveform resembling RV pressure.

pid regurgitation resembles the right ventricular pressure tracing. In the most extreme cases, the right atrial and ventricular pressure tracings are virtually superimposable, which is to be expected because the right atrium and ventricle are physiologically a common chamber in such cases.

The hemodynamic distinction between organic and functional tricuspid regurgitation is difficult. Generally, if the patient with severe tricuspid regurgitation has a right ventricular systolic pressure >60 mm Hg, the tricuspid regurgitation is functional, whereas if the right ventricular systolic pressure is 40 mm Hg, there is a substantial organic component. This distinction is of practical importance in terms of surgical correction, because functional tricuspid regurgitation will improve substantially solely with correction of the right ventricular hypertension (e.g., following balloon valvuloplasty or corrective surgery for mitral stenosis), whereas the patient with major organic tricuspid regurgitation may not survive cardiac surgery unless the operation includes tricuspid valve replacement or tricuspid annuloplasty.

Angiographic Assessment

The angiographic demonstration of tricuspid regurgitation is generally accomplished by right ventricular cineangiography in the right anterior oblique (RAO) projection, as discussed in Chapter 12. Some artificial tricuspid regurgitation is seen because of the presence of the catheter across the tricuspid valve, but this is usually minor. It is important to choose a catheter type, position, and injection rate that will avoid extrasystoles because a run of ventricular tachycardia makes it impossible to evaluate the degree of tricuspid regurgitation; these considerations are discussed in Chapter 14. There has been much experience with the Grollman, pigtail, and Eppendorf catheters situated in mid-RV or RV outflow tract, with injection rates of 12 to 18 mL/second depending on RV size and irritability. A scale of 1+ to 4+ is used to grade severity of tricuspid regurgitation using criteria of definition similar to those described for mitral regurgitation. In some circumstances, a right atrial cineangiogram in RAO projection can be used for assessment of tricuspid regurgitation; in this instance, a negative jet (unopacified blood) from RV to RA shows the regurgitation.

Cardiac catheterization protocol depends on the associated conditions.

TRICUSPID STENOSIS

Previously, this rare condition was seen only in patients with rheumatic heart disease and mitral stenosis. Today, however, stenosis of a prosthetic tricuspid valve (placed originally as treatment for tricuspid regurgitation) accounts for most of the cases seen in most major medical centers. The clinical diagnosis may be difficult, especially if the patient is in atrial fibrillation. Diagnosis is aided by the characteristic finding of an increased jugular venous pressure with blunting or absence of the y descent. One patient seen by me had severe stenosis of her native mitral, aortic, and tricuspid valves. This was a 43-year-old woman with a history of repeated bouts of rheumatic fever in childhood, whose major complaint was fatigue and "blackouts."

Hemodynamic Assessment

The sine qua non of tricuspid stenosis is a pandiastolic gradient across the tricuspid valve. The gradient is usually small (4 to 8 mm Hg) and may be missed unless a careful assessment is made. Two catheters (or a single catheter with a double lumen) and simultaneous measurement of RA and RV pressures should be used if there is any doubt about the presence of this condition. A careful RV to RA pullback using a standard catheter, however, will serve to confirm or eliminate this diagnosis with reliability in most cases. The tricuspid valve area is calculated using the formula given in Chapter 10. Tricuspid stenosis is usually of clinical and hemodynamic significance when the tricuspid valve area is less than 1.3 cm^2.

Angiographic Assessment

The valve is usually calcified and shows decreased mobility. There may be associated right atrial dilatation and some tricuspid regurgitation.

Cardiac catheterization protocol depends on associated lesions.

PULMONIC STENOSIS AND REGURGITATION

Pulmonic stenosis is essentially a congenital condition. Pulmonic regurgitation is usually functional and a consequence of severe pulmonary hypertension. When the pulmonary artery pressure exceeds 100 mm Hg systolic, there is usually some pulmonic regurgitation. This may lead to widening of the pulmonary artery pulse pressure and an increase in right ventricular end-diastolic pressure (RVEDP). Angiographic assessment of pulmonic regurgitation is difficult because the angiographic catheter lying across the pulmonic valve may cause artifactual regurgitation. Echocardiography is far superior to angiography in assessing pulmonic regurgitation.

Cardiac catheterization protocol depends on associated conditions.

RELATIVE STENOSIS OF PROSTHETIC VALVES

An unusual case of relative tricuspid stenosis, mitral stenosis, and aortic stenosis in a 60-year-old man is shown in Fig. 28.14 and illustrates an important point concerning function of prosthetic cardiac valves. This man had mitral valve replacement with a Harken disc valve in 1969 for rheumatic mitral regurgitation. He then did well until 1980, when he presented with left and right heart failure and was found at cardiac catheterization to have severe aortic and tricuspid regurgitation but normal function of the mitral prosthetic valve. Aortic valve replacement (Starr-Edwards prosthesis) and tricuspid valve replacement (porcine prosthesis) led to improvement, but over the following years he required large amounts of diuretic therapy to remain free of edema and pulmonary congestion. Echocardiographic assessment of his prosthetic valves demonstrated apparently normal function, and left ventricular contraction was vigorous.

Because of persistent left and right heart failure, cardiac catheterization was undertaken in 1985. The porcine tricuspid valve was crossed antegrade with a Swan-Ganz catheter, and the Starr-Edwards aortic prosthesis was crossed retrograde with a Sones catheter to obtain the pressure measurements shown in Fig. 28.14. As can be seen, significant pressure gradients were present across tricuspid, mitral, and aortic prostheses. A surprising finding, however, was an elevated cardiac output, measured by both Fick and thermodilution methods. Oxygen consumption index was 148 mL/minute per m^2 and arteriovenous oxygen difference was 29 mL O$_2$/L, giving a Fick cardiac index of 5 L/minute per m^2 and a cardiac output of 10 L/minute. Using the Gorlin formula (Chapter 10), the calculated aortic valve area was 1.3 cm^2, the mitral valve area was 1.6 cm^2, and the tricuspid valve area was 2.4 cm^2; these values were all consistent with the known effective orifice

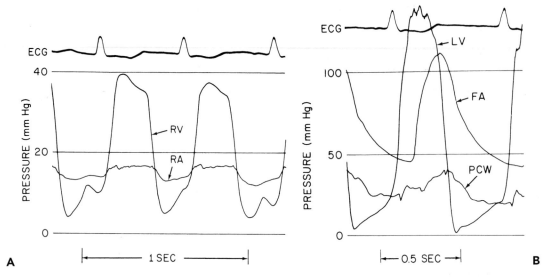

Figure 28.14 Pressure tracings in a 60-year-old man with high cardiac output and significant pressure gradients across normally functioning tricuspid, mitral, and aortic valve prostheses—**(A)** from the right ventricle (RV) and right atrium (RA); **(B)** from the left ventricle (LV), femoral artery (FA), and pulmonary capillary wedge (PCW) position.

areas of the particular prosthetic valves implanted and did not signify prosthetic valve dysfunction or stenosis. Thus, a high cardiac output state caused substantial pressure gradients to occur across the patient's three prosthetic valves, resulting in the clinical picture of biventricular failure. Thyroid function tests were normal, and a search for other causes of high-output state (e.g., arteriovenous fistula, Paget disease) was unrevealing. This patient responded nicely to thiamine supplementation, beta-blockade, and diuretic therapy with spironolactone and furosemide; evidence of high-output state receded and a vigorous diuresis ensued.

Catheter Passage Across Prosthetic Valves

As illustrated in the case just described, it has become routine to cross prosthetic valves with catheters in an attempt to assess their function or the function of other valves. Published reports have documented the safety of this procedure in many patients (24,25) with a variety of prosthetic valves. Based on our own experience and anecdotal experience reported to me by many others, we offer the following guidelines: First, porcine valves may be crossed retrograde or antegrade safely with a variety of catheters. For retrograde crossing of a porcine prosthetic valve in the aortic position, a pigtail catheter is generally highly effective. The pigtail catheter tip is rested on top of the valve's leaflets as they protrude into the aorta high above the sewing ring and is gently advanced until it prolapses into the left ventricular chamber. Antegrade crossing of a porcine tricuspid prosthesis is accomplished easily using a balloon-flotation catheter, as described in the preceding section. Retrograde crossing of a ball-valve (e.g., Starr-Edwards) prosthesis in

the aortic position may be accomplished easily using a 7F or 8F Sones catheter with or without guidewire assistance. The pigtail catheter also may be advanced into the left ventricle over a guidewire across a ball-valve prosthesis, but the wire should be reinserted for catheter withdrawal to avoid hooking the pigtail on the metal cage. Although some operators have crossed low-profile tilting-disc valve prostheses (e.g., Bjork-Shiley, St. Jude, Medtronic-Hall valve) retrograde without complications, instances where catheter entrapment occurred with retrograde crossing of such valves have been reported (26). Also, Dr. Viking Bjork has stated specifically that the Bjork-Shiley valve must not be crossed retrograde, based on his own large experience. When restudy has been required in his patients, a transseptal approach has been used. Accordingly, one should not attempt to cross a Bjork-Shiley valve or any low-profile disc valve prosthesis retrograde.

REFERENCES

1. Abbo KM, Carroll JD. Hemodynamics of mitral stenosis: a review. *Cathet Cardiovasc Diagn* 1994;Suppl 2:16–25.
2. Cequier A, Bonan R, Serra R, et al. Left-to-right atrial shunting after percutaneous mitral valvuloplasty: incidence and long-term hemodynamic follow-up. *Circulation* 1990;81:1190.
3. Braunwald E. Mitral regurgitation. Physiologic, clinical and surgical considerations. *N Engl J Med* 1969;281:425.
4. Braunwald E, Welch GH Jr, Morrow AG. The effects of acutely increased systemic resistance on the left atrial pressure pulse: a method for the clinical detection of mitral insufficiency. *J Clin Invest* 1958;37:35.
5. Brody W, Criley JM. Intermittent severe mitral regurgitation. Hemodynamic studies in a patient with recurrent acute left-sided heart failure. *N Engl J Med* 1970;183:673.
6. Baxley WA, Kennedy JW, Feild B, Dodge HT. Hemodynamics in ruptured chordae tendineae and chronic rheumatic mitral regurgitation. *Circulation* 1973;48:1288.

7. Pichard AD, et al. Large v waves in the pulmonary wedge pressure tracing in the absence of mitral regurgitation. *Am J Cardiol* 1982;50:1044.

8. Grose R, Strain J, Cohen MV. Pulmonary arterial v waves in mitral regurgitation: clinical and experimental observations. *Circulation* 1984;69:214.

9. Syed, Z, Salinger MH, Feldman T. Alterations in left atrial pressure and compliance during balloon mitral valvuloplasty. *Cathet Cardiovasc Intervent* 2004;61:571–579.

10. Fuchs RM, Heuser RP, Yin FCP, Brinker JA. Limitations of pulmonary wedge v waves in diagnosing mitral regurgitation. *Am J Cardiol* 1982;49:849.

11. Grossman W, et al. Lowered aortic impedance as therapy for severe mitral regurgitation. *JAMA* 1974;230:1011.

12. Snyder RW, Glamann DB, Lange RA, et al. Predictive value of prominent pulmonary arterial wedge v waves in assessing the presence and severity of mitral regurgitation. *Am J Cardiol* 1994; 73:568.

13. Dujardin KS, Enriquez-Sarano M, Bailey KR, Nishimura RA, Seward JB, Tajik AJ. Grading of mitral regurgitation by quantitative Doppler echocardiography. Calibration by left ventricular angiography in routine clinical practice. *Circulation* 1997;96:3409.

14. Croft CH, et al. Limitations of qualitative angiographic grading in aortic or mitral regurgitation. *Am J Cardiol* 1984;53:1593.

15. Solomon LW, Fusman B, Jolly N, Kim A, Feldman T. Percutaneous suture closure for management of large French size arterial puncture in aortic valvuloplasty. *J Invasive Cardiol* 2001; 13: 592–596.

16. Feldman T. Percutaneous suture closure for management of large French size arterial and venous puncture. *J Intervent Cardiol* 2000; 13:237–242.

17. Carabello BA, Barry WH, Grossman W. Changes in arterial pressure during left heart pullback in patients with aortic stenosis: a sign of severe aortic stenosis. *Am J Cardiol* 1979;44:424.

18. Feldman T, Carroll JD, Chiu YC. An improved catheter design for crossing stenosed aortic valves. *Cathet Cardiovasc Diagn* 1989; 16:279.

19. Fusman B, Faxon D, Feldman T: Hemodynamic rounds: transvalvular pressure gradient measurement. *Cathet Cardiovasc Intervent* 2001;53:553–561.

20. Omran H, Schmidt H, Hackenbroch M, et al. Silent and apparent cerebral embolism after retrograde catheterisation of the aortic valve in valvular stenosis: a prospective, randomised study. *Lancet* 2003;361:1241–1246.

21. Eltchaninoff H, Tron C, Cribier A. Percutaneous implantation of aortic valve prosthesis in patients with calcific aortic stenosis: technical aspects. *J Intervent Cardiol* 2003;16:515–521.

22. Cribier A, Eltchaninoff H, Tron C. Bauer F, et al. Early experience with percutaneous transcatheter implantation of heart valve prosthesis for the treatment of end-stage inoperable patients with calcific aortic stenosis. *J Am Coll Cardiol* 2004;43:698–703.

23. Mann T, McLaurin LP, Grossman W, Craige E. Assessing the hemodynamic severity of acute aortic regurgitation due to infective endocarditis. *N Engl J Med* 1975;293:108.

24. Kosinski EJ, Cohn PF, Grossman W, Cohn LH. Severe stenosis occurring in antibiotic sterilised homograft valves. *Br Heart J* 1978;40:194.

25. Rigaud M, et al. Retrograde catheterization of left ventricle through mechanical aortic prostheses. *Eur Heart J* 1987;8:689.

26. Kober G, Hilgermann R. Catheter entrapment in a Bjork-Shiley prosthesis in aortic position. *Cathet Cardiovasc Diagn* 1987; 13:262.

Profiles in Coronary Artery Disease

29

Jeffrey J. Popma   Judith L. Meadows

Atherosclerotic coronary artery disease (CAD) remains the most frequent cause of death in men and women in developed countries. Although it is well recognized that coronary atherosclerosis begins in one's late teens and early twenties (1), the clinical presentation of CAD may be delayed by decades and may be quite heterogeneous in its initial manifestation. The initial signs and symptoms of CAD may range from effort angina due to ischemia evident only caused by one or more fixed coronary stenoses, silent ischemia evident only on stress testing, or an acute coronary syndrome resulting from sudden plaque rupture of one or more previously hemodynamically insignificant coronary narrowings (2). Each atherosclerotic stenosis also has unique characteristics (such as calcification, total occlusion, or branch involvement) that may lead to technical challenges for revascularization using either coronary artery bypass surgery (CABG) or percutaneous intervention (PCI). The purpose of this chapter is to review several clinical profiles in patients with ischemic CAD and to relate these profiles to the strategies recommended for coronary arteriography and revascularization based on the current literature and published guidelines.

STABLE CORONARY ARTERY DISEASE

Case 1. A 45-year-old man, a former professional marathon runner, developed typical substernal chest discomfort 4 miles into his daily run. His chest pressure was relieved with slowing of his pace or with walking, and never developed at rest. Coronary risk factors included elevated total cholesterol and LDL-C levels (LDL-cholesterol, 150 mg/dL), a low HDL-C level (30 mg/dL), and normal serum triglycerides (140 mg/dL). His father developed a

myocardial infarction (MI) at age 50. There was no history of hypertension or diabetes mellitus. An exercise stress electrocardiogram demonstrated anterior wall ischemia (Fig. 29.1) and sestamibi scintigraphy showed a small to moderate-size anterior wall defect at a high workload (Fig. 29.2). Cardiac catheterization was performed and demonstrated two-vessel CAD involving the left anterior descending (LAD) artery and right coronary artery (RCA) vessels (Fig. 29.3). The left ventricular function was normal. Both the left anterior LAD and RCA vessels were treated with coronary stents. The patient has subsequently remained asymptomatic with a normal exercise capacity.

Indications for Coronary Arteriography and Percutaneous Revascularization

Coronary arteriography documents the presence or absence of CAD; identifies the location, number, and morphology of obstructive lesions; and guides referral for PCI or CABG in the event that revascularization is indicated (3). (See Chapter 11.) The American College of Cardiology/American Heart Association (ACC/AHA) Task Force on Coronary Angiography (3) and PCI (4) Class I indications for these procedures include patients with stable CAD who have severe angina despite medical treatment and as well as patients with less severe angina but high-risk criteria on noninvasive testing. Although this patient manifested his ischemia at a high workload, his desire to continue vigorous exercise warranted further invasive evaluation and revascularization.

Compared with medical therapy alone in patients with single-vessel CAD, PCI improves angina and reduces ischemia, although it does not reduce the frequency of

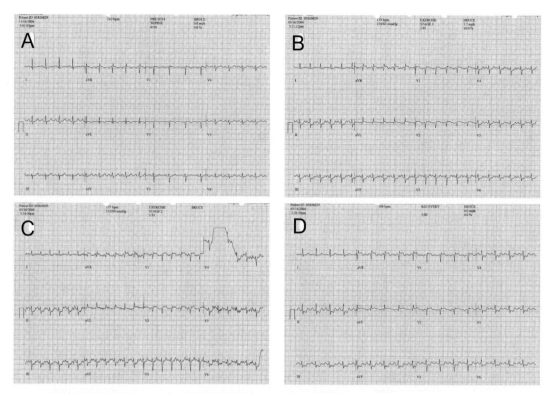

Figure 29.1 ECG exercise stress test demonstrating evidence of exercise-induced ischemia, likely in an anterior distribution. **A.** Pretest ECG is normal sinus rhythm. **B.** ECG during Bruce protocol stage 1 demonstrates 1-mm ST-segment elevation in leads V1-V2 with ST-segment depressions in the inferior and lateral leads. **C.** ECG during Bruce protocol stage 2 demonstrates 2-mm ST-segment elevation in leads V1-V2 with deepening of the ST-segment depressions in the inferior and lateral leads. **D.** At 5 minutes into recovery, there is persistence of the ST-segment changes. (Courtesy of Daniel Forman, M.D., Noninvasive Cardiac Laboratory, Brigham and Women's Hospital, Boston, MA.)

death or MI (5–7). Stable patients with multivessel coronary artery disease may benefit from revascularization, based on the Asymptomatic Cardiac Ischemia Pilot (ACIP) study that found a lower incidence of death or MI at 2 years when patients were treated with revascularization (4.7%) rather than angina-guided (12.1%) or ischemia-guided (8.8%) therapy ($P < .001$; 8). More than 50% of patients in this series underwent CABG.

In patients with multivessel CAD, both CABG and PCI have similar 1-year occurrence rates for death or MI, but patients undergoing PCI require more repeat procedures over the first year owing to restenosis (9). The Bypass And Revascularization Investigation (BARI) also found that diabetic patients assigned to PCI had a significantly ($P = .003$) worse survival rate (65.5%) than did diabetic patients assigned to CABG (80.6%; 10).

Coronary stenting is now used in >90% of PCIs, owing to reduced rates of emergency CABG and late recurrence compared with balloon angioplasty. Although long-term outcomes following bare metal coronary stenting were limited by clinical restenosis in ≤30% of patients, novel stents that elute drugs (i.e., sirolimus and paclitaxel) into the vessel wall have recently reduced recurrence rates by 70 to 80% compared with bare metal stents (11–13). As a

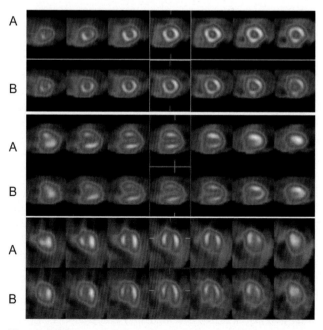

Figure 29.2 Exercise nuclear myocardial perfusion scan demonstrating anterior-apical perfusion defect at stress. **A.** Gated stress images. **B.** Gated rest images. (Courtesy of Marcelo F. Di Carli, Department of Nuclear Medicine, Brigham and Women's Hospital, Boston, MA.)

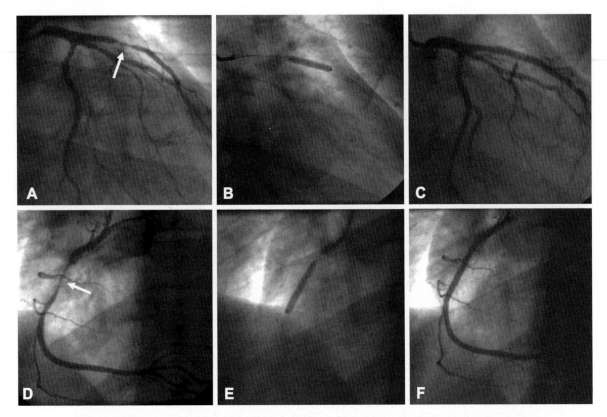

Figure 29.3 Coronary arteriography was performed and demonstrated two-vessel coronary artery disease. **A.** The midsegment of the LAD had a 90% stenosis that was concentric and tubular *(arrow)*. **B.** The mid-LAD was treated with a 3.5 mm × 23 mm Bx Velocity stent. **C.** This resulted in no residual stenosis and a step-up and step-down appearance indicating complete stent expansion. **D.** The midsegment of the mid-RCA had a diffuse 80% stenosis *(arrow)*. **E.** A 3.5 mm × 28 mm Bx Velocity stent was deployed in the midsegment. **F.** After stent placement, there was no residual stenosis and normal flow into the distal vessel.

result, there has been a paradigm shift toward the treatment of patients with complex, multivessel disease with drug-eluting stents rather than CABG (see Chapters 22 and 24). PCI was chosen in this nondiabetic patient because of the relatively focal stenoses treatable with bare metal stents. Although this procedure was performed prior to the availability of drug-eluting stents, a sustained long-term clinical benefit was achieved from stenting alone.

Medical Management

Following successful stenting, aspirin, 80 to 325 mg, should be given for 30 days to prevent subacute stent thrombosis, and then indefinitely for the secondary prevention of new MI. Clopidogrel, 75 mg daily, should also be given for 3 months after sirolimus-eluting stent placement (11–13) and for 6 months after paclitaxel-eluting stent placement. Extended clopidogrel up to nine months after PCI also reduces new ischemia events after PCI (14). Aggressive lipid-lowering therapy is indicated after PCI to prevent recurrent MIs (15). Beta-blocker therapy, ACE inhibition, and control of diabetes are also indicated in patients with established CAD after PCI.

ST-SEGMENT ELEVATION MYOCARDIAL INFARCTION (STEMI)

Case 2. A 60-year-old obese smoker was in good health until she developed substernal chest pain 3 days prior to admission; the pain lasted for 20 minutes and then resolved spontaneously. Two hours prior to admission, the patient's pain recurred, and she presented to the emergency department where electrocardiography showed ST-segment elevation in the inferior leads (Fig. 29.4). The patient was immediately given aspirin, unfractionated heparin, 5,000 units, and intravenous eptifibatide, 180 micrograms followed by a 2.0 μg/kg per minute infusion. Cardiac catheterization demonstrated a total occlusion of a large left circumflex coronary artery (Fig. 29.5). After wire crossing, the patient developed an elevated idioventricular rhythm (Fig. 29.6) associated with a fall in the systemic blood pressure from 134/82 mm Hg to 88/60 mm Hg. This rhythm was managed with fluid resuscitation and spontaneously reverted to normal sinus rhythm after 20 minutes. The left circumflex was predilated with a 2.5-mm balloon and was stented with a 3.5 mm × 33 mm sirolimus-eluting stent. Postdilatation was performed

A

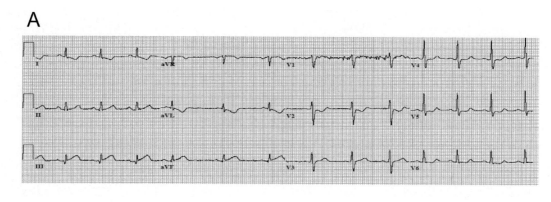

B

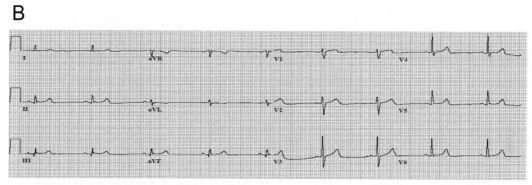

Figure 29.4 Inferior ST elevation myocardial infarction on ECG. **A.** On presentation with an acute inferior infarction, there are ST elevations in the inferior leads and T-wave inversions in the lateral leads. **B.** After percutaneous intervention of the large left circumflex, the ST segments normalize on the ECG.

using a 3.5-mm balloon, resulting in no residual stenosis and TIMI 3 flow into the distal vessel.

Indications for Coronary Arteriography and Percutaneous Revascularization

Primary PCI is more effective than thrombolytic therapy for the treatment of STEMI (see Chapter 22). A meta-analysis of 23 randomized trials showed that primary PCI reduce short-term mortality (7% versus 9% in thrombolytic patients; $P < .0002$), nonfatal reinfarction (3% versus 7% in thrombolytic patients; $P < .0001$), and the occurrence of stroke (1% versus 2% in thrombolytic patients; $P < .0004$; 16). These benefits have also been extended to bare metal and drug-eluting stents (17,18). Accordingly, ACC/AHA Class I recommendations for PCI as an alternative to thrombolytic therapy for STEMI include patients who can undergo PCI within 12 hours of symptom onset (or >12 hours if symptoms persist) by skilled operators (>75 cases per year) at institutions proficient in the performance of PCI (4,19). Recent studies have also shown that PCI for STEMI can be performed at institutions without on-site surgical facilities, provided careful selection criteria are followed and it is performed by experienced operators (20,21).

Technical Considerations

The "door-to-balloon" time is the most critical component of the invasive management of STEMI patients, and the

catheterization laboratory should be aware of the adage, "time is muscle" (22). Coronary arteriography of the non–infarct-related artery should be first performed, and a guiding catheter should be used for infarct-related artery angiography in anticipation of immediate PCI. In this case, the large distal left circumflex rather than the right coronary artery was the genesis of the inferior ST-segment elevation. The occlusion is generally soft, and a 0.014-inch soft-tipped wire should be tried initially. Once the occlusion is crossed, it is important to document the intraluminal position of the wire. There is usually a trickle of flow after wire crossing, or the balloon may be advanced and withdrawn in its deflated state to "Dotter" enough opening to permit distal contrast flow. Alternatively, a contrast injection may be performed through the distal tip of the coronary balloon catheter after it crosses the point of occlusion to document correct distal wire position. Reperfusion arrhythmias, including accelerated idioventricular rhythm and bradycardia, may occur with re-establishment of coronary perfusion, particularly with reperfusion of the right coronary artery. Atropine, 0.5 to 1.0 mg intravenously, and intravenous dopamine may be useful for rhythm and pressure support. Because laminar thrombus may not be appreciated by conventional angiography, it is important to size coronary stents appropriately to ensure complete stent strut apposition to the vessel wall. This is particularly true with the use of drug-eluting stents that require complete stent strut apposition for their antirestenotic effects.

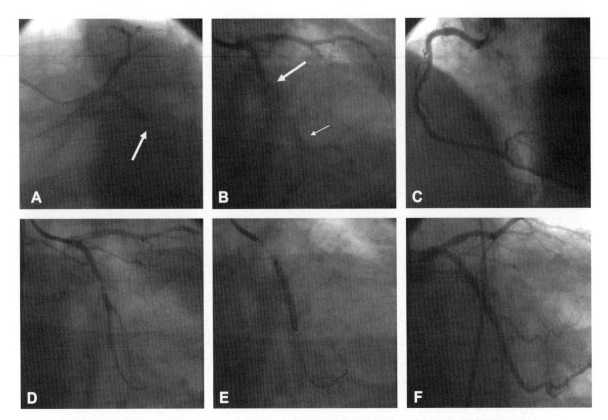

Figure 29.5 ST-segment elevation myocardial infarction. **A.** Although the EKG changes were located in the inferolateral leads, coronary arteriography demonstrated an occlusion of the midleft circumflex coronary artery *(arrow)*. **B.** A right anterior oblique projection with caudal angulation demonstrated the occlusion *(large arrow)* with faint filling into the distal left circumflex *(small arrow)*. **C.** The dominant right coronary artery had only minor lumen irregularities and was patent. **D.** After passage of a coronary guidewire across the coronary occlusion, reperfusion occurred. **E.** A 3.5 mm × 33 mm CYPHER stent was deployed in the midleft circumflex. **F.** The final angiogram demonstrated normal perfusion and no residual stenosis into a large left posterolateral branch. The EKG resolved to normal following coronary stenting.

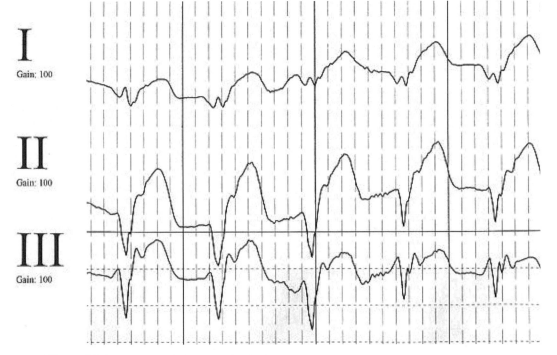

Figure 29.6 Accelerated idioventricular rhythm.

Medical Management

In patients with STEMI undergoing primary PCI, oral aspirin, 80 to 325 mg, and intravenous heparin should be given immediately with the diagnosis of STEMI. Pretreatment with clopidogrel may also be useful, but randomized trials in this setting are ongoing. Intravenous beta-blockers may be given to control hypertension and reduce recurrent ischemia. Glycoprotein IIb/IIIa (GP IIb/IIIa) inhibitors may also prevent recurrent ischemia, particularly if these agents can be administered prior to PCI (23,24).

NON–ST-SEGMENT ELEVATION MYOCARDIAL INFARCTION (NSTEMI)

Case 3. A 70-year-old man in good health developed substernal chest pressure at rest that was associated with shortness of breath. The baseline electrocardiogram on presentation to the emergency department demonstrated ST-segment depression in the anterior leads (Fig. 29.7). The troponin I was 0.6 mg per dL.

The patient was taken to the cardiac catheterization within 2 hours of presentation, and coronary arteriography demonstrated an ostial left anterior descending artery stenosis associated with TIMI 2 flow into the distal vessel (Fig. 29.8). Coronary stent placement using a 3.5 mm $\times$ 13 mm sirolimus-eluting CYPHER stent, resulting in no residual stenosis TIMI 3 flow into the distal vessel.

Indications for Coronary Arteriography and Percutaneous Revascularization

Coronary arteriography should be performed in patients who present with non-ST-elevation myocardial infarction or unstable angina (NSTEMI-UA) and who develop recurrent symptoms despite medical therapy or have markers of subsequent death or myocardial infarction (MI; 2) (see Chapter 11).

High-risk features include prolonged ongoing (>20 minutes) chest pain, pulmonary edema, worsening mitral regurgitation, dynamic ST-segment depression of 1 mm, elevated serum troponin levels, or hypotension. Intermediate- risk features include angina at rest (>20 minutes) relieved with rest or sublingual nitroglycerin, angina associated with dynamic ECG changes, recent-onset angina with a high likelihood of CAD, pathologic Q waves, ST-segment depression <1 mm in multiple leads, or age older than 65 years.

These recommendations are based on recent randomized clinical trials that suggest that many patients benefit from early revascularization by PCI or coronary bypass surgery (CABG), particularly in those with intermediate- and high-risk criteria for a recurrent infarction (2). These trials include the Fragmin and Fast Revascularization during InStability in Coronary artery disease (FRISC II) study (25), the Treat Angina with Aggrastat and Determine Cost of Therapy with an Invasive or Conservative Strategy (TACTICS-TIMI-18) study (26), and the British Heart Foundation Randomized Intervention Trial of Unstable Angina (RITA-3; 27). Collectively, these trials found that the occurrence of death and recurrent MI was lower in patients treated with a routine invasive strategy for cardiac catheterization and revascularization compared with patients in whom cardiac catheterization and revascularization was reserved for recurrent ischemia. The Intracoronary Stenting with Antithrombotic Regimen Cooling Off also found a benefit of an early (<6 hours) invasive strategy in 410 patients admitted with NSTEMI-UA who were randomized to a medical stabilization (aspirin, clopidogrel, tirofiban) for 72 to 120 hours before catheterization (median 86 hours) or to early intervention with intense antiplatelet coverage limited to <6 hours of pretreatment (median time to intervention: 2.4 hours). The 30-day composite event rate was significantly lower in patients with early intervention compared with those who were assigned to medical therapy before PCI (5.9% versus 11.6%, $P = .04$; 28). Subgroup analysis also showed

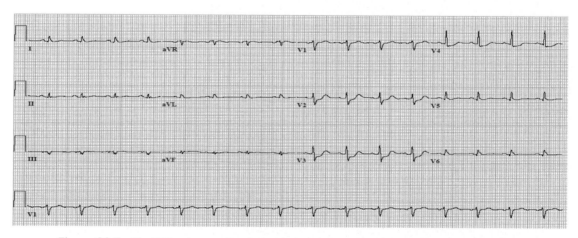

Figure 29.7 The EKG on presenting demonstrated anterior ST-segment depression in V_2-V_4 consistent with anterior wall ischemia.

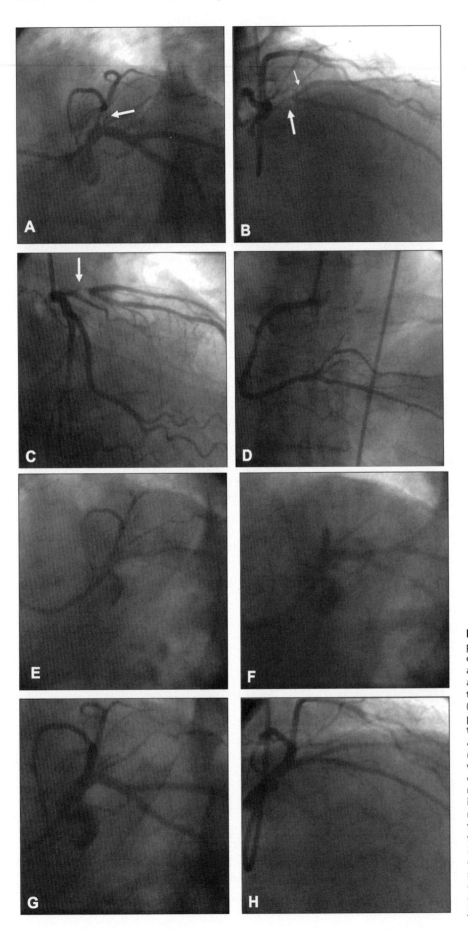

Figure 29.8 Coronary angiography in a patient with an anterior non–ST-segment elevation myocardial infarction. **A.** A left anterior oblique projection with caudal angulation demonstrates a 90% stenosis of the ostium of the left anterior descending (LAD; *arrow*). **B.** A right anterior oblique projection with cranial angulation shows the relationship of the stenosis *(large arrow)* to the origin of the diagonal branch *(small arrow)*. **C.** The right anterior oblique with caudal angulation also shows the ostial location of the LAD stenosis. **D.** The right coronary artery had only minor lumen irregularities in its midportion. **E.** A 3.5 mm × 13 mm CYPHER stent was placed in the origin of the LAD. **F.** Postdilatation of the stent was performed using a shorter 3.5-mm balloon. **G.** The left anterior oblique projection with caudal angulation shows the expansion of the stent without compromise of the side branch. **H.** This is confirmed in the right anterior oblique projection with cranial angulation.

consistent trends in favor of early intervention in patients who had positive troponin-T values, ST-segment depression, PCI, or CABG (28).

It should also be noted that patients with NSTEMI-UA can be treated safely with drug-eluting stents. The Rapamycin-Eluting Stent Evaluated At Rotterdam Cardiology Hospital (RESEARCH) registry compared 198 patients with NSTEMI-UA treated exclusively with drug-eluting stents with 301 patients with NSTEMI-UA treated with bare stents (29). The 30-day major adverse cardiac event rate was similar in both groups with stent thrombosis (29).

Technical Considerations

The ostial left anterior descending artery (LAD) and presence of a large, nondiseased diagonal branch with 15 mm of the LAD origin requires that the appropriate size and stent length be used to avoid compromise of the branch vessel. The angulation of the origin of the left circumflex was also favorable for ostial stent placement. Positioning of the stent is best performed in the left anterior oblique projection with caudal angulation, and 1 mm of stent can be left safely in the left main coronary artery to avoid inadequate coverage of the ostium. Postdilation should be performed to ensure complete stent expansion.

Medical Management

Patients with NSTEMI should be treated initially with aspirin, 75 to 325 mg, unfractionated or low–molecular-weight heparin, and a glycoprotein IIb/IIIa (GPIIb/IIIa) inhibitor in high-risk patients, administered within minutes to hours of clinical presentation. Pretreatment with clopidogrel, 300 to 600 mg, may be useful in preventing MI, particularly if the catheterization is delayed >24 hours (2). Aggressive lipid-lowering therapy also appears beneficial in patients with acute coronary syndromes (15).

BIFURCATION DISEASE

Case 4. A 55-year-old woman smoker presents with increasing angina at a reduced workload. Exercise stress testing demonstrates lateral wall ischemia in the left circumflex distribution (Fig. 29.9). Coronary angiography demonstrates a complex stenosis of the left circumflex at the origin of the obtuse margin branch (Fig. 29.10). Both branches are predilated and the parent left circumflex is stented with a 3.5 mm × 23 mm stent. The obtuse margin branch is recrossed, and a kissing balloon inflation is performed, resulting in no residual stenosis and TIMI 3 flow into the parent and branch vessel.

Technical Considerations

Various techniques have been proposed for the treatment of bifurcation lesions, depending on the size of the daughter branch, the presence of a stenosis within the daughter branch, the angle of the origin of the daughter branch from

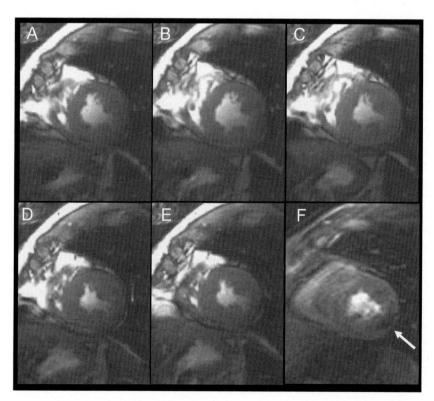

Figure 29.9 Dobutamine stress MRI demonstrating a lateral perfusion defect. **A.** At rest. **B–E.** Escalating dobutamine infusion with appropriate augmentation of all myocardial walls except for the basilar to midlateral wall. **F.** Perfusion imaging at peak dobutamine stress revealed a basilar to midlateral wall transmural perfusion defect *(arrow)*. (Courtesy of Raymond Kwong, M.D., Cardiovascular Imaging, Brigham and Women's Hospital, Boston, MA.)

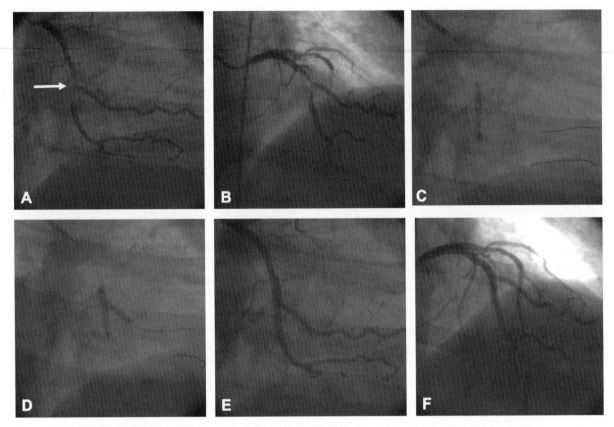

Figure 29.10 **A.** A right anterior oblique projection with caudal angulation demonstrates a 90% stenosis of the left circumflex at proximal and distal to the origin of a large obtuse marginal branch. **B.** A right anterior oblique projection with cranial angulation confirms the relationship of the circumflex stenosis and the obtuse marginal branch stenosis. **C.** A 3.5 mm × 23 mm stent was placed within the left circumflex. **D.** A simultaneous kissing balloon inflation was then performed with a 3.0-mm balloon in both the obtuse marginal branch and a left circumflex. **E.** The stent is well expanded and the side branch patent after stent placement. **F.** This is confirmed in a second view.

the parent vessel, and the presence of calcification within the bifurcation lesion. A primary concern in the treatment of bifurcation lesions is side-branch occlusion or compromise owing to "snowplow" shifting of plaque from the parent vessel lesion into the ostium of the daughter vessel. Treatment strategies to remove some of the plaque (debulking) have improved outcomes compared with balloon angioplasty alone (30). (See Chapter 22). However, with the advent of drug-eluting coronary stents (31), the treatment strategies have become more complex in an attempt to cover the entire bifurcation lesion with stent(s). (See Chapter 24). Depending on the specific anatomy, T-stenting, culotte stenting, V-stenting, Y-stenting, simultaneous kissing stents, and crush stenting may be used (32–34). Several studies suggest that routine stenting of both branches provides no incremental benefit over bailout stenting in the event of side-branch occlusion (35,36). If stents are placed in both the parent and daughter branch using any of these approaches, a final kissing balloon inflation does appear to reduce the late recurrence rate by simultaneously expanding the stents in both branches (33).

SAPHENOUS VEIN GRAFT DISEASE

Case 5. A 60-year-old man with a history of coronary artery disease and prior CABG presented with an acute inferior wall myocardial infarction. The EKG demonstrated an inferior wall myocardial infarction, manifest by ST-segment elevation of leads II, III, AvL (Fig. 29.11). Coronary arteriography demonstrated a patent left internal mammary artery (LIMA) to the LAD, patent SVG to the obtuse marginal and diagonal branches, an ostial left main and RCA occlusions, and a recently occluded SVG to the posterior descending artery (PDA; Fig. 29.12). The occluded SVG to the PDA was crossed with a 0.014-inch BMW wire, and a distal injection demonstrated abundant thrombus and a focal stenosis in the midportion of the SVG. A 0.014-inch FilterWire EZ (Boston Scientific, Natick, MA) was placed across the stenosis, and the FilterWire was deployed in a smooth portion of the SVG. A 5F AngioJet XVG catheter was used to remove the residual thrombus. Following this, two 3.5 mm × 33 CYPHER stents were placed in the proximal and mid SVG. The SVG was postdilated with a 4.0-mm postdilatation balloon. The FilterWire was then

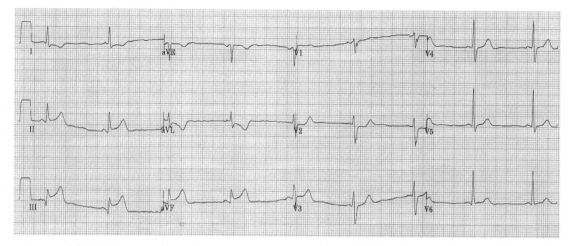

Figure 29.11 ECG demonstrating acute inferior ST elevation myocardial infarction.

removed, and normal flow was found in the distal RCA and its branches.

Indications for Coronary Arteriography and Percutaneous Revascularization

Even with excellent surgical techniques, SVGs are at risk for deterioration owing to progressive degeneration in the higher-pressure arterial environment. It is thus estimated that >50% of SVGs become diseased or occlude within the first decade after CABG. Repeat CABG for SVG failure, particularly when there is a patent LIMA to the LAD, is associated with lower success rates and less symptomatic benefit than the initial procedure. One recent series has suggested that PCI is preferable to repeat CABG in patients who develop recurrent symptoms after the first procedure (37).

Technical Considerations

The procedural success rate after balloon angioplasty of SVG lesions ranges from 84 to 92% (38–40), depending in part on the presence of graft degeneration, lesion location, and graft age of 36 months (38). The long-term success is limited by a high rate of restenosis or occlusion, even with the use of bare metal stents (41–44). In this case, a totally occluded graft was treated with distal protection, thrombectomy, and drug-eluting stents, techniques that may improve the long-term patency of these high-risk subjects, although long-term studies are limited in patients treated with drug-eluting stents.

The major risk of SVG intervention is the occurrence of distal embolization (45). Microvascular (arteriolar) spasm and dislodgement of platelet aggregates are also causes of periprocedural myocardial infarction (MI). Although glycoprotein IIb/IIIa inhibitors do not reduce embolic complications in patients with SVG intervention, embolic protection devices have been shown to reduce the incidence of these complications (see Chapters 22 and 23).

The degree of risk for embolization relates to the extent of SVG degeneration, which includes an estimate of the percentage of graft irregularity and ectasia, friability, presence of thrombus, and number of discrete or diffuse lesions (>50% stenosis) located within the graft. Although atherectomy and thrombectomy have been tried to prevent embolization (46), only the use of a distal protection device has resulted in a reduction of clinical events.

Two general classes of embolic protection devices have been approved for clinical use: occlusion systems that use a low-pressure balloon to occlude flow during intervention, and embolic entrapment filters that permit flow through the SVG during intervention but capture the debris within the distal filter. The PercuSurge Guardwire (Medtronic Vascular, Santa Rosa, CA) device is a low-profile system (0.014-inch guidewire) with a balloon that is inflated at low pressures to occlude flow once it is positioned distal to the target lesion (47). Any debris liberated by intervention remains trapped in the stagnant column of blood and is subsequently aspirated with a different catheter before the occlusion balloon is deflated to restore antegrade flow (47). The 801-patient SAFER trial, in which patients undergoing SVG intervention were randomized to stenting using this distal protection device versus a conventional guidewire, demonstrated a substantial reduction in 30-day major adverse clinical events (16.9 to 9.6%) and no reflow (8.3 to 3.3%) using the device (47). The EPI FilterWire (Boston Scientific, Natick, MA) is a 0.014-inch wire with a nitinol wire loop at its distal tip that contains an elliptical polyurethane filter with 100-micron pores. The FilterWire is delivered and removed with a 3.9F delivery and removal catheter. The FilterWire was compared with the PercuSurge Guardwire distal occlusion device in a randomized 656-patient trial. The distal filter was noninferior (equivalent or better) than the distal occlusion device with respect to 30-day major adverse cardiac events and thus is an acceptable

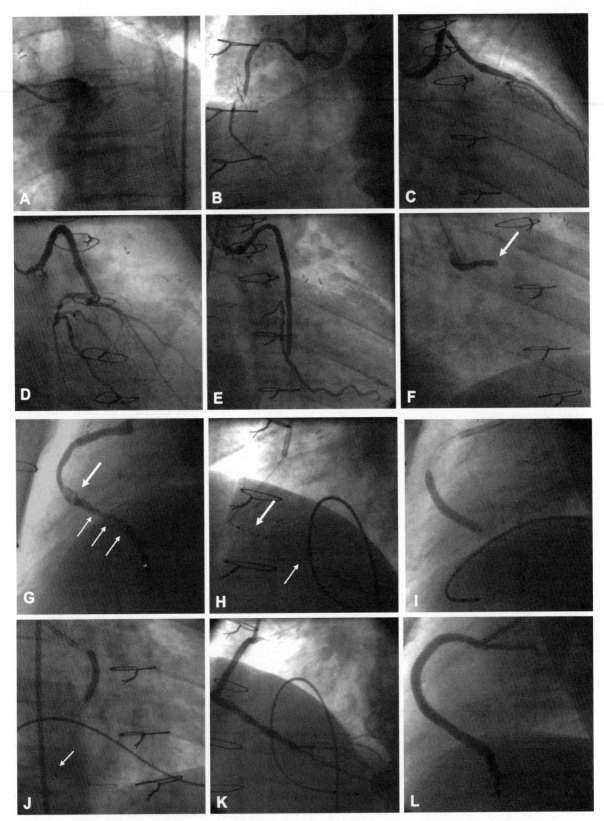

Figure 29.12 Saphenous vein graft intervention. **A.** The left main coronary artery is occluded at its origin. **B.** The right coronary artery is occluded and fills faintly by right-to-right bridging collaterals. **C.** A SVG to the diagonal branch is patent. **D.** A SVG to the ramus branch is patent. **E.** A SVG to an obtuse marginal branch is patient. **F.** The SVG to the posterior descending branch is acutely occluded *(arrow)*. **G.** After wire recanalization, a large thrombus is seen in the midsegment of the SVG *(large arrow)* that extends more distally within the SVG *(small arrows)*. **H.** An XVG AngioJet catheter *(large arrow)* is used to remove the thrombus after placement of a distal protection FilterWire *(small arrow)*. **I.** A 3.5 mm × 33 CYPHER stent is placed in the distal portion of the SVG. **J.** Another 3.5 mm × 33 CYPHER stent is positioned in the proximal portion of the SVG. **K.** After removal of the FilterWire, the left anterior oblique projection demonstrates patency of a cascade of posterior descending and posterolateral branches. **L.** Complete stent expansion is confirmed in the left lateral projection.

alternative (48). Given our inability to predict which patients will develop an embolic complication, embolic protection devices should be used in all suitable patients undergoing SVG intervention.

TOTAL CORONARY OCCLUSION

Case 6. A 59-year-old man with premature CAD, prior CABG, and multiple prior PCIs of the native vessel presented with severe exertional angina that developed with exercise and was relieved with rest, despite maximum medical therapy. Exercise stress testing demonstrated reversible inferior wall ischemia (Fig. 29.13). Coronary arteriography demonstrated a patent left internal mammary artery to the LAD and occluded SVGs to the diagonal branch and posterior descending branches. The native left coronary artery had a patent left circumflex coronary artery and diffuse disease of the LAD and diagonal branches. The right coronary artery was ectatic and was patent to the posterior descending artery. Just distal to the crux, there was a total occlusion of the distal continuation of the RCA (Fig. 29.14). A large right posterolateral branch was filled by left-to-right and right-to-left collaterals. Conventional coronary guidewires were unsuccessful in crossing the occlusion. The Intraluminal Therapeutics Safe Steer RF coronary guidewire was then used to cross the occlusion using optical coherence reflectometry guidance to confirm the intraluminal position of the guidewire and radiofrequency energy to cross the occluded segment (see Chapter 22). Once successful wire crossing was obtained, coronary stent placement was performed with normal flow into the large posterolateral branch.

Indications for Coronary Arteriography and Percutaneous Revascularization

Chronic total occlusions (CTOs) are present in 20 to 40% of patients undergoing angiography for the evaluation of CAD. The presence of a CTO is a frequent reason for referral to CABG in an effort to achieve a more complete revascularization. CTOs can cause severe effort angina because the distal myocardial bed may be viable owing to coronary collaterals. Effort angina occurs because the collaterals are inadequate to meet the increased oxygen requirement during exercise. Recanalization of CTOs has also been related to an improved late survival (49–52). A 10-year survival advantage associated with successful CTO treatment compared with failed CTO treatment (73.5 versus 65.1%; $P = .001$) was found in a study of 2,007 consecutive patients who underwent PCI for a CTO (50). When attempts at CTO intervention are unsuccessful, referral to coronary artery bypass surgery (CABG) becomes the sole remaining option.

Technical Considerations

Conventional angioplasty guidewires will successfully cross a CTO in 60 to 70% of patients, or more (53–56). In general, once the coronary guidewire is advanced into the distal lumen, coronary intervention can be completed with a combination of balloons and devices (see Chapter 22). Although debulking before stenting has a limited impact on late recurrence (57), excimer laser angioplasty or rotational atherectomy is occasionally required to facilitate advancement of balloons and stents across the occluded segment (58). Coronary stent placement has superior outcomes compared with balloon angioplasty alone for the

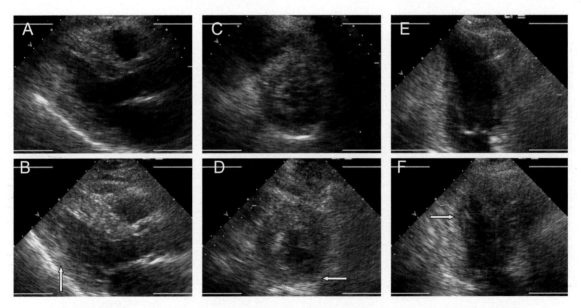

Figure 29.13 Stress echocardiogram demonstrating inferior-posterior hypokinesis with exercise. **A.** Parasternal long-axis rest. **B.** Parasternal long-axis stress. **C.** Parasternal short-axis rest. **D.** Parasternal short-axis stress. **E.** Apical two-chamber rest. **F.** Apical two-chamber stress. (Courtesy of Noninvasive Cardiac Laboratory, Brigham and Women's Hospital, Boston, MA.)

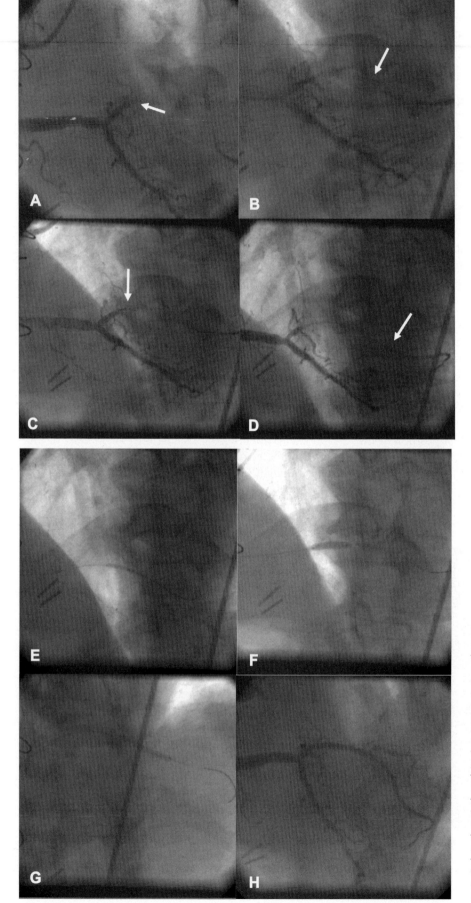

Figure 29.14 Recanalization of a total coronary occlusion. **A.** A flush occlusion of the distal continuation of the right coronary artery (arrow). **B.** Initial attempts at crossing the occlusion with a hydrophilic coronary guidewire result in the creation of a false lumen and parallel tract to the right posterolateral branch (arrow). **C.** The Intraluminal Therapeutics SafeSteer coronary guidewire was used to advance the wire into the true lumen using optical coherence reflectometry (arrow). **D.** Using this method, the guidewire is advanced into the distal portion of the right posterolateral branch. **E.** A 2.0-mm balloon was used to dilate the occlusion initially. **F.** This was followed by stent placement in the very distal right coronary artery. **G.** An additional balloon inflation was performed in the distal right posterolateral branch. **H.** The final angiographic result demonstrated no residual stenosis and normal flow into the distal vessel.

treatment of CTOs (59–65), and there is at least preliminary evidence that the use of drug-eluting stents reduces the late recurrence rate further (to <5%).

The inability to pass a guidewire through an occluded segment into the distal lumen is the major cause of failure in CTOs. If collaterals exist from a contralateral vessel, simultaneous injection may allow assessment of wire position in the distal lumen, particularly if ipsilateral collaterals are lost during advancement of the guidewire. Angiographic factors that predispose to failure to cross a chronic total occlusion include multivessel coronary artery disease (66) and unfavorable angiographic features including a blunt entry to the occlusion (67), long occlusions (67–69), presence of bridging collaterals (67,70), occlusion duration >180 days (67,69), and extensive calcification (68).

Better success in crossing chronic total occlusions has been achieved with stiffer, tapered-tip (to 0.010 inch), and hydrophilic-coated guidewires (68,71–74) advanced with extra support from a balloon catheter or small-caliber support catheter. Different guidewires may be helpful at different locations within the occlusion, using hydrophilic guidewires for coronary microchannels and stiffer-tipped guidewires to cross the distal fibrous cap of the occlusion. Although the risk for coronary perforation is increased with the use of these devices (75), the frequency of tamponade is <1 to 2%. The distal position of the wire should be confirmed using a distal contrast injection or visualization by collaterals before balloon inflation.

Several alternative devices have been evaluated as adjuncts to conventional wires in patients with CTOs (76), including the use of an excimer laser-tipped wire (77,78), the LuMend Front Runner (LuMend, Santa Clara, CA), 0.039-inch tipped by two blunt jaws, whose repetitive opening bluntly dissects across the occlusion (79), and the Safe-Cross wire (80). The Safe-Cross guidewire (Intraluminal Therapeutics, Carlsbad, CA) used in this case is a 0.014-inch guidewire containing a single optical fiber that carries a beam of low-coherence light. Optical coherence reflectometry (OCR) data discriminate whether plaque or organized vessel wall lie immediately ahead of the guidewire tip, and this information is used to decide whether to advance or redirect the wire tip (80–82). If only amorphous plaque is ahead of the wire, the reflection falls off rapidly, but if the tip of the wire is near the vessel wall, a secondary reflection from the organized collagen fibers is observed. If the fiber detects only plaque but cannot be advanced by mechanical force alone, the guidewire tip can be used to deliver a brief burst of radiofrequency energy to facilitate wire passage through the more fibrocalcific elements of the occlusion. In the Guided Radiofrequency Energy Ablation of Total Occlusion (GREAT) registry, 63 (54.3%) of 116 patients with CTOs refractory to conventional guidewire (10-minute fluoroscopy time attempt) were successfully recanalized with the Safe-Cross wire (80).

UNPROTECTED LEFT MAIN DISEASE

Case 7. A 70-year-old man with known severe occlusive peripheral vascular disease and chronic obstructive pulmonary disease (forced expiratory volume = 700 mL) developed pulmonary edema requiring intubation and ventilatory support. During an episode of atrial fibrillation with a rapid ventricular response, the patient developed deep precordial ST-segment depression and hypotension. Owing to ongoing ischemia despite maximal medical therapy and ongoing ventilator dependence, coronary arteriography was performed from the right radial approach. Diagnostic angiography demonstrated an 80% ostial left main disease (Fig. 29.15). Surgical consultation found that he was not a candidate for bypass owing to his severe pulmonary disease, and the left main lesion was corrected by balloon predilatation and implantation of a drug-eluting stent.

Indications for Coronary Arteriography and Revascularization

Patients with ongoing ischemia who are poor candidates for surgical revascularization can be considered for coronary arteriography and high-risk PCI.

Technical Considerations

The location of the stenosis within the left main coronary artery will generally determine the complexity of the PCI (see Chapters 22 and 24). Focal, ostial left main lesions can generally be treated with short, large-diameter stents with a minimum of peri-PCI ischemia. Coaxial guiding catheter support allows positioning of the proximal portion stent just 1 to 2 mm within the aorta and fully covering the ostial left main stenosis. Short, high-pressure balloon inflations minimize ischemia time and provide full stent expansion. Left main lesions involving the body and bifurcation of the left anterior descending (LAD) and left circumflex coronary artery generally require placing the distal portion of the stent within either the LAD, left circumflex, or both. In a series of 127 selected patients undergoing unprotected left main coronary artery stenting, angiographic restenosis was documented in 19 (19%) of 100 patients (83). The lumen diameter after stenting was significantly larger in the intravascular ultrasound (IVUS)-guided group ($P = .003$). The angiographic restenosis rate was significantly lower in the debulking/stenting group (8.3 versus 25%, $P = .034$). The reference artery size was the only independent predictor of angiographic restenosis. During 2-year follow-up, there were four deaths, but no nonfatal myocardial infarctions occurred. Recurrence rates have been improved with drug-eluting stents, but at this writing (see Chapter 24) unprotected left main intervention (especially of distal bifurcation lesions) should be reserved for patients who are at high risk for CABG.

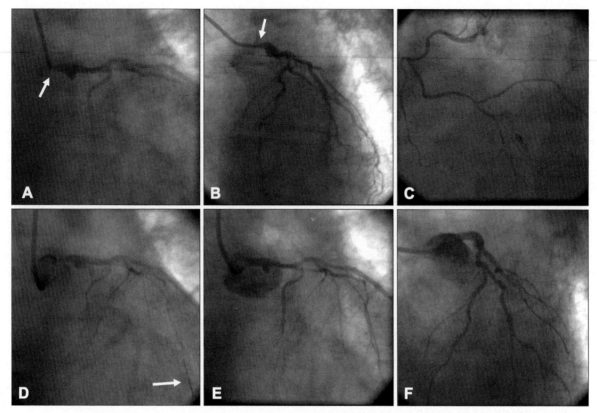

Figure 29.15 Unprotected left main intervention. **A.** A right anterior oblique projection demonstrates an 80% ostial stenosis of the origin of the left main coronary artery *(arrow).* **B.** The ostial left main stenosis is confirmed in the left anterior oblique with cranial angulation view *(arrow).* **C.** There is diffuse disease in the posterior descending artery. **D.** To avoid dampening, the guiding catheter is withdrawn into the aorta after the coronary guidewire is advanced into the distal left anterior descending. Stent positioning and deployment was performed with the guiding catheter withdrawn into the aorta. **E.** The right anterior oblique projection with caudal angulation shows full stent expansion in the left main. **F.** Stent expansion is confirmed in the left anterior oblique with cranial angulation.

The indications for coronary arteriography and revascularization will continue to evolve as newer techniques are developed. It is likely that the use of drug-eluting stents will be expanded into more complex patients and those with multivessel CAD, although the choice between catheter-based and surgical revascularization must be tailored for each patient based on clinical and angiographic features. Anticoagulation strategies (see Chapter 3) will also evolve with the addition of more novel regimens. In each case, the correction of the signal coronary lesion(s) must be followed by medical therapy to prevent stent thrombosis as well as aggressive lipid reduction and long-term aspirin to reduce the rate of lesion progression and new lesion development.

REFERENCES

1. Tuzcu E, Kapadia S, Tutar E, et al. High prevalence of coronary atherosclerosis in asymptomatic teenagers and young adults: evidence from intravascular ultrasound. *Circulation* 2001;103:2705–2710.
2. Braunwald E, Antman E, Beasley J, et al. ACC/AHA 2002 guideline update for the management of patients with unstable angina and non-ST-segment elevation myocardial infarction—summary article: a report of the American College of Cardiology/American Heart Association task force on practice guidelines (Committee on the Management of Patients With Unstable Angina). *J Am Coll Cardiol* 2002;40:1366–1374.
3. Scanlon P, Faxon D, Audet A, et al. ACC/AHA Guidelines for coronary angiography. *J Am Coll Cardiol* 1999;33:1756–1824.
4. Smith S, Dove J, Jacobs A, et al. ACC/AHA guidelines of percutaneous coronary interventions (revision of the 1993 PTCA guidelines)—executive summary. A report of the American College of Cardiology/American Heart Association Task Force on Practice Guidelines (committee to revise the 1993 guidelines for percutaneous transluminal coronary angioplasty). *J Am Coll Cardiol* 2001;37:2215–2239.
5. Parisi A, Folland E, Hartigan P. A comparison of angioplasty with medical therapy in the treatment of single-vessel coronary artery disease. Veterans Affairs ACME Investigators. *N Engl J Med* 1992;326:10–16.
6. Pitt B, Waters D, Brown W. Aggressive lipid lowering compared with angioplasty in stable coronary artery disease. *N Engl J Med* 1999;341:70–76.
7. RITA-2. Coronary angioplasty versus medical therapy: the second Randomised Intervention Treatment of Angina (RITA-2) trial. *Lancet* 1997;350:461–468.
8. Davies R, Goldberg A, Forman S. Asymptomatic Cardiac Ischemia Pilot (ACIP) study two-year follow-up: outcomes of patients randomized to initial strategies of medical therapy versus revascularization. *Circulation* 1997;95:2037–2043.
9. Pocock S, Henderson R, Rickards A, et al. Meta-analysis of randomized trials comparing coronary angioplasty with bypass surgery. *Lancet* 1995;346:1184–1189.

10. BARI Investigators. Influence of diabetes on 5-year mortality and morbidity in a randomized trial comparing CABG and PTCA in patients with multivessel disease: the Bypass Angioplasty Revascularization Investigation (BARI). *Circulation* 1997;96:1761–1769.

11. Moses J, Leon M, Popma J, et al. Sirolimus-eluting stents versus standard stents in patients with stenosis in a native coronary artery. *N Engl J Med* 2003;349:1315–1323.

12. Schofer J, Schluter M, Gershlick A, et al. Sirolimus-eluting stents for treatment of patients with long atherosclerotic lesions in small coronary arteries: double-blind, randomised controlled trial (E-SIRIUS). *Lancet* 2003;362:1093–1099.

13. Stone G, Ellis S, Cox D, et al. A polymer-based, paclitaxel-eluting stent in patients with coronary artery disease. *N Engl J Med* 2004;350:221–231.

14. Steinhubl S, Berger P, Mann J, et al. Early and sustained dual oral antiplatelet therapy following percutaneous coronary intervention: a randomized controlled trial. *JAMA* 2002;288:2411–2420.

15. Cannon C, Braunwald E, McCabe C, et al. Intensive versus moderate lipid lowering with statins after acute coronary syndromes. *N Engl J Med* 2004;350:1495–1504.

16. Keeley E, Grines C. Primary coronary intervention for acute myocardial infarction. *JAMA* 2004;291:736–739.

17. Schomig A, Kastrati A, Dirschinger J, et al. Coronary stenting plus platelet glycoprotein IIb/IIIa blockade compared with tissue plasminogen activator in acute myocardial infarction. Stent versus Thrombolysis for Occluded Coronary Arteries in Patients with Acute Myocardial Infarction Study Investigators. *N Engl J Med* 2000;343:385–391.

18. Kastrati A, Mehilli J, Dirschinger J, et al. Myocardial salvage after coronary stenting plus abciximab versus fibrinolysis plus abciximab in patients with acute myocardial infarction: a randomised trial. *Lancet* 2002;359:920–925.

19. Ryan T, Antman E, Brooks N, et al. 1999 Update: ACC/AHA guidelines for the management of patients with acute myocardial infarction. *J Am Coll Cardiol* 1999;34:889–911.

20. Aversano T, Aversano L, Passamani E, et al. Thrombolytic therapy vs primary percutaneous coronary intervention for myocardial infarction in patients presenting to hospitals without on-site cardiac surgery: a randomized controlled trial. *JAMA* 2002;287:1943–1951.

21. Wharton T, McNamara N, Fedele F, Jacobs M, Gladstone A, Funk E. Primary angioplasty for the treatment of acute myocardial infarction: experience at two community hospitals without cardiac surgery. *J Am Coll Cardiol* 1999;33:1257–1265.

22. Nallamothu B, Bates E. Percutaneous coronary intervention versus fibrinolytic therapy in acute myocardial infarction: is timing (almost) everything? *Am J Cardiol* 2003;92:824–826.

23. Montalescot G, Barragan P, Wittenberg O, et al. Platelet glycoprotein IIb/IIIa inhibition with coronary stenting for acute myocardial infarction. *N Engl J Med* 2001;344:1895–1903.

24. Stone G, Grines C, Cox D, et al. Comparison of angioplasty with stenting, with or without abciximab, in acute myocardial infarction. *N Engl J Med* 2002;346:957–966.

25. FRISC II. Invasive compared with non-invasive treatment in unstable coronary artery disease: FRISC II prospective randomised multcentre study. *Lancet* 1999;354:708–715.

26. Cannon C, Weintraub W, Demopoulos L, et al. Comparison of early invasive and conservative strategies in patients with unstable coronary syndromes treated with the glycoprotein IIb/IIIa inhibitor tirofiban. *N Engl J Med* 2001;344:1879–1887.

27. Fox K, Poole-Wilson P, Henderson R, et al. Interventional versus conservative treatment for patients with unstable angina or non-ST-elevation myocardial infarction: the British Heart Foundation RITA 3 randomised trial. Randomized Intervention Trial of unstable Angina. *Lancet* 2002;360:743–751.

28. Neumann F, Kastrati A, Pogatsa-Murray G, et al. Evaluation of prolonged antithrombotic pretreatment ("cooling-off" strategy) before intervention in patients with unstable coronary syndromes: a randomized controlled trial. *JAMA* 2003;290:1593–1599.

29. Lemos P, Lee C, Degertekin M, et al. Early outcome after sirolimus-eluting stent implantation in patients with acute coronary syndromes. Insights from the Rapamycin-Eluting Stent Evaluated At Rotterdam Cardiology Hospital (RESEARCH) registry. *J Am Coll Cardiol* 2003;41:2093–2099.

30. Dauerman HL, Baim DS, Cutlip DE, et al. Mechanical debulking versus balloon angioplasty for the treatment of diffuse in-stent restenosis. *Am J Cardiol* 1998;82:277–284.

31. Tanabe K, Serruys P, Degertekin M, et al. Fate of side branches after coronary arterial sirolimus-eluting stent implantation. *Am J Cardiol* 2002;90:937–941.

32. Di Mario C, Airoldi F, Reimers B, Anzuini A, Vilas DA, Colombo A. Bifurcational stenting. *Semin Intervent Cardiol* 1998;3:65–76.

33. Lefevre T, Louvard Y, Morice M, et al. Stenting of bifurcation lesions: classification, treatments, and results. *Cathet Cardiovasc Intervent* 2000;49:274–283.

34. Melikian N, Di Mario C. Treatment of bifurcation coronary lesions: a review of current techniques and outcome. *J Intervent Cardiol* 2003;16:507–513.

35. Al SJ, Berger P, Rihal C, et al. Immediate and long-term outcome of intracoronary stent implantation for true bifurcation lesions. *J Am Coll Cardiol* 2000;35:929–936.

36. Yamashita T, Nishida T, Adamian M, et al. Bifurcation lesions: two stents versus one stent—immediate and follow-up results. *J Am Coll Cardiol* 2000;35:1145–1151.

37. Morrison D, Sethi G, Sacks J, et al. Percutaneous coronary intervention versus repeat bypass surgery for patients with medically refractory myocardial ischemia: AWESOME randomized trial and registry experience with post-CABG patients. *J Am Coll Cardiol* 2002;40:1951–1954.

38. Platko W, Hollman J, Whitlow P, Franco I. Percutaneous transluminal angioplasty of saphenous vein graft stenosis: long-term follow-up. *J Am Coll Cardiol* 1989;14:1645–1650.

39. Webb J, Myler R, Shaw R, et al. Coronary angioplasty after coronary bypass surgery: Initial results and late outcome in 422 patients. *J Am Coll Cardiol* 1990;16:812–820.

40. Cote G, Myler R, Stertzer S, et al. Percutaneous transluminal angioplasty of stenotic coronary artery bypass grafts: 5 years' experience. *J Am Coll Cardiol* 1987;9:8–17.

41. Wong SC, Popma JJ, Pichard AD, et al. Comparison of clinical and angiographic outcomes after saphenous vein graft angioplasty using coronary versus 'biliary' tubular slotted stents. *Circulation* 1995;91:339–350.

42. Brener SJ, Ellis SG, Apperson-Hansen C, Leon MB, Topol EJ. Comparison of stenting and balloon angioplasty for narrowings in aortocoronary saphenous vein conduits in place for more than five years. *Am J Cardiol* 1997;79:13–18.

43. Savage MP, Douglas JS Jr, Fischman DL, et al. Stent placement compared with balloon angioplasty for obstructed coronary bypass grafts. Saphenous Vein De Novo Trial Investigators. *N Engl J Med* 1997;337:740–747.

44. Bhargava N, Kornowski R, Mehran R, et al. Procedural results and intermediate clinical outcomes after multiple saphenous vein graft stenting. *J Am Coll Cardiol* 2000;35:389–397.

45. Aueron F, Gruentzig A. Distal embolization of a coronary artery bypass graft atheroma during percutaneous transluminal coronary angioplasty. *Am J Cardiol* 1984;53:953–954.

46. Baumbach A, Oswald H, Kvasnicka J, et al. Clinical results of coronary excimer laser angioplasty: report from the European Coronary Excimer Laser Angioplasty Registry. *Eur Heart J* 1994;15:89–96.

47. Baim D, Wahr D, George B, et al. Randomized trial of a distal embolic protection device during percutaneous intervention of saphenous vein aorto-coronary bypass grafts. *Circulation* 2002;105:1285–1290.

48. Stone G, Rogers C, Ramee S, et al. Distal filter protection during saphenous vein graft stenting: technical and clinical correlates of efficacy. *J Am Coll Cardiol* 2002;40:1882–1888.

49. Yousef Z, Redwood S, Bucknall C, Sulke A, Marber M. Late intervention after anterior myocardial infarction: effects on left ventricular size, function, quality of life, and exercise tolerance: results of the Open Artery Trial (TOAT Study). *J Am Coll Cardiol* 2002;40:869–876.

50. Suero J, Marso S, Jones P, et al. Procedural outcomes and long-term survival among patients undergoing percutaneous coronary intervention of a chronic total occlusion in native coronary arteries: a 20-year experience. *J Am Coll Cardiol* 2001;38:409–414.

51. Dzavik V, Beanlands D, Davies R, et al. Effects of late percutaneous transluminal coronary angioplasty of an occluded infarct-related coronary artery on left ventricular function in patients with a recent (<6 weeks) Q-wave acute myocardial infarction (Total Occlusion Post-Myocardial Infarction Intervention Study [TOMIIS]—a pilot study). *Am J Cardiol* 1994;73:856–861.

52. Olivari Z, Rubartelli P, Piscione F, et al. Immediate results and one-year clinical outcome after percutaneous coronary interventions in chronic total occlusions: data from a multicenter, prospective, observational study (TOAST-GISE). *J Am Coll Cardiol* 2003;41:1672–1678.

53. Puma J, Sketch M, Tcheng J, et al. Percutaneous revascularization of chronic coronary occlusions: an overview. *J Am Coll Cardiol* 1995;26:1–11.

54. Ruocco N, Ring M, Holubkov R, Jacobs A, Detre K, Faxon D. Results of coronary angioplasty of chronic total occlusions (the National Heart, Lung, and Blood Institute 1985–1986 Percutaneous Transluminal Angioplasty Registry). *Am J Cardiol* 1992;69:69–76.

55. Bell MR, Berger PB, Bresnahan JF, Reeder GS, Bailey KR, Holmes DR Jr. Initial and long-term outcome of 354 patients after coronary balloon angioplasty of total coronary artery occlusions. *Circulation* 1992;85:1003–1011.

56. Safian R, McCabe C, Sipperly M, McKay R, Baim D. Initial success and long-term follow-up of percutaneous transluminal coronary angioplasty in chronic total occlusions versus conventional stenoses. *Am J Cardiol* 1988;61:23G–28G.

57. Gruberg L, Mehran R, Dangas G, et al. Effect of plaque debulking and stenting on short- and long-term outcomes after revascularization of chronic total occlusions. *J Am Coll Cardiol* 2000;35: 151–156.

58. Werner G, Buchwald A, Unterberg C, Voth E, Kreuzer H, Wiegand V. Recanalization of chronic total coronary arterial occlusions by percutaneous excimer-laser and laser-assisted angioplasty. *Am J Cardiol* 1990;66:1445–1450.

59. Sirnes P, Golf S, Myreng Y, et al. Stenting in Chronic Coronary Occlusion (SICCO): a randomized, controlled trial of adding stent implantation after successful angioplasty. *J Am Coll Cardiol* 1996;28:1444–1451.

60. Sirnes PA, Golf S, Myreng Y, et al. Sustained benefit of stenting chronic coronary occlusion: long-term clinical follow-up of the Stenting in Chronic Coronary Occlusion (SICCO) study. *J Am Coll Cardiol* 1998;32:305–310.

61. Buller C, Dzavik V, Carere R, et al. Primary stenting versus balloon angioplasty in occluded coronary arteries: the Total Occlusion Study of Canada (TOSCA). *Circulation* 1999;100:236–242.

62. Rubartelli P, Verna E, Niccoli L, et al. Coronary stent implantation is superior to balloon angioplasty for chronic coronary occlusions: six-year clinical follow-up of the GISSOC trial. *J Am Coll Cardiol* 2003;41:1488–1492.

63. Rubartelli P, Niccoli L, Verna E, et al. Stent implantation versus balloon angioplasty in chronic coronary occlusions: results from the GISSOC trial. Gruppo Italiano di Studio sullo Stent nelle Occlusioni Coronariche. *J Am Coll Cardiol* 1998;32:90–96.

64. Hoher M, Wohrle J, Grebe O, et al. A randomized trial of elective stenting after balloon recanalization of chronic total occlusions. *J Am Coll Cardiol* 1999;34:722–729.

65. Goldberg SL, Colombo A, Maiello L, Borrione M, Finci L, Almagor Y. Intracoronary stent insertion after balloon angioplasty of chronic total occlusions. *J Am Coll Cardiol* 1995;26: 713–719.

66. Ivanhoe RJ, Weintraub WS, Douglas JS Jr, et al. Percutaneous transluminal coronary angioplasty of chronic total occlusions. Primary success, restenosis, and long-term clinical follow-up. *Circulation* 1992;85:106–115.

67. Maiello L, Colombo A, Gianrossi R, et al. Coronary angioplasty of chronic occlusions: factors predictive of procedural success. *Am Heart J* 1992;124:581–584.

68. Noguchi T, Miyazaki MS, Morii I, Daikoku S, Goto Y, Nonogi H. Percutaneous transluminal coronary angioplasty of chronic total occlusions. Determinants of primary success and long-term clinical outcome. *Cathet Cardiovasc Intervent* 2000;49:258–264.

69. Stone GW, Rutherford BD, McConahay DR, et al. Procedural outcome of angioplasty for total coronary artery occlusion: an analysis of 971 lesions in 905 patients. *J Am Coll Cardiol* 1990;15: 849–856.

70. Kinoshita I, Katoh O, Nariyama J, et al. Coronary angioplasty of chronic total occlusions with bridging collateral vessels: immediate and follow-up outcome from a large single-center experience. *J Am Coll Cardiol* 1995;26:409–415.

71. Lefevre T, Louvard Y, Loubeyre C, et al. A randomized study comparing two guidewire strategies for angioplasty of chronic total coronary occlusion. *Am J Cardiol* 2000;85:1144–1147, A9.

72. Saito S, Tanaka S, Hiroe Y, et al. Angioplasty for chronic total occlusion by using tapered-tip guidewires. *Cathet Cardiovasc Intervent* 2003;59:305–311.

73. Corcos T, Favereau X, Guerin Y, et al. Recanalization of chronic coronary occlusions using a new hydrophilic guidewire. *Cathet Cardiovasc Diagn* 1998;44:83–90.

74. Bahl VK, Chandra S, Goswami KC, Manchanda SC. Crosswire for recanalization of total occlusive coronary arteries. *Cathet Cardiovasc Diagn* 1998;45:323–327; discussion 328.

75. Prati F, Di Mario C, Hamburger J, Gil R, von Birgelen C, Serruys P. Perforation of chronic total occlusion with laser guide wire followed by multiple stent deployment: usefulness of three-dimensional intracoronary ultrasound guidance. *Am Heart J* 1995; 130:1285–1289.

76. Turi Z. Total occlusion: old vs. new technology. *Cathet Cardiovasc Intervent* 2003;59:259–260.

77. Oesterle S, Bittl J, Leon M, et al. Laser wire for crossing chronic total occlusions: "learning phase" results from the U.S. TOTAL trial. Total Occlusion Trial With Angioplasty by Using a Laser Wire. *Cathet Cardiovasc Diagn* 1998;44:235–243.

78. Hamburger JN, Serruys PW, Scabra-Gomes R, et al. Recanalization of total coronary occlusions using a laser guidewire (the European TOTAL Surveillance Study). *Am J Cardiol* 1997;80:1419–1423.

79. Whitbourn R, Cincotta M, Mossop P, Selmon M. Intraluminal blunt microdissection for angioplasty of coronary chronic total occlusions. *Cathet Cardiovasc Intervent* 2003;58:194–198.

80. Baim D, Braden G, Heuser R, et al. Utility of the Safe-Cross-guided radiofrequency total occlusion crossing system in chronic coronary total occlusions (results from the Guided Radio Frequency Energy Ablation of Total Occlusions Registry Study). *Am J Cardiol* 2004;94:853–858.

81. Shammas N. Treatment of chronic total occlusions using optical coherent reflectometry and radiofrequency ablative energy: incremental success over conventional techniques. *J Invasive Cardiol* 2004;16:58–59.

82. Morales P, Heuser R. Chronic total occlusions: experience with fiber-optic guidance technology—optical coherence reflectometry. *J Intervent Cardiol* 2001;14:611–616.

83. Park S, Hong M, Lee C, et al. Elective stenting of unprotected left main coronary artery stenosis: effect of debulking before stenting and intravascular ultrasound guidance. *J Am Coll Cardiol* 2001;38: 1054–1060.

Profiles in Pulmonary Embolism and Pulmonary Hypertension

30

Samuel Z. Goldhaber　*Nils Kucher*　*Michael J. Landzberg*

Acute pulmonary embolism (PE) encompasses a wide spectrum of acuity, with varying prognoses and therapies. Most patients with acute PE maintain normal systolic arterial pressure and normal right ventricular function once therapeutic levels of anticoagulation are established. Unfortunately, some PE patients suffer clinical deterioration including death from right ventricular failure or the need for cardiopulmonary resuscitation, mechanical ventilation, pressors, thrombolysis, catheter thrombectomy, or surgical embolectomy (1).

Many patients with chronic thromboembolic hypertension (CTEPH) present with worsening dyspnea or fatigue and do not have a clear history of venous thromboembolism or an identifiable thrombophilic disorder. This condition often remains undiagnosed until an echocardiogram or chest computed tomogram (CT) shows right ventricular enlargement. Clinical outcome may improve with pulmonary thromboendarterectomy in combination with placement of a vena cava filter and indefinite-duration anticoagulation.

Most patients with idiopathic pulmonary arterial hypertension (IPAH) will suffer rapid clinical deterioration with right ventricular failure and death unless this condition is treated aggressively. Several new drugs are effective in improving symptoms and survival. This chapter will thus focus on diagnosis and management of patients with acute PE and pulmonary hypertension (see also Chapter 13).

ACUTE PULMONARY EMBOLISM

Diagnosis

Maintaining a high degree of clinical suspicion for PE is of paramount importance. The onset of symptoms may be sudden, gradual, or intermittent. The most common symptoms and signs are nonspecific: dyspnea, chest pain, tachypnea, and tachycardia. Usually, pulmonary embolism patients with pleuritic pain or hemoptysis have anatomically small emboli near the periphery of the lung, where nerve innervation is greatest and where pulmonary infarction is most likely to occur owing to poor collateral circulation. In contrast, patients with life-threatening PE often have a painless presentation characterized by profound dyspnea, syncope, or cyanosis.

PE should be suspected in a hypotensive patient when (1) there is evidence of, or there are predisposing factors for, venous thrombosis, and (2) there is clinical evidence of acute cor pulmonale (acute right ventricular failure) such as distended neck veins, an S3 gallop, a right ventricular heave, tachycardia, or tachypnea, especially if (3) there is electrocardiographic evidence of acute cor pulmonale manifested by a new S1-Q3-T3 pattern, new incomplete right bundle branch block, or right ventricular ischemia. Under such circumstances, a bedside echocardiogram is especially helpful.

Laboratory and Imaging Tests

Chest radiograph abnormalities include focal oligemia (Westermark sign), indicating massive central embolic occlusion, or a peripheral wedge-shaped density above the diaphragm (Hampton hump), indicating pulmonary infarction. An enlarged right descending pulmonary artery (Palla sign) is also a useful clue. Furthermore, the chest radiograph can help identify patients with other diseases, such as lobar pneumonia or pneumothorax, that can mimic pulmonary embolism.

The *electrocardiogram* helps to exclude acute myocardial infarction and to identify electrocardiographic manifestations of right-heart strain (2–4). The differential diagnosis of new right heart strain includes acute pulmonary embolism, acute asthma, or exacerbation of chronic bronchitis in patients with chronic obstructive pulmonary disease.

Unfortunately, the time-honored screening test of abnormal room air *arterial blood gases* is not helpful in triaging patients suspected of pulmonary embolism. Extensive analyses of the large PIOPED (Prospective Investigation of Pulmonary Embolism Diagnosis) database indicate that even sophisticated calculations of the alveolar-arterial oxygen difference do not differentiate patients with and without PE (5,6). Therefore, arterial blood gases should not be obtained as a screening test in patients suspected of pulmonary embolism.

An abnormally elevated level of enzyme-linked immunosorbent assay *(ELISA) plasma D-dimer* (>500 ng/mL) has a >90% sensitivity for identifying patients with PE proven by lung scan (7) or by angiogram (8). The plasma D-dimer is a specific derivative of cross-linked fibrin (Fig. 30.1). Although low plasma concentrations of D-dimers are sensitive for excluding PE, they are not specific. D-dimer levels remain elevated in patients for at least 1 week postoperatively and will also be abnormally high in patients with myocardial infarction, sepsis, or almost any other systemic illness. Therefore, the plasma D-dimer ELISA is best used in patients who present to the office or Emergency Department without coexisting acute systemic illness (9,10).

Ventilation-perfusion (V-Q) lung scanning has traditionally served as the principal diagnostic imaging test when the clinical suspicion for pulmonary embolism is high. The V-Q scan is most useful if it is clearly normal or if it demonstrates a pattern suggestive of a high probability for pulmonary embolism. Unfortunately, more than half of the patients with suspected PE have inconclusive scans (intermediate or low probability; 11). Currently, many institutions perform V-Q scanning only in patients with renal insufficiency, contrast allergy, or pregnancy.

Spiral chest CT scanning with contrast has virtually replaced lung scanning as the initial imaging test (12,12a). The latest generation of 16-slice detector scanners allows image acquisition with 1-mm resolution during a single breath-hold, enabling accurate detection of central, lobar, segmental, and subsegmental thrombi (13). Sensitivity and specificity for PE are >90% (14). The risk of recurrent venous thromboembolism in patients with suspected PE, in whom anticoagulation was withheld after a negative CT study, approximated 2% (15,15a). A similar recurrence rate has been reported in patients in whom anticoagulation was withheld after a negative pulmonary angiogram (16,17). Spiral chest CT is also useful for the rapid detection of alternative diagnoses, such as aortic dissection, pneumothorax, or pericardial tamponade.

Gadolinium-enhanced magnetic resonance (MR) angiography is accurate for PE diagnosis and avoids ionizing radiation or iodinated contrast agents. MR appears to be almost as sensitive and specific for PE as pulmonary angiography (18). However, in most institutions, MR has limited round-the-clock availability, and there is restricted monitoring, rendering this imaging modality unsuitable for hemodynamically unstable patients.

Venous ultrasound is usually accurate in diagnosing proximal leg deep venous thrombosis in *symptomatic outpatients* (19) and may serve as a useful surrogate for PE. However, almost two-thirds of PE patients have no venographic (20) or ultrasound evidence of leg deep venous thrombosis (21,22). Therefore, if clinical suspicion of pulmonary embolism is high, patients without clinical or imaging evidence of deep venous thrombosis should still be worked up for PE.

Echocardiography is most useful among hemodynamically unstable patients who appear to be too ill to be transported for an imaging study. If transthoracic echocardiographic images are technically inadequate, then transesophageal echocardiography may be considered (23). Rarely, echocardiography demonstrates a thrombus in the main pulmonary artery or at its proximal bifurcation. More often, bedside echocardiography will suggest PE if a constellation of findings indicates right heart failure, especially in the presence of regional systolic wall motion abnormalities (the McConnell

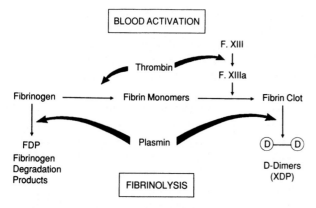

Figure 30.1 Plasma D-dimer is generated exclusively from plasmin breakdown of fibrin clot. The D-dimers can be measured by commercially available enzyme-linked immunosorbent assay (ELISA) kits. Plasma D-dimer ELISA is an excellent screening test for pulmonary embolism. Elevated levels are sensitive, and normal levels have a high negative predictive value for pulmonary embolism at angiography.

Sign; 24). In a patient with suspected massive PE and severe right ventricular dysfunction on the echocardiogram, initiation of reperfusion therapy, including thrombolysis, catheter fragmentation, or surgical embolectomy may be considered without obtaining time-consuming imaging tests (25). Echocardiography in this setting can also help to exclude other life-threatening conditions, such as ventricular septal rupture, aortic dissection, and pericardial tamponade. However, echocardiography is normal in about half of the patients with suspected PE and therefore is not a good screening test in hemodynamically stable patients.

Pulmonary angiography is warranted if the clinical suspicion for PE remains high after negative or equivocal noninvasive imaging studies, including contrast-enhanced chest CT, lung scanning, or venous ultrasound. The indications, technique, and complications of conventional pulmonary angiography are described in Chapter 13.

RISK STRATIFICATION

The classical approach for assessing risk in a PE patient has relied primarily on systemic arterial pressure. Patients with systolic blood pressure <90 mm Hg were started on pressors. If pressors failed to raise the systolic blood pressure to >90 mm Hg, thrombolysis or open surgical embolectomy was considered. This strategy delayed implementation of aggressive therapy. Consequently, patients had often passed the point of no return, with irreversible cardiogenic shock and multisystem organ failure. Contemporary risk stratification focuses on early detection of those patients who are at increased risk for adverse clinical events while

the systemic arterial pressure is preserved, prior to the development of cardiogenic shock (26).

On *physical examination*, tachycardia, tachypnea, and arterial hypotension suggest high risk. Clinical signs of right ventricular dysfunction include distended jugular veins, an accentuated pulmonic heart sound, a right ventricular heave, or a tricuspid regurgitation murmur.

The *Geneva Prognostic Index* (27) uses an eight-point scoring system and identifies clinical predictors of adverse clinical outcome: two points each for cancer and hypotension, and one point each for heart failure, prior DVT, arterial hypoxemia, and concomitant DVT. As points accumulate, prognosis worsens.

Although the *electrocardiogram* is neither sensitive nor specific for PE diagnosis, inverted T waves in the precordial leads and a QR pattern in V1 are strong predictors for adverse clinical events (3).

Echocardiography has emerged as the most important tool for risk assessment and treatment guidance because right ventricular dysfunction on the baseline echocardiogram is an independent predictor of early PE-related death (28). Right ventricular dysfunction is diagnosed in the presence of (1) right ventricular dilatation, defined as a right over left ventricular end-diastolic dimension ratio >0.6 in the parasternal view or >0.9 cm in the four-chamber view; (2) right ventricular systolic free wall hypokinesis; or (3) systolic pulmonary arterial hypertension, defined as a tricuspid regurgitant velocity >2.6 m/second (29). Indirect signs of right ventricular pressure overload are a flattened interventricular septum (Fig. 30.2), paradoxical systolic motion of the interventricular septum toward the left ventricle, or a dilated inferior vena cava without respiratory

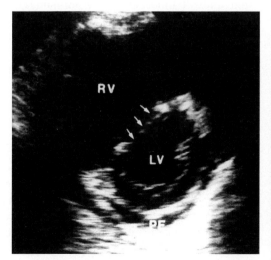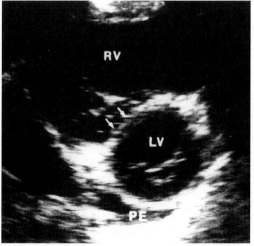

Figure 30.2 Parasternal short-axis views of the right ventricle (RV) and left ventricle (LV) in diastole *(left)* and systole *(right)*. There is diastolic and systolic bowing of the interventricular septum *(arrows)* into the left ventricle compatible with right ventricular volume and pressure overload, respectively. The right ventricle is appreciably dilated and markedly hypokinetic, with little change in apparent right ventricular area from diastole to systole. PE, small pericardial effusion. (Reprinted with permission from Come PC. Echocardiographic evaluation of pulmonary embolism and its response to therapeutic interventions. *Chest* 1992;101:151S.)

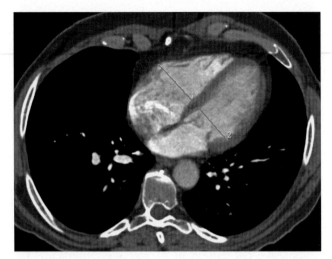

Figure 30.3 Two-dimensional reconstruction of a four-chamber view on multislice chest computed tomography in a patient with acute pulmonary embolism (PE). Right and left ventricular dimensions were measured by identifying the maximal distance between the ventricular endocardium and the interventricular septum, perpendicular to the long axis. In acute PE, a right over left ventricular dimension ratio >0.9 is associated with an increased risk for adverse clinical events.

variation. A patent foramen ovale identifies patients at risk for paradoxical embolism. Free-floating right heart thrombi increase the risk for adverse clinical events (30). Another noninvasive marker of adverse clinical events is right ventricular enlargement obtained from a reconstructed *chest CT* cardiac four-chamber view (Fig. 30.3; 31).

Cardiac biomarkers, including troponins and natriuretic peptides, have emerged as promising tools for risk assessment of patients with acute PE (Fig. 30.4). Cardiac troponins I and T are sensitive markers of myocardial necrosis. In acute PE, troponin levels correlate well with the extent of right ventricular dysfunction (31–35). In contrast to acute myocardial infarction, PE-related elevations of troponin

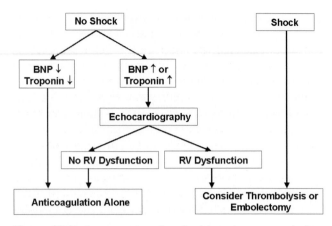

Figure 30.5 Incorporation of cardiac biomarker test results into the algorithm for the treatment for patients with acute pulmonary embolism. BNP, B-type natriuretic peptide; RV, right ventricular. (Reprinted with permission from Kucher N, Goldhaber SZ. Cardiac biomarkers for risk stratification of patients with acute pulmonary embolism. *Circulation* 2003;108:2193.)

levels are mild and of short duration. Myocardial ischemia and microinfarction owing to alterations in oxygen supply and demand of the failing right ventricle probably play a major role in the pathogenesis of troponin release.

The natriuretic peptides are useful prognostic markers for patients with congestive heart failure. Similar to cardiac troponins, elevations in B-type natriuretic peptide (BNP) or its prohormone, proBNP, are associated with right ventricular dysfunction in acute PE (36–40).

Troponins and natriuretic peptides have a high negative predictive value for in-hospital death (>97%; 36). In patients with normal biomarker levels, echocardiography need not generally be ordered because right ventricular function will almost always be normal (Fig. 30.5). Future studies will show whether cardiac biomarkers are useful for guiding treatment decisions. Abnormally elevated proBNP, BNP, or troponin levels may help select patients who benefit from further confirmation of right ventricular dysfunction by echocardiography.

ANTICOAGULATION

When PE is diagnosed or strongly suspected, anticoagulation therapy should be initiated immediately unless a contraindication exists. An intravenous bolus of unfractionated heparin (80 U/kg) followed by 18 U/kg per hour is the standard approach to initiate anticoagulation. The activated partial thromboplastin time (aPTT) should be followed at 6-hour intervals until it remains consistently in the therapeutic range of 1.5 to 2.5 times the upper limit of the normal range. Oral anticoagulation with warfarin can be started as soon as the aPTT is within the therapeutic range. Patients should receive at least 5 days of heparin while an adequate level of oral anticoagulation is established.

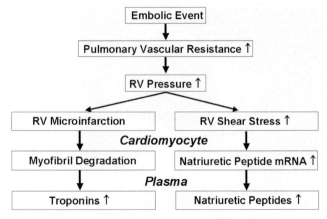

Figure 30.4 Mechanism of cardiac biomarker release in acute pulmonary embolism. (Reprinted with permission from Kucher N, Goldhaber SZ. Cardiac biomarkers for risk stratification of patients with acute pulmonary embolism. *Circulation* 2003;108:2192.)

Therapy with low–molecular-weight heparin (LMWH) is as safe and effective as therapy with unfractionated heparin in hemodynamically stable patients with acute PE (41,42). Extended 3-month monotherapy with enoxaparin without warfarin appears to be as effective and safe in the treatment of acute PE as unfractionated heparin bridged to warfarin (43). The Food and Drug Administration (FDA) has approved enoxaparin for outpatient treatment of symptomatic deep vein thrombosis with or without PE, as a bridge to warfarin.

Pentasaccharides, such as fondaparinux, are anti-Xa agents. They do not cause thrombocytopenia. Fondaparinux, 7.5 mg given subcutaneously once daily, is at least as effective and safe as unfractionated heparin (44). Ximelagatran, an oral direct thrombin inhibitor, is promising for the treatment of acute deep vein thrombosis (DVT) with or without PE. In a randomized trial of 2,489 patients with acute DVT, ximelagatran monotherapy was as effective and safe as enoxaparin bridged to warfarin (45).

In PE patients with transient risk factors, such as surgery or trauma, anticoagulation may be safely discontinued after 6 months. In other patients, indefinite-duration anticoagulation should be strongly considered. The intensity of long-term anticoagulation is controversial but will depend on the risk of both recurrent thromboembolic and bleeding events. In PREVENT (46), a double-blind randomized controlled trial of patients with idiopathic venous thromboembolism who had completed an average of 6 months of full-intensity warfarin, low-intensity warfarin (target International Normalized Ratio [INR] of 1.5 to 2.0) for an average of 2 years reduced the recurrence rate by two-thirds. In the ELATE study of 739 patients with idiopathic venous thromboembolism (47), indefinite-duration, full-intensity warfarin (target INR 2 to 3) was more effective than and as safe as indefinite-duration, low-intensity warfarin therapy (target INR 1.5 to 1.9). In the THRIVE III trial of 1,233 patients with venous thromboembolism who had completed 6 months of anticoagulation with warfarin, an additional 18 months of anticoagulation with ximelagatran (24 mg two times a day) reduced the recurrence rate significantly compared with placebo (48).

THROMBOLYSIS, CATHETER INTERVENTION, AND SURGICAL EMBOLECTOMY

Systemic *thrombolysis* is indicated in eligible patients with massive PE. Thrombolysis is effective up to 2 weeks after the onset of symptoms (Fig. 30.6; 49). The only contemporary FDA-approved thrombolytic regimen is a continuous intravenous infusion of 100 mg alteplase over 2 hours (50).

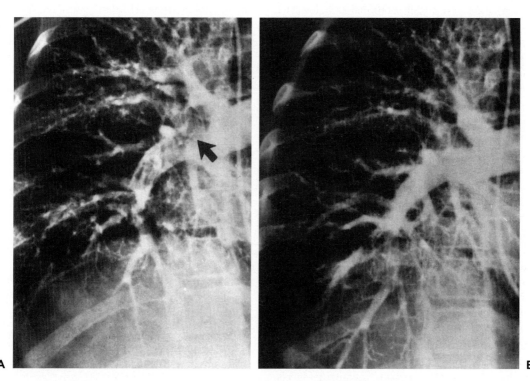

Figure 30.6 **A.** A large embolus is present in the right pulmonary artery *(arrow)*. **B.** After a 2-hour infusion of rt-PA through a peripheral vein, there is pronounced resolution, with only a small amount of residual thrombus in segmental branches. (Reprinted with permission from Goldhaber SZ, et al. Acute pulmonary embolism treated with tissue plasminogen activator. *Lancet* 1986;2:886.

In the largest randomized controlled trial of patients with submassive PE, heparin plus alteplase as a continuous infusion over 2 hours was compared with heparin alone (51). Alteplase markedly reduced adverse clinical events from 25 to 11%; these events were defined as in-hospital mortality or the need for cardiopulmonary resuscitation, mechanical ventilation, administration of vasopressors, secondary rescue thrombolysis, or surgical embolectomy. There was no significant increase in major or intracranial bleeding with alteplase among these carefully selected PE patients.

In submassive PE, thrombolysis remains controversial because a reduction in mortality with thrombolysis has not been shown. There are only 10 randomized PE trials of thrombolysis versus heparin alone, with a total of 717 patients. In overview (52), there is a trend toward reduction of mortality in favor of thrombolysis (relative risk 0.63, 95% confidence interval 0.32 to 1.23). However, thrombolysis was associated with a twofold increase in the hazard of major hemorrhage (relative risk 1.76, 95% confidence interval 1.04 to 2.98). Therefore, low-risk PE patients with preserved systemic arterial pressure and normal right ventricular function should not be treated with thrombolysis.

Catheter intervention is a promising alternative to thrombolysis or surgical embolectomy (53). The Greenfield suction embolectomy catheter is the only PE catheter device approved by the Food and Drug Administration (54). Thrombus fragmentation without embolectomy using balloon angioplasty (55) or a pigtail rotational catheter (56) has also been reported. Mechanical or rheolytic embolectomy devices, such as the AngioJet (Possis Medical, Minneapolis, MN) or Hydrolyser (Cordis, Warren, NJ) have been developed for indications other than PE but have been investigated in PE cohort studies (57). Catheter interventions can be combined with local or systemic thrombolysis.

Surgical pulmonary embolectomy should be considered in patients with massive PE and cardiogenic shock in the setting of (1) a high bleeding risk, (2) failed thrombolysis, (3) the presence of right atrial or ventricular thrombi, or (4) the need for other cardiac surgery, such as closure of an atrial septal defect or patent foramen ovale in a patient who has suffered a paradoxical embolism (53). The operation involves a median sternotomy, cardiopulmonary bypass, and deep hypothermia with circulatory arrest periods. Mortality in patients with cardiogenic shock who undergo emergency surgical embolectomy approximates 30% (58). If surgical embolectomy is performed prior to the onset of cardiogenic shock, the mortality rate may be lowered to about 10% (59).

The principal indications for *vena caval filter* placement are major contraindications to anticoagulation and recurrent venous thromboembolism despite therapeutic levels of anticoagulation. In the United States, a survey of 183 institutions found a high rate (24%) of vena caval filter insertion in patients with newly diagnosed acute deep vein

thrombosis (60). Unfortunately, patients with filters are more than twice as likely as nonfilter patients to require rehospitalization for deep vein thrombosis owing to formation of thrombus proximal to or on the proximal tip of the filter (61). Procedure-related complications are rare and include filter migration or improper filter positioning. Occasionally, the inferior vena cava may be completely obstructed by filter thrombosis.

Temporary filters have been placed in patients deemed at high risk for either thrombotic or bleeding events (62). Retrievable filters can be removed within several months or can be left in place because of a persistent contraindication to anticoagulation. Whenever possible, anticoagulation should be administered to prevent filter thrombosis.

Overall Management Strategy

Treatment decisions in patients with acute PE require rapid and accurate risk stratification (Fig. 30.7). In patients with cardiogenic shock, consider thrombolysis, catheter embolectomy, or surgical embolectomy. Management of patients with submassive PE may warrant early aggressive intervention. This will depend on the overall clinical state, cardiac biomarkers, and right ventricular size and function.

Case 1: Combined Approach of Suction Catheter Embolectomy and Thrombolysis in a Patient with Massive PE. A 78-year-old woman presented with marked shortness of breath, persistent hypotension (systemic arterial pressure 78/51 mm Hg), and right ventricular dilatation and hypokinesis on echocardiogram. Pulmonary angiogram showed a massive right pulmonary artery embolism as well as a small left lung volume because of a prior thoracoplasty to treat tuberculosis (Fig. 30.8A). She received heparin and placement of a Greenfield filter. Hypoxemia persisted despite ventilatory support. She developed melena on heparin. Cardiac surgeons felt she would not survive

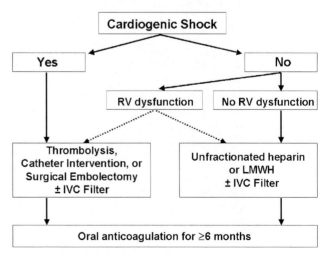

Figure 30.7 Suggested pulmonary embolism management strategy. RV, right ventricular; IVC, inferior vena caval; LMWH, low–molecular-weight heparin.

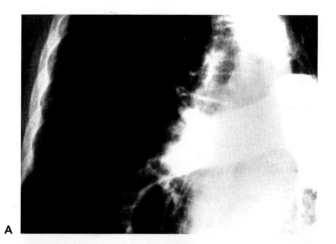

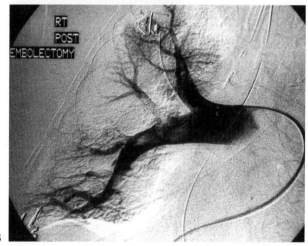

Figure 30.8 **A.** Massive right main pulmonary artery embolism in the presence of markedly diminished left lung volume owing to prior thoracoplasty. **B.** Digital subtraction pulmonary angiography immediately following combined suction catheter embolectomy and thrombolysis. There is an approximately 30% reduction in overall clot burden compared with the baseline angiogram **(A)**. (Reprinted with permission from Goldhaber SZ. Treatment of acute pulmonary embolism. In: Goldhaber SZ, ed. *Cardiopulmonary Diseases and Cardiac Tumors.* Vol III, Braunwald E, series ed. *Atlas of Heart Diseases.* Philadelphia: Current Medicine, 1995:3.1.)

surgical embolectomy because of the prior left lung thoracoplasty. Because of her hemodynamic compromise, with melena on heparin and surgical inoperability, aspiration thrombectomy was undertaken in the catheterization laboratory by Michael F. Meyerovitz, M.D., using the Meyerovitz technique. The right common femoral vein was accessed with a single wall puncture needle. A guidewire was advanced across the Greenfield filter. A 7F pigtail catheter was used with a tip-deflecting guidewire to enter the pulmonary artery. The catheter was exchanged for a 9F multipurpose coronary guiding catheter. Pressures were as follows: 18 mm Hg (mean) in the right atrium, 90/18 mm Hg in the right ventricle, and 90/40 mm Hg in the pulmonary artery. Suction catheter embolectomy removed both fresh and old clot from the pulmonary artery branches of the upper and lower right lobar arteries.

Systemic arterial hypotension persisted and, therefore, 50 mg of rt-PA was administered over 15 minutes through the pulmonary artery catheter. Pulmonary angiography then showed an approximately 30% reduction in the overall clot burden (Fig. 30.8B).

The procedure was complicated by a retroperitoneal bleed that was corrected with 12 units of packed red blood cells. The patient also developed pneumonia and acute respiratory distress syndrome. Nonetheless, her clinical picture gradually improved. She was successfully weaned from the ventilator and was transferred to a rehabilitation facility. Two years later, the patient wrote: "I am able to get around with a walker and portable canister of oxygen. I celebrated my 80th birthday last May, so I guess I'm a tough old bird."

Case 2: Failed Aspiration Thrombectomy Followed by Open Surgical Embolectomy. A 65-year-old dentist underwent right frontal craniotomy for resection of a malignant astrocytoma. He received venous thromboembolism prophylaxis with heparin 5,000 U subcutaneously twice daily and intermittent pneumatic compression boots. Nevertheless, on postoperative day 11, he developed pulmonary embolism with a systolic blood pressure of 100 mm Hg and severe right ventricular dysfunction on echocardiogram. A right (Fig. 30.9A) and left (Fig. 30.9B) pulmonary angiogram was done as a prelude to catheter aspiration embolectomy, which yielded only a small amount of thrombus (Fig. 30.9C) and did not improve his clinical condition. A bird's nest filter was then placed (Fig. 30.9D), and he was rushed to the operating room where a large volume of thrombus was removed from the right (Fig. 30.9E) and left pulmonary artery (Fig. 30.9F). He subsequently recuperated uneventfully and is clinically stable more than 2 years postoperatively. In his case, cardiac surgical backup during interventional angiography was crucial to ensure a successful outcome.

PULMONARY HYPERTENSION

Pulmonary hypertension represents a wide spectrum of diseases, with varying prognoses and therapies. It is diagnosed in the presence of an elevated mean pulmonary artery pressure $\geq$25 mm Hg at rest or $\geq$30 mm Hg during exercise. Many patients with pulmonary hypertension have passive elevation in pulmonary artery pressure owing to left ventricular diastolic dysfunction, indicated by an elevated left ventricular filling pressure. In 1998, the World Health Organization reclassified pulmonary hypertension (Table 30.1; 63). Pulmonary hypertension is common in patients with lupus erythematosus, scleroderma, and other collagen vascular disorders. Appetite suppressants have been reported as a cause of pulmonary hypertension. Pulmonary vein stenosis may cause pulmonary venous hypertension. Pulmonary hypertension may develop in patients with corrected congenital heart disease, mediastinal fibrosis, or following catheter ablation of pulmonary veins.

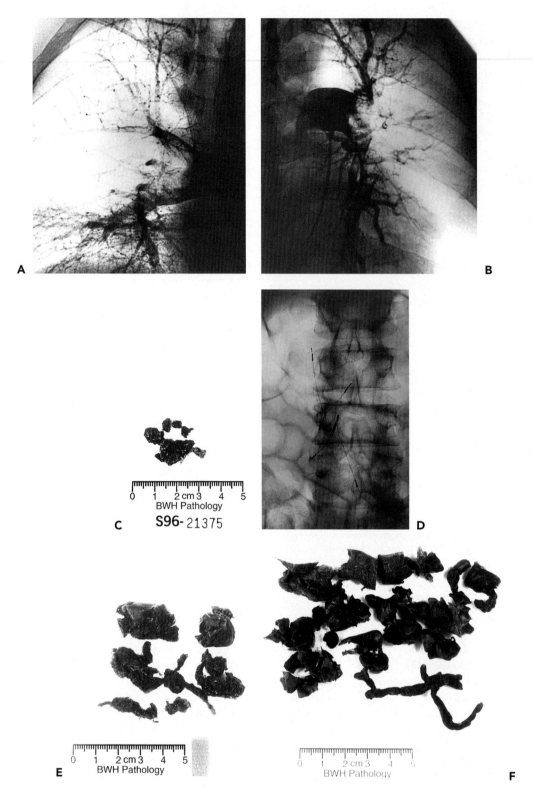

Figure 30.9 A. Massive right main pulmonary artery embolism. **B.** Massive left main pulmonary artery embolism. **C.** Several centimeters of thrombus removed in the Interventional Laboratory. **D.** Placement below the renal veins of a Bird's Nest Filter. **E, F.** Large amount of thrombus surgically extracted from the right and left pulmonary arteries, respectively.

TABLE 30.1

WHO CLASSIFICATION OF PULMONARY HYPERTENSION

1. Pulmonary arterial hypertension
   Idiopathic pulmonary arterial hypertension
   — Sporadic
   — Familial primary
   Associated with
   — Collagen vascular disease
   — HIV infection
   — Drugs or toxins
   — Portal hypertension
   — Congenital systemic to pulmonary shunts
   — Persistent pulmonary hypertension of the newborn
2. Pulmonary venous hypertension
3. Pulmonary hypertension associated with disorders of the respiratory system and/or hypoxemia
4. Pulmonary hypertension caused by chronic thrombotic and/or embolic disease
5. Pulmonary hypertension associated with miscellaneous diseases

Case 3: Management of Pulmonary Hypertension due to Congenital Pulmonary Vein Stenosis. A 28-year-old obese man presented for evaluation of progressive dyspnea, fatigue, and recurrent syncope. In addition to systemic hypertension, past medical history was significant for an unclear pulmonary vascular disease diagnosed in childhood, based on an abnormal ventilation perfusion scan and increased pulmonary artery pressures on right heart catheterization.

Chest CT revealed enlarged pulmonary arteries without filling defects. Echocardiography showed right ventricular dilatation with preserved systolic function. Catheterization showed severe pulmonary hypertension: right atrium 10, right ventricle 120/10, pulmonary artery 120/85/95, pulmonary wedge 35 to 40, transpulmonary gradient 15 to 20, and left ventricle 150/20 mm Hg.

Pulmonary capillary wedge angiography demonstrated stenoses of all pulmonary veins as they entered the mediastinal reflections. For pulmonary vein angiography, a trans-septal approach was used, via a modified 7 French pigtail catheter, injecting <15 mL contrast over 1 second. Gradients of 10 to 15 mm Hg were noted as the pulmonary veins entered the left atrium, with narrowing of all pulmonary veins to 2 to 4 mm maximal diameters compared with 6 to 10 mm more distally (Fig. 30.10A, B). Obstructions were sequentially dilated with balloons up to the adjacent vessel diameter, hand inflated for 1 to 5 seconds until the fluoroscopic waist disappeared, or until the balloon was fully expanded.

However, during the following 3 months, symptoms did not improve despite anticoagulation plus antihypertensive and diuretic therapy. Repeated catheterization documented

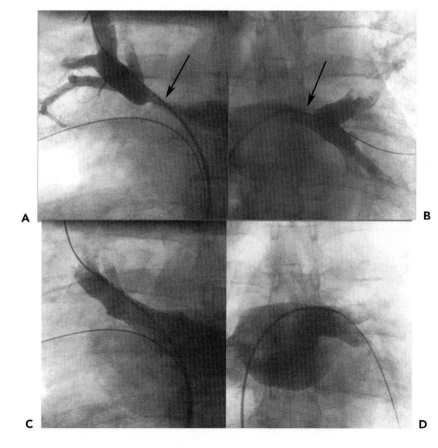

Figure 30.10 Isolated congenital pulmonary venous obstructions in a 28-year-old patient are demonstrated in the right upper (**A**) and the left (**B**) pulmonary veins. After stent implantation in the right upper pulmonary vein (**C**) and the left pulmonary veins (**D**), pulmonary artery pressures fell markedly, accompanied by improved pulmonary blood flow and right ventricular function.

pulmonary vein restenosis in all treated segments. Two 18-mm Palmaz stents were implanted within the right upper (Fig. 30.10C) and lower pulmonary veins on 12-mm and 9-mm balloons, respectively. A 30-mm Palmaz stent (Johnson and Johnson Medical Supply, Inc.) was implanted on a hand-inflated 14-mm balloon and postdilated with a 15-mm balloon, in the confluence of the left pulmonary veins (Fig. 30.10D). Over the ensuing 2 months, symptoms abated, and the 6-minute walk distance increased from 250 to 350 meters. The patient has returned to full activity without restriction. Repeated hemodynamics, performed at 6 years after stenting, revealed a cardiac output of >2.5 L/minute per m^2; pressure recordings were as follows: right atrium 6, right ventricle 40/6, pulmonary artery 40/20/28, pulmonary wedge and left ventricular end-diastolic pressure 10, aorta 128/75/85 mm Hg. No angiographic restriction to pulmonary venous flow was seen on pulmonary capillary wedge angiography.

Chronic Thromboembolic Pulmonary Hypertension (CTEPH)

In 3–4% of patients with acute PE, the thromboembolic burden does not resolve and causes CTEPH. Many patients who develop CTEPH have neither a prior history of documented venous thromboembolism nor an identifiable coagulopathy (64). Dyspnea with exertion and fatigue are common complaints. The nonspecific nature of these findings may substantially delay diagnosis.

Chest CT demonstrates chronic thrombi and may reveal other rare causes of pulmonary hypertension such as mediastinal fibrosis. Chest CT adds information to conventional angiography, including vessel wall thickness and the extent of pulmonary infarction, which may be helpful if potentially important surgery is considered. Optimal candidates for surgery are patients with functional class II or III who have proximal-type CTEPH, with preferential involvement of main and lobar pulmonary arteries.

Pulmonary thromboendarterectomy (64) involves a median sternotomy, cardiopulmonary bypass under deep hypothermia and circulatory arrest. Incisions are made in both pulmonary arteries. The surgeon creates an endarterectomy plane and then dissects endothelialized thrombus from as many involved pulmonary vessels as possible. The two major causes of postoperative mortality are inability to remove sufficient thrombotic material at the time of operation, resulting in persistent postoperative pulmonary hypertension and right ventricular dysfunction; and severe reperfusion lung injury. Overall mortality, which has continued to improve, is now <10% (65).

Repeated balloon angioplasty of the pulmonary arteries may be considered in patients who are not candidates for surgery, including patients with comorbidities or those with distal-type CTEPH (66,67). Lung transplantation is rarely performed, but can be considered in patients in whom thrombi are too distal to extract.

Case 4: Management of a Patient with Chronic Thromboembolic Pulmonary Hypertension, Proximal Disease. A 53-year-old man presented with gradually worsening dyspnea on exertion. He complained of fatigue and inability to work and pursue leisure activities without marked shortness of breath. Echocardiography showed a severely enlarged and somewhat hypertrophied right ventricle with moderately reduced systolic function. The left ventricle was relatively small with marked septal flattening and abnormal septal motion but preserved systolic function.

At age 25, he had suffered bilateral deep venous thrombosis of the legs, but did not receive a prolonged course of anticoagulation owing to a duodenal ulcer 3 years previously. At age 36, he presented with syncope accompanied by tachycardia and diaphoresis. His electrocardiogram was notable for atrial fibrillation and inverted T waves in leads V1 through V3. Five years later, he complained of exertional dyspnea. A lung scan showed perfusion defects that were of high probability for pulmonary embolism. At that time, his mean pulmonary artery pressure was 32 mm Hg, and a pulmonary angiogram was reportedly positive for pulmonary embolism. He was placed on warfarin.

Despite 12 years of anticoagulation, his dyspnea worsened to the point where he could not pursue the active lifestyle that he desired. Chronic pulmonary embolism was suspected, and he was referred for possible pulmonary thromboendarterectomy. Therefore, right heart catheterization and pulmonary angiography were repeated.

Catheterization demonstrated a right atrial pressure of 10 mm Hg, right ventricular pressure of 55/10 mm Hg, and pulmonary artery pressure of 55/28 mm Hg, with a mean pulmonary artery pressure of 35 mm Hg. Pulmonary angiography (Fig. 30.11A) revealed total occlusion of his left lower lobe pulmonary arteries. He underwent pulmonary thromboendarterectomy at Brigham and Women's Hospital. The surgeon endarterectomized multiple large thrombi that were chronic and laminated (Fig. 31.11B). The patient has subsequently done well and is no longer incapacitated in any way. He runs a factory and hunts and fishes in his leisure time.

Case 5: Management of a Patient with Chronic Thromboembolic Pulmonary Hypertension, Proximal and Distal Disease. A 57-year old woman presented with profound shortness of breath and right-sided pleuritic pain for 4 weeks, functional class IV. Past medical history included a history of recurrent deep vein thrombosis and PE and antiphospholipid antibodies. Four years previously, pulmonary angiography showed extensive PE of the right pulmonary artery. Signs of chronic embolism, including lumen irregularities and stenosis of the main pulmonary artery, were also noted (Fig. 30.12A). Pressures were as follows: right atrium 9, right ventricle 55/10, pulmonary artery 55/22/38, pulmonary wedge 10 mm Hg. At that time, an inferior vena caval filter was placed.

Now she was short of breath at rest. Pulse oximetry was 86% with 4 liters of supplemental oxygen. There was a right ventricular parasternal heave and a prominent pulmonary component of the second heart sound. Chest CT revealed complete occlusion of the right main pulmonary artery (Fig. 30.12B) and right atrial and right ventricular

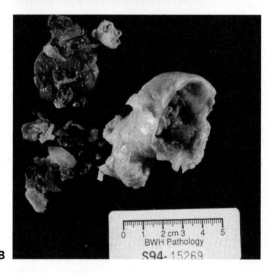

Figure 30.11 **A.** Left pulmonary arteriogram of a 53-year-old man with chronic pulmonary embolism causing total occlusion of left lower lobar pulmonary arteries. **B.** This patient underwent pulmonary thromboendarterectomy at Brigham and Women's Hospital, where large and extensive thrombi were surgically removed. The specimen contains laminated thrombus that is adherent to the endothelial wall of the endarterectomy.

enlargement (Fig. 30.12C). Right ventricular systolic dysfunction, dilatation, and pulmonary hypertension were confirmed using bedside echocardiography.

Right heart catheterization revealed the following pressures: right atrium 9 mm Hg, right ventricle 76/22, pulmonary artery 76/24/43, and pulmonary capillary wedge 4 mm Hg. Pulmonary thromboendarterectomy was performed on cardiopulmonary bypass, with aortic cross-clamping and circulatory arrest using repeated antegrade and retrograde cardioplegia. A pulmonary arteriotomy in the right main pulmonary artery was performed. Endarterectomy included complete thrombus extraction from the right main, lobar, and segmental pulmonary branches (Fig. 30.12D). The patient was discharged uneventfully on postoperative day 14.

Three months later, the symptoms improved moderately and her functional class improved from IV to II. Chest radiograph showed persistent enlargement of central pulmonary arteries, reduced vascularity in the right upper lung field, and a raised right-sided diaphragm (Fig. 30.12E).

Case 6: Management of a Patient with Chronic Thromboembolic Pulmonary Hypertension, Distal Disease. A 66-year old woman presented for evaluation of worsening dyspnea and fatigue, functional class III. She had ongoing therapy with warfarin for a history of idiopathic PE 1 year previously. Physical examination confirmed brachial cuff arterial blood pressure of 140/70 mm Hg, pulse 110, respirations 16 per minute, and jugular venous pressure 10 to 12 cm. Resting pulse oximetry was 92%, decreasing to 84% during 6 minutes walking. Baseline pulse oximetry rose to 98% with 4 liters supplemental oxygen. There was a right ventricular parasternal lift and hepatomegaly palpable three fingerbreadths below the right costal margin. Edema was present to the knees bilaterally.

Transaminases and bilirubin were twice the upper limit of normal. Six-minute walk distance was 160 meters. Chest CT showed diffuse obstructions of subsegmental pulmonary arteries.

Right heart catheterization revealed oximetric saturations of 74% in the superior vena cava, right atrium, right ventricle, and pulmonary artery. Pulse oximetry was 92% with 2 liters supplemental oxygen. Pressure recordings were as follows: right atrium 10, right ventricle 80/10, proximal pulmonary artery 80/30/45, pulmonary capillary wedge 10 mm Hg.

Superselective angiography was performed with a modified 7 French pigtail catheter, injecting 15 mL contrast in 1 second. Cutoffs, webs, and obstructions were diffuse, but most prominent in the lower lobe vessels (Figs. 30.13A and D). A highly maneuverable, soft 0.035-inch wire was used to facilitate entry into stenosed and occluded arteries. Medial and lateral basal segments of the right lower lobe were sequentially dilated with balloons, 75 to 100% vessel diameter, hand inflated for 1 to 5 seconds until the fluoroscopic waist disappeared or

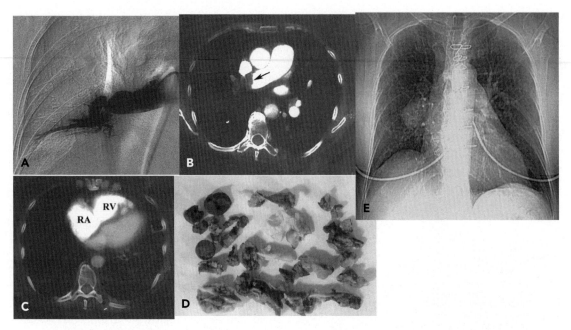

Figure 30.12 Selective cut-film pulmonary angiogram of the right pulmonary artery, with lumen irregularities and stenosis of the right main pulmonary artery **(A).** Note the rapid tapering of the lower lobe pulmonary artery, suggesting distal involvement. The right upper lobe pulmonary artery is completely occluded. Four years later, multislice chest CT demonstrates complete occlusion of the right main pulmonary artery (*arrow,* **B**). An axial image from the same CT study demonstrates right atrial (RA) and right ventricular (RV) enlargement **(C).** Surgically extracted thrombotic material from the right pulmonary artery **(D).** Chest radiograph showed persistent enlargement of the right pulmonary artery, reduced vascularity in the right upper lung field, and a raised right-sided diaphragm **(E).**

until the balloon was fully expanded. Follow-up catheterization at 6 weeks documented patency of previously dilated right lower lobe branches, without measurable gradient (Fig. 30.13D). Medial and lateral basal segments of the left lower lobe were approached and sequentially dilated with balloons 75 to 100% vessel diameter, until vessel size increased >50%, with improved angiographic transit time (Fig. 30.13C). Final pulmonary artery pressures were 38/20/28 mm Hg.

Four years after dilations, she had a 6-minute walking distance of 350 meters. Repeat catheterization confirmed patency of dilated pulmonary artery branches, with a pulmonary artery pressure <30% systemic levels.

Idiopathic Pulmonary Arterial Hypertension (IAPH)

IAPH, formerly known as primary pulmonary hypertension, is a disease affecting the pulmonary vasculature, resulting in pulmonary hypertension from no apparent cause. The annual incidence is about one to two cases per million. Prognosis among historical controls is poor. Before the era of modern therapy, the National Institutes of Health Registry estimated a median survival of 2.8 years (68). Survival rates used to be 68%, 48%, and 34% at 1, 3, and 5 years, respectively.

Endothelial dysfunction occurs early in the pathogenesis of IAPH (69,70). Disorganized endothelial cell proliferation results in the formation of glomeruloid structures known as plexiform lesions. In addition, endothelial and vascular smooth muscle cells mediators, including nitric oxide, prostacyclin, endothelin-1, thromboxane, vascular endothelial growth factor (VEGF), polyamines, and xanthine oxidoreductase contribute to vasoconstriction. Inflammation is an important component, mediated by increased levels of cytokines from lymphocytes and macrophages. Thrombotic lesions are common in patients with IAPH because the dysfunctional endothelium contributes to the hypercoagulable state. A genetic predisposition in 10% of patients with IAPH has been suggested. Although the spectrum of trigger factors is wide, infection with the human herpesvirus 8 may have an important role in pathogenesis (71).

Anticoagulation with warfarin (target INR 2.0 to 3.0) is standard therapy and improves survival in patients with IAPH (72). Calcium channel blockers, including long-acting nifedipine, amlodipine, or diltiazem, have been used the longest and are effective in about 10% of patients (Table 30.2; 72).

Continuous-infusion epoprostenol is the most effective therapy. Epoprostenol improves symptoms, exercise capacity, hemodynamics, and survival owing to its vasodilator, antithrombotic, and positive inotropic effects (73–76). Benefits are also observed in nonresponders to acute vasodilator challenge. The major drawback is that it is administered via a surgically implanted central line and delivered by an ambulatory infusion pump. Life-threatening

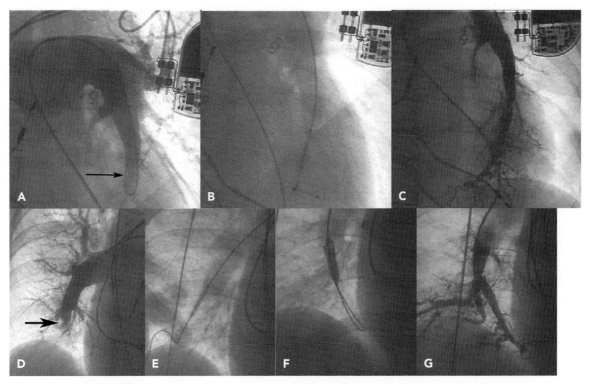

Figure 30.13 Subselective left **(A, B, C)** and right **(D, E, F, G)** lower lobe pulmonary angiographic images in a patient with distal chronic thromboembolic pulmonary hypertension. Matched cineangiograms **(A–G)** accompany images (see enclosed CD). Cutoffs of medial and lateral basal lower lobe vessels **(A, D)** were noted *(arrows)*. In serial sessions, highly maneuverable, soft-tipped 0.035-inch diameter wires were passed beyond the obstructions, and balloon dilations **(C, E, F)** were performed using angioplasty balloons sized 75 to 100% diameter of the native vessel. Balloon pulmonary angioplasty resulted in decrease of pulmonary artery pressure, pulmonary vascular resistance, and recruitment of medial and lateral basal lower lobe branches **(C, G)**.

rebound pulmonary hypertension may occur when the infusion is interrupted. Common side effects include flushing, headache, diarrhea, nausea, thrombocytopenia, and jaw discomfort.

The prostacyclin analog, treprostinil, has been recently approved by the FDA and is administered as a continuous subcutaneous infusion (77). Pain at the infusion site is common and limits its use.

The aerosolized analog, iloprost, is not available in the United States. It is effective in improving symptoms and exercise capacity (78,79). It needs to be inhaled up to 12 times per day owing to its short half-life. Oral prostacyclin derivatives, such as beraprost sodium, improve symptoms and exercise capacity but have no beneficial hemodynamic effects (80).

Bosentan, a nonselective endothelin receptor antagonist, was approved by the FDA for patients with functional class III or IV symptoms. It reduces major adverse clinical events, including death, lung transplantation, hospitalization, or the need for epoprostenol (81,82). Bosentan may elevate transaminase levels, which must be monitored periodically.

Sildenafil, an oral phosphodiesterase-5 inhibitor, increases cyclic guanosine monophosphate (GMP) similarly to nitric oxide. It appears to be highly effective in improving symptoms and hemodynamics, even when added to standard treatment (83–87).

Patients with less severe symptoms (functional class II or III) and less advanced hemodynamic alterations may be started on oral therapy, such as bosentan, sildenafil, or both. Functional class IV patients are usually treated with continuous-infusion epoprostenol. In addition to monitoring symptoms and hemodynamics, serial measurements of BNP may be helpful in guiding treatment decisions in patients with IAPH (88). Many patients will not respond to one regimen but will benefit from another. Drug combination therapy is becoming standard.

Case 7: Management of a Class III Patient with Primary Pulmonary Hypertension. A 21-year-old woman presented for evaluation of progressive dyspnea and fatigue, functional class III. There was no personal or family history of venous or arterial thrombosis, congenital heart or liver disease, or rheumatologic disease. The patient did not use oral contraceptives, stimulants, or diet medications.

Physical examination was remarkable for brachial cuff arterial blood pressure 100/80 mm Hg, pulse 110, respirations 16 per minute, and jugular venous pressure 14 cm. Resting pulse oximetry was 88%, decreasing to 80% with

TABLE 30.2

DRUGS FOR PULMONARY HYPERTENSION

Drug	Dose	Efficacy
Nifedipine Diltiazem	30–90 mg TID 60–240 mg TID	Improves symptoms and survival in 10–20% patients (72)
Bosentan (oral)	62.5 mg BID (4 weeks), then 125 mg BID	Improves symptoms and time to death, lung transplant, or hospitalization (81,82)
Sildenafil (oral)	50 mg TID	Improves symptoms and hemodynamics when added to standard therapy (83–87)
Beraprost (oral)	20–120 μg QID	Improves symptoms but not hemodynamics (80)
Epoprostenol (continuous IV via central line)	2.0–50.0 ng/kg per min, increments by 2 ng/kg per min	Improves symptoms and survival in responders and nonresponders to acute vasodilator challenge (73–76)
Treprostinil (continuous SC)	1.25–40 ng/kg per min, increments by 1.25 ng/kg per min	Improves symptoms and hemodynamics (77)
Iloprost (inhaled)	2.5–5.0 μg 6 or 12 times per day	Improves symptoms and hemodynamics (78,79)

6 minutes of walking. Baseline oximetry rose to 92% with 4 liters of supplemental oxygen. There was a diffuse prolonged right ventricular impulse over the sternum. The liver was enlarged and palpable two fingerbreadths below the right costal margin. Edema was present to the knees bilaterally.

Chest radiograph revealed enlarged pulmonary arteries with distal loss of vascularity. Contrast echocardiography revealed a patent foramen ovale with right-to-left shunt. Chest CT showed no proximal or distal obstruction of pulmonary arteries. Six-minute walk test distance was 170 meters.

At catheterization, she had severe pulmonary hypertension (Table 30.3). Pulmonary angiography showed decreased branching patterns (referred to as "pruning") of the distal pulmonary arteries, with slow transpulmonary transit time, without evidence of pulmonary arterial or venous obstruc-

tion. In addition, bilateral pulmonary arteriovenous malformations were noted (Fig. 30.14). The patient was a nonresponder to acute vasodilator testing with inhaled nitric oxide. Nevertheless, intravenous epoprostenol was begun via a central line. Her side effects included flushing, bone aches, and episodic catheter-related infection. One year after therapy was instituted, the epoprostenol dose was 50 ng/kg per minute. Her functional class improved from class III to II, and the 6-minute walk distance and hemodynamics also improved. However, epoprostenol-related bone pain required narcotics. Nosebleeds were increasingly frequent and required posterior packing on several occasions.

The endothelin antagonist, bosentan, was initiated at 62.5 mg orally twice daily and raised to 125 mg twice daily after 1 month. Over a 4-month period, epoprostenol was successfully tapered and then discontinued.

TABLE 30.3

HEMODYNAMICS IN A PATIENT WITH IDIOPATHIC PULMONARY ARTERIAL HYPERTENSION

	Baseline	At 12 Months	At 16 Months
Epoprostenol	—	50 ng/kg per min	—
Bosentan	—	—	125 mg BID
Six-minute walking distance, meters	170	245	255
Right atrial pressure, mm Hg	15	8	8
Pulmonary artery pressure, mm Hg	125/70/85	110/40/70	110/40/70
Aortic pressure, mm Hg	100/65/75	140/70/95	140/70/95
Pulmonary capillary wedge pressure, mm Hg	10	4	5
Cardiac index, L/min per m^2	2.3	2.8	2.8
Pulmonary resistance, Wood units	>30	22	23
Qp/Qs	0.8	1.0	1.0

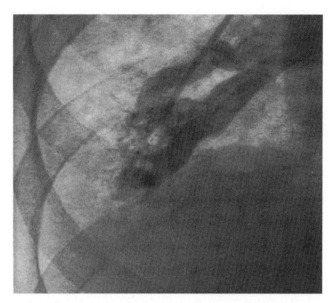

Figure 30.14 Right lower lobe subsegmental angiogram in a 21-year-old patient with idiopathic pulmonary arterial hypertension. Bilateral pulmonary arteriovenous fistulae were demonstrated, but given marked elevation in pulmonary vascular resistance, were not occluded.

REFERENCES

1. Goldhaber SZ. Pulmonary embolism. *Lancet* 2004;363:1295–1305.
2. Stein PD, Dalen JE, McIntyre KM, Sasahara AA, Wenger NK, Willis PW 3rd. The electrocardiogram in acute pulmonary embolism. *Prog Cardiovasc Dis* 1975;17:247–257.
3. Kucher N, Walpoth N, Wustmann K, Noveanu M, Gertsch M. QR in V1—an ECG sign associated with right ventricular strain and adverse clinical outcome in pulmonary embolism. *Eur Heart J* 2003;24:1113–1119.
4. Ferrari E, Imbert A, Chevalier T, Mihoubi A, Morand P, Baudouy M. The ECG in pulmonary embolism. Predictive value of negative T waves in precordial leads—80 case reports. *Chest* 1997;111:537–543.
5. Stein PD, Goldhaber SZ, Henry JW. Alveolar-arterial oxygen gradient in the assessment of acute pulmonary embolism. *Chest* 1995;107:139–143.
6. Stein PD, Goldhaber SZ, Henry JW, Miller AC. Arterial blood gas analysis in the assessment of suspected acute pulmonary embolism. *Chest* 1996;109:78–81.
7. Bounameaux H, Cirafici P, de Moerloose P, et al. Measurement of D-dimer in plasma as diagnostic aid in suspected pulmonary embolism. *Lancet* 1991;337:196–200.
8. Goldhaber SZ, Simons GR, Elliott CG, et al. Quantitative plasma D-dimer levels among patients undergoing pulmonary angiography for suspected pulmonary embolism. *JAMA* 1993;270: 2819–2822.
9. Dunn KL, Wolf JP, Dorfman DM, Fitzpatrick P, Baker JL, Goldhaber SZ. Normal D-dimer levels in emergency department patients suspected of acute pulmonary embolism. *J Am Coll Cardiol* 2002;40:1475–1478.
10. Brown MD, Rowe BH, Reeves MJ, Bermingham JM, Goldhaber SZ. The accuracy of the enzyme-linked immunosorbent assay D-dimer test in the diagnosis of pulmonary embolism: a meta-analysis. *Ann Emerg Med* 2002;40:133–144.
11. Value of the ventilation/perfusion scan in acute pulmonary embolism. Results of the prospective investigation of pulmonary embolism diagnosis (PIOPED). The PIOPED Investigators. *JAMA* 1990;263:2753–2759.
12. Schoepf UJ, Costello P, Goldhaber SZ. Spiral computed tomography for acute pulmonary embolism. *Circulation* 2004;109: 2160–2167.
12a. Goldhaber SZ. Multislice computed tomography for pulmonary embolism—a technological marvel. *N Engl J Med.* 2005;352: 1812–1814.
13. Schoepf UJ, Holzknecht N, Helmberger TK, et al. Subsegmental pulmonary emboli: improved detection with thin-collimation multi-detector row spiral CT. *Radiology* 2002;222:483–490.
14. Perrier A, Howarth N, Didier D, et al. Performance of helical computed tomography in unselected outpatients with suspected pulmonary embolism. *Ann Intern Med* 2001;135:88–97.
15. Donato AA, Scheirer JJ, Atwell MS, Gramp J, Duszak R Jr. Clinical outcomes in patients with suspected acute pulmonary embolism and negative helical computed tomographic results in whom anticoagulation was withheld. *Arch Intern Med* 2003;163: 2033–2038.
15a. Quiroz R, Kucher N, Zou KH, et al. Clinical validity of a negative computed tomography scan in patients with suspected pulmonary embolism: a systematic review. *JAMA* 2005;293:2012–2017.
16. van Beek EJ, Reekers JA, Batchelor DA, Brandjes DP, Buller HR. Feasibility, safety and clinical utility of angiography in patients with suspected pulmonary embolism. *Eur Radiol* 1996;6: 415–419.
17. Henry JW, Relyea B, Stein PD. Continuing risk of thromboemboli among patients with normal pulmonary angiograms. *Chest* 1995;107:1375–1378.
18. Oudkerk M, van Beek EJ, Wielopolski P, et al. Comparison of contrast-enhanced magnetic resonance angiography and conventional pulmonary angiography for the diagnosis of pulmonary embolism: a prospective study. *Lancet* 2002;359: 1643–1647.
19. Lensing AW, Prandoni P, Brandjes D, et al. Detection of deep-vein thrombosis by real-time B-mode ultrasonography. *N Engl J Med* 1989;320:342–345.
20. Hull RD, Hirsh J, Carter CJ, et al. Pulmonary angiography, ventilation lung scanning, and venography for clinically suspected pulmonary embolism with abnormal perfusion lung scan. *Ann Intern Med* 1983;98:891–899.
21. Mac Gillavry MR, Sanson BJ, Buller HR, Brandjes DP. Compression ultrasonography of the leg veins in patients with clinically suspected pulmonary embolism: is a more extensive assessment of compressibility useful? *Thromb Haemost* 2000;84:973–976.
22. Turkstra F, Kuijer PM, van Beek EJ, Brandjes DP, ten Cate JW, Buller HR. Diagnostic utility of ultrasonography of leg veins in patients suspected of having pulmonary embolism. *Ann Intern Med* 1997;126:775–781.
23. Pruszczyk P, Torbicki A, Kuch-Wocial A, Szulc M, Pacho R. Diagnostic value of transoesophageal echocardiography in suspected haemodynamically significant pulmonary embolism. *Heart* 2001;85:628–634.
24. McConnell MV, Solomon SD, Rayan ME, Come PC, Goldhaber SZ, Lee RT. Regional right ventricular dysfunction detected by echocardiography in acute pulmonary embolism. *Am J Cardiol* 1996;78:469–473.
25. Kucher N, Luder CM, Dornhofer T, Windecker S, Meier B, Hess OM. Novel management strategy for patients with suspected pulmonary embolism. *Eur Heart J* 2003;24:366–376.
26. Goldhaber SZ, Elliott CG. Acute pulmonary embolism, II: risk stratification, treatment, and prevention. *Circulation* 2003;108: 2834–2838.
27. Wicki J, Perrier A, Perneger TV, Bounameaux H, Junod AF. Predicting adverse outcome in patients with acute pulmonary embolism: a risk score. *Thromb Haemost* 2000;84:548–552.
28. Goldhaber SZ, Visani L, De Rosa M. Acute pulmonary embolism: clinical outcomes in the International Cooperative Pulmonary Embolism Registry (ICOPER). *Lancet* 1999;353:1386–1389.
29. Goldhaber SZ. Echocardiography in the management of pulmonary embolism. *Ann Intern Med* 2002;136:691–700.
30. Torbicki A, Galie N, Covezzoli A, Rossi E, De Rosa M, Goldhaber SZ. Right heart thrombi in pulmonary embolism: results from the International Cooperative Pulmonary Embolism Registry. *J Am Coll Cardiol* 2003;41:2245–2251.
31. Quiroz R, Kucher N, Schoepf UJ, et al. Right ventricular enlargement on chest computed tomography: prognostic role in acute pulmonary embolism. *Circulation* 2004;109:2401–2404.
32. Konstantinides S, Geibel A, Olschewski M, et al. Importance of cardiac troponins I and T in risk stratification of patients with acute pulmonary embolism. *Circulation* 2002;106:1263–1268.

33. Giannitsis E, Muller-Bardorff M, Kurowski V, et al. Independent prognostic value of cardiac troponin T in patients with confirmed pulmonary embolism. *Circulation* 2000;102:211–217.

34. Janata K, Holzer M, Laggner AN, Mullner M. Cardiac troponin T in the severity assessment of patients with pulmonary embolism: cohort study. *BMJ* 2003;326:312–313.

35. Kucher N, Wallmann D, Carone A, Windecker S, Meier B, Hess OM. Incremental prognostic value of troponin I and echocardiography in patients with acute pulmonary embolism. *Eur Heart J* 2003;24:1651–1656.

36. Kucher N, Goldhaber SZ. Cardiac biomarkers for risk stratification of patients with acute pulmonary embolism. *Circulation* 2003;108:2191–2194.

37. Kucher N, Printzen G, Doernhoefer T, Windecker S, Meier B, Hess OM. Low pro-brain natriuretic peptide levels predict benign clinical outcome in acute pulmonary embolism. *Circulation* 2003;107:1576–1578.

38. Kucher N, Printzen G, Goldhaber SZ. Prognostic role of brain natriuretic peptide in acute pulmonary embolism. *Circulation* 2003;107:2545–2547.

39. ten Wolde M, Tulevski, II, Mulder JW, et al. Brain natriuretic peptide as a predictor of adverse outcome in patients with pulmonary embolism. *Circulation* 2003;107:2082–2084.

40. Pruszczyk P, Kostrubiec M, Styczynski G, et al. N-terminal pro-B-type natriuretic peptide in patients with acute pulmonary embolism. *Eur Respir J* 2003;22:649–653.

41. Simonneau G, Sors H, Charbonnier B, et al. A comparison of low-molecular-weight heparin with unfractionated heparin for acute pulmonary embolism. The THESEE Study Group. Tinzaparine ou Heparine Standard: Evaluations dans l'Embolie Pulmonaire. *N Engl J Med* 1997;337:663–669.

42. Low-molecular-weight heparin in the treatment of patients with venous thromboembolism. The Columbus Investigators. *N Engl J Med* 1997;337:657–662.

43. Beckman JA, Dunn K, Sasahara AA, Goldhaber SZ. Enoxaparin monotherapy without oral anticoagulation to treat acute symptomatic pulmonary embolism. *Thromb Haemost* 2003;89: 953–958.

44. Buller HR, Davidson BL, Decousus H, et al. Subcutaneous fondaparinux versus intravenous unfractionated heparin in the initial treatment of pulmonary embolism. *N Engl J Med* 2003; 349:1695–1702.

45. Huisman MV, et al. Efficacy and safety of the oral direct thrombin inhibitor ximelagatran compared with current standard therapy for acute symptomatic deep vein thrombosis, with or without pulmonary embolism: a randomized, double-blind, multinational study (Abstract OC003). International Society on Thrombosis and Hemostasis 2003.

46. Ridker PM, Goldhaber SZ, Danielson E, et al. Long-term, low-intensity warfarin therapy for the prevention of recurrent venous thromboembolism. *N Engl J Med* 2003;348:1425–1434.

47. Kearon C, Ginsberg JS, Kovacs MJ, et al. Comparison of low-intensity warfarin therapy with conventional-intensity warfarin therapy for long-term prevention of recurrent venous thromboembolism. *N Engl J Med* 2003;349:631–639.

48. Schulman S, Wahlander K, Lundstrom T, Clason SB, Eriksson H. Secondary prevention of venous thromboembolism with the oral direct thrombin inhibitor ximelagatran. *N Engl J Med* 2003;349:1713–1721.

49. Daniels LB, Parker JA, Patel SR, Grodstein F, Goldhaber SZ. Relation of duration of symptoms with response to thrombolytic therapy in pulmonary embolism. *Am J Cardiol* 1997;80: 184–188.

50. Goldhaber SZ, Haire WD, Feldstein ML, et al. Alteplase versus heparin in acute pulmonary embolism: randomised trial assessing right-ventricular function and pulmonary perfusion. *Lancet* 1993;341:507–511.

51. Konstantinides S, Geibel A, Heusel G, et al. Heparin plus alteplase compared with heparin alone in patients with submassive pulmonary embolism. *N Engl J Med* 2002;347:1143–1150.

52. Thabut G, Thabut D, Myers RP, et al. Thrombolytic therapy of pulmonary embolism: a meta-analysis. *J Am Coll Cardiol* 2002;40:1660–1667.

53. Guidelines on diagnosis and management of acute pulmonary embolism. Task Force on Pulmonary Embolism, European Society of Cardiology. *Eur Heart J* 2000;21:1301–1336.

54. Greenfield LJ, Proctor MC, Williams DM, Wakefield TW. Long-term experience with transvenous catheter pulmonary embolectomy. *J Vasc Surg* 1993;18:450–457; discussion 457–458.

55. Handa K, Sasaki Y, Kiyonaga A, Fujino M, Hiroki T, Arakawa K. Acute pulmonary thromboembolism treated successfully by balloon angioplasty—a case report. *Angiology* 1988;39:775–778.

56. Schmitz-Rode T, Janssens U, Hanrath P, Gunther RW. Fragmentation of massive pulmonary embolism by pigtail rotation catheter: possible complication. *Eur Radiol* 2001;11:2047–2049.

57. Uflacker R. Interventional therapy for pulmonary embolism. *J Vasc Intervent Radiol* 2001;12:147–164.

58. Doerge H, Schoendube FA, Voss M, Seipelt R, Messmer BJ. Surgical therapy of fulminant pulmonary embolism: early and late results. *Thorac Cardiovasc Surg* 1999;47:9–13.

59. Aklog L, Williams CS, Byrne JG, Goldhaber SZ. Acute pulmonary embolectomy: a contemporary approach. *Circulation* 2002; 105:1416–1419.

60. Goldhaber SZ, Tapson VF. A prospective registry of 5,451 patients with ultrasound-confirmed deep vein thrombosis. *Am J Cardiol* 2004;93:259–262.

61. White RH, Zhou H, Kim J, Romano PS. A population-based study of the effectiveness of inferior vena cava filter use among patients with venous thromboembolism. *Arch Intern Med* 2000;160:2033–2041.

62. Offner PJ, Hawkes A, Madayag R, Seale F, Maines C. The role of temporary inferior vena cava filters in critically ill surgical patients. *Arch Surg* 2003;138:591–594; discussion 594–595.

63. Rich S. Primary pulmonary hypertension. Executive summary from the World Symposium on Primary Pulmonary Hypertension 1998. World Health Organization, available at www.who.int/ncd/cvd/pph.htm, date last accessed 4/14/05.

64. Fedullo PF, Auger WR, Kerr KM, Rubin LJ. Chronic thromboembolic pulmonary hypertension. *N Engl J Med* 2001;345: 1465–1472.

65. Jamieson SW, Kapelanski DP, Sakakibara N, et al. Pulmonary endarterectomy: experience and lessons learned in 1,500 cases. *Ann Thorac Surg* 2003;76:1457–1462; discussion 1462– 1464.

66. Feinstein JA, Goldhaber SZ, Lock JE, Ferndandes SM, Landzberg MJ. Balloon pulmonary angioplasty for treatment of chronic thromboembolic pulmonary hypertension. *Circulation* 2001; 103:10–13.

67. Pitton MB, Herber S, Mayer E, Thelen M. Pulmonary balloon angioplasty of chronic thromboembolic pulmonary hypertension (CTEPH) in surgically inaccessible cases. *Rofo Fortschr Geb Rontgenstr Neuen Bildgeb Verfahr* 2003;175:631–634.

68. Rich S, Dantzker DR, Ayres SM, et al. Primary pulmonary hypertension. A national prospective study. *Ann Intern Med* 1987; 107:216–223.

69. Rich S, McLaughlin VV. Endothelin receptor blockers in cardiovascular disease. *Circulation* 2003;108:2184–2190.

70. Budhiraja R, Tuder RM, Hassoun PM. Endothelial dysfunction in pulmonary hypertension. *Circulation* 2004;109:159–165.

71. Cool CD, Rai PR, Yeager ME, et al. Expression of human herpesvirus 8 in primary pulmonary hypertension. *N Engl J Med* 2003;349:1113–1122.

72. Rich S, Kaufmann E, Levy PS. The effect of high doses of calcium-channel blockers on survival in primary pulmonary hypertension. *N Engl J Med* 1992;327:76–81.

73. Barst RJ, Rubin LJ, Long WA, et al. A comparison of continuous intravenous epoprostenol (prostacyclin) with conventional therapy for primary pulmonary hypertension. The Primary Pulmonary Hypertension Study Group. *N Engl J Med* 1996;334: 296–302.

74. McLaughlin VV, Genthner DE, Panella MM, Rich S. Reduction in pulmonary vascular resistance with long-term epoprostenol (prostacyclin) therapy in primary pulmonary hypertension. *N Engl J Med* 1998;338:273–277.

75. McLaughlin VV, Shillington A, Rich S. Survival in primary pulmonary hypertension: the impact of epoprostenol therapy. *Circulation* 2002;106:1477–1482.

76. Sitbon O, Humbert M, Nunes H, et al. Long-term intravenous epoprostenol infusion in primary pulmonary hypertension: prognostic factors and survival. *J Am Coll Cardiol* 2002;40: 780–788.

77. McLaughlin VV, Gaine SP, Barst RJ, et al. Efficacy and safety of treprostinil: an epoprostenol analog for primary pulmonary hypertension. *J Cardiovasc Pharmacol* 2003;41:293–299.

78. Hoeper MM, Schwarze M, Ehlerding S, et al. Long-term treatment of primary pulmonary hypertension with aerosolized iloprost, a prostacyclin analogue. *N Engl J Med* 2000;342: 1866–1870.

79. Olschewski H, Simonneau G, Galie N, et al. Inhaled iloprost for severe pulmonary hypertension. *N Engl J Med* 2002;347: 322–329.

80. Galie N, Humbert M, Vachiery JL, et al. Effects of beraprost sodium, an oral prostacyclin analogue, in patients with pulmonary arterial hypertension: a randomized, double-blind, placebo-controlled trial. *J Am Coll Cardiol* 2002;39: 1496–1502.

81. Channick RN, Simonneau G, Sitbon O, et al. Effects of the dual endothelin-receptor antagonist bosentan in patients with pulmonary hypertension: a randomised placebo-controlled study. *Lancet* 2001;358:1119–1123.

82. Rubin LJ, Badesch DB, Barst RJ, et al. Bosentan therapy for pulmonary arterial hypertension. *N Engl J Med* 2002;346:896–903.

83. Sastry BK, Narasimhan C, Reddy NK, Raju BS. Clinical efficacy of sildenafil in primary pulmonary hypertension: a randomized, placebo-controlled, double-blind, crossover study. *J Am Coll Cardiol* 2004;43:1149–1153.

84. Ghofrani HA, Rose F, Schermuly RT, et al. Oral sildenafil as long-term adjunct therapy to inhaled iloprost in severe pulmonary arterial hypertension. *J Am Coll Cardiol* 2003;42:158–164.

85. Michelakis E, Tymchak W, Lien D, Webster L, Hashimoto K, Archer S. Oral sildenafil is an effective and specific pulmonary vasodilator in patients with pulmonary arterial hypertension: comparison with inhaled nitric oxide. *Circulation* 2002;105: 2398–2403.

86. Michelakis ED, Tymchak W, Noga M, et al. Long-term treatment with oral sildenafil is safe and improves functional capacity and hemodynamics in patients with pulmonary arterial hypertension. *Circulation* 2003;108:2066–2069.

87. Wilkens H, Guth A, Konig J, et al. Effect of inhaled iloprost plus oral sildenafil in patients with primary pulmonary hypertension. *Circulation* 2001;104:1218–1222.

88. Leuchte HH, Holzapfel M, Baumgartner RA, et al. Clinical significance of brain natriuretic peptide in primary pulmonary hypertension. *J Am Coll Cardiol* 2004;43:764–770.

31

Profiles in Cardiomyopathy and Congestive Heart Failure

James C. Fang   *Andrew C. Eisenhauer*

Heart failure is a chronic progressive condition that arises when the heart cannot provide adequate cardiac output to meet the systemic metabolic demands or cannot accommodate the venous return without elevation of filling pressure. This process may be initiated by any primary insult to the myocardium: infarction, excessive loading, or a frank disorder of the heart muscle itself—a cardiomyopathy. Cardiomyopathies are generally divided into three categories: dilated, restrictive, and hypertrophic. Alternatively, some authorities have divided patients based on whether the clinical syndrome is owing to abnormal systolic function, or to normal systolic function with abnormal diastolic filling (i.e., a restrictive or hypertrophic cardiomyopathy, also known as "diastolic heart failure"). Abnormal diastolic function is also seen with constrictive pericardial disease, but is not a disorder of the heart muscle per se (see Chapter 32).

Heart failure is in part due to the adverse effects of ongoing neurohormonal activation. There is a fairly good correlation between clinical manifestations and the hemodynamic profile, and the most recent classification system emphasizes the progression of hemodynamic and neurohumoral stages, rather than the traditional New York Heart Association (NYHA) functional classification (which may wax and wane over time). Patients thus evolve from being at risk for developing heart failure (stage A), to structural heart disease (stage B), to symptomatic heart failure (stage C), and finally to medically refractory heart failure (stage D; 1). Therapy is driven by both symptoms and the stage of disease and may include diuretic, vasodilator, and inotropic therapies that target the hemodynamic derangements of heart failure (low output, high resistance, elevated filling pressures) and thereby improve symptoms. Antagonism of the adrenergic and renin-angiotensin systems also helps to prevent further injury to the myocardium and thereby slow the progression of heart failure.

Cardiac catheterization is performed in patients with heart failure for several reasons: (1) to assess etiology, (2) to define both resting and exercise hemodynamic status, and (3) to evaluate therapeutic interventions. In most patients with heart failure, all three goals can usually be addressed in a single procedure. The hemodynamic profile is generally characterized in the supine state, where resting and exercise conditions can be studied (see Chapter 15), although some centers prefer measurements in the upright state, especially if exercise is being used for diagnostic or prognostic purposes. After the hemodynamic assessment has been completed, angiography should be performed to define the coronary anatomy. Clinical criteria such as the presence or absence of angina are poor predictors of the presence or absence of clinically relevant coronary artery disease (2). Ventriculography should also be considered to assess systolic function, mitral regurgitation, and ventricular size and shape, although most patients will have had echocardiographic assessment prior to catheterization. If sufficient coronary artery disease is not present to explain the degree of ventricular dysfunction, an endomyocardial biopsy should be considered to help to define the etiology, especially when a specific diagnosis is suspected on clinical grounds (3). (See Chapter 20.)

TABLE 31.1

CAUSES OF DILATED CARDIOMYOPATHIES (IN ORDER OF DECREASING FREQUENCY)

Idiopathic cardiomyopathy
  Familial
  Viral
Ischemic heart disease
Myocarditis
  Chagas
  Enteroviruses (i.e., Coxsackie A/B)
  Sarcoid
  HIV
  Drugs (i.e., anthracyclines)
Alcohol
Cocaine
Peripartum
Rheumatologic disorders (i.e., lupus)
Endocrine disorders (i.e., pheochromocytoma, hypothyroidism)

DILATED CARDIOMYOPATHY

There are many potential causes of dilated cardiomyopathy (Table 31.1). The noninvasive clinical assessment may suggest a specific diagnosis such as sarcoidosis or Chagas disease, but in most instances the cause will remain undefined (i.e., idiopathic). Idiopathic cardiomyopathy most likely represents the sequelae of prior myocarditis (4) or a genetic mutation (5). Only a few etiologies have patho-

gnomonic histologic findings, but endomyocardial biopsy may be helpful in confirming or excluding those diseases. In 1,230 patients who underwent endomyocardial biopsy at the Johns Hopkins Hospital for unexplained heart failure, only 15% had a specific histologic diagnosis (3), but using the results of the endomyocardial biopsy in combination with clinical information, a specific cause was eventually determined in 50% of the patients. Similarly, cardiac catheterization including coronary angiography is recommended for most patients with new-onset heart failure from dilated cardiomyopathy, since the noninvasive assessment of ischemic heart disease can be misleading (2), and heart failure from ischemia is one of the few etiologies reversible (by revascularization assuming sufficient myocardial viability is present; 4–7). Ventriculography also allows assessment of mitral regurgitation and dyskinesis, both of which can be targeted surgically (Fig. 31.1).

Invasive hemodynamic assessment is also important, since the physical examination may underestimate the degree of congestion (8) and noninvasive methods are limited in accuracy (9). Although baseline hemodynamic profiles are not unique to particular cardiomyopathies (10), definition of the hemodynamic profile can be used to optimally titrate vasodilators and diuretics (11). In some instances, this tailored management adjusted with an indwelling Swan-Ganz catheter over 48 hours can obviate the need for cardiac transplantation (12). Furthermore, a detailed hemodynamic profile provides prognostic information (13,14). In a consecutive series of 152 advanced heart failure patients referred to UCLA for cardiac

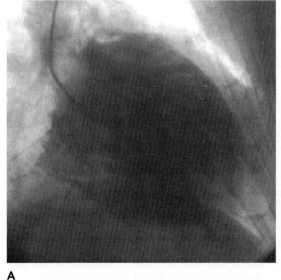
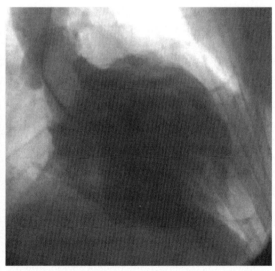

A   **B**

Figure 31.1   Left ventriculography in dilated cardiomyopathy at end-diastole **(A)** and end systole **(B).** This patient sustained an anterior myocardial infarction several years prior to presentation owing to single-vessel left anterior descending disease. The ventricle is now diffusely hypokinetic with a dyskinetic anterior wall. Postinfarct remodeling accounts for the enlargement of the ventricle and hypokinesis in the other (noninfarcted) territories. The lack of significant mitral regurgitation probably explains his relatively preserved exercise capacity.

TABLE 31.2

SERIAL HEMODYNAMICS IN CHRONIC HEART FAILURE OWING TO AN IDIOPATHIC DILATED CARDIOMYOPATHY

Year	RA	PCW (mean and V wave)	PA	CO	PVR	MAP	SVR
2000 (first diagnosis)	10	15	36/13/24	4.5	160	70	1067
2003 (baseline)	5	15/25	36/13/24	4.4	167	70	1181
2003 (exercise)		32/48	73/28/51	9.3	163		
2004 (baseline)	9	25/35	53/22/37	2.5	234	75	2112
2004 (nitroprusside)	5	16/20	30/16/22	4.5	107	60	978

RA, right atrial; PCW, pulmonary capillary wedge; PA, pulmonary artery; MAP, mean arterial pressure (mm Hg); CO, cardiac output (liters per minute); SVR, systemic vascular resistance, in dyne-sec-cm (exponent minus 5).

transplantation, the presenting capillary wedge pressure (mean of 28 mm Hg) was not predictive of survival, but the ability to reduce the pulmonary capillary wedge pressure to <16 mm Hg by the end of the hospitalization was predictive of outcome with a 1-year survival of 83% (compared with 38% if the filling pressures could not be so lowered by the end of hospitalization). The effect was independent of the final cardiac index achieved (13).

Responses to exercise, vasodilators, and inotropes are also optimally assessed with invasive hemodynamic measurements, although it should be noted that hemodynamics may improve significantly in the absence of drug therapy over time presumably due to favorable changes in adrenergic tone. In 21 patients who had their hemodynamics serially assessed over a 24-hour period, the cardiac index (CI) rose by an average of 0.23 L/minute per m^2 and the left ventricular filling pressure decreased by 5.9 mm Hg (15). Some patients even had spontaneous improvements that rivaled the effects of oral and intravenous vasodilator therapies. Postprandial improvements were also seen, confirming the importance of studying patients in the fasting state.

Case 1: Progressive Dyspnea in a Patient With Dilated Cardiomyopathy. A 50-year-old man presented with worsening exertional dyspnea, 4 years after presenting with new-onset heart failure. Evaluation at that time included compensated hemodynamics, normal coronary angiography, and an ejection fraction of 10% with an end-diastolic dimension of 7.2 cm plus moderately severe mitral regurgitation. An endomyocardial biopsy demonstrated myocyte hypertrophy and interstitial fibrosis. With an ACE inhibitor, a beta-blocker, digoxin, and diuretics, he improved to NYHA II, and cardiac transplantation was deferred because of his preserved functional capacity and a maximal oxygen consumption of 17 mL/kg per minute. One year ago, repeat right heart catheterization demonstrated compensated hemodynamics at baseline but significant increases in wedge and pulmonary pressures with exercise. Biventricular pacing with an implantable cardiac defibrillator improved his symptoms and increased his oxygen consumption to 19 mL/kg per minute.

Over the past few weeks, however, he developed increasing dyspnea and orthopnea despite an augmented diuretic regimen. Repeat cardiopulmonary exercise testing demonstrated a fall in his oxygen consumption to 15 mL/kg per minute, and he was readmitted for transplant evaluation. Repeat right heart catheterization demonstrated elevated pressures that were responsive to acute vasodilator therapy with nitroprusside and were reproduced with oral vasodilators and diuretics (see Table 31.2). He returned to NYHA II, and cardiac transplantation was again deferred.

Illustrative Points. Ambulatory patients with dilated cardiomyopathies are usually characterized by a relatively low normal resting cardiac output and a modest elevation in both right- and left-sided filling pressures. In advanced heart failure, the systemic vascular resistance rises significantly in response to the reduced cardiac output and neurohormonal response and may be quite elevated despite a reduced systolic blood pressure of 80 to 100 mm Hg. In 1,000 consecutive patients with chronic heart failure electively referred for transplantation (mean ejection fraction [EF] 22%, end-diastolic dimension 7.3 cm, NYHA class 3.4), the initial right atrial pressure was 11 ± 7 mm Hg, the pulmonary capillary wedge pressure was 25 ± 9 mm Hg, the pulmonary arterial (PA) systolic pressure was 50 ± 16, the cardiac index was 2.1 ± 0.7 liter/minute per m^2, and the systemic vascular resistance was 1,610 ± 610 dynes·sec·cm^{-5} (16). The right atrial (RA) pressure is typically 50 to 60% of the pulmonary capillary wedge (PCW) pressure and often correlates with left-side filling pressures regardless of heart failure etiology or tricuspid regurgitation. In the series of patients reported by Drazner (16), the positive predictive value of a RA >10 mm Hg for a PCW >22 was 88% (Fig. 31.2). The PCW usually corresponds with the PA systolic pressure (usually 50% of the PA systolic) as well as the PA diastolic pressure (PAD; usually within 1 to 2 mm Hg of PCW) as long as pulmonary vascular resistance is <2 Wood units (17). Right ventricular pressure can also be used to estimate the PAD, since right ventricular pressure closely approximates pulmonary end-diastolic pressure at the time of pulmonary valve opening (maximal right ventricular dP/dt (Fig. 31.3; 17).

TABLE 31.3

RESTING AND EXERCISE HEMODYNAMICS AFTER CARDIAC TRANSPLANTATION

Parameter	Rest	Exercise
Right atrial pressure (mm Hg)	6 ± 2	14 ± 7
Pulmonary artery pressure (mm Hg)	18 ± 3	32 ± 9
Pulmonary capillary wedge pressure (mm Hg)	10 ± 3	20 ± 6
Cardiac output (L/min)	5.0 ± 0.9	9.9 ± 1.7
Stroke volume (mL)	55 ± 9	77 ± 13
Heart rate (bpm)	90 ± 11	122 ± 18
Mean arterial pressure (mm Hg)	91 ± 12	102 ± 14
Systemic vascular resistance (Wood)	17.7 ± 4.0	9.3 ± 2.4

Hosenpud JD, Morton MJ. Physiology and hemodynamic assessment of the transplanted heart. In: *Cardiac Transplantation.* 164–189.

Pulmonary hypertension is also common in dilated cardiomyopathy and is predictive of prognosis. In patients with dilated cardiomyopathy and myocarditis, every 5 mm Hg rise in the mean pulmonary artery pressure increased mortality, with a relative hazard ratio of 1.85 (1.50 to 2.29; 10). In most patients, the pulmonary vascular resistance will be modestly elevated but still less than 2.5 Wood units. In other patients, more severe pulmonary hypertension and increases in pulmonary vascular resistance may be present if the heart failure is chronic or associated with significant mitral regurgitation or concurrent pulmonary disease (see later transplant case presentation).

Advanced heart failure in dilated cardiomyopathy is characterized by biventricular failure. The right atrial pressure waveform will demonstrate steep x and y descents indicative of severe volume overload and right ventricular systolic and diastolic dysfunction (Fig. 31.4A). Lack of the normal inspiratory fall (or an actual increase) in the right atrial pressure, i.e., the Kussmaul sign, is also common as the result of pericardial constraint in the massively dilated heart, significant tricuspid regurgitation, and right ventricular diastolic dysfunction. The y descent is typically very steep as a result of concomitant tricuspid regurgitation and poor right atrial compliance from excessive volume overload. The right ventricular diastolic waveform may also demonstrate a prominent y descent during rapid early diastolic filling, which becomes more prominent during inspiration (Fig. 31.4B). The pulmonary capillary wedge

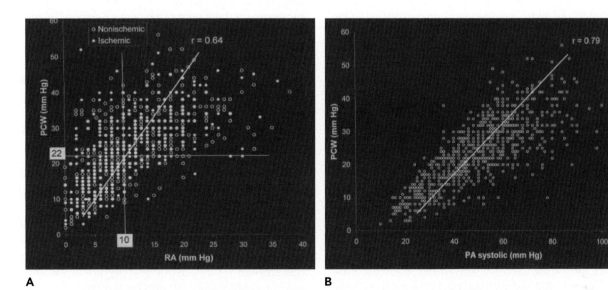

A   **B**

Figure 31.2 The relationship between **(A)** right atrial (RA) and pulmonary capillary wedge (PCW) pressure and **(B)** pulmonary capillary wedge pressure and pulmonary artery (PA) systolic pressure in 1,000 consecutive patients with chronic heart failure. (Reproduced with permission from Drazner MH, et al. Relationship between right and left-sided filling pressures in 1000 patients with advanced heart failure. *J Heart Lung Transplant* 1999;18:1126.)

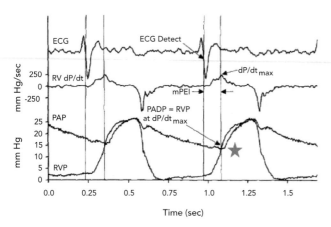

Figure 31.3 The pulmonary artery diastolic (PAD) pressure can be estimated from the right ventricular pressure (RVP) tracing since PAD is equal to right ventricular pressure at the maximal dP/dt (see *asterisk*). (Reproduced with permission from Reynolds DW, et al. Measurement of pulmonary artery diastolic pressure from the right ventricle. *J Am Coll Cardiol* 1995;25:1176.)

pressure may demonstrate a prominent V wave that may exceed twice the magnitude of the post A-wave pressure owing to reduced left atrial compliance, even in the absence of severe mitral regurgitation (Fig. 31.4C). The V wave may even be discernible in the pulmonary arterial waveform (Fig. 31.4E). The left ventricular pressure tracing is characterized by an elevation in pressure throughout early diastole. The systolic left ventricular waveform may be triangular owing to the reduced + and − dP/dt, and there may be loss of the normal improvement in dP/dt with increasing heart rate (Bowditch treppe effect). The arterial waveform demonstrates a narrow pulse pressure (pulsus parvus), which may be <25% of the systolic pressure when the cardiac index falls below 2.2 liters/minute per m² (8). In severe heart failure, there may also be pulsus alternans (Fig. 31.4D), owing to oscillations in myocardial contractility with cyclic changes in cytosolic calcium (18,19).

A common misconception about dilated cardiomyopathy is that elevated filling pressures are required to maximize preload-sensitive contractility (Starling's law). Severe left ventricular dysfunction can be well tolerated with well-compensated hemodynamics, concomitant satisfactory functional capacity comparable to transplantation (20), and reasonable long-term survival. In fact, a low ejection fraction alone is not an indication for cardiac transplantation for either morbidity or mortality reasons (21). In patients with dilated cardiomyopathy, stroke volume, stroke work index, and cardiac output can be maximized at pulmonary capillary wedge pressures as low as 10 mm Hg (Fig. 31.5; 22), and there is no justification for insufficient diuresis and dyspnea resulting from inadequate lowering of filling pressures. In 754 consecutive patients with chronic heart failure referred electively for cardiac transplantation, tailored doses of vasodilators and diuretics increased the cardiac index from 2.1 ± 0.7 to 2.6 ± 0.6 L/minute per m² despite a fall in the pulmonary capillary

wedge pressure from 25 ± 9 to 16 ± 6 mm Hg. In part, this improvement in forward cardiac output despite significant reduction of filling pressures is due to a decrease in mitral regurgitation caused by favorable changes in ventricular, atrial, and mitral annular geometry. This change can cause an increased forward stroke volume rather than an increase in total stroke volume (23,24). Left ventricular myocardial systolic performance can also improve due to elimination of right ventricular volume overload (7) whereas myocardial diastolic performance can improve due to reduced myocardial turgor that follows decreased venous congestion (25).

In general, optimization of hemodynamics is best achieved with intravenous vasodilators and diuretics rather than inotropic support. Vasodilator therapy takes advantage of the inverse relationship between resistance and output (Fig. 31.6) and is especially effective when systemic vascular resistance is >2,000 dynes·sec·cm⁻⁵. Once an optimal hemodynamic profile is achieved, the effects of intravenous vasodilators such as nitroprusside are easily replaced by oral vasodilators like ACE inhibitors (26), hydralazine, and nitrates. Intravenous nitroprusside (27,28) can be used even in the presence of relative hypotension (systolic blood pressure <100 mm Hg) if the hypotension is the result of low cardiac output and high vascular resistance. If clinically significant ischemia is present, intravenous nitroglycerin is preferred over nitroprusside owing to considerations of coronary steal. Intravenous nitroglycerin and nesiritide (29,30) can also be used to acutely improve the hemodynamics, especially when pulmonary hypertension and high central venous pressures are present.

The use of inotropic agents to optimize hemodynamics becomes limited by the inability to replace the direct inotropic effects with oral vasodilators. Clinical trials have suggested a worsening of mortality with intermittent use of inotropes for the longitudinal management of heart failure (31), but some patients may still require inotropic support despite attempts to tailor their hemodynamics with vasodilators and diuretics. Such patients in general will be bridged to more definitive treatments such as mechanical support or cardiac transplantation. Inotropic agents, such as phosphodiesterase inhibitors (i.e., milrinone) or beta agonists (i.e., dobutamine), will increase contractility (+dP/dt) and also decrease early and late diastolic pressures through their lusitropic (−dP/dt) effects (Fig. 31.7; 32). Milrinone is also a vasodilator, which can augment the cardiac output over and above its direct inotropic action (33).

In chronic heart failure, hemodynamic goals include a right atrial pressure <10 mm Hg, pulmonary capillary wedge pressure <15 mm Hg, and a systemic vascular resistance of <1,200 dynes·sec·cm⁻⁵, maintaining a systolic blood pressure >80 mm Hg or higher to avoid lightheadedness (12). Cardiac output can be measured reliably with the thermodilution technique in advanced heart failure, even in the presence of moderate to severe tricuspid

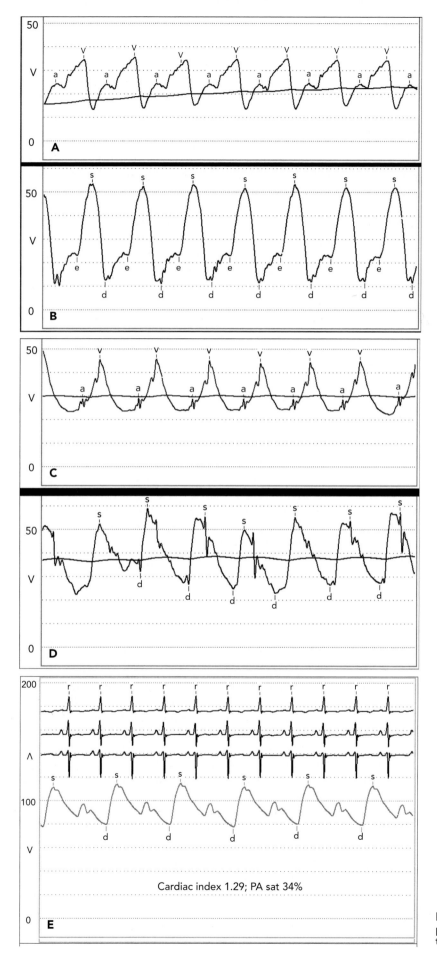

Cardiac index 1.29; PA sat 34%

Figure 31.4 Hemodynamic findings in decompensated heart failure from dilated cardiomyopathy. (See text for discussion.)

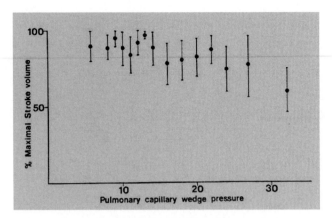

Figure 31.5 Maximal stroke volumes can be achieved at low filling pressures in advanced heart failure from dilated cardiomyopathy. (Reproduced with permission from Stevenson LW, et al. Maintenance of cardiac output with normal filling pressures in patients with dilated heart failure. *Circulation* 1986;74:1303.)

regurgitation (34,35). It may even be preferred over the Fick method with assumed (rather than measured) oxygen consumption. It is rare that hemodynamic monitoring is required for >72 hours to tailor hemodynamics in chronic heart failure, but some chronic monitoring is better than relying solely on measurements in the catheterization laboratory (15). Because hemodynamic goals are tailored and achieved in the supine position, the tolerability of an oral vasodilator regimen should be assessed after 24 hours of ambulation. With careful attention to volume status and vasodilators in follow-up, these hemodynamic profiles can also be maintained for months and years.

Exercise hemodynamic responses can be used to delineate the cause of persistent dyspnea, especially when resting hemodynamics are unremarkable or to assess cardio-

vascular reserve and prognosis (36). (See Chapter 15.) Most laboratories are not equipped to perform upright exercise protocols, so supine exercise strategies are often used. At the Brigham and Women's Hospital, we favor supine bicycling (with a specially designed bicycle) or arm exercise (by having the patient "bench press" saline or sandbags placed in both hands) until the patient becomes breathless or fatigued. We generally target at least a 50% increase in heart rate. Dramatic elevations in the pulmonary capillary wedge pressure and pulmonary arterial pressure with exercise despite "normal" or compensated hemodynamics at rest will confirm heart failure as the cause of exercise intolerance in such patients. Characteristically, a prominent V wave will also be present and will reflect worsening mitral regurgitation as well as poor atrial and ventricular compliance (Fig. 31.8). Cardiovascular reserve, by assessing the cardiac output response to exercise, is also used by some centers to assess prognosis, especially when the oxygen consumption is modestly reduced in the 10 to 18 mL/kg per minute range. At low levels of exertion, an increase in left ventricular end-diastolic volume and filling pressure are the primary determinants of stroke volume through the Starling mechanism. At high levels of exertion, tachycardia is accompanied by a decrease in end-diastolic volume despite a progressive increase in filling pressure, so that stroke volume must be maintained by a decrease in end-systolic volume. Beyond this point, increases in cardiac output are entirely due to increases in heart rate because the stroke volume is fixed. The lower limit of normal for the exercise cardiac output response is five times oxygen consumption (L/minute) plus 3 L/minute (37). To make these measurements, the laboratory must be equipped with either a treadmill or stationary bicycle and have the capacity to measure oxygen consumption simultaneously (36).

HEART TRANSPLANTATION

Despite the radical nature of replacing the human heart with another, the cardiac allograft has emerged as an effective way of restoring essentially normal cardiovascular function in end-stage heart failure. However, the transplanted heart is subject to a number of post-transplant factors that can influence cardiac function including denervation, organ preservation/ischemic injury, myocardial rejection, donor/recipient size mismatch, allograft coronary artery disease, and hypertension/ventricular hypertrophy. Initially, the transplanted heart also demonstrates a restrictive hemodynamic profile that resolves over days to weeks (38,39), although less dramatic abnormalities in diastolic function may persist (40-43, and Table 31.3). Resting contractility and ejection fraction are relatively normal (44), but total blood volume, cardiac volume, and end-systolic wall stress increase even if myocardial mass is unchanged (38). In general, mild impairment of ventricular functional reserve

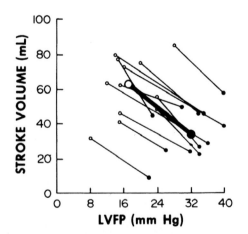

Figure 31.6 The effects of acute administration of nitroprusside on left ventricular filling pressures (LVFP) and stroke volume in patients with advanced heart failure. Maximal stroke volume is preserved at pulmonary capillary wedge pressures as low as 10 mm Hg. (Reproduced with permission from Guiha NH, et al. Treatment of refractory heart failure with infusion of nitroprusside. *N Engl J Med* 1974;291:587.)

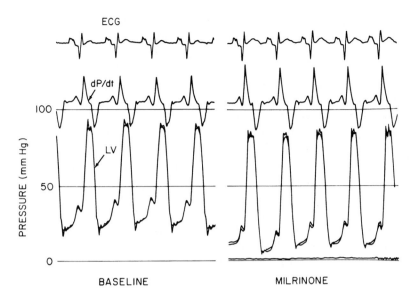

Figure 31.7 The hemodynamic effects of an inotropic agent, milrinone, in dilated cardiomyopathy. Milrinone increases contractility (positive dP/dt), improves lusitropy (negative dP/dt), and lowers preload (decreased left ventricular end-diastolic pressure [LVEDP]). The improvement in systolic and diastolic function occurs without an increase in systolic blood pressure. (Reproduced with permission from Baim DS, et al. Evaluation of a new bipyridine inotropic agent—milrinone—in patients with severe congestive heart failure. *N Engl J Med* 1983; 309:748.)

is present but demonstrable only with maximal exercise stress and may be in part a result of decreases in coronary flow reserve (45). The primary limitation in maximal cardiac output is due to the denervated heart having a blunted heart rate response, and the Frank-Starling mechanism is exhausted early in the response to supine (46,47) and upright exercise (48). This is partially offset by an increased sympathetic sensitivity, with dependence on circulating catecholamines for an adequate but delayed chronotropic exercise response (49).

Although left ventricular responses to hypertension and acute increases in afterload are normal after cardiac transplantation, the denervated heart does not tolerate hypoten-

sion well, presumably because of lack of ventricular compliance and reflex sympathetic tone. Denervation also leads to several other clinically relevant hemodynamic abnormalities in addition to the obvious loss of cardiac pain sensation. Efferent parasympathetic denervation of the heart leads to a resting tachycardia of 90 to 110 beats per minute (bpm), lack of heart rate variability, and the ineffectiveness of atropine and digoxin; efferent sympathetic denervation leads to blunted and delayed increases in heart rate in response to physiologic stress. Afferent denervation results in dysregulation of sodium and water homeostasis as well as abnormalities in peripheral vascular responses (50).

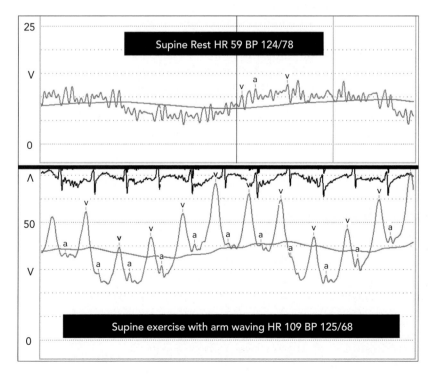

Figure 31.8 Effects of exercise on hemodynamics in dilated cardiomyopathy. Note development of prominent V wave and dramatic increase of pulmonary capillary wedge pressure with exercise. This effect was achieved with supine arm exercise (moving bags of saline up and down while supine) resulting in an almost twofold increase in heart rate (HR). The patient had an ejection fraction of 20%, an end-diastolic dimension of 7 cm, and moderately severe mitral regurgitation at rest. The lack of V waves and normal wedge pressure at rest are indicative of the chronic nature of the regurgitation. BP, blood pressure.

Right ventricular function is critical in the early post-transplant period. The normal right ventricle cannot accommodate significant acute pressure overload (51), and nowhere is this more apparent than in the post–cardiac transplant setting. Acute right heart failure accounts for 50% of all peri– and post–cardiac transplant complications and is a leading cause of early allograft failure and death. Not surprisingly, an elevated preoperative pulmonary vascular resistance predicts early postoperative death from acute right heart failure (52–54), and severe fixed pulmonary hypertension is a contraindication to cardiac transplantation.

Case 2: Assessing Pulmonary Vascular Resistance Prior to Transplantation. A 45-year-old woman with a 30-pack-year smoking history is transferred with advanced heart failure for consideration of heart transplantation following an anterior myocardial infarction 2 years earlier. She had three hospitalizations in the past year for heart failure and was readmitted 3 days prior to transfer after stabilization on lisinopril, carvedilol, digoxin, and furosemide. Pulmonary evaluation was remarkable for mild obstructive pulmonary disease. Acute vasodilator testing in the catheterization lab with various agents demonstrated reversible pulmonary hypertension, and she was considered acceptable for transplantation (see Table 31.4).

However, repeat catheterization 3 months later demonstrated recurrent severe pulmonary hypertension. Because of relative hypotension, milrinone was used to assess pulmonary vasoreactivity. Bolus milrinone did lower the pulmonary vascular resistance to an acceptable extent, and she was maintained on continuous intravenous milrinone while awaiting transplantation.

Illustrative Points. Pulmonary hypertension, defined as a pulmonary artery systolic pressure >30 mm Hg or mean pulmonary artery pressure of >20 mm Hg, is a common complication of heart failure and can contribute to its morbidity. Resting pulmonary vascular resistance predicts exercise tolerance in heart failure and is inversely correlated with oxygen consumption in these patients (55,56). In fact, exercise capacity is better predicted by right ventricular ejection fraction rather than the left ventricular ejection fraction, reflecting the role of pulmonary vascular resistance in limiting exercise capacity in heart failure (57).

In heart failure, the elevated left ventricular end diastolic pressure results in a passive or reactive increase in the pulmonary venous pressure and a consequent increase in the upstream pulmonary arterial pressure. These passive changes may also be accompanied by an increase in the transpulmonary gradient (mean PA minus mean PCW) reflected by increases in pulmonary vascular resistance (PVR) and right ventricular afterload. These changes in PVR in heart failure are mediated by alterations in pulmonary smooth muscle vascular tone as well as by structural changes in the pulmonary vessels. Changes in smooth muscle tone are generally reactive and reversible over the course of hours to days, but structural remodeling of the pulmonary vascular tree is likely fixed and reversible only over the course of months to years.

Pulmonary hypertension becomes a concern in the pretransplant setting when the pulmonary artery systolic pressure is >60 mm Hg, the transpulmonary gradient is >15 mm Hg, and/or the pulmonary vascular resistance is >4 Wood units (320 dynes·sec·cm^{-5}). Although in the Bethesda consensus conference on heart transplantation, PVR >6 to 8 Wood units was considered high risk (21), most centers do not use a fixed cutoff value for an acceptable PVR. In fact, in some patients with severe pulmonary hypertension who have successfully undergone heart transplantation or long-term ventricular assist device support, pulmonary pressures have returned to normal (39,58). Therefore, it is essential to ensure that pretransplant elevations in PVR are reversible. If so, specific chronic interventions such as continuous inotropic support or a ventricular assist device (VAD) may be required to keep their PVR low while patients await transplantation. This reduces the risk of allograft right ventricular failure in the early transplant course.

Costard-Jackle and Fowler at Stanford reported the predictive value of acute testing of pulmonary vasoreactivity with nitroprusside in 301 consecutive cardiac transplant candidates. The 3-month post-transplant mortality in this cohort was high in those candidates with a baseline PVR >2.5 Wood units (or 200 dynes·sec·cm^{-5}; 17.9% versus 6.9% for PVR <2.5 Wood units). Using graded incremental doses of nitroprusside in patients with either a PVR

TABLE 31.4

CHANGES IN PULMONARY VASCULAR RESISTANCE TO VARIOUS MANEUVERS

Condition	RA	PCW	PA	TPG	CO	PVR	SVR
Baseline	10	15	60/24/35	20	3.6	400	1666
Nitroprusside	5	20	40/24/30	10	4.5	178	1067
Milrinone	9	15	55/22/32	17	5.3	257	830

RA, right atrial; PCW, pulmonary capillary wedge; PA, pulmonary artery; TPG, transpulmonary gradient; CO, cardiac output; PVR, pulmonary vascular resistance; SVR, systemic vascular resistance (units are the same as Table 31.2.)

TABLE 31.5

AGENTS THAT CAN BE USED TO ASSESS PULMONARY VASOREACTIVITY

Agent	PVR	PAmean	PCW	CI	SVR	Notes
Nitroprusside	↓36%	↓23%	↓27%	↑30%	↓31%	Titrated in 25–50 µg/min increments
Milrinone	↓31%	↓12%	↓16%	↑42%	↓30%	50 µg/kg intravenous bolus
Nitric oxide	↓47%	NC	↑24%	↓9%	NC	80 ppm over 10 min
Prostaglandin E1	↓47%	↓21%	↓13%	↑23%	↓31%	Titrated in incremental doses of 0.02, 0.05, 0.10, 0.20, 0.30 µg/kg per min
Adenosine	↓41%	NC	↑12%	↑9%	NC	100 µg/kg per min

PVR, pulmonary vascular resistance; PA, pulmonary artery mean; PCW, pulmonary capillary wedge; CI, cardiac index; SVR, systemic vascular resistance; NC, no change.

>2.5 Wood units or a PA systolic pressure >40 mm Hg, the hemodynamic response was predictive of outcome. If the PVR could be decreased to <2.5 Wood units without hypotension (>85 mm Hg), the 3-month mortality was only 3.8%. In contrast, if the PVR could not be reduced to <2.5 Wood units or only at the expense of hypotension, the mortality was high (40.6 and 27.5%, respectively). In addition, in their series, all patients who died of right heart failure were in these latter two groups (59).

When used to assess pretransplant pulmonary vasoreactivity, nitroprusside should be started at 25 to 50 µg/kg and increased in 25 µg/kg increments every 5 minutes with reassessment of the pulmonary vascular resistance after each change in dose. Cardiac output is best assessed with thermodilution in this setting since it is more practical than trying to measure resting oxygen consumption repeatedly. Smaller increments or slower titration schemes should be considered when left ventricular filling pressures are low (<10 mm Hg).

Various other agents have been used to assess the reversibility of pulmonary hypertension (Table 31.5), although the mechanism by which PVR falls differs between agents. High-flow oxygen should be considered first, especially if the baseline arterial saturation is <95%. Nitroprusside, an endothelium-independent nitric oxide donor, decreases PVR by both decreasing the transpulmonary gradient and increasing the cardiac output (60,61). Dobutamine and other inotropes increase pulmonary blood flow with subsequent recruitment of parallel vessels in the pulmonary circulation and produce flow-mediated vasodilation (62). Bolus milrinone is simple and attractive since it avoids the need for titration and potential hypotension intrinsic to nitroprusside use (63). Using 50 µg/kg over 1 minute via a systemic vein, the peak lowering of PVR occurs within 5 to 10 minutes and is not associated with changes in systemic blood pressure or heart rate. Milrinone lowers the PVR by approximately 30% with a concomitant significant increase in the cardiac output but with little change in the transpulmonary gradient.

Selective pulmonary vasodilators are also attractive alternative pulmonary vasodilators since they presumably lack the systemic hypotensive effects of traditional vasoactive agents. For example, inhaled nitric oxide lowers PVR by decreasing the transpulmonary gradient and increasing the left ventricular filling pressure without significant changes in cardiac output or mean PA pressure (64–66). Although not useful for chronic therapy owing to its short half-life and potential toxicity, it has been used for assessing pulmonary vasoreactivity in cardiac transplant candidates (67), supporting high-risk surgical patients undergoing coronary bypass or valve replacement (68), and treating right ventricular dysfunction after heart transplantation or implantation of a ventricular assist device (69,70). When left ventricular function is normal, the increase in left ventricular filling from increased volumetric flow across the pulmonary circulation can be easily accommodated without significant symptomatic increases in the filling pressure. However, when left ventricular diastolic function is not normal and baseline filling pressures are elevated, the increase in pulmonary blood flow can result in further increases in left ventricular filling pressure in a noncompliant ventricle and may produce alveolar pulmonary edema (71). Adenosine (72) and prostaglandin E1 (73) produce similar effects (Table 31.5). Endothelin antagonists also appear to selectively vasodilate the pulmonary circulation (74) and have been used in primary forms of pulmonary hypertension when left ventricular function is normal (75). However, oral endothelin antagonists in heart failure do not appear to be beneficial in clinical trials, and these agents have not been used for acute testing of pulmonary vasoreactivity.

Case 3: Tricuspid Regurgitation (TR) After Cardiac Transplantation. A 56-year-old man presented for routine surveillance endomyocardial biopsy 1 week following cardiac transplantation for an idiopathic dilated cardiomyopathy. He had been awaiting cardiac transplantation in the hospital on intravenous milrinone, which had decreased his pulmonary vascular resistance from 340 to 200 dynes·sec^{-1}·cm^{-5}. A bicaval anastomosis was used during transplantation with an ischemic time of 150 minutes. Postoperatively, he required atrial pacing for sinus node dysfunction and prolonged inotropic and pressor support. His weight was 5 kg greater than his preoperative weight. Routine three-drug immunosuppression had been initiated without difficulty.

At right heart catheterization (Fig. 31.9), his right atrial pressure waveform was ventricularized consistent with severe TR. The right ventricular waveform was also characterized by a steep rapid early filling wave and an elevated end-diastolic pressure. Left-sided filling pressures were nor-

mal. The cardiac output was 4 L/minute, and the PVR was 180 dynes·sec·cm^{-5}. Echocardiography confirmed normal left ventricular systolic function without mitral regurgitation and severe TR in a hypokinetic, dilated RV.

Illustrative Points. Within days of transplantation, hemodynamics demonstrate evidence of right ventricular (RV) systolic and diastolic dysfunction characterized by the presence of a rapid y descent (greater in magnitude than the x descent), lack of an inspiratory decline in the right atrial pressure (the Kussmaul sign), and sometimes ventricularization of the atrial waveform suggestive of significant tricuspid regurgitation (Fig. 31.10). The right ventricular tracing is marked by a steep rapid filling wave and elevation of the end-diastolic pressure. The pulmonary capillary wedge pressure may demonstrate a prominent V wave (as much as twofold greater than the atrial wave) in the absence of sig-

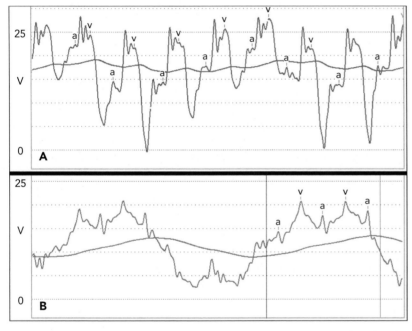

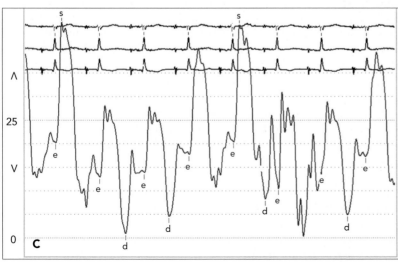

Figure 31.9 Severe tricuspid regurgitation early after cardiac transplantation. **A.** Right atrial waveforms are ventricularized consistent with severe tricuspid regurgitation. **B.** Pulmonary capillary wedge pressure is normal without V waves. **C.** Right ventricular waveforms suggest severe volume overload and dip and plateau phenomenon in absence of constrictive pericarditis.

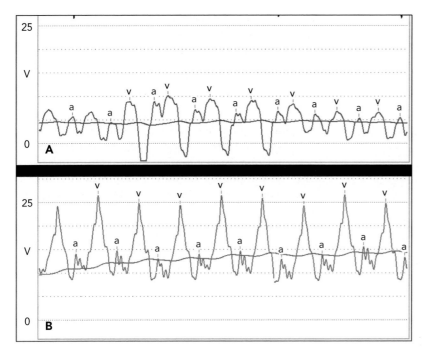

Figure 31.10 Typical hemodynamics after transplantation. This patient underwent uncomplicated transplantation 2 months prior. Echocardiography demonstrated mild right ventricular enlargement and dysfunction and normal left ventricular function with trivial mitral regurgitation. **A.** Kussmaul sign with dramatic Y descents notable in right atrial tracing and suggestive of right ventricular dysfunction in absence of constrictive pericarditis. **B.** V waves are prominent despite lack of significant mitral regurgitation and reflect poor left atrial compliance. No rejection was seen on biopsy.

nificant mitral regurgitation and reflects a volume-overloaded state and a poorly compliant left atrium and ventricle. Volume loading or leg raising may also bring out similar findings after transplantation if initial resting hemodynamics are normal and reflect the often occult nature of this restrictive picture (76). These hemodynamics usually improve with time, although the pace of improvement is variable. Bhatia et al. reported that left and right filling pressures decline within weeks with concomitant decreases in PVR and TR despite persistent RV enlargement (Table 31.6; 39). Evidence of elevated right ventricular end diastolic pressures is unusual late after transplant in the absence of severe TR. If present, consideration should be given to constrictive pericarditis, albeit rare in the posttransplant setting (77).

Tricuspid regurgitation early after transplantation is common. Generally, it is a secondary phenomenon and a reflection of right ventricular dilation and dysfunction, which is universal after transplantation. In this setting, right ventricular dysfunction is a consequence of ischemic injury, increased pulmonary vascular resistance, and volume overload.

Therapy for right ventricular failure should include prolonged intravenous inotropic support, aggressive volume control, and pulmonary vasodilators, such as nitric oxide. With appropriate treatment, even severe degrees of tricuspid regurgitation can resolve. In rare instances, tricuspid valve repair or replacement may be necessary. However, aggressive pharmacologic therapy and appropriate diuresis should be exhausted first, which may take days to weeks.

Tricuspid regurgitation late after transplantation is usually the consequence of bioptome injury to the tricuspid valve or allograft coronary artery disease. Some centers have been able to decrease the incidence of this problem by placing the biopsy sheath across the tricuspid valve to avoid inadvertent injury to the valve apparatus (78). Tricuspid regurgitation is also more frequent with the traditional biatrial anastomotic technique and less frequent with the more contemporary operation using a bicaval anastomosis (79). Rejection also appears to be a risk factor for late TR (80). Indications for surgery are similar to the nontransplant state and should be entertained if significant exercise capacity declines or if right heart failure becomes refractory to diuretics (81).

TABLE 31.6

HEMODYNAMIC CHANGES AFTER CARDIAC TRANSPLANTATION

Variable	Preop	2 Weeks	3 Months	1 Year
Right atrial pressure (mm Hg)	15 ± 5	9 ± 4	8 ± 4	7 ± 4
Mean pulmonary artery pressure (mm Hg)	38 ± 9	22 ± 5	21 ± 7	19 ± 5
Pulmonary wedge pressure (mm Hg)	30 ± 8	14 ± 5	13 ± 5	12 ± 4
Cardiac output (L/min)	3.5 ± 1.1	—	—	6.3 ± 1.5
PVR (dynes·sec^{-1}·cm^{-5})	213 ± 113	—	—	99 ± 36

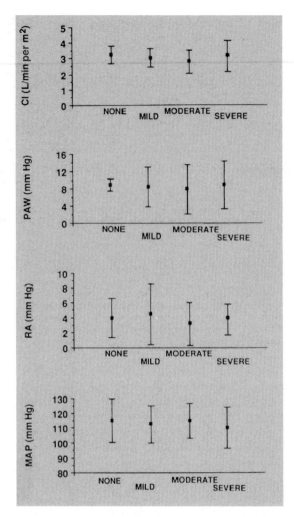

Figure 31.11 Hemodynamic profiles of the transplanted heart do not predict the presence, absence, or severity of rejection. MAP, mean arterial pressure; RA, right atrial; PAW, Pulmonary artery wedge pressure; CI, cardiac index. (Reproduced with permission from Uretsky, BF. *Physiology of the Transplanted Heart.* Cardiovasc Clin. 1990;20(2):41.)

Myocardial rejection is usually asymptomatic and is rarely predictable from hemodynamic abnormalities (Fig. 31.11), even when rejection is severe (82). Because rejection is most common in the first year after transplantation, biopsies are frequent and are used to guide the titration of the immunosuppressive regimen (see Chapter 20). As time from transplant lengthens, rejection becomes less common and biopsy frequency declines. Some centers stop routine surveillance biopsies after the second year because rejection is uncommon. In our center, annual biopsies are still performed regardless of time since transplant, significant transplant rejection, although rare, can still be seen years later (83,84).

VENTRICULAR ASSIST DEVICES

When advanced heart failure cannot be stabilized despite maximal medical therapy (typically involving inotropic

and vasoactive agents and/or intra-aortic balloon counterpulsation), surgically implantable ventricular assist devices (VADs) can be used as bridges to cardiac transplantation or to myocardial recovery and even as a permanent solution to end-stage heart disease (i.e., destination therapy; see also Chapter 21). Implantable VADs have been in clinical use since 1986 and are now used in >25% of patients eventually undergoing transplantation because donor shortages have forced longer and longer waiting times to transplantation. Several devices are currently approved for bridge-to-transplant, but only the HeartMate XVE LVAS is currently approved for destination therapy. One percutaneous device, the TandemHeart pVAD, is approved for cardiogenic shock (see Chapter 21). The currently approved devices primarily provide pulsatile flow, but continuous flow pumps are now in clinical trials.

As bridges to transplant, surgically implantable VADs are effective bridges to successful transplantation with two-thirds of patients making it to transplant and a post-transplant survival that is comparable with patients who have not required pretransplant VAD support. Complications of VADs include device failure (primarily motor bearing wear and inflow valve incompetence), infection, bleeding, thromboembolism (particularly stroke), and immunosensitization of the pretransplant candidate.

In the acute setting, the hemodynamic profile of a VAD candidate will be a cardiac index <2.0 L/minute per m^2, pulmonary capillary wedge pressure >20 mm Hg, and systolic blood pressure <80 mm Hg, despite inotropic/pressor agents and/or the need for intra-aortic balloon counterpulsation. In chronic heart failure, these hemodynamic criteria do not need to be met, but most patients will be inotrope dependent (85). In these patients, VAD support allows for nutritional and physical rehabilitation to occur, allows pulmonary vascular resistance to fall, and allows discharge of patients with long anticipated wait times to transplantation pressure. Clinical considerations at the time of implantation include the proposed clinical end point (i.e., recovery, transplant, and destination), need for biventricular support, and predicted surgical mortality in the postsurgical period.

The assessment in the catheterization laboratory prior to LVAD implantation should include coronary angiography to assess right ventricular blood supply (to ensure adequate right ventricular function when only LVAD is planned) as well as right atrial pressure and pulmonary vascular resistance. A right atrial pressure >20 mm Hg and a transpulmonary gradient >16 mm Hg predict right ventricular failure after LVAD placement (86) and should trigger consideration of biventricular VAD support. However, in patients with significant pulmonary vascular resistance but right atrial pressures <10 mm Hg, LVAD therapy alone can suffice and will eventually lead to normalization of the pulmonary vascular resistance.

Various centers use specific protocols when assessing the potentially dysfunctional VAD (87,88). In our center,

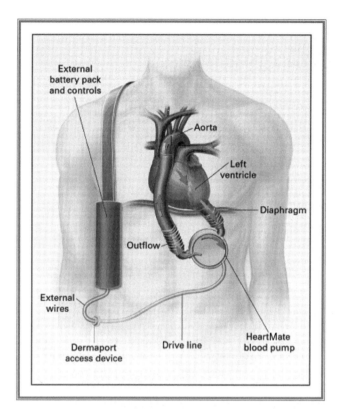

Figure 31.12 Representative configuration of an implantable ventricular assist device (see text for discussion). (Reproduced with permission from Goldstein DJ, Oz Mc, Rose EA. Implantable left ventricular assist devices. N Engl J Med 1998, 339:1522–33.)

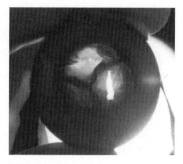

Still frames of inflow regurgitation from echo

A   **B**

Figure 31.13 Echocardiographic assessment of left ventricular assist device (LVAD) function. **A.** LVAD inflow valvular regurgitation can be seen as a regurgitant Doppler signal at the os of the inflow cannula at the left ventricular apex. **B.** Tear in inflow valve leaflet seen after explant resulted in VAD regurgitation.

post-VAD patients routinely undergo right heart catheterization to assess pulmonary vascular resistance 1, 3, and 6 months after surgery. Left and right heart hemodynamics with device fluoroscopy is also performed if clinical and/or echocardiographic assessment suggests device dysfunction. Appreciation of the VAD anatomy is also crucial before invasive hemodynamic assessment of the patient with VAD support. The inflow cannula is typically placed in the ventricular apex but may be placed in the atrium, especially if bridge to recovery is anticipated. The outflow graft is usually anastomosed to the anterior aspect of the great artery (aorta or pulmonary artery) several centimeters above the native outflow valve (Fig. 31.12). Depending on the device and body size, the pump itself is either placed within the abdomen or extracorporeally connected by percutaneous tubing.

Case 4: LVAD Dysfunction. A 67-year-old man presented with complaints that his LVAD rate had suddenly risen from a baseline rate of 70 bpm to 100 bpm in the automatic mode. A Thoratec HeartMate LVAD had been placed 9 months earlier due to advanced heart failure from coronary artery disease and complicated by severe pulmonary hypertension despite inotropic and vasodilator therapy. He had returned to part-time employment and was awaiting cardiac transplantation at home. While having dinner, he had noted the sudden rise in the rate of his device. In response to this change, he switched the LVAD mode from automatic to fixed

(at 50 bpm), but switched back because the fixed mode was associated with light-headedness and dyspnea. On exam, he appeared well without pallor. His blood pressure was 145/76 with a LVAD rate of 100 and an atrioventricular (AV) paced intrinsic heart rate of 100. His venous pressures were 10 cm of water and he was breathing comfortably. His lung and precordial exam demonstrated normal VAD sounds. The liver was not enlarged; no pedal edema was present, and he had warm extremities. Laboratories demonstrated no evidence for hemolysis, but the serum creatinine had risen from 1.5 to 2.0 mg/dL and the serum sodium had fallen from 138 to 133 mg/dL. Echocardiography confirmed the presumptive diagnosis of inflow valvular regurgitation with lack of left ventricular decompression, regular opening of the aortic valve, and evidence of a regurgitant flow signal in the apical outflow graft (Fig. 31.13).

Cardiac catheterization was performed to confirm the diagnosis and assess the pulmonary vascular resistance in light of recurrent heart failure despite the LVAD. The hemodynamics are shown in Table 31.7. The wedge pressure is elevated from baseline (normally post-LVAD, the wedge pressure should be <10 mm Hg) and increases further with limiting the VAD rate by switching the device to the fixed rate mode at 80 bpm. The VAD flow is 7.3 L/minute, but the cardiac output assessed by thermodilution is 5.5 L/minute (Table 31.7). (Normally, the measured cardiac output may be greater than the VAD flow or output by as much as 1 L/minute owing to the contribution of the native ventricle. In contrast, a VAD output greater than the measured cardiac output suggests inflow regurgitation.)

An end-hole multipurpose catheter was placed in the left ventricle retrograde across the aortic valve and placed into the os of the inflow valve, demonstrating the presence of "VAD" V waves and thus confirming the echocardiographic diagnosis (Fig. 31.14). The VAD V wave was not appreciated until the catheter was moved from the body of the ventricle to the os of the inflow cannula (Fig. 31.15).

Illustrative Points. The primary limitation to long-term support with implantable VADs is mechanical device

TABLE 31.7

THE HEMODYNAMICS OF INFLOW VALVULAR REGURGITATION

Conditions	VAD Flow (L/min)	CO (TD) (L/min)	RA (mm Hg)	PCW (mm Hg)	PA (mm Hg)	PVR (d·s·cm^{-5})
Baseline post LVAD	5.0	4.8	5	11	33/10/21	160
Auto rate	7.3	5.5	9	15	41/17/27	174
Fixed rate	6.4	—	—	20	46/21/32	160

VAD, ventricular assist device; CO (TD), cardiac output (thermodilution); RA, right atrial; PCW, pulmonary capillary wedge; PA, pulmonary artery; PVR, pulmonary vascular resistance; LVAD, left ventricular assist device.

failure. In the REMATCH trial, which randomized 129 advanced heart failure patients to the HeartMate electric LVAD or optimal medical therapy, 35% of patients experienced device failure over 24 months of follow-up and 10 of 68 patients required device replacement (89). Inflow valve regurgitation is the most common type of device failure; it is characterized by a rapid increase in the baseline output of the LVAD in the automatic mode and can occur within months of device implantation (87). Outflow obstruction may also occur, especially if the outflow graft conduit becomes kinked. At our institution, we have had a case of fungal endocarditis obstructing the outflow valve. The bearings used in the electrically driven rotor may also wear with time, and this dysfunction is usually discovered from device alarms and examination of the air vent filter for trace metals. Although echocardiographic studies are initially used to diagnose LVAD dysfunction, right and left heart catheterization is recommended to confirm the diagnosis (89a).

In general, the VAD pump cycle is asynchronous to the native heart's rhythm. The VAD fills passively from the ventricle via a unidirectional porcine valve. In the auto rate mode, the pump ejects when the pumping chamber is at least 90% filled (or 75 mL of the 83 mL chamber with a HeartMate LVAD) to deliver a relatively constant stroke volume. It therefore is responsive to physiologic demands and preload; it will speed up or slow down according to the preload received. If the patient is hypovolemic, the VAD auto rate will slow to allow time for the device to fill. If the patient is hypervolemic, the VAD auto rate will increase to

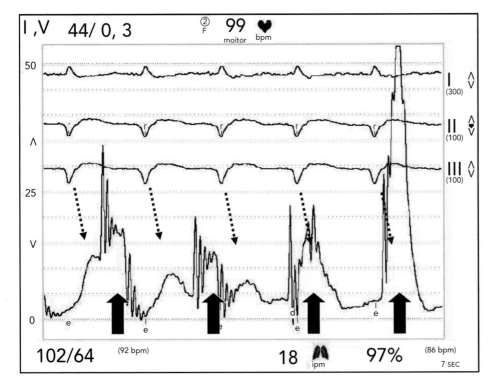

Figure 31.14 Hemodynamic waveforms taken from inside the inflow cannula of a ventricular assist device with inflow valvular regurgitation. *Dotted arrows* indicate native left ventricular systolic pressure. Native left ventricular systolic pressures are less than the aortic diastolic pressure and do not result in aortic valve opening. The *solid arrows* indicate the VAD ejecting retrograde into the ventricle across the incompetent VAD inflow valve (a VAD V wave).

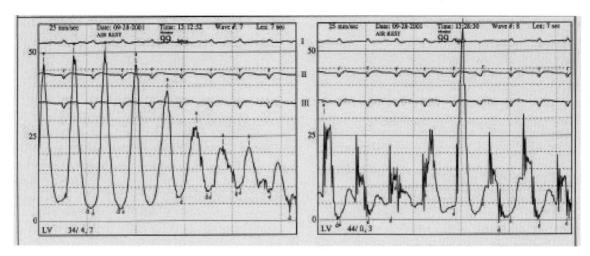

Figure 31.15 Left ventricular hemodynamics in a patient with left ventricular assist device (LVAD) inflow valvular regurgitation. VAD V wave is not apparent in main body of ventricle until catheter is moved to the os of the inflow cannula. (See text for discussion.)

accommodate the increase in filling. In the fixed rate mode, the device pumps at the preset rate independent of loading conditions. In the normally functioning LVAD, the native aortic valve opens only occasionally if at all and is dependent on the variable preload and afterload the ventricle encounters as the synchrony with the LVAD pump cycle varies (Fig. 31.16). This is actually a desired feature to prevent thromboembolism from the aortic root.

Inflow valvular regurgitation is characterized by an increase in VAD pumping rate in the auto rate mode as the device attempts to keep up with the regurgitating volume.

Unlike the human heart, the VAD cannot dilate over time, so the forward stroke volume cannot be increased and the output of the device is increased by increasing its rate. In the automatic mode, the VAD may not be able to keep pace with the regurgitant preload and the pulmonary capillary wedge pressure can rise. The wedge pressure in the fixed rate mode will also rise, especially if the rate is set too low since there will be not be adequate decompression of the ventricle. Left ventricular hemodynamics may demonstrate a V wave, especially if an end-hole catheter is placed within the os of the inflow cannula (Fig. 31.14). With inflow valvular regurgitation, the ventricle is incompletely unloaded and inadequately decompressed because of the regurgitant volume, and systolic pressures in the ventricle will open the aortic valve frequently (Fig. 31.17). Finally, ventriculography can be useful since it may

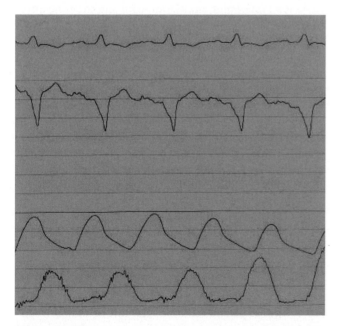

Figure 31.16 Left ventricular hemodynamics in a patient without inflow valvular regurgitation. In the adequately decompressed ventricle with left ventricular assist device (LVAD) support, the native left ventricle will only intermittently generate systolic pressure great enough to open the aortic valve. **Top.** Tracing is femoral arterial waveform. **Bottom.** Tracing is from catheter in left ventricle.

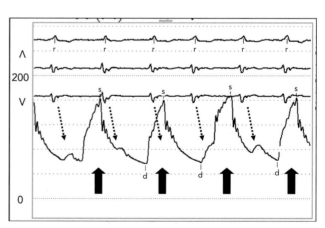

Figure 31.17 Arterial waveform in a patient with an inadequately decompressed ventricle despite left ventricular assist device (LVAD) support. *Dotted arrows* demonstrate native left ventricular ejection discernible in the arterial waveform. *Solid arrows* indicate arterial pressure generated from LVAD. (See text for further discussion.)

demonstrate a negative contrast effect from the regurgitating volume.

Therapy for this type of dysfunction is inflow valve or VAD replacement. If the patient is awaiting transplantation but is stable without heart failure, recurrent renal insufficiency, or persistent pulmonary hypertension despite the regurgitation, replacement can be safely deferred for eventual transplantation.

GIANT CELL MYOCARDITIS

Unexplained heart failure from systolic dysfunction is a common clinical problem in the catheterization laboratory, and the decision to proceed to endomyocardial biopsy is often debated. (In Chapter 20, the role of endomyocardial biopsy is discussed in greater detail.) Although many potential diagnoses can be made by endomyocardial biopsy, myocarditis is probably the most common distinct histopathologic diagnosis. Although the positive predictive value of the endomyocardial biopsy for myocarditis is high, the negative predictive value is low (90,91), which has tempered the enthusiasm for the procedure in many catheterization laboratories. Furthermore, conventional immunosuppressive therapies appear ineffective (92), sustaining the argument that therapy is unlikely to change on the basis of biopsy findings. Yet, the diagnosis of myocarditis in certain situations is important, especially when specific types of myocarditis can be identified.

Case 5: Giant Cell Myocarditis. A 39-year-old woman without significant prior medical history presented with 1 month of cough, dyspnea, weakness, and nausea. She denied fever, sick contacts, or chest pain. In the emergency room, she was pale, cool, and confused. Her blood pressure was 75/60, her heart rate was 140 and irregular, and she was tachypneic. The chest radiograph demonstrated pulmonary edema without cardiomegaly, and the electrocardiogram was notable for low volts and rapid atrial fibrillation. Urgent echocardiography demonstrated a nondilated left ventricle but a dilated right ventricle, severe biventricular dysfunction, and moderate mitral and tricuspid regurgitation. She was brought urgently to the cath lab where an intra-aortic balloon was inserted and angiography demonstrated normal coronary arteries. Hemodynamics were notable for a right atrial pressure of 22, pulmonary capillary wedge pressure of 26 with V waves to 40, and a cardiac index of 1.3 L/minute per m^2. An endomyocardial biopsy was obtained. The following day, biventricular assist devices were placed owing to persistent shock despite maximal inotropic/vasopressor support, mechanical ventilation, and an intra-aortic balloon pump. The endomyocardial biopsy revealed diffuse giant cell myocarditis with multifocal areas of healing injury. Over the course of 2 weeks, she was treated with immunosuppressive agents with significant improvement in her ventricular function.

Following a successful VAD weaning trial, the ventricular assist devices were successfully explanted and she was eventually discharged to rehabilitation with normal ventricular systolic function.

Illustrative Points. The presence of cardiogenic shock in the absence of myocardial infarction or extensive coronary artery disease should elicit a consideration of fulminant myocarditis (see later discussion) and obtaining an endomyocardial biopsy. In fact, viral myocarditis may mimic acute myocardial infarction (93). The initial size and geometry of the dysfunctional ventricle may also be clues to the chronicity of the myocardial inflammation since lack of dilation and sphericity implies an acute-onset cardiomyopathy. The rapidly progressive nature of heart failure culminating in shock is characteristic of giant cell myocarditis although other forms of myocarditis, i.e., including lymphocytic, may also present in this manner (94). Giant cell myocarditis, in particular, is important to identify because of its natural history and implications for therapy (95). It can be diagnosed only histologically since it may clinically mimic other types of myocarditis and may even be confused histologically with cardiac sarcoidosis. In a multicenter registry of 63 patients with this disorder, the rate of death or cardiac transplantation was 89% with a median survival of only 5.5 months from the onset of symptoms. Compared with lymphocytic myocarditis, giant cell myocarditis is more likely to be associated with ventricular tachycardia, heart block, more severe depression in ventricular function, and a worse prognosis (92,96). Afflicted patients tend to be relatively young (mean age 44 in registry), Caucasian (88% in registry), and previously healthy. There is an interesting association with autoimmune disorders, especially Crohn disease and ulcerative colitis, implying a unifying autoimmune pathogenesis. The pathophysiology appears dependent on CD-4 positive T lymphocytes, and an experimental Lewis rat model has been created using autoimmunization against myosin (97). Treatment with immunosuppression with either azathioprine or cyclosporine may extend survival to as long as a year although corticosteroids alone do not appear to have any impact. However, the treatment of choice is cardiac transplantation, but a high early postoperative mortality that approaches 15% should be anticipated. Even more disheartening is the disease may recur in the transplanted heart (98). In the multicenter registry, 9 of 35 patients who underwent transplantation developed biopsy evidence of recurrence on average 3 years after transplantation, but most did not develop recurrent heart failure.

Lymphocytic myocarditis is a more common myocarditis and quite lethal with a 1-year mortality of 15 to 20% (99,100). It is presumed to be viral in etiology, although this hypothesis has been difficult to prove. The utility for searching for this entity in new-onset dilated cardiomyopathy remains unclear, especially since the yield for a pathologic diagnosis is highly variable (ranging from 0 to 63% in 30 studies) and specific therapy remains undefined

(92). In the Myocarditis Treatment Trial, using a consensus panel of experienced cardiac pathologists, only 214 of 2,233 patients with unexplained heart failure had histopathologic evidence of myocarditis. The yield may be increased if biopsies are limited to those individuals with symptoms of 6 months or less (94).

Despite these limitations, histologic evidence of myocarditis can prove useful, especially for predicting prognosis. A clinicopathologic classification was developed at the Johns Hopkins Hospital that combines histologic evidence of myocarditis with specific features of the clinical course (see Chapter 20 for a more extensive discussion). In this classification system, fulminating myocarditis is defined by severe hemodynamic compromise requiring vasopressors (>5 μg/kg per minute of dopamine or dobutamine) or a left ventricular assist device. In addition, at least two of three clinical criteria are required: fever, a viral prodrome of less than 2 weeks before hospitalization, and the distinct onset of heart failure symptoms (fatigue, dyspnea, or new-onset edema). Fulminant myocarditis is also characterized by a greater degree of right heart failure and a lower systemic vascular resistance when compared with acute myocarditis despite similar pulmonary capillary wedge pressures and cardiac outputs (99). The presence of significant pulmonary hypertension appears to be especially lethal in myocarditis, with an almost twofold increase in mortality (RR 1.85, CI 1.50 to 2.29) for every 5 mm Hg increase in mean pulmonary artery pressure (10). Fortunately, a fulminating course is a relatively uncommon clinical manifestation of myocarditis (15 of 147 myocarditis patients in the Hopkins series). Fulminant myocarditis should be contrasted with the more common form of myocarditis (so-called acute myocarditis), which is characterized by a less distinct onset, a more indolent course, and lack of spontaneous recovery.

Ironically, a distinct clinical course consistent with fulminant myocarditis predicted a good prognosis with a transplant free survival of 93% after 11 years (99). Concomitant with clinical recovery and improvement in left ventricular function is long-term survival if the patient can be successfully supported with either mechanical or pharmacologic means during cardiovascular collapse. Interestingly, immunosuppression does not appear to improve survival in this situation.

DIASTOLIC HEART FAILURE AND RESTRICTIVE CARDIOMYOPATHIES

Heart failure when left ventricular systolic function is normal (HF-nEF), commonly referred to as *diastolic heart failure*, is often a difficult clinical entity to diagnose. The traditional physiologic definition states that filling of the left ventricle to a normal end-diastolic volume occurs only at higher-than-normal end-diastolic pressures, i.e., that there is a leftward and upward shift of the end-diastolic

pressure-volume relationship. In clinical practice, it is defined by the presence of heart failure symptoms (effort intolerance, dyspnea, peripheral edema) in the absence of significant systolic dysfunction. When the diagnosis of HF-nEF is made on clinical grounds, it rarely requires confirmation with the traditional physiologic definition. When diagnostic uncertainty exists, however, the physiologic definition is often sought to confirm the clinical impression.

One of the more common clinical errors is to attribute exertional intolerance or signs of heart failure to the heart before other diagnoses (restrictive lung disease, pericardial processes, pulmonary hypertension, and anemia) have been sufficiently excluded. Only then can the diagnosis of HF-nEF be established, and the distinction between primary or intrinsic conditions (such as restrictive cardiomyopathies) versus secondary or reactive conditions (such as hypertensive heart disease) be made. If primary diastolic dysfunction is a consideration in the absence of an explanation such as significant hypertension or renal insufficiency, cardiac catheterization should be considered to exclude coronary artery disease and pericardial constriction, two imitators of a restrictive cardiomyopathy. If these are not present and restriction is documented by hemodynamics, an endomyocardial biopsy should be performed to assess its etiology. Primary restrictive cardiomyopathies are characterized pathophysiologically by diastolic dysfunction owing to an infiltrative disorder in the absence of a physiologic loading condition (i.e., hypertension) that might lead to reactive ventricular hypertrophy or fibrosis. Hemodynamically, there is impedance to ventricular filling, impaired relaxation, relatively fixed end-diastolic volumes, and biatrial enlargement. Examples include infiltrative conditions, such as amyloid, hemochromatosis, and sarcoidosis, as well as rarer conditions, such as idiopathic restrictive cardiomyopathy, endomyocardial fibrosis, and Fabry disease.

In contrast, secondary HF-nEF denotes diastolic dysfunction that occurs as the consequence of excessive preload (i.e., renal failure) and/or afterload (i.e., hypertension). This type of HF-nEF is more common than restrictive cardiomyopathies and is sometimes referred to as diastolic heart failure, as mentioned above. It was recently concluded that abnormalities in diastolic function are sufficient to explain the primary pathophysiologic process. Zile et al. demonstrated a longer time constant for isovolumic-pressure decline (tau) and a shift up and to the left in the end-diastolic pressure volume relationship comparing a group of middle-aged men with a history of HF-nEF without hypertrophy with age-matched controls (Fig. 31.18; 101). Yet, epidemiologic studies consistently show that most patients with HF-nEF are predominantly elderly (median age >70 years), female (60 to 70%), hypertensive, and diabetic. These observations suggest that it is likely a subset of patients with HF-nEF, i.e., the Zile cohort, have a primary abnormality of LV filling as a type of restrictive

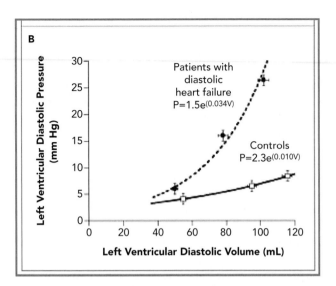

Figure 31.18 Leftward and upward shift of the end-diastolic pressure-volume relationship in men with a history of heart failure but normal systolic function (see text for discussion). (Reproduced with permission from Zile MR, et al. Diastolic heart failure—abnormalities in active relaxation and passive stiffness of the left ventricle. *N Engl J Med* 2004;350:1953.)

cardiomyopathy, whereas the more common elderly hypertensive women with HF-nEF more likely have abnormalities of diastolic function that reflect a reactive or secondary response of ventricular form and function to a more primary insult such as vascular stiffness (102–104). In addition, volume expansion, renal dysfunction, and anemia (105) may also play important roles in disease pathogenesis and progression in such patients, constituting more amenable targets for therapy than trying to improve diastolic stiffness itself. .

In clinical practice, demonstrating diastolic abnormalities by either noninvasive or invasive means may not be necessary to make the diagnosis of these secondary forms of HF-nEF. Most patients with a history of HF-nEF will have some type of demonstrable abnormality of diastolic function by either invasive or noninvasive means that serves to confirm rather than establish the diagnosis (106). Furthermore, since the type of diastolic abnormality is not uniform, the clinical utility of documenting diastolic dysfunction is less clear. In fact, diastolic abnormalities are not uncommon in asymptomatic individuals (107). In a study of 2,042 randomly selected residents from Olmstead county, diastolic dysfunction (defined by echocardiographic criteria) was common (28.1%), yet less than half of those affected had any history of heart failure.

Case 6: Amyloid Heart Disease. A 60-year-old man presented with persistent heart failure and weight loss. He had suffered an inferior myocardial infarction and had undergone right coronary stenting 5 years previously. He began to experience dyspnea and recurrent angina 6 months ago and had undergone repeat cardiac catheteri-

zation at that time. Coronary angiography demonstrated a new high-grade ulcerated plaque in the proximal circumflex and a widely patent previously stented right coronary artery. Ventriculography demonstrated an ejection fraction of 40% with no mitral regurgitation or wall motion abnormalities. Hemodynamics were remarkable for decompensated heart failure: RA 12/12/10, RV 55/11, PA 55/27/36, PCW 30, CI 1.4 (Fig. 31.19). He underwent circumflex stenting and was admitted for heart failure management. He returned 24 hours later with stent thrombosis, which was successfully treated with repeat angioplasty.

He continued to have severe fatigue, weight loss, and exertional angina. He was intolerant of angiotensin-converting enzyme inhibitors (ACEI) owing to hypotension and excessive azotemia. He had recently developed atrial fibrillation and had undergone a left popliteal arterial thrombectomy for an acutely painful cold left foot. There had been no history of hypertension or diabetes, but he had only recently stopped smoking and drinking alcohol.

On exam, he was chronically ill with a blood pressure (BP) of 85/70, a heart rate of 95 and irregular, breathing comfortably. Multiple ecchymoses were noted. His venous pressures were elevated at 12 cm of water with weak carotid upstrokes. His lungs were dull in the bases. His cardiac exam revealed distant heart sounds without gallop or murmur. His liver was enlarged and pulsatile, but the abdomen was without frank ascites. The extremities were tepid to touch and without significant edema.

Electrocardiography demonstrated atrial fibrillation, low limb voltage, a rightward axis, and prior inferior myocardial infarction (IMI; Fig. 31.20). Echocardiography was notable for severe concentric hypertrophy, myocardial speckling, a mild decrease in left ventricular function, and biatrial enlargement (Fig. 31.21). Fat pad aspirate and duodenal biopsy were negative for amyloid, but a serum protein electrophoresis demonstrated a monoclonal spike consistent with multiple myeloma. Endomyocardial biopsy demonstrated myocyte hypertrophy, separation of myofibrils by infiltrating amyloid protein, and green birefringence with congo red consistent with amyloid (Fig. 31.22). Bone marrow confirmed multiple myeloma. Melphalan and prednisone were initiated, which transiently improved his symptoms, but he died 3 months later. At autopsy, classic "wax drippings" lined the left atrium, confirming endocardial deposition of amyloid protein (Fig. 31.22).

Illustrative Points. In patients with heart failure and preserved systolic function, simultaneous right and left heart hemodynamics should be measured to distinguish restrictive heart disease from pericardial constriction. If there is primary diastolic heart failure, an endomyocardial biopsy should be performed, especially if the hemodynamics are not diagnostic of constriction. In clinical practice, restrictive physiology is most likely encountered in the context of previous mediastinal radiation, diabetes, "burned out"

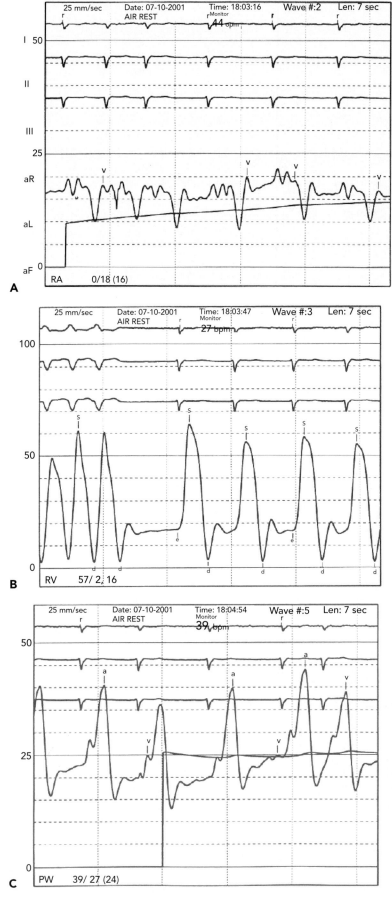

Figure 31.19 Hemodynamics of amyloidosis, a restrictive cardiomyopathy. The elevated right atrial pressure, Kussmaul sign, and prominent Y descents **(A)** as well as the dip and plateau in the right ventricular tracing **(B)** are indicative of severe right ventricular dysfunction and not constriction. Prominent V waves **(C)** are present in the wedge tracing despite the lack of mitral regurgitation and reflect the volume overload in the stiff atrium, characteristic of amyloid. Classically, the involvement of the left ventricle is greater than the right and simultaneous assessment of right and left ventricular end-diastolic pressures show LVEDP – RVEDP > 5 mm Hg. Severe pulmonary hypertension is also consistent with restrictive heart disease **(D)**. Also note prominent A wave in left ventricular end-diastolic pressure **(E)**. Respirophasic ventricular systolic concordance **(F)** is more consistent with restrictive heart disease, even if other hemodynamic findings are suggestive of constrictive pericarditis. The ventricular systolic pressures both fall with inspiration (*black arrows*) and peak with expiration (*crosshatched arrows*).

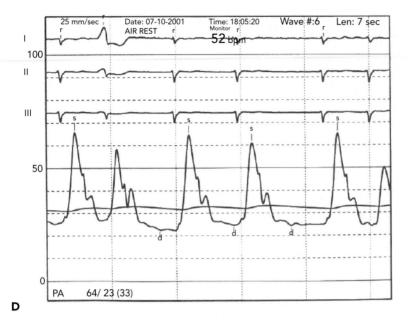

D

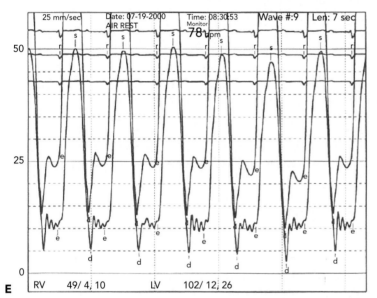

E

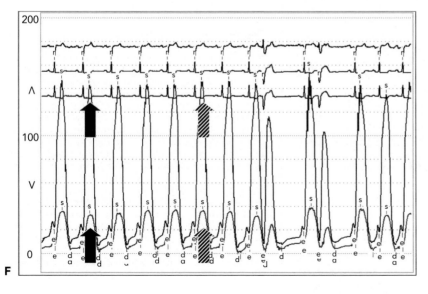

F

Figure 31.19   *(continued)*

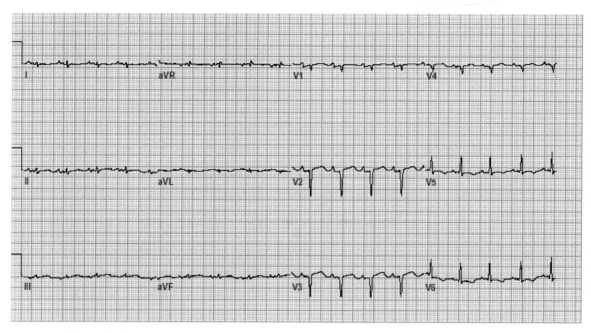

Figure 31.20 Electrocardiogram of a patient with amyloid. Classic findings include low limb lead voltage but preserved precordial voltage, nonspecific ST changes, P wave prominence, and pseudoinfarct pattern with precordial Q waves.

hypertrophic cardiomyopathy, anthracyclines, and amyloidosis. In general, true restrictive cardiomyopathies such as idiopathic restrictive cardiomyopathy, storage diseases (i.e., hemochromatosis and Fabry disease), and endomyocardial fibrosis are quite rare, and are described further in Chapter 20.

The hemodynamics of restrictive heart disease (Fig. 31.19) classically demonstrate advanced right heart failure and poor left atrial compliance (large V waves). A rapid early filling wave in the end diastolic pressure tracing

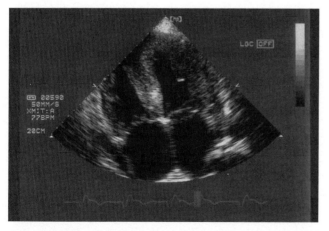

Figure 31.21 Echocardiogram of a patient with amyloid. Note low normal sized ventricular cavity, severe hypertrophy despite low limb voltage on EKG, biatrial enlargement, speckling pattern of myocardium, slow myocardial relaxation, and restrictive mitral inflow pattern. (Images courtesy of Carolyn Ho, M.D.)

(square root sign), dramatic x and y descents (M or W sign), and the Kussmaul sign may also be present. Traditionally, restrictive processes affect the left ventricle to a greater extent than the right ventricle and the LVEDP will be greater than the RVEDP. Severe pulmonary hypertension may be present in contrast to constrictive pericarditis, which typically produces only modest pulmonary hypertension (i.e., <50 mm Hg). Unfortunately, most of these hemodynamic characteristics are not specific enough to distinguish the restrictive profile from constrictive pericarditis. Hurrell et al. notes that interventricular dependence through the demonstration of respirophasic systolic ventricular dissociation is more reliable in separating cases of constriction from restriction (108).

Amyloidosis is caused by the fibrillar deposition of insoluble amyloid (meaning starch or cellulose) proteins into various organs, causing dysfunction and ultimately death (109). There are three forms of amyloidosis defined by the type of amyloid protein deposited. In *primary amyloidosis* (AL), the most common form, monoclonal light-chain immunoglobulins (Bence Jones proteins) are generated by plasma cells, which become deposited in the heart and kidney resulting in heart failure and nephrotic syndrome. In *secondary or reactive amyloidosis* (SAA), the amyloid protein is serum amyloid A, an acute phase reactant, which is produced in response to untreated chronic inflammatory illnesses such as tuberculosis and rheumatoid arthritis. Although renal insufficiency and hepatosplenomegaly are common, heart failure is very rare. *Familial amyloidosis* (ATTR) is caused by transthyretin, a thyroxine transport protein capable of forming beta-pleated

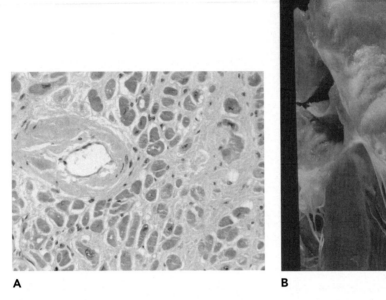

A   B

Figure 31.22 Endomyocardial biopsy of patient with amyloid. **A.** Even without congo red stain-ing, amyloid is suggested by separation of myofibrils and infiltration of blood vessels by pink amor-phous proteinaceous material. Hypertrophy notably absent as well. **B.** At autopsy, left atrial walls appear leathery and waxy, consistent with endocardial deposition of amyloid protein. (Photographs courtesy of Gayle Winters, M.D.)

fibrillar sheets. Depending on the type of transthyretin, the clinical syndrome may be familial or associated with aging. Heart failure tends to be less severe with both peripheral and autonomic neuropathies dominating the picture. In clinical practice, only AL and ATTR are of concern since SAA is rare in the absence of some untreated chronic infec-tious or inflammatory disease.

Amyloid heart disease is a common cause of true restric-tive cardiomyopathy and should be considered in any patient with primary HF-nEF. Angina may also be present, even in the absence of obstructive coronary disease. Noninvasive clinical clues include echocardiographic evi-dence of biatrial enlargement, pseudohypertrophy, speck-ling of the myocardium, small ventricular cavities, and restrictive mitral inflow profiles (see echo images). Electrocardiography may demonstrate low limb lead volt-age, Q waves/pseudoinfarct pattern, and various levels of AV block (Fig. 31.20). Atrial fibrillation is common as well and reflects both the consequences of chronically elevated atrial pressures and atrial infiltration by amyloid. The cardiovascu-lar exam is dominated by signs of right heart failure with ele-vation in venous pressures, rapid y descents, an inspiratory increase in venous distension (Kussmaul sign), and hepatomegaly. The diagnostic evaluation begins with high clinical suspicion and a tissue diagnosis of an affected organ system. The heart should be biopsied if heart failure is pre-sent. A bone marrow biopsy to assess plasma cell abundance and serum and urine immunofixation electrophoresis

should also be obtained, especially if the biopsy confirms the presence of amyloid. Primary amyloidosis is uniformly fatal with a mean survival <6 months if heart failure is present.

Therapy is generally limited owing to the physiology of restrictive heart disease. Cardiac output is essentially heart rate dependent since stroke volumes are small and fixed and cannot be increased with vasodilator therapy. For this rea-son, beta-blockers and calcium channel blocking agents are extremely poorly tolerated and not recommended. These negative inotropic agents are often recommended in dia-stolic heart failure to increase diastolic filling, but it is often at the expense of increased rather than decreased filling pres-sures and fewer stroke volumes per minute. Amyloid, in par-ticular, appears to get worse with calcium channel blockers, which are often initiated for treatment of diastolic dysfunc-tion (110,111). In amyloidosis, orthostatic hypotension is also common and limits tolerability of vasodilators, which further complicates hemodynamic therapy. Digoxin is con-traindicated because of an idiopathic sensitivity to toxicity (112). Finally, thromboembolic complications are common and attributable to the thrombogenicity of amyloid protein on the endocardial atrial surfaces (seen at pathology as wax-like drippings). Most patients should be anticoagulated if contraindications do not exist. In primary amyloidosis, ther-apy is directed at the malignant plasma clones. Chemo-therapy with melphalan and prednisone is palliative; heart and bone marrow transplantation have been successfully performed when heart failure is present.

HYPERTROPHIC CARDIOMYOPATHY

Hypertrophic cardiomyopathy (HCM) is a common autosomal dominant genetic disorder that affects 1 in every 500 adults. More than 200 familial and sporadic mutations in 11 genes have been described. The most common mutations occur in the genes for the β-myosin heavy chain, troponin I, and myosin-binding protein C. It is clinically recognized when there is left ventricular hypertrophy in the absence of an identifiable stimulus such as hypertension or aortic stenosis. Recent advances in molecular genetics now make genetic confirmation and preclinical diagnosis possible.

The clinical manifestations of HCM (dyspnea, angina, syncope, and sudden death) are due to complex interrelated conditions, which include diastolic dysfunction, myocardial ischemia, dynamic outflow obstruction, mitral regurgitation, and arrhythmias. Although classically defined by dynamic outflow obstruction caused by asymmetric hypertrophy of the interventricular septum, the hemodynamic derangements are very heterogeneous and of variable severity. In fact, most patients do not have this physiology, are minimally symptomatic, and have an excellent survival. The natural history may also be complicated by atrial fibrillation, concomitant coronary artery disease, endocarditis, and left ventricular systolic dysfunction (so-called "burnt out" HCM). It is also important to distinguish true provocable gradients from catheter entrapment, which can lead to an artificial outflow gradient (113), and HCM from other conditions that may also lead to intracavitary gradients (e.g., subaortic membranes, concentrically hypertrophied ventricles in the setting of acute distal anterior myocardial infarction, tako-tsubo syndrome, intense inotropic stimulation, and mitral valve replacement without resection of the native anterior leaflet). Similarly, concentric (e.g., in aortic stenosis or hypertension) or localized apical (a spadelike left ventricle with large negative T waves) left ventricular hypertrophy without intracavitary obstruction (113,114), must be distinguished from the more common hypertrophic obstructive cardiomyopathy discussed below.

The most dramatic hemodynamic feature of HCM is the dynamic intraventricular pressure gradient. In the setting of vigorous contraction of the basal aspect of an asymmetrically hypertrophied interventricular septum, there is obstruction to ejection in the left ventricular outflow tract. Because the outflow tract becomes narrowed, blood flow necessarily becomes accelerated in this region and the anterior leaflet of the mitral valve is sucked into the outflow tract from a Venturi effect. This phenomenon exacerbates the outflow obstruction and also contributes to mitral regurgitation. However, extensive variability and heterogeneity of this phenomenon is common among affected patients and even within the same patient over time. In fact, many patients with HCM do not have a systolic pressure gradient at rest but can have one provoked with the Valsalva maneuver, an extrasystole, a potent systemic vasodilator (amyl nitrate), or with inotropic stimulation.

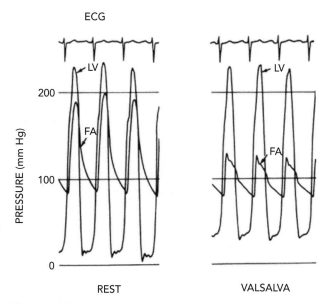

Figure 31.23 Left ventricular (LV) and femoral artery (FA) pressure tracings in a patient with hypertrophic cardiomyopathy (HCM). Valsalva maneuver produces a marked increase in the gradient, as well as a change in the femoral arterial pressure waveform to a spike-and-dome configuration.

The dynamic outflow obstruction leads to a characteristic arterial pressure waveform described as a spike-and-dome configuration, which is most apparent in the proximal aorta and transmitted to some extent to the peripheral pulses. The early spike is owing to rapid ventricular ejection from the hypercontractile myocardium, and the pressure dip and subsequent doming of the pulse reflect the dynamic outflow obstruction. It is most evident following conditions that increase the dynamic gradient, such as an extrasystole or the Valsalva maneuver (Fig. 31.23). The narrowing in pulse pressure of the spike-and-dome arterial waveform is known as the Brockenbrough-Braunwald sign (Fig. 31.24; 115). The fall in pulse pressure is felt to be due to worsening obstruction in the setting of augmented contractility from increased systolic calcium loading in the cardiac myocytes. Diastolic dysfunction is also an important hallmark of HCM (116,117) and is often evident in the contour of the left ventricular diastolic pressure tracing (Fig. 31.25). These diastolic abnormalities can be altered by calcium channel blockade (116,118,119), although caution should be taken with verapamil since its vasodilator effect may outweigh its lusitropic effect (120).

Ventriculography typically demonstrates a hypercontractile state, ventricular hypertrophy, and a small ventricular cavity. Dynamic outflow obstruction may even be visible as a swan neck deformity in a banana-shaped ventricle, which becomes distorted from large, displaced papillary muscles. In this setting, significant mitral regurgitation will be present as a result of the Venturi effect. In patients with apical hypertrophic cardiomyopathy (113), the left ventricle shows marked thickening of its anteroapical wall, giving

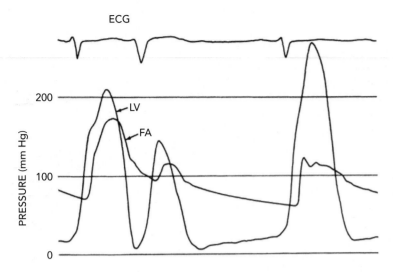

Figure 31.24 Hemodynamic findings in obstructive hypertrophic cardiomyopathy (HCM). Following an extrasystole, there is an increase in gradient and development of a spike-and-dome configuration in the arterial pressure waveform. The arterial pulse pressure clearly narrows in the postextrasystolic beat compared with the beat before the extrasystole. This narrowing of pulse pressure is known as the Brockenbrough-Braunwald sign. LV, left ventricular; FA, femoral artery.

the ventricle a spade-shaped appearance. Coronary angiography may demonstrate marked systolic compression of septal branches of the left anterior descending artery (121) and a "sawfish" systolic narrowing of the left anterior descending artery (122).

Therapy for HCM is directed toward the hemodynamic derangements. Beta-blockers and calcium channel blockers are the cornerstones of pharmacologic therapy and act to decrease contractility, reduce outflow obstruction, and improve diastolic function. Because of its potent negative inotropic property, disopyramide can also be effective. However, its use is often limited by its anticholinergic side effects and the risk of proarrhythmia. Maintenance of A-V synchrony with arrhythmia control is also critical. When pharmacologic therapies fail to improve symptoms, surgical or catheter-based approaches are indicated to relieve outflow obstruction and decrease mitral regurgitation.

Case 7: Alcohol Septal Ablation in a Patient With HCM. A 51-year-old man with HCM was referred for medically refractory symptoms of angina, dyspnea, and exertional light-headedness. Despite escalating doses of metoprolol, he remained symptomatic. Verapamil and disopyramide were not tolerated. His examination was consistent with dynamic outflow obstruction, with a spike-and-dome carotid pulse and murmurs of outflow obstruction and mitral regurgitation that increased with the strain phase of Valsalva. An echocardiogram showed significant asymmetric hypertrophy (septum 23 mm, posterior wall 19 mm), modest mitral regurgitation with systolic anterior motion of the anterior leaflet, and a resting gradient of 55 mm Hg that increased to 79 mm Hg with Valsalva.

At catheterization, a >100 mm Hg outflow gradient and classic findings of obstructive HCM were demonstrable with a pigtail catheter in the left ventricular apex and with RV pacing. Three mL of absolute alcohol into the first septal perforator decreased the gradient to <30 mm Hg (Fig. 31.26).

The creatine phosphokinase peaked at 1,200 units the following day. He was discharged on the third hospital day without heart block or arrhythmia. At follow-up 2 years later, he remained free of symptoms.

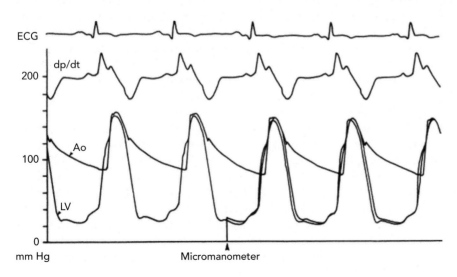

Figure 31.25 Abnormal left ventricular (LV) diastolic pressure waveform in a patient with hypertrophic cardiomyopathy (HCM). There is no resting systolic gradient. Impairment of diastolic relaxation is suggested by the abnormal LV diastolic pattern and the (-) dP/dt. Fluid-filled and micromanometer LV tracings are both shown. Ao, aorta.

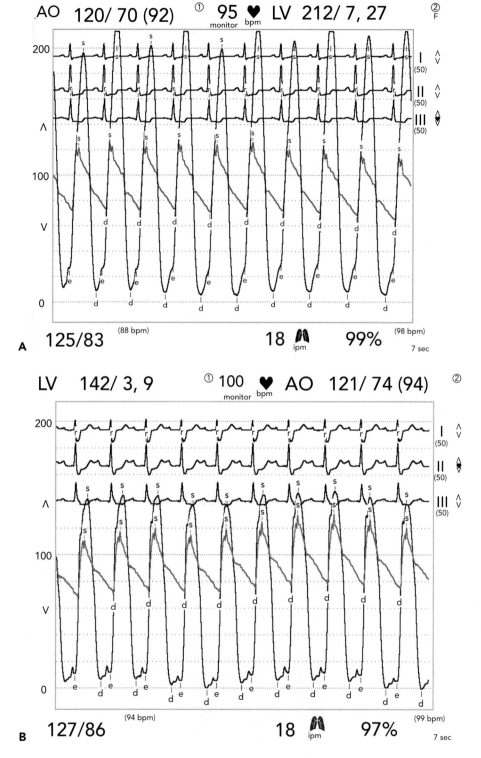

Figure 31.26 Outflow gradient in hypertrophic cardiomyopathy (HCM) decreased by alcohol septal ablation. **A.** Resting gradient of >100 mm Hg is present with pigtail catheter in left ventricular apex and coronary guide assessing aortic pressure. **B.** Resting gradient is significantly decreased following alcohol infusion and is almost immediately apparent. Also note change in aortic waveform from spike-and-dome configuration to more normal waveform after decrease in gradient following alcohol septal ablation.

Illustrative Points. Surgical myomectomy to thin the interventricular septum is an effective therapy for HCM when dynamic outflow obstruction is present. In 1995, Sigwart reported a catheter-based approach to thinning the hypertrophied septum by selectively infarcting the septum with ethanol using the septal perforators (123). Since that

initial report, several investigators have confirmed the effectiveness of alcohol septal ablation (124–129), and the procedure appears to be at least comparable with surgical myomectomy for relief of symptoms (130). In addition to the relief of outflow obstruction, septal ablation may also decrease ventricular mass and improve diastolic function over time, presumably by relieving the stimulus for hypertrophy (i.e., outflow obstruction; 131,132). An important limitation to alcohol septal ablation is the lack of long-term follow-up data. This issue may be quite relevant, since the creation of a myocardial infarction may lead to late heart block and ventricular arrhythmias. In contrast, surgical myomectomy has been performed safely for more than 20 years with excellent long-term survival.

Appropriate patient selection is paramount. Unfortunately, clearly agreed on indications are still evolving. It is important to counsel patients that septal ablation should be considered primarily when medical therapy has been exhausted, since long-term outcomes are unknown. Although other investigators have found that age alone does not predict response (129), we have found that relatively young and otherwise healthy patients with exertional dyspnea are those most likely to benefit. When there are other comorbidities, such as atherosclerosis and pulmonary disease, relief of symptoms becomes less predictable despite relief of hemodynamic obstruction. It is not necessary for symptomatic patients to have a significant outflow tract gradient at rest to benefit from ablation (133), although the initial reports have used a resting gradient of 30 mm Hg.

Complications can occur and include immediate (126) and late AV block (134), injury to the left anterior descending artery, unplanned infarction of nontarget tissue (135,136), ventricular septal defects, and late ventricular tachycardia (137). Although immediate heart block is common (20 to 30% of cases), need for permanent pacing is relatively uncommon, and ventricular tachycardia is rare. In patients at high risk for sudden death (i.e., family history of sudden death, syncope, significant hypertrophy), postprocedural permanent pacing and implantable defibrillators are strongly recommended. Other complications are not unique to septal ablation and include stroke, arrhythmias, infection, endocarditis, and cardiac perforation.

Alcohol Septal Ablation—Technique

Careful hemodynamic assessment with left and right heart catheterization, coronary angiography, and ventriculography should precede any attempt at alcohol septal ablation. The presence of advanced multivessel coronary artery disease is usually a contraindication to performing septal ablation. Angiography also allows for identification of suitable target septal perforators, preferably a large first septal perforator. Ventriculography is useful for determining the degree of mitral regurgitation and location of the dynamic outflow obstruction. Suitable echocardiography is also essential for safe and effective septal ablation (125). If supine transthoracic images are not adequate, transesophageal echocardiography with anesthesia support should be considered.

We prefer to monitor pressures continuously with a 5F pigtail catheter in the LV apex and a 7F coronary guide to assess the proximal pressure. Although straight end-hole catheters are often recommended to determine the precise

location of a gradient, we find that they carry an unacceptable risk of perforation or entrapment and are more likely to create ventricular arrhythmias. Options include an end-hole-only pigtail, or an end-and-side-hole pigtail advanced to the LV apex. If only a minimal or no resting gradient is present, maneuvers (Valsalva, ventricular pacing, extrasystoles, or inotropic agents) should be used to provoke a gradient. In this situation, we prefer the use of continuously infused dobutamine because the hemodynamic response to septal ablation can be followed during the procedure. The inability to elicit any gradient is a contraindication to the procedure. Because the development of bradycardia from high-degree AV block is common, we ensure that a pacing wire can be passed into the right ventricle. An activated clotting time (ACT) of 250 to 300 seconds should be maintained with heparin.

Concomitant contrast echocardiography is used to determine the most appropriate septal perforator for ethanol infusion by showing echo contrast localization in the area of maximal septal bulge when the target septal is injected. A short 1.5- to 2.0-mm over-the-wire (OTW) coronary balloon is placed and inflated in the candidate septal perforator over a guidewire (we prefer a highly angulated hydrophilic guidewire). A contrast injection through the guide catheter is used to confirm that only the septal perforator is obstructed (Fig. 31.27). The guidewire is then

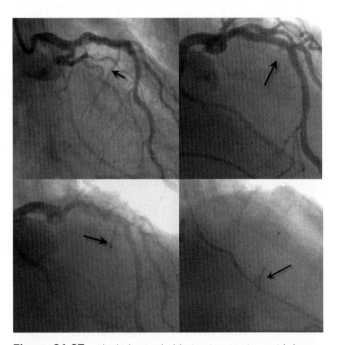

Figure 31.27 Alcohol septal ablation in a patient with hypertrophic cardiomyopathy (HCM). Right anterior oblique cranial coronary angiography shows **(top left)** baseline appearance of the first septal perforator (*arrow*, not shown was clear "milking" of that branch during systole owing to the compression of septal contraction), **(bottom left)** inflation of angioplasty balloon in that branch, **(bottom right)** contrast injection via balloon central lumen, and **(top right)** final result with obliteration of septal perforator is now occluded but without compromise or embolization of the left anterior descending artery.

removed and dilute Optison (1:10) is injected through the balloon lumen to echocardiographically visualize the septal territory perfused by the target septal perforator. The area of outflow obstruction should be opacified with little spillover to other areas. Often, when the correct septal perforator is chosen, myocardial ischemia from balloon inflation will be sufficient to reduce the gradient—a sensitive sign that alcohol ablation will be effective.

If Optison injection confirms appropriate placement, a small amount of dilute radiographic contrast is infused through the inflated balloon to confirm stasis in the septal branch. One to 4 mL of dehydrated ethanol USP is then infused slowly over several minutes through the balloon lumen (larger volumes or more rapid infusion may distribute ethanol through collaterals to other areas of the myocardium, causing more extensive myocardial necrosis). Glass or special solvent-resistant plastic syringes are needed for the ethanol. The QRS complex will usually widen and premature ventricular contractions (PVCs) are common. Various degrees of AV block may occur. Mild to moderate chest discomfort is usual (and severe in some) and should be treated with narcotics. Throughout the course of balloon inflation, the patency of the downstream LAD should be monitored with occasional contrast injection through the guiding catheter. Once the outflow tract gradient is abolished, the alcohol infusion can be terminated, and a small amount of chaser contrast injected to stain the treated area of the septum (this contrast will persist after balloon deflation). The balloon may be deflated and removed 5 to 10 minutes after completion of the ethanol injection. If the gradient is not adequately reduced, consideration then can be given to repeating the process in an adjacent septal perforating branch, bearing in mind that each additional amount of alcohol increases the risk of AV block.

If there is any evidence of AV block (other than first degree) following the procedure, a temporary pacing wire should be placed. Even if AV block does not occur during the procedure, permanent pacing should be considered since conduction abnormalities and syncope may develop days later. The creatinine phosphokinase will typically peak the day after the ablation and often reaches 1,000 to 1,500. Patients should be maintained on aspirin indefinitely.

REFERENCES

1. Hunt SA, et al. ACC/AHA guidelines for the evaluation and management of chronic heart failure in the adult: executive summary. A report of the American College of Cardiology/American Heart Association Task Force on Practice Guidelines (Committee to revise the 1995 Guidelines for the Evaluation and Management of Heart Failure). *J Am Coll Cardiol* 2001;38:2101–2113.
2. Hare JM, et al. Ischemic cardiomyopathy: endomyocardial biopsy and ventriculographic evaluation of patients with congestive heart failure, dilated cardiomyopathy and coronary artery disease. *J Am Coll Cardiol* 1992;20:1318–1325.
3. Felker GM, et al. Underlying causes and long-term survival in patients with initially unexplained cardiomyopathy. *N Engl J Med* 2000;342:1077–1084.
4. Kawai C. From myocarditis to cardiomyopathy: mechanisms of inflammation and cell death: learning from the past for the future. *Circulation* 1999;99:1091–1100.
5. Kamisago M, et al. Mutations in sarcomere protein genes as a cause of dilated cardiomyopathy. *N Engl J Med* 2000;343:1688–1696.
6. Cohn L, et al. Use of the augmented ejection fraction to select patients with left ventricular dysfunction for coronary revascularization. *J Thorac Cardiovasc Surg* 1976;72:835–840.
7. Louie HW, et al. Ischemic cardiomyopathy. Criteria for coronary revascularization and cardiac transplantation. *Circulation* 1991;84(5 suppl):III290–295.
8. Stevenson LW, et al. The limited reliability of physical signs for estimating hemodynamics in chronic heart failure. *JAMA* 1989;261:884–888.
9. Dokainish H, et al. Optimal noninvasive assessment of left ventricular filling pressures: a comparison of tissue Doppler echocardiography and B-type natriuretic peptide in patients with pulmonary artery catheters. *Circulation* 2004;109:2432–2439.
10. Cappola TP, et al. Pulmonary hypertension and risk of death in cardiomyopathy: patients with myocarditis are at higher risk. *Circulation* 2002;105:1663–1668.
11. Stevenson LW. Tailored therapy before transplantation for treatment of advanced heart failure: effective use of vasodilators and diuretics. *J Heart Lung Transplant* 1991;10:468–476.
12. Stevenson LW, et al. Efficacy of medical therapy tailored for severe congestive heart failure in patients transferred for urgent cardiac transplantation. *Am J Cardiol* 1989;63:461–464.
13. Stevenson LW, et al. Importance of hemodynamic response to therapy in predicting survival with ejection fraction less than or equal to 20% secondary to ischemic or nonischemic dilated cardiomyopathy. *Am J Cardiol* 1990;66:1348–1354.
14. Nohria A, et al. Clinical assessment identifies hemodynamic profiles that predict outcomes in patients admitted with heart failure. *J Am Coll Cardiol* 2003;41:1797–1804.
15. Packer M, et al. Hemodynamic changes mimicking a vasodilator drug response in the absence of drug therapy after right heart catheterization in patients with chronic heart failure. *Circulation* 1985;71:761–766.
16. Drazner MH, et al. Relationship between right and left-sided filling pressures in 1000 patients with advanced heart failure. *J Heart Lung Transplant* 1999;18:1126–1132.
17. Reynolds DW, et al. Measurement of pulmonary artery diastolic pressure from the right ventricle. *J Am Coll Cardiol* 1995;25:1176–1182.
18. Diaz ME, et al. Sarcoplasmic reticulum calcium content fluctuation is the key to cardiac alternans. *Circ Res* 2004;94:650–656.
19. Surawicz B, et al. Cardiac alternans: diverse mechanisms and clinical manifestations. *J Am Coll Cardiol* 1992;20:483–499.
20. Stevenson LW, et al. Exercise capacity for survivors of cardiac transplantation or sustained medical therapy for stable heart failure. *Circulation* 1990;81:78–85.
21. Mudge GH, et al. 24th Bethesda conference: Cardiac transplantation. Task Force 3: recipient guidelines/prioritization. *J Am Coll Cardiol* 1993;22:21–31.
22. Stevenson LW, et al. Maintenance of cardiac output with normal filling pressures in patients with dilated heart failure. *Circulation* 1986;74:1303–1308.
23. Stevenson LW, et al. Afterload reduction with vasodilators and diuretics decreases mitral regurgitation during upright exercise in advanced heart failure. *J Am Coll Cardiol* 1990;15:174–180.
24. Rosario LB, et al. The mechanism of decrease in dynamic mitral regurgitation during heart failure treatment: importance of reduction in the regurgitant orifice size. *J Am Coll Cardiol* 1998;32:1819–1824.
25. Watanabe J, et al. Effects of coronary venous pressure on left ventricular diastolic distensibility. *Circ Res* 1990;67:923–932.
26. Davis R, et al. Treatment of chronic congestive heart failure with captopril, an oral inhibitor of angiotensin-converting enzyme. *N Engl J Med* 1979;301:117–121.
27. Guiha NH, et al. Treatment of refractory heart failure with infusion of nitroprusside. *N Engl J Med* 1974;291:587–592.
28. Yin FC, et al. Effect of nitroprusside on hydraulic vascular loads on the right and left ventricle of patients with heart failure. *Circulation* 1983;67:1330–1339.

29. Abraham WT, et al. Systemic hemodynamic, neurohormonal, and renal effects of a steady-state infusion of human brain natriuretic peptide in patients with hemodynamically decompensated heart failure. *J Card Fail* 1998;4:37–44.

30. Intravenous nesiritide vs nitroglycerin for treatment of decompensated congestive heart failure: a randomized controlled trial. *JAMA* 2002;287:1531–1540.

31. Felker GM, et al. Inotropic therapy for heart failure: an evidence-based approach. *Am Heart J* 2001;142:393–401.

32. Baim DS, et al. Evaluation of a new bipyridine inotropic agent—milrinone—in patients with severe congestive heart failure. *N Engl J Med* 1983;309:748–756.

33. Ludmer PL, et al. Separation of the direct myocardial and vasodilator actions of milrinone administered by an intracoronary infusion technique. *Circulation* 1986;73:130–137.

34. Hamilton MA, et al. Effect of tricuspid regurgitation on the reliability of the thermodilution cardiac output technique in congestive heart failure. *Am J Cardiol* 1989;64:945–948.

35. Rubin SA, et al. Accuracy of cardiac output, oxygen uptake, and arteriovenous oxygen difference at rest, during exercise, and after vasodilator therapy in patients with severe, chronic heart failure. *Am J Cardiol* 1982;50:973–978.

36. Chomsky DB, et al. Hemodynamic exercise testing. A valuable tool in the selection of cardiac transplantation candidates. *Circulation* 1996;94:3176–3183.

37. Higginbotham MB, et al. Regulation of stroke volume during submaximal and maximal upright exercise in normal man. *Circ Res* 1986;58:281–291.

38. Tischler MD, et al. Serial assessment of left ventricular function and mass after orthotopic heart transplantation: a 4-year longitudinal study. *J Am Coll Cardiol* 1992;19:60–66.

39. Bhatia SJ, et al. Time course of resolution of pulmonary hypertension and right ventricular remodeling after orthotopic cardiac transplantation. *Circulation* 1987;76:819–826.

40. Paulus WJ, et al. Deficient acceleration of left ventricular relaxation during exercise after heart transplantation. *Circulation* 1992;86:1175–1185.

41. Greenberg ML, et al. Long-term hemodynamic follow-up of cardiac transplant patients treated with cyclosporine and prednisone. *Circulation* 1985;71:487–494.

42. Stinson EB, et al. Hemodynamic observations one and two years after cardiac transplantation in man. *Circulation* 1972;45:1183–94.

43. Hosenpud JD, et al. Abnormal exercise hemodynamics in cardiac allograft recipients 1 year after cardiac transplantation. Relation to preload reserve. *Circulation* 1989;80:525–532.

44. Borow KM, et al. Left ventricular contractility and contractile reserve in humans after cardiac transplantation. *Circulation* 1985;71:866–872.

45. Vassalli G, et al. Reduced coronary flow reserve during exercise in cardiac transplant recipients. *Circulation* 1997;95:607–613.

46. Pope SE, et al. Exercise response of the denervated heart in long-term cardiac transplant recipients. *Am J Cardiol* 1980;46:213–218.

47. Pflugfelder PW, et al. Cardiac dynamics during supine exercise in cyclosporine-treated orthotopic heart transplant recipients: assessment by radionuclide angiography. *J Am Coll Cardiol* 1987;10:336–341.

48. Kao AC, et al. Central and peripheral limitations to upright exercise in untrained cardiac transplant recipients. *Circulation* 1994;89:2605–2615.

49. Givertz MM, et al. Long-term sequential changes in exercise capacity and chronotropic responsiveness after cardiac transplantation. *Circulation* 1997;96:232–237.

50. Mohanty PK, et al. Impairment of cardiopulmonary baroreflex after cardiac transplantation in humans. *Circulation* 1987;75:914–921.

51. Guyton AC, et al. The limits of right ventricular compensation following acute increase in pulmonary circulatory resistance. *Circ Res* 1954;2:326–332.

52. Kirklin JK, et al. Pulmonary vascular resistance and the risk of heart transplantation. *J Heart Transplant* 1988;7:331–336.

53. Erickson KW, et al. Influence of preoperative transpulmonary gradient on late mortality after orthotopic heart transplantation. *J Heart Transplant* 1990;9:526–537.

54. Griepp RB, et al. Determinants of operative risk in human heart transplantation. *Am J Surg* 1971;122:192–197.

55. Franciosa JA, et al. Pulmonary versus systemic hemodynamics in determining exercise capacity of patients with chronic left ventricular failure. *Am Heart J* 1985;110:807–813.

56. Butler J, et al. Pulmonary hypertension and exercise intolerance in patients with heart failure. *J Am Coll Cardiol* 1999;34:1802–1806.

57. Di Salvo TG, et al. Preserved right ventricular ejection fraction predicts exercise capacity and survival in advanced heart failure. *J Am Coll Cardiol* 1995;25:1143–1153.

58. Martin J, et al. Implantable left ventricular assist device for treatment of pulmonary hypertension in candidates for orthotopic heart transplantation-a preliminary study. *Eur J Cardiothorac Surg* 2004;25:971–977.

59. Costard-Jackle A, et al. Influence of preoperative pulmonary artery pressure on mortality after heart transplantation: testing of potential reversibility of pulmonary hypertension with nitroprusside is useful in defining a high risk group. *J Am Coll Cardiol* 1992;19:48–54.

60. Leier CV, et al. Central and regional hemodynamic effects of intravenous isosorbide dinitrate, nitroglycerin and nitroprusside in patients with congestive heart failure. *Am J Cardiol* 1981;48:1115–1123.

61. Corin WJ, et al. The relationship of afterload to ejection performance in chronic mitral regurgitation. *Circulation* 1987;76:59–67.

62. Coddens J, et al. Effects of dobutamine and/or nitroprusside on the pulmonary circulation in patients with pulmonary hypertension secondary to end-stage heart failure. *J Cardiothorac Vasc Anesth* 1993;7:321–325.

63. Givertz MM, et al. Effect of bolus milrinone on hemodynamic variables and pulmonary vascular resistance in patients with severe left ventricular dysfunction: a rapid test for reversibility of pulmonary hypertension. *J Am Coll Cardiol* 1996;28:1775–1780.

64. Semigran MJ, et al. Hemodynamic effects of inhaled nitric oxide in heart failure. *J Am Coll Cardiol* 1994;24:982–988.

65. Loh E, et al. Cardiovascular effects of inhaled nitric oxide in patients with left ventricular dysfunction. *Circulation* 1994;90:2780–2785.

66. Hare JM, et al. Influence of inhaled nitric oxide on systemic flow and ventricular filling pressure in patients receiving mechanical circulatory assistance. *Circulation* 1997;95:2250–2253.

67. Kieler-Jensen N, et al. Inhaled nitric oxide in the evaluation of heart transplant candidates with elevated pulmonary vascular resistance. *J Heart Lung Transplant* 1994;13:366–375.

68. Rich GF, et al. Inhaled nitric oxide selectively decreases pulmonary vascular resistance without impairing oxygenation during one-lung ventilation in patients undergoing cardiac surgery. *Anesthesiology* 1994;80:57–62; discussion 27A.

69. Argenziano M, et al. Randomized, double-blind trial of inhaled nitric oxide in LVAD recipients with pulmonary hypertension. *Ann Thorac Surg* 1998;65:340–345.

70. Rajek A, et al. Inhaled nitric oxide reduces pulmonary vascular resistance more than prostaglandin E(1) during heart transplantation. *Anesth Analg* 2000;90:523–530.

71. Bocchi EA, et al. Inhaled nitric oxide leading to pulmonary edema in stable severe heart failure. *Am J Cardiol* 1994;74:70–72.

72. Haywood GA, et al. Adenosine infusion for the reversal of pulmonary vasoconstriction in biventricular failure. A good test but a poor therapy. *Circulation* 1992;86:896–902.

73. Murali S, et al. Utility of prostaglandin E1 in the pretransplantation evaluation of heart failure patients with significant pulmonary hypertension. *J Heart Lung Transplant* 1992;11(4 pt 1):716–723.

74. Givertz MM, et al. Acute endothelin A receptor blockade causes selective pulmonary vasodilation in patients with chronic heart failure. *Circulation* 2000;101:2922–2927.

75. Rubin LJ, et al. Bosentan therapy for pulmonary arterial hypertension. *N Engl J Med* 2002;346:896–903.

76. Young JB, et al. Evolution of hemodynamics after orthotopic heart and heart-lung transplantation: early restrictive patterns persisting in occult fashion. *J Heart Transplant* 1987;6:34–43.

77. Roca J, et al. Constrictive pericarditis after heart transplantation: report of two cases. *J Heart Lung Transplant* 1995;14:1006–1010.

78. Williams MJ, et al. Biopsy-induced flail tricuspid leaflet and tricuspid regurgitation following orthotopic cardiac transplantation. *Am J Cardiol* 1996;77:1339–1344.

79. Aziz TM, et al. Orthotopic cardiac transplantation technique: a survey of current practice. *Ann Thorac Surg* 1999;68:1242–1246.

80. Aziz TM, et al. Risk factors for tricuspid valve regurgitation after orthotopic heart transplantation. *Ann Thorac Surg* 1999;68:1247–1251.

81. Chan MC, et al. Severe tricuspid regurgitation after heart transplantation. *J Heart Lung Transplant* 2001;20:709–717.

82. Hosenpud JD, et al. Lack of progressive "restrictive" physiology after heart transplantation despite intervening episodes of allograft rejection: comparison of serial rest and exercise hemodynamics one and two years after transplantation. *J Heart Transplant* 1990;9:119–123.

83. Winters GL, et al. Natural history of focal moderate cardiac allograft rejection. Is treatment warranted? *Circulation* 1995;91:1975–1980.

84. Winters GL, et al. Immediate evaluation of endomyocardial biopsies for clinically suspected rejection after heart transplantation. *Circulation* 1994;89:2079–2084.

85. Stevenson LW, et al. Left ventricular assist device as destination for patients undergoing intravenous inotropic therapy: a subset analysis from REMATCH (Randomized Evaluation of Mechanical Assistance in Treatment of Chronic Heart Failure). *Circulation* 2004;110:975–981.

86. Nakatani S, et al. Prediction of right ventricular dysfunction after left ventricular assist device implantation. *Circulation* 1996;94 (9 suppl):II216–221.

87. Horton SC, et al. Left ventricular assist device malfunction: a systematic approach to diagnosis. *J Am Coll Cardiol* 2004;43 (9):1574–1583.

88. Ferns J, et al. Evaluation of a patient with left ventricular assist device dysfunction. *ASAIO J* 2001;47:696–698.

89. Rose EA, et al. Long-term mechanical left ventricular assistance for end-stage heart failure. *N Engl J Med* 2001;345:1435–1443.

89a. Horton SC, Khodaverdian R, Chatelain P, et al. Left ventricular assist device malfunction an approach to diagnosis by echocardiography. *J AM Coll Cardiol* 45:1435–1440.

90. Hauck AJ, et al. Evaluation of postmortem endomyocardial biopsy specimens from 38 patients with lymphocytic myocarditis: implications for role of sampling error. *Mayo Clin Proc* 1989;64:1235–1245.

91. Chow LH, et al. Insensitivity of right ventricular endomyocardial biopsy in the diagnosis of myocarditis. *J Am Coll Cardiol* 1989;14:915–920.

92. Cooper LT Jr, et al. Immunosuppressive therapy for myocarditis. *N Engl J Med* 1995;333:1713–1714.

93. Dec GW Jr, et al. Viral myocarditis mimicking acute myocardial infarction. *J Am Coll Cardiol* 1992;20:85–89.

94. Lieberman EB, et al. Clinicopathologic description of myocarditis. *J Am Coll Cardiol* 1991;18:1617–1626.

95. Cooper LT Jr, et al. Idiopathic giant-cell myocarditis—natural history and treatment. Multicenter Giant Cell Myocarditis Study Group Investigators. *N Engl J Med* 1997;336:1860–1866.

96. Davidoff R, et al. Giant cell versus lymphocytic myocarditis. A comparison of their clinical features and long-term outcomes. *Circulation* 1991;83:953–961.

97. Kodama M, et al. Rat dilated cardiomyopathy after autoimmune giant cell myocarditis. *Circ Res* 1994;75:278–284.

98. Grant SC. Recurrent giant cell myocarditis after transplantation. *J Heart Lung Transplant* 1993;12(1 pt 1):155–156.

99. McCarthy RE 3rd, et al. Long-term outcome of fulminant myocarditis as compared with acute (nonfulminant) myocarditis. *N Engl J Med* 2000;342:690–695.

100. Grogan M, et al. Long-term outcome of patients with biopsy-proved myocarditis: comparison with idiopathic dilated cardiomyopathy. *J Am Coll Cardiol* 1995;26:80–84.

101. Zile MR, et al. Diastolic heart failure—abnormalities in active relaxation and passive stiffness of the left ventricle. *N Engl J Med* 2004;350:1953–1959.

102. Burkhoff D, et al. Heart failure with a normal ejection fraction: is it really a disorder of diastolic function? *Circulation* 2003;107:656–658.

103. Kawaguchi M, et al. Combined ventricular systolic and arterial stiffening in patients with heart failure and preserved ejection fraction: implications for systolic and diastolic reserve limitations. *Circulation* 2003;107:714–720.

104. Mitchell GF, et al. Pulsatile hemodynamics in congestive heart failure. *Hypertension* 2001;38:1433–1439.

105. Klapholz M, et al. Hospitalization for heart failure in the presence of a normal left ventricular ejection fraction: results of the New York Heart Failure Registry. *J Am Coll Cardiol* 2004;43:1432–1438.

106. Zile MR, et al. Heart failure with a normal ejection fraction: is measurement of diastolic function necessary to make the diagnosis of diastolic heart failure? *Circulation* 2001;104:779–782.

107. Redfield MM, et al. Burden of systolic and diastolic ventricular dysfunction in the community: appreciating the scope of the heart failure epidemic. *JAMA* 2003;289:194–202.

108. Hurrell DG, et al. Value of dynamic respiratory changes in left and right ventricular pressures for the diagnosis of constrictive pericarditis. *Circulation* 1996;93:2007–2013.

109. Falk RH, et al. The systemic amyloidoses. *N Engl J Med* 1997;337:898–909.

110. Gertz MA, et al. Selective binding of nifedipine to amyloid fibrils. *Am J Cardiol* 1985;55(13 pt 1):1646.

111. Gertz MA, et al. Worsening of congestive heart failure in amyloid heart disease treated by calcium channel-blocking agents. *Am J Cardiol* 1985;55(13 pt 1):1645.

112. Rubinow A, et al. Digoxin sensitivity in amyloid cardiomyopathy. *Circulation* 1981;63:1285–1288.

113. Yamaguchi H, et al. Hypertrophic nonobstructive cardiomyopathy with giant negative T waves (apical hypertrophy): ventriculographic and echocardiographic features in 30 patients. *Am J Cardiol* 1979;44:401–412.

114. Kitaoka H, et al. Comparison of prevalence of apical hypertrophic cardiomyopathy in Japan and the United States. *Am J Cardiol* 2003;92:1183–1186.

115. Brockenbrough EC, et al. A hemodynamic technic for the detection of hypertrophic subaortic stenosis. *Circulation* 1961;23:189.

116. Lorell BH, et al. Improved diastolic function and systolic performance in hypertrophic cardiomyopathy after nifedipine. *N Engl J Med* 1980;303:801–803.

117. Stewart S, et al. Impaired rate of left ventricular filling in idiopathic hypertrophic subaortic stenosis and valvular aortic stenosis. *Circulation* 1968;37:8–14.

118. Lorell BH. Use of calcium channel blockers in hypertrophic cardiomyopathy. *Am J Med* 1985;78:43–54.

119. Bonow RO, et al. Effects of verapamil on left ventricular systolic function and diastolic filling in patients with hypertrophic cardiomyopathy. *Circulation* 1981;64:787–796.

120. Epstein SE, et al. Verapamil: its potential for causing serious complications in patients with hypertrophic cardiomyopathy. *Circulation* 1981;64:437–441.

121. Pichard AD, et al. Septal perforator compression (narrowing) in idiopathic hypertrophic subaortic stenosis. *Am J Cardiol* 1977;40:310–314.

122. Brugada P, et al. "Sawfish" systolic narrowing of the left anterior descending coronary artery: an angiographic sign of hypertrophic cardiomyopathy. *Circulation* 1982;66:800–803.

123. Sigwart U. Non-surgical myocardial reduction for hypertrophic obstructive cardiomyopathy. *Lancet* 1995;346:211–214.

124. Faber L, et al. Intraprocedural myocardial contrast echocardiography as a routine procedure in percutaneous transluminal septal myocardial ablation: detection of threatening myocardial necrosis distant from the septal target area. *Cathet Cardiovasc Intervent* 1999;47:462–466.

125. Faber L, et al. Echo-guided percutaneous septal ablation for symptomatic hypertrophic obstructive cardiomyopathy: 7 years of experience. *Eur J Echocardiogr* 2004;5:347–355.

126. Lakkis NM, et al. Echocardiography-guided ethanol septal reduction for hypertrophic obstructive cardiomyopathy. *Circulation* 1998;98:1750–1755.

127. Seggewiss H. Current status of alcohol septal ablation for patients with hypertrophic cardiomyopathy. *Curr Cardiol Rep* 2001;3:160–166.

128. Chang SM, et al. Predictors of outcome after alcohol septal ablation therapy in patients with hypertrophic obstructive cardiomyopathy. *Circulation* 2004;109:824–827.

129. Gietzen FH, et al. Transcoronary ablation of septal hypertrophy for hypertrophic obstructive cardiomyopathy: feasibility, clinical benefit, and short term results in elderly patients. *Heart* 2004;90:638–644.

130. Qin JX, et al. Outcome of patients with hypertrophic obstructive cardiomyopathy after percutaneous transluminal septal myocardial ablation and septal myectomy surgery. *J Am Coll Cardiol* 2001;38:1994–2000.

131. Park TH, et al. Acute effect of nonsurgical septal reduction therapy on regional left ventricular asynchrony in patients with hypertrophic obstructive cardiomyopathy. *Circulation* 2002;106: 412–415.

132. Mazur W, et al. Regression of left ventricular hypertrophy after nonsurgical septal reduction therapy for hypertrophic obstructive cardiomyopathy. *Circulation* 2001;103:1492–1496.

133. Gietzen FH, et al. Role of transcoronary ablation of septal hypertrophy in patients with hypertrophic cardiomyopathy, New York Heart Association functional class III or IV, and outflow obstruction only under provocable conditions. *Circulation* 2002;106: 454–459.

134. Kern MJ, et al. Delayed occurrence of complete heart block without warning after alcohol septal ablation for hypertrophic obstructive cardiomyopathy. *Cathet Cardiovasc Intervent* 2002;56:503–507.

135. Parham WA, et al. Apical infarct via septal collateralization complicating transluminal alcohol septal ablation for hypertrophic cardiomyopathy. *Cathet Cardiovasc Intervent* 2003;60:208–211.

136. Nagueh SF, et al. Images in cardiovascular medicine. Avoiding papillary muscle infarction with myocardial contrast echocardiographic guidance of nonsurgical septal reduction therapy for hypertrophic obstructive cardiomyopathy. *Circulation* 2004;109: e27–28.

137. McGregor JB, et al. Monomorphic ventricular tachycardia: a late complication of percutaneous alcohol septal ablation for hypertrophic cardiomyopathy. *Am J Med Sci* 2004;328:185–188.

Profiles in Pericardial Disease

32

John F. Robb   Roger J. Laham[a]

The pericardium covers and contains the heart and thereby has important anatomic and physiologic functions. It consists of both a visceral and a parietal component, each composed of an inner layer of mesothelial cells covering an underlying fibrosa. The visceral pericardium is attached to the heart by loose connective tissue and surrounds the epicardial fat pads and coronary arteries. At the pericardial reflections, it extends onto the pulmonary veins, superior and inferior vena cavae, and several centimeters of proximal pulmonary artery and aorta, before folding around to continue as the parietal (or free) pericardium. The parietal pericardial then envelops the heart and visceral pericardium as a separate 1- to 2-mm-thick layer. The pericardial space lies between the visceral and parietal layers and normally contains 15 to 35 mL of serous pericardial fluid—an ultrafiltrate of plasma. If outward pressure is exerted by chronic pericardial effusion or cardiac chamber dilation, the pericardial layers can stretch slowly over time, but over shorter periods, the pericardium behaves as a fixed-capacity sac. Both the parietal and visceral pericardium are supplied by nerves, arteries, and lymphatics and are metabolically active, producing prostaglandin E, eicosanoids, prostacyclin, and growth factors. Inflammatory cytokines, complement myocardial cellular enzymes, and other factors may appear in the pericardial fluid in response to inflammation or transmural myocardial ischemia and necrosis and may affect the underlying myocardium, cardiac nerves, and coronary arteries (1).

The pericardial pressure is usually subatmospheric (-5 to $+5$ mm Hg) and tracks with intrathoracic pressure during the respiratory cycle (1). During inspiration, intrapleural pressure and pericardial pressure fall more than systemic venous pressure, augmenting the right atrial filling gradient and right ventricular stroke output. In contrast, the falling intrapleural pressure during inspiration reduces pulmonary venous pressure, and thus decreases the left atrial filling gradient and left ventricular filling. Together with an increase in left ventricular afterload (owing to an increase in the relative difference between left ventricular end-diastolic and aortic pressure), this reduces left ventricular stroke output during inspiration. These effects are reversed during expiration. Under normal conditions, the hemodynamic effects of respiration thus cause cyclical changes in ventricular stroke output that are nearly 180° out of phase between the right and left ventricles.

The parietal pericardium also contributes to the diastolic compliance characteristics of the heart, especially over the thin-walled atrial and right ventricular chambers (2,3). The pericardium thus limits acute cavity dilation in situations such as right ventricular infarction, massive pulmonary embolism, and acute aortic insufficiency. If excess pericardial fluid accumulates in the pericardial space beyond its limited capacity to stretch, the pericardial pressure rises and begins to progressively compress the underlying cardiac chambers. Since this pressure is applied equally to all chambers, a rising pericardial pressure couples the diastolic behavior of the left and right ventricles together and creates ventricular interdependence whereby changes in pressure and volume in one ventricle thus produce changes in diastolic filling, contraction, and relaxation in the other ventricle (1). For example, acute increases in right ventricular size (such as in right ventricular infarction or pulmonary embolism) will increase the intrapericardial pressure, cause an increase in the stiffness

---

[a] Drs. Beverly Lorrell and William Grossman contributed material for this chapter in previous editions.

of both ventricles, and reduce their compliance. Whenever right ventricular diastolic pressure exceeds left ventricular diastolic pressure, the common external pericardial constraint can cause the intraventricular septum to shift leftward and impede left ventricular filling.

Pericardial disease can manifest as fluid accumulation owing to injury or inflammation (pericardial effusion, possibly leading to pericardial tamponade) or as progressive thickening of the parietal and/or visceral pericardium (possibly leading to pericardial constriction). Either tamponade or constriction impedes diastolic filling, elevates right and left heart diastolic pressures, and reduces cardiac output, but these two processes differ significantly in the pattern of diastolic filling impairment during each cardiac cycle and the hemodynamic response to respiration. There are thus distinctive echocardiographic and hemodynamic profiles for tamponade versus constriction, and for constriction as opposed to restrictive cardiomyopathy in which impaired left ventricular diastolic filling is owing to reduced myocardial compliance without pericardial involvement (see also Chapter 20).

PERICARDITIS, PERICARDIAL EFFUSION, AND TAMPONADE

Discussion of the myriad of causes of pericarditis and pericardial effusion are beyond the scope of this chapter, but suffice it to say that virtually any pathologic process can affect the pericardium (4) and cause a detectable pericardial effusion whenever the rate of accumulation of pericardial contents (transudate, exudate, pus, blood, or gas) exceeds the reabsorption ability of the pericardium. The most common causes of pericardial effusion are idiopathic pericarditis (presumably viral), trauma (including iatrogenic catheter injury to the cardiac chambers or vessels), malignant, post-myocardial infarction, uremic, connective tissue disease/ autoimmune, myxedema and radiation (5,6). Infectious or purulent pericarditis is most commonly caused by *Staphylococcus aureus*, followed by other Gram-positive organisms, fungal or mycobacterial infections (7,8). Myocarditis and pericarditis frequently coexist, and elevations of cardiac troponin levels can be seen in both (9). Acute pericardial injury of any type can also trigger an autoimmune process that can lead to continued or recurrent effusion.

Patients with acute pericarditis often experience sharp, aching, or pressurelike precordial pain that is worsened by cough, inspiration and, recumbency. Pain may radiate to the shoulders (1) and may be confused with angina or acute myocardial infarction, particularly since the ECG may show diffuse concave ST-segment elevation. One distinguishing feature, however, is the concomitant depression of the PR segment depression and the absence of reciprocal ST depression. A pericardial friction rub and fever may be present, but rigors or spiking fevers should raise the

concern of purulent pericarditis. The mainstay of diagnosis is echocardiography, which clearly shows an effusion. Fluid first accumulates posteriorly and then extends anteriorly. Small effusions have <10 mm clear space between the heart and parietal pericardium, moderate effusions have a 10- to 20-mm gap, and large effusions have a >20-mm gap. The size of the effusion correlates roughly with prognosis (10). Effusions may be loculated (partitioned) by nonuniform fibrous adhesions that form between the parietal and visceral pericardium, a pattern typically observed after cardiac surgery. Echocardiography also reveals the extent to which the pericardial pressure is compromising cardiac function, showing early diastolic collapse of the right ventricle as pericardial pressure transiently exceeds intracavitary pressure. In idiopathic pericarditis, the effusion usually resolves spontaneously or after symptomatic treatment with nonsteroidal anti-inflammatory agents and sometimes colchicine (11) or corticosteroids.

Chronic idiopathic effusions may also persist without symptoms or signs of tamponade despite effusion, and volumes >500 mL may be followed conservatively with serial echocardiograms if asymptomatic (12). On the other hand, significant pericardial effusion with even early signs of hemodynamic compromise is usually an indication for prompt drainage (pericardiocentesis, or surgical subxiphoid window placement). By the time the classic bedside findings of jugular venous distension and pulsus paradoxus (fall in systolic arterial pressure on normal inspiration) develop, only a small further accumulation of fluid separates the patient from frank hemodynamic collapse.

PERICARDIOCENTESIS

The main pericardial procedure performed in the catheterization laboratory is needle puncture and catheter drainage of pericardial fluid—pericardiocentesis. Diagnostic pericardiocentesis may be performed to evaluate the etiology of pericarditis, particularly for suspected purulent or tuberculous pericarditis, persistence or recurrence of a large effusion, or a high suspicion of malignant effusion without a tissue diagnosis from the primary site. The diagnostic yield for pericardial fluid analysis is quite low, with as few as 6% of diagnostic procedures and 29% of therapeutic procedures yielding useful information (13–15). Diagnostic yield tends to be higher in large pericardial effusions (16).

Pericardial fluid always should be sent for cell count; Gram, AFB, and special stains; cultures (aerobic, anaerobic, AFB, fungal), and cytology. Although differentiation between an exudate and a transudate can be accomplished with fluid protein and LDH levels, such differentiation is of dubious value as the timing of sampling and effects of treatment may alter values, and there is poor sensitivity and specificity with significant overlap between the exudative and transudative groups (15). Since most effusions are serosanguineous or hemorrhagic, fluid appearance is not useful in differentiating various etiologic groups with the exception of purulent fluid that is specific but not sensitive for infection. As long as adequate samples are obtained, fluid cytology has 92–95% sensitivity and 100% specificity for malignant pericardial effusion, although nonmalignant effusions are also common in patients with underlying malignancy. There are no specific pericardial fluid findings for postpericardiotomy syndrome, radiation or uremic pericarditis, hypothyroidism, or trauma. Special circumstances may require additional analysis for the following: viral cultures for viral infection, fluid cholesterol level in myxedema, fat studies for chylopericardium, latex fixation for rheumatoid antigen, gamma globulin complexes and fluid complement levels for rheumatoid arthritis, fluid antinuclear antibody levels for systemic lupus erythematosus, as well as tuberculosis stains or and cultures, fluid adenosine deaminase (17) or polymerase chain reaction (18) for tuberculosis. Purulent pericarditis may be associated with a low pH, high protein levels, glucose levels <35 mg/dL, and elevated leukocyte counts in the range of 6,000 to 240,000/mm^3 (7,19).

The diagnostic yield may be increased by retrieval of pericardial tissue by a surgical pericardial biopsy performed via thoracotomy, subxiphoid incision, or thoracoscopy. Percutaneous pericardial biopsy (assisted by pericardioscopy) has lead to a specific diagnosis in 49 to 53% of patients in several limited series (20,21). The pericardioscopy technique is not widely available and requires surgical or 16F percutaneous pericardial access. In hemorrhagic effusion, obtaining adequate parietal pericardial visualization may require 2 to 3 days of active drainage, replacement of pericardial effusion with saline, and instillation of 100 to 300 mL of air (21). Several small uncontrolled series suggest that this approach may increase the likelihood of obtaining a definitive diagnosis in patients with large recurrent pericardial effusions and in patients in whom there is a strong clinical suspicion of malignant pericarditis or tuberculous pericarditis. In a prospective series of 141 patients with unexplained pericardial effusions who underwent 142 surgical pericardioscopy including cytological fluid analysis, visualization of the pericardium, and guided biopsy, a specific etiologic cause (neoplastic, infected purulent, or sterile radiation-induced effusion) was identified in 49%, whereas 51% were considered idiopathic. Of note, an unrecognized cause not detected by pericardioscopy-biopsy was subsequently discovered in 4% (22). No deaths were attributable to pericardioscopy but in-hospital mortality was 5.6% related to underlying disease.

In another series, 35 patients with pericardial effusion owing to inflammatory disease underwent pericardioscopy, and pericardial biopsies were performed. Diagnosis of viral pericarditis, lymphocytic perimyocarditis, bacterial pericarditis, and antibody-mediated autoreactive pericarditis were obtained; however, it was unclear if this resulted in a change of management strategy (23). The same authors reported a series of 14 patients with idiopathic pericarditis and 15 patients with malignant pericarditis who underwent percutaneous pericardioscopy with both pericardial and epicardial biopsy from a registry of 136 patients undergoing pericardiocentesis. In this experience, subxiphoid pericardiocentesis and sampling of fluid for cytology, immunologic studies, and culture was performed first, followed by evacuation of pericardial fluid, replacement of warmed clear sterile saline in the pericardial sac, and introduction of both rigid and flexible pericardioscopes. Both epicardial biopsies and pericardial biopsies were obtained with a resterilizable bioptome, after site selection by both pericardioscopy and biplane fluoroscopy, before the saline was evacuated. In this series of patients with proven malignant pericarditis, fluid cytology was diagnostic in 71% and epicardial biopsy was diagnostic in 80% (24,25).

In a more recent study by Seferovc, 49 patients with a large pericardial effusion underwent parietal pericardial biopsy using fluoroscopy or pericardioscopy guidance (for more extensive sampling). Diagnostic efficiency was improved by extensive sampling (4 to 20 biopsies) compared with a single biopsy (40% versus 8.3%, $P < .05$; 26) In our experience and in several series of pericardiocentesis in patients with malignant effusion, cytologic examination is positive in about 80 to 85% of cases and false-negative cytologic analysis is rare in carcinomatous pericarditis (as opposed to malignant involvement by lymphoma or mesothelioma). In the era of molecular diagnostic tools, a clear role for diagnosis pericardioscopy and directed pericardial and/or epicardial biopsy is not yet defined relative to cytologic examination of recovered fluid.

Therapeutic pericardiocentesis is indicated for any sign or symptom of tamponade, limiting dyspnea (16), symptoms of compression of surrounding structures such as lung or esophagus, and acute hemopericardium with circulatory compromise following a catheter-based or surgical intervention. The diagnosis of early tamponade is usually made echocardiographically. Hemodynamically, the diagnosis of tamponade is made if there is identical elevation of left- and right-sided diastolic pressures with loss of the y descent in a patient with pericardial effusion. Note however, that pericardiocentesis is contraindicated for hemopericardium or tamponade in the presence of a diagnosed ascending aortic dissection, as it can accelerate bleeding and shock (27), making immediate surgery preferable in this circumstance. Another particular example in which emergency pericardiocentesis is required is when catheter injury to a cardiac chamber or vessel produces acute hemopericardium. This may happen as the result of temporary pacemaker placement in the right ventricle, passage of a stiff right heart catheter, endomyocardial biopsy, transseptal puncture, retrograde crossing of a stenotic aortic valve with a straight guidewire, coronary atherectomy or high-pressure stent dilation, or passage of a stiff hydrophilic guidewire into a small coronary branch in a patient receiving a glycoprotein IIb/IIIa platelet antagonist.

The patient may complain of chest pain, followed by progressive hypotension and tachycardia. Bradycardia may also appear owing to stimulation of the vagal nerve by blood in the pericardium, but the hypotension persists after the bradycardia has been resolved by atropine administration. Careful fluoroscopy of the right and left heart borders may show that the normal pulsations of the heart have been replaced by an immobile tense pericardial shadow, and right heart catheterization may show the classic hemodynamic findings described below as well as inability to advance the right heart catheter fully to the right atrial border. Urgent pericardiocentesis may be lifesaving in this situation. When the cause of bleeding into the pericardium is injury to a coronary artery, either placement of a fabric-covered stent or coil embolization of a small bleeding distal branch may be required. Ongoing bleeding after initial drainage and reversal of anticoagulation, however, usually warrants emergency surgery.

Pericardiocentesis: Technique

At most centers, pericardiocentesis is performed in the cardiac catheterization laboratory using a combination of echocardiographic and fluoroscopic guidance. It is helpful to obtain a two-dimensional echocardiogram just prior to the procedure to document the presence, location, and size of the effusion; to determine the presence of loculation or significant stranding; and to determine the location on the body surface where the effusion lies closest to the surface and at which the fluid depth overlying the heart is maximal (28). Once an entry location is selected, the echo can indicate the optimal direction for needle passage and the approximate depth of needle insertion that will be required. Some centers have reported pericardiocentesis using echocardiographic guidance alone (29), but we have found that access to pressure measurement, continuous ECG and vital sign monitoring, and fluoroscopy with the ability to inject radiographic contrast in the cardiac catheterization laboratory to be preferable, particularly in difficult or challenging cases, in patients with small or localized effusions or when complications ensue. It is important to have access to adequate ancillary support and other technologies in hemodynamically unstable patients, unless an emergency requires a bedside procedure (30). Performing the procedure in the catheterization laboratory in conjunction with right heart pressure measurement is also required if the diagnosis of effusive-constrictive pericarditis is suspected, the effusion is small or loculated, or if the patient is hemodynamically unstable.

The patient torso is propped up to a level of about 45° using a bolster or other mechanism, and the transducers are zeroed to the level of the heart in this position. The subxiphoid approach is classic: a skin nick is made 1 to 2 cm below the costal margin just to the left of the xiphoid process, to allow the needle to miss the ribs. The desired needle path is generally toward the posterior aspect of the left shoulder, passing anterior to or through the anterior

capsule of the liver, and entering the pericardial space overlying the right ventricle. Echocardiography from the subxiphoid window is thus very useful to confirm the optimal direction toward the pericardial entry point and the approximate depth below the skin. When this geometry is unfavorable—as in posterior effusions or patients with large body habitus—apical or low parasternal intercostal puncture sites are potential alternatives. Since echocardiography does not image through air (and to avoid pneumothorax), sites with significant intervening lung should be excluded; care should be taken in the parasternal approach to avoid the internal mammary artery that runs 3 to 5 cm from the parasternal border, and also the neurovascular bundle at the lower margin of each rib.

After a sterile prep and appropriate draping, the skin and subcutaneous tissues are infiltrated with lidocaine with a small-gauge needle along the proposed path of entry. We then usually use a 5- to 8-cm, 18-gauge needle attached to a 10-mL syringe filled with saline or lidocaine and inserted following the echo-determined trajectory. As the needle is advanced, the syringe is alternately aspirated to determine pericardial space entry and injected to deliver more local anesthesia along the route. If a three-way stopcock is interposed between the syringe and the needle, it can be used to connect to a pressure manifold via a fluid-filled extension tube. Classically, electrocardiographic monitoring of the needle (by attaching its shaft to the V lead of the ECG system using a sterile alligator clip) was used to provide an additional measure of safety: the ST segment recorded from the needle should be isoelectric during advancement, but dramatic elevation of the ST segment appears if the needle contacts the right ventricular epicardium. The needle must be withdrawn slightly until ST elevation resolves to minimize the chance of right ventricular puncture or laceration. Use of a properly grounded ECG system is imperative to avoid introducing leakage currents through the needle. Recently, we have started using a blunt-tip epicardial needle (Tuohy-17) to minimize risk of right ventricular puncture. This technique may be also modified to enable access of the normal pericardium for drug delivery and epicardial mapping (see below; 31,32).

When the needle enters the pericardial space, a distinct pop is usually felt and it is possible to aspirate fluid. We then turn the interposed stopcock to display intrapericardial pressure, which should be superimposable on the simultaneously displayed right atrial pressure from the right heart catheter. The waveform should emphatically not resemble that of right ventricular pressure (Figs. 32.1, 32.2). If the pericardial needle tip displays a right ventricular waveform, the tip is quickly but smoothly withdrawn under continuous hemodynamic monitoring until the overlying pericardial space is entered. Entry of the pericardial space can be confirmed by injection of radiographic contrast, agitated saline echo contrast, or the advancement of an 0.035-inch J wire in the characteristic path wrapping around the heart. An 8F dilator is then introduced over the

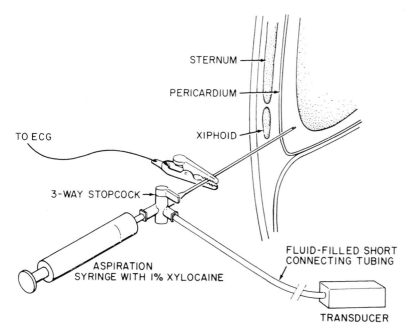

Figure 32.1 Diagram showing the subxiphoid approach to pericardiocentesis. A hollow, thin-walled, 18-gauge needle is connected via a three-way stopcock to an aspiration syringe filled with 1% Xylocaine and to a short length of fluid-filled tubing connected to a pressure transducer. A sterile V lead of an electrocardiographic recorder may be attached to the metal needle hub. The needle is advanced until pericardial fluid is aspirated or an injury current appears on the V-lead electrocardiographic recording. Once fluid is aspirated, the stopcock is turned so that needle-tip pressure is displayed against simultaneously measured right atrial pressure from a right heart catheter. When needle-tip position within the pericardial space is confirmed, a J-tipped guidewire is passed through the needle into the pericardial space, the needle is removed, and a catheter with end and side holes is advanced over the guidewire and subsequently connected via the three-way stopcock to both its transducer and the syringe. This permits, first, thorough drainage of the pericardial effusion using a catheter rather than a sharp needle, and second, documentation that tamponade physiology is relieved when right atrial pressure falls and intrapericardial pressure is restored to a level at or below zero.

guidewire, followed by a drainage catheter (straight or pigtail shaped, with multiple side holes). If difficulty is encountered in advancing the drainage catheter, the dilator can be reintroduced and used to substitute an extra-stiff J wire for better support. We usually attach a 50-mL syringe and three-way stopcock to the drainage catheter, connecting an extension tube from the other port of the three-way stopcock to a drainage bag or vacuum bottle. This allows

fluid to be aspirated into the syringe and transferred to the bottle. Removal of as little as 50 mL is often sufficient to relieve frank tamponade and improve hemodynamics. After removal of 100 to 200 mL of fluid, it is informative to remeasure the pericardial and right atrial pressure before resuming aspiration.

When fluid can no longer be aspirated, fluoroscopy should show that the previously immobile cardiac silhouette

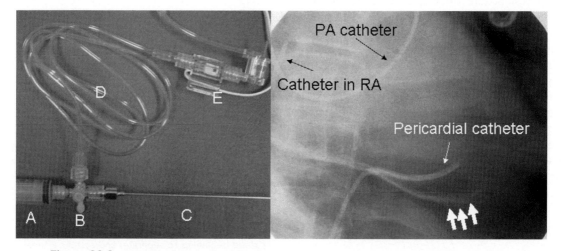

Figure 32.2 Diagram showing the subxiphoid approach to pericardiocentesis. **Left.** Needle set up with syringe (A), three-way stopcock (B), needle (C; we currently use the Tuohy-17 blunt-tip needle), pressure tubing (D), pressure transducer (E). **Right.** The patient had an existing PA catheter. A high-fidelity catheter is placed in the right atrial (RA) for simultaneous pericardial-RA recording. The needle is slowly inserted through the skin toward the pericardial space under echocardiographic or fluoroscopic guidance and ECG monitoring. When fluid is aspirated, the stopcock is turned to display intrapericardial pressure. The mean pericardial and right atrial pressure are simultaneously displayed and recorded. If cardiac tamponade is present, both pericardial pressure and RA pressures will be virtually equal, with nearly identical waveforms. The needle's position in the pericardial space may be confirmed by slow injection of 5 to 10 mL of radiocontrast (large arrows). If in the pericardial space, this contrast will slowly dissipate and outline the beating heart as a negative contrast object within. The needle is then used to place a guidewire to wrap around the heart, over which a drainage catheter is positioned in the pericardial space.

now exhibits a normal pulsation pattern, and a repeat echocardiogram should show only minimal posterior effusion. Occasional patients will experience pericardial pain when the effusion is tapped dry. Parenteral narcotic analgesics and benzodiazepines can be administered, and if the pain is severe, 50 mL of pericardial fluid, sterile saline, or 10 to 20 mL of 1% Xylocaine can be reintroduced to help ease the pain. The patient should be laid flat and a final set of pericardial and right heart pressures measured. As shown in Fig. 32.3, the abnormal physiology of cardiac tamponade is relieved if: (a) pericardial pressure falls to a level ≤0 mm Hg and separates from the right atrial pressure; (b) right atrial pressure itself falls to the normal range and exhibits return of the normal diastolic y descent (indicating restoration of normal rapid atrial emptying and early ventricular diastolic filling); and (c) any pulsus paradoxus is relieved. In previously hypotensive patients, systemic arterial pressure usually rises in association with an increase in mixed venous oxygen content, indicative of an increase in cardiac output. Failure of pericardial pressure to fall close to 0 indicates that the reference height of the transducers is incorrect or that free or loculated pericardial fluid is still under pressure. If the pericardial pressure falls appropriately but the right atrial pressures remain elevated with prominent x and y descents, the diagnosis of effusive-constrictive pericarditis must be entertained, with an ongoing element of constriction after the tamponade physiology has been relieved.

We then sew the drainage catheter in place attached to a sterile fluid path (stopcock, syringe, and drainage bag) to allow the postprocedure nursing staff to periodically attempt additional aspiration. Sterility must be tightly maintained with this technique, because regularly interrupting the integrity of the drainage circuit may introduce infectious agents. Other institutions rely on continuous or intermittent suction applied via a water-seal device. The pericardial catheter is removed when the drainage has decreased to <25 to 50 mL per 24 hours and there is no echocardiographic evidence of reaccumulation of fluid. Subsequently, periodic echo reassessment for fluid reaccumulation should be performed. Larger effusions may benefit from slightly more prolonged drainage, but >48-hour dwell time should be avoided to reduce the risk of infection (33).

Pericardiocentesis: Complications

The safety and success of percutaneous pericardiocentesis is related to the choice of entry site as well as to the size of the effusion. Pericardiocentesis is most likely to be uncomplicated if both anterior and posterior echo-free spaces of at least 10 mm (29). In smaller effusions, there is an increased risk of cardiac injury, so pericardiocentesis should usually be avoided in minimally symptomatic patients with small incidental effusions, unless there is clear echocardiographic evidence of hemodynamic compromise. The risk is also increased in patients who are anticoagulated with warfarin,

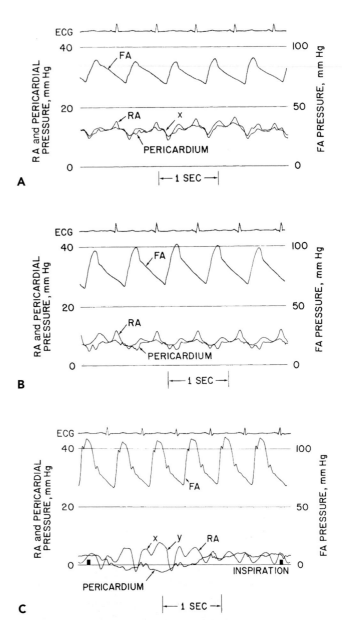

Figure 32.3 Simultaneous right atrial (RA) and intrapericardial pressure (scale 0 to 40 mm Hg) and femoral artery (FA) pressure (scale 0 to 100 mm Hg) recorded in a patient with cardiac tamponade. **A.** Recordings before pericardiocentesis show the presence of systemic hypotension and the elevation and equalization of the RA and intrapericardial pressures. Note that a systolic x descent is present, but the diastolic y descent is absent, suggesting that RA emptying in early diastole is impeded because of cardiac compression by the pericardial effusion. **B.** After aspiration of 100 mL of pericardial fluid, RA and intrapericardial pressures have fallen and are beginning to separate, and systolic arterial hypertension has improved compared with baseline. **C.** After aspiration of a total of about 300 mL of pericardial fluid, tamponade physiology is relieved, as evidenced by (a) restoration of intrapericardial pressure to zero, (b) restoration of RA pressure to a normal level, and (c) reappearance of the diastolic y descent in the RA waveform, indicative of the relief of cardiac compression in early diastole. Note the negative fluctuation in intrapericardial pressure during inspiration, accompanied by an increased steepness in the fall of RA pressure during the x and y descents. Although this degree of fluid aspiration completely relieved tamponade physiology, an additional 1,500 mL of fluid was removed from the pericardial space.

so pericardiocentesis should be deferred if possible until the international normalized ratio (INR) is within normal range. If hemodynamic status demands urgent pericardiocentesis in the patient with elevated INR, fresh frozen plasma should be administered in the catheterization suite immediately after catheter access to the pericardium is achieved by an expert operator and drainage is initiated (to avoid conversion of a free hemorrhagic effusion into mixture of fluid and gelatinous clot).

A series of 960 consecutive pericardiocenteses performed at the Mayo Clinic (30) included 9.6% performed for cardiac perforation complicating catheter-based procedures. Using echocardiographically guided pericardiocentesis, tamponade was relieved in 99% and further pericardial drainage was required in only 18%. But pericardiocentesis can cause complications that include laceration of a chamber wall or laceration of a coronary artery or vein, which can result in hemopericardium, worsening tamponade, or circulatory collapse. Perforation of the ventricular myocardium with just the needle usually does not result in significant bleeding and is usually well tolerated, but reflex hypotension can occur. Ventricular and atrial arrhythmias may occur as a result of mechanical irritation from the needle, guidewire, or catheter, but are usually transient and not life threatening. Pneumothorax can occur as the result of entry into the pleural space, and laceration of the liver or penetration of the stomach, colon, or spleen have also been described as complications of pericardiocentesis via the subxiphoid route. Right and left ventricular failure, pulmonary edema, and exacerbation of bleeding from an ascending aortic dissection have been described following pericardiocentesis (27,34–37)

Case 1: Pericardial Tamponade. A 55-year-old man presented with unstable angina. Severe stenoses in the proximal and mid LAD were stented, but a shelflike step-up was seen within the stented segment. That area was postdilated at 16 atm, with vessel perforation noted immediately on deflation (Fig. 32.4). Hypotension ensued, and the 3.0-mm balloon was reinflated to block the vessel as emergent subxiphoid pericardiocentesis was performed. The contralateral femoral artery was punctured to allow introduction of an 8F XB3.5 guiding catheter, through which a second BMW wire was advanced to the distal vessel. The 3.0-mm balloon was deflated and removed through the initial 6F guiding catheter as a 3.0 × 16 Jomed covered stent was advanced to span the area of perforation. Delivery of the stent and postdilation at 18 atm sealed the perforation. The cardiac surgeons were present in the catheterization laboratory and agreed with continued nonoperative management, given that bleeding had been stopped and the vessel was patent. No further pericardial problems were noted, and the drain came out the next day. The patient did have moderate myocardial infarction (MI) owing to occlusion of diagonals, but the stent remained open at restudy day 3, and the patient went home on day 4.

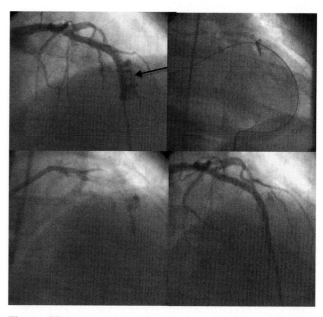

Figure 32.4 Coronary perforation and management. **Top left.** Immediately after 18 atm postdilation of a mid-LAD stent through a 6F catheter, coronary perforation with free extravasation of contrast was noted *(arrow)*. **Top right.** The patient became hypotensive within minutes, and the angioplasty balloon was reinflated within the area of perforation to seal the leak as pericardiocentesis was performed via the subxiphoid route. **Bottom left.** Via the contralateral groin, an 8F guiding catheter was engaged in the left coronary ostium, and a wire and Jomed covered stent were advanced to the point of perforation. **Bottom right.** After this stent was deployed, there was no further extravasation, and the heparin was not reversed as the platelet glycoprotein IIb/IIIa receptor blocker was continued to protect the patency of the stents that had been placed in the right coronary artery and proximal LAD prior to the perforation. LAD, left anterior descending.

CONSTRICTIVE PERICARDITIS

Constrictive pericarditis is a symmetrical process in which scarring of both the parietal and visceral pericardial layers constrains all cardiac chambers. Localized constriction may rarely produce external compression and stenosis of the mitral and tricuspid valves (38). In the chronic stage of constriction, pericardial calcification may develop, but absence of calcification can be seen in more recent constriction despite severe hemodynamic compromise. Although tuberculosis was once the most important cause of constrictive pericarditis, the most common causes of constrictive pericarditis today are recurrent idiopathic or viral pericarditis, delayed constriction after mediastinal radiation therapy (sometimes years later), and pericarditis after open heart surgery (39–41). Less common causes include any cause of acute pericarditis including neoplasm, septic pericarditis including opportunistic AIDS-related infections, chronic renal failure, post–myocardial infarction syndrome (Dressler), drugs, and connective tissue or autoimmune disorders. Some patients with acute pericarditis may develop transient mild pericardial constriction that resolves spontaneously within a few months of the initial illness (42). Constrictive pericarditis should be considered in any patient with unexplained jugular venous distension, systemic edema, hepatic congestion, and dyspnea. It should also be considered in the postoperative heart surgery patient who has unexplained tachycardia, low cardiac output, and venous congestion in the first months after surgery.

The clinical features of constrictive pericarditis reflect the physiologic effects produced as the constricting pericardium restricts cardiac filling and causes the gradual development of systemic venous and pulmonary venous hypertension followed by reduction of cardiac output. In patients in whom right and left atrial pressures are elevated in the range of 10 to 18 mm Hg, symptoms and signs of systemic venous congestion predominate. These include leg edema, postprandial discomfort, hepatic congestion, and ascites. As right and left heart filling pressures become elevated to a level of 18 to 30 mm Hg, exertional dyspnea and orthopnea appear, and pleural effusions may develop. As stroke volume falls, compensatory increases in systemic resistance and sinus tachycardia develop, which initially help maintain cardiac output and systemic blood pressure at rest, although the inability to augment cardiac output during exercise causes exertional fatigue and dyspnea. As resting cardiac output then begins to fall, severe lethargy and cardiac cachexia may occur.

The electrocardiogram usually shows reduced voltage and diffuse ST-T wave abnormalities that may be mistaken for ischemic coronary artery disease. Atrial fibrillation is present in about 10% of patients. The chest roentgenogram may show a small, normal, or modestly enlarged cardiac silhouette with redistribution of pulmonary flow or pleural effusions. The finding of pericardial calcification on the lateral projection may be present in about 50% of cases. Pericardial thickening, when present, is best demonstrated by cine and gated magnetic resonance imaging (MRI) and computed tomography (CT) with and without contrast enhancement (4). The mean normal pericardial thickness in adults is 1.2 ± 0.8 mm (two standard deviations [SD])—a pericardial thickness >3.5 mm indicates pathologic thickening, whereas any thickness >6 mm is specific for pericardial constriction. The finding of a pathologic increase in pericardial thickening supports the diagnosis, but does not demonstrate that constrictive physiology is present; conversely, hemodynamically significant constriction can be present with a tough but minimally thickened pericardium. CT or MR may also demonstrate small deformed ventricles, dilated left atrium, and dilated venae cavae. Measurement of pericardial thickness can also be achieved by transesophageal echocardiography (43), which may show pericardial thickening, dilatation of the superior and inferior vena cavae, diastolic flattening of the posterior ventricular wall, and abrupt cessation of ventricular dimension change in early diastole.

Right and left heart catheterization and angiography should be performed in every patient with suspected constrictive pericarditis (a) to confirm the presence of constrictive physiology and assess its severity before consideration

of pericardiectomy; (b) to assist in differentiating pericardial disease from restrictive cardiomyopathy; (c) to exclude major coexisting causes of right atrial hypertension, such as severe pulmonary hypertension; and (d) to exclude rare instances of localized constriction causing external valvular constriction or pinching of the epicardial coronary arteries. Endomyocardial biopsy (see below and Chapter 20) is sometimes useful in excluding a restrictive cardiomyopathy before surgical exploration for pericardial stripping is contemplated.

Both pericardial constriction and cardiac tamponade increase ventricular interdependence (see above), in which filling of one ventricle limits simultaneous filling of the other ventricle owing to the shared mechanical constraint of the pericardium and the interventricular septum. The pericardial constraint of the left and right ventricles in cardiac tamponade is coupled by uniform liquid pressure on the heart, whereas it is uncoupled in constriction given regional differences in surface pressure (44). Coupled constraint (tamponade) produces greater ventricular interdependence, so that increased inspiratory filling of the right ventricle results in highly coupled reduction in filling of the left ventricle (hence the occurrence of pulsus paradoxus), whereas uncoupled constraint (constriction) has a more modest effect on ventricular interdependence but more prominently reduces the effective elastance of the thin-walled right ventricle (hence the Kussmaul sign, an increase in right atrial pressure during inspiration; 45). This provides a framework for understanding the steady state and respiratory-related events that are detected by complementary echo-Doppler and hemodynamic evaluations in constrictive pericarditis and cardiac tamponade.

The right and left ventricular pressures should be measured simultaneously at equisensitive gains, with meticulous attention to zeroing, calibration and elimination of waveform damping. In constrictive pericarditis with elevated atrial pressures, early diastolic filling of the ventricles is unimpeded and abnormally rapid, but late diastolic filling is abbreviated and halts abruptly when total cardiac volume expands to the volume limit set by the stiff pericardium. This is reflected in the diastolic dip-and-plateau pattern in the right and left ventricular waveforms. Right and left ventricular diastolic pressures are typically equalized or nearly so. In the right atrial waveform, a prominent and rapid diastolic y descent is followed by a steep A wave and a blunted systolic x descent because the atrium is attempting to eject blood into a right ventricle that is already filled to capacity. In the right or left atrial waveform, the x and steep y descents impart to the characteristic M or W configuration (Fig. 32.5). Right and left atrial pressures may differ if coexisting mitral or tricuspid regurgitation is present associated with a large V wave in either atrium. In a patient with constriction and superimposed hypovolemia, a rapid volume challenge of 1,000 mL normal saline solution may be useful to unmask the hemodynamics of constrictive pericarditis. Tachycardia, inadequate

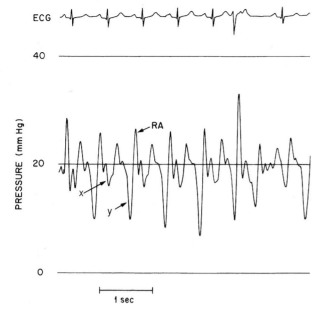

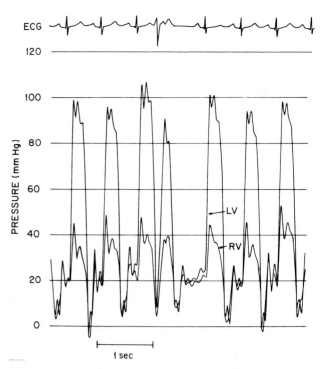

Figure 32.5 Right atrial (RA) pressure recording from a patient with constrictive pericarditis. Note the prominent y descent in the right atrial waveform, which indicates that the RA emptying is rapid and unimpeded in early diastole. The nadir of the y descent corresponds with the abrupt cessation of early diastolic ventricular filling. The prominent x and y descents give the RA waveform its characteristic M- or W-shaped appearance in constrictive pericarditis. The mean value of the RA pressure is more than twice normal, at 18 to 20 mm Hg.

Figure 32.6 Left ventricular (LV) and right ventricular (RV) pressures recorded simultaneously in the patient with constrictive pericarditis shown in Fig. 32.5 illustrate technical pitfalls in evaluation of pressure tracings. The presence of resting tachycardia partially obscures evaluation of the diastolic waveforms, and underdamping of the LV pressure transducer system accentuates an undershoot of LV pressure in early diastole and an overshoot during atrial contraction. A long diastole following a premature beat permits the recognition of equilibration of LV and RV diastolic pressures and the appreciation of a dip-and-plateau configuration of the ventricular waveforms.

transducer zeroing, and transducer underdamping may obscure the evaluation of diastolic waveforms (Fig. 32.6).

Examination of respiratory fluctuations in hemodynamics is an important component of the cardiac catheterization for constriction. In severe pericardial constriction, negative intrathoracic pressure during inspiration is not communicated to the intrapericardial space and the right heart. There is typically little respiratory variation in right atrial pressure. This contrasts with both normal subjects and patients with cardiac tamponade who demonstrate a fall in systemic venous and right atrial pressures during inspiration. In extreme cases, systemic venous pressure increases during inspiration (Kussmaul sign), as illustrated in Fig. 32.7; 45). Using micromanometer pressure measurements, Hurrell et al. (46) reported that discordance of right and left ventricular systolic pressures during respiration is an indicator of increased ventricular interdependence in constrictive pericarditis. As illustrated in Fig. 32.8, the inspiratory augmentation of right heart filling, stroke output, and right ventricular systolic pressure occur simultaneously with a fall in left ventricular systolic pressure, which results from an inspiratory fall in intrathoracic and pulmonary venous pressures and a reduction of left heart filling and stroke volume. This finding helps distinguish patients with surgically proven constrictive pericarditis from patients with other causes of heart failure. In addition, Hurrell (46) found a respiratory gradient of left ventricular pressure to pulmonary capillary wedge pressure

that correlated with the Doppler examination of respiratory fluctuations in mitral inflow velocity. An inspiratory reduction or reversal of pulmonary capillary wedge pressure to early left ventricular diastolic pressure was found in constrictive pericarditis, but not uniformly in other causes

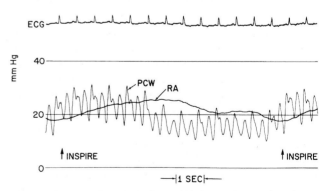

Figure 32.7 Right atrial (mean, RA) and pulmonary capillary wedge (phasic, PCW) pressure tracings from a patient with constrictive pericarditis. An *arrow* marks the beginning of the inspiratory phase of each respiratory cycle. Note that the mean right atrial pressure increases during inspiration (Kussmaul sign). The PCW pressure is out of phase with RA pressure and begins to fall during inspiration as RA pressure is rising.

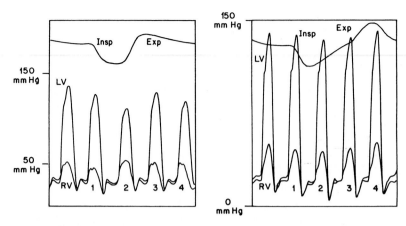

Figure 32.8 Respiratory (insp and exp) changes in left ventricular (LV) and right ventricular (RV) pressures measured with micromanometer catheters in a patient with constrictive pericarditis **(left)** and in a patient with restrictive cardiomyopathy **(right).** Peak inspiration is indicated in beat 2 in each cardiac cycle. In the patient with constrictive pericarditis **(left),** there is a discordant change in LV and RV systolic pressures during respiration: LV systolic pressure falls to its minimum value during peak inspiration simultaneously with an increase in RV systolic pressure to its highest value in the cardiac cycle. These findings indicate the presence of ventricular interdependence owing to the constricting pericardium, and suggest that as LV filling and stroke volume decreases, there is a corresponding increase in RV filling and stroke volume. In contrast, in the patient with cardiomyopathy **(right),** there are concordant changes in LV and RV pressures during respiration. (Adapted from Hurrell DG, Nishimura RA, Higano ST, et al. Value of dynamic respiratory changes in left and right ventricular pressures for the diagnosis of constrictive pericarditis. *Circulation* 1996;93:2007.)

of heart failure. This finding was less sensitive and specific for constriction than the right ventricle–left ventricle discordance noted above.

Stroke volume is almost always reduced in patients with constrictive pericarditis, but resting cardiac output may be preserved owing to tachycardia. Studies of atrial pacing in patients with constrictive pericarditis showed that increases in heart rate up to about 140 beats per minute increased cardiac output in the presence of unchanged stroke volume and ventricular filling pressure (47). After pericardiectomy, when ventricular filling was no longer impeded and confined to early diastole, atrial pacing caused a normal pattern of improvement in cardiac output at higher heart rates. In advanced constrictive pericarditis, resting cardiac index is depressed in association with systemic arterial vasoconstriction and arterial hypotension. In the absence of extensive coexisting myocardial fibrosis, left ventricular ejection fraction is usually normal or increased, and both isovolumic and ejection phase indices of contractile function (e.g., peak dP/dt) are preserved (46,48). The important exception to this are those patients with extensive coexisting myocardial fibrosis, which is a complication of radiation-induced pericardial constriction, or conditions in which infiltrative processes such as amyloid may involve both pericardium and myocardium (49).

When pericardial thickening is not evident, it is important to distinguish constrictive pericarditis from restrictive cardiomyopathy, which may produce similar clinical, hemodynamic, and echocardiographic findings. Doppler flow velocity studies in constrictive pericarditis typically show an exaggerated inspiratory increase in tricuspid flow velocity and a reduction in mitral flow velocity (>25% inspiratory reduction in mitral flow velocity) that may also be seen in tamponade, but is usually absent in restrictive cardiomyopathy. Tissue Doppler, which measures displacement and velocities of left ventricular motion, usually shows high or normal early diastolic velocity in patients with constrictive pericarditis, whereas these are usually reduced in restrictive cardiomyopathy. In addition, pulmonary venous flow by transesophageal echocardiography shows greater pulmonary venous peak systolic flow velocity in constrictive pericarditis compared with restrictive cardiomyopathy (50). Because none of these echo measurements have perfect discriminatory ability, they need to be taken in the context of the clinical presentation and hemodynamic findings (see below).

Coronary angiography should be performed as part of the cardiac catheterization evaluation of constrictive pericarditis. In addition to defining significant occult atherosclerotic coronary artery disease, the angiogram can detect the rare problem of external pinching or compression of the coronary arteries by the constricting pericardium prior to pericardiectomy (51). Studies indicate that pericardial constriction limits coronary flow reserve measured by adenosine-induced hyperemia and causes abrupt cessation and rapid deceleration of the normal pattern of early diastolic flow velocity (52). Left ventriculography may not be required during cardiac catheterization if a current high-quality imaging study (echocardiography, gated CT, or MRI) has defined global and regional left ventricular ejection fraction and volumes and excluded significant coexisting valvular heart disease.

Treatment

Medical management is purely palliative with control of edema and arrhythmias. The definitive treatment of constrictive pericarditis is surgical pericardiectomy, which should be reserved for symptomatic patients, in whom there are typical noninvasive imaging and hemodynamic findings. An experienced cardiovascular surgical team should perform a complete visceral and parietal pericardiectomy, facilitated by the ability to mobilize the heart on cardiopulmonary bypass. Outcome is excellent in patients in whom the operation is performed early in the disease before development of dense epicardial fibrosis that is less amenable to resection, end-stage depression of rest cardiac output, and poor organ perfusion. For example, a recent surgical series of 21 patients from a major tertiary center reported no perioperative mortality, mean postoperative hospital stay of 7 days, and return to functional NYHA Class I in all patients (53). Mayo Clinic studies of 58 patients showed that abnormalities of diastolic filling detected by Doppler mitral flow velocity signals were present in about 40% of patients 3 months after pericardiectomy, with approximately 34% showing abnormalities at 21 months post (54). Most patients improve quickly postoperatively with diuresis and resolution of edema and hepatic congestion. Others recover more slowly over months, but atrial arrhythmias may persist. Poorer surgical outcome is predicted by inadequate pericardial resection, inability to relieve epicardial constriction with scoring or meshing of the epicardium (55), uncorrected coronary disease, older age, after radiation pericarditis, and with peripheral organ failure (56).

Case 2: Constrictive Pericarditis. A 59-year-old man was admitted for cardiology evaluation after 4 years of progressive peripheral edema, which had recently become resistant to increasing doses of oral diuretics. For the 2 weeks prior to hospital admission, he had noted increasing fatigue and dyspnea on exertion and orthopnea, increasing abdominal girth, increasing leg and scrotal edema, and a rapid weight gain of at least 15 pounds. Physical examination showed a chronically ill appearing white male with dyspnea at rest. Blood pressure (BP) was 140/95; the heart rate was irregular and 150 beats per minute. The chest showed dullness at both bases, and heart sounds were distant. The cardiac exam showed an irregular tachycardia with distant heart sounds, and no rubs, gallops, or murmurs were appreciated. His abdomen was distended with ascites and an enlarged liver and mild right upper quadrant tenderness. There was marked scrotal edema. Extremities showed significant pitting edema to the level of the groin with chronic venous stasis changes of the skin of his legs bilaterally. Laboratory examination was normal (including

thyroid function) except for mild elevation of total bilirubin and liver transaminases.

Echocardiography showed biatrial dilation, moderate hypokinesis of the ventricles with a left ventricular ejection fraction of 35%, and no regional wall motion abnormalities. There was +1 mitral regurgitation, +1 tricuspid regurgitation with an estimated right ventricular systolic pressure of 29 mm Hg by Doppler. There was a thickened pericardium with "railroad tracking" around the left ventricular apex and right ventricular free wall.

Cardiac catheterization revealed equalization of diastolic pressures with a left ventricular end-diastolic pressure (LVEDP) of 22 mm Hg, a mean pulmonary capillary wedge pressure of 22 mm Hg, a pulmonary artery pressure of 29/22 mm Hg, and a right atrial pressure of 21 mm Hg. The mean right atrial pressure increased with inspiration (Kussmaul sign), and the right and left ventricular diastolic pressures were equal. The resting tachycardia and atrial fibrillation obscured the evaluation of the x and y descents in the right atrial pressure tracing. (See Figs. 32.5 through 32.7.) Cardiac output and index measured by thermodilution were reduced at 3.7 L/minute and 1.7 L/minute per m², respectively. Coronary angiography showed normal right dominant coronary arteries. Left ventriculography showed a normal-sized left ventricle with a calculated ejection fraction of 42% and calcification of the anterolateral, apical, and inferior pericardium (Fig. 32.9).

The patient underwent pericardial stripping, during which the pericardium was described as thickened, heavily calcified, and having the consistency of bone. The parietal pericardium was densely adherent to the epicardium. The calcified anterior pericardium was removed piecemeal after identifying and preserving the phrenic nerves. The right atrium was entered inadvertently, requiring the institution

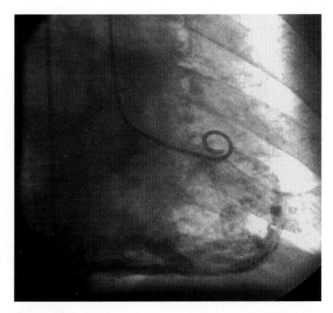

Figure 32.9 Left ventriculography. Note pericardial calcification.

of cardiopulmonary bypass and repair. Histology showed focal fibrosis, calcification, and chronic inflammation with aggregates of lymphocytes and mesothelial cells. Routine stains and cultures were negative, as was cytology.

Postoperatively, the patient maintained sinus rhythm, but required pharmacologic inotropic and pressure support for several days. He required intravenous diuretics and thoracentesis, but eventually diuresed 15 kg over the next week, and his peripheral edema largely resolved. By 3 months after surgery, he resumed normal activities and within 3 months was able to walk several miles a day without symptoms. He remained free of edema on reduced doses of once-daily furosemide and free of atrial fibrillation on Quinaglute and digoxin.

EFFUSIVE-CONSTRICIVE PERICARDITIS

Failure of right atrial pressure to fall to normal levels following pericardiocentesis for tamponade suggests that a coexisting cause of right atrial hypertension is present. Persistent elevation of right atrial pressure with appearance of a prominent y descent and a dip-and-plateau pattern in the right ventricular waveform suggest the presence of effusive-constrictive pericarditis. In this condition, relief of cardiac tamponade unmasks significant residual visceral pericardial constriction (57,58). The jugular venous pulse may resemble that of constriction, with prominent x and y descent, rather than blunting of the y descent that typically occurs in tamponade (59). Diastolic pressures remain equalized between the right and left heart after pericardiocentesis. Effusive-constrictive pericarditis is important to recognize and diagnose, since definitive treatment requires extensive visceral and parietal pericardiectomy (60). The most common causes are idiopathic, malignancy, radiation, rheumatoid arthritis, and tuberculosis.

Case 3: Effusive-Constrictive Pericarditis. A 29-year-old female was admitted to the hospital complaining of posi-

tional chest pain, progressive dyspnea on exertion, and orthopnea. She complained of orthostatic dizziness and had a resting tachycardia of 120 beats per minute. Two years earlier, she had been diagnosed with stage IV nodular sclerosing Hodgkin's disease with a large mediastinal mass. Chemotherapy resulted in diminution of the mediastinal mass but new disease activity developed in several bony locations, which was treated by high-dose chemotherapy and an autologous peripheral stem cell rescue. A CT of the chest 3 months prior to admission had revealed a partial response, with reduction in the size of the mediastinal mass and a normal pericardium, with no pericardial effusion (Fig. 32.10A).

Physical exam revealed her BP to be 90/60, with a pulsus paradoxus of 18 mm Hg and elevated jugular venous pressure of 18 cm water without an apparent Kussmaul sign. There was +1 edema of the lower extremities bilaterally. An echocardiogram revealed normal chamber dimensions with normal global and segmental ventricular function. A moderate anterior and posterior pericardial effusion with minimal inferior and apical effusion and right ventricular and right atrial diastolic collapse was noted. There was >50% variation in tricuspid valve inflow velocities and >30% variation in mitral valve inflow velocities by Doppler consistent with tamponade physiology. There was a homogeneous echogenic mass, >12 mm in thickness, seen encasing the heart in multiple views. Bedside right atrial pressure measure via a central line showed a mean of 25 mm Hg with a prominent y descent and an inspiratory increase in mean pressure. Chest CT revealed a large mediastinal mass encasing the heart and a moderate pericardial effusion (Fig. 32.10B), with a clear decrease in pericardial volume compared with the previous CT 4 months earlier.

Subxiphoid pericardiotomy was performed surgically; 200 mL of serous fluid was returned and a pericardial drain placed. Pericardial biopsy revealed histiocytoid cells and mixed inflammatory infiltrate consistent with nodular-sclerosing Hodgkin lymphoma. Her right atrial pressure

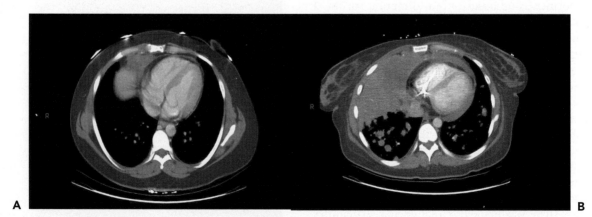

Figure 32.10 **A.** Computed tomography (CT) of the chest 3 months prior to admission. Note the normal pericardial thickness and lack of effusion. **B.** CT of the chest on admission. Note the mass in the right hemithorax, scattered masses throughout the lung fields, thickened and encased pericardium, decreased pericardial cross sectional area, and small pericardial effusion.

dropped from 25 to 18 mm Hg with removal of the peri-cardial fluid, but she remained hypotensive and dyspneic, despite adequate filling pressures. After discussions with the patient, family, and oncologists, a decision was made to forgo more aggressive therapy and comfort measures were initiated. The patient expired 1 week later.

RESTRICTIVE CARDIOMYOPATHY

The differentiation between constrictive pericarditis and restrictive cardiomyopathy is often difficult but important, because only the former can be effectively treated with peri-cardiectomy. In restrictive cardiomyopathy, there is an abnormality of diastolic function, and the ventricular walls are noncompliant and resist filling. Systolic function is usu-ally preserved. The most common etiologies of restrictive cardiomyopathy are idiopathic, amyloidosis, sarcoidosis, endomyocardial fibrosis, radiation, and anthracycline toxi-city (see Chapter 20). Less common causes are familial; scleroderma; pseudoxanthoma elasticum; diabetic; storage diseases such as Gaucher, Hurler, Fabry, and glycogen storage disease; hemochromatosis, carcinoid, hypereosinophilia, metastatic cancers, and drugs. The clinical features of restrictive cardiomyopathy are often similar to those of con-strictive pericarditis (61)—both disorders manifest impaired ventricular diastolic filling and elevated diastolic pressures with symptoms of congestive heart failure such as exercise intolerance, weakness, and fatigue. Central venous pressure is elevated with peripheral edema, liver enlarge-ment, ascites, and anasarca in advanced cases. Stroke vol-ume is fixed or reduced in both, although systolic contrac-tile function may be essentially normal. In both disorders, patients may complain of chest and neck discomfort during exertion that may be related to impaired coronary reserve and/or neck vein distension. In both disorders, the electro-cardiogram commonly shows abnormal voltage and ST-T wave abnormalities, and atrial fibrillation may occur.

Echocardiography may show thickening of the left ven-tricular wall and an increase in ventricular mass. Patients with restrictive cardiomyopathy have an increased early left ventricular filling velocity (E), a decreased atrial filling veloc-ity (A), with E/A ratios ≥2, and a decreased isovolumic relax-ation time (62). Tissue Doppler, which measures displace-ment and velocities of left ventricular motion, usually shows normal early diastolic velocity in patients with constrictive pericarditis versus reduced velocities in restrictive cardiomy-opathy. Color M-mode Doppler spatial velocity distribution using the slope of the first aliasing contour shows a slower slope in constrictive pericarditis than in restrictive car-diomyopathy (50). In addition, pulmonary venous flow by transesophageal echocardiography shows peak systolic pulmonary venous flow velocity is less than diastolic flow velocity in restrictive cardiomyopathy, and there is reversal of diastolic flow after atrial contraction with inspiration in the hepatic and pulmonary veins (62). Measurement of

pericardial thickening may be accomplished by trans-esophageal echocardiography (43), CT, or MRI, and if pres-ent, favors constrictive pericarditis. None of these echo measurements has perfect discriminatory ability; all need to be taken in the context of the clinical presentation and hemodynamic findings. On the other hand, echocardio-graphic findings of thickened cardiac valves, a granular sparkling appearance of the myocardium, and the presence of thickened ventricular walls with reduced electrocardio-graphic R-wave voltage suggest the presence of an infiltra-tive process such as amyloid, but their absence does not exclude the presence of restrictive cardiomyopathy (62).

In most cases, careful attention to hemodynamics at car-diac catheterization can permit identification of the patient whose symptoms of congestive failure are owing to restric-tive cardiomyopathy. Right and left ventricular diastolic pressures should be recorded simultaneously at equisensi-tive gains. Right atrial pressure is usually elevated and has a prominent y descent followed by a rapid rise with an M- or W-shaped waveform as in constrictive pericarditis. The res-piratory variation in right atrial pressure may be lacking, and the y descent may become steeper with inspiration. Diastolic pressures in both ventricles may be elevated, with a dip-and-plateau configuration, but left ventricular dia-stolic pressure is usually higher than right ventricular dia-stolic pressure. There is usually concordance in the fall of right and left ventricular systolic pressures with inspiration (46). Supine exercise usually causes elevation of left greater than right ventricular diastolic pressures. Pulmonary hyper-tension is usually more common and more severe in restrictive cardiomyopathy than in constrictive pericarditis, and pulmonary systolic pressures >45 to 50 mm Hg are common. However, in cohorts of patients with constrictive pericarditis versus restrictive cardiomyopathy, there is fre-quently overlap in these measurements between individu-als in each group (46).

In some but not all patients with restrictive cardiomy-opathy, the diastolic filling pattern differs from that of con-strictive pericarditis. Using frame-by-frame angiographic or radionuclide analysis of ventricular filling, one pattern in restrictive cardiomyopathy is a slow early diastolic filling rate compared with normal. This sluggish pattern of early diastolic filling sharply contrasts with the explosively rapid but abbreviated early diastolic filling pattern in constrictive pericarditis (63,64). However, other patients with restrictive cardiomyopathy exhibit an excessively rapid and abbrevi-ated early diastolic filling pattern similar to constrictive pericarditis. Importantly, insights from noninvasive studies have shown that this "restrictive" pattern of atrioventricular valve inflow and diastolic filling is not specific for restrictive cardiomyopathy. It can be observed in other forms of car-diomyopathy besides restrictive cardiomyopathy in the set-ting of high left atrial pressure and can be modified or abol-ished by reduction in preload (65,66). Thus, the diagnosis of restrictive cardiomyopathy requires careful clinical judg-ment and integration of both noninvasive imaging data and hemodynamic analyses. A clinical history suggestive of pericarditis makes a diagnosis of constrictive pericarditis more likely, as does a history of tuberculosis, trauma, or cardiac surgical procedures. No diagnostic technique is totally reliable in differentiating these two entities, and in some patients the only reliable way to make the diagnosis is to perform pericardiectomy (62).

Since pericardiectomy is a major procedure (especially the dissection of the adherent visceral pericardium free from the myocardium), further certainty is desirable before surgery in equivocal cases. Whereas the diagnostic yield of endomyocardial biopsy is low in the evaluation of patients with dilated cardiomyopathy, showing a specific etiologic diagnosis is obtained in <10% of patients, and a treatable process is found in about 2% (63), biopsy does play an important role in the evaluation of the symptomatic patient with potential constriction versus restrictive cardiomyopathy (67,68). Myocardial biopsy is valuable in making a definitive diagnosis in patients with restrictive cardiomyopathy owing to amyloid as well as other specific causes such as myocarditis, metabolic storage disease, and hemochromatosis. In patients with cardiac irradiation injury in which both pericardium and myocardium may be involved, the documentation of extensive myocardial fibrosis and myocyte dropout should temper the decision to proceed to surgical pericardiectomy (67; see also Chapter 20).

OTHER CONDITIONS ASSOCIATED WITH CONSTRICTIVE PHYSIOLOGY

As noted at the beginning of this chapter, the normal pericardium functions restrain cardiac dilatation and couple the function of both ventricles in conditions in which the pericardium has not expanded to accommodate an increase in cardiac or effusion volume. In the presence of normal cardiac volumes and low filling pressures, cardiac volumes dynamically fluctuate during respiration and with changes in posture within the loose lubricated pericardial sac with minimal pericardial constraint and minimal ventricular interaction. However, as right ventricular volume increases to a level associated with a diastolic pressure of about 10 to 12 mm Hg, pericardial constraint appears and ventricular interdependence increases. Ventricular interdependence can be recognized when increments in ventricular diastolic pressure cause a similar gain in diastolic pressure of the opposite ventricle, and when respiratory filling of one ventricle causes marked reduction of filling of the opposite chamber. This phenomenon has been shown to be important in dilated cardiomyopathy, in which reductions in elevated right heart filling result in the augmentation of left ventricular filling via ventricular interaction (66).

Acute right ventricular infarction in humans (69) and experimental animal models may cause constrictive physiology with right ventricular dilation, elevation and

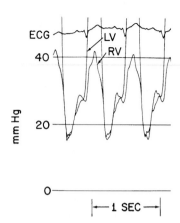

Figure 32.11 Simultaneous right ventricular (RV) and left (LV) pressure tracings recorded in a patient with several-week history of severe tricuspid insufficiency. Note that RV and LV end-diastolic pressures are markedly elevated (approximately 28 mm Hg) with virtual identity of pressures throughout diastole. RV systolic pressure is minimally increased, an indication that the elevation of RV diastolic pressure is not caused primarily by pulmonary hypertension. These findings suggest a restraining effect of the intact normal pericardium with increased ventricular interdependence in the presence of subacute volume overload of the right ventricle.

equilibration of right and left ventricular pressures, a dip-and-plateau ventricular waveform, and reduced right ventricular pulse pressure. Right ventricular volume overload owing to subacute tricuspid regurgitation with an intact pericardium can also cause increased pericardial constraint and ventricular interdependence, as illustrated in Fig. 32.11. In a classic paper, Bartle and Hermann (70) reported that acute and subacute mitral regurgitation can cause a striking hemodynamic pattern suggestive of pericardial constriction. Acute pulmonary embolism, with secondary right ventricular dilatation and moderate pulmonary hypertension in the setting of a nonhypertrophied right ventricle, can also result in constrictive physiology owing to pericardial constraint.

OTHER PERICARDIAL PROCEDURES

Percutaneous Balloon Pericardiotomy

Percutaneous balloon pericardiotomy is an alternative approach to the treatment of cardiac tamponade in patients with large recurrent malignant effusions (71) or idiopathic effusions that have recurred or not abated after prolonged catheter drainage (e.g., >100 mL/day after three days of catheter drainage). Of patients who undergo pericardiocentesis for malignant effusion, 66% of these patients have recurrence after simple drainage by pericardiocentesis (72,73). In comparison, in most series of cardiac tamponade not related to malignant effusion, pericardiocentesis with prolonged catheter drainage (33) was effective without further intervention in >80% of patients. An analysis by Vaitkus (74) suggests that balloon pericardiostomy, surgical pericardiectomy, pleuropericardial window, and subxiphoid window are all superior in terms of freedom from recurrence to repeat simple pericardiocentesis, instillation of sclerosing agents, radiation, or prolonged catheter drainage. Patients with recurrent tamponade from malignant effusions usually have a limited life span and are often poor surgical candidates.

An alternative to a subxiphoid window is percutaneous balloon pericardiotomy. The technique begins with pericardiocentesis via the subxiphoid approach. After pericardiocentesis, approximately 20 mL of contrast is injected to aid visualization of the pericardial space. An 0.035-inch J-tip guidewire is then introduced and looped in the pericardium. The pericardiocentesis catheter is withdrawn, the tract is dilated with a 10F dilator, and a 10F to 12F sheath inserted under fluoroscopy. A 20-mm-diameter by 3- to 4-cm-long dilating balloon (e.g., Mansfield, Z-Med) is advanced over the guidewire. The balloon is positioned to straddle the pericardial border, and the sheath is withdrawn to uncover the balloon. The balloon is slightly inflated to define a waist at the parietal pericardial border as illustrated in Fig. 32.12, and then fully expanded to create a rent in the pericardium. Depending on the stiffness of the pericardium, the balloon may "watermelon seed" into the pericardium and require strong countertraction. In thin patients, the skin and subcutaneous tissues may need to be retracted inferiorly to avoid dilating through the skin. If the 20-mm balloon cannot be successfully inflated, we have found that moving to a 12- or 18-mm balloon may allow dilation, with subsequent upsizing of the balloon to 20 to 22 mm in diameter. Balloon dilatation across the pericardium tends to cause severe pain, and adequate prophylactic narcotic analgesics should be administered prior to inflation to minimize discomfort.

The balloon is removed, pericardial catheter reintroduced, and about 10 mL of contrast may be injected to confirm free exit of fluid through the rent in the pericardium. Any remaining fluid is evacuated, and the catheter placed to drainage for 24 hours or until the catheter drainage is less <50 to 75 mL/24 hours. Sometimes more than one site must be dilated to ensure rapid emptying of the pericardial space, or the balloon pericardiostomy may need to be repeated for recurrent tamponade. Chest roentgenography must be performed within 24 hours to evaluate for left pleural effusion, which is common, or pneumothorax, which is uncommon. Echocardiography should be performed 48 hours after catheter removal to confirm resolution of the pericardial effusion.

Modifications of the procedure include use of an Inoue balloon catheter. In 11 patients who underwent Inoue balloon pericardiotomy for treatment of recurrent large effusion, the procedure was successful in 10 patients (91%), who remained free of recurrent effusion for a follow-up period of 4 months (75). It has been established that balloon pericardiotomy causes drainage and absorption of fluid within the peritoneal cavity and the pleura (71,76). Given the experience with subxiphoid surgical pericardial window, it is unlikely that the communication between the pericardium and pleura or peritoneum produced by balloon pericardiectomy stays open for the long term (77) as inflammatory fusion of the opposed parietal and visceral pericardium occurs over time and obliterates the potential space.

A multicenter registry of 130 patients undergoing balloon pericardiotomy has been reported (78). The procedure was performed without major complications in all patients; minor complications included fever, which occurred with lesser frequency later in the series when prophylactic antibiotics were routinely administered. There

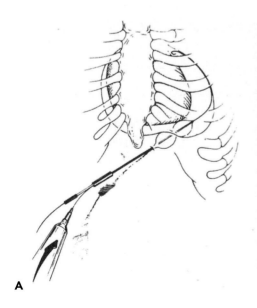

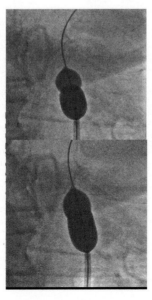

A   **B**

Figure 32.12 A. Illustration of the percutaneous balloon pericardiotomy technique. After partial drainage of the pericardium using a pericardial catheter, an 0.038-inch stiff J-tip wire is introduced into the pericardial space. A 3-cm-long dilating balloon is then advanced over the guidewire to straddle the parietal pericardial membrane and is manually inflated to create a rent in the pericardium. **B.** Still frames from a percutaneous balloon pericardiotomy. (From Ziskind AA, Pearce AC, Lemmon CC, et al. Percutaneous balloon pericardiotomy for the treatment of cardiac tamponade and large pericardial effusions: description of technique and report of the first 50 cases. *J Am Coll Cardiol* 1993;21:1.)

was no recurrence of pericardial effusion or need for surgery in 85% of patients followed for a mean of 5.0 ± 5.8 months. After percutaneous balloon pericardiotomy, 15% required chest tube placement for pleural effusion. In a recent series of 94 patients treated with subxiphoid pericardiotomy for cardiac tamponade of which 64% were malignant effusions, the procedure was successful in all patients with no operative deaths and associated with a rate of recurrent tamponade of 1.1% in comparison with a recurrence rate of 30% in a nonrandomized concurrent series of 23 patients managed with percutaneous catheter pericardiocentesis (79). In patients with recurrent malignant effusion, there are multiple small series that discuss the use of intrapericardial sclerosing agents, but there are no prospective randomized series that compare the risks and benefits of catheter pericardiocentesis with and without instillation of sclerosing agents.

Case 4: Balloon Pericardiotomy. A 54-year-old man with lung adenocarcinoma that had been treated with chemotherapy, radiation therapy, and right lobectomy with chronic left pleural effusion (chest tube in place), developed a large pericardial effusion with echocardiographic evidence of pericardial tamponade (right atrial and right ventricular collapse). He underwent pericardiocentesis showing a pericardial pressure of 23 mm Hg, with relief of tamponade physiology after drainage of more than 500 mL of serosanguineous fluid. Two weeks later, however, symptoms recurred and echocardiography showed reaccumulation of pericardial effusion and signs of tamponade. Right heart catheterization showed a mean right atrial pressure of 16 mm Hg, mean PCW pressure of 22 mm Hg, and mean pericardial pressure of 15 mm Hg with some separation of pericardial and right atrial pressures. Cardiac index was mildly depressed at 2.4 L/minute per m^2, with a 15 mm Hg paradox.

After needle pericardiocentesis and removal of 100 mL of bloody fluid, the pericardial pressure decreased to 0 mm Hg with little change in the right atrial (RA) pressure. Balloon pericardiotomy (Fig. 32.13) was performed by advancing a guidewire through the drainage catheter, predilating with a 4.0×40 mm balloon, and final dilation with inflation of the 15 mm $\times$ 40 mm balloon straddling the pericardial edge. The pericardial waist resolved fully, and the balloon was exchanged for a drainage catheter left in overnight. The cardiac index improved to 3.4 L/minute per m^2, and repeat echocardiography at 1 month showed no reaccumulation of pericardial fluid.

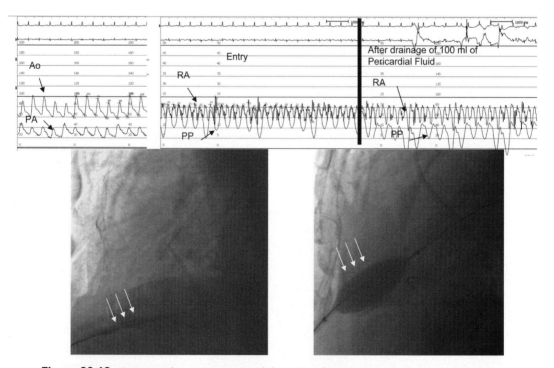

Figure 32.13 Patient with recurrent pericardial tamponade undergoing balloon pericardiotomy. **Top left.** Aortic (Ao) and pulmonary artery pressure tracing showing narrow pulse pressure and a paradoxical pulse on Ao pressure tracing. **Top middle.** Right atrial (RA) and pericardial pressure (PP) displayed simultaneously, showing an elevated PP with some separation of pericardial and right atrial pressure unlike initial tap, which showed equalization. **Top right.** Post removal of 100 mL of bloody fluid, PP decreased significantly. At end of procedure, PP decreased further and became negative. **Bottom left.** the pericardium and tract were dilated with a small balloon (predilation), which is often not necessary with newer low-profile peripheral balloons. **Bottom right.** The pericardium is dilated with a larger balloon (15 $\times$ 40 mm) to achieve an adequate pericardiotomy. Balloons as large as 20 mm in diameter can be used in larger patients.

Therapeutic Intrapericardial Intervention

The pericardial mesothelium actively secretes and metabolizes bioactive molecules, including prostaglandins, nitric oxide, atrial natriuretic peptide, and endothelin-1 that have the potential to modulate cardiac performance via paracrine signaling (80). In addition, growth factors with the potential to modify underlying myocyte and smooth muscle cell growth appear to be diffusible between cardiac tissue and the pericardial space and concentrated in pericardial fluid. Fujita and coworkers (81) demonstrated that concentrations of basic fibroblast growth factor (bFGF) are about 10-fold higher in the pericardial fluid of patients with unstable angina compared with patients with nonischemic heart disease, raising the possibility that growth factors concentrated in the pericardial space may mediate collateral blood vessel growth in humans. Thus, the pericardial space may serve as a potential drug delivery reservoir bathing the cardiac structures with increased myocardial delivery and reduced systemic recirculation (82,83). In addition, intrapericardial delivery of FGF-2 has been shown to result in functional angiogenesis in animal models of acute (84) and chronic myocardial ischemia (85), and percutaneous intrapericardial drug administration in patients with normal pericardium (and in the absence of significant pericardial effusion) has been shown to be feasible (31,32,86–89). In addition, presence of an epicardially located accessory bypass tract or ventricular tachycardia focus may necessitate epicardial mapping, which may be performed by pericardial access (90).

For these reasons, there is interest in the development of techniques for minimally invasive access of the pericardial space in patients without pericardial effusions for sampling of pericardial fluid; intrapericardial drug delivery of growth factors, gene therapy vectors, and drugs that may modify arrhythmias and myocardial perfusion; and epicardial mapping. There are three major techniques for access of the normal pericardium. The simplest is carried out using the subxiphoid blunt-tip needle approach. This is done by using a combination of a blunt-tip needle (Tuohy-17), pressurized saline flow (to push away the RV wall on pericardial entry), electrocardiographic (ST-segment elevation) and fluoroscopic guidance (injection of contrast; 91). Entry of the pericardial space is suspected after an increase in the saline flow through the intraflow system and confirmed by the injection of 1 mL of diluted contrast under fluoroscopy. A soft floppy-tip 0.025-inch guidewire is then advanced to the pericardial space, and the needle is exchanged for a pericardial catheter. A second technique involves transatrial pericardial access and enables access of the pericardial space via the right atrial appendage (82). A catheter is used to pierce the right atrial appendage. Pericardial access is then confirmed by placement of a radiopaque guidewire under fluoroscopy. A third technique uses the subxiphoid approach using the PerDUCER device. A stab incision is made in the subxiphoid area and a 17F angled cannula, with preloaded guidewire, is advanced into the mediastinal space. After cannula removal, a 19F sheath/dilator is inserted over the wire. The device is positioned over the pericardial cavity; the pericardium is captured by suction, and a bleb is formed within a side hole on the PerDUCER tip. A sheathed needle is advanced, puncturing the isolated bleb of pericardium allowing pericardial access (92,93). Further developments and widespread use will await the identification of therapeutic agents with proven clinical benefit. A potential disadvantage of pericardial drug delivery is the potential for poor endocardial penetration (83).

ANOMALIES OF THE PERICARDIUM

Congenital anomalies of the pericardium may cause confusion during cardiac catheterization and angiography unless their characteristic features are recognized. Pericardial cysts, which are filled with clear fluid, are usually located at the right costophrenic angle and come to attention as unexplained protrusion of the right heart border on the chest roentgenogram or during fluoroscopy at cardiac catheterization. Rarely, cysts may cause chest pain or right ventricular outflow obstruction (94). Although most can be managed conservatively, large pericardial cysts located at the costophrenic angle can be decompressed by percutaneous aspiration under fluoroscopic guidance (95).

Congenital pericardial defects are rare and mostly occur in males, with associated congenital abnormalities of the heart and lungs in up to 30% of patients. Isolated congenital absence of the pericardium encompasses a range from a small foramen to complete absence. Total absence of the pericardium is extremely rare and usually not associated with symptoms. Complete absence of the left side of the pericardium is more common, and patients may be referred to cardiac catheterization because of stabbing sharp chest pain that is occasionally positional (96), palpitations, or dyspnea. These patients have prominent apical impulses that displace with body position, electrocardiographic findings of right axis deviation and clockwise displacement of the precordial transition zone, chest roentgenogram findings of a leftward displacement of the heart with loss of right heart border, and a "tongue" of lung interposed between the main pulmonary artery and aortic knob. Echocardiographic findings mimic right ventricular volume overload with enlarged right ventricle and abnormal septal motion, and the left atrial appendage is laterally displaced. This anomaly can be accurately diagnosed with cardiac MRI (97,98). Smaller atrial left-sided pericardial defects are uncommon; however, cardiac catheterization and angiography can be helpful. These patients frequently complain of chest pain and are at risk for sudden death owing to herniation and strangulation of the heart or left atrial appendage through the defect. Echocardiographic findings are similar to above, and the left atrial appendage is laterally displaced. A definitive diagnosis can be made by CT or MRI, with a myocardial crease caused by the edge of the pericardium considered a high-risk feature (98,99). Partial right-sided pericardial defects can also be accompanied by severe chest pain related to inspiratory herniation of the right atrium (100).

REFERENCES

1. Spodick DH. *The Pericardium, A Comprehensive Textbook.* New York: Marcel Dekker, 1997.
2. Tyberg JV, Smith ER. Ventricular diastole and the role of the pericardium. *Hertz* 1999;15:354–361.
3. Hammond HK, et al. Heart size and maximal cardiac output are limited by the pericardium. *Am J Physiol* 1992;263:H1675–H1681.
4. LeWinter MM, Kalabani S. *Pericardial Diseases in Heart Disease,* 7th ed. Zipes DP, Libby P, Bonow R, Braunwald E, eds. New York: WB Saunders, 2005.
5. Sagrista-Sauleda J, et al. Clinical clues to the causes of large pericardial effusions. *Am J Med* 2000;109:95.
6. Corey GR, et al. Etiology of large pericardial effusions. *Am J Med* 1993;95:209.
7. Rubin RH, Moellering RC. Clinical, microbiologic and therapeutic aspects of purulent pericarditis. *Am J Med* 1975;59:68.
8. Klacsman PG, Bulkley BH, Hutchins GM. The changed spectrum of purulent pericarditis: an 86 year autopsy series in 200 patients. *Am J Med* 1977;63:666.
9. Imazio M, Demichelis B, et al. Cardiac troponin I in acute pericarditis. *J Am Coll Cardiol* 2003;42:2144.
10. Merce J, et al. Should pericardial drainage be performed routinely in patients who have large pericardial effusion without tamponade? *Am J Med* 1998;105:106–109.
11. Adler Y, et al. Colchicine treatment for recurrent pericarditis: a decade of experience. *Circulation* 1998;97:2183–2185.
12. Sagrista-Sauleda J, et al. Long term follow-up of idiopathic chronic pericardial effusion. *N Engl J Med* 1999;341:2054–2059.
13. Permanyer-Miralda G, Sagrista-Sauleda J, Soler-Soler J. Primary acute pericardial disease: a prospective series of 231 consecutive patients. *Am J Cardiol* 1985;56:623.
14. Malmou-Mitsi VD, Zioga AP, Agnantis J. Diagnostic accuracy of pericardial fluid cytology: an analysis of 53 specimens from 44 consecutive patients. *Diagn Cytopathol* 1996;15:197–204.
15. Myers DG, Meyers RE, Prendergast TW. The usefulness of diagnostic tests on pericardial fluid. *Chest* 1997;111:1213–1221.
16. Corey GR, et al. Etiology of large pericardial effusions. *Am J Med* 1993;95:209.
17. Koh KK, et al. Adenosine deaminase and carcinoembryonic antigen pericardial effusion diagnosis, especially in suspected tuberculous pericarditis. *Circulation* 1994;89:2728–2735.
18. Seino Y, et al. Tuberculous pericarditis presumably diagnosed with polymerase chain reaction analysis. *Am Heart J* 1993;126:249–251.
19. Goodman LJ. Purulent pericarditis. *Curr Treat Options Cardiovasc Med* 2000;2:343–350.
20. Nugue O, et al. Pericardioscopy in the etiologic diagnosis of pericardial effusion in 141 consecutive patients. *Circulation* 1996;94:1635.
21. Seferovic PM, et al. Diagnostic value of pericardial biopsy. Improvement with extensive sampling enabled pericardioscopy. *Circulation* 2003;107:978–983.
22. Seferovic PM, Ristic AD, Maksimovic R, et al. Diagnostic value of pericardial biopsy: Improvement with extensive sampling enabled by pericardioscopy. *Circulation* 2003;107:978–983.
23. Maisch B, et al. Pericardioscopy and epicardial biopsy–new diagnostic tools in pericardial and perimyocardial disease. *Eur Heart J* 1994;15(suppl C):68–73.
24. Maisch B, et al. Intrapericardial treatment of inflammatory and neoplastic pericarditis guided by pericardioscopy and epicardial biopsy–results from a pilot study. *Clin Cardiol* 1999;22:I17–22.
25. Maisch B, et al. Intrapericardial treatment of inflammatory and neoplastic pericarditis guided by pericardioscopy and epicardial biopsy - results from a pilot study. *Clin Cardiol* 1999;22(suppl I):17.
26. Mebazaa A, et al. Potential paracrine role of the pericardium in the regulation of cardiac function. *Cardiovasc Res* 1998;40:332.
27. Isselbacher EM, Cigarroa JE, Eagle KA. Cardiac tamponade complicating aortic dissection: is pericardiocentesis harmful? *Circulation* 1994;90:2375.
28. Tsang TSM, et al. Echocardiographically guided pericardiocentesis: evolution and state of the art technique. *Mayo Clin Proc* 1998;73:647–652.
29. Seward JB, et al. 500 consecutive echo-directed pericardiocenteses. *J Am Coll Cardiol* 1992;19(suppl A):356A
30. Tsang TSM, et al. Rescue echocardiographically guided pericardiocentesis for cardiac perforation complicating catheter-based procedures. *J Am Coll Cardiol* 1998;32:1345.
31. Mannam AP, et al. Safety of subxyphoid pericardial access using a blunt-tip needle. *Am J Cardiol* 2002;89:891–893.
32. Laham R, Simons M, Hung D. Subxyphoid access of the normal pericardium: a novel drug delivery technique. *Cathet Cardiovasc Diagn* 1999;47:109–111.
33. Tsang SM, et al. Outcomes of clinically significant idiopathic pericardial effusion requiring intervention. *Am J Cardiol* 2003;91:704–707.
34. Uemura S, et al. Acute left ventricular failure with pulmonary edema following pericardiocentesis for cardiac tamponade—a case report. *Jpn Circ J* 1995;59:55–59.
35. Hamaya Y, et al. Severe circulatory collapse immediately after pericardiocentesis in a patient with chronic cardiac tamponade. *Anesth Analg* 1993;77:1278–1281.
36. Wolfe MW, Edelman ER. Transient systolic dysfunction after relief of cardiac tamponade. *Ann Intern Med* 1993;119:42–44.
37. Vandyke WH, et al. Pulmonary edema after pericardiocentesis for cardiac tamponade. *N Engl J Med* 1983;309:595–596.
38. Pi, RG, Tarazi R, Wong S. Constrictive pericarditis causing extrinsic mitral stenosis and a left heart mass. *Clin Cardiol* 1996;19:517–519.
39. Cameron J, et al. The etiologic spectrum of constrictive pericarditis. *Am Heart J* 1987;113:354.
40. Mehta A, Mehta M, Jain AC. Constrictive pericarditis. *Clin Cardiol* 1999;22:334–344.
41. Tuna IC, Danielson GK. Surgical management of pericardial diseases. *Cardiol Clin* 19990;84:683–696.
42. Sagrista-Saudeda J, et al. Transient cardiac constriction: an unrecognized pattern of evolution in effusive acute idiopathic pericarditis. *Am J Cardiol* 1987;59:961.
43. Ling LH, et al. Pericardial thickness measured with transesophageal echocardiography: feasibility and potential clinical usefulness. *J Am Coll Cardiol* 1997;29:1317.
44. Takata M, et al. Coupled vs uncoupled pericardial constraint: effects on cardiac chamber interactions. *J Appl Physiol* 1997;83:1799.
45. Shabetai R, et al. The hemodynamics of cardiac tamponade and constrictive pericarditis. *Am J Cardiol* 1970;26:480.
46. Hurrell DG, et al. Value of dynamic respiratory changes in left and right ventricular pressures for the diagnosis of constrictive pericarditis. *Circulation* 1996;93:2007.
47. Chandrashekhar Y, et al. Rate-dependent hemodynamic responses during atrial pacing on chronic constrictive pericarditis before and after surgery. *Am J Cardiol* 1993;72:615.
48. Gaasch WH, Peterson KL, Shabetai R. Left ventricular function in chronic constrictive pericarditis. *Am J Cardiol* 1974;34:107.
49. Kern MJ, Lorell BH, Grossman W. Cardiac amyloidosis masquerading as constrictive pericarditis. *Cathet Cardiovasc Diagn* 1982;8:629.
50. Rajagopalan N, et al. Comparison of new Doppler echocardiographic methods to differentiate constrictive pericardial disease and restrictive cardiomyopathy. *Am J Cardiol* 2001;87:86–94.
51. Goldberg E, et al. Diastolic segmental coronary artery obliteration in constrictive pericarditis. *Cathet Cardiovasc Diagn* 1981;7:197.
52. Akasaka T, et al. Phasic coronary flow characteristics in patients with constrictive pericarditis: comparison with restrictive cardiomyopathy. *Circulation* 1997;96:1874–1881.

53. Trotter MC, et al. Pericardiectomy for pericardial constriction. *Am Surg* 1996;62:304.
54. Senni M, et al. Left ventricular systolic and diastolic function after pericardiectomy in patients with constrictive pericarditis: Doppler echocardiographic findings and correlation with clinical status. *J Am Coll Cardiol* 1999;33:1182.
55. Kao CL, Chang JP. Modified method for epicardial constriction: the electric waffle procedure. *J Cardiovasc Surg* 2001;42:643–646.
56. Tirilomis T, et al. Pericardiectomy for chronic constrictive pericarditis: risks and outcome. *Eur J Cardiothorac Surg* 1994;8:487–492.
57. Hancock EW. Subacute effusive-constrictive pericarditis. *Circulation* 1971;43:183.
58. Sagrista-Sauleda J, et al. Effusive-constrictive pericarditis. *N Engl J Med* 2004;350:469–475.
59. Shabeti R. *The Pericardium.* Boston: Kluwer Academic Press, 2003.
60. Walsh TJ, et al. Constrictive epicarditis as a cause of delayed or absent response to pericardiectomy. *J Thorac Cardiovasc Surg* 1982;83:126.
61. Benotti JR, et al. The clinical profile of restrictive cardiomyopathy. *Circulation* 1980;61:1206.
62. Kushwaha SS, Fallon JT, Fuster V. Restrictive cardiomyopathies. *N Engl J Med* 1997;336:267.
63. Tyberg TI, et al. Left ventricular filling in differentiating restrictive amyloid cardiomyopathy and constrictive pericarditis. *Am J Cardiol* 1981;47:791.
64. Aroney CN, et al. Differentiation of restrictive cardiomyopathy from pericardial constriction: assessment of diastolic function of radionuclide angiography. *J Am Coll Cardiol* 1989;13:1007.
65. Little WC, et al. Evaluation of left ventricular diastolic function from the pattern of left ventricular filling. *Clin Cardiol* 1998;21:5.
66. Atherton JJ, et al. Restrictive left ventricular filling patterns are predictive of diastolic ventricular interaction in chronic heart failure. *J Am Coll Cardiol* 1998;31:413.
67. Mason JW, O'Connell JB. Clinical merit of endomyocardial biopsy. *Circulation* 1989;79:971–979.
68. Schoenfield MH, et al. Restrictive cardiomyopathy versus constrictive pericarditis: role of endomyocardial biopsy in avoiding unnecessary thoracotomy. *Circulation* 1987;75:1012.
69. Lorell BH, et al. Right ventricular infarction. *Am J Cardiol* 1979;43:465.
70. Bartle SH, Hermann HJ. Acute mitral regurgitation in man. Hemodynamic evidence and observations indicating an early role for the pericardium. *Circulation* 1967;36:839.
71. Ziskind AA, et al. Percutaneous balloon pericardiotomy for the treatment of cardiac tamponade and large pericardial effusions: description of technique and report of the first 50 cases. *J Am Coll Cardiol* 1993;21:1.
72. Celermajer DS, et al. Pericardiocentesis for symptomatic malignant pericardial effusion. *Med J Aust* 1991;154:19–22.
73. Markiewicz W. Cardiac Tamponade in medical patients. *Am Heart J* 1986;111:1138–1142.
74. Vaitkus PT, Herrmann HC, LeWinter MM. Treatment of malignant pericardial effusion. *JAMA* 1994;272:59–64.
75. Chow WH, et al. Inoue balloon pericardiotomy for patients with recurrent pericardial effusion. *Angiology* 1996;47:57.
76. Bertrand O, Legrand V, Kulburtus H. Percutaneous balloon pericardiotomy: a case report and analysis of mechanism of action. *Cathet Cardiovasc Diagn* 1996;38:180.
77. Sugimoto JT, et al. Pericardial window: mechanisms of efficacy. *Ann Thor Surg* 1990;50:442–445.
78. Ziskind AA, et al. Final report of the percutaneous balloon pericardiotomy registry for the treatment for effusive pericardial disease. *Circulation* 1994;90(suppl I):I-21.
79. Allen KB, et al. Pericardial effusion: subxiphoid pericardiotomy versus percutaneous catheter drainage. *Ann Thorac Surg* 1999;67:437.
80. Horkay F, et al. Presence of immunoreactive endothelin-1 and atrial natriuretic peptide in human pericardial fluid. *Life Sci* 1998;62:267.
81. Fujita M, et al. Elevated basic fibroblast growth factor in pericardial fluid of patients with unstable angina. *Circulation* 1996; 94:610
82. Laham RJ, et al. Intrapericardial delivery of fibroblast growth factor-2 induces neovascularization in a porcine model of chronic myocardial ischemia. *J Pharmacol Exp Ther* 2000;292:795–802.
83. Laham RJ, et al. Intrapericardial administration of basic fibroblast growth factor: myocardial and tissue distribution and comparison with intracoronary and intravenous administration. *Cathet Cardiovasc Intervent* 2003;58:375–381.
84. Uchida Y, et al. Angiogenic therapy of acute myocardial infarction by intrapericardial injection of basic fibroblast growth factor and heparan sulfate: an experimental study. *Am Heart J* 1995;130:1182–1188.
85. Landau C, et al. Intrapericardial basic fibroblast growth factor induces myocardial angiogenesis in a rabbit model of chronic ischemia. *Am Heart J* 1995;129:924–931.
86. Verrier RL, et al. Transatrial access to the normal pericardial space: a novel approach for diagnostic sampling, pericardiocentesis, and therapeutic interventions. *Circulation* 1998;98:2331–2333.
87. Waxman S, et al. Preclinical safety testing of percutaneous transatrial access to the normal pericardial space for local cardiac drug delivery and diagnostic sampling. *Cathet Cardiovasc Intervent* 2000;49:472–477.
88. Pulerwitz TC, et al. Transatrial access to the normal pericardial space for local cardiac therapy: preclinical safety testing with aspirin and pulmonary artery hypertension. *J Intervent Cardiol* 2001;14:493–498.
89. March KL, et al. Efficient in vivo catheter-based pericardial gene transfer mediated by adenoviral vectors. *Clin Cardiol* 1999; 22:I23–29.
90. Schweikert RA, et al. Percutaneous pericardial instrumentation for endo-epicardial mapping of previously failed ablations. *Circulation* 2003;108:1329–1335.
91. Sosa E, et al. Endocardial and epicardial ablation guided by nonsurgical transthoracic epicardial mapping to treat recurrent ventricular tachycardia. *J Cardiovasc Electrophysiol* 1998;9:229–239.
92. Maisch B, Ristic AD, Rupp H, Spodick DH. Pericardial access using the PerDUCER and flexible percutaneous pericardioscopy. *Am J Cardiol* 2001;88:1323–1326.
93. Seferovic PM, et al. Initial clinical experience with PerDUCER device: promising new tool in the diagnosis and treatment of pericardial disease. *Clin Cardiol* 1999;22:I30–35.
94. Ng AF, Olak J. Pericardial cyst causing right ventricular outflow tract obstruction. *Ann Thorac Surg* 1997;63:1147.
95. Peterson DR, Zatz LM, Popp RL. Pericardial cyst ten years after acute pericarditis. *Chest* 1975;67:719.
96. Nasser WK. Congenital absence of the left pericardium. *Am J Cardiol* 1970;26:466.
97. Gatzoulis MA, et al. Isolated congenital absence of the pericardium: clinical presentation, diagnosis, and management. *Ann Thoracic Surg* 2000;69:1209–1215.
98. Marani SD, et al. Congenital absence of the left pericardium: nuclear magnetic and other imaging techniques. *Am J Noninvasive Cardiol* 1992;6:304–312.
99. Gassner I, Judmaier W, Fink C. Diagnosis of congenital pericardial defects, including a pathognomic sign for dangerous apical ventricular herniation on magnetic resonance imaging. *Br Heart J* 1995;74:60–66.
100. Minocha GK, Falicov RE, Nijensohn E. Partial right-sided congenital pericardial defect with herniation of right atrium and right ventricle. *Chest* 1979;76:484.

Profiles in Congenital Heart Disease

33

Michael J. Landzberg   Robert J. Sommer

Congenital heart disease has grown more common in the adult catheterization laboratory due to increasing survival of patients with lesions surgically corrected in childhood and to the increasing availability of catheter-based treatments for lesions that do not present until adulthood. Some basic issues regarding catheterization in patients with congenital heart disease have been reviewed in Chapter 6, and some of the interventional techniques have been reviewed in Chapter 27. This Profiles chapter presents a series of real-world cases illustrating some of these principles.

ADULT WITH PULMONIC STENOSIS

Case 1: A 72-year-old woman presented with a loud murmur since birth and several years of progressive shortness of breath. Pulse oximetry showed an arterial oxygen saturation of 90 to 91% at baseline, falling into the mid-80s during a stress test. A transthoracic echo demonstrated valvar pulmonary stenosis with a peak instantaneous gradient of approximately 115 mm Hg. A bubble contrast injection was positive for a right-to-left shunt at the atrial level, consistent with a diagnosis of patent foramen ovale (PFO).

In the cath lab under intravenous sedation, an 8 French sheath was placed in the femoral vein, and a 5 French sheath was placed in the femoral artery. A multipurpose catheter was advanced from the femoral vein to obtain right-sided pressures and saturations and to cross the PFO to obtain left-sided data. Oxygen saturation in the pulmonary veins was 96% (room air) with a simultaneous aortic saturation of 89%, defining a right-to-left shunt. Right atrial (RA) and left atrial (LA) filling pressures were elevated with the mean right atrial pressure 2 to 3 mm Hg higher than the left. (RA mean, 15 mm Hg; LA mean, 12 mm Hg).

There was severe right ventricular (RV) hypertension, consistent with the echocardiographic gradient (RV pressure, 130/15), with mildly elevated pulmonary artery (PA) pressure (Fig. 33.1). There were no additional obstructions at the branch PAs. There was no mitral stenosis and no obstruction of the left ventricular outflow or aortic arch. Coronary angiography showed no obstructive disease.

A Berman catheter was placed in the right ventricle and a right ventricular angiogram was performed. The ventricle was severely hypertrophied with preserved systolic function. The pulmonary valve was thin and doming, with a jet of contrast seen through the small orifice of the doming valve (Fig. 33.2). There was post-stenotic dilatation of the main pulmonary artery (MPA) and the left pulmonary artery (LPA), with the right pulmonary artery (RPA) dilated to a lesser extent. This is typical as the high-velocity flow is directed into the LPA (Fig. 33.3). During systole, there was dynamic subvalvar muscular (infundibular) narrowing of the outflow tract.

We elected to dilate the pulmonic valve with an Inoue balloon technique (see Chapters 25 and 28). An Inoue balloon was selected with a maximum inflation diameter a few millimeters larger than the measured valve annulus, but was prepared with only enough volume to expand to the size of the annulus. A stiff exchange-length 0.032-inch guidewire was advanced through a multipurpose catheter into the distal LPA. The Inoue was straightened and introduced through a 14 French sheath at the femoral vein. The balloon was advanced over the wire to the right atrium, where the straightening rod was removed to ease passage through the two valves. (In some cases, manipulation through the tricuspid valve and the RV outflow tract can be facilitated by partial inflation of the balloon.) Once in the MPA, the distal portion of the balloon was inflated and pulled back against

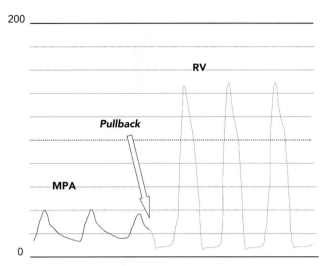

Figure 33.1 Pullback across the stenotic pulmonary valve. Systolic pressure increases simultaneously with change in diastolic pressure tracing, indicating a gradient at the valve. The peak-to-peak gradient was >100 mm Hg. MPA, main pulmonary artery; RV, right ventricle.

the valve tissue. The proximal portion and middle waist were inflated. There was a pop as the indentation of the valve on the balloon was eliminated. The stiff guidewire provided with the Inoue was advanced through the balloon to the LPA. A side-arm valve was added to the back of the catheter, and a pressure transducer was attached to the side port of the valve. The balloon was then withdrawn, over the wire, back into the RV to assess the residual gradient. (Had the valve not been opened adequately, additional volume

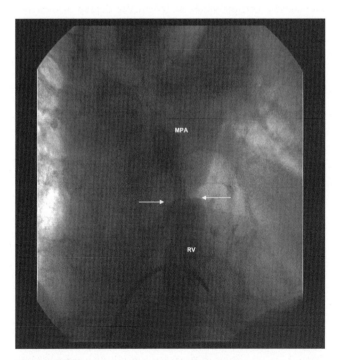

Figure 33.2 Doming pulmonary valve leaflets in early systole and the jet of contrast emerging into the MPA from the stenotic valve orifice. MPA, main pulmonary artery; RV, right ventricle.

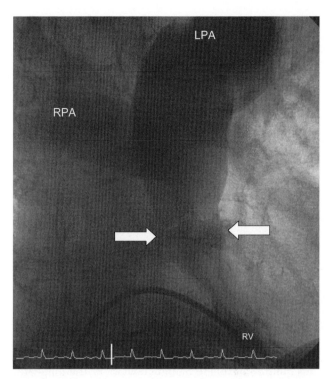

Figure 33.3 Right ventricular angiogram demonstrating the dilated PA branches and the subvalvar narrowing of the outflow tract. *White arrows* indicate the level of the valve annulus. RPA, right pulmonary artery; LPA, left pulmonary artery; RV, right ventricle.

could have been added to the balloon to perform another inflation at a larger balloon diameter.)

On pullback, an increase in the gradient across the RV outflow tract was noted. However, closer inspection of the pullback tracing revealed that the gradient had shifted from the level of the valve to the subvalvar (infundibular) area (Fig. 33.4). On pullback 1, from the MPA into the RV,

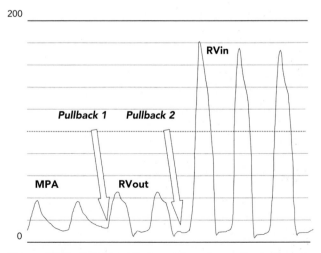

Figure 33.4 Following dilation of the valve, pullbacks from the main pulmonary artery (MPA) to right ventricular (RV) outflow tract show little residual systolic gradient and a large degree of intra-ventricular obstruction.

the diastolic tracing confirmed that the catheter was in a ventricular chamber, with virtually no systolic gradient across the valve. Pullback 2, identified that the systolic gradient was located within the ventricular chamber, at the subvalvar level.

Arterial saturations fell acutely into the mid-80s following valvuloplasty. A repeat angiogram revealed markedly improved mobility of the valve leaflets with a larger valve orifice (Fig. 33.5). However, there was profound dynamic obstruction at the level of the valve (Fig. 33.6). The patient was hydrated intravenously and started on an intravenous beta-blocker infusion. Over 10 to 15 minutes, oxygen saturations rose to the mid-90s, as the gradient fell to 50 to 55 mm Hg. Over the subsequent 6 weeks, the peak instantaneous gradient by Doppler decreased to <20 mm Hg, arterial saturations normalized, and oral beta-blocker therapy was discontinued.

Discussion. Valvar pulmonary stenosis (PS) is far less common in the adult population than in children and young adults, but when left untreated into adulthood, it can cause significant symptoms. Unlike valvar aortic stenosis, the pulmonary valves do not generally calcify and are thus quite amenable to balloon dilatation. The long-term follow-up of repaired valvar PS, by surgical or balloon valvuloplasty, demonstrates that in most cases it is a highly successful, if not curative, procedure (1). Late valvar insufficiency may also cause symptoms of shortness of breath on exertion, but is more frequently a product of surgical intervention (2).

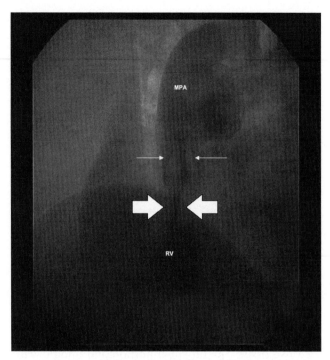

Figure 33.6 Following dilation of the valve, there is severe sub-valvar dynamic outflow obstruction *(thick arrows)*. The *thin arrows* denote the level of the valve leaflets. MPA, main pulmonary artery; RV, right ventricle.

Severe infundibular stenosis after valvuloplasty, which has been termed the "suicide" right ventricle (3) in surgical series, is physiologically identical to subaortic obstruction with asymmetric septal hypertrophy: Hypovolemia and increased inotropic states augment the degree of obstruction, which is typically a product of long-standing PS with RV hypertrophy. The cyanosis in this patient occurred as a result of right-to-left shunt across the patent foramen ovale, driven by long-standing RV hypertrophy and reduced RV diastolic compliance sufficient to elevate RA pressures and open the PFO flap.

In children, in whom most PS repairs are performed, standard valvuloplasty balloons are very effective, and also inexpensive. In adults and in teenagers, the size of the valve annulus is such that a double-balloon technique is often required to obtain enough dilating force and diameter. The Inoue balloon can be selected to larger diameters and is variable in its inflation size, so that a larger inflation size can be used without needing to change catheters (4).

Balloon valvuloplasty is a highly effective and extremely safe catheter intervention. It should be considered the procedure of choice for valvar PS.

COARCTATION OF THE AORTA

Case 2: A 32-year-old man presented with poorly controlled hypertension and bilateral lower extremity claudication. He had been using long-term beta-blocker and ACE

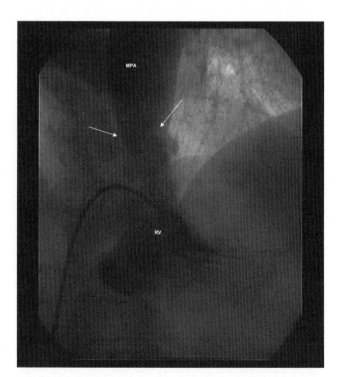

Figure 33.5 Marked improvement in valvar excursion after balloon dilation (compare with Fig. 33.2). *White arrows* denote tips of valve leaflets. MPA, main pulmonary artery; RV, right ventricle.

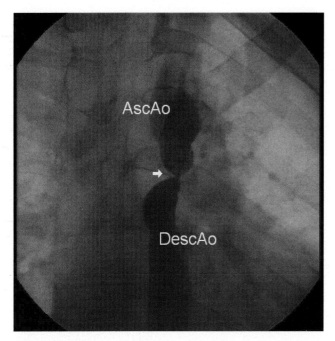

Figure 33.7 Discrete, severe coarctation of the aorta *(white arrow)*. AscAo, ascending aorta; DescAo, descending aorta.

inhibition therapy, with continued poor blood pressure control and slightly impaired renal function. Blood pressure in the right arm was 165/90, with no palpable femoral pulses and a blood pressure of 75/40 in the lower extremities. There was an apical click, a soft systolic murmur, and a diastolic decrescendo murmur. MRI revealed a discrete coarctation of the aorta approximately 2 cm distal to the left subclavian artery.

Under intravenous propofol sedation, sheaths were placed in the femoral artery and vein. Right-sided hemodynamics were obtained, but a pigtail catheter advanced from the femoral artery and would not pass around the aortic arch. A floppy-tipped wire was then manipulated through a multipurpose catheter around the aortic arch, after which the pigtail catheter was readvanced over the wire and an ascending angiogram was performed (Fig. 33.7). With a proximal aortic isthmus diameter of 18 mm and a distal

descending aortic measurement of approximately 21 mm, the minimum dimension at the coarctation site was approximately 2.5 mm. The angiogram also demonstrated filling of the descending aorta from intercostal and internal mammary collaterals.

A stiff wire with a hand-formed loop was advanced through the pigtail catheter around the arch to the ascending aorta, and a pigtail catheter was removed. A 10 French Mullins sheath was advanced over the wire to the descending aorta. Simultaneous pressure tracings were obtained from the pigtail catheter in the ascending aorta and the sheath in the descending aorta (Fig. 33.8). The pigtail catheter was removed, and the long sheath was advanced through the coarctation to the ascending aorta. A balloon-dilatable Palmaz iliac stent (Johnson & Johnson) was mounted on a 10-mm balloon catheter and advanced through the sheath to the level of the coarctation site. The sheath was withdrawn into the descending aorta, and an angiographic injection was performed through the side port of the Mullins sheath to position the stent. The balloon was inflated rapidly, expanding the stent to 10 mm (Figs. 33.9, 33.10).

The pigtail catheter was replaced, and repeat simultaneous pressures were measured (Fig. 33.11). There was a small residual gradient through the stent, but the ascending aortic pressure was markedly reduced, with increase in descending aortic pressure to a normal range. Because of the initial small diameter of the coarctation segment, we elected to do full dilation in two stages. The sheaths were removed, and hemostasis was obtained. Six months later, the patient returned with a small persistent gradient, though with improved blood pressure (BP) control and elimination of the symptoms in his lower extremities. From a femoral access, 15- and then 18-mm balloons (Figs. 33.12, 33.13) were used sequentially to redilate the stent to equal the size of the proximal aorta, abolishing the residual pressure gradient.

Discussion. De novo diagnosis of coarctation in the adult population is uncommon, but patients who have had previous aortic coarctation surgery may have residual obstruction at surgical sites. Any patient with hypertension should have examination of the lower extremity pulses,

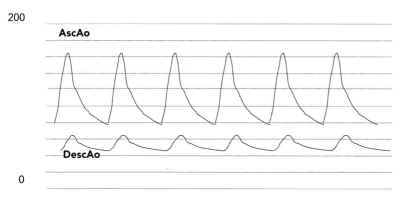

Figure 33.8 Simultaneous pressure tracings from ascending aorta (AscAo) and descending aorta (DescAo), pre–stent implant.

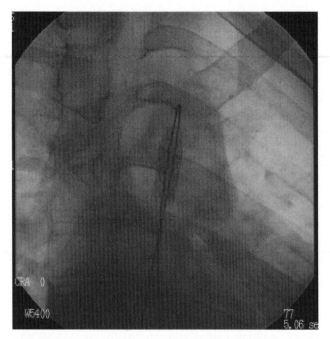

Figure 33.9   Initial inflation of balloon-mounted stent at site of coarctation.

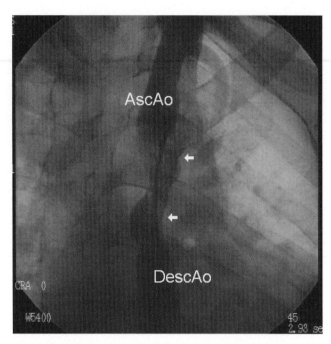

Figure 33.10   Repeat angiogram after initial stent inflation. AscAo, ascending aorta; DescAo, descending aorta.

and four extremity pressures should be checked to rule out this disease. In children who have not reached full adult size, surgery is often the preferred therapy for native coarctation, although there are a number of centers performing primary balloon angioplasty. For recurrent coarctation after surgical repair in children, however, balloon angioplasty is accepted as the procedure of choice, when feasible. Stenting is generally not used in children given the need for ongoing growth, but has become widely accepted in adults with coarctation (5,6). Stenting appears to provide more control in dilating the coarcted segment and eliminates the need for oversizing of the balloon with attendant risks of aortic rupture, tear, or dissection.

In this case, owing to the small size of the native vessel, we elected to perform the dilation in a staged approach. We limited the initial stent size to four to five times the initial diameter of the coarctation lesion, and then brought

the patient back at 6 months (with presumptive healing of the stent site) for full expansion.

Stent placement is also possible in more proximal lesions, such as coarctations that involve the transverse arch and isthmus, and may impinge on the left subclavian or even the carotid vessels. Lesions in each of these locations have been successfully treated with stent angioplasty without adverse neurologic events or arm ischemia (7). A multicenter registry of balloon-assisted stent dilation of aortic coarctation is being collected to highlight experience, safety, and efficacy of this technique. Some interventionalists have endorsed the use of covered stents to reduce the risk of acute aortic injury, but these systems are currently more bulky, require larger sheaths, and more frequently lead to femoral arterial compromise, so they are best reserved for a salvage option in the event of vascular rupture or dissection.

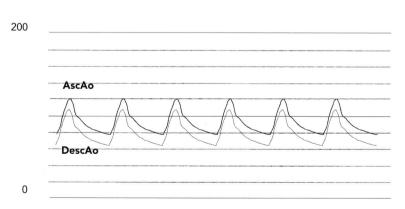

Figure 33.11   Simultaneous pressure tracings from ascending aorta (AscAo) and descending aorta (DescAo), post–initial stent implant.

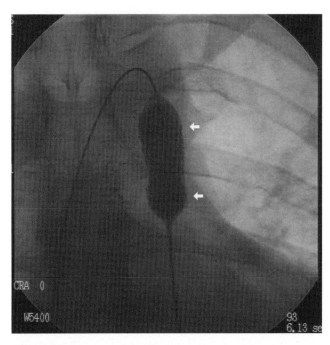

Figure 33.12 Subsequent inflation of stent at follow-up cath. *White arrowheads* mark extent of the stent.

ATRIAL SEPTAL DEFECT

Case 3: A 43-year-old woman with no past medical history presented with increasing shortness of breath on exertion. Oxygen saturation was normal by pulse oximetry. An echocardiogram revealed a dilated right atrium and right

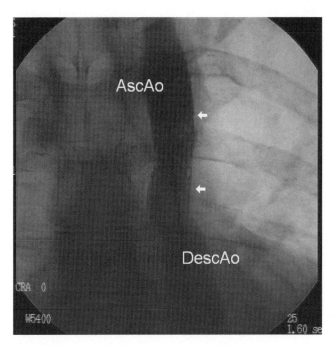

Figure 33.13 Angiographic assessment of aortic contour after final dilation. *White arrowheads* mark extent of the stent. AscAo, ascending aorta; DescAo, descending aorta.

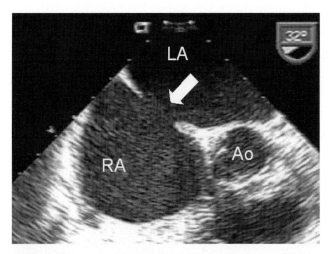

Figure 33.14 Transesophageal image of secundum atrial septal defect *(white arrow)*. RA, right atrium; LA, left atrium; Ao, aorta.

ventricle with a tricuspid regurgitation velocity of approximately 3.8 cm/second, and transesophageal echo revealed a 1.7-cm atrial septal defect with predominantly left-to-right shunting (Fig. 33.14).

The patient was taken to the cardiac catheterization lab, and two sheaths were placed in the right femoral vein under local anesthesia and conscious sedation. Through the first, an intracardiac echo (ICE) catheter (Acuson, Siemens), was passed to the right atrium for imaging the septum. Through the second sheath, a multipurpose catheter was used to perform hemodynamic measurements. There was only moderate pulmonary hypertension (PA pressure, 54/14 with simultaneous aortic pressure of 140/78). The calculated Qp/Qs ratio was 2.3:1 with an indexed pulmonary vascular resistance of 3.2 Units (see Chapter 9).

The multipurpose catheter was then used to cross the atrial septal defect and was manipulated to the left upper pulmonary vein. A stiff guidewire was passed to the pulmonary vein. A balloon sizing catheter was advanced over the wire to straddle the defect and was inflated until flow stopped by ICE (Fig. 33.15). At that point, the diameter of the waist on the balloon catheter was 19 mm. Circumferential septal rims were adequate (as assessed by echo), and a 20-mm Amplatzer Septal Occluder (AGA Medical, Minneapolis, MN) was selected (Fig. 33.16). The balloon catheter was removed, and a 9 French Mullins sheath was advanced over the wire and into the left atrium. The Amplatzer device was collapsed and advanced through the delivery sheath until the left atrial side opened in the left atrium and was pulled back toward the septum (Fig. 33.17). When the left atrial occluder was adjacent to the septum, the middle waist and right atrial side were opened, and the device allowed to return to its native shape. In this case, because of the deficient retroaortic rim, the device appears splayed out somewhat over the aortic root (Fig. 33.18), but is in good position with no residual shunt. The

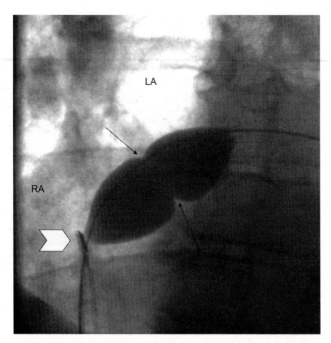

Figure 33.15 Fluoroscopic image of balloon sizing of atrial septal defect (ASD). Device size selection is based on the stretched diameter of the defect (between the *thin black arrows*). The white arrowhead indicates the ICE imaging catheter. RA, right atrium; LA, left atrium.

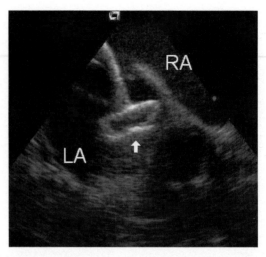

Figure 33.17 Intracardiac echo images of delivery of Amplatzer device, left atrial (LA) occluder opened *(white arrow)* and being pulled back toward the septum. RA, right atrium.

device was released without difficulty, sheaths were removed, and the patient was discharged 4 hours later.

Discussion. Transcatheter closure of atrial septal defects (ASDs) has become well accepted, with reasonable demonstrated safety and efficacy. A small potential for thrombus formation and device erosion of the atrial wall exist and

will require further study (8,9). There are some anatomic variants of ASD that remain unsuitable for the currently available devices. There is also substantial controversy surrounding patient selection for ASD. Most natural history studies of atrial septal defects preceded the modern echo era and generally included patients who were symptomatic and had larger defects. With the routine use of transesophageal echo, smaller defects are more likely to be identified in asymptomatic patients. It is not known whether the presence of such smaller ASDs actually affects survival or is associated with any additional morbidity.

Standard of care supports closure of an ASD in any age patient with dilated right-sided cardiac chambers and a significant left-to-right shunt. When the ASD is small, and the RV is not dilated, no intervention is typically warranted (except in the patient who is at risk for, or has suffered, paradoxical embolization). There are also issues regarding

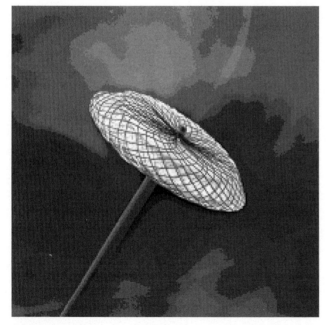

Figure 33.16 Amplatzer Septal Occluder (AGA Medical, Minneapolis, MN).

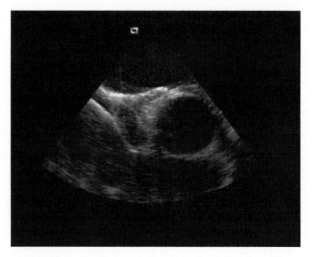

Figure 33.18 Intracardiac echo images of Amplatzer device in its final position. Anterior edges of device are splayed out over the aortic root.

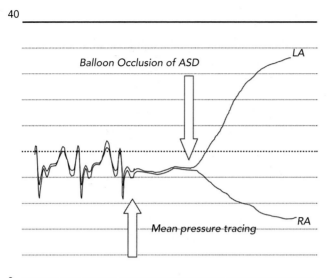

Figure 33.19 Simultaneous right atrial (RA) and left atrial (LA) tracings. Temporary balloon occlusion of an atrial septal defect (ASD) in a patient with left ventricular dysfunction and a large left–to-right shunt. Mean LA pressure rises sharply, with elimination of the LA pop-off, suggesting that the LV is too sick to tolerate closure of ASD.

patients with severe pulmonary hypertension related to a larger ASD (10), as well as in the primary pulmonary hypertension population (11), where the presence of an atrial level shunt may actually improve survival when indexed pulmonary vascular resistance exceeds 14 Units. Most of these patients have some degree of right-to-left shunting at the atrial level with associated cyanosis, owing to RV dysfunction, and closing the atrial septal defect eliminates the pop-off route for the right heart. By forcing all systemic venous return through the RV and into the high-resistance pulmonary arteriolar bed, the RV may fail in more rapid fashion than if the ASD had been left alone. In the patient discussed above, RV systolic pressures were less than one-half of systemic levels in the setting of a large left-to-right shunt, making the patient suited for closure despite elevation of PA pressure.

Rarely, an ASD with left-to-right shunting will be newly discovered in a patient with left ventricular (LV) myocardial dysfunction presenting with progressive congestive heart failure. It can be difficult to determine, noninvasively, whether the LV myocardial disease or the left-to-right shunt is responsible for the patient's symptoms. Similar to the patient with pulmonary hypertension, the ASD in this case allows a pop-off for the left atrium and sharing of diastolic properties between right and left hearts. (In the setting of a right ventricular infarction, however, right-to-left shunting may take place, with resulting systemic arterial desaturation.) In such a patient, we may test occlude the ASD with the balloon sizing catheter (with a second catheter through the defect into the LA). If the LA pressure remains in a relatively physiologic range (mean <25 mm Hg), and there are no symptoms of pulmonary edema, the defect can be closed.

Typically such patients appear to return to baseline LA pressures within a few days after closure. If mean LA pressure rises acutely with balloon occlusion >30 to 35 mm Hg, however, pulmonary venous congestion, acute pulmonary edema, and systemic desaturation may occur, indicating that the LV may be too compromised in its current state to allow ASD closure (Fig. 33.19).

After transcatheter ASD closure, all previously symptomatic patients tend to notice improvement in exercise tolerance. Objective measures of exercise capacity have corroborated these clinical observations, though in uncontrolled fashion (12,13). Transcatheter closure of atrial septal defects is now an established therapy within the mainstream of interventional cardiology for congenital heart disease and is an excellent alternative to open heart surgery in most affected persons.

POST–MYOCARDIAL INFARCTION VENTRICULAR SEPTAL RUPTURE SHUNT REDUCTION

Case 4: A 72-year-old man, s/p prior coronary artery bypass grafting, with diabetes, a single kidney with renal failure, hypertension, and hypercholesterolemia presented 72 hours after first onset of chest pain, with pulmonary edema and cardiogenic shock, requiring mechanical ventilatory and circulatory support. A harsh systolic murmur prompted echocardiography, which noted mildly reduced global LV systolic function, with a posteroinferior ventricular septal rupture.

Catheterization allowed implantation of intra-aortic balloon counterpulsation. Oximetric measure revealed superior vena cava (SVC) saturation of 57%, PA saturation 88%, aortic saturation 98%, and Qp/Qs greater than 3, with systemic cardiac index <1.5 L/minute per m². Coronary angiography and assessment of coronary grafts revealed only a mid obtuse marginal branch subtotal occlusion, which, after joint discussion between the medical and surgical teams, was revascularized with stent implantation. Given his medical comorbidities, the decision was made to pursue a percutaneous approach to ventricular septal rupture closure.

After trans-septal puncture from a right femoral venous approach, a balloon end-hole catheter was passed from LA to LV and guided through the ventricular septal rupture to the RV and PA, where a 280-cm guidewire was inserted to maintain this position. The guidewire was snared via a catheter placed from the ipsilateral femoral vein and retrieved out through the second sheath, to create an "arteriovenous" guidewire loop through the ruptured septum (Fig. 33.20).

Localized angiography within the ruptured segment was performed using a side-hole angiographic catheter advanced over the guidewire (Fig. 33.21). The ruptured segment was estimated to have a minimal diameter of 25 mm, and a 38-mm CardioSEAL occlusion device (NMT Medical,

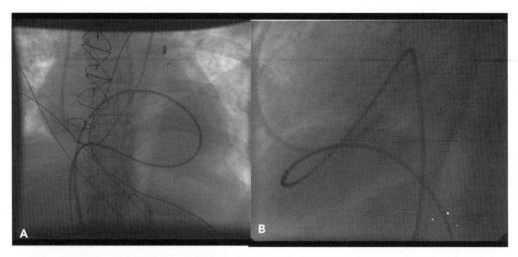

Figure 33.20 Arteriovenous guidewire loop, imaged in orthogonal views (**A** and **B**) allows passage of catheters to and within the ventricular septal ruptured area to facilitate anatomic delineation and potential implantation of closure device.

Boston, MA) was chosen for implantation via a 12 French delivery system. A long sheath was placed from a venous approach, in this case using the trans-septal access from RA to LA to LV to RV, to allow passage of the device-delivery system to the sheath tip and subsequent complete expansion of the distal device arms within the RV. With traction on the expanded RV occluder, the device conformed to the septal and apical surfaces within the RV (Fig. 33.22). (The other approach that has been used in posterior-inferior ventricular septal defect (VSD) closure is retrograde place-

ment of a balloon flotation catheter in the LV, passage across the VSD, with sharing of the guidewire from an internal jugular puncture.) The device was centered within the ruptured segment, and proximal arms were allowed to expand on the LV side of the rupture (Fig. 33.23). Appropriate positioning was confirmed via fluoroscopy; the device was released and demonstrated stable positioning, with reduction of shunt flow (Fig. 33.24).

Oximetry performed immediately postimplantation revealed SVC saturation 68%, PA saturation 78%, aortic

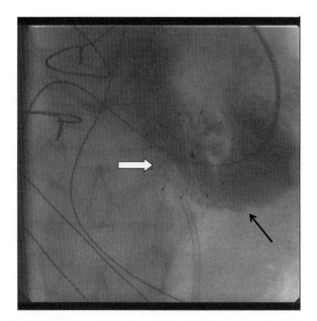

Figure 33.21 Localized angiography of the ruptured septum allows delineation of the defect (*black arrow*), as well as proximity of the ventricular surfaces and adjacent structures. A 38-mm CardioSEAL occlusion device is noted on the patient's chest surface (*white arrow*) to serve as a sizing reference.

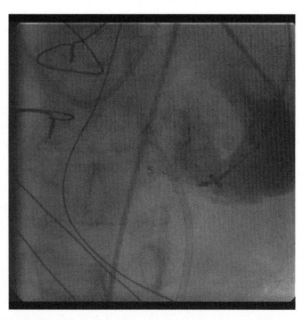

Figure 33.22 Deployment of CardioSEAL distal device arms, fully expanded and conforming with septal and apical right ventricular surfaces, within the ruptured segment.

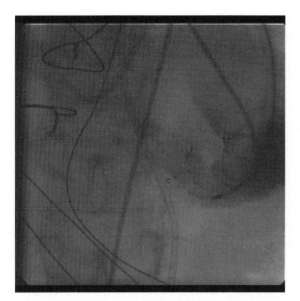

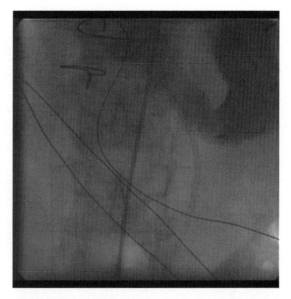

Figure 33.23 Deployment of CardioSEAL proximal device arms, fully expanded and conforming with septal and apical right ventricular surfaces, within the ruptured segment.

Figure 33.24 CardioSEAL occlusion device implantation within 25 mm posteroinferior to ventricular septal rupture, demonstrating persistence of shunt flow though markedly reduced in size.

saturation 98%, Qp/Qs 1.5, with improved systemic cardiac index. Intra-aortic balloon counterpulsation was continued for 36 hours and subsequently discontinued, as was mechanical ventilation. The patient returned home on posthospitalization day 7 and remained in functional class II symptoms 1 year after presentation. Minimal shunting is still visualized by echocardiography, with mildly reduced global LV systolic function.

Discussion. Despite advances in the management of acute coronary syndromes, rupture of the interventricular septum remains one of the most threatening mechanical complications of myocardial infarction (14). Surgical strategies emphasizing total exclusion of infarcted regions of the ventricular septum and closure of the defect carry very high risk. Based on the experience with percutaneous closure of congenital VSDs in the late 1980s to early 1990s (15), it was suggested that (1) use of left ventricular approach be used to intubate the defect (to ensure positioning through the widest aspect of the passage), (2) use of femoral venous entry for trans-septal access to the left ventricle (to decrease intraprocedural, catheter-induced, aortic regurgitation, and allowing for potential for either transvenous or transarterial device delivery, as appropriate by defect location), (3) local contrast injection angiography be used within the defect, and (4) maintenance of position be ensured with secure extra-long stiff wires (to best enable delivery system and device passage to, and within, the defect). Double-umbrella devices appear adequate to the closure of muscular VSDs given their ability to (1) have differing conformations (flattening against the interventricular septum, or remaining partially expanded, to provide for best defect occlusion), (2) be applied from either a RV or LV approach, to allow for safest and most secure device deployment, and (3) be retrieved or repositioned with relative ease and safety.

Closure of post–myocardial infarction ventricular septal ruptures offers additional challenges to those seen with congenital muscular VSD closure (16). The defects are typically complex tears through the necrotic septum, with poorly aligned entry and exit sites on LV and RV surfaces. Continuing necrosis and scar retraction lead to defect expansion over the first days to weeks. Our experience with transcatheter ventricular septal rupture closure with double-umbrella devices highlights technical feasibility in nearly all patients. However, device evolution, to allow larger device size and the ability to autoadjust to defect expansion over the first weeks after implantation, is necessary to permit potential for longer-term success in acutely ruptured segments. Increasing experience with this technique is expected to extend its application from limited centers and to allow more rigorous comparison of safety and efficacy to currently practiced surgical therapies.

PATENT DUCTUS ARTERIOSUS

Case 5: A 3-year-old asymptomatic child presented with a soft continuous murmur that was not previously appreciated. Transthoracic echo imaging with Doppler color flow mapping showed a patent ductus arteriosus (PDA), with a continuous high-velocity flow jet entering the MPA adjacent to the bifurcation of the branch PAs (Fig. 33.25).

The patient was taken to the cardiac catheterization laboratory, where femoral artery and femoral venous sheaths were placed under intravenous sedation. The patient had normal right-sided pressures. There was slight widening in the aortic pulse pressure (aorta, 90/45), consistent with the diastolic runoff of flow from the aorta into the pulmonary artery (with physiology similar to that seen in patients with

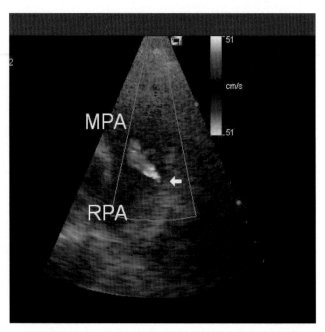

Figure 33.25 Jet of flow into pulmonary artery seen by flow mapping in a patient with a patent ductus arteriosus. *White arrow* denotes origin of flow. MPA, main pulmonary artery; RPA, right pulmonary artery.

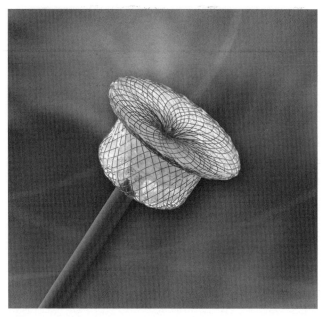

Figure 33.27 Amplatzer Duct Occluder. Wide aortic retention disk and slightly tapered body, which fits into and occludes the funnel of the patent ductus arteriosus (PDA).

aortic regurgitation.) The calculated Qp/Qs ratio was estimated at 2:1, though it is difficult to assess these flows accurately in the presence of a PDA (there is no location distal enough from the shunt source to obtain a true mixed sample). An aortic angiogram was taken in anteroposterior (AP) and lateral projections (Fig. 33.26). This revealed a

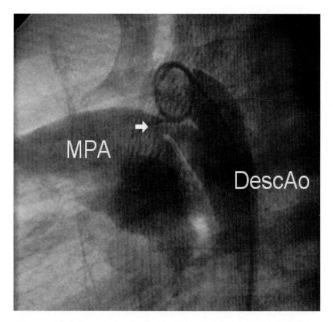

Figure 33.26 Aortic angiogram in the lateral projection (90° left anterior oblique [LAO]). The funnel of the patent ductus arteriosus (PDA) is well demonstrated, with its narrowest portion at the main pulmonary artery (MPA) insertion *(white arrow)*. DescAo, descending aorta.

type A PDA (17), with a wide aortic ampulla and a 3-mm minimum dimension at the MPA end of the funnel. Based on these images, we elected to use an Amplatzer Duct Occluder (AGA Medical, Minneapolis, MN; Fig. 33.27). The device size was chosen such that the PA end of the device exceeded the MPA dimension of the PDA by 2 to 3 mm.

A multipurpose catheter was manipulated to the MPA from the femoral vein, and a floppy-tipped torque wire (0.035 inch) was advanced through the PDA into the descending aorta. A delivery sheath was advanced from the femoral vein over the wire into the descending aorta. The device was loaded into the sheath and was advanced out the end of the sheath, opening only the retention disk in the aorta. The sheath was then withdrawn until the disk lodged firmly against the aortic ampulla of the PDA (Fig. 33.28). As traction was maintained against the aortic ampulla, the delivery sheath was slowly withdrawn, which allowed the body of the device to open within the funnel of the PDA (Fig. 33.29). As is quite common in patients with larger PDAs, there was a small residual shunt, through the mesh of the device, immediately after implantation. Within 10 to 15 minutes, all flow had stopped and the PDA was completely closed (Fig. 33.30). The patient was discharged home 5 hours later.

Discussion. Patent ductus arteriosus can be discovered at any age, and may present with significant congestive heart failure in infants (especially premature infants), in whom surgical intervention is generally preferable. In older children with small ductus (<2 mm in diameter), coil embolization remains the preferable closure device (18). For PDAs >2.0 mm, the Amplatzer Duct Occluder is being used with increasing frequency (19).

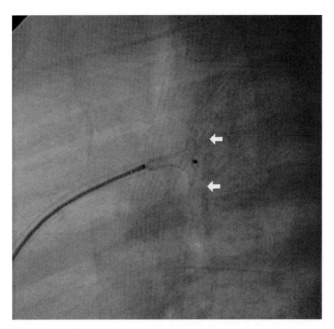

Figure 33.28 Retention disk opened in descending aorta and pulled back against mouth of the patent ductus arteriosus (PDA). The remainder of the device is still collapsed inside the delivery sheath. *White arrows* denote the edges of the retention disk.

Although older children very rarely present with symptoms, adults with previously undiagnosed PDA may manifest symptoms as they age, and diastolic runoff into the pulmonary artery reduces aortic diastolic pressure and coronary perfusion (20). Therefore, patients with nonobstructive coronary artery disease may have angina in the presence of even a small PDA. Alternatively, patients who have had small shunts for many decades may become symptomatic as the left ventricular compliance changes as

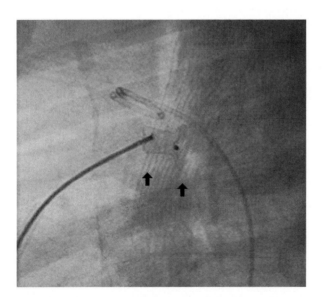

Figure 33.29 The Amplatzer device fully deployed, prior to release. The *black arrows* indicate the fully expanded length of the device within the patent ductus arteriosus (PDA).

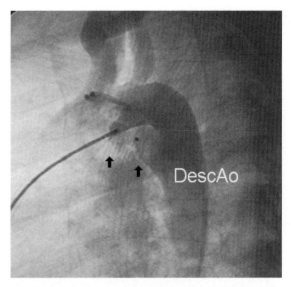

Figure 33.30 Amplatzer Duct Occluder well positioned within the funnel of the patent ductus arteriosus (PDA) as marked by the *black arrows*. DescAo, descending aorta.

part of the normal aging process. With the onset of systemic hypertension, PDA flow may increase and the left ventricular volume load may cause high-output failure. The result is exercise intolerance, similar to a patient with aortic or mitral valve regurgitation. Infective endocarditis remains a risk throughout life if the PDA is not closed and is the principal touted reason for closing a PDA in children. In older adults without clinical symptoms who also have valvar regurgitation or other cardiac lesions that require antibiotic prophylaxis, the benefit of closing a small PDA is less clear.

CORONARY ARTERIOVENOUS FISTULA

Case 6: A 47-year-old premenopausal woman without atherosclerotic risk factors presented with episodic mid-chest ache, atypical for angina. Since childhood, symptoms had occurred in a nonuniform fashion both at rest and with extreme exertion. A continuous cardiac murmur along the right sternal border had been noted since birth, but the patient had been active in high school and collegiate sports and had carried two uncomplicated pregnancies to term. A recent change in primary care provider had led to an evaluation with cardiac echo, which found increased right- and left-sided chamber dimensions, as well as an abnormal velocity jet in the right atrium, near the os of the coronary sinus, but excluded septal defect or patent ductus arteriosus. Nuclear exercise scintigraphy was remarkable for resting hypoperfusion in the anteroapical and inferior distributions of the left ventricle, without redistribution at rest.

Left and right heart catheterization was performed. There were normal intracardiac and arterial pressures, but

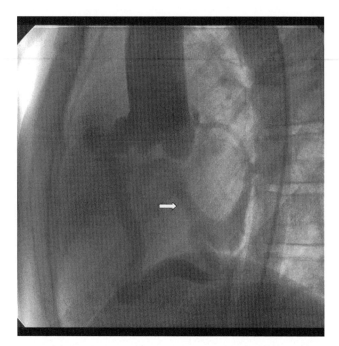

Figure 33.31 Nonselective aortography, noting right coronary artery arteriovenous fistula, emptying into the coronary sinus (*arrow*).

oximetry showed an SVC saturation of 75%, with a step-up to 85% in the RA, RV, and both PAs. The calculated Qp/Qs was 1.7. Selective left coronary angiography demonstrated a normal left coronary artery without obstruction. However, it was difficult to fully opacify the dominant right coronary system. Nonselective ascending aortography showed a markedly dilated right coronary

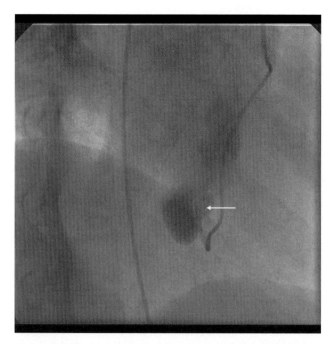

Figure 33.32 Angiography within the dilated right coronary arteriovenous fistula, noting a region of nonopacification near the os of the coronary sinus (*arrow*), suggesting a membranous obstruction.

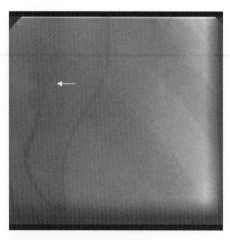

Figure 33.33 A steel occlusion coil has been extruded into the obstructed exit site of the arteriovenous fistula (*arrow*).

artery, with the presence of an arteriovenous fistula originating in the distal coronary and emptying into the coronary sinus (Fig. 33.31). The distal RCA vasculature was again not well seen (see Chapter 11). The right coronary artery was engaged with a guiding catheter, through which a 5 French thin-walled steerable catheter was advanced into the distal vessel over a soft-tipped steerable guidewire. Angiography of the distal coronary noted a region of relative stenosis of the fistula near the os of the coronary sinus (Fig. 33.32), with evidence of membranous obstruction at that site.

A steel vascular occlusion coil, chosen to be 1-mm greater than the size of the dilated arteriovenous fistula at the site of the presumed membranous obstruction, was extruded through the catheter positioned at the site, and angiography confirmed stable position (Fig. 33.33). Subsequent coronary angiography distally revealed closure of the defect with visualization of the small RCA vessels for the first time during the procedure (Fig. 33.34).

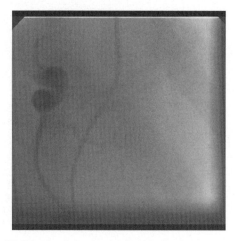

Figure 33.34 Opacification of the distal right coronary arterial branches are noted immediately on occlusion of the arteriovenous fistula.

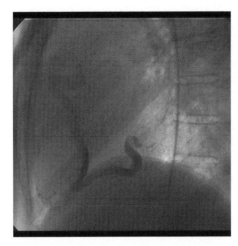

Figure 33.35 Selective proximal right coronary artery angiography. The arteriovenous fistula is occluded, with filling of the distal branches noted.

Proximal right coronary arterial injection confirmed occlusion of the arteriovenous fistula, with normal filling of the distal right coronary arterial branches (Fig. 33.35). No residual oximetric shunt was detectable. Postprocedure nuclear scintigraphy revealed normal rest and exercise perfusion, though occasional atypical chest pain continues to occur.

Discussion. Coronary arteriovenous fistulae may occur from either congenital or acquired causes, with passage of blood from the coronary arterial tree to any cardiac chamber, pulmonary artery, or systemic or pulmonary vein, competing with perfusion of the distal myocardial capillary tree (see Chapter 11). Though highly variable in structure, fistulae are typically thin-walled, dilated, and follow a serpiginous course. Most have a single drainage site in the right heart, though multiple exit sites may be seen. Left-to-right shunting occurs from the aortic level to the right heart, resulting in biventricular volume loading, although most smaller fistula do not produce measurable shunts (fistula flow of 100 to 200 mL/minute is large compared with coronary flow to the myocardium but small compared with the cardiac output of 4 to 5 liters).

Symptomatic patients typically complain of dyspnea and less often of myocardial ischemia, though the presence and nature of symptoms have not been correlated with size of shunt or fistula, nor drainage site. Symptoms of left atrial hypertension (dyspnea, development of atrial fibrillation) owing to high-volume shunting have been reported. Less symptomatic patients have long-term survival similar to unaffected individuals. Fistula repair may be indicated in the setting of documented ischemic or shunt-related symptoms, but surgical repair may be difficult owing to the typically distal and serpiginous nature of such fistulae (making exit sites difficult to identify and reach) in affected older patients.

Transcatheter approach to coronary arteriovenous fistula closure allows accurate definition of fistula origin, potential for temporary fistula occlusion (with a balloon end-hole catheter) to allow angiography of distal vasculature, and closure of the fistula via an endovascular approach with a variety of occlusion devices (21). The fate of the native, thin-walled proximal epicardial coronary artery (previously at high flow and now at lower flow owing to fistula occlusion) appears to be good, though long-term follow-up post–endovascular fistula occlusion has not been reported.

REFERENCES

1. Hayes CJ, Gersony WM, Driscoll DJ, et al. Second natural history study of congenital heart defects. Results of treatment of patients with pulmonary valvar stenosis. *Circulation* 1993;87 (suppl):I-28–37.
2. O'Connor BK, Beekman RH, Lindauer A, Rocchini A. Intermediate-term outcome after pulmonary balloon valvuloplasty: comparison with a matched surgical control group. *J Am Coll Cardiol* 1992;20:169–173.
3. Thapar MK, Rao PS. Significance of infundibular obstruction following balloon valvuloplasty for valvar pulmonic stenosis. *Am Heart J* 1989;118:99–103.
4. Chen CR, Cheng TO, Huang T, et al. Percutaneous balloon valvuloplasty for pulmonic stenosis in adolescents and adults. *N Engl J Med* 1996;335:21–25.
5. Suarez de Lezo J, Pan M, Romero M, et al. Balloon-expandable stent repair of severe coarctation of aorta. *Am Heart J* 1995;129: 1002–1008.
6. Bulbul ZR, Bruckheimer E, Love JC, Fahey JT, Hellenbrand WE. Implantation of balloon-expandable stents for coarctation of the aorta: implantation data and short-term results. *Cathet Cardiovasc Diagn* 1996;39:36–42.
7. Recto MR, Elbl F, Austin E. Use of the new IntraStent for treatment of transverse arch hypoplasia/coarctation of the aorta. *Cathet Cardiovasc Intervent* 2001;53:499–503.
8. Krumsdorf U, Ostermayer S, Billinger K, et al. Incidence and clinical course of thrombus formation on atrial septal defect and patient foramen ovale closure devices in 1,000 consecutive patients. *J Am Coll Cardiol* 2004;43:302–309.
9. FDA Website: http://www.accessdata.fda.gov/scripts/cdrh/cfdocs/ cfMAUDE/search.CFM (last accessed May 23, 2005).
10. Steele PM, Fuster V, Cohen M, Ritter DG, McGoon DC. Isolated atrial septal defect with pulmonary vascular obstructive disease—long-term follow-up and prediction of outcome after surgical correction. *Circulation* 1987;76:1037–1042.
11. Kerstein D, Levy PS, Hsu DT, Hordof AJ, Gersony WM, Barst RJ. Blade balloon atrial septostomy in patients with severe primary pulmonary hypertension. *Circulation* 1995;91:2028–2035.
12. Giardini A, Donti A, Specchia S, et al. Recovery kinetics of oxygen uptake is prolonged in adults with an atrial septal defect and improves after transcatheter closure. *Am Heart J* 2004;147: 910–914.
13. Giardini A, Donti A, Formigari R, et al. Determinants of cardiopulmonary functional improvement after transcatheter atrial septal defect closure in asymptomatic adults. *J Am Coll Cardiol* 2004;43:1886–1891.
14. Crenshaw BS, Granger CB, Birnbaum Y, et al. Risk factors, angiographic patterns, and outcomes in patients with ventricular septal defect complicating acute myocardial infarction. GUSTO-I Trial Investigators. *Circulation* 2000;101:27–32.
15. Bridges ND, Perry SB, Keane JF, et al. Preoperative transcatheter closure of congenital muscular ventricular septal defects. *N Engl J Med* 1991;324:1312–1317.
16. Landzberg MJ, Lock JE. Transcatheter management of ventricular septal rupture after myocardial infarction. *Semin Thorac Cardiovasc Surg* 1998;10:128–132.

18. Krichenko A, Benson LN, Burrows P, et al. Angiographic classification of the isolated, persistently patent ductus arteriosus and implications for percutaneous occlusion. *Am J Cardiol* 1989;63: 877–880.

19. Pass RH, Hijazi Z, Hsu DT, Lewis V, Hellenbrand WE. Multicenter USA Amplatzer patent ductus arteriosus occlusion device trial: initial and one-year results. *J Am Coll Cardiol* 2004;44:513–519.

20. Harada K, Toyono M, Tamura M. Effects of coil closure of patent ductus arteriosus on left anterior descending coronary artery blood flow using transthoracic Doppler echocardiography. *J Am Soc Echocardiogr* 2004;17:659–663.

21. Armsby L, Keane JF, Sherwood MC, et al. Management of coronary artery fistulae. Patient selection and results of transcatheter closure. *J Am Coll Cardiol* 2002;39:1029–1032.

Profiles in Aortic and Peripheral Vascular Disease

34

Stephen R. Ramee   *José A. Silva*   *Christopher J. White*

Over the past decade, an increasing number of interventional cardiologists have expanded their clinical practice beyond purely coronary procedures to also include peripheral vascular intervention. The peripheral diagnostic techniques have been reviewed in Chapter 14, and the basic interventional techniques have been reviewed in Chapter 26. This Profiles section gives actual case examples, following the same head-to-foot organization used in the previous peripheral vascular chapters.

AORTIC ARCH AND CAROTID ARTERY ANGIOPLASTY

Vertebral Artery Angioplasty

Revascularization of the vertebral arteries is indicated only for patients with symptoms of vertebrobasilar insufficiency, namely, dizziness, visual disturbances, and confusion or coma. However, there is little correlation between severity of stenosis affecting these vessels and the presence of symptoms (1). Some patients may experience few or no symptoms despite severe stenosis, whereas others may experience profound symptoms despite only moderate stenosis. This poor correlation stems from the fact that the posterior fossa receives blood supply from the contralateral vertebral artery and from the carotid artery system through the posterior communicating arteries. Consequently, assessment of a patient with significant stenosis of a vertebral artery should always involve evaluating the patency of the contralateral vertebral artery, the dominance of the diseased vertebral artery, and the amount of blood supplied to the vertebrobasilar system by the carotid arteries.

Depending on the location of the stenosis, treatment options to revascularize the vertebral arteries may include balloon angioplasty with or without stent placement (2–6), surgery with transplantation of the vertebral arteries onto the carotid artery, or bypass grafting from the subclavian to the vertebral artery (7). Lesions located in the ostium or the proximal portion of the vertebral artery can be approached percutaneously (2–6). As is the case for other aorto-ostial lesions (saphenous vein grafts, right coronary arteries, or renal arteries), stenting should be strongly considered to minimize elastic recoil. Lesions located more distally may be treated with balloon angioplasty with provisional stenting, depending on the angiographic results and the tortuosity of the vessel. Distal vertebral artery lesions are much more difficult to access and more prone to dissection. In particular, those at the vertebrobasilar junction and in the basilar artery itself have a higher complication rate and are the most prone to dissection, occlusion, perforation, and stroke (8–10).

In a prospective study from our institution (6), 16 patients and 20 lesions (18 ostial, 1 proximal, and 1 mid-vertebral) were treated with 22 stents for indications including: diplopia ($n = 1$), dizziness ($n = 10$), transient ischemic attack of the vertebrobasilar system ($n = 3$), and asymptomatic angiographic stenosis ($n = 2$). Angiographic success (<20% residual diameter stenosis and freedom from in-hospital death, stroke, or emergent surgery) was achieved in all patients, although one patient had a 5-minute transient ischemic attack 1 hour postprocedure with a patent stent. At a mean follow-up of 491 ± 387 days, all patients were alive, and 15 of 16 patients (94%) were free of recurrent symptoms. One patient developed symptomatic in-stent restenosis 6 months after the procedure, which was successfully treated with balloon angioplasty. *Endoluminal stenting thus can be performed safely and effectively, with a low complication rate and a durable clinical success, in selected patients, particularly those with atherosclerotic lesions of the vertebral arteries located in the ostium or the proximal portion of the vessel.*

Case 1. This patient is a 66-year-old man who presented with recurrent episodes of orthostatic dizziness associated with diplopia but not light-headedness over a 2-month period. He had known atherosclerotic disease including prior myocardial infarction, coronary artery bypass surgery, carotid stenting, and lower extremity percutaneous intervention. Physical examination revealed a right carotid bruit and a right supraclavicular bruit. The neurologic examination was normal, and color-flow Doppler examination of the carotid and vertebral vessels revealed no significant carotid stenosis. There were, however, high velocities noted at the origin of both vertebral arteries consistent with stenosis with antegrade flow. He was referred for aortic arch, cerebral, and vertebral angiography and possible intervention.

He was pretreated with clopidogrel and aspirin. Diagnostic angiography was performed using digital subtraction with a 4F Berenstein catheter and revealed 80%

stenosis of the right vertebral artery, a left vertebral artery that ended in the posterior inferior cerebellar artery, and noncritical carotid artery stenosis. Right vertebral artery intervention was performed in the following manner: The 4F Berenstein catheter was advanced into the right subclavian artery with an extra-stiff 0.035-inch hydrophilic wire, which was exchanged for a 0.035-inch extra-stiff exchange wire. Over the extra-stiff wire, a 6F short femoral sheath and a 6F JR4 coronary guiding catheter were advanced into the right subclavian artery. The right vertebral ostium was engaged and after baseline angiography (Fig. 34.1A), a 0.014-inch coronary guidewire was inserted into the vertebral artery and positioned at the base of the skull. The lesion was stented directly using a 4.0 mm × 12 mm balloon expandable coronary stent at 12 atmospheres (atm). Poststent angiography (Fig. 34.1B) revealed no residual stenosis or dissection. The patient had complete resolution of his symptoms at 1-year follow-up.

Illustrative Points. The vertebral arteries arise from the right and left subclavian artery just proximal to and opposite the internal mammary arteries. They converge to form the basilar artery, which supplies the brainstem (pons, medulla, and midbrain), cerebellum, and posterior cerebral arteries (supplying the visual cortex). They may also supply collaterals to the middle and anterior cerebral arteries via the posterior communicating arteries in patients with critical carotid artery stenosis. To have neurologically symptomatic ischemia, both vertebral arteries (or the basilar artery itself) must be involved, unless (as in this case) one artery ends before it reaches the basilar. A corollary is that

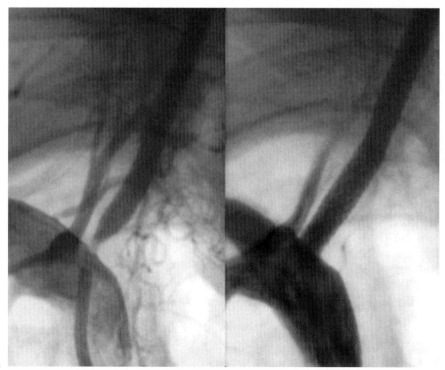

A   **B**

Figure 34.1   A. Selective injection of the right vertebral artery through a 6F guiding catheter demonstrating ostial stenosis. **B.** Poststenting, there is excellent filling of the vertebral artery and no residual ostial stenosis.

only one artery usually needs to be treated to relieve the vertebral ischemia.

Carotid Angioplasty

Most patients with internal carotid atherosclerotic are asymptomatic (11,12), but even asymptomatic patients with 75% or greater stenoses have a 2 to 5% risk of stroke during the first year. If there is concomitant plaque ulceration, the risk of stroke increases to 7.5% per year (13). Several large cooperative randomized trials have shown that surgical intervention with carotid endarterectomy (CEA) improves the natural history of this disease compared with aspirin therapy. The North American Symptomatic Carotid Endarterectomy Trial (NASCET) suggested that patients with *symptomatic* internal carotid artery (ICA) of 50% or greater will benefit from CEA (14). In this trial, the risk of ipsilateral stroke was 26% at 2 years (i.e., 13% per year) for patients with symptomatic stenoses of 70 to 99% treated medically, compared with a 9% risk of stroke in the surgical group during this 2-year period (i.e., 4.5% per year). This translates into a relative risk reduction of 65% for the surgically treated patients. The Asymptomatic Carotid Atherosclerosis Study (ACAS) found that patients with an *asymptomatic* stenosis of 60% or greater treated by endarterectomy had a 5.8% absolute risk reduction of fatal or nonfatal ipsilateral stroke (15) over 5 years. But the inclusion criteria for these trials were quite narrow, leading to exclusion of most of the patients screened. There are many patients with high-risk carotid lesions who do not meet the criteria established for enrollment in those studies and for whom the indications and risks of CEA are not established. Although the published mortality in the NASCET trial was thus 0.6%, the mortality of the universe of Medicare CEA patients was 3% during the same period (16).

Carotid stenting is now available as an alternative to both medical and surgical management. Several studies have been published in which stenting was carried out with a very acceptable degree of safety and with excellent acute and 6-month outcomes (17–24). Furthermore, a landmark trial (Stenting and Angioplasty with Protection in Patients at High Risk for Endarterectomy, SAPPHIRE) compared carotid stenting with distal protection favorably with endarterectomy in high-risk surgery patients (25). A total of 723 patients were enrolled in this trial, with 156 randomized to carotid stenting with distal protection, 151 randomized to endarterectomy, and 416 patients treated in a nonrandomized registry (409 stent, 7 surgery). The 30-day stroke/death/myocardial infarction (MI) rate for the randomized patients was significantly lower in the carotid stent group (5.8%) compared with the surgical group (12.6%, $P < .05$). In the nonrandomized registry patients, the 30-day stroke, death, or MI rate was 7.8% for stents and 14.7% for surgery, without the 5.3% rate of cranial nerve injury seen in the surgical group This trial provides strong support that stent placement with distal protection may

TABLE 34.1

PATIENTS AT HIGH RISK FOR ENDARTERECTOMY WHO ARE CANDIDATES FOR ANGIOPLASTY AND STENTING

1. Significant medical comorbidity
2. Recurrent stenosis after carotid endarterectomy
3. Contralateral carotid artery occlusion
4. Radiation-induced stenosis
5. Surgically difficult to access high-cervical stenosis
6. Aorto-ostial lesions
7. Tracheotomy

now be the procedure of choice in patients at increased risk for surgery (Table 34.1; 22–25).

Case 2. This 80-year-old woman presented with right hemispheric transient ischemic attacks (TIAs) manifest by left-sided weakness. Her history includes hyperlipidemia, three-vessel coronary artery disease, a permanent pacemaker, and prior coronary percutaneous intervention. At the time of evaluation, she had stable angina. Her physical examination was remarkable for a harsh right carotid bruit and a normal neurologic exam. Carotid duplex examination revealed 80 to 99% stenosis of the right internal carotid artery and 40 to 59% stenosis of the left internal carotid artery. Carotid angiography confirmed a 90% right internal carotid stenosis and 50% left internal carotid stenosis. Vertebral angiography was unremarkable, and she was referred for carotid angioplasty and stenting.

After pretreatment with aspirin and clopidogrel, and 5,000 units of intra-arterial heparin, carotid stenting was performed under a protocol for patients at high risk for carotid endarterectomy. A 5F Vitek catheter and an extra-stiff 0.035-inch Glidewire were used to engage the right external carotid artery. The Glidewire was exchanged for an extra-stiff Amplatz exchange wire, and the 6F shuttle sheath was inserted into the right common carotid artery over the wire in the external carotid artery. Angiography was performed using digital subtraction, with anteroposterior (AP) and lateral views of the common carotid bifurcation and the cerebral circulation. The right internal carotid artery had a 90% stenosis just after the common carotid bifurcation (Fig. 34.2A). The lesion was crossed with an Angio Guard distal embolic protection device (see Chapter 23), and the lesion was predilated with a 4.0 × 30 mm balloon. A 9.0 × 40 mm nitinol stent was then deployed across the carotid bifurcation. The stent was postdilated to 12 atm using a 5.0 mm × 2 cm coronary balloon, after which the distal protection device was retrieved and final angiography was performed. There was 30% residual stenosis at the angioplasty site (Fig. 34.2B). Postprocedure, the patient developed transient hypotension that responded to volume expansion, atropine, and α-agonists. She has remained asymptomatic at 1 year with no evidence of restenosis by carotid duplex examination.

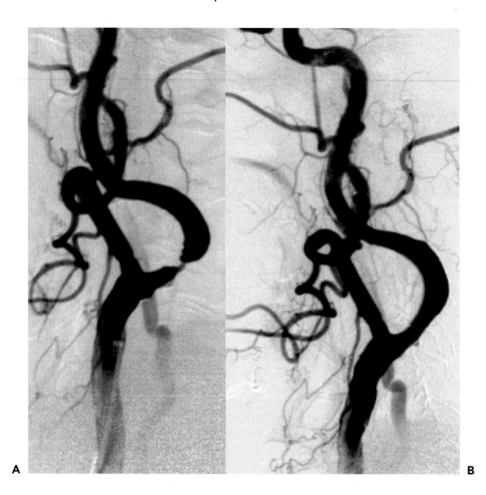

A   B

Figure 34.2   A. A lateral digital subtraction angiogram of the common carotid artery and its branches demonstrates minor plaquing in the common carotid just before the bifurcation and critical stenosis of the right internal carotid artery 1.0 cm beyond the bifurcation. **B.** After stenting, there is still 10–20% residual stenosis in the internal carotid artery. Aggressive dilating and trying to achieve a perfect result is not recommended because of the risk of distal embolization and stroke.

Illustrative Points. Treatment of both symptomatic and asymptomatic carotid artery is no longer experimental! More than seven pivotal trials (including one randomized controlled trial [RCT]) comparing CEA with carotid stenting (25) have been completed in the United States, with 30-day stroke and mortality rates in high-risk surgical patients rivaling the best results with endarterectomy. Patients are candidates for carotid stenting if they are high risk for carotid endarterectomy, including those with inaccessible carotid lesions (high internal carotid or aorto-ostial common carotid), contralateral carotid occlusion, prior ipsilateral endarterectomy, permanent tracheostomy, radiation fibrosis, or high medical comorbidity.

Self-expanding stents are preferred for the carotid bifurcation because of the risk of crushing balloon-expandable stents by external forces. There are two carotid stent systems (embolic protection plus self-expanding stent) currently approved by the FDA, with more expected over the next 12 to 18 months. They can be delivered through either a 6F sheath or an 8F guiding catheter. The nonkinking 6F sheaths have an outer diameter that is approximately the same as an 8F guiding catheter, so the size of the access site hole is similar in both. *Unlike coronary artery stenting, the goal after carotid stenting does not require obtaining a perfect angiographic result.* Because the main risk of this carotid

intervention is distal embolization given the large plaque burden, great care is taken to avoid manipulating the carotid artery any more than is necessary to achieve a smooth flow channel of reasonable diameter. Using this technique of underdilation of self-expanding stents gives a restenosis rate of <10% (20), and major complications are not seen from covering the ostium of the external carotid artery (although the status of the other vessels needs to be considered).

Hypotension post–carotid stenting may signify bleeding from the access site (see Chapter 3), but is commonly seen owing to stretching of the carotid sinus by the stent. This generally responds to volume expansion, although atropine and α-agonists are used when volume expansion alone is not sufficient.

Intracranial Angioplasty

Several studies have shown that intracranial disease can be viewed as a marker of extensive cerebrovascular and systemic atherosclerotic disease, particularly coronary artery disease (26). Although the traditional risk factors for development of atherosclerotic disease, particularly tobacco abuse and hypertension, also affect the intracranial circulation (27), some authors have suggested that intracranial atherosclerosis is especially prevalent in Black Americans and Asians (28,29).

The incidence of stenotic lesions located in the intracranial ICA, the intracranial vertebrobasilar system, and the proximal middle cerebral artery is far less than that of extracranial carotid and vertebral atherosclerosis. In one study from the Mayo Clinic, of 1,000 consecutive patients undergoing angiography, 19% had moderate to severe intracranial ICA stenosis and 29% had mild intracranial ICA stenosis (26). The most common location is the intracranial portion of the ICA (49%; particularly the intracavernous portion), followed by the middle cerebral artery (20%), posterior cerebral artery (11%), distal vertebral and basilar arteries (11%) and anterior cerebral artery (9%; 30). These lesions are responsible for 5 to 10% of all ischemic strokes (31).

The prognosis of symptomatic patients with intracranial stenosis is well characterized, particularly for lesions involving the ICA and middle cerebral artery. In one study (32), 58 patients with intracranial ICA stenosis were followed for 30 months. Forty-three percent of the patients suffered a cerebrovascular accident or died at this follow-up, mostly owing to a cardiac event or stroke. In another study (33), 72 patients with stenosis or occlusion involving the anterior circulation were randomized to medical treatment or extracranial-intracranial bypass surgery. The stroke rate was 36% in the patients randomized to medical treatment and 38% in the patients randomized to surgery. A comparable fate has been observed in patients with symptomatic intracranial lesions of the posterior circulation (34). Because of the current technical limitations of angioplasty for intracranial stenosis, this form of treatment should be reserved for patients who have failed medical treatment (10,35–37). Based on retrospective data, warfarin appears to be superior to aspirin (34); however, this has not been confirmed prospectively.

Compared with angioplasty of the extracranial carotid and vertebral arteries, angioplasty of the intracranial portion of these vessels is technically more difficult and carries a higher complication rate. In one study of 17 patients and 22 vessels treated with balloon angioplasty, procedural success was obtained in 82% (10). There were two strokes during angioplasty, for a 30-day morbidity rate of 9.1% per treated vessel and 11.7% per case. The average preangioplasty stenosis was 72 ± 8%, and postangioplasty stenosis was 43 ± 24%. Interestingly, at 6-month angiographic follow-up, further angiographic improvement was observed (37 ± 21%) in 8 patients and 12 vessels, suggesting a process of positive remodeling.

Stent placement for intracranial carotid arteries has also been reported with encouraging results (37–39). We recently reported our results of 15 patients with symptomatic intracranial carotid ($n = 10$) or vertebrobasilar ($n = 5$) atherosclerotic lesions with balloon angioplasty and provisional stenting (40). Stand-alone angioplasty was performed in 10 patients and stenting was attempted in 6 patients, in whom the device was successfully delivered in 5. Technical success

(residual stenosis of <50%) and clinical success (technical success and in-hospital freedom from death and stroke) with ongoing 30-day event-free survival were obtained in all patients. Interestingly, 8 patients (53%) showed improvement in a chronic neurologic deficit believed to be permanent prior to the procedure—hence the term *brain angina*. At 1-year follow-up, one patient died. Of the 14 patients still alive, 13 (93%) remained free from TIA or stroke.

We conclude that intracranial angioplasty with provisional stenting is a feasible treatment option for symptomatic patients with stenosis of the intracranial portion of the carotid or vertebrobasilar arterial circulation. Whether the new more flexible stents will improve the outcome of angioplasty in the intracranial circulation and change the natural history of the disease will have to be determined in larger controlled studies.

Case 3. This 35-year-old woman presented with a 2-month history of left hemispheric stroke manifest by aphasia and right-sided weakness. After her stroke, she sustained three more transient episodes of right-sided weakness and aphasia; consistent with TIAs in the same distribution. Magnetic resonance imaging (MRI) demonstrated a stroke in the left middle cerebral artery (MCA) distribution, and magnetic resonance arteriography (MRA) revealed high-grade bilateral MCA stenosis. Her exam was remarkable for expressive aphasia. She was referred by neurology to interventional cardiology and neuroradiology for evaluation and treatment. This was done in a collaborative manner by the interventional cardiologist and interventional neuroradiologist.

Four-vessel selective cerebral angiography was performed using a 4F Berenstein catheter. This revealed critical left MCA, M1 branch, stenosis (Fig. 34.3A) and a normal right MCA (in contradiction to the MRA findings). There were no collaterals from the vertebral artery, indicating an absence of the left posterior communicating artery. Intervention was then performed by advancing a multipurpose 6F coronary guiding catheter over an Amplatz exchange wire into the distal extracranial left internal carotid artery (ICA) just below the base of the skull. Using a coronary manifold and road mapping, a hydrophilic coronary guidewire (Whisper wire) was advanced through the intracranial carotid artery and across the critical stenosis in the left MCA. The lesion was then dilated using a 2.0 × 15 mm coronary balloon at 10 atm. Angiography revealed an excellent balloon result, so the guidewire was removed and angiography was repeated. Because of a small dissection at the site of the lesion (Fig. 34.3B), we attempted to pass a coronary stent; however, this would not traverse the bony siphon. Hemostasis was obtained with a closure device. Her symptoms of aphasia improved but did not resolve completely, and she was discharged the following morning on acetylsalicylic acid (ASA, aspirin) and clopidogrel.

Case 4. This 63-year-old patient was referred by her neuroradiologist because of recurrent episodes of dizziness, weakness, and diplopia 10 days after suffering a posterior

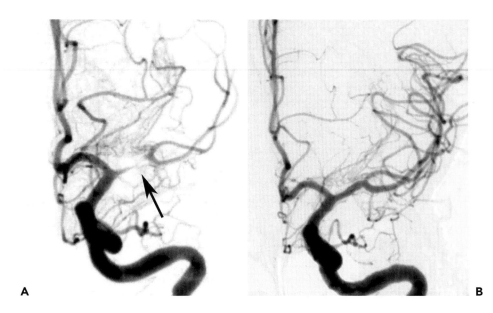

Figure 34.3 **A.** Critical stenosis *(arrow)* of the left M1 segment of the middle cerebral artery. **B.** After balloon angioplasty, there is a small dissection that does not appear to be flow limiting. The small superior side branches arising from the M1 segment are the lenticulostriate arteries. Occlusion of these small end arteries by stenting can lead to a large stroke.

circulation stroke. Her exam was consistent with cerebellar stroke (unable to stand, diplopia, and weakness). MRI showed pontine and basal ganglia infarction with ischemia in the visual cortex. MRA revealed high-grade stenosis of the basilar artery.

After premedication with ASA and clopidogrel, angiography was performed with a 6F headhunter catheter, demon-strating critical stenosis of the midbasilar artery (Fig. 34.4A) with stenosis in the V4 segment (intracranial portion) of the left vertebral artery. Intervention was performed initially using a 6F guiding catheter and a hydrophilic coronary wire, which was then exchanged for a conventional coronary guidewire. The lesion was dilated with a monorail 3.0 × 15 mm coronary balloon at 8 atm, with a 20% residual

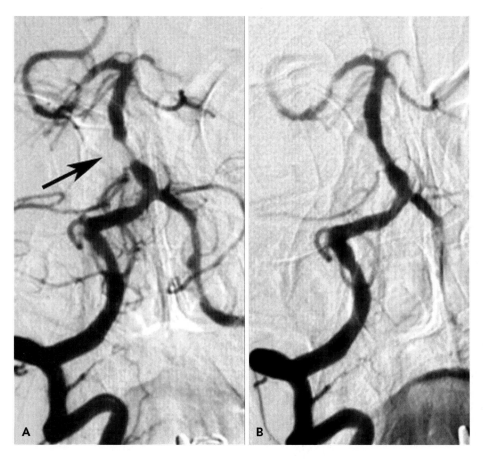

Figure 34.4 **A.** Intracranial angioplasty. Critical stenosis in the basilar artery located just distal to the anterior inferior cerebellar artery. **B.** After balloon angioplasty with a coronary system, showing significant improvement.

stenosis (Fig. 34.4B). Stenting was not performed because of the pontine branches that arise from the basilar artery at the point of the stenosis. The patient had no subsequent events and remains asymptomatic at 2 years.

Illustrative Points. Intracranial angioplasty is a field in its infancy where collaboration between neurology, neuroradiology, and the interventionist is important. These two cases illustrate how patients with recurrent focal symptoms in the same vascular distribution should be referred for angiography even if the duplex examination shows no cervical carotid stenosis. Lesions of the aorto-ostial common carotid artery and the high internal carotid, including intracranial carotid or vertebral arteries, can be missed by carotid duplex examination and other noninvasive imaging methods. Computerized Tomographic Angiography (CTA) and MRA may also undercall or overestimate the percent diameter stenosis—angiography remains the gold standard. The role of platelet glycoprotein IIb/IIIa receptor inhibitors has some theoretic basis, but has not been established in this patient population. Stenting is performed in a provisional manner because, first, many lesions are not stentable with current devices given tortuosity in the target vessel, and second, side-branch occlusion of the small branches, especially of M1 (lenticulostriate arteries) and the basilar artery (pontine perforators), can lead to a major stroke.

Case 5. This previously healthy 63-year-old woman presented to a community hospital with an acute anterior wall MI treated with percutaneous coronary intervention (PCI) and abciximab 3 days ago. Her course was complicated by atrial fibrillation for which she was treated with amiodarone with subsequent conversion to sinus rhythm. Two days post-PCI, she developed sudden onset of right-sided hemiplegia and dense aphasia. Her cardiologist administered rt-PA 50 mg and transferred her by helicopter to the stroke center where she underwent immediate angiography at 3 hours, demonstrating occlusion of the M2 segment (first bifurcation) of the left MCA (Fig. 34.5A). Because this lesion most likely represented an embolus of some age, meaning it is likely to be organized thrombus, thrombolysis and balloon angioplasty are not likely to be successful.

Intervention was performed using the concentric retrieval system. A 7F balloon-tipped guiding catheter was advanced to the distal ICA at the base of the skull. A Whisper wire was advanced through the concentric microcatheter across the occlusion in the left MCA. The wire was replaced with the concentric retrieval system. The thrombus was entangled in the coils of the retrieval device (Fig. 34.5B), then was withdrawn under fluoroscopic guidance while aspirating through the balloon-tipped guiding catheter into the guide. Angiography demonstrated recanalization of the occlusion

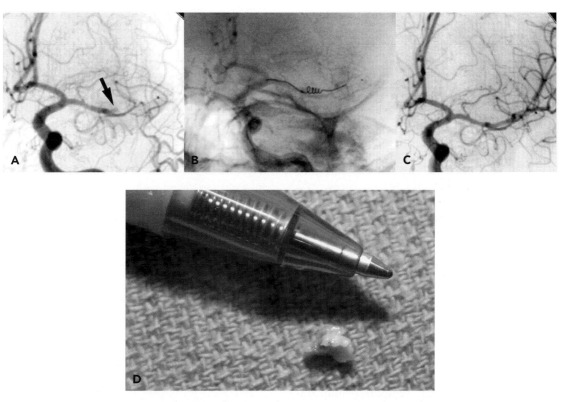

Figure 34.5 A. Occlusion of the distal left M1 branch of the middle cerebral artery (MCA) in a woman with embolic stroke due to atrial fibrillation. **B.** Positioning of the concentric retrieval system in the occlusion. **C.** Angiographic appearance after clot removal with no residual stenosis. **D.** The clot that was removed (below the ballpoint pen for reference) was small, fibrous, organized, and had trabeculation similar to that found in the left atrial appendage.

with no residual stenosis or thrombus (Fig. 34.5C). The aspirate revealed a large, white, organized thrombus with trabeculation resembling the inside of the left atrial appendage (Fig. 34.5D top). The patient developed sudden and dramatic resolution of her hemiplegic symptoms over the next 12 hours and had no residual deficit the next morning. She was treated with aspirin, clopidogrel, and warfarin to prevent further embolization.

Illustrative Points. This case illustrates the potential importance of cardiologists being able to prevent, diagnose, and treat stroke. Rapid recognition and treatment are essential because patients with stroke for over 3 hours do not benefit from systemic thrombolysis, and patients greater than 6 hours after the onset rarely benefit from any intervention. Occlusion of the major branches of the MCA does not usually respond to intravenous lysis, and this patient, in particular, had a contraindication to lysis, namely, the arterial puncture treated with manual compression 72 hours earlier. Catheter-based intervention with balloons, stents, and retrieval devices is still investigational, but has become the treatment of choice in our institution for strokes between 3 and 6 hours old or major strokes (MCA or basilar distribution) of any age. With proper patient selection and technique, the outcome of catheter-based intervention in patients who are not candidates for lysis can be as good as for those who receive lysis. This procedure should be done only in collaboration with neurologists and neuroradiologists, because the anatomy, pathology, and treatment are different than that of acute MI. Intracranial hemorrhage, the most common serious complication of stroke intervention, is usually fatal if it occurs in this setting.

Subclavian and Brachiocephalic Artery Angioplasty

Significant subclavian artery stenosis has been found to be approximately 2% in the general population and 7% in patients with risk factors for atherosclerotic disease in a recent large study (41). The stenosis is usually focal and located in the proximal portion of the vessel, before the origin of the vertebral and internal mammary artery. The left subclavian artery is involved three to four times more frequently than the right. Although atherosclerotic disease is by far the most common cause of subclavian artery stenosis, unusual conditions such as Takayasu arteritis, fibromuscular dysplasia, giant cell arteritis, radiation-induced occlusive disease, and the thoracic outlet syndrome may affect this vessel and cause significant stenosis (42–47; see Chapter 14).

The clinical manifestations of subclavian artery stenosis include upper extremity ischemic symptoms with arm claudication related to exercise or from embolization to the digits (48). Subclavian steal syndrome occurs as a result of flow reversal in the vertebral artery, leading to symptoms of vertebrobasilar insufficiency (49,50). In the

coronary-subclavian steal syndrome, there is reversal of flow in an internal mammary graft as a result of a proximal subclavian stenosis, which may cause symptoms of myocardial ischemia (51,52).

Before the advent of percutaneous revascularization techniques, surgery was considered the standard treatment for this condition. Techniques included transthoracic procedures, carotid-subclavian bypass, and axilloaxillary bypass—all carrying significant morbidity and mortality. Hadjipetru et al. (53) recently reviewed the outcomes of 52 surgical studies with 2,496 patients. The technical success was 96% (range: 75 to 100%) and the complication rate was 16 ± 11% (range: 0 to 43%) with a mortality rate of 2 ± 2% (range: 0 to 11%) and a stroke rate of 3 ± 4% (range: 0 to 14%). At a mean follow-up of 51 ± 25 months, recurrence of symptoms occurred in 16 ± 14%.

Balloon angioplasty for subclavian artery stenosis can be carried out with high technical success as an alternative to surgery (54–57). Stenting, when used in addition to balloon dilation, may reduce the risk of embolization and achieve anatomically and physiologically superior results. In the study of Hadjipetru (53), the published series of patients treated with stents were also summarized. Of 108 patients treated with these devices, technical success was obtained in 97 ± 4%, with adverse events in 6 ± 5%. In a multicenter registry involving eight centers, stenting of the subclavian artery was successful in 98.5% of patients, and a TIA occurred in only one (0.5%) patient.

Based on the current available data, percutaneous revascularization with balloon angioplasty followed by stent placement appears to yield superior results with fewer complications than surgery for the treatment of significant stenoses of the subclavian arteries. Stenting is thus often considered the treatment of choice these lesions.

Case 6. This 66-year-old woman presented with a chief complaint of left arm claudication. She stated that she had a history of progressive pain and weakness in her left arm that was associated with the symptom of the room "spinning around her" during left arm exertion. Symptoms were especially prominent while washing the dishes and folding laundry. She had a history of hypertension, hyperlipidemia, and diabetes. Her blood pressure was 180/90 in the right arm and 130/60 in the left arm. Her left radial pulse was weak. Duplex scanning revealed reversal of flow in the left vertebral artery. Coronary angiography by the referring physician revealed nonobstructive coronary disease. Angiography of the left subclavian artery revealed 90% stenosis of the left subclavian artery proximal to the left internal mammary artery (Fig. 34.6A). The vertebral vessel filled in a retrograde manner.

The patient underwent percutaneous intervention using a 6F long sheath, which was inserted into the left subclavian artery over an extra-stiff 0.035-inch guidewire that had been placed across the stenosis. The peak translesional gradient was measured to be 50 mm Hg. The lesion was

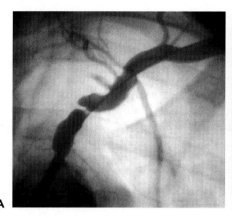 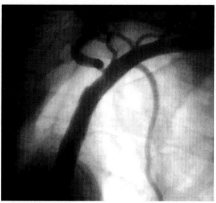

Figure 34.6 **A.** Critical stenosis in the left subclavian artery *(arrow)*, which supplies both the left vertebral (underfilled) and left internal mammary artery as well as the axillary artery. There is ostial disease in the subclavian artery as well. **B.** After placing tandem balloon-expandable Palmaz stents in the left subclavian artery, there is normalization of flow to the left vertebral and left axillary arteries. The left vertebral has a 50% ostial stenosis, which was not treated.

predilated using a 6 × 20 mm balloon over an extra-stiff coronary 0.014-inch guidewire. A 6 × 17 mm balloon-expandable stent was then advanced across the lesion and deployed at 12 atm. A second 7 × 17 mm balloon-expandable stent was deployed at the ostium at 16 atm. Final angiography was performed revealing restoration of antegrade flow into the left vertebral artery (Fig. 34.6B). The pressure gradient across the lesion was abolished.

Illustrative Points. Subclavian artery stenosis can present with claudication, critical limb ischemia, or subclavian steal syndrome. This patient's symptoms and examination were classic for the lesion that was found. In patients with prior left internal mammary artery (LIMA) to coronary artery bypass surgery, angina may be the presenting symptom. The surgical treatment of this lesion by carotid to subclavian bypass has a mortality of 5% and a major morbidity (mainly cardiac) of approximately 25%. In a multicenter registry (57), the treatment of these patients with stents has a major morbidity of <1% and a restenosis rate of 10%. The same technique is used to perform aorto-ostial stenting of the carotid and brachiocephalic arteries. Balloon-expandable stents are preferred in this location because of the ability to precisely position them at the ostium without compromise of important side branches.

THORACIC AORTIC INTERVENTION

Coarctation of the Aorta

Patients with long-standing coarctation of the aorta have an increased risk for development of coronary artery disease, aortic dissection, and pseudoaneurysm formation (58). The treatment of native coarctation of the aorta has traditionally been surgical. Although this procedure is effective in obliterating the pressure gradient and relieving symptoms, the incidence of restenosis and aneurysm formation is not negligible, ranging from 5% to as high as 50% (59–63). Percutaneous catheter-based procedures have emerged as a feasible alternative to surgical treatment

in selected patients (see also Chapters 14, 27, and 33). Several studies have shown that balloon angioplasty can be carried out with a high technical success and a low complication rate (64–69). There is still controversy as to whether balloon angioplasty or surgery is the treatment of choice for native coarctation of the aorta, but most investigators agree that balloon angioplasty is a better treatment for postoperative coarctation (70,71).

Most published studies have found that angioplasty was highly effective in reducing the pressure gradient (64–71). In one study of 43 patients with native coarctation of the aorta, the pressure gradient was reduced from 69 ± 24 mm Hg before angioplasty to 12 ± 8 mm Hg after angioplasty (65). There were no procedural deaths, but 7% developed an aneurysm at follow-up (range: 1 to 10 years), and 7% developed recurrent coarctation at 12-month angiographic follow-up. In another study of 90 patients with recurrent coarctation, the pressure gradient was reduced from 31 ± 21 mm Hg to 8 ± 9 mm Hg (68). In 11 patients (12%), the procedure failed to reduce the pressure gradient to <20 mm Hg (procedure failure). There were two neurologic events and one death. At 12-month follow-up, 72% remained free from need for reintervention. On the other hand, some investigators have not found significant differences in treating native or recurrent coarctation with balloon angioplasty (69).

The use of endoluminal stents to minimize the elastic recoil, improve the immediate hemodynamic results, and possibly decrease the recurrence of coarctation has been investigated (72,73). In one study (72), nine patients were treated with stenting (seven patients had had a previous operation or balloon dilation). Reduction in gradient across the coarctation and increase in diameter of the narrow segment occurred immediately after stent implantation. At a median follow-up of 13 months, residual gradient across the stented segment remained low in eight patients. One patient required redilation of the stent. In a more recent series of 32 patients with coarctation of the aorta (23 patients had postoperative recurrent coarctation and 9 patients had native coarctation) treated with endovascular stents, the mean systolic pressure gradient was decreased from 31 to 1.8 mm Hg (73). At 1.5 years of follow-up, eight patients required repeated stent dilation, and the only complication was stent migration in one case.

The indications for the use of endoluminal stents in coarctation of the aorta is still uncertain, but on the basis of this limited but encouraging experience, it has been suggested that potential indications for these devices include the following: hypoplasia of the isthmus or transverse aortic arch, tortuous coarctation with misalignment of the proximal with distal aortic segment, which are difficult to treat surgically, and recurrent aortic coarctation or small aneurysm after previous surgical or balloon therapy (74).

Case 7. This 70-year-old woman presents with severe hypertension on multiple medications and asymptomatic two-vessel coronary artery disease. Her examination was remarkable for a systolic bruit between the scapulae, a 50 mm Hg gradient between her arm and leg blood pressure, and weak but symmetrical pulses in her lower extremities. She was referred for intervention rather than surgery because of her age and concomitant coronary disease. The coarctation was crossed with a multipurpose catheter and floppy Glidewire. Angiography revealed an 80% stenosis in the aorta just distal to the left subclavian artery with post-stenotic dilatation (Fig. 34.7A), with a 60 mm Hg peak systolic gradient across the coarctation. Intravascular ultrasound (IVUS) demonstrated the aorta to be 18 mm in diameter proximal to the coarctation and 25 mm in diameter distal to the coarctation. Angiographic measurements

were also obtained. Using an extra-stiff 0.035-inch wire, a long 12F sheath was advanced across the coarctation. A transvenous pacemaker was placed in the right ventricle (RV) and asynchronous rapid ventricular pacing was begun at 180 beats per minute (bpm) to reduce left ventricular ejection and thus forward flow in the aorta. Using the sheath to protect the stent as it crossed the lesion, the coarctation was stented directly with a 12 × 36 mm stent mounted on a 16 mm × 4.0 cm balloon (Fig. 34.7B). Angiography revealed underdilation of the stenosis with a persistent gradient of 18 mm Hg, so a 20 × 40 mm balloon was used to postdilate the balloon-expandable stent. Angiography (Fig. 34.7C), IVUS, and pressure gradients all confirmed correction of the coarctation.

Illustrative Points. Coarctation of the aorta usually presents with hypertension proximal to the coarctation. In some patients with long-standing coarctation, congestive heart failure can result from chronic pressure overload. When treating coarctation of the aorta with endovascular techniques, IVUS is recommended to accurately size the vessel and avoid overdilation of the aorta, which can lead to serous dissection, rupture, or death. Self-expanding stents tend to migrate into the distal ectatic aorta, making balloon-expandable stents preferable. The use of rapid ventricular pacing effectively stops the cardiac output for a few moments to allow proper placement of the stent without distal migration during systole. The maximum diameter of this balloon-expandable stent is 20 mm, and considerable

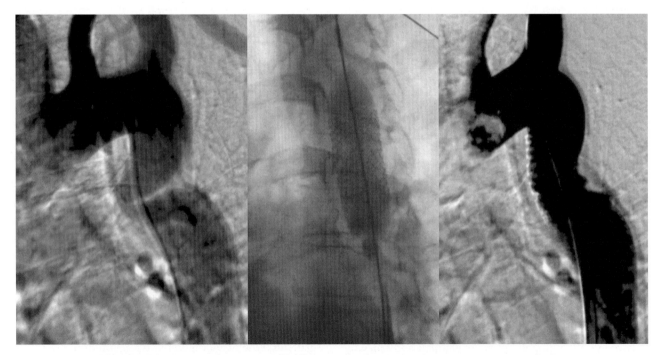

Figure 34.7 A. A typical coarctation just distal to the left subclavian artery seen by digital subtraction angiography with a pigtail catheter located in the aortic arch. **B.** Poststenting with a balloon-expandable stent, there is minimal residual stenosis compared with the isthmus (proximal part) of the coarctation. It is important to size the balloon by measuring the vessel proximal to the coarctation rather than distal to reduce the risk of the serious complications of dissection and rupture.

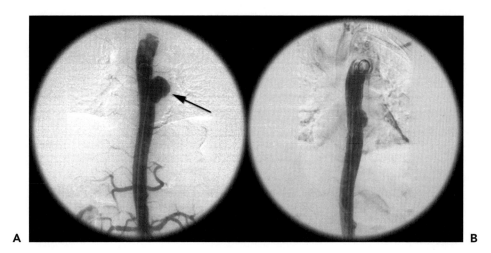

Figure 34.8 **A.** Digital subtraction aortography of the descending thoracic aorta demonstrates a saccular aneurysm *(arrow)*. **B.** After placement of an oversized, self-expanding endoluminal graft, there is no evidence of graft leaking. There is ectasia at the site of the aneurysm owing to expansion of the prosthesis into the aneurysm. This appearance is expected. Oversizing is necessary with self-expanding stents and endoluminal grafts to ensure good apposition of the stent or graft to the vessel wall.

shortening occurs at this diameter, so careful positioning is important. Postsurgical correction coarctations are less likely to develop dissection and rupture with balloon angioplasty than native or virgin coarctations.

Endoluminal Thoracic Aneurysm Repair

The prevalence of thoracic aneurysms is difficult to determine because of under-reporting of these aneurysms in U.S. mortality statistics. In Sweden, in a stable urban population with an autopsy rate of 83%, the incidence of thoracic aortic aneurysm between 1958 and 1985 was 489 per 100,000 autopsies in 65-year-old men and 670 per 100,000 autopsies in 80-year-olds (75).

The prognosis of untreated thoracic aneurysms is poor. In three large studies, which included 264 patients with thoracic aneurysms who did not undergo surgery at the time of diagnosis, rupture of the aneurysm was the most common cause of death, ranging from 42 to 70% (76–78) of mortality, with a 5-year survival rate ranging from 13 to 39%.

In general, patients with aneurysms >5.0 to 5.5 cm in the ascending aorta, >5.5 to 6.0 cm in the aortic arch, or >5.0 to 6.0 cm in the descending aorta should undergo surgical intervention (79). But given the high prevalence of cardiovascular disease in this patient population, surgical treatment carries a significant mortality—12% when the procedure is performed electively, or as high as 50% when the procedure is performed emergently (76,80). Similarly, stroke and spinal cord injury are frequent complications of surgical treatment (79).

Endovascular stent grafts have been described as an alternative to surgical treatment for descending thoracic aortic aneurysms in selected patients (81,82). Dake et al. (82) reported experience in 13 patients with descending thoracic aortic aneurysm with a mean diameter of 6.1 cm (range, 5 to 8 cm). Technical success was obtained in all 13 patients. There were no deaths, paraplegia, or stroke at 11.6 months of follow-up, and there was complete thrombosis of the thoracic aortic aneurysm surrounding the stent graft

in 12 patients. One patient with extensive chronic dissection required open surgical graft placement because of progressive dilation of the arch. Following submission of their paper, 20 additional patients with 23 thoracic aneurysms underwent endovascular stent grafts, with success in 21 cases and 2 deaths in patients from multiorgan failure (1 preceded by paraplegia). Although the experience is still limited, endovascular stent grafts appear to be a promising alternative to surgery for the treatment of thoracic aortic aneurysms in selected patients.

Case 8. This 58-year-old Hispanic man was referred from South America with an asymptomatic 6-cm saccular descending thoracic aneurysm (Fig. 34.8A). He was treated by endovascular means using a femoral cutdown and a self-expanding nitinol endoluminal graft during a procedure that lasted <1 hour. Following deployment of the graft, there was still a bulge of graft material into the aneurysm owing to a lack of external support on the graft, with no evidence of leaking (Fig. 34.8B).

Illustrative Points. Although this is a very promising and exciting area for endovascular intervention, the nonsurgical treatment of these aneurysms is still in its infancy. Because standard surgical repair carries with it a high morbidity and mortality as stated above, investigators are anxiously awaiting the development of an endovascular solution to this problem. Of note, the most likely cause of this type of saccular aneurysm of the thoracic aorta is infection, especially salmonellosis, not atherosclerosis.

CELIAC AND MESENTERIC ARTERY ANGIOPLASTY

Mesenteric artery stenosis is relatively common, with a prevalence of 17% in patients older than 70 years of age (83). Despite the prevalence of this condition, chronic mesenteric ischemia is an uncommon cause of chronic abdominal pain, with a reported prevalence in approximately one case per 100,000 population (84). This is because symptoms do not usually occur until all three mesenteric vessels are stenotic or occluded: the celiac trunk, the superior mesenteric artery (SMA), and the inferior mesenteric artery (IMA). The stomach and upper half of the duodenum (the foregut) are supplied by the celiac trunk. The lower half of the duodenum, jejunum, ileum, cecum appendix, ascending colon, and proximal two-thirds of the transverse colon (the midgut) are supplied by the SMA. The lower third of the transverse colon, sigmoid colon, descending colon, sigmoid colon, rectum, and the upper part of the anal canal (the hindgut) are supplied by the IMA.

Not only is there significant communication among these three vessels, but there is also significant collateral flow to the mesenteric circulation from other aortic branches such as the lumbar intercostal, middle sacral, mammary, and internal iliac arteries. Thus, the clinical syndrome of chronic mesenteric ischemia usually develops as a result of critical stenosis or occlusion of two or more of the celiac artery, SMA, or IMA. Over 90% of the cases of chronic mesenteric ischemia are owing to atherosclerosis, usually extensions of aortic atheroma rather than intrinsic disease of the mesenteric branches.

Abdominal pain is the most frequent symptom, with some series reporting this manifestation in all patients (84–86). Other symptoms include weight loss, diarrhea, nausea, vomiting, and constipation. The abdominal pain is usually postprandial and cramping, localized in the epigastrium or midabdomen. Over 80% of the patients note the relationship of pain with food intake (85,86). A significant percentage of patients may have concomitant coronary or peripheral vascular disease (87), so this should be considered a risk factor for development of this condition.

The traditional treatment for chronic mesenteric ischemia has been surgical. Because stenosis of the mesenteric branches is frequently focal, limited to the ostium and/or the very proximal portion of the vessel, percutaneous, catheter-based techniques of revascularization have been explored and appear to be a feasible alternative to surgery in selected patients. An analysis of 11 published studies with 126 patients treated with balloon angioplasty (88) revealed a mean initial technical success of 86% (range: 38 to 100%). After exclusion of technical failures, the clinical success rate (resolution of symptoms) was 90%. At a follow-up of ≤101 months, the primary and secondary clinical success was 76% and 92%. Major complications occurred in 6% of the patients, and the 30-day mortality was 3%.

Endovascular stenting of the mesenteric branches appears to be safe and effective in selective patients. We recently reported our results of 61 patients with chronic mesenteric ischemia treated with endovascular stent placement, including 81 mesenteric arteries (47 celiac, 24 SMA , 8 IMA, 1 vein graft, and 1 common hepatic artery; 89). Angiographic success (<30% diameter stenosis), clinical

success (angiographic success without in-hospital death or need for surgery), and symptom relief were obtained in 98%, 97%, and 91% the patients, respectively. At a mean follow-up of 35 ± 23 months, 11 patients died. Anatomical follow-up was obtained in 88% of the patients with CT angiography, angiography, or ultrasound, revealing a restenosis (>50% diameter stenosis) rate of 26% per vessel and 43% per patient; however, only 10 patients (17%) developed recurrence of symptoms and were successfully treated with a second percutaneous intervention. Although experience is still limited, catheter-based techniques of revascularization such as balloon angioplasty with or without stenting appears a promising alternative to surgical intervention in selective patients with chronic mesenteric ischemia.

Case 9. This 32-year-old woman, a heavy smoker, had a 9-month history of postprandial midepigastric pain with a 5-lb weight loss and bloating. She denied anorexia; however, she stopped eating to avoid the recurrence of the pain. On examination, she was cachectic, weighing only 110 lb, and appeared chronically ill. She had an epigastric bruit and diminished tibial and dorsalis pedis pulses bilaterally. An extensive GI workup including upper and lower endoscopy; small bowel follow-through; CT scan of the abdomen; ultrasound of the gallbladder, liver, and spleen; complete blood count; and serum chemistries was negative. She was referred for abdominal aortography and selective celiac and mesenteric angiography, performed through brachial artery access using a 4F multipurpose catheter. The superior mesenteric artery and inferior mesenteric artery were occluded. Figure 34.9A demonstrates high-grade stenosis of the celiac trunk. This lesion was crossed with a 0.014-inch angioplasty guidewire through a 6F multipurpose guide, and was directly stented with a 6 × 28 Guidant balloon-expandable stent. It was postdilated with a 7-mm balloon at 12 atm. Final angiography (Fig. 34.9B) demonstrated no residual stenosis. The gradient was reduced from 60 mm Hg to less than 5 mm Hg. The patient's symptoms were immediately relieved, and 2 months later she had regained 20 lb.

Case 10. This 49-year-old woman has a history of chronic postprandial abdominal pain with a 40-lb weight loss. Diagnostic angiography revealed occlusion of the celiac and IMA, with 99% stenosis in the SMA (Fig. 34.10A). Using a 6F multipurpose guiding catheter and a coronary angioplasty guidewire, the lesion was predilated with a 3.0-mm coronary balloon, stented with a 4.0 × 25 mm coronary stent, and postdilated with a 5.0 × 20 mm balloon. Final angiography (Fig. 34.10B) revealed no residual stenosis. The patient had immediate relief of her symptoms.

Illustrative Points. These are classic cases of chronic mesenteric ischemia. The diagnosis is usually missed in the early stages because of the myriad causes of abdominal pain. Profound weight loss with postprandial abdominal pain is the hallmark of this condition. Symptoms do not usually occur unless there is stenosis or occlusion of two or

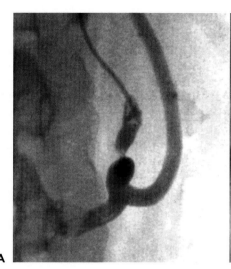 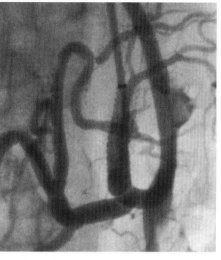

Figure 34.9 **A.** Angiography of the celiac artery demonstrating high-grade stenosis of the mid-celiac before intervention. **B.** After stenting, there is no residual stenosis. The stent is placed so that several millimeters of stent extend into the aorta since this is an ostial lesion.

more of the three vessels (celiac, SMA, IMA). The traditional management of this condition has been surgical, but mesenteric ischemia lends itself very nicely to an endovascular approach since the lesions are usually ostial and ideal for balloon-expandable stents. Furthermore, by the time the diagnosis is made, the patients are usually cachectic and not ideal surgical candidates. Most patients are treated with aspirin and clopidogrel for 3 to 6 months post–peripheral stenting.

RENAL ARTERY ANGIOPLASTY

Renal artery stenosis is common in patients with known coronary or peripheral atherosclerotic disease (90,91; see also Chapters 14 and 26). In one study of 196 patients undergoing cardiac catheterization for presumptive coronary artery disease, the prevalence of significant (>50%) renal artery disease was 18%, and when coronary artery disease was confirmed in 152 patients, the prevalence was

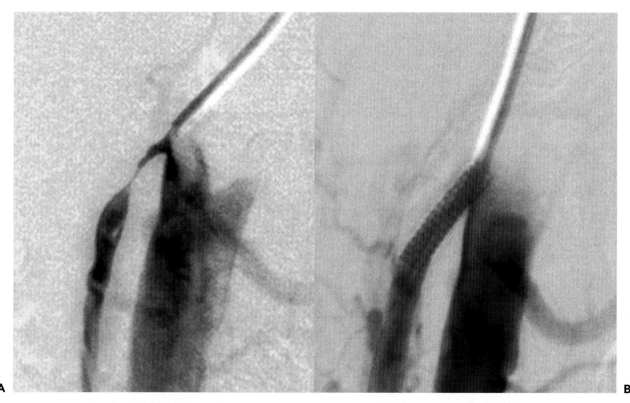

Figure 34.10 **A.** Angiography reveals subtotal occlusion of the origin of the superior mesenteric artery (SMA). The celiac and inferior mesenteric are occluded (not shown). **B.** Poststenting, there is normal flow and no residual stenosis.

22% (90). Some investigators have reported a >60% prevalence of renal artery stenosis in patients with concomitant peripheral vascular disease and hypertension (92). For this reason, many cardiac catheterization laboratories perform screening renal angiography in patients undergoing cardiac catheterization for atherosclerotic coronary disease, particularly if there is arterial hypertension or a baseline creatinine >1.5 mg/dL.

Significant hemodynamic obstruction of the renal blood flow causes renovascular hypertension by activation of the renin angiotensin system, and consequent production of angiotensin I and II, causing systemic hypertension and fluid retention. The diagnosis of renovascular hypertension should be suspected in patients with onset of hypertension <35 years and >55 years, malignant or refractory hypertension, renal failure, resistant hypertension, coronary or peripheral atherosclerosis, an abdominal bruit, or a unilateral small kidney, and in patients who develop azotemia with angiotensin-converting enzyme (ACE) inhibitor therapy (93). The noninvasive test of choice for evaluating renal artery stenosis is the renal duplex ultrasound examination (94). Captopril renal artery scintigraphy is a sensitive and specific test for demonstrating unilateral renal artery stenosis (95); however, the incidence of a false-negative test is substantial in patients with parenchymal disease or bilateral renal artery stenosis, which occurs in approximately one-third of the patients. Renal vein renin assays have been used in the past; however, many antihypertensive medications such as beta-blockers may interfere with the release of renin, and the patients need to withhold these medications prior to the test, making it impractical (96). MRA is used as a screening test in many centers, although there can be falsely positive and falsely negative findings.

Surgical revascularization of atherosclerotic renal artery stenosis is an effective treatment for renovascular hypertension (97), but carries an operative mortality of 3% as well as complications such as bypass graft thrombosis and nephrectomy in 4% of the cases (98,99). Percutaneous transluminal renal angioplasty has been recognized as the treatment of choice for fibromuscular dysplasia (100–102) and is an accepted treatment for selected patients with renal artery stenosis causing renovascular hypertension and/or renal insufficiency (100,103). However, atherosclerotic aorto-ostial renal artery lesions are particularly difficult to treat with balloon angioplasty alone because they are prone to significant vascular recoil leading to a restenosis rate of approximately 50% over 6 months (104). On the other hand, endovascular stents can scaffold such lesions and minimize the elastic recoil. Several studies have shown a significantly greater acute gain in luminal diameter and better angiographic results with renal artery stenting compared with balloon angioplasty alone (105–107). In a study of 76 patients and 92 renal arteries treated with primary stenting, technical success was obtained in 100%, with a restenosis rate at 6

months of 25% (106). Blum et al. (108) treated 74 renal artery stenoses with endovascular stents. Technical success was achieved in 100% of the vessels, and the restenosis rate at 12-month follow-up was 11%. The renal function remained unchanged in all patients, but in 62% of the patients, there was significant improvement of blood pressure and in 16% the blood pressure normalized. In one study, balloon-expandable stents were placed in 100 patients and 133 renal arteries (109). Angiographic success was obtained in 132 of 133 (99%) of the lesions. At 6-month follow-up, the systolic blood pressure was reduced from 173 ± 25 to 147 ± 12 mm Hg ($P < .001$) and the diastolic blood pressure was reduced from 88 ± 17 to 76 ± 12 mm Hg ($P < .001$). At a mean angiographic follow-up of 8.7 ± 5.0 months, the restenosis rate was 19%. Renal function after stent placement showed no significant change in serum creatinine.

Stenting for renal artery stenosis also appears to have a beneficial effect in patients with refractory unstable angina and congestive heart failure (110). In 48 patients with unstable angina ($n = 23$) or congestive heart failure ($n = 25$) who had hypertension refractory to medical therapy and significant unilateral ($n = 30$) or bilateral ($n = 18$) renal artery stenosis, stenting significantly improved the blood pressure and functional class at 24-hour and 6-month follow-up. The dramatic improvement seen in this group of patients was independent of the concomitant performance of a coronary angioplasty procedure.

In summary, the incidence of renal artery stenosis in patients with poorly controlled hypertension and atherosclerotic cardiovascular disease ranges from 20 to 30%. These patients should be identified at the time of diagnostic cardiac catheterization. The treatment of renal artery stenosis has a dramatic impact on the hypertension control and appears to have a beneficial effect in the treatment of refractory unstable angina and congestive heart failure. Considering the treatment alternatives for atherosclerotic renal artery stenosis causing medically refractory hypertension and/or renal insufficiency, stent placement is the current treatment of choice.

Case 11. This 77-year-old female with known coronary artery disease and angina has a history of long-standing hypertension and diastolic dysfunction. Despite three antihypertensive medications, her blood pressure was 200/95. Her physical examination and laboratory data were normal. A color flow duplex Doppler examination suggested unilateral right renal artery stenosis. At the time of diagnostic coronary angiography, renal angiography was also performed, revealing fibromuscular dysplasia of the midright renal artery and ostial atherosclerosis (Fig. 34.11A). Balloon angioplasty was performed on the area of fibromuscular dysplasia with a 5.0-mm balloon and 0.035-inch Wholey wire. The ostium was treated with a balloon-expandable stent (Fig. 34.11B). She was discharged the next morning on only one antihypertensive medication with a blood pressure of 145/70 mm Hg.

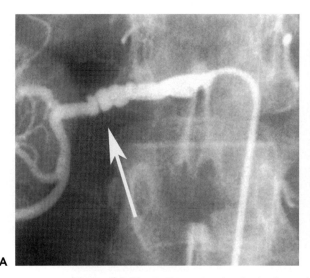
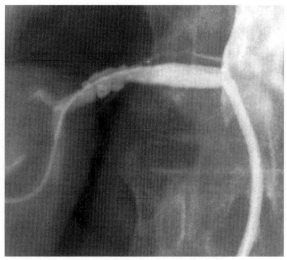

Figure 34.11   A. This patient has both atherosclerotic ostial stenosis and fibromuscular dysplasia. The typical appearance of fibromuscular dysplasia *(arrow)* is a corrugation of the vessel. This is diagnostic of fibromuscular dysplasia, but not of renovascular hypertension. **B.** The corrugated appearance of the vessel does not change after balloon angioplasty; however, the ostial lesion has been successfully stented. Stenting of the fibromuscular disease is reserved for persistent hypertension after balloon angioplasty.

Illustrative Points. Fibromuscular dysplasia (FMD) is commonly found in young adults, especially women, but the condition can persist into later life. This interesting case illustrates the combination of two classical lesions: atherosclerotic renal artery ostial stenosis and FMD of the midrenal artery. The angiographic appearance of a corrugated vessel is diagnostic of FMD, and the renal artery is the most common location for this abnormality. The finding of fibromuscular dysplasia is not diagnostic of renovascular hypertension, but the noninvasive screening tests and selective renal vein renin analysis also lack sensitivity and specificity for this condition. In a patient with FMD who is hypertensive despite medical therapy, balloon angioplasty is indicated, and the lesion usually responds to balloon angioplasty alone, without the need for stenting. Ostial renal artery stenosis owing to atherosclerosis does not respond to balloon angioplasty and does require stenting. In this hypertensive patient, both treatments were used to treat the specific lesions that were found with clinical success.

Case 12. This 73-year-old man was referred for evaluation and treatment of uncontrolled hypertension and ischemic cardiomyopathy with congestive heart failure and five hospital admissions for coronary heart failure (CHF) over the past 12 months. His blood pressure was 179/96 on four antihypertensive medications: Diltiazem 300 mg every day, metoprolol 200 mg every day, Cardura 2 mg every day, and Dyazide. He underwent coronary artery bypass surgery 12 years previously. There were no audible abdominal bruits. His blood urea nitrogen (BUN) was 23 mg/dL and creatinine 1.4 mg/dL. Because he was unstable, noninvasive studies were deferred and he underwent cardiac catheterization and renal angiography. Nonselective

renal angiography was obtained with an AP abdominal aortogram (Fig 34.12.A). This demonstrated bilateral severe aorto-ostial renal artery stenosis and no significant coronary artery stenoses. The left renal artery was engaged with a 5F IMA catheter, and selective angiography was performed. Renal artery stenting was performed using peripheral balloons and biliary stents. The right renal stent was dilated with a 7.0-mm balloon, and the left renal stent with an 8.0-mm balloon. Final angiography revealed no significant stenosis (Fig. 34.12B). The patient remains asymptomatic without recurrent hospitalizations on Dyazide and metoprolol 50 mg every day 5 years after renal stenting.

Illustrative Points. As this case illustrates, not all patients with bilateral severe renal artery stenosis have renal insufficiency or audible bruits. It also illustrates how the lesions of renal artery stenosis are often aortic plaque that encroaches on the renal ostia rather than plaque originating in the renal arteries themselves. Notice how diseased the abdominal aorta is in this patient. For this reason, the authors strongly recommend selective cannulation of the renal arteries using a diagnostic 4F to 6F catheter rather a larger guiding catheter to minimize the risk of distal atheroembolism. Furthermore, as this case also illustrates, bilateral renal artery stenosis can be easily treated at one session using the same catheters and balloons. Given the fact that we have an excellent low-risk treatment for atherosclerotic renovascular hypertension, *one wonders whether it is ethical NOT to study the renal arteries in patients with atherosclerosis and hypertension undergoing cardiac catheterization.*

Case 13. This 62-year-old woman has a history of chronic hypertension and back pain. Abdominal radiographs demonstrated a calcified mass in the left abdomen, and an

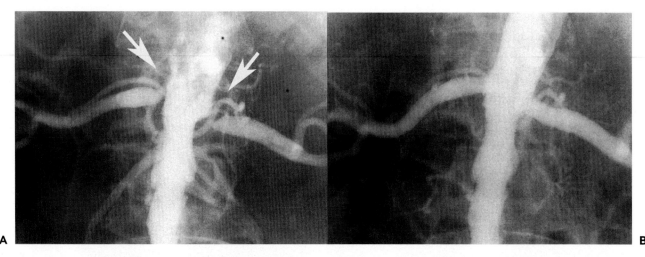

Figure 34.12   A. Bilateral aorto-ostial renal artery stenosis *(arrows)* as demonstrated by cineangiography at the time of cardiac catheterization. Notice the diffuse atherosclerotic involvement of the infrarenal aorta. **B.** Aortogram of the same patient immediately after bilateral stent implantation.

ultrasound confirmed the presence of a left renal artery aneurysm (Fig. 34.13A) and bilateral renal fibromuscular dysplasia. She was referred for endovascular therapy. In collaboration with neuroradiology, the left renal artery aneurysm was treated first using coiling techniques that are familiar to neuroradiologists. A 6F hockey stick guiding catheter was placed in the ostium of the left renal artery. A 0.014-inch floppy hydrophilic wire was placed in the body of the aneurysm and a Transit catheter was advanced into the aneurysm body. Multiple long hydrophilic coils (HydroCoils) were deployed through the transit catheter (20 mm × 20 cm, 18 × 20 cm, 14 × 20 cm) to obliterate the aneurysm sac. The FMD in the main renal artery branches was then dilated with a 6.0-mm balloon,

and a Magic Wallstent was placed across the aneurysm neck to keep the coils in place. The FMD in the contralateral renal artery was also dilated with a balloon alone. At 18 months, she remains off antihypertensive medications and has had no enlargement of her aneurysm.

Illustrative Points. The surgical treatment of renal artery aneurysms is nephrectomy. Although there are no large, randomized, prospective trials since this condition is rather rare, it makes sense to try to preserve renal function whenever possible, especially in patients with bilateral disease. Collaboration with other specialties, in this case neuroradiology, is essential in planning such a case because they are the true experts when it comes to treating small vessel aneurysms nonsurgically.

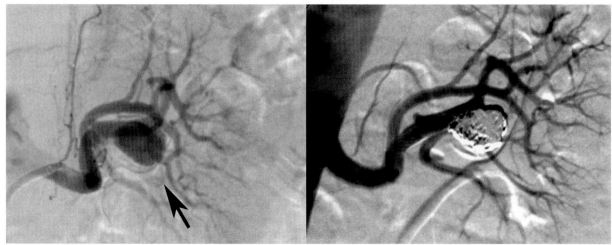

Figure 34.13   A. One of the unusual manifestations of fibromuscular dysplasia (FMD) is aneurysm formation as shown by the *arrow.* This aneurysm is well within the parenchyma of the kidney. **B.** After coiling, the aneurysm no longer fills with blood or contrast.

AORTOILIAC ANGIOPLASTY

Angioplasty has proved to be an effective technique for the treatment of aortoiliac occlusive atherosclerotic disease. Nevertheless, angioplasty should be performed *only in symptomatic patients* (111), or in patients with aortoiliac arterial occlusive disease prior to insertion of an intra-aortic balloon pump for high-risk coronary revascularization procedures or cardiogenic shock (112). The ideal candidates for aortoiliac angioplasty are patients with discrete stenosis. The technical success and 5-year patency rate of iliac angioplasty are related to many factors, including lesion length, adequacy of distal runoff, presence of occlusion or stenosis, and presence of diabetes (113–115). Based on this, the American Heart Association, in the Guidelines for Peripheral Percutaneous Transluminal Angioplasty of the Abdominal Aorta and Lower Extremity Vessels (111), stratified lesions according to the degree of complexity. Category 1 iliac lesions are concentric uncalcified stenoses <3 cm long. Category 2 lesions are calcified stenoses 3 to 5 cm long or eccentric stenoses <3 cm long. Category 3 lesions are stenoses 5 to 10 cm long or occlusions <5 cm long after thrombolytic therapy. Category 4 lesions are stenoses >10 cm long, occlusions >5 cm, extensive bilateral disease, or iliac stenoses in patients with abdominal aortic aneurysms. Although some consensus panels recommend that category 4 lesions should be treated surgically, there are very little data to support this recommendation, and in experienced hands even the most complex iliac lesions can be treated with interventional techniques. The overall technical success for categories 1 and 2 lesions is 95%. The 5-year patency rate is 80 to 85% for categories 1 to 2 lesions compared with a patency of 65 to 75% for category 3 lesions. A very similar classification applies for aortic lesions with a technical success of aortic angioplasty 90% for category 1 (<2 cm [111]).

Endovascular stents have been introduced in the treatment of aortoiliac atherosclerotic disease in an attempt to overcome the acute procedural complications such as abrupt occlusion and long-term restenosis rate. Several studies have suggested that the procedural success with these devices is as high (or higher) and the restenosis rate lower than balloon angioplasty alone (116–119). However, comparative studies between these two catheter-based approaches are scarce in the literature. Bosh et al. (120) performed a meta-analysis of six percutaneous transluminal angioplasty (PTA) studies (1,300 patients) with eight stent placement studies (816 patients). The technical success was higher for the stent patients (96% versus 91%, $P < .05$). The complication and mortality rates were similar for the two groups. The 4-year primary patency rate for stenosis (77% versus 65%) and occlusions (61% versus 54%) in patients with claudication was statistically higher in the stent-treated group. The 4-year primary patency rate for stenosis (67% versus 53%) and occlusions (53% versus 44%) in patients with critical ischemia was also statistically higher in patients treated with endovascular stents.

Until large prospective randomized trials comparing PTA versus stenting are available, whenever possible stenting should be the treatment of choice for aortoiliac arterial occlusive disease with surgery reserved for those patients who are not candidates for intervention.

Case 14. This 77-year-old hypertensive man complained of bilateral lower extremity fatigue with exercise and can walk less than 100 ft before stopping. He also complained of calf claudication. Resting relieved his symptoms. He also had severe hypertension. His examination was remarkable for diminished bilateral femoral and lower extremity pulses. His ankle-to-brachial index (ABI) was 0.5 bilaterally, and his BUN and creatinine were normal. Angiography revealed severe bilateral common iliac stenoses with extensive collaterals (Fig. 34.14A) and bilateral renal artery stenosis.

Bilateral common femoral artery access was obtained, and the lesions were crossed with hydrophilic guidewires. Two 35-cm-long 6F sheaths were advanced across the lesions bilaterally, and both common iliac arteries were dilated simultaneously with 7 × 40 mm balloons. Stents were then deployed, using 7 × 40 mm balloon-expandable stents bilaterally. Following this, the renal arteries were also stented with balloon-expandable stents.

Illustrative Points. This case is an example of the systemic nature of atherosclerosis and how a global approach to the diagnosis and management of these patients is important for providing optimal care. The iliac arteries are treated first to preserve vascular access for the other procedures. The renal arteries were treated at the same time; however, staging of these procedures is also a very reasonable choice, especially if the patient has renal insufficiency. Furthermore, this case demonstrates how valuable it is for cardiologists to possess the knowledge and skill to perform iliac intervention to prevent iliofemoral complications and to preserve access for peripheral, renal, and coronary intervention. Iliac stenting can be performed safely in patients before undergoing intra-aortic balloon counterpulsation during coronary intervention (112). It is important that the stent be well expanded to prevent the balloon catheter from catching on the stent.

FEMOROPOPLITEAL AND PROFUNDA FEMORIS ANGIOPLASTY

Femoropopliteal Angioplasty

Atherosclerotic occlusive disease is three to five times more common in the femoropopliteal artery than in the iliac artery. Among the femoropopliteal artery, occlusions are three times more frequent than stenosis, a distribution that is reversed in the aortoiliac system (121,122). Furthermore, most occlusions are long, which often precludes the use of angioplasty in many of these patients (121).

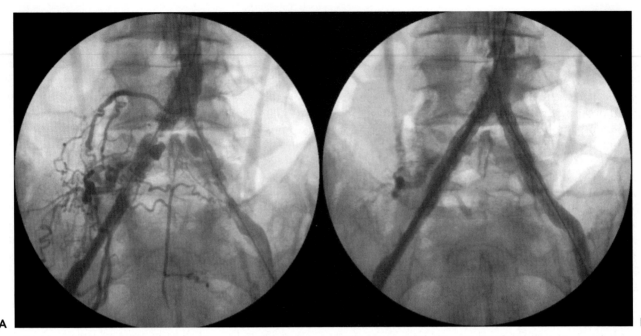

Figure 34.14   A. Severe bilateral common iliac stenosis with collaterals from the inferior mesenteric artery (IMA) and lumbar arteries to the right internal iliac. **B.** Poststenting with balloon-expandable stents. Notice the absence of collaterals and persistent filling of the right internal iliac artery.

Only symptomatic patients must be considered for percutaneous revascularization of the femoropopliteal artery (111). As is the case for the aortoiliac system, the technical success and the long-term patency rate vary according to the lesion characteristics. Treatment of short occlusions (<5 cm) and/or stenoses yield better results than treatment of long stenoses (>10 cm) and occlusions (111). The presence of patent runoff vessels correlates with long-term benefits, reflected in the improved outcome in patients with milder symptoms (114,123,124). Significant residual stenosis after angioplasty correlates with a poor long-term outcome (124), and absence of diabetes correlates with an improved patency rate (111).

In a study of 236 patients who underwent conventional balloon angioplasty in 254 femoral or popliteal arteries, procedural success was obtained in 96% (123,125). At 1-month follow-up, 88.8% of the procedures were considered successful (determined by an improved clinical grade and noninvasive vascular laboratory measurements). The success rate was 62.5% at 1-year follow-up and only 38% at 4-year follow-up. In this study, the most important independent predictors of long-term success, using multivariate analysis, were adequate distal runoff and lesion stenosis (rather than occlusion). Adar et al. (126) reviewed several published studies and found an early patency rate of 89% with a 3-year patency rate of 62% for patients with intermittent claudication compared with an early patency rate of 77% and a 3-year patency rate of 43% for limb salvage.

Although the long-term patency rate of femoropopliteal angioplasty is not as favorable as in PTA of the aortoiliac

system, particularly when treating long or occluded lesions, percutaneous revascularization is an alternative to surgery in selected patients or may complement surgical treatment in patients with more extensive disease. In contrast with the favorable impact of endovascular stents on patency rate in the aortoiliac system, these devices have not shown to improve the late patency rate when implanted in the femoropopliteal system. A European prospective study (127) showed that conventional femoropopliteal PTA has a 1-year primary patency rate (65%) equivalent to that of femoropopliteal Wallstent secondary patency rate (69%). In this study, early clinically significant restenosis was 38% and early thrombosis was 19% in the stent group. Another large prospective U.S. study showed similar lack of benefits with stents (128). On the other hand, the use of IntraCoil stents for significant stenoses of the femoropopliteal arteries appears promising. A pilot study of 93 patients with stenosis or occlusion (29%) of these vessels showed a 9-month target vessel revascularization of 82% (Fig. 34.15; 129). Likewise, a recent prospective randomized trial of drug-eluting, self-expanding coated stents with sirolimus for femoropopliteal stenosis showed significant inhibition of intimal proliferation compared with noncoated stents at 6-month follow-up (130). The preliminary, unpublished results of these drug-eluting femoral stents at 9 and 12 months are disappointing, however. Because no studies have shown a clear advantage of stent placement over conventional balloon angioplasty in the femoropopliteal system, most experts recommend that stents should be reserved for cases of suboptimal results, flow-limiting dissection, or abrupt occlusions after balloon angioplasty.

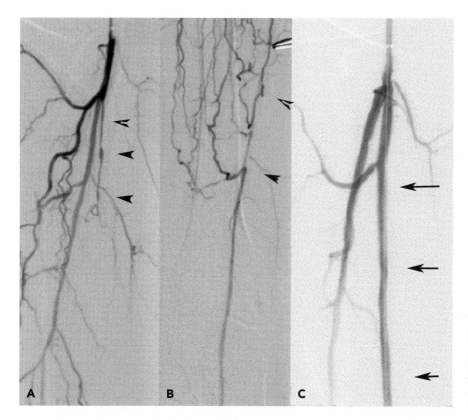

Figure 34.15 **A.** Long occlusion of the right superficial femoral artery before intervention *(arrows)*. **B.** Reconstitution of the distal superficial femoral artery (SFA) via collaterals from the profunda or deep femoral artery. **C.** Following recanalization and stenting *(arrows)*, there is a widely patent lumen.

Case 15. This 79-year-old woman with multiple sclerosis was referred with nonhealing ulcers in her right lower extremity, which she uses to transfer from wheelchair to bed. She was scheduled for amputation, but came for a second opinion. Her ABI was 0.4, and she had faint Doppler signals in both tibial arteries. Angiography revealed SFA occlusion with patent tibial vessels. She was scheduled for recanalization of the chronically occluded SFA, for limb salvage.

Access was obtained in the left common femoral artery (CFA) with a crossover 6F sheath using an extra-stiff Glidewire for support. Angiography was performed revealing an occlusion of the right SFA (Fig. 34.16 A and B). The lesion was crossed with a glide catheter and a straight and angled extra-stiff Glidewire. Balloon dilation failed to restore flow, so three self-expanding nitinol stents were deployed in a staggered manner and dilated with a 6 × 100 mm balloon. This restored normal flow to the lower extremity and foot. She successfully had limb salvage.

Illustrative Points. Most patients with SFA disease present with claudication. This patient was asymptomatic except for trauma to her legs that led her to have nonhealing ulcers. The decision to amputate is a difficult one; however, if a patient still uses her leg to walk or transfer from wheelchair to bed, then limb salvage is justified. The long length of stents in this SFA mandates close follow-up with duplex ultrasound and long-term aspirin and clopidogrel. There is no demonstrated role for platelet glycoprotein inhibitors at this time.

Profunda Femoris Artery Angioplasty

The profunda femoris artery (PFA) is an essential vessel for maintaining limb patency when occlusive atherosclerotic disease affects other vascular territories of the same limb. The profunda femoris artery not only provides the primary blood supply to the tissues of the thigh, but is also the most important collateral vessel for bypassing an obstructed or occluded superficial femoral artery (131–134). Historically, significant occlusive disease of the PFA has been treated surgically. However, atherosclerosis of the PFA is usually focal, preferentially involving the origin and the very proximal portion of the vessel in most limbs (135), making a percutaneous catheter-based approach an attractive alternative to surgical profundoplasty.

There are a handful of studies in the literature that have suggested that balloon angioplasty is a feasible alternative to surgery in selective patients (136–139). In a study from our institution (140), PFA balloon angioplasty was performed in 31 patients and 32 limbs with severe ischemia (41% had Fontaine class 2B, and 59% had Fontaine class 3 or 4). The superficial femoral artery was occluded in 20 limbs (62%). In 22 limbs (69%), an additional vessel was treated. Procedural success was attained in 91% of the limbs. The ABI increased from 0.5 ± 0.2 at baseline to 0.73 ± 0.2 after intervention ($P < .01$). In-hospital limb salvage in 30 survivors was 94% and the in-hospital amputation-free and revascularization-free survival was 90%. At a mean follow-up of 34 ± 20 months, no patients underwent amputation

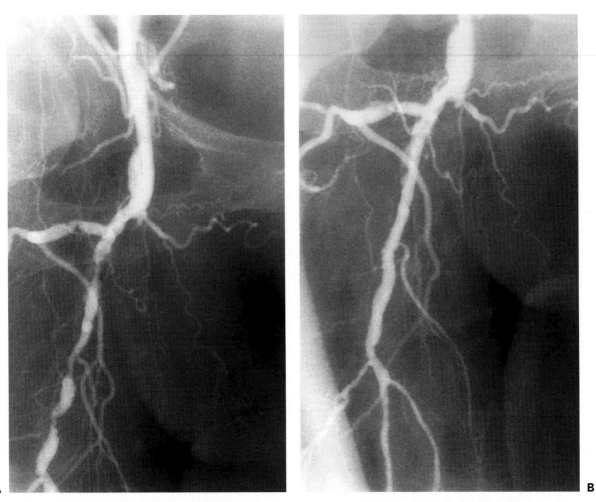

A   **B**

Figure 34.16 **A.** Severe, diffuse atherosclerotic involvement of the infrainguinal vessels. The superficial femoral artery (SFA) is occluded, and the profunda femoris is diffusely diseased. Involvement of the profunda femoris is typical in patients with long-standing diabetes. **B.** After rotational atherectomy and balloon angioplasty, an excellent angiographic result.

and five additional patients died. Freedom from revascularization of the 25 survivors was 88%. At follow-up, 88% had Fontaine class 1 or 2A , and only 12% had Fontaine class 2B or 3 ($P < .001$ compared with baseline). Based in our results as well as previous studies, we conclude that percutaneous revascularization of the profunda femoris artery is a safe and effective alternative to surgical treatment.

Case 16. This 65-year-old woman with coronary artery disease, bilateral carotid endarterectomy, and bilateral renal artery stenting presents with a 1-year history of progressive, Fontaine class 2B claudication in both lower extremities, worse on the left. She has known chronic bilateral SFA occlusion. The femoral pulses were normal, but the tibial pulses were weak and monophasic on the right and absent on the left. The ABI was 0.3 on the right and not obtainable on the left. Angiography performed at the referring institution revealed occlusion of the proximal SFA and serial high-grade stenoses of the left profunda femoris (Fig. 35.17A). Using contralateral retrograde femoral access, a 6F contralateral sheath was advanced to the left

external iliac artery. Baseline angiography was performed, and the lesion was crossed with a 0.035-inch Wholey wire; however, a 4 × 20 mm balloon could not be advanced across the lesions. The wire was exchanged for a floppy rotablator wire, and rotational atherectomy was performed on all three profunda femoris lesions using a 1.75-mm followed by a 2.25-mm burr (see Chapter 23). The lesions were then dilated with the 4 mm × 2 cm balloon at 6 atm. Postangioplasty angiography demonstrated a widely patent profunda femoris, and the ABI increased to 0.4 on the left (Fig. 35.17B). The patient was discharged with relief of his claudication the following morning.

Illustrative Points. The two most important arteries for maintaining a viable leg are the common femoral artery and the profunda femoris. The SFA is often occluded; however, in the presence of a patent profunda, the limb usually remains viable. In patients with chronic SFA occlusion and lesions of the common femoral or profunda, revascularization of these vessels can restore the patient to his or her previous mild level of symptoms even without revascularizing

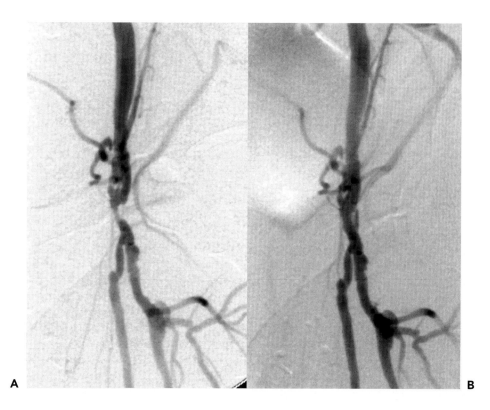

Figure 34.17 A. Critical stenosis in the left common femoral artery with moderate superficial femoral artery (SFA) origin stenosis at baseline. **B.** Postintervention, excellent filling of both the SFA and profunda with no persistent angiographic stenosis.

the chronically occluded SFA. This case also demonstrates that the use of coronary equipment and techniques can permit peripheral angioplasty success in otherwise undilatable lesions. Another option in this patient would have been to use coronary wires and balloons to cross and dilate the lesions; however, by debulking the lesions with rotablator in patients with lower extremity ischemia, it is easier to achieve an acceptable balloon result with lower pressure and less risk of dissection. The acute clinical success and limb salvage rate using the rotablator for undilatable lesions is >90%.

Common Femoral Artery Angioplasty

Atherosclerotic obstructive disease of the common femoral artery (CFA) is an infrequent clinical problem. This may be owing to an infrequent occurrence of this condition and/or to a low rate of detection of peripheral athero-occlusive disease (141–143).

Traditionally, surgical endarterectomy with or without patch angioplasty has been the preferred technique for CFA revascularization (144–147). Percutaneous revascularization of the CFA has rarely been described in the literature (148). We recently reported our experience of percutaneous transluminal intervention in 20 consecutive patients (21 limbs) with CFA lesions causing symptomatic limb ischemia (149). In 12 limbs, concurrent additional percutaneous intervention proximal or distal to the target CFA lesion were performed. Angiographic success was obtained in 100%, with procedural success (angiographic success

without a major in-hospital complications) in 90% and clinical success (procedural success and in-hospital improvement by at least one Fontaine functional class) in 81% of the limbs. The in-hospital Fontaine class improved by at least one functional class in 17 of 19 patients (90%), and the overall in-hospital event-free survival was 90% (18 of 20 patients). At follow-up (11.4 ± 6 months), the overall event-free survival was 90% (18 of 20 patients), and 17 of 19 patients (89%) continue to show improvement by at least one functional (Fontaine) class.

Case 17. A 66-year-old man with a history of coronary artery disease (CAD), coronary artery bypass graft (CABG), hypertension, and peripheral vascular disease with iliac bifurcation stenting and known bilateral SFA stenosis presented with severe left lower extremity claudication at 50 ft that was symptom limiting. His femoral pulse was normal, but his popliteal and tibial pulses could be detected only by Doppler, with an ABI of 0.3 on the left. Because of the iliac bifurcation stents, access was obtained through the brachial artery. Abdominal angiography revealed critical stenosis in the left common femoral artery with SFA occlusion (Fig. 34.15A). Angulated views were obtained using digital subtraction angiography (DSA). A 90 cm long × 6 cm sheath was inserted via the brachial artery into the abdominal aorta. Through this sheath, a 6.0 × 20 mm balloon and extra-stiff Glidewire were used to cross and dilate the lesion in the left CFA. The angiographic result of this PTA was excellent (Fig. 34.15B) and there was no gradient, so stenting was deferred. Hemostasis was obtained manually, and the patient was discharged in 6 hours without claudication.

Illustrative Points. Reports of atherosclerotic disease of the CFA and the treatment options available are uncommon in the literature (148). However, the recognition and management of CFA lesions is critical for the invasive/interventional cardiologist because this is the most commonly used site for vascular access.

Vascular insufficiency was confirmed at the office with an abnormal ABI, and the diagnosis of CFA stenosis was made at the time of angiography. The stenosis was treated successfully with PTA alone, and stenting was avoided. Stenting is a last resort in the CFA because of its necessity as a site for vascular access, as well as concerns regarding flexion of the joint, stent fracture, and the durability of vessel patency after percutaneous intervention. For this reason, we advocate the use of endovascular stents only after failed balloon angioplasty (provisional stent placement). Although obstructive disease of the CFA may occur as an isolated finding, it more frequently occurs in association with disease of other vascular territories, particularly the superficial femoral artery.

INFRAPOPLITEAL ANGIOPLASTY

The traditional indications for infrapopliteal angioplasty have been ischemic rest pain, ischemic ulceration, or gangrene (111). However, severe claudication that prevents minimal ambulation and patients with moderate to severe claudication undergoing femoropopliteal PTA have been advocated by some investigators as acceptable indications (150–154). It is possible that with the advent of small-profile balloons, improvement in technique, and increased operator experience, the use of tibial angioplasty will not be limited to the above-mentioned indications.

Some centers have reported tibial angioplasty to be an integral component in the treatment of limb salvage, which has led to a dramatic decrease in the amputation rate (152,153). Dorros et al. (151) reported an acute clinical and lesion success rate of 95% and 91% in 417 cases with critical limb ischemia or claudication. Significant complications (death, emergent bypass surgery, distal embolization, compartment syndrome, or amputation) occurred in 3%. At hospital discharge, 96% of their patients were clinically improved. The same investigators reported the long-term outcome of 284 critically ischemic limbs (154). The in-hospital clinical success (relief of rest pain or improvement of blood flow) was 95%. At the 5-year follow-up, clinically 91% of the limbs were salvaged, 8% required bypass surgery, and 9% required significant amputation. Hanna et al. (155) reported their results of infrapopliteal PTA for limb salvage in 29 diabetic patients. Technical success (<20% residual stenosis) was achieved in 26 patients (90%), and clinical success (avoidance of amputation and achievement of wound healing) at 12-month follow-up was obtained in 23 patients (79%).

Balloon angioplasty of the infrapopliteal vessels is an effective technique for treating patients with distal atherosclerotic occlusive disease. It has been used mainly in patients with limb-threatening ischemia and multisegment disease. Appropriate anatomic selection is a key factor in maximizing the benefit of the technique.

Case 18. This 65-year-old man with a 100-pack-a-year smoking history presented with a nonhealing ulcer of the second digit on his left lower extremity. He denies trauma to this extremity. He has a past history of severe coronary artery disease and peripheral vascular disease and had undergone bilateral SFA angioplasty 7 years earlier for symptom-limiting claudication. At that time, he had an 80% stenosis of his left tibioperoneal trunk, but this was not treated because his claudication was relieved by treatment of the SFA lesions alone. His ABI was 0.4 on the left, 0.8 on the right. Right common femoral access was obtained, and a pigtail catheter was used to perform bilateral aortography and runoff using digital subtraction and stepping of the table. Selective left lower extremity angiography was performed from the contralateral access using an IMA catheter and a Glidewire, demonstrating critical stenosis in the tibioperoneal trunk and occlusion of the posterior and anterior tibial vessels with single-vessel peroneal runoff (Fig. 34.18A). The IMA catheter was exchanged over an extra-stiff wire for a 6F multipurpose coronary guiding catheter, which was advanced to the distal popliteal artery. The lesions were crossed and dilated using a 0.014-inch extra-support wire and a 3.0 mm × 4.0 cm coronary balloon. Provisional stenting with a 3.0 × 8 mm coronary balloon-expandable stent was performed because of a suboptimal balloon result (Fig. 35.18B). The final angiogram revealed an excellent angiographic result (Fig. 35.18C). The patient was discharged on aspirin, clopidogrel, and antibiotics and follow-up at weekly intervals until he had complete healing of his ulcer. His ABI improved to 0.9 on the left. He continues to smoke, but now can walk to the store to buy cigarettes.

Illustrative points. The primary indication for tibial angioplasty in chronic lower extremity ischemia is critical limb ischemia, defined as rest pain, nonhealing ulcers, or gangrene. As this case demonstrates, critical limb ischemia requires stenosis or occlusion of all three infrapopliteal vessels, unlike coronary artery disease in which single-vessel involvement can cause severe symptoms or even death. In some centers with excellent results, tibial intervention is also offered to patients with severe claudication, but this is not the norm. Typically, claudication improves with treatment of the proximal stenoses (i.e., iliac and femoral) even in the presence of untreated severe tibial disease, as was illustrated by this man's course 7 years ago. Once critical limb ischemia is present, the interventionist and surgeon both attempt to provide pulsatile flow to the extremity, since the chances of healing are very low in the absence of pulsatile flow. The introduction of low-profile coronary systems into the periphery has greatly improved the success rate of infrapopliteal intervention. Stenting is not performed routinely in these lesions, but a prudent

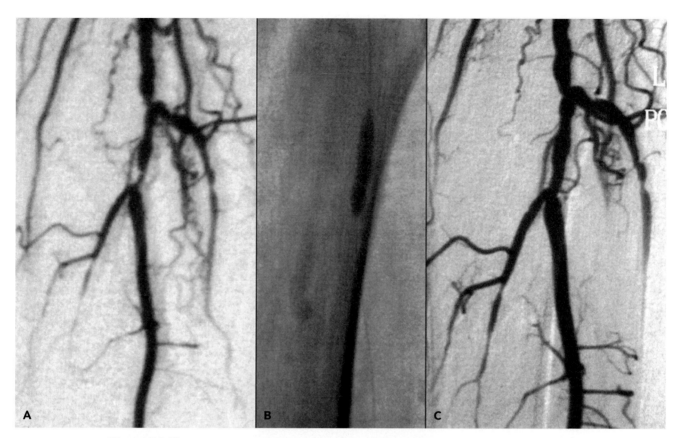

Figure 34.18 **A.** Single-vessel peroneal patency with high-grade stenosis in the tibioperoneal trunk. **B.** Because of a suboptimal percutaneous transluminal angioplasty (PTA) result, a balloon-expandable stent is deployed. **C.** Completion angiogram showing excellent angiographic result. Digital subtraction angiography (DSA) is a very useful technique when doing tibial intervention.

strategy of provisional stenting with antiplatelet therapy appears to be beneficial in cases such as this one. The surgical procedure of choice for critical limb ischemia is a distal vein bypass, which has a limb salvage rate of 70% and a 5-year patency of <50%. The important goal here is to heal the ulcer. Restenosis, if it occurs, may in fact be asymptomatic and does not require treatment. The role of drug-eluting stents in this location, while promising, has not been defined.

PERCUTANEOUS TREATMENT OF ACCESS SITE COMPLICATIONS

Access site complications are the most common complication of percutaneous intervention and include dissection, thrombosis, abrupt occlusion, rupture, bleeding, and pseudoaneurysm. The most serious of these complications, retroperitoneal bleeding and acute limb ischemia, are also life threatening (see Chapter 3). The following cases will illustrate how these complications can be managed percutaneously (156). Bear in mind, however, that in the hands of the inexperienced operator, these treatments may not be technically possible, so vascular surgery consultation or referral to an experienced interventionist may be prudent and necessary.

Case 19. This 64-year-old woman underwent uncomplicated percutaneous coronary intervention from the left common femoral artery (CFA) after failed right CFA access owing to inability to pass the guidewire up the external iliac. Four hours post-PCI, she was noted to be hypotensive and diaphoretic. Examination revealed a pulse of 90 bpm, cool clammy extremities, and fullness, guarding, and tenderness in the right lower quadrant (RLQ). The left lower quadrant (LLQ) and left CFA access sites were unremarkable. A clinical diagnosis of retroperitoneal hemorrhage was made and manual compression was applied. Her ACT was normal, and she had not received IIb/IIIa inhibitors. She was taken urgently back to the catheterization laboratory for angiography and intervention.

Angiography from the left common femoral artery with an IMA catheter across the aortic bifurcation revealed bleeding at the right external iliac/common femoral artery junction, the aborted access site (Fig. 34.19A). An extra-stiff 0.035-inch guidewire was placed in the right SFA, and a contralateral 6F Sheath was inserted. The bleeding site was tamponaded internally with an 8 × 40 mm balloon at 4 atm. Despite several long inflations of 5 minutes each, the bleeding continued. A 9 × 30 mm Wallgraft was deployed across the bleeding site in the distal external iliac and CFA without a sheath by using bony landmarks and roadmapping features (Fig. 34.19B). Angiography demonstrated cessation of bleeding. Hemostasis in the left CFA was obtained with a closure device. She was treated with clopidogrel and aspirin for 6 months. There were no sequelae.

Illustrative Points. This case demonstrates the quickest, and in our opinion, the optimal way to manage vascular access bleeding. The diagnosis of retroperitoneal bleeding is a clinical one and usually does not require CT scanning. "Ramee's Triad" of *ipsilateral lower quadrant fullness, tenderness, and guarding in a patient with hypotension postangiography is diagnostic of retroperitoneal bleeding.* The initial management of the patient includes manual compression over the common femoral puncture site and evaluation of the patient's hemostatic competence (ACT, prothrombin time (PT) if on warfarin, and platelet count). The most critical question is, "How can you tell if the bleeding has stopped?" CT scanning does not give you this information, and

duplex scanning also cannot tell the difference between free bleeding and a pseudoaneurysm, or contained bleeding. *In the hypotensive patient, we recommend return to the angiography suite if a skilled peripheral interventionist is available to use a combination of balloon inflation, thrombin injection, and/or stent graft deployment to manage hemorrhage. In a center without skilled peripheral interventionists, manual compression and urgent surgical consultation are warranted.*

Case 20. The patient is a 60-year-old man with a previous aortobifemoral bypass (AFB) graft who had diagnostic coronary and carotid angiography at a community hospital with manual compression of the CFA and was transferred to our institution for carotid stenting. On presentation, he complained of a cold, painful right lower extremity since the diagnostic angiogram 3 days earlier. On examination, he had ecchymosis without hematoma over the right groin and an absent pulse. Doppler exam revealed an absent common femoral pulse and monophasic Doppler signals in the feet. Duplex ultrasound confirmed our suspicion

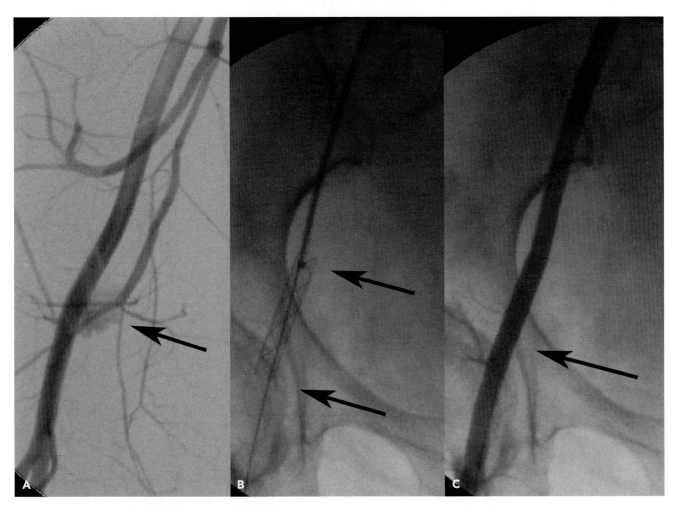

Figure 34.19 **A.** Site of bleeding is identified *(arrow)* by using digital subtraction angiography (DSA). A small amount of visible extravascular bleeding correlates with severe, life-threatening hemorrhage. **B.** Deployment of a Wallgraft just above the femoral head. **C.** Site of bleeding *(arrow)* is no longer visible after Wallgraftdeployment.

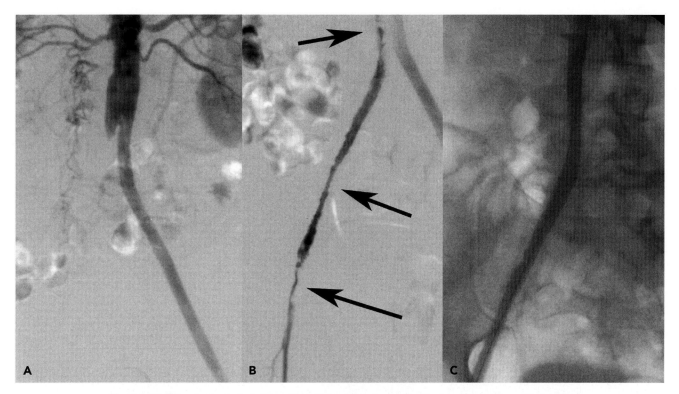

Figure 34.20 **A.** Occluded right-sided limb of the aortobifemoral graft. **B.** After mechanical thrombectomy, multiple high-grade stenoses remain in the graft and native vessel *(arrows).* **C.** Post-PTA and stenting, a widely patent graft and viable lower extremity.

that he had occluded the right limb of his aortobifemoral graft. Angiography was performed from the left brachial artery with a diagnostic catheter (Fig. 34.20A) demonstrating occlusion of the proximal right limb of the AFB graft.

The occlusion was traversed with an extra-stiff Glidewire and multipurpose catheter. An extra-support coronary guidewire was placed in the distal profunda, over which a coronary AngioJet rheolytic thrombectomy catheter (see Chapter 23) was inserted through a coronary multipurpose guiding catheter. Figure 34.20B demonstrates DSA of the high-grade stenosis that remains at the CFA and in the graft itself after thrombus removal. These lesions were dilated and stented, resulting in normalization of the pulse in the lower extremity and relief of the ischemia (Fig. 34.20C).

Illustrative Points. One cannot overemphasize the necessity of checking pulses postprocedure. This patient suffered an iatrogenic complication that was not recognized, despite his complaints, that was life and limb threatening. The *mortality* from acute limb ischemia is 20%. The cause of the complication was placement of a catheter across a critical but occult common femoral stenosis, leading to stasis during the procedure and thrombosis during manual compression. Although this complication may not be preventable, it is treatable by either mechanical thrombectomy (as in this case) or surgical thrombectomy with or without patch angioplasty or bypass. *Remember that when acute limb ischemia happens after a catheter-based procedure, there is usually an underlying vascular stenosis that becomes occluded*

during the procedure or during hemostasis. Unless this stenosis is relieved, recurrent thrombosis will occur.

Case 21. A 60-year-old man underwent PCI followed by suture closure of the common femoral access site. Forty-eight hours later, he returned with complaints of right lower extremity weakness and claudication. His pulses had been normal pre-PCI, and his CFA was normal on preclosure angiography. Post-PCI, his pulses were noted in the medical record to be diminished but present. On examination, he had absence of his right common femoral and tibial pulses, which were monophasic by Doppler. Color flow Doppler demonstrated subtotal occlusion of the right CFA.

The preliminary diagnosis was acute common femoral artery occlusion, so the patient underwent emergent angiography via the left common femoral artery using a 6F IMA diagnostic catheter (Fig. 34.21A). The lumen is narrowed and irregular with a filling defect. This appearance may represent dissection or suturing of the posterior wall to the anterior wall of the lumen. The lesion was crossed with difficulty with an angled hydrophilic 0.035-inch wire and 6 × 20 mm PTA balloon through a 6F crossover sheath. Despite multiple balloon inflations, the appearance never changed, so an 8 × 29 mm Wallstent was deployed, positioned so it would be below the inguinal ligament. It was dilated to 14 atm, and angiography demonstrated no residual stenosis (Fig. 34.21B). Hemostasis was obtained with a suture closure device in the left CFA.

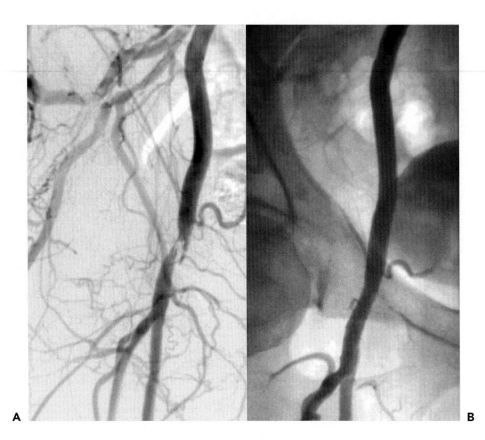

A

B

Figure 34.21 A. The site of occlusion is where the Perclose was deployed. This appearance may indicate dissection or suturing of the posterior wall of the vessel to the anterior wall. **B.** After stent deployment, limb viability is preserved.

Illustrative Points. Abrupt occlusion can occur regardless of one's choice of access site hemostasis, as these two cases (i.e., cases 20 and 21) illustrate. The importance of postprocedure evaluation of the peripheral pulses again cannot be underestimated. When dealing with suture-based or collagen-based occlusions, one must keep in mind that in addition to dissection and thrombosis, one must also consider suturing of the posterior wall (as in this case) or intravascular deployment of collagen. The operator in this case attempted PTA alone repeatedly without success before placing a stent, because the CFA is a site of extreme mobility and stent fracture is always a possibility. The placement of the stent below the inguinal ligament rather than across it will minimize the long-term risk of stent fracture in this case. Repeat access in this patient's stented right CFA is possible, but will require a high CFA stick, preferably with fluoroscopic guidance. The surgical alternative, open repair of the vessel, is associated with more acute morbidity, but the long-term outcome of each has not been compared. The placement of a stent does not compromise surgery at this site, as such stents are easily removed if subsequent operation is required.

Case 22. This 67-year-old man underwent diagnostic angiography with manual compression for hemostasis 3 days prior to presentation with a painful swelling at his access site. Physical examination revealed an exquisitely tender, pulsatile mass over the right CFA with ecchymosis. Duplex

ultrasound confirmed the presence of a right CFA pseudoaneurysm (PSD). The patient was scheduled for elective PCI of his coronary with percutaneous closure of the PSD. Using left CFA access, angiography was performed using a 6F crossover sheath with 30° of right anterior oblique (RAO) angulation, demonstrating the angiographic appearance of a PSD (Fig. 34.22A). The PSD sac was entered percutaneously perpendicular to the skin with the 18-gauge needle used for access and roadmapping technique. When pulsatile flow appeared through the needle, a syringe of contrast was injected to confirm the location in the PSD sac (Fig. 34.22B). A tuberculin syringe with 1,000 U thrombin USP in one mL of saline was attached to the needle and injected very slowly. Interval angiography was performed until the PSD was obliterated. Total thrombin injected was 400 U or 0.4 mL, and procedure time was 10 minutes. The patient was then heparinized and PCI was successfully performed.

Illustrative Points. The arterial pathology of access site bleeding and pseudoaneurysm are the same: a hole in the artery from the sheath. The only difference in the two is that in the PSD the connective tissue surrounding the artery has contained the bleeding, whereas in hemorrhage, the bleeding continues. Ultrasound-guided thrombin injection has been shown to be effective in treating PSD, and in patients who are not undergoing additional angiographic procedures, is our preference (156). Whether using duplex ultrasound or fluoroscopy, it is

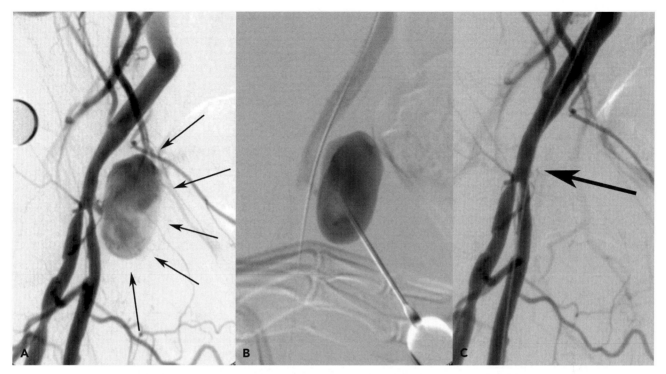

Figure 34.22 **A.** The angiographic appearance of a pseudoaneurysm sac (outlined by *arrows*). The hole in the artery is between the sac and the common femoral artery. **B.** Using roadmapping and fluoroscopy, a needle is inserted percutaneously into the pseudoaneurysm sac. Once pulsatile flow is obtained, contrast is injected to confirm location, followed by very slow injection of thrombin a tenth of a cc at a time. **C.** Final angiography demonstrates closure of the hole in the common femoral artery and obliteration of the pseudoaneurysm *(arrow)*.

critical to document proper placement of the needle and to *inject the thrombin very slowly* to avoid intravascular injection and acute limb ischemia. Manual compression has been abandoned because it causes severe pain and is unreliable. Surgery is rarely needed and reserved for refractory cases.

REFERENCES

1. Connors JJ III. Other extra cranial locations amenable to angioplasty and stenting. In: Connors JJ III, Wojak JC, eds. *Interventional Neuroradiology. Strategies and Practical Techniques.* Philadelphia: WB Saunders, 1999:484–499.
2. Schutz H, Yeung HP, Chiu MC, et al. Dilation of vertebral-artery stenosis. *N Engl J Med* 1981;304:732.
3. Motarjeme A, Keifer JW, Zuska AJ. Percutaneous transluminal angioplasty of the vertebral arteries. *Radiology* 1981;139:715–717.
4. Storey GS, Marks MP, Dake M, et al. Vertebral artery stenting following percutaneous transluminal angioplasty. Technical note. *J Neurosurg* 1996;84:883–887.
5. Feldman RL, Rubin JJ, Kuykendall RC. Use of coronary Palmaz-Schatz stent in the percutaneous treatment of vertebral artery stenoses. *Cathet Cardiovasc Diagn* 1996;38:312–315.
6. Jenkins JS, White CJ, Ramee SR, et al. Vertebral artery stenting. *Cathet Cardiovasc Intervent* 2001;54:1–5.
7. Smith RB III. The surgical treatment of peripheral vascular disease. In: Hurst JW, Schlant RC, Rackley CZ, Sonnenblick EH, Wenger NK, eds. *The Heart*, 7th ed. New York: McGraw-Hill, 1992:2235–2236.
8. Terada T, Higashida R, Halbach VV, et al. Transluminal angioplasty for atherosclerotic disease of the distal vertebral and basilar arteries. *J Neurol Neurosurg Psychiatry* 1996;60:377–381.
9. Takis C, Kwan ES, Pessin MS, Jacobs DH, Caplan LR. Intracranial angioplasty: experience and complications. *Am J Neuroradiol* 1997;18:1661–1668.
10. Clark WM, Barnwell SL, Nesbit G, et al. Safety and efficacy of percutaneous transluminal angioplasty for intracranial atherosclerotic stenosis. *Stroke* 1995;26:1200–1204.
11. Norris JW, Zhu CZ, Bornstein NM, et al. Stroke risk of asymptomatic carotid stenosis. *Stroke* 1991;22:1485–1490.
12. O'Holleran LW, Kennelly MM, McClurken M, et al. Natural history of asymptomatic carotid plaque: five-year follow-up study. *Am J Surg* 1987;154:659–662.
13. Autret A, Pourcelot L, Saudeau D, et al. Stroke risk in patients with carotid stenosis. *Lancet* 1987;1:888–890.
14. North American Symptomatic Carotid Endarterectomy Trial Collaborators. Beneficial effect of carotid endarterectomy in symptomatic patients with high-grade carotid stenosis. *N Engl J Med* 1991;325:445–453.
15. Executive Committee for the Asymptomatic Carotid Atherosclerosis Study. *JAMA* 1995;237:1421–1428.
16. Hsia DC, Krushat WM, Moscoe LM. Epidemiology of carotid endarterectomies among Medicare beneficiaries. *J Vasc Surg* 1992;16:201–208.
17. Roubin GS, Yadav S, Iyer SS, Vitek J. Carotid stent-supported angioplasty: a neurovascular intervention to prevent stroke. *Am J Cardiol* 1996;78(suppl 3A):8–12.
18. Diethrich EB, Ndiaye M, Reid DB. Stenting in the carotid artery: initial experience in 110 patients. *J Endovasc Surg* 1996;3:76–79.
19. Dorros G: Complications associated with extracranial carotid artery interventions. *J Endovasc Surg* 1996;3:166–170.
20. Yadav, Roubin GS, Vitek J, et al. Elective stenting of extracranial arteries. *Circulation* 1997;95:376–381.
21. Yadav, Roubin GS, Vitek J, et al. Late outcome after carotid angioplasty and stenting. *Circulation* 1996;94(suppl I):I-58.
22. Diethrich EB. Indications for carotid artery stenting: A preview of the potential derived from early clinical experience. *J Endovasc Surg* 1996;3:132–139.

23. Joint Officers of the Congress of Neurological Surgeons and the American Association of Neurological Surgeons: carotid angioplasty and stents: an alternative to carotid endarterectomy. *Neurosurgery* 1997;40:344–345.

24. Wholey MH, Wholey M, Bergeron P, et al. Current global status of carotid artery stent placement. *Cathet Cardiovasc Diagn* 1998;44:1–6.

25. Yadav JS, Wholey MH, Kuntz RE, et al. Protected carotid-artery stenting versus endarterectomy in high-risk patients. *N Engl J Med* 2004;351:1493–1501.

26. Marzewski DJ, Furlan AJ, St Louis PS, et al. Intracranial internal carotid artery stenosis: longterm prognosis. *Stroke* 1982;13:821–824.

27. Ingall TJ, Homer D, Baker HL, et al. Predictors of intracranial carotid artery arteriosclerosis. Duration of cigarette smoking and hypertension are more powerful than serum lipid levels. *Arch Neurol* 1991;48:687–691.

28. Caplan LR, Gorelick PB, Hier DB. Race, sex and occlusive cerebrovascular disease: a review. *Stroke* 1986;17:648–655.

29. Leung SY, Ng THK, Yuen ST, et al. Patterns of cerebral atherosclerosis in Hong Kong Chinese. Severity in intracranial and extracranial vessels. *Stroke* 1993;24:779–786.

30. Akins PT, Pilgram TK, Cross DT, Moran CJ. Natural history of stenosis from intracranial atherosclerosis by serial angiography. *Stroke* 1998;29:433–438.

31. Sacco RL, Kargman DE, Gu Q, et al. Race-ethnicity and determinants of intracranial atherosclerotic cerebral infarction. The Northern Manhattan Stroke Study. *Stroke* 1996;26:14–20.

32. Craig DR, Meguro K, Watridge C, et al. Intracranial carotid artery stenosis. *Stroke* 1980;13:825–828.

33. The EC/IC Bypass Study Group: failure of extracranial/intracranial arterial bypass to reduce the risk of ischemic stroke. Results of an international randomized trial. *N Engl J Med* 1985;313:1191–1200.

34. Chimowitz MI, Kokkinos J, Strong J, et al. The warfarin-aspirin symptomatic intracranial disease study. *Neurology* 1995;45:1488–1493.

35. Higashida RT, Tsai FY, Halbach VV, et al. Transluminal angioplasty for atherosclerotic disease of the vertebral and basilar arteries. *J Neurosurg* 1993;78:192–198.

36. Higashida RT, Tsai FY, Halbach VV, et al. Cerebral percutaneous transluminal angioplasty. *Heart Dis Stroke* 1993;2:497–502.

37. Dorros G, Cohn JM, Palmer LE. Stent deployment resolves a petrous carotid artery angioplasty dissection. *Am J Neurovasc Radiol* 1998;19:392–394.

38. Feldman RL, Trigg L, Gaudier J, Galat J. Use of coronary Palmaz-Schatz stent in percutaneous treatment of an intracranial carotid stenosis. *Cathet Cardiovasc Diagn* 1996;38:316–319.

39. Gomez CR, Vitek JJ, Roubin GS. Stenting of intracranial carotid artery. *J Endovasc Surg* 1998;5(suppl 1):I-12.

40. Ramee SR, Dawson R, McKinley, et al. Provisional stenting for symptomatic intracranial stenosis, using a multidisciplinary approach: acute results, unexpected benefit, and one-year outcome. *Cathet Cardiovasc Intervent* 2001;52:457–467.

41. Shadman R, Criqui MH, Bundens WP, et al. Subclavian artery stenosis: prevalence, risk, factors, and association with cardiovascular diseases. *J Am Coll Cardiol* 2004;44:18–23.

42. Perace WM, Yao JST. Upper extremity ischemia: overview. *Sem Vasc Surg* 1990;3:207–212.

43. Pokrowsky AV. Nonspecific aortoarteritis. In: Rutherford RB, ed. *Vascular Surgery*, 3rd ed. Philadelphia: WB Saunders, 1989.

44. Iwai T, Konno S, Hiejima K, et al. Fibromuscular dysplasia in the extremities. *J Cardiovasc Surg* 1985;26:496–501.

45. Joyce JW. The giant cell arteritides: diagnosis and the role of surgery. *J Vasc Surg* 1986;3:827–833.

46. Kretschmer G, Niederle B, Polterauer P, et al. Irradiation-induced changes in the subclavian and axillary arteries after radiotherapy for carcinoma of the breast. *Surgery* 1986;99:658–663.

47. Scher LA, Veith FJ, Samson RM, et al. Vascular complications of the thoracic outlet syndrome. *J Vasc Surg* 1986;3:565–568.

48. Bryan AJ, Hicks E, Lewis MH. Unilateral digital ischemia secondary to embolization from subclavian atheroma. *Ann Coll Surg Eng* 1989;71:140–142.

49. Reivich M, Holling HE, Roberts B, Toole JF. Reversal of blood flow through the vertebral artery and its effects on the cerebral circulation. *N Engl J Med* 1961;265:878–885.

50. Fields WS, Lemak NA. Joint study of extracranial arterial occlusion. VII. Subclavian steal—a review of 168 cases. *JAMA* 1972;222:1139–1143.

51. Granke K, Van Meter CH Jr, White CJ, Ochsner JL, Hollier LH. Myocardial ischemia caused by postoperative malfunction of an internal mammary coronary artery graft. *J Vasc Surg* 1990;11:659–664.

52. Olsen CO, Dunton RF, Maggs PR, Lahey SJ. Review of coronary-subclavian steal following internal mammary artery-coronary artery bypass surgery. *Ann Thorac Surg* 1988;46:675–678.

53. Hadjipetru P, Cox S, Piemonte T, Eisenhauer A. Percutaneous revascularization of atherosclerotic obstruction of aortic arch vessels. *J Am Coll Cardiol* 1999;33:1238–1245.

54. Bachman DM, Kim RM. Transluminal dilation for subclavian steal syndrome. *AJR Am J Roentgenol* 1980;135:995–996.

55. Burke DR, Gordon RL, Mishkin JD, et al. Percutaneous transluminal angioplasty of subclavian arteries. *Radiology* 1987;164:699–704.

56. Insall RL, Lambert D, Chamberlain J, et al. Percutaneous transluminal angioplasty of the innominate, subclavian and axillary arteries. *Eur J Vasc Surg* 1990;4:591–595.

57. Jain SP, Ramee SR, Ansel GM, et al. Endoluminal stenting of subclavian and innominate artery: acute and long term results from a multicenter stent registry [abstract]. *Circulation* 1998;98:I-484.

58. Ralph-Edwards AC, Williams WG, Coles JC, et al. Reoperation for recurrent aortic coarctation. *Ann Thorac Surg* 1995;60:1303–1307.

59. Johnson MC, Canter CE, Strauss AW, Spray TL. Repair of coarctation of the aorta of the aorta in infancy: comparison of surgical and balloon angioplasty. *Am Heart J* 1993;125:464–468.

60. Kron IL, Flanagan TL, Rheuban KS, et al. Incidence and risk of reintervention after coarctation repair. *Ann Thorac Surg* 1990;49:920–926.

61. Beekman RH, Rocchini AP, Behrendt DM, Rosenthal A. Reoperation for coarctation of the aorta. *Am J Cardiol* 1981;48:1108–1114.

62. Bromberg BI, Beekman RH, Rocchini AP, et al. Aortic aneurysm after patch aortoplasty repair of coarctation: prospective analysis of prevalence, screening tests and risks. *J Am Coll Cardiol* 1989;14:734–741.

63. Beekman RH, Rocchini AP, Behrendt DM, et al. Long-term outcome after repair of coarctation in infancy: subclavian angioplasty does not reduce the need for reoperation. *J Am Coll Cardiol* 1986;8:1406–1411.

64. Giovanni JV, Lip GYH, Osman K, et al. Percutaneous balloon dilation of aortic coarctation in adults. *Am J Cardiol* 1996;77:435–439.

65. Fawzy ME, Sivanandam V, Galal O, et al. One- to ten-year follow-up results of balloon angioplasty of native coarctation of the aorta in adolescents and adults. *J Am Coll Cardiol* 1997;30:1542–1546.

66. Lababidi Z. Percutaneous balloon coarctation angioplasty: long-term results. *J Intervent Cardiol* 1992;5:57–61.

67. Beekman RH, Rocchini AP, Dick M, et al. Percutaneous balloon angioplasty for native coarctation of the aorta. *J Am Coll Cardiol* 1987;10:1078–1084.

68. Yetman AT, Nykanen D, McCrindle BW, et al. Balloon angioplasty of recurrent coarctation: a 12-year review. *J Am Coll Cardiol* 1997;30:811–816.

69. McCrindle BW, Jones TK, Morrow WR, et al. Acute results of balloon angioplasty of native coarctation versus recurrent aortic obstruction are equivalent. *J Am Coll Cardiol* 1996;28:1810–1817.

70. Anjos R, Quershi SA, Rosenthal E, et al. Determinants of hemodynamic results of balloon dilation of aortic recoarctation. *Am J Cardiol* 1992;69:665–671.

71. Rao PS, Wilsson AD, Chopra PS. Immediate and follow-up results of balloon angioplasty of postoperative recoarctation in infants and children. *Am Heart J* 1990;120:1315–1320.

72. Ebeid MR, Prieto LR, Latson LA. Use of balloon-expandable stents for coarctation of the aorta: initial results and intermediate-term follow-up. *J Am Coll Cardiol* 1997;30:1847–1852.

73. Johnston TA, Grifka RG, Jones TK. Endovascular stents for the treatment of coarctation of the aorta: acute results and follow-up experience. *Cathet Cardiovasc Intervent* 2004;62:499–505.

74. Rao PS. Stents in treatment of aortic coarctation. *J Am Coll Cardiol* 1997;30:1853–1855.

75. Svensjo S, Bengtsson H, Bergqvist D. Thoracic and thoracoabdominal aortic aneurysm and dissection: an investigation based on autopsy. *Br J Surg* 1996;83:68–71.

76. Pressler V, McNamara JJ. Thoracic aortic aneurysm: natural history and treatment. *J Thorac Cardiovasc Surg* 1980;79:489–498.

77. Bickerstaff LK, Pairolero PC, Hollier LH, et al. Thoracic aortic aneurysms: a population-based study. *Surgery* 1982;92:1103–1108.

78. Perko MJ, Norgaard M, Herzog TM, Olsen PS, Schroeder TV, Pettersson G. Unoperated aortic aneurysms: a survey of 170 patients. *Ann Thorac Surg* 1995;59:1204–1209.

79. Kouchoukos NT, Dougenis D. Surgery of the thoracic aorta. *N Engl J Med* 1997;336:1876–1888.

80. Moreno-Cabral CE, Miller DC, Mitchell RS, et al. Degenerative and atherosclerotic aneurysms of the thoracic aorta: determinants of early and late surgical outcome. *J Thorac Cardiovasc Surg* 1984;88:1020–1032.

81. Mitchell RS, Dake MD, Sembra CP, et al. Endovascular stent graft repair of thoracic aneurysm. *J Thorac Cardiovasc Surg* 1996;11:1054–1052.

82. Dake M, Miller C, et al. Transluminal placement of endovascular stent-graphs for the treatment of descending thoracic aortic aneurysms. *N Engl J Med* 1994;331:1729–1734.

83. Hansen KJ, Wilson DB, Craven TE, et al. Mesenteric artery disease in the elderly. *J Vasc Surg* 2004;40:45–52.

84. Marston A. Diagnosis and management of intestinal ischaemia. *Ann R Coll Surg Engl* 1972;50:29–41.

85. Harward TR, Brooks DL, Flynn TC, Seeger JM. Multiple organ dysfunction after mesenteric artery revascularization. *J Vasc Surg* 1993;18:459–469.

86. Calderon M, Reul GJ, Gregoric ID, et al. Long-term results of the surgical management of symptomatic chronic intestinal ischemia. *J Cardiovasc Surg* 1992;33:723–728.

87. Schwartz LB, Gewertz BL. Chronic mesenteric arterial occlusive disease: clinical presentation and diagnostic evaluation. In: Perler BA, Becker GJ, eds. *Vascular Intervention. A Clinical Approach.* New York: Thieme, 1998:517–523.

88. Matsumoto AH, Angle JF, Tegtmeyer CJ. Mesenteric angioplasty and stenting for chronic mesenteric ischemia. In: Perler BA, Becker GJ, eds. *Vascular Intervention. A Clinical Approach.* New York: Thieme, 1998:545–556.

89. Silva JA, White CJ, Ramee SR, et al. Endovascular stent placement for the treatment of chronic mesenteric ischemia. (Submitted).

90. Jean WJ, Al-Bittar I, Xwicke DL, Port SCO, et al. High incidence of renal artery stenosis in patients with coronary artery disease. *Cathet Cardiovasc Diagn* 1994;32:8–10.

91. Olin JW, Melia M, Young JR, Graor RA, Risius B. Prevalence of atherosclerosis renal artery stenosis in patients with atherosclerosis elsewhere. *Am J Med* 1990;88:46N–51N.

92. Eyler WR, Clark GJ, Rian RL, Menninger DE. Angiography of the renal areas including a comparative study of renal arterial stenosis with and without hypertension. *Radiology* 1962;78:879–892.

93. White CJ, Ramee SR, Collins TJ, Jenkins JS. Renal artery stent placement. *J Endovasc Surg* 1998;5:71–77.

94. Olin JW, Young JR, DeAnna S, Grubb M, Childs MB. The utility of duplex ultrasound scanning of the renal arteries for diagnosing significant renal artery stenosis. *Ann Inter Med* 1995;122:833–838.

95. Meir GH, Sumpio B, Black HR, Gusberg RJ. Captopril renal scintigraphy: an advance in the detection and treatment of renovascular hypertension. *J Vasc Surg* 1990;11:770–777.

96. Working Group on Renovascular Hypertension. Detection, evaluation, and treatment of renovascular hypertension. Final report. *Arch Intern Med* 1987;145:820–829.

97. Weibull H, Bergqvist D, Bergentz SE, et al. Percutaneous transluminal angioplasty versus reconstruction of atherosclerotic renal artery stenosis: a prospective randomized study. *J Vasc Surg* 1993;18:841–852.

98. Hansen KJ, Starr SM, Sands RE, et al. Contemporary surgical management of renovascular disease. *J Vasc Surg* 1992;16:319–331.

99. Novick AC, Ziegelbaum M, Vidt DG, et al. Trends in surgical revascularization for renal artery disease. *JAMA* 1987;257:498–495.

100. Derkx F, Schalekamp M. Renal artery stenosis and hypertension. *Lancet* 1994;344:237–239.

101. Archibald GR, Beckmann CF, Libertino JA. Focal renal artery stenosis caused by fibromuscular dysplasia: treatment by percutaneous transluminal angioplasty. *Am J Radiol* 1988;151:593–596.

102. Cluzel P, Raygnaud A, Beyssen B, Pagny JV, Gaux JC. Stenosis of renal branch arteries in fibromuscular dysplasia: results of percutaneous transluminal angioplasty. *Radiology* 1994;193:227–232.

103. Losinno F, Zuccala A, Busato F, Zucchelli P. Renal artery angioplasty for renovascular hypertension and preservation of renal function: long-term angiographic and clinical follow-up. *Am J Radiol* 1994;162:853–857.

104. Weibull H, Bergqvist D, Jonsson K, Hulthen L, et al. Long-term results after percutaneous transluminal angioplasty of atherosclerotic renal artery stenosis: the importance of intensive follow-up. *Eur J Vasc Surg* 1991;291–301.

105. Dorros G, Prince C, Mathiak L. Stenting of a renal artery stenosis achieves better relief of the obstructive lesion than balloon angioplasty. *Cathet Cardiovasc Diagn* 1993;29:191–198.

106. Dorros G, Jaff M, Jain A, Dufek C, Mathiak L. Follow-up of primary Palmaz-Schatz stent placement for atherosclerotic renal artery stenosis. *Am J Cardiol* 1995;75:1051–1055.

107. Rees CR, Palmaz JC, Becker GJ, Ehrman KO, et al. Palmaz stent in atherosclerotic stenoses involving the ostia of the renal arteries: preliminary report of a multicenter study. *Radiology* 1991;181:507–514.

108. Blum U, Krumme B, Flugel P, et al. Treatment of ostial renal-artery stenoses with vascular endoprostheses after unsuccessful balloon angioplasty. *N Engl J Med* 1997;336:459–465.

109. White CJ, Ramee SR, Collins TJ, Jenkins JS, Escobar A, Shaw D. Renal artery stent placement: utility in lesions difficult to treat with balloon angioplasty. *J Am Coll Cardiol* 1997;30:1445–1450.

110. Khosla S, White CJ, Collins TJ, Jenkins JS, Shaw D, Ramee SR. Effects of renal artery stent implantation in patients with renovascular hypertension presenting with unstable angina or congestive heart failure. *Am J Cardiol* 1997;80:363–366.

111. Pentecost MJ, Criqui MH, Dorros G, et al. Guidelines for peripheral percutaneous transluminal angioplasty of the abdominal aorta and lower extremity vessels. A statement for health professionals from a special writing group of the councils on cardiovascular radiology, arteriosclerosis, cardio-thoracic and vascular surgery, clinical cardiology, and epidemiology and prevention, the American Heart Association. *Circulation* 1994;89:511–531.

112. Cooper CJ, Moore JA, Burket MW, et al. Intraaortic balloon pump insertion after percutaneous revascularization in patients with aortoiliac stenosis. *Circulation* 1998;98(suppl I):I-444.

113. Kwasnik EM, Siouffi SY, Jay ME, Khuri SF. Comparative results of angioplasty and aortofemoral bypass in patients with symptomatic iliac disease. *Arch Surg* 1987;122:288–291

114. Cambria RP, Faust G, Gusberg R, et al. Percutaneous angioplasty for peripheral arterial occlusive disease: correlates of clinical success. *Arch Surg* 1987;122:283–287.

115. Stokes KR, Strunk HM, Campbell DR, et al. Five-year results of iliac and femoropopliteal angioplasty in diabetic patients. *Radiology* 1990;174:977–982.

116. Vorwerk D, Gunther RW, Schurman K, Wendt G. Aortic and iliac stenoses: follow-up results of stent placement after insufficient balloon angioplasty in 118 cases. *Radiology* 1996;198:45–48.

117. Vorwerk D, Gunther RW, Schurmann K, et al. Primary stent placement for chronic iliac artery occlusions: follow-up results in 103 patients. *Radiology* 1995;194:745–749.

118. Strecker EPK, Hagen B, Liermenn D, et al. Iliac and femoropopliteal vascular occlusive disease treated with flexible tantalum stents. *Cardiovasc Intervent Radiol* 1993;16:158–164.

119. Spijkerboer AM. Peripheral angiography and angioplasty. *Curr Opin Radiol* 1992;4:81–87.

120. Bosch JL, Hunin K MGM. Meta-analysis of the results of percutaneous transluminal angioplasty and stent placement for aortoiliac occlusive disease. *Radiology* 1997;204:87–96.

121. Martin EC. Transcatheter therapies in peripheral and noncoronary vascular disease. *Circulation* 1991;(suppl):I1–I5.
122. Martin EC. The impact of angioplasty: a perspective. *J Vasc Intervent Radiol* 1992;3:511–514.
123. Johnston KW, Rae M, Hogg-Johnston SA, et al. Five-year results of a prospective study of percutaneous transluminal angioplasty. *Ann Surg* 1987;206:403–413.
124. Capek P, McLean GK, Berkowitz HD. Femoropopliteal angioplasty: factors influencing longterm success. *Circulation* 1991;83(suppl):170–180.
125. Johnston KW. Femoral and popliteal arteries: reanalysis of results of balloon angioplasty. *Radiology* 1992;183:767–771.
126. Adar R, Critchfield GC, Eddie DM. A confidence profile analysis of the results of femoropopliteal percutaneous transluminal angioplasty in the treatment of lower-extremity ischemia. *J Vasc Surg* 1989;10:57–67.
127. Do D, Triller J, Walpoth BH, et al. A comparison study of self-expandable stents vs balloon angioplasty alone in femoropopliteal artery occlusions. *Cardiovasc Intervent Radiol* 1992;15:306–312.
128. Martin EC, Katzen BT, Benenati JF, et al. Multicenter trial of the Wallstent in the iliac and femoral arteries. *J Vasc Intervent Radiol* 1995;6:843–849.
129. Ansel GM, Botti CF Jr, George BS, Kazienko BT. Clinical results for the training-phase roll-in patients in the IntraCoil femoropopliteal stent trial. *Cathet Cardiovasc Intervent* 2002;56:450–451.
130. Duda SH, Pusich B, Richter G, et al. Sirolimus-eluting stents for the treatment of obstructive superficial femoral artery disease. *Circulation* 2002;106:1505–1509.
131. Leeds FH, Gilfillan RS. Importance of the profunda femoris artery in the revascularization of the ischemic limb. *Arch Surg* 1961;82:25–31.
132. Morris GC Jr, Edwards E, Cooley DA, Crawford ES, De Bakey ME. Surgical importance of the profunda femoris artery. *Arch Surg* 1961;82:32–37.
133. Waibel PP, Wolff G. The collateral circulation in occlusions of the femoral artery: an experimental study. *Surgery* 1966;60:912–918.
134. Bernhard VM, Ray LI, Millitello JP. The role of angioplasty of the profunda femoris artery in revascularization of the ischemic limb. *Surg Gynecol Obstet* 1976;142:840–844.
135. Beales JSM, Adcock FA, Frawley JS, et al. The radiological assessment of disease of the profunda femoris artery. *Br J Radiol* 1971;44:854–859.
136. Motarjame A, Keifer JW, Zuska AJ. Percutaneous transluminal angioplasty of the deep femoral artery. *Radiology* 1980;135:613–617.
137. Waltman AC. Percutaneous transluminal angioplasty: iliac and deep femoral arteries. *AJR Am J Roentgenol* 1980;135:921–925.
138. Dacie JE, Daniell SJN. The value of percutaneous transluminal angioplasty of the profunda femoris artery in threatened limb loss and intermittent claudication. *Clin Radiol* 1991;44:311–316.
139. Varty K, London NJM, Ratliff DA, Bell PRF, Bolia A. Percutaneous angioplasty of the profunda femoris artery: a safe and effective endovascular technique. *Eur J Vasc Surg* 1993;7:483–487.
140. Silva JA, White CJ, Ramee SR, et al. Percutaneous profundoplasty in the treatment of severe lower extremity ischemia: immediate results and clinical follow-up. *J Endovasc Ther* 2001;8:75–82.
141. Mavor GE. The patterns of occlusion in atheroma of lower limb arteries. The correlation of clinical and arteriographic findings. *Br J Surg* 1964;5:352–364.
142. Haimovici H. Patterns of atherosclerotic lesions of the lower extremity. *Arch Surg* 1967;95:918–933.
143. Hirsch AT, Criqui MH, Treat-Jacobson D, et al. Peripheral arterial disease detection awareness, and treatment in primary care. *JAMA* 2001;286:1317–1324.
144. Archie JP Jr, Feldtman RW. Common femoral artery atherosclerotic occlusion. Difficult to diagnose but easy to treat. *Am Surg* 1982;48:339–340.
145. McGovern PJ Jr, Stark KR, Kaufman JL, Rosenberg N. Management of common femoral artery occlusion. A report of ten cases. *J Cardiovasc Surg* 1987;28:38–41.
146. Mukherjee D, Inahara T. Endarterectomy as the procedural of choice for atherosclerotic occlusive lesions of the common femoral artery. *Am J Surg* 1989;157:498–500.
147. Springhorn ME, Kinney M, Littooy FN, et al. Inflow atherosclerotic disease localized to the common femoral artery: treatment and outcome. *Ann Vasc Surg* 1991;5:234–240.
148. Johnston KW, Rae M, Hogg-Johnston SA, et al. 5-year results of a prospective study of percutaneous transluminal angioplasty. *Ann Surg* 1987;206:403–412.
149. Silva JA, White CJ, Quintana HA, Collins TJ, Jenkins JS, Ramee SR. Percutaneous revascularization of the common femoral artery for the treatment of limb ischemia. *Cathet Cardiovasc Intervent* 2004;62:230–233.
150. Horvath W, Oertl M, Haidinger D. Percutaneous transluminal angioplasty of crural arteries. *Radiology* 1990;177:565–569.
151. Dorros G, Jaff MR, Murphy KJ, Mathiak L. The acute outcome of tibioperoneal vessel angioplasty in 417 cases with claudication and critical limb ischemia. *Cathet Cardiovasc Diagn* 1998;45:251–256.
152. Veith FJ, Gupta SK, Wengerten KR, et al. Changing arteriosclerotic disease patterns and management strategies in lower-limb-threatening ischemia. *Ann Surg* 1990;212:402–414.
153. Veith FJ, Gupta SK, Samson RH, et al. Progress in limb salvage by reconstructive arterial surgery combined with new or improved adjunctive procedures. *Ann Surg* 1981;194:386–401.
154. Dorros G, Jaff MR, Dorros AM, et al. Tibioperoneal (outflow lesion) angioplasty can be used as primary treatment in 235 patients with critical limb ischemia. Five-year follow-up. *Circulation* 2001;104:2057–2062.
155. Hanna GP, Fujise K, Kjellgren O, et al. Infrapopliteal transcatheter interventions for limb salvage in diabetic patients: importance of aggressive interventional approach and role of transcutaneous oximetry. *J Am Coll Cardiol* 1997;30:664–669.
156. Samal AK, White CJ, Collins TJ, Ramee SR, Jenkins JS. *Cathet Cardiovasc Intervent* 2001;53:259–263.

Index

A

AAA. See Abdominal aorta aneurysm (AAA)
Abciximab, 61–63
  dose, 65t
  for PCI, 61
Abciximab Before Direct Angioplasty and
    Stenting in Myocardial Infarction
    Regarding Acute and Long-term
    follow-up (ADMIRAL), 62
Abdominal aorta, 263–264, 582–592
  access, 585
  anatomy of, 263
  balloon inflation, 586
  complications, 586
  diagnostic angiography, 585–586
  periprocedural care, 586
  renal arteries, 582–583
  stent deployment, 586
Abdominal aorta aneurysm (AAA), 582
Abdominal aortic disease
  clinical manifestations of, 263–264
Abdominal aortography, 257f, 261f, 264
ABI. See Ankle brachial index (ABI)
Ablative laser techniques, 476–480
  calcified lesions, 479–480
  catheter delivery systems, 477
  in-stent restenosis, 480
  laser generation, 476
  laser-tissue interactions, 476–477
  procedure, 478
  pulsed excimer laser, 477f
  results, 478
  total occlusions, 479
  undilatable lesions, 478–480
ACC. See American College of Cardiology
    (ACC)/American Heart Association
    (AHA)
Access site complications
  percutaneous treatment of, 781–785
Accreditation Council for Graduate
    Medical Education (ACGME)
  training guidelines, 10
Acculink for Revascularization of Carotids
    in High Risk Patient, 578
Acetylcholine, 216
Acetylcysteine, 54
  dose, 68t
Acetyl salicylic acid (ASA)
  allergic reactions to, 57
  for cardiac catheterization, 55–56
  guidelines for, 57
ACGME. See Accreditation Council for
    Graduate Medical Education
    (ACGME)
ACIP. See Asymptomatic Cardiac Ischemia
    Pilot (ACIP)

ACS Multi-Link Stent Clinical Equivalence
    in De Novo Lesions Trial
    (ASCENT), 503t
Acute aortic dissection
  aortic fenestration, 572f
Acute coronary syndrome, 381
Acute limb ischemia
  clinical categories of, 563t
Acute myocardial infarction (AMI),
    358–360
  coronary stents, 532–534
  phasic flow-velocity signals, 361f
  primary angioplasty for, 458f
Acute pulmonary embolism, 677–679,
    738
  arterial blood gases, 678
  chest radiograph, 678
  diagnosis, 677
  echocardiography, 678–679
  electrocardiogram, 678
  ELISA, 678
  gadolinium-enhanced magnetic
    resonance angiography, 678
  imaging tests, 678–679
  laboratory tests, 678–679
  spiral chest CT scans, 678
  venous ultrasound, 678
  ventilation-perfusion lung scanning,
    678
Acute right ventricular infarction, 738
Acute subvalvar (infundibular)
    obstruction, 609
Additional Value of NIR Stents
    for Treatment of Long
    Coronary Lesions (ADVANCE)
    trial, 527
Adenosine
  assessing pulmonary vasoreactivity,
    703t
  for coronary flow studies, 349t
  dose, 66t, 70t
  inducing coronary hyperemia, 346
ADMIRAL. See Abciximab Before Direct
    Angioplasty and Stenting in
    Myocardial Infarction Regarding
    Acute and Long-term follow-up
    (ADMIRAL)
Adolescents
  congenital obstructive lesions
    percutaneous balloon pulmonary
    valvuloplasty, 608–609
ADRC. See Automatic dose rate control
    (ADRC)
Adriamycin
  cardiotoxicity
    endomyocardial biopsy, 407

ADVANCE. See Additional Value of NIR
    Stents for Treatment of Long
    Coronary Lesions (ADVANCE) trial
Afterload, 315–316
Afterload mismatch, 324
AHA. See American College of Cardiology
    (ACC)/American Heart Association
    (AHA)
AIMI. See AngioJet Rheolytic
    Thrombectomy in Patients
    Undergoing Primary Angioplasty
    for Acute Myocardial Infarction
    (AIMI) trial
Air kerma, 14
  defined, 15t
Alcohol septal ablation, 720–721
Allen test
  modified, 98f
Allergic reactions
  to acetyl salicylic acid, 57
  with coronary angiography, 201
    premedication for, 201
  with diagnostic catheterization, 52–53
  to iodinated contrast agents, 52
A-Med percutaneous ventricular assist
    device, 424f, 425
American College of Cardiology
    (ACC)/American Heart
    Association (AHA)
  angioplasty guidelines, 455–456
  cardiac catheterization indications
    guidelines, 5
  cardiac catheterization laboratory
    guidelines, 11t
  freestanding cardiac catheterization
    labs, 9
  lesion classification system, 448t
AMETHYST trial, 487
AMI. See Acute myocardial infarction
    (AMI)
Amiodarone
  dose, 66t
Amipaque, 32
Amplatz catheters, 189f, 193f
Amplatz curves, 435
Amplatz device, 750
Amplatzer Duct Occluder, 628f, 754f, 755f
Amplatzer Muscular VSD, 624f
Amplatzer PFO Occluder, 620f
Amplatzer Septal Occluder, 622f
Amrinone
  dose, 69t
  influencing myocardial contractility,
    316t
Amyloid heart disease, 712–714, 715f
  endomyocardial biopsy, 716f

Amyloidosis, 715
  hemodynamics of, 713f–714f
Anaphylactoid reactions. *See* Allergic
    reactions
Anatomic variants, 204
Aneurysm. *See also* Abdominal aorta
    aneurysm (AAA)
  aortic
    aortic angiography, 261
    CT angiography, 255f
  endoluminal thoracic, 769
  pulmonary artery, 249–250
  saccular
    thoracic aorta, 769f
  thoracic aortic, 261, 571
Angina
  pacing-induced, 295
  unstable
    cardiac catheterization for, 5
    IABP, 422
Angiographically silent disease, 374f
Angiographic blood flow estimation,
    341–345
Angiographic projections, 207f
Angiographic room, 24
  equipment
    quality assurance, 24
Angiography. *See also* Coronary
    angiography; Pulmonary
    angiography
  bypass graft
    catheters, 194f
  digital subtraction
    aortic stenosis, 589f
    with pulmonary arterial injections,
      239
  internal mammary, 196f
  mitral regurgitation, 644
  noninvasive, 254–255
  peripheral, 254
  saphenous vein graft, 195f
Angiography Versus IVUS-Directed stent
    placement (AVID), 377
Angioguard, 486
AngioJet Rheolytic Thrombectomy in
    Patients Undergoing Primary
    Angioplasty for Acute Myocardial
    Infarction (AIMI) trial, 481–482
Angiomax
  dose, 65t
  guidelines for, 61
  during PCI, 56t, 60–61
Angioplasty. *See also* Percutaneous balloon
    angioplasty
  angiography, 367f
  aortoiliac, 775
    complications of, 591–592
  balloon
    limitations of, 492–494
    replacement by stenting, 462f
  brachiocephalic artery, 766–767
  candidates for, 761t
  carotid, 579–580, 761–762
  carotid balloon, 577f
  celiac artery, 769–774, 771f
  coronary system, 434, 434f
  femoropopliteal, 775–777

focused force, 438
  guidelines, 455–456
  infrapopliteal, 780–781
  intracranial, 762–766, 764f
  LIMA, 460f
  mesenteric artery, 769–774, 771f
  percutaneous transluminal coronary, 5
  profunda femoris artery, 777–779
  pulsed excimer laser, 478
  sensor-guidewire use, 345
  subclavian, 766–767
  training, 462
  vertebral arteries, 759–761, 760f
Angioscopy, 379–382
  clinical experience, 381–382
  image interpretation, 380–381
  imaging systems, 379–380
AngioSeal, 94, 95f
Angiovist (Berlex), 31
  structure, 32f
Angled pigtail catheters, 91f
Angulated views
  geometry of, 207f
Ankle brachial index (ABI), 272
Anomalous coronary takeoff
  brachial approach to, 114
Antecubital fossa
  anatomy of, 108f
Antegrade femoral artery puncture, 256f
Anterior projection (AP), 38
Anterior tibial artery (AT), 270
Anteroposterior diameter
  measurement of, 141f
Anticoagulants
  contraindicating interventional
    cardiology, 7
Anticoagulants in the secondary
    prevention of events in coronary
    thrombosis (ASPECT) trial, 378
Aorta. *See also* Abdominal aorta;
    Coarctation of the aorta; Thoracic
    aorta
  iliac
    revascularization, 566t
  infrarenal
    revascularization, 566t
    MRA, 255f
  perforation with diagnostic
    catheterization, 51
Aortic aneurysm
  aortic angiography, 261
  CT angiography, 255f
Aortic arch, 573–574
  angioplasty, 759–767
Aortic diagnosis, 571–573
Aortic dissection, 261–262
  acute
    aortic fenestration, 572f
Aortic pressure, 319f
  central, 142f, 144f
    measurement of, 143f
Aortic regurgitation, 653–656, 654f, 655f
  acute *vs.* chronic, 655, 655t
  angiographic assessment, 655–656
  catheterization protocol, 656
  hemodynamic assessment, 654
  premature mitral valve closure, 654

Aortic stenosis, 647–653, 647t, 648f
  angiographic assessment, 649
  aortic valve replacement, 652–653
  with appreciable cardiomegaly, 652
  Carabello sign, 648–649
  cardiac output with mean aortic systolic
    pressure gradient, 177f
  catheterization protocol, 649–653
  digital subtraction angiography, 589f
  femoral artery, 180f
  hemodynamic assessment, 647–648
  left ventricular pressure tracings, 178f
  with low cardiac output
    assessment of, 181–182
  MRI ventriculogram, 232f
  neonatal critical, 612–613
  nitroprusside infusion in, 182t
  percutaneous valve replacement and
    repair, 558
  pressure gradients in, 179f
  pressure recordings, 650f
  without appreciable cardiomegaly,
    650–652
Aortic valve area
  calculation of, 177–181
    example, 178–180
    pitfalls, 181
    pullback hemodynamics, 181
    transducer calibration, 181
Aortic valve prosthesis, 658f
Aortic valvuloplasty. *See* Balloon aortic
    valvuloplasty
Aortobifemoral graft, 783f
Aortography, 254
Aortoiliac angioplasty, 775
  complications of, 591–592
Aortoiliac disease
  stents for, 589–590
  thrombolytic therapy, 590
Aortoiliac obstructive disease, 588–589
Aortoiliac percutaneous transluminal
    angioplasty
  with surgery, 591
Aortopulmonary (bronchial) collaterals,
    628
AP. *See* Anterior projection (AP)
Apical left ventricular puncture, 103–104,
    104f
APV. *See* Average peak velocity (APV)
Aramine
  dose, 70t
ARAS. *See* Atherosclerotic renal artery
    stenosis (ARAS)
Area length method, 306
Arrhythmias
  atrial, 631
  with cardiac ventriculography, 230
  malignant ventricular
    with endomyocardial biopsy, 404
  supraventricular
    with endomyocardial biopsy, 404
Arterial blood gases
  acute pulmonary embolism, 678
Arterial occlusive disease. *See also*
    Peripheral arterial occlusive disease
    (PAD)
  lower extremities, 270–271

Arterial pressure waveform
  transformation, 146f
Arterial Revascularization Therapies Study
  II (ARTS II), 527, 528f
Arterial venous fistula
  with endomyocardial biopsy, 405
Arteriography
  carotid, 266–268
  pulmonary
    balloon-tipped catheters, 237
    pigtail catheters, 237
  renal
    atherosclerotic renal artery stenosis,
      269
  vertebral, 264–265
Arteriovenous difference, 148–149
Arteriovenous fistula
  with diagnostic catheterization, 45–46
Arteriovenous guidewire loop, 752f
Arteriovenous oxygen difference, 153–154
  related to cardiac index, 149f
Artery. *See also* individual artery(ies)
  angiograms, 359f
  FFR, 359f
ARTS II. *See* Arterial Revascularization
  Therapies Study II (ARTS II)
ASA. *See* Acetyl salicylic acid (ASA)
Ascending aortic pressure waveform,
  142f
ASCENT. *See* ACS Multi-Link Stent Clinical
  Equivalence in De Novo Lesions
  Trial (ASCENT)
ASD. *See* Atrial septal defect (ASD)
ASO. *See* Atherosclerosis obliterans (ASO)
ASPECT. *See* Anticoagulants in the
  secondary prevention of events in
  coronary thrombosis (ASPECT) trial
Aspirin
  with cardiac catheterization, 55–56
  with coronary stents, 507–508
  dose, 65t
  during PCI, 56t
  with percutaneous balloon angioplasty,
    440, 442
Asymptomatic Cardiac Ischemia Pilot
  (ACIP), 456
AT. *See* Anterior tibial artery (AT)
Atenolol
  dose, 67t
Atherectomy, 467–488. *See also* Directional
  coronary atherectomy (DCA); High-
  speed mechanical rotational
  atherectomy
  extraction, 462
  IVUS, 376
  rotational, 462
Atherectomy devices
  in coronary stents implantation, 507
Atheromatous plaque
  compression, 443
    redistribution, 443
  distal embolization, 443
  microembolization, 443
Atherosclerosis
  carotid arteries, 265–266
  diffuse
    assessment of, 358

Atherosclerosis obliterans (ASO), 263–264
Atherosclerotic occlusive disease,
  263–264
Atherosclerotic renal artery stenosis
  (ARAS), 268–269, 583–584
  renal arteriography, 269
Atrial arrhythmias, 631
  with diagnostic catheterization, 48–49
Atrial extrasystole
  with diagnostic catheterization, 48
Atrial fibrillation, 643f
  with diagnostic catheterization, 48–49
Atrial flutter
  with diagnostic catheterization, 48–49
Atrial pacing
  clinical use of, 301–302
Atrial pacing tachycardia, 298f
Atrial septal defect (ASD), 167–168, 622f,
  749–751, 749f, 750f, 751f
  pathophysiology of, 617
  transcatheter closure, 621–622
Atrial septal defect secundum
  diagnostic catheterization
    indications for, 120t
Atrial septal defect sinus primum
  diagnostic catheterization
    indications for, 120t
Atrial septal defect sinus venosus
  diagnostic catheterization
    indications for, 120t
Atrial septum
  anatomy of, 616
Atrioventricular canal defect
  diagnostic catheterization
    indications for, 120t
Atrioventricular malformation (AVM)
  pulmonary, 629f
Atrium
  left
    congenital heart disease, 122
    retrograde catheterization of, 113f
  right
    intracardiac echo from within, 102f
Atropine sulfate
  dose, 66t
Automatic dose rate control (ADRC), 20
Average peak velocity (APV), 345
AVID. *See* Angiography Versus IVUS-
  Directed stent placement (AVID)
AVM. *See* Atrioventricular malformation
  (AVM)
AVOXimeter 1000, 153

B

Balanced dominant circulation, 204
Balloon angioplasty. *See also* Percutaneous
  balloon angioplasty
  branch pulmonary artery stenosis,
    610–611
  branch vessel occlusion, 450f
  vs. coronary stents, 525t
  limitations of, 492–494
  replacement by stenting, 462f
Balloon aortic valvuloplasty, 552–558,
  554f, 556f
  calcific aortic stenosis, 553
  clinical results, 556–558

complications, 556–558
  elderly, 557f
  improved aortic orifice area, 553
  indications for, 553t
  long-term results, 558
  noncalcific aortic stenosis, 553
  technique, 553–556
Balloon compliance characteristics, 438
Balloon counterpulsation. *See* Intraaortic
  balloon counterpulsation (IABP)
Balloon expandable stents, 463
Balloon flotation catheters
  flow-directed, 111
Balloon mitral angioplasty. *See*
  Percutaneous balloon mitral
  valvuloplasty
Balloon pericardiotomy
  percutaneous, 738–740, 739f, 740f
Balloon-tipped catheters
  pulmonary arteriography, 237
  for pulmonary arteriography, 237
Balloon *vs.* Optimal Atherectomy Trial
  (BOAT), 469
Barbiturates
  influencing myocardial contractility,
    316t
BARI. *See* Bypass Angioplasty
  Revascularization Investigation
  (BARI) study
Basilar artery, 575
BAT. *See* Bivalirudin Angioplasty Trial
  (BAT)
Beam modulation, 16f
Belgium Netherlands stent (BENESTENT),
  493, 494f, 524
Benadryl
  for cardiac catheterization, 55
  dose, 68t
  for premedication prior to contrast
    agents, 52
BENESTENT. *See* Belgium Netherlands
  stent (BENESTENT)
Beraprost
  for PPH, 690t
Berenstein catheters, 267
Berlex, 31
  structure, 32f
Berman Balloon catheters, 238
Bernoulli equation, 339f
BES, 503t
BeStent, 496f
Bicycle ergometer exercise, 291f
Bicycle exercise
  supine
    dilated cardiomyopathy, 290t
Bidirectional shunts
  calculation of, 168
Bifurcation disease, 667–668
Biodegradable stents, 496
BiodivYsio stent in controlled trial
  (DISTINCT), 499f, 503t
Bioptomes
  modern, 397
Biotronik Tensum stents, 498
Bird's Nest filters, 237
Bivalirudin
  PCI, 56t

Bivalirudin (Angiomax)
    dose, 65t
    guidelines for, 61
    during PCI, 56t, 60–61
Bivalirudin Angioplasty Trial (BAT), 60
Blood flow measurement, 148–161
Blood/intima (luminal) border, 372
Blood lactate, 297f
Blood oxygen saturation
    in right heart, 163–164
Blue digit syndrome
    stents for, 574f
BOAT. See Balloon vs. Optimal
        Atherectomy Trial (BOAT)
Body surface area
    calculating, 150f
Bosentan
    for PPH, 689, 690, 690t
Boston Scientific SYMBIOT stents, 500f
Bracco, 31
    structure, 32f
Bracco-Squibb Acist device, 190f
Brachial arteriotomy
    suture repair of, 115f
Brachial artery
    isolation of, 109f, 110f
Brachial cutdown, 107–117
    catheter selection, 111
    hand numbness, 117
    indications for, 107
    instruments for, 108f
    preprocedure evaluation, 107–108
    radial pulse loss, 117
    right heart catheter advancement,
        111–113
    special techniques, 114
    troubleshooting, 117
    vessel repair and aftercare, 114–117
Brachiocephalic artery angioplasty,
        766–767
Brachytherapy, 30–31
Brachytherapy devices, 462
Bradyarrhythmias
    with diagnostic catheterization, 49
Branch pulmonary artery stenosis,
        609–611
    balloon angioplasty, 610–611
    bladed cutting balloons, 611
    intravascular stents, 611
Branch vessel occlusion
    balloon angioplasty, 450f
Bridging collaterals, 213f
Brockenbrough system, 102f
Bronchial collaterals, 628
BSC/EPI FilterWire, 484f
Bumetanide (Bumex)
    dose, 69t
Bumex
    dose, 69t
Bundle branch block
    with diagnostic catheterization, 49
BX Stent, 496f
Bypass Angioplasty Revascularization
        Investigation (BARI) study, 455
    numerical coding system, 203f
Bypass graft angiography
    catheters, 194f

C
CABG. See Coronary artery bypass graft
        (CABG)
CAD. See Coronary artery disease (CAD)
CADILLAC. See Controlled Abciximab and
        Device Investigation to Lower Late
        Angioplasty Complications
        (CADILLAC)
Caffeine
    influencing myocardial contractility,
        316t
Calcium blocking agents
    influencing myocardial contractility,
        316t
Calcium chloride
    dose, 69t
Calcium salts
    influencing myocardial contractility,
        316t
Cannulated coronary venous system,
        345f
Can Routine Ultrasound Improve Stent
        Expansion (CRUISE) trial, 377
CAPTIVE trial, 486
CAPTURE. See Chimeric c7E3 Fab
        Antiplatelet Therapy in Unstable
        Angina Refractory to standard
        treatment (CAPTURE)
Carabello sign
    aortic stenosis, 648–649
Cardiac allograft vasculopathy, 212
Cardiac Assist TandemHeart system, 424f
Cardiac catheterization. See also Left heart
        catheterization
    acetyl salicylic acid, 55–56
    adjunctive pharmacology for, 55–71
    anxiety with, 55
    aspirin for, 55–56
    complications of, 36–71, 37t
    contraindications to, 7t
    death in course of, 39
    diazepam for, 55
    diphenhydramine for, 55
    first documented, 4f
    in fontan physiology, 630–631
    history of, 3–12
    hypotension with, 54
    indication for, 5–7
    indications for, 5
    laboratory guidelines, 11t
    laboratory pharmacology
        at Brigham and Women's Hospital,
        65t–71t
    pain with, 55
    practice standards, 3–12
    procedure, 12
    respiratory insufficiency with, 55
    retained equipment with, 55
    volume overload with, 54–55
Cardiac catheterization facility, 9–12
    director, 11–12
    hospital vs. freestanding, 9
    laboratory caseload, 11
    outpatient, 9–10
    physician caseload, 11, 11t
    quality assurance, 11–12
    training standards, 10–11

Cardiac catheterization labs
    coronary Doppler flow velocity, 347f
    freestanding
        guidelines for, 9
Cardiac hypertrophy, 327
Cardiac output
    determination of, 150–151
    factors influencing, 149–150
    lower limits of, 148
    measurement errors, 154–155
    upper limits of, 149
Cardiac transplantation. See Heart
        transplantation
Cardiac ventriculography, 222–232
    analysis, 228–229
    arrhythmias with, 230
    complications, 230–231
    contrast materials
        complications, 231
    fascicular block, 230
    filming projection and technique,
        227–228
    hazards, 230–231
    injection catheters, 222–224
    injection rate and volume, 225–226
    injection site, 224–225
    mitral regurgitation, 229
    pigtail catheters, 222–223
Cardiogenic shock
    IABP, 420–421
Cardiomyopathy. See also Hypertrophic
        cardiomyopathy (HCM)
    restrictive, 711–716, 737–738
Cardiopulmonary support systems (CPS),
        412
CardioSEAL devices, 620f, 752f, 753f
CardioSEAL Septal Occluder, 619f
Carotid and Vertebral Artery Transluminal
        Angioplasty Study (CAVATAS) trial,
        578
Carotid angioplasty, 579–580, 761–762
Carotid arteries, 265–268, 576–578
    anatomy of, 265
    angioplasty, 759–767
    extracranial atherosclerosis, 265–266
    internal
        color duplex image, 267f
    puncture with endomyocardial biopsy,
        405
    stenosis, 581f
    stents, 576f
Carotid arteriography, 266–268
Carotid balloon angioplasty, 577f
Carotid endarterectomy (CEA), 577
Carotid revascularization
    stroke prevention, 578t
Carotid stenting, 580t
Castillo curves, 111
Catecholamines
    influencing myocardial contractility,
        316t
Catheter impact artifacts, 145
Catheter-induced coronary spasm, 218
Catheterization. See also Cardiac
        catheterization; Diagnostic
        catheterization; Femoral
        artery/vein catheterization

left heart
  alternative sites for, 97–104
  axillary artery percutaneous entry, 97
  brachial artery percutaneous entry, 97
  radial artery percutaneous entry,
    97–100
percutaneous femoral arterial and
    venous
  regional anatomy, 81f
transradial
  complications, 99
  equipment, 99, 99t
trans-septal, 4
  equipment for, 102f
  from right femoral vein, 101
Catheters, 257–258. *See also* Pigtail
    catheters
  Amplatz, 189f, 193f
  balloon flotation
    flow-directed, 111
  balloon-tipped
    pulmonary arteriography, 237
    for pulmonary arteriography, 237
  Berenstein, 267
  Cobra, 258f
  Cook NIH Torcon blue, 224
  Cordis NIH, 224
  for coronary angiography, 189f
  Davies, 267
  dilatation
    percutaneous balloon angioplasty,
      437–438
    size, 439
  electrical conductance, 232
  Eppendorf, 224
  7F Berman Balloon, 238
  flow-directed balloon flotation, 111
  8F Sones I
    insertion into brachial artery, 110f
  Gensini, 223f
  Goodale-Lubin, 111, 111f
  Grollman, 238, 238f
  Gruentzig, 436
  guiding
    deep engagement, 435f
    percutaneous balloon angioplasty,
      434–435
  Headhunter, 258f, 267
  hockey stick, 194f, 435
  IABP, 413
  injection
    cardiac ventriculography, 222–224
  internal mammary, 194f
  Judkins
    spasm, 217f
  Judkins left, 189f
  Judkins right, 189f
  Kawai flexible endomyocardial biopsy,
    397f
  left heart, 111f
    advancing, 113–114
    brachial cutdown, 111
    used from femoral approach, 91f
  left ventricular conductance, 232f
  Lehman, 223f
  midcavitary position, 224f
  multielectrode impedance, 309f

multipurpose, 194f, 258f, 435
NIH, 223f, 224
Nyman, 238f
original dilatation, 436
over-the-wire (OTW), 437
pacing, 294–295
perfusion balloon, 438f
peripheral angiographic, 258f
Proxis proximal protection, 484f
pulmonary embolism, 681–683
right heart, 111f
  advancing from right atrium to
    pulmonary artery, 112f
  advancing from right atrium to
    ventricle, 88f
  brachial cutdown, 111
right-sided heart, 85f
Simmons, 258f, 267
Sones, 111, 111f, 113, 189f, 199f, 200f,
    223, 223f
SOS-omni, 258f
Swan-Ganz, 85f, 113
Teflon Gensini, 91f
tennis racket, 258f
van Aman, 238
ventriculographic, 223f
Voda, 435
VTK, 267
Wexler, 194f
Catheter-tip spasm, 216
Catheter-transducer system, 138f
Catheter whip artifacts, 145
CAVATAS. *See* Carotid and Vertebral Artery
    Transluminal Angioplasty Study
    (CAVATAS) trial
Caves-Schulz bioptome, 396, 396f
CCD. *See* Charge-coupled device (CCD)
CEA. *See* Carotid endarterectomy (CEA)
Celiac artery angioplasty, 769–774, 771f
CE-MRA. *See* Contrast-enhanced MRA
    (CE-MRA)
Central aortic pressure, 142f, 144f
  measurement of, 143f
Cerebral artery
  middle
    occlusion of, 765f
Cerebrovascular accidents
  from diagnostic catheterization, 41–42
CFA. *See* Common femoral artery (CFA)
CFR. *See* Coronary flow reserve (CFR)
Charge-coupled device (CCD), 22
Children
  diagnostic catheterization
    death as complication of, 39
  radiation
    induced neoplasms, 27
Chimeric c7E3 Fab Antiplatelet Therapy in
    Unstable Angina Refractory to
    standard treatment
    (CAPTURE), 62
Cholesterol embolization, 586
Chronic heart failure, 697f
Chronic limb ischemia
  clinical categories of, 564t
Chronic thromboembolic pulmonary
    hypertension, 245–246, 248f
  angiographic findings in, 248t

Chronic thromboembolic pulmonary
    hypertension (CTEPH), 686–688,
    687f, 689f
Cimetidine, 58
  for coronary angiography allergic
    reactions, 201
  for premedication prior to contrast
    agents, 52
Cinefluorographic system
  acquisition (cine), 20
  cine camera, 21
  DICOM PACS, 22–24
  feedback, 20
  flat-panel x-ray detectors, 22
  fluoroscopy, 20
  focal spot, 19
  generator, 18, 18f
  image detection, 20
  image display and processing, 22
  image framing, 21f
  imaging modes, 19
  operation of, 17–24
  patient size and dose, 20f
  radiation production and control, 18
  video, 22
  x-ray beam filtration and shaping, 19
  x-ray detection and recording, 20–22
  x-ray image intensifier, 21, 21f
  x-ray tubes, 18–19, 19f
Cine left ventriculography, 226
Circumflex arteries
  left
    ostia of, 204
Cisatracurium besylate (Nimbex)
  dose, 68t
CK-MB. *See* Creatine kinase myocardial
    band (CK-MB)
CLASSICS. *See* Clopidogrel Aspirin Stent
    International Cooperative Study
    (CLASSICS)
Clopidogrel
  with bleeding, 58
  for coronary artery disease, 662
  with coronary stents, 508
  dose, 65t
  PCI, 56t
  during PCI, 56t
  with percutaneous balloon angioplasty,
    440, 442
  pretreatment with, 57, 57f
Clopidogrel Aspirin Stent International
    Cooperative Study (CLASSICS),
    508
Clopidogrel in Unstable Angina Recurrent
    Events (CURE), 56, 58
Coarctation of the aorta, 259–261,
    614–616, 746–748, 747f, 748f,
    749f
  aortography, 570f
  diagnostic catheterization
    indications for, 120t
  pediatric technique, 614
  pre-stent implant, 615f
  results, 614–615
  stent angioplasty, 615–616
Cobra catheters, 258f
Collateral pathways, 213f

Collateral quantitative assessment
catheterization lab, 361–368
COMBAT trial, 470
Common femoral artery (CFA), 270, 592, 592f
angioplasty, 779–780, 779f
revascularization, 566t
Complete AV block
with diagnostic catheterization, 49
Complete heart block
with diagnostic catheterization, 49
Complications, 767–769, 768f
Congenital cath lab, 605
Congenital heart disease, 118–128, 605–631, 744–757
angiographic projections, 125t
angiography, 125–126
confounding physiologic abnormalities in, 119t
cyanosis, 127
diagnostic catheterization
indications for, 120t
Down syndrome, 126
oximetry, 122–125
pregnancy, 126
pressure measurement, 122–125
special circumstances, 126–128
surgical repairs, 119t
vascular access, 119–122
Congenital lesions
with shunts, 616
Congenital mitral stenosis, 616
Congenital obstructive lesions, 605–611
percutaneous balloon pulmonary
valvuloplasty, 607–609
adolescents, 608–609
complications, 609
pediatric modifications, 608
Congenital pulmonary venous
obstruction, 685f
Connective tissue disorders, 262–263
Conray, 31
structure, 32f
CONSERVE, 503t
Constrictive pericarditis, 731–736
pulmonary capillary wedge, 733f
right atrial pressure, 733f
treatment, 735–736
ventricular pressure, 733f, 734f
Continuous-infusion method, 155
Continuous Quality Improvement
cardiac catheterization facility, 12
Contractility indices
left ventricular systolic performance, 320t
Contrast agents, 258–259
adverse effects of, 200–201
inadequate injection of, 217
structure, 32f
superselective injection of, 217–218
Contrast-enhanced MRA (CE-MRA), 255
Contrast-induced nephropathy, 53, 258
Contrast ventriculography
alternatives to, 231–323
respiration during
patient instructions, 227

Controlled Abciximab and Device
Investigation to Lower Late
Angioplasty Complications
(CADILLAC), 534
Cook NIH Torcon blue catheters, 224
Cordis Angioguard filter, 484f
Cordis Hydrolyser, 480–481
Cordis NIH catheters, 224
Coronary anatomy, 202–204, 203f
Coronary angiography, 187–219
adverse effects of, 200–201
allergic reactions, 201
premedication for, 201
allergic reactions with, 201
angiographic views, 204–205
brachial approach, 199–200
contraindications to, 7t
current indications for, 187–188
femoral approach, 189–198
catheter insertion and flushing, 189–190
free arterial grafts, 193–194
gastroepiploic graft cannulation, 197–198, 198f
internal mammary cannulation, 193–196
left coronary ostium cannulation, 191–193
pressure waveform damping and ventricularization, 190–191
right coronary ostium cannulation, 193
saphenous vein cannulation, 193–194
history, 188–189
injection technique, 201–202, 202f
left anterior oblique projection, 205–207
left lateral projections, 207–208
lesion quantification, 208–210
posteroanterior projections, 207–208
pressure tracings, 191f
radial approach, 199–200
renal dysfunction with, 53–54
right anterior oblique projection, 205
selective, 4
stenosis, 202–210
Coronary angioplasty system, 434, 434f
Coronary arteriography
saphenous vein graft disease, 669
ST-segment elevation myocardial
infarction (STEMI), 663
total coronary occlusion, 671
unprotected left main disease, 673
Coronary arteriovenous fistula, 755–757, 756f, 757f
Coronary artery. See also Right coronary
artery (RCA)
left
coronary collaterals, 212f
native, 487–488
occluded collateralized, 364f
perforation of, 450–451
Coronary artery bypass graft (CABG), 585f
brachial cutdown, 114
Coronary artery disease (CAD), 660–674
clopidogrel for, 662

congenital heart disease, 127–128
coronary arteriography, 662f
coronary arteriography indications, 660–661
medical management, 662
nonatherosclerotic, 211–217
percutaneous revascularization
indications, 660–661
stable, 660–662
Coronary artery dissection
after excimer laser angioplasty, 479f
Coronary artery fistula, 214f
Coronary artery obstruction
left
coronary collaterals, 212f
Coronary Artery Surgery Study, 39
Coronary atherectomy, 467–488. See also
Directional coronary atherectomy
(DCA)
Coronary blood flow
case studies in, 367
regulation of, 337–340
Coronary blood flow measurements
clinical applications of, 355–361
Coronary calcification, 374f
Coronary circulation
regulation of, 338t
Coronary collaterals, 210, 211f
Coronary debulking, 470
Coronary Doppler flow velocity, 347–349
Coronary fistula, 211, 628
Coronary flow reserve (CFR), 340f, 340t, 351f, 353f
measurement of, 347–354
Coronary flow velocity, 362f
Coronary hyperemia, 345–346
adenosine inducing, 346
Coronary intervention
deferral of, 355–356
Coronary origin and distribution
congenital variants of, 218–219
Coronary pressure, 354f
Coronary resistances, 337f
Coronary Revascularization Using
Integrilin and Single Bolus
Enoxaparin (CRUISE), 59
Coronary sinus adenosine, 297
Coronary sinus cannulation technique, 344–345
Coronary spasm, 215f
Coronary stenosis, 209f
myocardial blood flow, 209f
Coronary stents, 492–534. See also Stents
in acute myocardial infarction, 532–534
adjunct pharmacotherapy, 507–508
after failed balloon angioplasty, 523–524
in aorto-ostial lesions, 529
aspirin with, 507–508
vs. balloon angioplasty, 525t, 526f
balloon-expandable vs. self-expanding, 499–500
bare metal
vs. balloon angioplasty, 529t, 532f, 533t
vs. DES, 528t
implantation of, 506t

randomized studies, 499t
  vs. stent trials, 500–502
bare metal restenosis
  brachytherapy, 511t
in bifurcation lesions, 529–531, 530f
vs. bypass grafts
  randomized trials, 514t
carbon-coated
  randomized studies, 499t
in chronic total occlusion, 528–529
classification of, 495
clinical outcomes, 523–534
coatings, 498, 498t
complications of, 508–513
composition of, 495–498
configuration of, 496–497
coronary perforation, 512–513
covered, 499
design of, 495–502
development of, 492–494
diabetes mellitus, 527
direct, 506–507
early designs of, 496f
embolization, 512
future directions, 534
glycoprotein IIb/IIIa inhibitors
    with, 508
guide catheter selection, 502
guidewire catheter selection, 502
historical perspectives, 492–494
implantation technique, 502–507, 505t
    plaque modification during, 507
    in small vessels, 524–526
    technical aspects of, 502–507
infectious endarteritis, 513
in long lesions, 527
modular, 498
multicellular, 497–498
in multivessel disease, 527
outcomes, 502–506
overcoming limitations of, 494
PCI, 661
for PCI, 661
potential drug carrier vehicles, 515t
real-world, 524
restenosis, 510–511
in saphenous vein grafts, 532
selection of, 502–506, 505t
side-branch occlusion, 511–512
slotted tubes, 497–498
stainless steel *vs.* stent trials, 503t
vs. surgical revascularization, 513
thrombosis, 508–509, 509f
in unprotected left main lesions, 531
wire coils, 497
Coronary vasodilation
  mediators of, 338t
Coronary vasodilator reserve (CVR), 338,
    345, 352f
  abnormal, 216–217
Coronary vasomotion, 337f
Coronary vasospasm, 213–216
Coronary venous efflux, 343–344
Coronary venous oximetry thermodilution
    flow, 344f
Costs
  IVUS, 379

CPK. *See* Creatinine phosphokinase (CPK)
CPS. *See* Cardiopulmonary support
    systems (CPS)
Creatine kinase myocardial band (CK-MB)
    following directional coronary
    atherectomy, 469
Creatinine phosphokinase (CPK), 449
CrossFlex LC Stent, 496f
CRUISE study. *See* Coronary
    Revascularization Using Integrilin
    and Single Bolus Enoxaparin
    (CRUISE)
CRUISE trial. *See* Can Routine Ultrasound
    Improve Stent Expansion (CRUISE)
    trial
Crush stent technique, 530
CTEPH. *See* Chronic thromboembolic
    pulmonary hypertension
    (CTEPH)
Culotte stent technique, 530
Cumulative dose
  defined, 15t
CURE. *See* Clopidogrel in Unstable Angina
    Recurrent Events (CURE)
Curved Kelly forceps, 109
Cutdown technique, 4
CVR. *See* Coronary vasodilator reserve (CVR)
Cyanosis
  congenital heart disease, 127
Cypher stents, 517, 518
  malapposition, 523
  randomized trials of, 519t
  restenosis, 522
  vs. TAXUS, 520

D
Damping, 139f
  defined, 134t
Danish multicenter stent study
    (DANSTENT), 504t
DAP. *See* Dose-area product (DAP)
Davies catheters, 267
Davis double-end soft tissue retractors,
    108f
DCA. *See* Directional coronary
    atherectomy (DCA)
DeBakey classification, 262
Decompensated heart failure
  from dilated cardiomyopathy, 699f, 700f
Deep femoral artery (DFA), 270
Deep venous thromboembolism
  with diagnostic catheterization, 44f
Deltatrac II, 152
DES. *See* Drug-eluting stents (DES)
Device failures, 451
DFA. *See* Deep femoral artery (DFA)
Diabetes mellitus
  coronary stents, 527
  PAD, 272
DIABETES trial, 518
Diagnostic catheterization
  allergic reactions, 52–53
  arrhythmias with, 47–49
  bradyarrhythmias with, 49
  cerebrovascular complications, 41–42
  conduction disturbances with, 47–49
  death as complication of, 37–39

left main disease, 38
left ventricular dysfunction, 38
prior bypass, 39
valvular heart disease, 38
great vessels perforation with, 50–51
heart perforation with, 50–51, 50f
infection with, 51–52
local vascular complications, 42–47
MI as complication of, 39–41
Diastolic distensibility *vs.* compliance,
    325f
Diastolic filling period (DFP)
  left ventricular pressure tracings, 174f
Diastolic function, 324–330
Diastolic heart failure, 711–716
Diastolic left ventricular regional wall
    motion, 330f
Diastolic left ventricular wall thinning,
    330
Diazepam (Valium)
  for cardiac catheterization, 55
Diffuse atherosclerosis
  assessment of, 358
Diffuse reflectance NIR spectroscopy, 386,
    388
Digital image receptors, 22f
Digitalis glycosides
  influencing myocardial contractility,
    316t
Digital subtraction, 308
Digital subtraction angiography (DSA)
  aortic stenosis, 589f
  with pulmonary arterial injections, 239
Digital surgery, 257
Digoxin
  dose, 70t
Dilatation catheters
  percutaneous balloon angioplasty,
    437–438
  size, 439
Dilated cardiomyopathy, 695–700, 695f
  biopsy diagnosis, 408t
  decompensated heart failure from, 699f,
    700f
  endomyocardial biopsy, 407
  etiology, 695t
  exercise, 701f
  idiopathic, 696t
  milrinone for, 701f
  progressive dyspnea in, 696–698
  supine bicycle exercise, 290t
Diltiazem, 215, 216f
  dose, 67t, 71t
  influencing myocardial contractility,
    316t
  for PPH, 690t
Diphenhydramine (Benadryl)
  for cardiac catheterization, 55
  dose, 68t
  for premedication prior to contrast
    agents, 52
Diprivan
  dose, 68t
Directional coronary atherectomy (DCA),
    462, 467–476, 468f
  bifurcation lesions, 469, 470f
  deep wall resection, 469

Directional coronary atherectomy (DCA)
(*continued*)
device description, 467–468
in-stent restenosis, 470, 471f
new approaches to, 470
procedure, 468
results, 468–469
tissue analysis, 469
Direct stenting, 441
Direct thrombin antagonists
with percutaneous balloon angioplasty,
440
Direct thrombin inhibitors (DTI), 60–61
DIRP. *See* Dose at the interventional
reference point (DIRP)
Dissections, 376f
Distal Embolic Protection During Primary
Angioplasty in Acute Myocardial
Infarction (EMERALD), 487
Distal filters, 486–487
Distal occlusion systems (Guardwire),
483–484
Distal protection devices, 462
DISTINCT. *See* BiodivYsio stent in
controlled trial (DISTINCT)
Dobutamine (Dobutrex)
dose, 69t
Dobutamine stress magnetic resonance
imaging, 667f
Dobutrex
dose, 69t
Dofetilide
dose, 66t
Dominant circulation
left, 203–204
Dopamine
dose, 69t
Doppler average peak velocity, 353f
Doppler frequency shift, 347
Doppler ultrasound
intracoronary physiologic
measurements, 357
Dorsalis pedis (DP) artery, 270
Dose (x-ray)
defined, 15, 15t
measuring points, 16f
Dose-area product (DAP)
defined, 15t
Dose at the interventional reference point
(DIRP)
defined, 15t
Dosimetry
definitions, 15t
Douglas bag, 152
Down syndrome
congenital heart disease, 126
DP. *See* Dorsalis pedis (DP) artery
DRASTIC. *See* Dutch Renal Artery Stenosis
Intervention Cooperative Study
(DRASTIC)
Drug-eluting stents (DES), 378, 513–523, 515f
components of, 515–516
failed, 516, 520–523
proven, 516–518, 518–520
restenosis after, 520–522, 522f
thrombosis, 523
in unprotected left main lesions, 531

DSA. *See* Digital subtraction angiography
(DSA)
DTI. *See* Direct thrombin inhibitors (DTI)
Dual antiplatelet therapy, 495f
Ductus arteriosus
congenital heart disease, 122
Duet device, 94, 95f
Duet Stent, 496f
Dutch Renal Artery Stenosis Intervention
Cooperative Study (DRASTIC), 583
Dynamic exercise, 283–292
exercise factor, 285
exercise index, 284–285
left ventricular diastolic function,
286–287, 287f
left ventricular failure
in cardiac catheterization lab, 287–290
oxygen uptake and cardiac output, 284,
284f
supine
with mitral stenosis, 291t
systemic and pulmonary arterial
pressure and heart rate, 285
upright *vs.* supine, 285–286
Dynamic exercise test
performing, 291–292
Dyspnea
progressive
in dilated cardiomyopathy, 696–698

E
Echocardiographic scoring system for
mitral stenosis, 544t
EDRF. *See* Endothelium-derived relaxation
factor (EDRF)
Effective dose
defined, 15t
Effusive-constrictive pericarditis, 736–737,
736f
Ehlers-Danlos syndrome, 263
8F Sones I catheters
insertion into brachial artery, 110f
Ejection fraction, 307–308
defined, 320
left ventricles
normal values, 310t
Ejection phase indices, 319–320
left ventricular systolic performance,
320t
Elderly
balloon aortic valvuloplasty, 557f
Electrical conductance catheters, 232
Electrical strain gauge, 138–139
Electrochemical fuel-cell method, 164
Electromechanical mapping, 231
Electronic calipers, 374
Embolism. *See also* Acute pulmonary
embolism; Pulmonary embolism
with cardiac ventriculography, 230–231
Embolization protection devices,
483–488
EMERALD. *See* Distal Embolic Protection
During Primary Angioplasty in
Acute Myocardial Infarction
(EMERALD)
Enalapril
dose, 70t

Endarterectomy
high risk for, 761t
End-diastolic volume
left ventricles
normal values, 310t
Endocardial staining
with cardiac ventriculography, 230
Endoluminal thoracic aneurysm repair,
769
Endomyocardial biopsy, 395–409
Adriamycin cardiotoxicity, 407
complications, 404–405
dilated cardiomyopathy, 407
equipment for, 398t
femoral vein approach, 400
femoral vein approach-preformed
sheath, 402–403
future, 409
historical approaches, 395–396
indications, 406t
internal jugular access, 397–399
left ventricular-femoral artery preformed
sheath, 403
methods, 400–403
myocarditis, 408–409
postprocedure care, 405
restrictive *vs.* constrictive disease, 409
right internal jugular preformed sheath,
402
right internal jugular venous approach,
400–402
right subclavian vein access, 400
technique, 397–403
transplant rejection, 406–407
Endothelium-derived relaxation factor
(EDRF), 451
End pressure artifacts, 145
End-systolic volume
left ventricles
normal values, 310t
omega-length, 321–322
Enhanced Suppression of the Platelet
IIb/IIIa Receptor with Integrilin
Therapy (ESPIRIT), 62, 509f
Enoxaparin
for acute coronary syndrome, 59–60
EPIC. *See* Evaluation of IIb/IIIa platelet
receptor antagonist in Preventing
Ischemic Complications (EPIC)
Epinephrine
dose, 68t, 69t
for premedication prior to contrast
agents, 53
EPISTENT. *See* Evaluation of Platelet
IIb/IIIa Inhibition in Stenting Trial
(EPISTENT)
Epoprostenol (Flolan)
dose, 71t
for PPH, 690t
Eppendorf catheters, 224
Eptifibatide, 61–63
dose, 65t
during PCI, 56t
for PCI, 61
ERBAC. *See* Excimer, Rotablator, Balloon
Angioplasty for Complex Lesions
(ERBAC)

Ergonovine testing, 216
Erythrityl tetranitrate, 161, 161f
Esmolol
  dose, 67t
ESPIRIT. *See* Enhanced Suppression of the
    Platelet IIb/IIIa Receptor with
    Integrilin Therapy (ESPIRIT)
Ethanol
  influencing myocardial contractility,
    316t
European TOTAL Surveillance Study, 479
Evaluation of IIb/IIIa platelet receptor
    antagonist in Preventing Ischemic
    Complications (EPIC), 62
Evaluation of Platelet IIb/IIIa Inhibition in
    Stenting Trial (EPISTENT), 62, 509f
Excimer, Rotablator, Balloon Angioplasty
    for Complex Lesions (ERBAC),
    473–475
Excimer lasers, 462
Exercise. *See also* Dynamic exercise
  bicycle ergometer, 291f
  dilated cardiomyopathy, 701f
  isometric, 292–293
    hemodynamic response, 293
Exercise-induced ischemia, 661f
External metallic clips, 95
EXTRA, 503t
Extracardiac shunts
  transcatheter embolization of, 625
Extracranial carotid percutaneous
    transluminal angioplasty
    stenting, 579t
Extraction atherectomy, 462
Extraction reserve, 148–149
Extremities, 563t. *See also* Lower extremities
  acute ischemia
    clinical categories of, 563t
  chronic ischemia
    clinical categories of, 564t
  ischemia
    with PAD, 272

F
Familial amyloidosis, 715
Fascicular block
  with cardiac ventriculography, 230
Fatigue syndrome
  with mitral stenosis, 640
7F Berman Balloon catheters, 238
Femoral artery. *See also* Common femoral
    artery (CFA); Superficial femoral
    artery (SFA)
  antegrade puncture, 256f
  aortic stenosis, 180f
  catheterizing left heart from, 89–93
  deep, 270
  puncture, 87–89
  right
    entry of, 90f
Femoral artery thrombosis
  with diagnostic catheterization, 42–43,
    43f
Femoral artery/vein catheterization,
    79–96
  catheter selection, 91–92
  crossing aortic valve, 92–93

heparin, 91
left heart
  contraindications to, 96
local anesthesia, 80
patient preparation, 79–80
puncture closure devices, 94–95, 95f
puncture site control following sheath
    removal, 93–96
puncture site selection, 80
Femoral pseudoaneurysm
  with diagnostic catheterization, 47f
Femoral vascular complications
  with diagnostic catheterization, 46f
Femoral vein
  catheterization, 79–96
    right heart from, 84–87, 86f
  puncture, 80–84
  right
    trans-septal catheterization, 101
  right common, 236
Femoral venous thrombosis
  with diagnostic catheterization, 43
Femoropopliteal angioplasty, 775–777
Fentanyl
  dose, 67t
  for interventional cardiology, 9
FFR. *See* Fractional flow reserve (FFR)
Fibromuscular dysplasia (FMD), 583,
    584f, 773f, 774f
Fick oxygen method, 151–152, 155
Fick's principle, 4, 8
  illustration of, 151, 151f
Field of view (FOV), 19
FilterWire, 484f, 486
FilterWire EXRandomized Evaluation
    (FIRE) trial, 486, 487
FIM. *See* First-In-Man (FIM)
First-In-Man (FIM), 517
FlexStent
  Gianturco-Roubin, 497
Flolan
  dose, 71t
  for PPH, 690t
Flow-directed balloon flotation catheters,
    111
Flow measuring guidewires, 442
Flow ratio, 168
Flow velocity
  coronary artery, 350f
  measurements of, 345–347
Flumazenil (Romazicon)
  dose, 67t
Fluorescence spectroscopy, 388
Fluoroscopy
  pregnancy, 28
Focused force angioplasty, 438
Fontan physiology
  cardiac catheterization in, 630–631
  hemodynamic evaluation, 631
Forssmann's technique, 4
Fossa ovalis
  fluoroscopic landmarks for localizing,
    101
Fourier analysis, 135f
  defined, 134t
Four-port coronary manifold, 190f
FOV. *See* Field of view (FOV)

Fractional flow reserve (FFR)
  formulas to predict, 356f
  pressure derived, 348f
Freestanding cardiac catheterization labs
  guidelines for, 9
Frequency response
  characteristics evaluation, 137–138
  desirable, 136
  deterioration of, 144–145
Frequency response curves, 136f
Frequency response of pressure
    measurement system
  defined, 134t
Fundamental frequency
  defined, 134t
Furosemide (Lasix)
  dose, 69t

G
Gantry, 24
Gensini catheters, 223f
GFX stents, 496f, 498
Giant cell arteritis, 262
Giant cell myocarditis, 710–711
Gianturco coil embolization, 626f
Gianturco-Roubin
  FlexStent, 497, 523
  stents
    original configuration of, 493f
Gianturco-Roubin II (GR-II), 498
  randomized trial, 497, 497t, 503t
  stent, 502
Glucagon
  dose, 69t
Glycoprotein IIb/IIIa inhibitors
  with coronary stents, 508
  guidelines for, 64
  meta-analysis, 63f
  outcomes, 63t
  and thrombocytopenia, 63–64
Glycosides
  influencing myocardial contractility,
    316t
Gold-coated stents
  clinical trials of, 496t
Goodale-Lubin catheters, 111, 111f
Gorlin formula
  alternatives to, 181
Great vessels
  aortogram, 260f
  perforation with diagnostic
    catheterization, 50–51
Greenfield filters, 237
Grieshaber wire self-retaining retractor,
    108f
GR-II. *See* Gianturco-Roubin II (GR-II)
Grollman catheters, 238, 238f
Grossman method of
  brachial cutdown
    vessel repair and aftercare, 116, 116f
Gruentzig catheters, 436
Guardwire, 483–484
Guidewires, 257–258
  angioplasty, 345
  arteriovenous, 752f
  buddy wire, 436
  coronary stents, 502

Guidewires (*continued*)
flow measuring, 442
high-speed mechanical rotational
atherectomy, 471
hydrophilic, 436
modern, 436
percutaneous balloon angioplasty,
436–437
pressure measuring, 442
probing force, 436
sensor-tipped, 345–347
sensory angioplasty, 346t
shaft support, 436
Guidewire thermodilution blood flow
technique, 349–350
Guiding catheters
deep engagement, 435f
percutaneous balloon angioplasty,
434–435

H

Halsey needle holder, 108f
Halstead curved mosquito hemostats,
108f
Halstead straight mosquito hemostats, 108f
Harmonic
defined, 134t
HCM. *See* Hypertrophic cardiomyopathy
(HCM)
Headhunter catheters, 258f, 267
Heart
perforation with diagnostic
catheterization, 50–51
Heart block
with endomyocardial biopsy, 404
Heart disease
structural, 5
Heart failure
chronic, 697f
decompensated
from dilated cardiomyopathy, 699f,
700f
diastolic, 711–716
end-diastolic pressure-volume, 712f
left ventricular filling pressure, 700f
with normal left ventricular systolic
function, 288f
HeartMate, 427f
HeartMate XVE LVAS, 706
Heart rate, 336
Heart transplantation, 700–706
assessing pulmonary vascular resistance
prior to, 702
hemodynamic changes after, 704t
hemodynamic profiles after, 706f
hemodynamics after, 697t
Heart valve prosthesis
percutaneous, 651f
Hematomas
with diagnostic catheterization, 43
Hemodynamic data, 124f
Heparin, 498. *See also* Low molecular
weight heparin (LMWH);
Unfractionated heparin (UFH)
contraindicating interventional
cardiology, 7–8
dose, 65t

Heparin-induced thrombocytopenia,
53
Heparin induced thrombocytopenia or
thrombosis syndrome (HITTS), 440
Hepatic vein
congenital heart disease, 121
Hexabrix, 32
structure, 32f
High-speed mechanical rotational
atherectomy (Rotablator), 470–472
assembly, 472f
bifurcation lesions, 475
burr, 471f, 472t
calcified lesions, 475
contraindications, 475f
device description, 470–471
guidewires, 471
in-stent restenosis, 474f, 476
jailed side branches, 475
mechanisms of, 473
ostial lesions, 476
procedure, 471–472
resistant calcified lesions, 475f
results, 473–475
undilatable lesions, 475–476
HITTS. *See* Heparin induced
thrombocytopenia or thrombosis
syndrome (HITTS)
Hockey stick catheters, 194f, 435
Hurthle manometer, 135f
Hybrid resistance units (HRU), 157–158
Hydration
dose, 68t
Hydrophilic plastic-covered guidewires,
436
Hypaque (Nycomed), 31
structure, 32f
Hypertension. *See* Primary pulmonary
hypertension (PPH); Pulmonary
hypertension
Hypertrophic cardiomyopathy (HCM),
717–721, 717f, 718f, 719f, 720f

I

IABP. *See* Intraaortic balloon
counterpulsation (IABP)
Ibutilide
dose, 66t
ICA. *See* Internal carotid artery (ICA)
IEC. *See* International Electrotechnical
Commission (IEC)
Iliac aorta
revascularization, 566t
Iliac artery
laceration with diagnostic
catheterization, 45f
occlusions of, 565f
pelvic arteriogram, 275f
selective angiography, 275
Iloprost
for PPH, 689, 690t
Image intensifiers, 257
vs. flat panel detectors
zoom differences, 23f
Image noise, 17
Image quality
exposure parameters, 17

Image receptor dose, 17f
Impella Recover system, 424–425, 424f
Indicator dilution methods, 155–156
Infants
thoracic aorta
coarctation of, 565
Infectious endarteritis
coronary stents, 513
Inferior ST elevation myocardial
infarction, 669f
Inflation pressure, 438
Inflow valvular regurgitation
hemodynamics of, 708f
Infrapopliteal angioplasty, 780–781
Infrapopliteal arteries, 595–596
stenosis, 597f
Infrarenal aorta
revascularization, 566t
Infundibular obstruction, 609
acute, 609
Injection catheters
cardiac ventriculography, 222–224
Innominate arteries (*see also*
Brachiocephalic), 573–574
Input signal
pressure, 133
Integrilin and Enoxaparin Randomized
Assessment of Acute Coronary
Syndrome Treatment (INTERACT),
59
Intermittent claudication
with PAD, 272
Internal carotid artery (ICA)
color duplex image, 267f
Internal mammary angiography, 196f
Internal mammary artery
via brachial cutdown, 114
left subclavian stenosis in, 197f
Internal mammary catheters, 194f
International Electrotechnical
Commission (IEC)
Interventional Fluoroscopic Safety
standard, 16
Interpretation
mistakes in, 217–219
Interventional cardiology, 5–9, 10
board exam, 10t
contraindications to, 7–8
fentanyl for, 9
MI as complication of, 40–41
midazolam for, 9
patient preparation, 8–9
premedication for, 8–9
protocol design, 8
research, 7
selection of, 8
Interventional fluoroscope
scatter isodose curves, 31f
Intervention cardiac ventriculography,
229
Intraaortic balloon counterpulsation
(IABP), 412–413
angiography during counterpulsation,
416
bridge to cardiac transplantation, 422
cardiogenic shock, 420–421
catheters, 413

clinical results, 419–420
complications, 417
counterpulsation, 414–416
emergent CABG for failed PCI, 422
enhanced external counterpulsation, 422–423
high risk CABS/weaning, 412–422
indications and contraindications for, 417–418, 418t, 419t
inflation and deflation timing, 416f
left ventricular support, 423–424
long term circulatory support, 425–427
manufacturers, 413t
patient management, 417
percutaneous coronary intervention, 419–420
percutaneous insertion, 413–414
sheathless insertion, 414
short-term circulatory support, 423–424
unstable angina, 422
uses of, 420t
weaning from, 417
Intracardiac shunt lesions, 616–629
Intracardiac shunts
left-to-right
detection of, 163–164
right-to-left, 170–172
angiography, 171–172
oximetry, 172
Intracoronary Doppler flow velocity, 361–364
Intracoronary pressure
cath lab, 364–365
measurements of, 345–347
Intracoronary stenting and angiographic results strut thickness effect on restenosis outcome (ISAR-STEREO), 504t
Intracranial angioplasty, 762–766, 764f
Intraluminal filling defects, 244f
Intramyocardial injection
with cardiac ventriculography, 230
Intravascular contrast agents, 31–33
Intravascular imaging techniques, 371–391
Intravascular magnetic resonance imaging, 390–391
experimental data, 390–391
future, 391
limitations, 391
safety, 391
systems and procedures, 390
Intravascular thermography, 388–390, 390f
clinical experience, 389
experimental data, 389
future, 389–390
imaging systems, 388–389
limitations, 389
procedures, 388–389
safety, 389
Intravascular ultrasound (IVUS), 371–379, 522
arterial disease, 374–379
atherectomy, 376
balloon angioplasty, 376
costs, 379

diagnostic applications, 375
future directions, 381
image, 373f
imaging systems, 371–372
interpretation, 372–373
interventional applications, 381–382
intervention guide, 376
intravenous
future directions, 381
limitations, 381
mechanical, 372
quantitative assessment, 373–374
safety, 379, 381
stents, 376–378
usage, 379
Intravenous GP IIB/IIIa inhibitors, 61–63
Invasive cardiology, 10
Iodinated contrast agents
allergic reaction to, 52
Iodine, 31
Iodixanol (Visipaque), 32, 53
structure, 32f
Iohexol (Omnipaque), 32, 238–239
structure, 32f
Iopamidol (Isovue), 32, 238–239
structure, 32f
Iothalamic acid (Conray), 31
structure, 32f
Ioversol (Optiray), 32
structure, 32f
Ioxaglate (Hexabrix), 32
structure, 32f
Ioxilan (Oxilan), 32
Iris scissors, 108f
ISAR-STEREO. *See* Intracoronary stenting and angiographic results strut thickness effect on restenosis outcome (ISAR-STEREO)
Ischemia
acute limb
clinical categories of, 563t
chronic limb
clinical categories of, 564t
exercise-induced, 661f
myocardial, 326–327
with coronary angiography, 201
percutaneous balloon angioplasty, 456
Isometric exercise, 292–293
hemodynamic response, 293
Isopaque, 31
structure, 32f
Isoproterenol
dose, 66t
Isovolumic indices, 316–318
Isovolumic pressure decay, 327
Isovue, 32, 238–239
structure, 32f
IVUS. *See* Intravascular ultrasound (IVUS)

J
Jomed JOSTENT, 500f
Judkins and Amplatz curves, 435
Judkins catheters
spasm, 217f
Judkins left catheters, 189f
Judkins right catheters, 189f
Judkins technique, 192f, 193

K
Kawai flexible endomyocardial biopsy catheters, 397f
Kawasaki disease, 212
Kensey Nash Triactiv system, 485–486
Kissing balloon technique, 450
Konno biopsy technique, 396
Konno Bioptome, 396
Kugel collaterals, 213f
Kussmaul sign, 697

L
Labetalol
dose, 67t
LAO. *See* Left anterior oblique (LAO) projection
Lasix
dose, 69t
Left anterior descending arteries
contrast injection, 363f
ostia of, 204
stenosis, 365f–366f
Left anterior oblique (LAO) projection, 227–228
Left atrium
congenital heart disease, 122
retrograde catheterization of, 113f
Left circumflex arteries
ostia of, 204
Left coronary artery obstruction
coronary collaterals, 212f
Left dominant circulation, 203–204
Left heart catheterization
alternative sites for, 97–104
axillary artery percutaneous entry, 97
brachial artery percutaneous entry, 97
radial artery percutaneous entry, 97–100
Left heart catheters, 111f
advancing, 113–114
brachial cutdown, 111
used from femoral approach, 91f
Left internal mammary artery (LIMA)
angioplasty, 460f
Left subclavian artery
stenosis in, 767f
Left-to-right intracardiac shunts
detection of, 163–164
Left-to-right shunts, 170f
angiography, 170
calculation of, 167
detection of, 167
early recirculation, 170
oximetry detection of, 165f
quantification of, 167
Left ventricles
echocardiographic visualization of, 231
ellipsoid reference figure, 305f
normal values, 310t
pressure volume curves, 311
pressure volume diagram, 312f
retrograde catheterization of, 113f
wall stress, 310–311, 311f
Left ventricular assist devices (LVAD), 412, 707f, 709f
dysfunction of, 707–709
Left ventricular casts, 308f

Left ventricular chamber
  pressure tracings, 179f
Left ventricular conductance catheters,
  232f
Left ventricular diastolic distensibility
  pressure volume relationship, 324–325
Left ventricular diastolic performance
  normal values, 327t
Left ventricular diastolic relaxation rate
  indices of, 327–328
Left ventricular ejection fraction, 324f
Left ventricular end diastolic pressure
  (LVEDP), 300f, 315
  postpacing rise in, 300
Left ventricular function
  with upright bicycle exercises, 289
Left ventricular hypertrophy (LVH)
  MRI ventriculogram, 232f
Left ventricular mass, 309–310
Left ventricular outflow tract
  anatomy and physiology, 611–612
  obstruction, 611–614
  transcatheter, 612
Left ventricular pressure, 137f, 144f, 180f
  aortic stenosis, 180f
  micromanometer recordings of, 317f
  signals, 145f
  volume loops, 322f
  volume plots, 321f
Left ventricular rate of pressure fall, 329f
Left ventricular regional area change, 330f
Left ventricular systolic performance, 320t
Left ventriculogram
  right anterior oblique projection, 305f
Lehman catheters, 223f
Lesion risk scores, 448f
Levophed
  dose, 70t
Lidocaine
  dose, 66t
LIMA. See Left internal mammary artery
  (LIMA)
Limbs. See Extremities
LMWH. See Low molecular weight heparin
  (LMWH)
Lower extremities, 269–276, 592–599
  anatomy of, 269–274
  angiography, 274–276
  arterial occlusive disease, 270–271
  arteries
    MRA, 274
  arteriogram, 271f
  bypass grafts, 596–597
Low molecular weight heparin (LMWH)
  dose, 65t
  guidelines for, 60
  with PCI, 56t, 59–60
  with percutaneous balloon angioplasty,
    440
Lumbar aortic puncture, 100
Luminal border, 372
LVAD. See Left ventricular assist devices
  (LVAD)
LVEDP. See Left ventricular end diastolic
  pressure (LVEDP)
LVH. See Left ventricular hypertrophy
  (LVH)

M

MACE. See Major adverse clinical event
  (MACE)
Magnesium sulfate
  dose, 66t
Magnetic resonance angiography (MRA)
  contrast enhanced, 255
  phase contrast, 255
  time-of-flight, 254–255
Magnetic resonance imaging (MRI)
  dobutamine stress, 667f
  intravascular, 390–391
  ventriculography, 231
Main pulmonary artery (MPA)
  pullbacks from, 745f
Major adverse clinical event (MACE), 60
Malignant ventricular arrhythmias
  with endomyocardial biopsy, 404
Mammary artery
  internal
    left subclavian stenosis in, 197f
Marfan syndrome, 263
Matrix VSG system, 94
Mayo clinic risk score for mortality after
  coronary intervention, 40f
MBG. See Myocardial blush grade (MBG)
MCA. See Middle cerebral artery (MCA)
MDCT. See Multidetector CT (MDCT)
Mechanical intravascular ultrasound,
  372
Mechanical thrombectomy, 480–485
  cut-and-aspirate devices, 480
  pharmacologic strategies, 480
  procedure, 481
  results, 481–483
  Venturi-Bernoulli suction, 480–481
Mechanical transducers, 372
Media/adventitia border, 372
Median nerve injury, 117
MedNova filter device, 484f
Medtronic Interceptor Filter, 484f
Meglumine, 32
Menghini needle, 395
Mercedes Benz lesion, 470f
Mesenteric arteries, 586–587
  angioplasty, 769–774, 771f
  stenosis, 776f
Metabolic rate meter (MRM), 152
Metal stents, 57f
Metaraminol (Aramine)
  dose, 70t
Methylergonovine, 215
Metoprolol
  dose, 67t
Metrizamide (Amipaque), 32
Metrizoic acid (Isopaque), 31
  structure, 32f
MI. See Myocardial infarction (MI)
Microcirculatory resistance (R3), 338
Micromanometers, 146–147
Micropuncture apparatus, 399f
Microvascular disease, 340t
Midazolam (Versed)
  for interventional cardiology, 9
Middle aortic syndrome, 264
Middle cerebral artery (MCA)
  occlusion of, 765f

Milrinone (Primacor)
  assessing pulmonary vasoreactivity, 703t
  for dilated cardiomyopathy, 701f
  dose, 69t
  influencing myocardial contractility,
    316t
Mitral regurgitation, 226f, 641–647, 642f,
    643f, 738
  angiography, 644
  cardiac ventriculography, 229
  catheterization protocol, 645
  with degenerative etiology, 646–647
  exercise hemodynamics, 642–644
  hemodynamic assessment, 642–644
  hemodynamic findings, 292f
  physiology, 641–642
  regurgitant fraction, 644
  v-waves, 642
Mitral stenosis, 637–641, 638f
  cardiac output and mean diastolic
    pressure, 175f
  catheterization protocol, 638–639
  congenital, 616
  with fatigue syndrome, 640
  natural history, 639f
  pulmonary wedge pressure, 175f
  second stenosis, 638
  with severe pulmonary hypertension,
    640–641
  valve area calculation, 174–175
Mitral valve area
  alignment mismatch, 176
  calculation pitfalls, 175–176
  calibration errors, 176–177
  cardiac output determination, 177
  early diastasis, 177
Mitral valve prolapse
  left ventriculography, 228f
Modern bioptomes, 397
Modern guidewires, 436
Modified Allen test, 98f
Morphine sulfate
  dose, 67t
MPA. See Main pulmonary artery (MPA)
MRA. See Magnetic resonance angiography
  (MRA)
MRI. See Magnetic resonance imaging
  (MRI)
MRM. See Metabolic rate meter (MRM)
Mucocutaneous lymph node syndrome,
  212
Mullins sheath, 103
Multidetector CT (MDCT), 255
Multielectrode impedance catheters, 309f
Multipurpose catheters, 194f, 258f, 435
Muscle bridges, 211, 214f
Myocardial blood flow, 335–340
  cardiac cath lab, 341
Myocardial blush grade (MBG), 343
Myocardial bridges, 219
Myocardial contractility, 316, 336
  hormones and drugs influencing, 316t
  left ventricular isovolumic indices, 318f
Myocardial hibernation, 335
Myocardial infarction (MI). See also Acute
    myocardial infarction (AMI)
  biplane left ventriculogram, 227f

with diagnostic catheterization, 39–41
Q-wave, 448
Myocardial ischemia, 326–327
with coronary angiography, 201
Myocardial metabolism
measurement of, 340–341
Myocardial oxygen consumption, 336f,
336t
Myocardial oxygen supply
and demand relationship, 335–340
determinants of, 337
Myocardial systolic function, 315–324
Myocardial wall tension, 336–337
Myocarditis
endomyocardial biopsy, 408–409

N
N-acetyl cysteine, 54
dose, 68t
Naloxone hydrochloride
dose, 68t
NASCET. See North American
Symptomatic Carotid
Endarterectomy Trial (NASCET)
Native coronary artery intervention,
487–488
Natural frequency
defined, 134t
Neonatal critical aortic stenosis, 612–613
Neonatal critical pulmonary stenosis,
605–607
Neo-Synephrine
dose, 70t
Nerve paresis
with endomyocardial biopsy, 405
Nicardipine
dose, 71t
Nifedipine
influencing myocardial contractility, 316t
for PPH, 690t
NIH catheters, 223f, 224
Nimbex
dose, 68t
NIR Stent, 496f
NIRVANA, 503t
Nitric oxide
assessing pulmonary vasoreactivity, 703t
Nitroglycerin
dose, 70t
Nitroprusside, 215
in aortic stenosis, 182t
assessing pulmonary vasoreactivity, 703t
dose, 70t, 71t
Nonatherosclerotic coronary artery disease,
211–217
Noninvasive angiography, 254–255
Non-ST-segment elevation myocardial
infarction (NSTEMI), 666–667
coronary angiography, 666–667, 667f
medical management, 667
percutaneous revascularization,
666–667
technical considerations, 667
Norcuron
dose, 68t
Norepinephrine (Levophed)
dose, 70t

Normal coronary flow velocity, 350
North American Symptomatic Carotid
Endarterectomy Trial (NASCET),
266, 577, 761
NSTEMI. See Non-ST-segment elevation
myocardial infarction (NSTEMI)
Nycomed, 31
structure, 32f
Nyman catheters, 238f

O
Occluded collateralized coronary artery, 364f
OCT. See Optical coherence tomography
(OCT)
Olympus bioptome, 397f
Omnipaque, 32, 238–239
structure, 32f
Ondansetron
dose, 69t
Optical coherence tomography (OCT),
381–386, 384f
clinical experience, 385
drug eluting stents, 385f
experimental data, 383–384
future, 386
imaging systems and procedures,
381–382
limitations, 385–386
safety, 385–386
Optimal damping
defined, 134t
Optiray, 32
structure, 32f
Oral intake
with percutaneous balloon angioplasty,
440
Oral platelet ADP-receptor antagonist
with percutaneous balloon angioplasty,
440
Original dilatation catheters, 436
Orthogonal projections, 306
Ostial first obtuse marginal branch lesion,
367f
Ostial RCA rotastents, 474f
Outcomes data
cardiac catheterization facility, 12
Over-the-wire (OTW) catheters, 437
Oxilan, 32
structure, 32f
Oximetric data, 124f
Oximetry
limitations of, 168–169
Oximetry run, 163–165, 167f, 168f
Oxygen consumption, 152–153
measurement of, 152f
Oxygen content, 153
calculation of, 154f
expected value of, 169t

P
Pacemaker lead
fractured, 56f
Pacing catheters, 294–295
Pacing-induced angina, 295
Pacing stress test, 294–295
electrocardiographic changes in
response to, 295–297, 296f

hemodynamic changes during, 298–301
myocardial metabolic changes induced
by, 297–298
regional wall motion abnormalities, 301
thallium scintigraphy, 301
Pacing tachycardia, 293–302
vs. exercise stress, 294
hemodynamic effects, 293–294
left ventricular pressure volume, 299f
Paclitaxel elution, 520f
from durable polymer, 518–520
vs. TAXUS, 521t
PAD. See Peripheral arterial occlusive
disease (PAD)
Palmaz-Schatz stents, 494f, 497
creation of, 493
Palmaz stents, 497
original configuration of, 493f
Papaverine, 111
for coronary flow studies, 349t
inducing coronary hyperemia, 346
Papillary muscle rupture
left ventriculography, 228f
PARAGON. See Platelet IIb/IIIa
antagonism for the reduction of
acute coronary syndrome events in
the global organization network
(PARAGON)
Partial anomalous pulmonary vein return,
250
Patent ductus arteriosus (PDA), 625–638,
753–755, 754f, 755f
Amplatzer duct occluder, 627
aortic angiography, 261
coil occlusion, 627
complications, 627–628
transcatheter closure of, 626–627
Patent foramen ovale (PFO), 618f
closure technique, 619
diagnostic catheterization
indications for, 120t
intracardiac echocardiography, 617
pathophysiology of, 616–617
special techniques, 619–621
TEE, 617–618
transcatheter closure of, 617
Patient instructions
radiation, 29
respiration during contrast
ventriculography, 227
PAVM. See Pulmonary arteriovenous
malformation (PAVM)
PCI. See Percutaneous coronary
intervention (PCI)
PC-MRA. See Phase contrast MRA (PC-MRA)
PDA. See Patent ductus arteriosus (PDA)
Peak dP/dt and end-diastolic volume,
322–323
Peak filling rate (PFR), 328–329
Peak skin dose
defined, 15t
Pelvis, 269–276
anatomy of, 269–274
angiography, 274–276
arteriogram, 259f, 271f, 275
PercuSurge distal occlusion aspiration
embolic protection system, 457

PercuSurge Guardwire, 483–484, 485
Percutaneous balloon angioplasty,
     433–464, 781f
  abrupt closure, 447–449
  acute results, 445–446
  aspirin with, 440
  asymptomatic with ischemia, 456
  bare metal stents, 454f
  brachial approach, 440
  brachytherapy, 454
  clopidogrel, 440
  complications, 446–451
  coronary artery dissection, 447
  coronary dissection, 444f, 445f
  dilatation catheters, 437–438
  drug-eluting stents, 454
  equipment, 434–436
  femoral approach, 440
  finances, 461–462
  guidewires, 436–437
  guiding catheters, 434–435
  healing response to, 451–454
  history of, 433–434, 434f
  indications, 455–461
  left main intervention, 461
  long-term results, 454–455
  with low molecular weight heparin,
     440
  mechanism of, 443–445, 444f
  mild stable angina, 456
  moderate stable angina, 456
  mortality predictors, 446t
  PCI, 455f
  postprocedure management, 442–443
  prior coronary bypass surgery, 457–459
  procedure, 439–442
  radial approach, 440
  regulations, 461–462
  restenosis, 451f, 452f, 453f
  revascularization, 455
  ST-elevation myocardial infarction,
     456–457
  total coronary occlusion, 459–461
  unstable angina, 456
Percutaneous balloon mitral valvuloplasty,
     160, 543–551, 546f, 548f, 549f
  complications, 551
  contraindications, 544
  immediate results, 549–550
  Inoue balloon technique, 545–549
  long-term hemodynamic results, 550,
     550t
  mechanisms of, 543
  patient selection for, 543–544
     anatomic factors in, 544–545
  vs. surgery, 550–551
  technique, 545
Percutaneous balloon pericardiotomy,
     738–740, 739f, 740f
Percutaneous cardiopulmonary support
  intraaortic balloon counterpulsation,
     423
Percutaneous coronary intervention (PCI),
     5, 508
  abciximab, 61
  antithrombotics during, 56t
  bivalirudin during, 56t

brachial cutdown, 114
  Cleveland Clinic, 449f
  clopidogrel, 56t
  coronary stents for, 661
  low molecular weight heparin, 56t,
     59–60
Percutaneous femoral arterial and venous
     catheterization
  regional anatomy, 81f
Percutaneous heart valve prosthesis, 651f
Percutaneous needle, 82f
Percutaneous revascularization, 564f
Percutaneous technique, 4
Percutaneous transluminal angioplasty
     (PTA)
  aortoiliac
     with surgery, 591
  extracranial carotid
     stenting, 579t
Percutaneous transluminal coronary
     angioplasty (PTCA), 5
  history of, 433
Percutaneous valve replacement and
     repair, 558–559
Perfusion balloon catheters, 438f
Pericardial disease, 725–742
Pericardial effusion, 726
Pericardial tamponade, 731
Pericardiocentesis, 726–731, 730f, 731f
  complications, 730–731
  technique, 728–730, 729f
Pericarditis, 726
  constrictive, 731–736
  effusive-constrictive, 736–737
Pericardium
  anomalies of, 741–742
Peripheral angiographic catheters, 258f
Peripheral angiography, 254
Peripheral arterial occlusive disease (PAD),
     270–272, 272–273
  arterial duplex ultrasonography, 273
  diabetes mellitus, 272
  graft surveillance, 273–274
  native vessel arterial duplex
     ultrasonography, 273
  physical examination, 273
  pulse volume recordings, 273
  risk factors for, 272
  segmental limb series, 273
Peripheral imaging techniques, 254
Peripheral intervention, 562–599
Peripheral vascular disease, 759–785
  invasive therapy for, 563t
  percutaneous intervention
     training and credentialing for, 599
Perivascular landmarks, 373f
Peroneal artery, 270
PFO. See Patent foramen ovale (PFO)
PFR. See Peak filling rate (PFR)
Phase contrast MRA (PC-MRA), 255
Phenylephrine (Neo-Synephrine)
  dose, 70t
Phytis Medical Devices Diamond Flex
     stents, 498
Pigtail catheters, 91f, 111, 223f, 225f, 238,
     238f, 258f
  angled, 91f

cardiac ventriculography, 222–223
  central aortic pressure, 92f
  for coronary angiography, 189
  crossing aortic valve, 93f
  original Judkins design, 223
  pulmonary arteriography, 237
  for pulmonary arteriography, 237
PIOPED. See Prospective Investigation of
     Pulmonary Embolism Diagnosis
     (PIOPED)
Plain old balloon angioplasty (POBA),
     462–463
Plaque
  detection of, 381–382
Platelet Glycoprotein IIb/IIIa in Unstable
     Angina: Receptor Suppression
     Using Integrilin Therapy
     (PURSUIT), 62
Platelet glycoprotein IIb/IIIa receptor
     blockers
  balloon angioplasty, 450f
Platelet IIb/IIIa antagonism for the
     reduction of acute coronary
     syndrome events in the global
     organization network (PARAGON),
     502, 503t
Pneumothorax
  with endomyocardial biopsy, 404–405
POBA. See Plain old balloon angioplasty
     (POBA)
Poiseuille's Law, 156–157
Polyarteritis nodosa, 212
Polytetrafluoroethylene (PTFE), 499
  stent grafts, 500f
  vs. bare metal stents, 501t
Popliteal artery, 270, 593–594
  revascularization, 567t–570t
Possis AngioJet, 481, 481f, 482f
Posterior tibial artery (PT), 270
Postmyocardial infarction ventricular
     septal rupture shunt reduction,
     751–753
Postprocedure care
  tissue processing, 405–409
PPH. See Primary pulmonary hypertension
     (PPH)
Practical pressure transducer system
  for catheterization laboratory, 139–141,
     140f
Prednisone
  for coronary angiography allergic
     reactions, 201
  dose, 68t
  for premedication prior to contrast
     agents, 52
Pregnancy
  congenital heart disease, 126
  fluoroscopy, 28
  radiation, 27–28
Preload, 315–316
Premedication
  for allergic reactions with coronary
     angiography, 201
  for coronary angiography allergic
     reactions, 201
  for interventional cardiology, 8–9
  prior to contrast agents, 52

Preserved ejection fraction
  MRI ventriculogram, 232f
Pressure derived fractional flow reserve, 348f
Pressure measurement, 133–147
  artifacts, 144–146
  balancing errors, 146
  calibration errors, 146
  errors, 144–146
  terminology, 134t
  zero level errors, 146
Pressure measuring devices, 133–136
  damping, 135–156
  frequency response, 134–135
  natural frequency, 135–156
  sensitivity, 133–134
Pressure measuring guidewires, 442
Pressure volume analysis, 318–324
Pressure waveforms, 144f
  physiologic characteristics of, 141–143
Pressure waves
  defined, 133, 134t
  transforming into electrical signals, 138–139
PressureWire, 349
PRIDE. See Protection during Saphenous Vein Graft Intervention to Prevent Distal Embolization (PRIDE)
Primacor
  assessing pulmonary vasoreactivity, 703t
  for dilated cardiomyopathy, 701f
  dose, 69t
  influencing myocardial contractility, 316t
Primary amyloidosis, 715
Primary pulmonary hypertension (PPH), 246–247, 248f, 688–691, 691f
  diltiazem for, 690t
  hemodynamics in, 690t
  nifedipine for, 690t
Prinzmetal angina, 213
Procainamide
  dose, 66t
Profunda femoris artery, 592–593
  angioplasty, 777–779
  revascularization, 566t
Progressive dyspnea
  in dilated cardiomyopathy, 696–698
Projections
  inadequate number of, 217
Propofol (Diprivan)
  dose, 68t
Propranolol
  dose, 67t
Prospective Investigation of Pulmonary Embolism Diagnosis (PIOPED), 239, 243
Prostaglandin E1
  assessing pulmonary vasoreactivity, 703t
Prostar, 94, 95f
Prosthetic valves
  catheter passage across, 658
  relative stenosis of, 657–658
Protection during Saphenous Vein Graft Intervention to Prevent Distal Embolization (PRIDE), 486, 487

Protein-losing enteropathy, 631
Provocative test, 215, 216
Proximal occlusion systems, 487
Proxis inflation device and catheter hub system, 484f
Proxis proximal protection catheters, 484f
Pseudoaneurysm
  with diagnostic catheterization, 44
  femoral
    with diagnostic catheterization, 47f
  left ventriculography, 228f
Pseudoaneurysm sac, 785f
PT. See Posterior tibial artery (PT)
PTA. See Percutaneous transluminal angioplasty (PTA)
PTCA. See Percutaneous transluminal coronary angioplasty (PTCA)
PTFE. See Polytetrafluoroethylene (PTFE)
Pulmonary angiography, 234–252
  anatomy, 234–235
  catheters for, 238f
  complications, 239–240, 240t
  contraindications, 239–240
  contrast agents, 238–239
    injection rates, 239t
  foreign bodies, 251–252
  hemodynamic measurements, 235–240, 236t
  imaging modes, 239
  inflammation, 250–251
  interpretation, 242–244
  procedure, 235–240
  rare indications for, 247–252
  validity, 242–244
  venous access, 236–239
Pulmonary arteriography
  balloon-tipped catheters, 237
  pigtail catheters, 237
Pulmonary arteriovenous
    malformation (PAVM), 247–248, 249f, 250f
Pulmonary artery, 688f. See also Branch pulmonary artery stenosis
  anatomy, 234–235
  aneurysm, 249–250
  catheterization, 237f
    techniques, 237–238
  diastolic pressure, 698f
  main
    pullbacks from, 745f
  neoplasms, 250
  perforation with diagnostic catheterization, 51
  perfusion segments, 236f
  pressure tracing, 251f
  segmental arterial anatomy, 235f
  stenosis, 248–249, 250f, 251f
Pulmonary atresia
  diagnostic catheterization indications for, 120t
Pulmonary atrioventricular malformation, 629f
Pulmonary blood flow
  calculation of, 165–166
Pulmonary capillary wedge pressure, 143
Pulmonary capillary wedge tracing
  mitral valve area, 175–176

Pulmonary embolism, 240–245, 243f, 677–691, 680f, 681f, 683f, 684f. See also Acute pulmonary embolism
  anticoagulation, 680–681
  arterial blood gas analysis, 241
  cardiac biomarkers, 680, 680f
  catheter fragmentation, 245, 246f, 247f
  catheters, 681–683
  contrast-enhanced chest computed tomography, 241–242
  contrast venography, 242
  CT, 241f
  D-Dimer, 240–241
  diagnosis, 240–241, 242, 242f
    with diagnostic catheterization, 43
  echocardiography, 242, 679–680
  electrocardiography, 240
  embolectomy, 245
  with endomyocardial biopsy, 405
  gadolinium-enhanced magnetic resonance angiography, 242
  Geneva Prognostic Index, 679
  hemodynamic characteristics, 244–245
  interventional devices for, 247t
  management, 682–683, 682f
  natriuretic peptides, 680
  nonimaging tests, 240–241
  noninvasive imaging tests, 241–242
  physical examination, 679
  right atrial curves, 245f
  right heart pressure tracings, 244f
  risk stratification, 679–680
  surgical embolectomy, 681–683
  thrombolysis, 681–683
  troponins, 680
  venous ultrasonography, 242
  ventilation perfusion scanning, 241
Pulmonary fistulas, 628–629
Pulmonary hypertension, 245–246, 683–691
  with congenital pulmonary vein stenosis, 685–686
  drugs for, 690t
  severe
    mitral stenosis with, 640–641
  WHO classification of, 685t
Pulmonary stenosis, 607f
  adolescents, 607
  children, 607
  neonatal critical, 605–607
Pulmonary thromboendarterectomy
  for CTEPH, 686
Pulmonary vascular disease
  with congenital central shunts, 159–160
  congenital heart disease, 127
  with mitral stenosis, 160
Pulmonary vascular resistance, 159
Pulmonary vasoreactivity
  assessment of, 703t
Pulmonary vein stenosis, 248–249
Pulmonary ventricular failure
  congenital heart disease, 127
Pulmonic regurgitation, 657
Pulmonic stenosis, 657, 744–746, 745f, 746f

Pulmonic valves area
    calculation, 181
Pulmonic valvuloplasty, 551–552
    clinical results, 552
    complications, 552
    pathophysiology, 551
    technique, 551–552
Pulsed excimer laser, 477f
    angioplasty, 478
PURSUIT. *See* Platelet Glycoprotein
        IIb/IIIa in Unstable Angina:
        Receptor Suppression Using
        Integrilin Therapy (PURSUIT)

Q

Quantitative analysis (QA), 257
Quantum mottle, 17
Q-wave myocardial infarction, 448

R

R3. *See* Microcirculatory resistance (R3)
Rad
    defined, 15
Radial artery
    anatomy of, 98f
Radial sheaths, 99
Radiation
    annual effective dose, 25, 25f
    beam collimation, 28–29
    beam orientation, 30
    biologic effects, 24–30
    cancer, 25
    clinical dose monitoring, 29
    clinical measurement of, 15–16
    deterministic effects, 25–26, 26t
    dose management, 28
    equipment selection, 28
    exposure, 14
    gantry positioning, 28
    heritable abnormalities, 25
    induced injuries
        time line, 27f
    induced neoplasms, 26–27
    multiple procedures, 29
    patient consent, 29
    patient education, 29
    patient management, 28
    patient risks, 26–27
    patient size *vs.* dose, 28
    pregnancy, 27–28
    scattered, 17
    skin injuries, 26
    staff exposure reduction, 30
    staff monitoring, 30
    staff safety, 29–30
        exposure reduction, 30
        staff safety
            deterministic effects, 30
        stochastic effects, 29–30
    stochastic effects, 25
    technique selection, 28
Radiation induced coronary stenosis, 212
Radiocontrast nephropathy (RCN), 33
Radiographic imaging, 256
Radiologic equipment, 257
Radiometer OSM2, 153
Radius Stent, 496f

Raman spectroscopy, 388
Randomized Evaluation in PCI Linking
        Angiomax to Reduced Clinical
        Events (REPLACE-2), 60–61, 457
Ranitidine (Zantac)
    dose, 68t
    for premedication prior to contrast
        agents, 52
RAO. *See* Right anterior oblique (RAO)
        projection
Rapamycin Eluting Stent Evaluated At
        Rotterdam Cardiology Hospital
        (RESEARCH), 522
RAS. *See* Renal artery stenosis (RAS)
Rated burst pressure, 438
Ratio-1.5 ionic compounds, 31
RCA. *See* Right coronary artery (RCA)
RCN. *See* Radiocontrast nephropathy (RCN)
rCVR. *See* Relative coronary flow velocity
        reserve (rCVR)
Reactive amyloidosis, 715
Reactive hyperemia, 346
Reflectance oximetry, 154f
Reflected waves
    factors influencing magnitude of, 143f
    physiologic characteristics of, 141–142
Regional diastolic dysfunction, 329–330
Regional left ventricular wall motion,
        311–313, 312f
Registry Study to Evaluate the NeuroShield
        Bare-Wire Cerebral Protection
        System and X-Act Stent, 578
Regurgitant fraction, 307–308
Relative coronary flow velocity reserve
        (rCVR), 350–352, 353f
Renal arteries, 268–269
    abdominal aorta, 582–583
    abdominal aortogram, 270f
    anatomy of, 268
    angioplasty, 771–774
    atherosclerotic stenosis, 268–269,
        583–584
        renal arteriography, 269
    balloon angioplasty, 587f
Renal arteriography
    atherosclerotic renal artery stenosis,
        269
Renal artery stenosis (RAS), 582–583,
        774f
    revascularization, 585t
Renal insufficiency
    with coronary angiography, 201
RENEWAL, 504t
Renografin (Bracco), 31
    structure, 32f
REPLACE-2. *See* Randomized Evaluation in
        PCI Linking Angiomax to Reduced
        Clinical Events (REPLACE-2)
RESEARCH. *See* Rapamycin Eluting Stent
        Evaluated At Rotterdam Cardiology
        Hospital (RESEARCH)
Resistance
    calculations, 123f
Respiration
    during contrast ventriculography
        patient instructions, 227
Respiratory quotient (RQ), 153

Restrictive cardiomyopathy, 711–716,
        737–738
Retinal artery embolization, 41
Retroperitoneal bleeding
    with diagnostic catheterization, 43, 45f
Reverse crush technique, 530
Reverse remodeling, 427
Rheolytic thrombectomy, 481f, 485f
Rheolytic thrombectomy, 482f
Rheumatic heart disease, 656f
Right anterior oblique (RAO) projection,
        38, 227–228
Right atrium
    intracardiac echo from within, 102f
Right common femoral vein, 236
Right coronary artery (RCA)
    anomalous origin of
        CT, 205f
    chronic total occlusion, 460f
    circumflex from, 204
        anomalous origin of, 206f
    guiding catheter dissection of, 51f
    pleating artifact, 218f
Right dominant circulation, 202–203
Right femoral artery
    entry of, 90f
Right femoral vein
    trans-septal catheterization from, 101
Right heart catheters, 85f, 111f
    advancing from right atrium to
        pulmonary artery, 112f
    advancing from right atrium to ventricle,
        88f
    brachial cutdown, 111
Right-to-left intracardiac shunts,
        170–172
    angiography, 171–172
    oximetry, 172
Right ventricular infarction
    acute, 738
Right ventricular outflow enlargement
    congenital heart disease, 127
Right ventricular outflow tract
    congenital obstructive lesions of,
        605–606
Right ventricular volumes, 306
Rigid calcified lesion
    dilatation of, 439f
Road mapping, 257
ROBUST trial, 480
Roentgen
    defined, 14
Romazicon
    dose, 67t
Rotablator, 470–476. *See also* High-speed
        mechanical rotational atherectomy
        (Rotablator)
Rotastents, 475, 507f
    ostial RCA, 474f
Rotational atherectomy, 462
RQ. *See* Respiratory quotient (RQ)
Rubicon filter, 484f, 487

S

SAA. *See* Secondary amyloidosis (SAA)
Saccular aneurysm
    thoracic aorta, 769f

SAFER. *See* Saphenous Vein Graft Angioplasty Free of Emboli Randomized (SAFER)
Saphenous Vein Graft Angioplasty Free of Emboli Randomized (SAFER), 457, 485, 487
Saphenous vein grafts (SVG)
  angiography, 195f
  coronary stents, 532
  disease, 668–671, 670f
    coronary arteriography, 669
    percutaneous revascularization, 669
    technical considerations, 669–671
  intervention, 459f
  restenosis, 457
  stents
    embolic material, 484f
SAPPHIRE. *See* Stenting and Angioplasty with Protection in Patients at High Risk for Endarterectomy (SAPPHIRE) trial
SAVED. *See* Small Saphenous Vein Graft Disease (SAVED)
Scalpel, 108f
Scattered radiation, 17
SCORES, 503t
Seafood allergy
  premedication prior to contrast agents, 52
Secondary amyloidosis (SAA), 715
SECURE. *See* Study to evaluate carotid ultrasound changes in patients treated with ramipril and vitamin E (SECURE) trial
SECURITY, 581
Seldinger technique, 83f
Selective coronary angiography, 4
Semple technique, 104
Sensitivity of pressure measurement system
  defined, 134t
Sensor-guidewire
  angioplasty, 345
SensorMedics Deltatrac II, 153
Sensor-tipped guidewires, 345–347
Sensory angioplasty guidewires, 346t
SEP. *See* Systolic ejection period (SEP)
Separation energy loss, 339
Serial stenoses, 354–355
Severe pulmonary hypertension
  mitral stenosis with, 640–641
SFA. *See* Superficial femoral artery (SFA)
Shunt
  calculations, 123f
  congenital heart disease, 122
  detection and quantification, 163–172
  oximetric detection and quantification, 169t
Sildenafil
  for PPH, 689, 690t
Simmons catheters, 258f, 267
Simpson Fox Hollow device, 470
Simultaneous kissing stents, 530
Simultaneous pressure-flow velocity relationships, 355
Single-injection method, 155

SIRIUS Trial, 518, 526f
Sirolimus-eluting stents, 517f, 518f
Sirolimus elution
  from durable polymer, 516–518
Skin dose
  defined, 15t
Small Saphenous Vein Graft Disease (SAVED), 457
SMART, 503t
Snowplow effect, 450
Sodium bicarbonate
  dose, 67t
Sones catheters, 111, 111f, 113, 189f, 199f, 200f, 223, 223f
Sones I catheters
  insertion into brachial artery, 110f
Sones method, 199–200
Sorin Carbostent, 498
SOS-omni catheters, 258f
Spectroscopy, 386–388
  diffuse reflectance NIR, 386, 388
  experimental data, 387–388
  fluorescence, 388
  future, 388
  imaging systems and procedures, 387
  limitations, 388
  Raman, 388
  safety, 388
Spider view, 206
Stable angina
  cardiac catheterization for, 5
    indications for, 6t
Stanford biopsy sheath, 397f
Stanford (Caves-Schulz) bioptome, 396, 396f
Stanford classification, 262
ST elevation myocardial infarction (STEMI), 439, 662–665, 663f, 664f
  cardiac catheterization for, 5
  coronary arteriography, 663
  medical management, 665
  percutaneous revascularization, 663
  technical considerations, 663
Stenosis resolution pressure, 441
Stenotic valve orifice area
  aortic valve area, 177–181
  calculation of, 173–183
  Gorlin formula, 173–174
  mitral valve area, 174–177
  valve resistance, 182–183
Stenting and Angioplasty with Protection in Patients at High Risk for Endarterectomy (SAPPHIRE) trial, 578, 581
Stents, 377f, 762f. *See also* Coronary stents; Drug-eluting stents (DES)
  abdominal aorta, 586
  aortoiliac disease, 589–590
  balloon expandable, 463
  biodegradable, 496
  Biotronik Tensum, 498
  Boston Scientific SYMBIOT, 500f
  candidates for, 761t
  carotid arteries, 576f, 580t
  clinical outcomes of, 358f
  crush, 530

  culotte, 530
  Cypher, 517, 518
    malapposition, 523
    randomized trials of, 519t
    restenosis, 522
    vs. TAXUS, 520
  direct, 441
  GFX, 496f
  Gianturco-Roubin
    original configuration of, 493f
  gold-coated
    clinical trials of, 496t
  IVUS detected problems, 377f, 378f
  metal, 57f
  Palmaz, 497
    original configuration of, 493f
  Palmaz-Schatz, 494f, 497
    creation of, 493
  Phytis Medical Devices Diamond Flex, 498
  saphenous vein graft
    embolic material, 484f
  simultaneous kissing, 530
  sirolimus-eluting, 517f, 518f
  TAXUS, 518
  two balloon-expandable, 462
Straight iris forceps, 108f
Strain gauge
  defined, 134t
Strain gauge pressure, 139f
STRESS, 493, 494f, 524
Stress, 661f
Stress shortening relationships, 323–324
Stress testing. *See also* Pacing stress test
  during cardiac catheterization, 283–302
Strokes
  from diagnostic catheterization, 41–42
Stroke work, 318–321
Structural heart disease, 5
Study to evaluate carotid ultrasound changes in patients treated with ramipril and vitamin E (SECURE) trial, 486
Subclavian angioplasty, 766–767
Subclavian arteries, 264–265, 573–574, 573t
  arteriography, 264–265
  disease manifestation, 264
  left
    stenosis in, 767f
  revascularization, 573f
  stents, 574f
Subclavian arteriogram, 265f
Subclavian artery puncture
  with endomyocardial biopsy, 405
Subpulmonary left ventricle
  congenital heart disease, 122
Subvalvar (infundibular) obstruction
  acute, 609
Subvalvar pulmonary stenosis, 605, 606f
Suction thrombectomy, 483
Superficial femoral artery (SFA), 270, 593–594, 594f, 597f, 599f
  stenosis, 274f
Superior vena cava
  congenital heart disease, 121–122
Superior vena cava syndrome, 261

Superior Yield of the New Strategy of Enoxaparin, Revascularization and Glycoprotein IIb/IIIa inhibitors (SYNERGY), 60
Superselective cannulation
  ostial stenosis masking during, 218f
Supine bicycle exercise
  dilated cardiomyopathy, 290t
Supine dynamic exercise
  with mitral stenosis, 291t
Supravalvar pulmonary stenosis, 605
Supraventricular arrhythmias
  with endomyocardial biopsy, 404
Sure Stat, 94
SVG. *See* Saphenous vein grafts (SVG)
Swan-Ganz catheters, 85f, 113
Syndrome of diffuse cholesterol embolization, 41
SYNERGY. *See* Superior Yield of the New Strategy of Enoxaparin, Revascularization and Glycoprotein IIb/IIIa inhibitors (SYNERGY)
Systemic AV fistulas, 628
Systemic blood flow
  calculation of, 166, 166t
Systemic cholesterol embolization
  with cardiac catheterization, 54
Systemic vascular resistance, 159
Systemic ventricular heart failure
  congenital heart disease, 127, 128t
Systolic ejection period (SEP)
  left ventricular pressure tracings, 174f
Systolic pressure amplification
  in periphery, 145–146

T

TAA. *See* Thoracic aortic aneurysm (TAA)
Tachycardia
  pacing, 293–302
    vs. exercise stress, 294
    hemodynamic effects, 293–294
    left ventricular pressure volume, 299f
Takayasu arteritis, 250, 262
Tako-tsubo heart, 230f
Tamponade, 50, 451, 726
Tandem heart
  intraaortic balloon counterpulsation, 423–424
TandemHeart pVAD, 706
TARGET. *See* Tirofiban and ReoPro Give Similar Efficacy Trial (TARGET)
TAXUS, 518, 527, 534
  vs. Cypher stent, 520
  malapposition, 523
TAXUS II, 378, 520
TAXUS IV, 526, 526f
Teflon Gensini catheters, 91f
Temporal cell arteritis, 262
Tennis racket catheters, 258f
Terry needle, 395
Tetralogy of Fallot
  diagnostic catheterization
    indications for, 120t
Thallium scintigraphy
  pacing stress test, 301

Therapeutic intrapericardial intervention, 741
Thermodilution method, 156
Thermodilution technique, 343f
Thienopyridines, 57–58
  with coronary stents, 507–508
  guidelines for, 58
Thoracic aneurysm
  endoluminal, 769
Thoracic aorta, 259–263, 565–573
  anatomy of, 259
  aneurysm, 571
  coarctation of, 565–573
  disorders of, 259–263
  intervention, 767–769
  revascularization of, 566t–570t
  saccular aneurysm, 769f
Thoracic aortic aneurysm (TAA), 261
Thoracic aortography, 263
Thrombectomy. *See also* Mechanical thrombectomy
  rheolytic, 481f, 482f, 485f
  suction, 483
  ultrasonic, 483
Thrombectomy devices, 462
Thrombocytopenia
  with abciximab, 64f
  with glycoprotein IIb/IIIa inhibitors, 63–64
  heparin-induced, 53
Thromboembolic pulmonary hypertension
  chronic, 245–246, 248f
    angiographic findings in, 248t
Thrombolysis in myocardial infarction (TIMI)
  blush score, 342–343
  flow grades, 341, 341t
  frame count
    anatomic landmarks for, 342f
    reference values for, 342t
Thrombosis
  coronary stents, 508–509, 509f
  drug-eluting stents (DES), 523
  femoral artery
    with diagnostic catheterization, 42–43, 43f
  femoral venous
    with diagnostic catheterization, 43
Thumb dressing forceps, 108f
Thyroid hormone
  influencing myocardial contractility, 316t
Tibial artery
  anterior, 270
  posterior, 270
Tibioperoneal trunk (TPT), 270
Ticlopidine, 58
  with coronary stents, 508
  dose, 65t
  during PCI, 56t
Time constant of relaxation, 327–328
Time-of-flight magnetic resonance angiography (TOF-MRA), 254–255
TIMI. *See* Thrombolysis in myocardial infarction (TIMI)

Tirofiban, 61–63
  dose, 66t
Tirofiban and ReoPro Give Similar Efficacy Trial (TARGET), 61–62
Tissue plasminogen activator (tPA), 451
TOF-MRA. *See* Time-of-flight magnetic resonance angiography (TOF-MRA)
Total anomalous pulmonary venous return
  diagnostic catheterization
    indications for, 120t
Total coronary occlusion, 671–673
  coronary arteriography, 671
  percutaneous revascularization, 671
  revascularization, 672f
  technical considerations, 671–672
Total occlusion, 219
Total occlusion crossing devices, 462
Total pulmonary resistance, 159
Toxilan (Oxilan)
  structure, 32f
tPA. *See* Tissue plasminogen activator (tPA)
TPT. *See* Tibioperoneal trunk (TPT)
Transducer balancing
  defined, 134t
Translesional pressure derived fractional flow reserve
  measurement, 352–354
Transposition of great arteries
  diagnostic catheterization
    indications for, 120t
Transradial catheterization
  complications, 99
  equipment, 99, 99t
Trans-septal catheterization, 4
  equipment for, 102f
  from right femoral vein, 101
Trans-septal puncture, 100–103
  regional anatomy for, 100f
Treppe phenomenon, 317
Treprostinil
  for PPH, 689, 690t
Tricuspid insufficiency, 738f
Tricuspid regurgitation, 226f, 656–657, 705, 738
  after heart transplantation, 703–704, 704f
  angiographic assessment, 656–657
  hemodynamic assessment, 656
Tricuspid stenosis, 657
Tricuspid valves area
  calculation, 181
Tri-iodobenzoic acid, 31
Trinitroglycerin, 216f
T-stent technique, 530
Two balloon-expandable stents, 462

U

UFH. *See* Unfractionated heparin (UFH)
Ultrasonic thrombectomy, 483
Umbilical vessels
  congenital heart disease, 119–121
Unfractionated heparin (UFH)
  guidelines for, 59
  during PCI, 58–59
  with percutaneous balloon angioplasty, 440

Unprotected left main disease, 673–674
    coronary arteriography, 673
    revascularization, 673
    technical considerations, 673–674
Unstable angina
    cardiac catheterization for, 5
    IABP, 422
Urokinase, 480

V
Valium
    for cardiac catheterization, 55
Valvar aortic stenosis, 612
Valvar pulmonary stenosis, 605
    diagnostic catheterization
        indications for, 120t
Valve orifice are determination, 176t
Valvular heart disease, 637–658
    evaluation of, 290–291
    percutaneous therapies for, 543–559
Valvular stenosis
    evaluation of, 290–291
Valvuloplasty. *See* Balloon aortic
    valvuloplasty; Percutaneous
    balloon mitral valvuloplasty;
    Pulmonic valvuloplasty
Van Aman catheters, 238
Variant angina, 213
    vs. focal spasm, 216
Vasa vasora collaterals, 213f
Vascular access, 256–257
Vascular resistance
    clinical measurement of, 156–157
    clinical use of, 158
    estimation of, 157–158
    normal values for, 158t
    related to pressure flow, 157
Vascular sheath, 84f
Vasculitides, 262
Vasodilated coronary pressure flow
    relationships, 339f
Vasodilator drugs
    assessment of, 160–161
Vasodilator testing, 249t
Vasopressin
    dose, 70t
VasoSeal, 94, 95f
VBI. *See* Vertebral-basilar insufficiency (VBI)
Vecuronium bromide (Norcuron)
    dose, 68t

Vein. *See* individual vein
Vein Graft AngioJet Study (VeGAS 1),
    481–482
Velocity of circumferential fiber
    shortening, 320
Vena-Tech filters, 237
Venous hematoma
    with endomyocardial biopsy, 405
Venovenous collaterals, 629
Ventilation-perfusion lung scanning
    acute pulmonary embolism, 678
Ventricular assist devices, 706–710, 708
    A-Med percutaneous, 424f, 425
    implantable, 707f
Ventricular diastolic chamber
    distensibility, 326, 326t
Ventricular diastolic pressure-volume,
    325f
Ventricular fibrillation
    with diagnostic catheterization, 48
Ventricular perforation
    with endomyocardial biopsy, 404
Ventricular premature beats (VPB)
    with diagnostic catheterization, 47–48
Ventricular pressure curve, 135f, 319f
Ventricular puncture
    apical left, 103–104, 104f
Ventricular septal defect, 623
    diagnostic catheterization
        indications for, 120t
    left ventriculography, 228f
    muscular closure, 624
    oximetry run, 168
    transcatheter closure, 623–624
Ventricular volumes, 304–313
    biplane formula, 305–306
    magnification correction, 306–307
    regression equations, 307, 307t
    single plane formula, 306
    technical considerations, 304–307
Ventricular wall motion, 313f
Ventriculographic catheters, 223f
Ventriculography
    contrast
        alternatives to, 231–323
    intervention cardiac, 229
    MRI, 231
Verapamil, 215
    dose, 67t, 71t
    influencing myocardial contractility, 316t

Versed
    for interventional cardiology, 9
Versed
    dose, 67t
Vertebral arteries, 264–265, 575
    angioplasty, 759–761, 760f
    stents, 576f
Vertebral arteriography, 264–265
Vertebral-basilar insufficiency (VBI)
    symptoms of, 575t
Vieussens collaterals, 213f
Vim-Silverman needle, 395
Visipaque, 32, 53
    structure, 32f
Voda catheters, 435
Volume-derived indices of relaxation,
    328–329
VPB. *See* Ventricular premature beats
    (VPB)
VTK catheters, 267

W
Wallstent, 496f
Wall thickness
    left ventricles
        normal values, 310t
Wedge pressure, 142–143
Wexler catheters, 194f
Wheatstone bridge, 138
    defined, 134t
    strain gauge connection of, 140f
WIN, 503t
Woven dacron Goodale-Lubin, 85f

X
X-rays
    dose, 14–15
    image formation, 16
    physics, 14–17
    production, 16

Y
Yellow plaque, 380f

Z
Zantac
    dose, 68t
    for premedication prior to contrast
        agents, 52